Molecular Nephrology

Kidney Function in Health and Disease

Molecular Nephrology

Kidney Function in Health and Disease

edited by

Detlef Schlöndorff
Ludwig-Maximilians University Munich
Munich, Germany

Joseph V. Bonventre
Harvard Medical School, Massachusetts Institute of Technology, and Massachusetts General Hospital
Boston, Massachusetts

Marcel Dekker, Inc. **New York • Basel • Hong Kong**

Library of Congress Cataloging-in-Publication Data

Molecular Nephrology : kidney function in health and disease / edited
by Detlef Schlöndorff, Joseph V. Bonventre.
p. cm.
Includes index.
ISBN 0-8247-9508-3 (hardcover : alk. paper)
1. Kidneys—Molecular aspects. 2. Kidneys—Disease—Molecular
aspects. I. Schlöndorff, Detlef II. Bonventre, Joseph V.
[DNLM: 1. Kidney—physiology. 2. Kidney Diseases—
physiopathology. WJ 301 M7185 1995]
QP249.M656 1995
612.4'63—dc20
DNLM/DLC
for Library of Congress 95-23371
CIP

The publisher offers discounts on this book when ordered in bulk quantities. For more information, write to Special Sales/Professional Marketing at the address below.

This book is printed on acid-free paper.

Marcel Dekker, Inc.
270 Madison Avenue, New York, New York 10016

Current printing (last digit):
10 9 8 7 6 5 4 3 2 1

PRINTED IN THE UNITED STATES OF AMERICA

To Barbara, Sophie, and Johannes Schlöndorff,
and Kristie, Joanna, and Andrew Bonventre,
and in memory of Vincent Bonventre

Preface

Molecular Nephrology is the first book to define kidney development, structure, function, and pathology primarily from a molecular viewpoint. It is not intended to compete with the many excellent textbooks of nephrology, but rather to complement them and provide the reader with an overview of the molecular basis of nephrology. The modern techniques of molecular and cellular biology and immunology allow us to assign specific functions to specific molecules and to identify molecular mechanisms of diseases. As a consequence of the application of these techniques to nephrology, impressive progress has been made in our understanding of renal physiology and pathophysiology. It was our goal as editors to convey this information to a broad readership and to make the text useful for students, residents, clinicians, and investigators. Therefore, the chapters are purposely short and, we hope, "palatable" for the nonexpert wanting to obtain an overview of the topic.

Some brief examples ranging from developmental issues to renal diseases and physiology may illustrate how the progress in nephrology is based on advances in molecular and cellular biology. Fundamental to our understanding of normal and abnormal renal development is an understanding of the orderly sequence of events that occurs as each set of developmentally regulated genes is activated at the appropriate time to result in the distinctive and varied phenotype of vascular and tubular elements of the kidney. An excellent example of how the identification and characterization of a developmental gene lead to better understanding of normal renal development and disease is the Wilms' tumor gene. Wilms' tumor is responsible for pediatric kidney cancer arising in 1 of 10,000 children and is thought to originate in the cells of the metanephric blastema. The gene responsible for at least some forms of Wilms' tumor, *WT-1*, encodes a transcription factor whose expression is developmentally regulated in the kidney. When techniques of homologous recombination have been used to inactivate *WT-1*, homozygously deleted mice die within the second week of fetal development with an absence of both kidneys and gonads, implicating *WT-1* as a critical gene in the normal development of these organs. This demonstrates the power of molecular techniques that result in the ability to engineer animals in which a specific gene is inactivated or overexpressed and that provide a way of identifying the functional significance of that gene's expression. It also illustrates how a developmental gene can be involved in a disease process.

The lack of precise etiological understanding of numerous renal diseases has limited our therapeutic approaches. If the molecular basis of renal diseases could be identified, then more specific therapies could be designed. Such advances in identifying the etiology of renal dysfunction have indeed been made. For example, the occurrence of Goodpasture's syndrome in renal transplants of patients with familial nephritis allowed the identification of both the antigen for Goodpasture syndrome and the genetic defect for familial nephritis in the α_5 chain of collagen type IV. Obviously this would not have been possible without the cloning of the various collagen genes.

Very recently, the gene for the major form of adult polycystic kidney disease was identified thanks to new molecular genetic techniques that were in part developed for the Human Genome Project. While the function of the mutated gene for adult polycystic kidney disease remains to be defined, the identification of the gene will now clarify its in vitro expression, the characterization of its protein structure, biochemistry, and function, and its distribution within various tissues, including the kidney. This knowledge will then allow the design of novel therapies, which may be directed toward altering the expression of the mutated gene.

In the case of nongenetic, inflammatory, and fibrosing renal diseases, considerable progress has also been made. For example, the role of various cytokines, their molecular regulation, and their effects have been defined. The prominent role of TGF-β in renal fibrosis has been identified and has allowed the design of novel therapeutic avenues in experimental models of glomerular disease. It is hoped that this is only the beginning of experimental approaches that will ultimately result in specific molecular therapies for renal diseases.

Molecular characterization of growth factors, such as insulin-like growth factors, epidermal growth factor, and their receptors, has allowed us to study how these molecules are involved in normal kidney growth as well as in abnormal mitogenesis, mesangial proliferation, and glomerular scarring. In addition, their role in the repair phase of ischemic acute renal failure and the recognition that this in part recapitulates renal development have had a profound effect on the understanding of renal regeneration. This new information may now provide paradigms for developing approaches to the treatment of this costly kidney disease in hospitalized patients.

Molecular techniques have also added greatly to our understanding of basic aspects of electrolyte and other solute transport as genes for transmembrane pumps, exchangers, and channels have been identified. In some cases this has led to fundamental insight into the processes controlling kidney reabsorptive mechanisms, in a way not possible using the physiological and pharmacological tools that nephrologists have depended on in the past.

The cloning of hormone receptors, such as those for calcitonin, parathyroid hormone, vasopressin, and angiotensin, offers opportunities to study at a molecular level the structural features of ligand receptor interactions, identify mutations in these receptors, and characterize downstream effectors in cellular signaling cascades. It also provides a means for the design of receptor antagonists that can be used in pharmacological studies and in therapy. For example, the cloning of the vasopressin receptor and its characterization in the kidney have provided an opportunity to understand diseases such as X-linked congenital nephrogenic diabetes insipidus and autosomal recessive congenital nephrogenic diabetes insipidus. This, together with the cloning of the water channel, provides tools not only for understanding basic mechanisms of water transport across cells, but also for development of therapeutic receptor antagonists. In the case of the molecular characterization of the angiotensin receptors, the therapeutic promise of a receptor antagonist has been fulfilled. The angiotensin receptor antagonist already expands our therapeutic armamentarium for the treatment of hypertension and perhaps other disease states as well, such as congestive heart failure.

Understanding how changes in the *milieu intérieur* influence the regulation of genes in the kidney is also an important component of molecular nephrology. For example, the characterization of the regulatory pathways involved in hypoxia-induced erythropoetin gene expression has implications not only for the expression of this important renal hormone, but also for other genes that may be regulated through local changes in oxygen tension or the cellular redox potential.

Finally, a great hope of molecular nephrology will be realized when we are able to influence the expression of specific genes in particular renal cell types in a therapeutic attempt to alter the phenotype and correct or ameliorate cellular defects. Approaches to "gene therapy" are being attempted with various techniques using viral and nonviral vector approaches. This field is in its infancy, but will likely lead to the ability of the nephrologist to approach renal disease with an entirely novel therapeutic perspective.

The editors and contributors invite the readers to join them in the excitement of the race to keep up with this information explosion. Finally, however, our success as nephrologists will be measured not simply by the amount of basic information we accumulate, but by how well we translate this information into clinically useful forms and therapies to better the lot of our patients.

Detlef Schlöndorff
Joseph V. Bonventre

Contents

Molecular Nephrology

Kidney Function in Health and Disease

1
Developmental Control Genes

Gregory R. Dressler
Howard Hughes Medical Institute and University of Michigan, Ann Arbor, Michigan

INTRODUCTION

The development of a complete mammalian organism from a single fertilized egg requires a complex genetic program that is encoded by embryonic genes expressed in specific tissues at precise intervals. If these embryonic genes can be identified and their mechanisms of action determined, real insights into fundamental biological processes such as signal transduction, cell proliferation, apoptosis, and oncogenesis will surely be at hand. The genetic basis of development determines not only the lineage pathways of specialized cell types—that is, how cells differentiate from their progenitors and when their developmental fates become restricted—but also the structural organization, or pattern formation, of whole tissues for particular species. In fact, many species share common cell lineage pathways, although they are structurally quite different. How this genetic information is stored and processed is a fundamental question in developmental biology.

In considering the development of a single organ, such as the kidney, many of the principles driving embryogenesis of the whole organism also apply. The kidney consists of specialized cell types located within a three-dimensional architectural framework. This implies a coordinate system with spatial cues that convey positional information to cells before or during differentiation along the cell lineage pathways. The embryonic development of the kidney has been described in great detail (1). Through the pioneering work of Grobstein (2) and Saxen (3), it is clear that the initiation of kidney development occurs when the ureteric bud, an outgrowth of the Wolffian duct, induces the metanephric mesenchyme. Reciprocally, the mesenchyme induces the ureteric bud to branch repeatedly, thus generating the collecting ducts. Upon induction, the mesenchyme forms aggregates adjacent to the tips of the branching ureter that undergo a sequence of defined morphological transformations to generate the renal vesicle, the S-shaped body, and finally the mature nephron. Although many of the changes in gene expression that accompany the conversion of kidney mesenchyme to epithelium are well described (4), the inductive signals and underlying genetic basis of renal epithelial development remain to be determined. Furthermore, the role of developmental regulatory genes in regenerating renal epithelium and in renal carcinomas must also be addressed.

It is valuable to first introduce some basic principles of development and how they may apply to the study of the kidney. I would also like to discuss how known developmental regulatory genes were identified through mutation analyses in other organisms and how mammalian counterparts to these regulatory genes were identified. Subsequent chapters of this text will introduce many other genes that regulate specific events during the development of the kidney. Genes encoding transcription factors (i.e., proteins capable of potentiating transcription of other genes) clearly play a major role in the specification of cell types. However, the potential of cell surface adhesion molecules, extracellular matrix, and intracellular signaling molecules to drive morphogenic events is also becoming apparent.

SOME FUNDAMENTAL CONCEPTS IN DEVELOPMENTAL BIOLOGY

No matter what organisms is under investigation, developmental biologists share a common set of formulations that they believe underlie basic mechanisms of morphogenesis. For a more detailed description of developmental systems and concepts, the reader is referred to several excellent texts (5,6). Much has been learned by observing the development of embryos and detailing the anatomical structures over time. In fact, a historical association between anatomy and embryology was grounded in principle because anatomists, who wished to describe structure, began to examine embryos to better understand how structural organization came to be. However, histological observation has limits, as it is only a static picture of an extremely dynamic process. With the development of fate-mapping techniques, the ability to follow the cell lineage pathways to determine the origin of tissues was at hand. Fate mapping requires the marking of a cell or group of cells so that their progeny can be observed over time. Cells can be marked by microinjecting a tracer dye, by making chimeric embryos (such as quail/chick) where the different cells can be distinguished morphologically, or by introducing new genetic material with retroviruses. Embryos such as the frog or chick are particularly useful for generating fate maps as they are easily accessible and develop rapidly. More recently, the cell lineages of the kidney mesenchyme have been fate-mapped using a beta-galactosidase transducing retrovirus in kidney organ cultures (7). These experiments clearly demonstrate that mesenchymal cells are not restricted in their developmental potential prior to induction; rather, they differentiate into all epithelial cell types of the nephron. Fundamental to developing a fate map and following cell lineage pathways is the ability to distinguish different cell types along the lineage pathways with a set of specific markers. Antibodies against cell-type–specific antigens are particularly useful, although other distinctive morphological features can also be used. In the kidney, markers against different nephron segments have been described (8). Lectins such as wheat germ or peanut agglutinin bind specifically to the glomerular epithelium, whereas proximal and distal tubules can be stained with antibodies against brush-border antigens and Tamm-Horsfall protein respectively. The distribution of functional proteins involved in acid-base homeostasis can also be used to distinguish cell types. For example, the potassium-ATPase is found exclusively in the terminal nephron segments, including the connecting and collecting tubules (9).

Morphogens are external factors that influence the developmental program of cells by inducing differentiation, cell movement, polarization, cell patterning, or any other distinctive change in cellular properties. They can be small inorganic molecules, such as lithium or ammonium chloride, or large protein complexes. Morphogens can act over distances by diffusion through extracellular space, or locally by cell-cell contact or association with the extracellular matrix. Among the best characterized morphogens are the activins, a fibroblast growth factor–like protein able to induce mesoderm formation in frogs (10,11), and retinoic acid, a vitamin A derivative with a variety of inducing activities (12,13).

Induction is the ability of one cell type or tissue, the inducer, to change the developmental potential of another responding tissue. The concepts of induction have evolved from the classic experiments by Spemann and Mangold (14), who first proposed the idea of a central organizer—a group of cells from the blastopore lip that could alter the developmental fate of surrounding tissue and induce a second body axis after transplantation to an ectopic site in the newt embryo. Induction of the kidney mesenchyme by the ureteric bud is a secondary inductive event, as the mesenchymal cells are already restricted in their developmental potential to making only nephrons. Heterologous inducers, such as spinal cord (15), do not alter the developmental fate of the kidney mesenchyme; they merely provide the stimulus for the initiation of the renal mesenchyme-to-epithelium conversion. The inductive signals are still not well defined, although they do not appear to be diffusible morphogens. In the transfilter induction assay, cellular processes permeate the filter and are necessary for transducing the induction signal (16). Mesenchymal cells located near the inducing tissue apparently do not have the capacity to transmit the inducing signals to more distal mesenchyme (17), suggesting that these inducing cellular processes from the ureter may permeate far into the mesenchyme.

Positional information is the ability of cells to differentiate along certain lineages based on their immediate environment, or position, with respect to other cells. Modern genetic analyses in the fruit fly, *Drosophila*, have revealed elegant molecular mechanisms for storing and transmitting positional information along the coordinate axes of the embryo. In its simplest form, positional information along an axis can be delineated by a single morphogen, secreted at one pole and allowed to diffuse, so that any given coordinate has a unique concentration of morphogen. Such is the case in the developing chick limb bud, where the zone of polarizing activity is a source of retinoic acid and transplantation to ectopic sites results in duplication of digits and alterations in developmental gene expression (18,19).

A more recently developed concept that may have direct implications for kidney development is the community effect described during frog muscle cell differentiation (20,21). Cells taken from the early to middle gastrula were transplanted to a mesodern-inducing environment and would differentiate into muscle cells if taken as a group, whereas single cells would not differentiate. Only if the single muscle precursor cell was taken from a late gastrula did it have the capacity to differentiate in isolation. These experiments indicate that the number of cells and the timing of induction are critical for tissue differentiation. In the kidney transfilter induction system, a critical number of mesenchymal cells are required to generate tubules after induction.

GENETIC REGULATORY NETWORKS FROM *DROSOPHILA* TO HUMANS

The concept of common regulatory genes among very dissimilar organisms is based in part on the premise that a complex system designed to organize billions of cells in time and space would, once perfected, evolve and adapt to individual organisms by altering the eventual targets of regulation and not the fundamental controllers. For example, a mechanisms that translates a morphogen gradient into a segmented pattern of gene expression may be used repeatedly in different species to define separate body axes, be they longitudinal, dorsal-ventral, or proximal-distal along the limbs. Thus, it has proven possible for investigators to exploit the experimental advantages of different organisms—such as the genetics of *Drosophila*, tissue transplantation in frog and chick, and gene transfer and mutations in mouse—to address similar developmental questions.

Developmental biology is indebted to the many *Drosophila* geneticists who have laid the foundation for modern genetic analyses through mutational analyses and gene cloning. A thorough review of early *Drosophila* embryogenesis would fill a large textbook, so the reader is referred to a number of recent reviews covering particular aspects (22–24). It is useful, though, to summarize a few widely applicable principles. The adult fly is clearly segmented along the longitudinal axis and consists of three head, three thoracic, and nine abdominal segments. The delineation of the anterior-posterior axis of the *Drosophila* embryo occurs through the interpretation of two opposing protein gradients, with maximal concentrations at either end (25,26). These morphogen gradients activate a genetic hierarchy that progressively segments the embryo into increasingly smaller units. In a landmark report by Nuesslein-Volhard and Wieschaus (27), this segmentation gene hierarchy was deduced by examining developmental mutations that deleted adjacent groups of segments, every other segment, or parts of every segment before any of the genes responsible had been identified at the molecular level. It must be stressed that many of the segmentation genes are also expressed in the nervous system, where they can specify the developmental fates of specific neurons (28). In fact, these neurodevelopmental expression patterns and functions may be even more conserved across species (29) than the segmentation functions.

Once the body plan is segmented, the individual fate, or identity of each segment is specified by the homeotic genes. The process of homeosis is defined as the transformation of one body part into another (30), and that is precisely what deregulation of a single homeotic gene can produce. By misexpressing the homeotic gene *Antennaepedia*, the fly sprouts legs from the head at a position normally reserved for antennae (31). Similarly, misexpression of the *Ultrabithorax* gene transforms the third thoracic segment into the second, resulting in an additional pair of wings (32,33). Upon cloning many homeotic and segmentation genes from *Drosophila*, DNA sequence comparisons revealed a very similar protein coding sequence, called the homeobox, with a characteristic helix-turn-helix structure, indicative of a DNA-binding protein (34,35). The DNA-binding characteristics and crystallographic structure of several homeodomains have now been determined (36,37), and all the available data point to a transcription-potentiating function, although specific downstream target genes are still few and far between.

The remarkable conservation of the homeodomain among *Drosophila* developmental control genes led many investigators to search for mouse and human homologues. Not only were the protein-coding sequences found in all vertebrate species but the linear gene order along the chromosomes and the relationships of anterior-posterior expression pattern were also conserved (38–40). Figure 1 outlines the homeotic genes of *Drosophila*, the corresponding *HOX* genes of the mouse, and the anterior limits of their expression patterns. Note the linearity along the four *HOX* gene clusters and the anterior limits of gene expression. Through the successful application of homologous recombination technology in mouse embryonic steam cells (41), several *HOX* genes have been mutated in the mouse, and the resultant phenotypes clearly demonstrate a master regulatory function during mammalian development (42–44). Interestingly, the developmental abnormalities in *HOX* mutant mice are primarily restricted to the expression domains unique for that particular gene, with respect to the more 5′ or posterior gene on the cluster. Thus many cells and tissues that express a particular *HOX* gene are unaffected in the null mutants, underscoring the principle that gene expression patterns may be much broader than the functional requirement for the gene product. In fact, there is no need to develop complex transcription suppression mechanisms if that gene product is not detrimental to the normal growth and differentiation of a particular cell type.

A search for mammalian homologues of segmentation genes identified the murine *Pax* gene family (see Table 1) by virtue of their sequence similarity to the paired domain sequence found in at least three *Drosophila* segmentation genes (58). Some of the mouse *Pax* genes are indeed expressed in a periodic pattern in segmented structures, such as *Pax-1* in the vertebral column and *Pax-2* and *Pax-8* in the segmented tubules of the mesonephrons. As in *Drosophila*, most of the *Pax* genes are also expressed in the developing neural tube, which, in mammals, is partitioned primarily in the transverse plane. It has been proposed that the unique but overlapping patterns of *Pax* gene expression

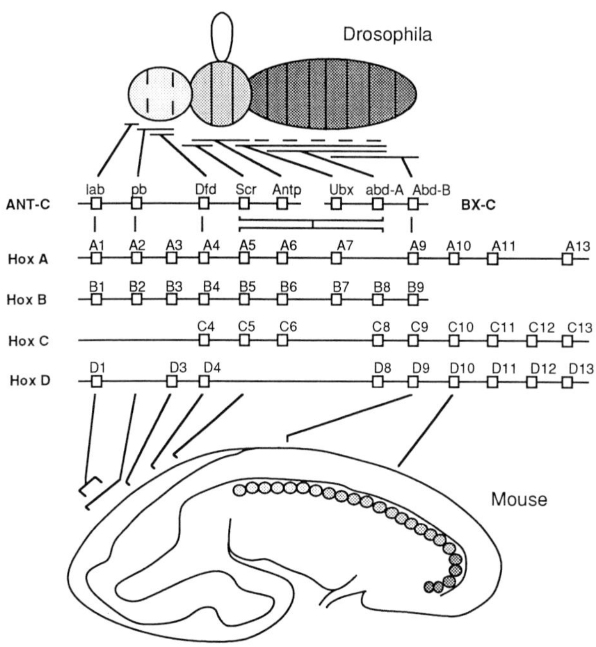

Figure 1 Homeotic genes of *Drosophila* and their mammalian counterparts. The *Drosophila* homeotic genes map to the Antennapedia complex (ANT-C) and the Bithorax complex (BX-C). The expression domains of individual genes are delineated by the horizontal lines. In mouse, there are four *Hox* gene clusters (A to D), as defined by the new standard nomenclature (86). The anterior limit of the *Hox* gene expression domains are delineated by the vertical lines. The *Drosophila* and mouse genes are colinear, such that *labial* (*lab*) is most homologous to *HoxA1*, *Deformed* (*Dfd*) is most homologous to *Hox-A4*, and *Abdominal B* (*Abd-B*) is most homologous to *Hox-A9*. (Adapted from Refs. 87 and 88.)

Table 1 The *Pax* Gene Family

Gene	Chromosome Mouse	Chromosome Human	Expression pattern	Mutations (mouse/human)	Ref.
Pax-1	2	20p	Vertebral column, thymus	*Undulated*	45
Pax-2	19	10q	Neural tube, kidney		46, 47
Pax-3	1	2q	Neural crest, neural epithelium	*Splotch*/Waardenburg syndrome	48
Pax-4	6	7	Pseudogene?		49
Pax-5	4	9p	Neural tube, B cells, kidney		50
Pax-6	2	11p	Neural tube, optic cup	*Small eye*/aniridia	51, 52
Pax-7	4	1p	Neural tube, muscle		53
Pax-8	2	2q	Neural tube, kidney		54, 55
Pax-9	12	14q			56, 57

during neurogenesis may help to pattern the central nervous system by delineating specific subpopulations of neurons (59).

There are a number of mutations in mouse and human that serve to underline the importance of *Pax* genes as developmental regulators. A point mutation in the DNA binding domain of *Pax-1* results in the mouse *undulated* phenotype (60), characterised by enlarged intervertebral discs and small vertebral bodies. The *Pax-3* gene has been associated with the mouse *Splotch* mutation (61) and the human equivalent. Waardenburg syndrome (62,63), both of which affect the development of the neural crest cells and neural tube. The mouse *Small eye* (64) and human aniridia (52) syndromes are the result of mutations or deletions in the *Pax-6* gene. Although *Pax* genes were initially identified based on homology to *Drosophila* segmentation genes, their mammalian expression patterns reveal common features that transcend segmentation per se. Both *Pax-1* and *Pax-2* are expressed in cells that appear to aggregate and form boundaries with adjacent nonexpressing cells. *Pax-3*, *6*, and *7* also define boundaries, or cell types, in the undifferentiated neural epithelium. If one important aspect of segmentation is to distinguish like cells from their neighbors by promoting like cell adhesion, thus excluding dissimilar cells, the mammalian *Pax* genes may have retained some of the morphogenic function of *Drosophila* segmentation genes whose primary functions are to define boundaries of segments in the mesoderm and specify cell phenotypes in the neuroectoderm.

THE MOLECULAR BIOLOGY OF *PAX* PROTEINS

The mammalian *Pax* gene family includes at least nine members that are, unlike the *Hox* genes, not linked genetically. The map positions of both human and mouse *Pax* genes are listed in Table 1. Structurally, the individual members of the *Pax* gene family can be further divided into subfamilies of genes that are more or less similar based on sequence and expression patterns (49). Thus, *Pax-3* and *Pax-7* are most homologous outside the paired domain and contain a second conserved sequence, the paired-type homeodomain with a classical helix-turn-helix structure. A third conserved region common to most *Pax* genes is the octapeptide found downstream of the paired domain. *Pax-6* and *Pax-4* also contain the homeodomain but not the conserved octapeptide and constitute a second subfamily. *Pax-1* and *Pax-9* have only the paired domain and octapeptide and are expressed in similar tissues of the vertebral column. The *Pax-2*, *Pax-5*, and *Pax-8* genes contain a paired domain, an octapeptide sequence, and only the first helix of a paired homeodomain. These three genes also have many similar features to their respective expression patterns in the neural tube and developing kidney. From what little is known about the genomic structure, some of the *Pax* genes span over 100 kb with multiple exons, including introns within both the paired domain and the paired-type homeodomain.

The factors activating *Pax* genes and the DNA regulatory sequences that promote correct spatial and temporal expression remain to be determined. However, in the developing neural tube, it is clear that external signals from inducing tissues, such as the notochord, influence the boundaries of expression along the dorsal-ventral axis. In an elegant series of transplantation experiments, Goulding et al. (65) transplanted notochord tissue adjacent to developing chick neural tube such that a second ventral floor plate was induced and ectopic ventral motor neurons were generated. The changes in *Pax-3*, *Pax-7*, and *Pax-6* expression evident in the neural epithelium occured prior to neural differentiation; thus the signals emanating from the transplanted notochord may redirect the developmental potential of undifferentiated cells through the altered expression of *Pax* genes. The *Pax-2* gene expression pattern in the developing neural tube is also altered in response to signals from the notochord (66), but this may be a more indirect effect, because *Pax-2* is expressed in the differentiating neural cells and not in the pluripotent neuroepithelium (67). In the kidney, *Pax-2* is activated shortly after induction and thus may be one of the first nuclear transcription factors regulated by the inducing signals emanating from the ureteric bud.

The *Pax* genes encode DNA-binding proteins capable of potentiating transcription, and they most probably exert their developmental effects by activating a battery of cell-type–specific genes. The paired domain alone, from the *Drosophila paired* protein, could bind DNA independent of the homeodomain found at the C terminus of that protein (68). Using the binding sequence of *paired* as a starting point, target DNA sequences for the Pax-1 protein were optimized by changing nucleotides flanking a GTTCC core sequence (69). The undulated mutant allele of *Pax-1*, which has a point mutation and amino acid substitution in the paired domain, was unable to bind the target sequence with the same efficiency. Thus, the molecular basis of the undulated phenotype is most probably due to insufficient DNA binding of the mutant Pax-1 protein.

The *Pax-5* gene was cloned independently by virtue of its DNA-binding capacity (50) and its conserved paired domain sequence (49). *Pax-5* is identical to the B-cell–specific transcription factor BSAP, which is expressed in differentiating B cells but not in terminally differentiated plasma cells (50). The CD19 gene, which encodes a transmembrane receptor, is the one of the targets of activation by the Pax-5 protein. Thus, the binding of *Pax-5* to the CD19 promoter and recognition site represents the best model for paired domain/nucleic acid interactions. It appears that the N- and C-terminal domains interact independently with two elements of the bipartite recognition sequence (70), as diagramed schematically in Fig. 2. At the protein level, the bipartite nature of the paired domain is reflected by a more homologous N-terminal region, approximately 80% over 70 amino acids, and a less homologous C-terminal region, 40–60% over 60 amino acids, among the different members of the *Pax* gene family. The disparate levels of conservation may indicate binding of the N-terminal domain to a consensus-type sequence and binding of the C-terminal part of the paired domain to a more heterogenous protein-specific DNA sequence. In any event, characterization of the interactions among *Pax* genes and nucleic acids is still in its infancy and clearly requires the identification of more genes directly under the control of Pax proteins.

DEVELOPMENTAL CONTROL GENES OF THE KIDNEY

Since the development of the kidney organ culture system over 40 years ago, the kidney has proven to be an excellent model for embryonic induction and epithelial differentiation. Later chapters of

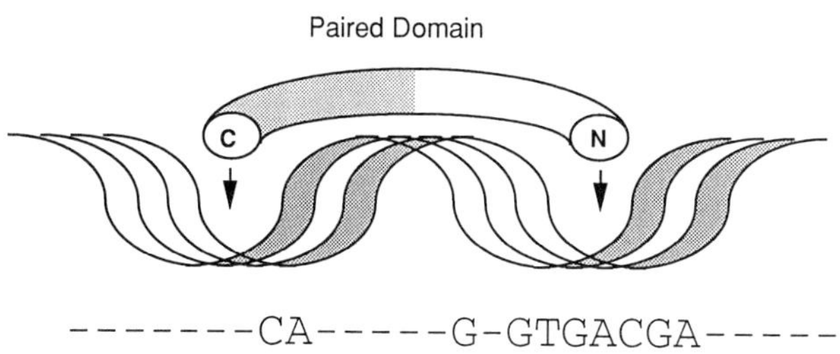

Figure 2 Model of paired domain interaction with DNA. Using the *Pax-5* paired domain as a prototype, Czerny et al. (70) proposed a bipartite recognition sequence that interacts with the N- and C-terminal domains independently. The recognition sites are located in adjacent major grooves of the DNA helix and the consensus nucleotide sequence is shown below.

this text will discuss in detail much of what is known about cell adhesion, cell-cell interactions, and cell-matrix interactions during kidney development. I would like to focus on potential regulatory factors that may control the development and patterning of the early embryonic kidney after induction.

Much of the work in my own lab has focused on the function of *Pax-2* during early kidney development. The *Pax-2* gene encodes a DNA-binding transcription factor expressed in the developing kidney and neural tube. The transient expression pattern of *Pax-2* and the experimental amenability of the kidney had made this an attractive system for addressing basic questions of morphogenesis. Expression of *Pax-2* is detected in the epithelial components of the pro- and mesonephros and persists in the ureteric bud, an outgrowth of the mesonephric duct. However, it is the activation and suppression of *Pax-2* in the metanephric mesenchymal cells that is most intriguing. Both by in situ hybridization (46) and using *Pax-2*–specific antibodies (71), expression is first detected in the induced mesenchymal cells and in the aggregates of mesenchyme that surround the tips of the branching ureter (Fig. 3). Activation of *Pax-2* expression cannot be detected in the mesenchyme of a mutant mouse strain that fails to induce the adult kidney (66). Thus, *Pax-2* activation in the mesenchyme is dependent upon induction by the ureter and may be the first detectable marker for the induced mesenchyme. Using antisense oligonucleotides designed to inhibit Pax-2 protein synthesis, in vitro organ culture experiments demonstrated a clear requirement for *Pax-2* during the initial mesenchymal condensation phase shortly after induction (72). It is likely that *Pax-2* functions at the beginning of a genetic cascade that ultimately specifies the conversion of kidney mesenchyme to epithelium.

The expression of *Pax-2* persists in the early mesenchymal derivatives, the renal vesicle, the comma-shaped body, and in the distal portion of the S-shaped body. However, downregulation of *Pax-2* first becomes evident in the proximal part of the S-shaped body as the visceral glomerular epithelium matures. With the maturation of the proximal and distal convoluted tubules, *Pax-2* suppression is complete in the mesenchyme-derived epithelium, although the ureter-derived collecting ducts continue to express low levels of the Pax-2 protein. Suppression of *Pax-2* is required for the glomerular and tubular epithelium to mature, as experiments deregulating the gene in transgenic mice have demonstrated (73). As shown in Fig. 4, this persistent expression of *Pax-2*, under the control of a human cytomegalovirus promoter element in mice, produces abnormal kidneys with a phenotype similar to that of congenital nephrotic syndrome. *Pax-8* and *Pax-5* are also expressed in the kidney and, together with *Pax-2*, constitute a subfamily of homologous genes. However, it is unlikely that these genes are functionally redundant. The existing mutations for *Pax-1*, *3*, and *6* are not complemented by their homologous subfamily members and are, in fact, haploid-insufficient. Thus, there is a strict quantitative requirement for Pax protein levels in specific embryonic tissues. By elucidating the mechanism of action of the Pax-2 protein and its interactions with other developmental regulators, our understanding of kidney development and the fundamental process of morphogenesis will surely be advanced.

The ability to create mutations in the mouse germline has identified several other key factors in early kidney development. Human genetic analysis has pointed to the Wilms' tumor suppressor gene (*WT1*) as a regulator of kidney mesenchyme proliferation and differentiation. The properties of *WT1* and its relation to Wilms' tumor will be discussed in subsequent chapters. However, a mouse *WT1* mutation was created by homologous recombination in embryonic stem cells and the subsequent phenotype was rather surprising (74). *WT1* homozygous mutant mice completely failed to induce the kidney and died in utero due to other unrelated complications. Ureteric bud outgrowth was limited in the embryo and the metanephric mesenchyme lost the capacity to respond to induction even using a normal ureter in vitro. Thus, *WT1* plays a very early role in the uninduced kidney mesenchyme. The loss of heterozygosity at *WT1*, associated with familial Wilms' tumor, probably occurs in a very small number of kidney mesenchyme cells after induction, at a time when these cells are highly proliferative. It would be interesting to transplant mouse *WT1* mutant mesenchymal cells into a wild-type newborn kidney. Perhaps then the oncogenic suppressor role of *WT1* would become evident.

Several known oncogenes are expressed in cell type–specific ways during kidney development. Members of the *myc* family show partially overlapping but unique expression patterns in the embryonic kidney (75). Whereas C-*myc* is expressed in the undifferentiated mesenchymal cell, N-*myc* is activated in the induced mesenchyme and persists in the early derivatives thereof before decreasing. In the ureter, L-*myc* is predominant. In fact, mutating the N-*myc* gene by homologous recombination

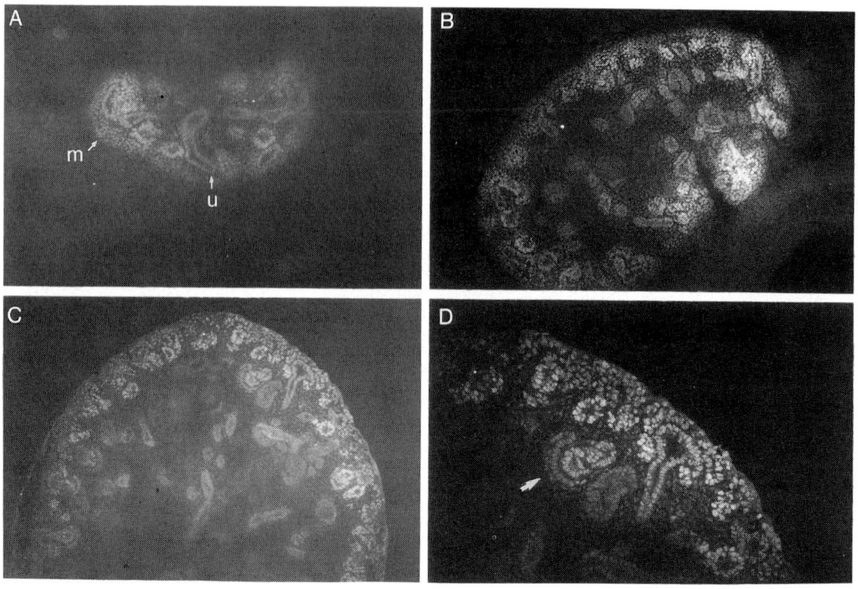

Figure 3 Expression of the *Pax-2* gene in developing kidney. Immunostaining with *Pax-2*–specific antibodies on frozen sections of mouse embryos. (A) At 12 days gestation, *Pax-2* expression is activated in mesenchymal aggregates (m) adjacent to the ureteric bud epithelium (u). (B) At 14 days gestation, *Pax-2* expression is widespread in the developing tubules and in the collecting ducts. (C) By 17 days gestation, the kidney consists of an outer nephrogenic zone, where mesenchyme proliferation and induction is still ongoing, and a more developed inner region where nephrogenesis has progressed. *Pax-2* expression is still evident in the induced mesenchyme and its early derivatives, but the mature renal epithelium has repressed *Pax-2* expression. The ureter-derived collecting ducts, however, still show low levels of *Pax-2* expression. (D) Higher magnification of C, showing *Pax-2* expression in condensing mesenchyme and ureter buds. Note decrease of expression in proximal part of S-shaped body (arrow).

results in the failure of the kidney epithelium to develop fully (76). Other organs with epithelial components are similarly affected, indicating that N-*myc* may be required for the proliferation of the epithelium after induction but prior to terminal differentiation. Multiple *Hox* genes are expressed in the posterior intermediate mesoderm before the nephric cord is fully differentiated, and *Hox* gene expression persists in the differentiated kidney. Perhaps the most interesting *Hox* expression pattern is that of *Hox-B7* (*Hox-2.3*), which is coincident with the generation of mesonephric and metanephric epithelium (77).

Growth factors and receptors are also intimately involved in developmental decision making during kidney development and are discussed in more detail in subsequent chapters. The low-affinity nerve growth factor is expressed on the kidney mesenchymal cells and appears to be required for induction in vitro (78). Also, it is worth noting that because of the potential for ligands and receptors to be directly involved with inductive signaling, oncogenes encoding receptor tyrosine kinases (79,80) have also been implicated in kidney development. The major receptors of interest would include c-*ret*, c-*met*, c-*ros*, and the epithelial growth factor (EGF) receptor. Recently, Schuchardt et al. (81) have mutated the c-*ret* gene in mouse and the resultant phenotype includes a near complete absence of kidneys. Since c-*ret* is expressed at the tips of the ureter buds, it is worth speculating that this receptor may be the target for ureter branching and proliferation signals emanating from the induced mesenchyme cells. The ligand for c-*met*, hepatocyte growth factor, or scatter factor is expressed in the metanephric mesenchyme, whereas the receptor is found on the ureter bud epithelium (82). Thus, c-*met* could receive growth-potentiating signals from the induced mesenchyme. The *ros*-1 receptor tyrosine kinase is also expressed just at the tips of the ureter bud (83,84), in a pattern similar to that of c-*ret*.

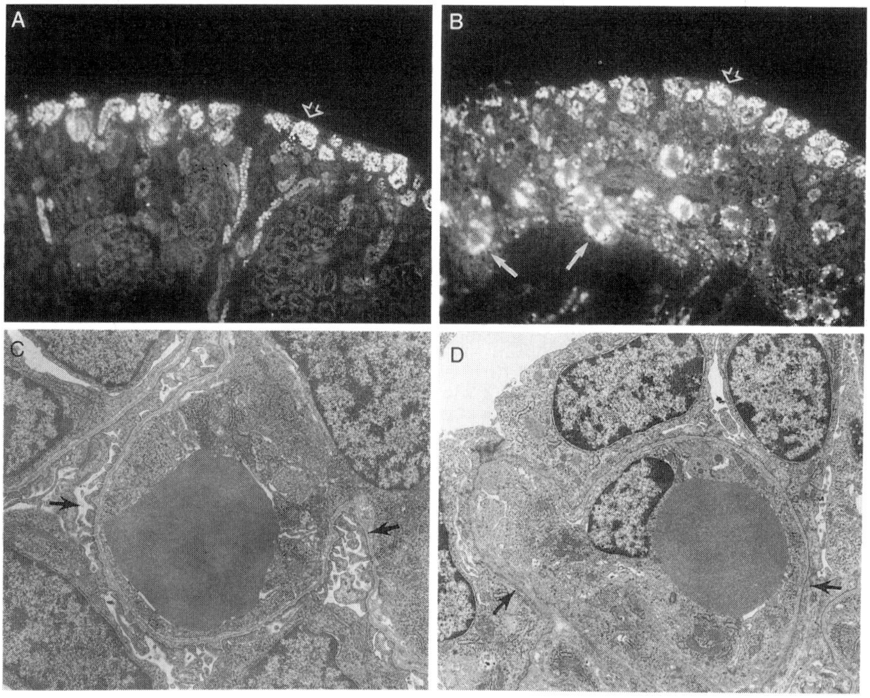

Figure 4 *Pax-2* suppression is required for normal kidney development. The *Pax-2* gene was fused to a strong promoter and introduced into transgenic mice (73). Antibody staining against *Pax-2* is shown in the normal (A) and transgenic (B) 1-day-old kidney. Note the *Pax-2*–expressing cells around the glomerulus of transgenic mice (arrows). Endogenous *Pax-2* expression is still very apparent in the nephrogenic zone at this time (open arrows, A and B). Newborn mice expressing the transgene had severe kidney abnormalitites, including proteinuria, elevated BUN, and hyperkalemia. Electron microscopy revealed a complete absence of foot processes (arrows) in the podocyte cells of the glomeruler epithelium in transgenic mice (D) compared to normal litter mates (C). The phenotype is characteristic of human congenital nephrotic syndromes. (Electron microscopy micrographs courtesy of Dr. J. E. Wilkinson.)

The number and types of developmental regulatory proteins is steadily increasing as more genes are revealed. Oncogenes originally identified by their transforming potential clearly have developmental functions. Growth factors and their receptors also constitute a large family of morphogenic proteins that can function as autocrine and paracrine regulators of proliferation and differentiation. With the power of gene mapping and chromosome walking, many of the genes responsible for developmental mutations in mouse and human have been identified and others are at hand. Moreover, it is not unusual for regulatory proteins to be expressed in multiple tissues, as the biochemistry of function may depend on specific interactions with other proteins or DNA target sequences. However, the embryonic expression pattern of a gene does not necessarily dictate a required function in each tissue, since there is no evolutionarty pressure to eliminate the expression of gene as long as it is not detrimental (85).

CONCLUSIONS

There is a resurgence in developmental biology, fueled by modern genetic and molecular methods and a renewed appreciation for the encompassing role developmental mechanisms play in normal and abnormal cellular processes. We are at the beginning of a long investigative journey and must decipher large volumes of genetic information to identify the key control genes from the many others that are merely along for the ride. Unfortunately, the ability to analyze the functions of the gene products has not kept pace with the rapid cloning and sequencing of new developmentally expressed genes.

The kidney has proved to be an excellent model for the study of inductive interactions and cellular differentiation. The genetic bases underlying the morphogenesis of renal epithelium are now being addressed in a variety of ways that will illuminate not only fundamental developmental mechanisms but also the pathological basis of renal diseases.

ACKNOWLEDGMENTS

I thank Dervla Mellerick for helpful discussions and critical reading of the manuscript. I also thank Uwe Rothenpieler and Larry Patterson for helping me to appreciate kidney anatomy and function.

Many of the references are review articles designed to help readers who wish to pursue individual topics. Due to the broad nature of this chapter, I was unfortunately unable to cite all the original references for each topic.

REFERENCES

1. Saxen, L. Organogenesis of the kidney. In: Barlow PW, Green PB, White CC, eds. Developmental and Cell Biology Series. Vol. 19. Cambridge University Press, 1987.
2. Grobstein C. Trans-filter induction of tubules in mouse metanephrogenic mesenchyme. Exp Cell Res 1956; 10:424–440.
3. Saxen I, Koskimies O, Lahti A, et al. Differentiation of kidney mesenchyme in an experimental model system. Adv Morphol 1968; 7:251–293.
4. Ekblom P. Developmentally regulated conversion of mesenchyme to epithelium. FASEB J 1989; 3:2141–2150.
5. Slack JMW. From Egg to Embryo. Oxford, UK: Oxford University Press, 1991.
6. Gilbert SF. Developmental Biology, 3d ed. Sunderland, MA: Sinauer Associates, 1991.
7. Herzlinger D, Koseki C, Mikawa T, Al-Awqati Q. Metanephric mesenchyme contains multipotent stem cells whose fate is restricted after induction. Development 1992; 114:565–572.
8. Ekblom P, Miettinen A, Virtanen I, et al. In vitro segregation of the metanephric nephron. Dev Biol 1981; 84:88–95.
9. Doucet A, Marsy S. Characterization of K-ATPase activity in distal nephron: Stimulation by potassium depletion. Am J Physiol 1987; 253:F418–F423.
10. Smith JC. Mesoderm induction and mesoderm inducing factors in early amphibian development. Development 1989; 105:665–677.
11. Slack JM, Tannahill D. Mechanism of anteroposterior axis specification in vertebrates: Lessons from the amphibians. Development 1992; 114:285–302.
12. Bryant SV, Gardiner DM. Retinoic acid, local cell-cell interactions, and pattern formation in vertebrate limbs. Dev Biol 1992; 152:1–25.
13. Brockes JP. Retinoids, homeobox genes and limb morphogenesis. Neuron 1989; 2:1285–1294.
14. Spemann H, Mangold H. Uber Induktion von Embryonalanlagen durch Implantation artfremder Organisatoren. Arch Mikrosk Anat Entw Mech 1924; 100:599–638.
15. Sariola H, Ekblom P, Henke-Fahle S. Embryonic neurons as in vitro inducers of differentiation of nephrogenic mesenchyme. Dev Biol 1989; 132:271–281.
16. Wartiovarra J, Nordling S, Lehtonen E, Saxen L. Transfilter induction of kidney tubules: Correlation with cytoplasmic penetration into nucleopore filters. J Embryol Exp Morphol 1974; 31:667–682.
17. Saxen L, Saksela E. Transmission and spread of embryonic induction: II. Exclusion of an assimilatory transmission mechanism in kidney induction. Exp Cell Res 1971; 66:369–377.
18. Tickle C. Retinoic acid and chick limb bud development. Development 1991; 1:113–121.
19. Izpisua-Belmonte JC, Duboule D. Homeobox genes and pattern formation in the vertebrate limb. Dev Biol 1992; 152:26–36.
20. Gurdon JB. A community effect in animal development. Nature 1988; 336:772–774.
21. Gurdon JB, Kato K, Lemaire P. The community effect, dorsalization and mesoderm induction. Curr Opin Genet Dev 1993; 3:662–667.
22. St Johnston D, Nuesslein-Volhard C. The origin of pattern and polarity in the *Drosophila* embryo. Cell 1992; 68:201–219.

23. Carroll SB. Zebra patterns in fly embryos: Activation of stripes or repression of interstripes? Cell 1990; 60:9–16.
24. Lawrence PA. The Making of a Fly: The Genetics of Animal Design. Cambridge, MA: Blackwell Scientific Publications, 1992.
25. Driever W, Nuesslein-Volhard C. The bicoid protein determines position in the *Drosophila* embryo in a concentration dependent manner. Cell 1988; 54:95–104.
26. Wang C, Lehman R. *Nanos* is the localised posterior determinent in *Drosophila*. Cell 1991; 66:637–647.
27. Nuesslein-Volhard C, Wieschaus E. Mutations affecting segment number and polarity in *Drosophila*. Nature 1980; 287:795–801.
28. Patel NH, Schafer B, Goodman CS, Holmgren R. The role of segment polarity genes during *Drosophila* neurogenesis. Genes Dev 1989; 3:890–904.
29. Patel NH, Ball EE, Goodman CS. Changing role of *even-skipped* during the evolution of insect pattern formation. Nature 1992; 357:339–342.
30. Bateson W. Materials for the Study of Variation Treated with Especial Regard to Discontinuity in the Origin of Species. London: Macmillan Press, 1894. London.
31. Kaufman TC, Seeger MA, Olsen G. Molecular and genetic organization of the antennapedia gene complex of *Drosophila* melanogaster. Adv Genet 1990; 27:309–362.
32. Lewis EB. A gene complex controlling segmentation in *Drosophila*. Nature 1978; 276:565–570.
33. Pfeifer M, Karch F, Bender W. The bithorax complex: Control of segmental identity. Genes Dev 1987; 891–898.
34. McGinnis W, Levine MS, Hafen E, et al. A conserved DNA sequence in homeotic genes of the *Drosophila* antennapedia and bithorax complexes. Nature 1984; 308:428–433.
35. Scott MP, Weiner AJ. Structural relationships among genes that control development: Sequence homology between *Antennapedia*, *Ultrabithorax*, and *fushi tarazu* loci of *Drosophila*. Proc Natl Acad Sci USA 1984; 81:4115–4119.
36. Gehring W, Muller M, Affolter M, et al. The structure of the homeodomain and its functional implications. Trends Genet 1990; 6:323–329.
37. Kissinger C, Liu B, Martin-Blanco E, et al. Crystal structure of the engrailed homeodomain-DNA complex at 2.8A resolution: A framework for understanding homeodomain-DNA interactions. Cell 1990; 63:579–590.
38. Graham A, Papalopolu N, Krumlauf R. The murine and *Drosophila* homeobox gene complexes have common features of organization and expression. Cell 1989; 57:367–378.
39. Duboule D, Dolle P. The structural and functional organization of the murine HOX gene family resembles that of *Drosophila* homeotic genes. EMBO J 1989; 8:1497–1505.
40. Dressler GR, Gruss P. Anterior boundries of Hox gene expression in mesoderm derived structures correlate with the linear gene order along the chromosome. Differentiation 1989; 41:193–201.
41. Capecchi MR. Altering the genome by homologous recombination. Science 1989; 244:1288–1292.
42. Chisaka O, Capecchi M. Regionally restricted developmental defects resulting from targeted disruption of the mouse homeobox gene *hox-1.5*. Nature 1991; 350:473–479.
43. Lufkin T, Dierich A, LeMeur M, et al. Disruption of the *hox-1.6* homeobox gene results in defects in a region corresponding to its rostral domain of expression. Cell 1991; 66:1105–1119.
44. Le Mouellic H, Lallemand Y, Brulet P. Homeosis in the mouse induced by a null mutation in the *Hox-3.1* gene. Cell 1992; 69:251–264.
45. Deutsch U, Dressler GR, Gruss P. *Paxl*, a member of a paired box homologous murine gene family, is expressed in segmented structures during development. Cell 1988; 53:617–625.
46. Dressler GR, Deutsch U, Chowdhury K, et al. *Pax2*, a new murine paired box containing gene and its expression in the developing excretory system. Development 1990; 109:787–795.
47. Eccles MR, Wallis LJ, Fidler AE, et al. Expression of the *Pax2* gene in human fetal kidney and Wilms' tumor. Cell Growth Diff 1992; 3:279–289.
48. Goulding MD, Chalepakis G, Deitsch U, et al. *Pax-3*, a novel murine DNA binding protein expressed during early neurogenesis. EMBO J 1991; 10:1135–1147.
49. Walther C, Guenet JL, Simon D, et al. Pax: A multigene family of paired box-containing genes. Genomics 1991; 11:424–434.
50. Adams B, Doerfler P, Aguzzi A, et al. *Pax-5* encodes the transcription factor BSAP and is expressed in B lymphocytes, the developing CNS, and the adult testis. Genes Dev 1992; 6:1589–1607.
51. Walther C, Gruss P. *Pax-6*, a murine paired box gene, is expressed in the developing CNS. Development 1991; 113:1435–1449.
52. Ton CCT, Hirvonen H, Miwa H, et al. Positional cloning and characterization of a paired box and homeobox-containing gene from the aniridia region. Cell 1991; 67:1059–1074.
53. Jostes B, Walther C, Gruss P. The murine paired box gene, *Pax7*, is expressed specifically during the development of the nervous and muscular system. Mech Dev 1991; 33:27–38.

54. Plachov D, Chowdhury K, Walther C, et al. *Pax8*, a murine paired box gene expressed in the developing excretory system and thyroid gland. Development 1990; 110:643–651.
55. Pooleev A, Fickenscher H, Mundlos S, et al. *Pax8*, a human paired box gene: Isolation and expression in developing thyroid, kidney, and Wilms' tumors. Development 1992; 116:611–623.
56. Wallin J, Mizutani Y, Imai K, et al. A new Pax gene, *Pax-9*, maps to mouse chromosome 12. Mammal Gen 1993; 4:354–358.
57. Stapleton P, Weith A, Urbanek P, et al. Chromosomal localization of seven PAX genes and cloning of a novel family member, *Pax-9*. Nature Genet 1993; 3:292–298.
58. Bopp D, Burri M, Baumgartner S, et al. Conservation of a large protein domain in the segmentation gene *paired* and in functionally related genes of *Drosophila*. Cell 1986; 47:1033–1040.
59. Deutsch U, Gruss P. Murine paired domain proteins as regulator factors of embryonic development. Semin Dev Biol 1991; 2:413–424.
60. Balling R, Deutsch U, Gruss P. *Undulated*, a mutation affecting the development of the mouse skeleton, has a point mutation in the paired box of Pax1. Cell 1988; 55:531–535.
61. Epstein DJ, Vekemans M, Gros P. *splotch* (Sp^{2H}), a mutation affecting development of the mouse neural tube, shows a deletion within the paired homeodomain of Pax3. Cell 1991; 67:767–774.
62. Baldwin CT, Hoth CF, Amos JA, et al. An exonic mutation in the HuP2 paired domain gene causes Waardenburg's syndrome. Nature 1992; 355:637–638.
63. Tassabehji M, Read AP, Newton VE, et al. Waardenburg's syndrome patients have mutations in the human homologue of the *Pax-3* paired box gene. Nature 1992; 355:635–636.
64. Hill RE, Favor J, Hogan BLM, et al. Mouse *small eye* results from mutations in a paired-like homeobox-containing gene. Nature 1992; 354:522–525.
65. Goulding MD, Lumsden A, Gruss P. Signals from the floor plate regulate the region specific expression of two Pax genes in the developing spinal cord. Development 1993; 117:1001–1016.
66. Phelps DE, Dressler GR. Aberrant expression of *Pax-2* in *Danforth's short tail* (Sd) mice. Dev Biol 1993; 157:251–258.
67. Pueschel A, Westerfield M, Dressler GR. Comparitive analysis of Pax-2 protein distributions during neurulation in mice and zebrafish. Mech Dev 1992; 38:197–208.
68. Treisman J, Harris E, Desplan C. The paired box encodes a second DNA-binding domain in the paired homeo-domain protein. Genes Dev 1991; 5:594–604.
69. Chalepakis G, Fritsch R, Fickenscher H, et al. The molecular basis of the undulated/Pax-1 mutation. Cell 1991; 66:873–884.
70. Czerny T, Schaffner G, Busslinger M. DNA sequence recognition by Pax proteins: Bipartite structure of the paired domain and its binding site. Genes Dev 1993; 7:2048–2061.
71. Dressler GR, Douglass EC. *Pax-2* is a DNA binding protein expressed in embryonic kidney and Wilms' tumor. Proc Natl Acad Sci USA 1992; 89:1179–1183.
72. Rothenpieler UW, Dressler GR. *Pax-2* is required for mesenchyme to epithelium conversion during kidney development. Development 1993; 119:711–720.
73. Dressler GR, Wilkinson JE, Rothenpieler UW, et al. Deregulation of *Pax-2* expression in transgenic mice generates severe kidney abnormalities. Nature 1993; 362:65–67.
74. Kreidberg JA, Sariola H, Loring JM, et al. Jaenisch R WT-1 is required for early kidney development. Cell 1993; 74:679–691.
75. Mugrauer G, Ekblom P. Contrasting expression patterns of three members of the myc family of protooncogenes in the developing adult mouse kidney. J Cell Biol 1991; 112:13–25.
76. Stanton BR, Perkins AS, Tessarollo L, et al. Loss of *N-myc* function results in embryonic lethality and failure of the epithelial component of the embryo to develop. Genes Dev 1992; 6:2235–2247.
77. Kress C, Vogels R, De Graaff W, et al. *Hox2.3* upstream sequences mediate lacZ expression in intermediate mesoderm derivatives of transgenic mice. Development 1990; 109:775–786.
78. Sariola H, Saarma M, Sainio K, et al. Dependence of kidney morphogenesis on the expression of nerve growth factor receptor. Science 1991; 254:571–573.
79. Pawson T, Bernstein A. Receptor tyrosine kinases: Genetic evidence for their role in Drosophila and mouse development. Trends Genet 1990; 6:350–356.
80. Birchmeier C, Sonnenberg E, Weidner KM, Walter B. Tyrosine kinase receptors in the control of epithelial growth and morphogenesis during development. BioEssays 1993; 15:185–189.
81. Schuchardt A, D'Agati V, Larsson-Blomberg L, et al. The c-ret tyrosine kinase gene is required for the development of the kidney and the neteric nervous system. Nature 1994; 367:380–383.
82. Sonnenberg E, Meyer D, Weidner KM, Birchmeier C. Scatter factor/hepatocyte growth factor and its receptor, the c-met tyrosine kinase, can mediate a signal exchange between mesenchyme and epithelia during mouse development. J Cell Biol 1993; 123:223–225.
83. Sonnenberg E, Goedecke A, Walter B, et al. Transient and locally restricted expression of the *ros1* protooncogene during mouse development. EMBO J 1991; 10:3693–3702.

84. Tessarollo L, Nagarajan L, Parada LF. *C-ros*: the vertebrate homolog of the sevenless tyrosine kinase receptor is tightly regulated during organogenesis in mouse embryonic development. Development 1992; 115:11–20.
85. Erickson HP. Gene knockouts of c-src, transforming growth factor b1, and tenascin suggest superfluous, nonfunctional expression of proteins. J Cell Biol 1993; 120:1079–1081.
86. Scott MP. Vertebrate homeobox gene nomenclature. Cell 1992; 71:551–553.
87. McGinnis W, Krumlauf R. Homeobox genes and axial patterning. Cell 1992; 68:283–302.
88. Krumlauf R. Evolution of the vertebrate Hox homeobox genes. BioEssays 1992; 14:245–252.

2
Early Response Genes and Renal Growth

Dean A. Kujubu
University of Pennsylvania School of Medicine and Philadelphia Veteran Affairs Medical Center, Philadelphia, Pennsylvania

Leon G. Fine
University College London Medical School, Rayne Institute, London, England

INTRODUCTION

To establish a coordinated program of growth and development and maintain tissue integrity in the adult organism, cell growth must be under stringent control. Studies on cultured cells have led to the identification of growth factors that stimulate a program of cell differentiation or proliferation. Interaction of these growth factors with responsive cells initiates a cascade of intracellular signaling events, culminating in the expression of genes the products of which are required for either cell proliferation or differentiation. The initial collection of genes induced as a results of growth-factor stimulation are termed "early response genes," "immediate early genes," or "primary response genes." The induction of these genes occurs due to the activation of preexisting transcriptional machinery and is independent of de novo protein synthesis. The cDNAs for a number of these genes have been cloned and sequenced from several different cell systems (1). Predicted amino acid sequences indicate that these genes encode transcription factors and transcriptional activators, cytokines, enzymes, and proteins of as yet unknown function. A brief list of early response genes commonly studied is included in Table 1.

Examination of early response gene expression has proven useful as a tool to dissect differences in intracellular signaling processes. Expression of early response genes depends on the appropriate ligand-receptor interactions, the triggering of intracellular signaling mechanisms, and the activation of preexisting transcriptional machinery. Since all early response genes can be induced by several mechanisms, observing gene expression does not implicate any one particular signaling pathway. However, failure to observe gene expression in response to a stimulus in a given cell type suggests that a block exists in the cellular events leading to transcription. This approach has defined differences in ligand-responsive cells and ligand-nonresponsive variants in culture (2), and, with the use of specific inhibitors, has implicated particular signaling pathways in mediating gene expression (3).

Early response gene expression has also been used to define differences between biological processes. Although many of these genes, which are expressed in mitogen-induced cell proliferation, are identical to those expressed in growth-factor–mediated differentiation, distinct differences can be observed, suggesting that differentiation and proliferation are distinguishable in regard to their earliest nuclear events (4). Moroever, differences in the relative patterns of induction for early response genes are seen in responses to different mitogenic stimuli (2), suggesting that the combined expression of these genes may be crucial in mediating responses specific to a given ligand (1).

The above approach has been used to study renal growth, which is not a simple process (5). Given the heterogeneity of cell types and the complexity of functions they perform in the kidney, it is not surprising that a growth stimulus for one cell type may not be a stimulus for others. Signals for glomerular hypertrophy are distinct from those for tubular hypertrophy. Renal growth may involve

Table 1 Frequently Studied Early Response Genes

Name	Function
c-*fos*	Transcription factor
c-*jun*	Transcription factor
egr-1	Transcription factor
c-*myc*	Transcription factor
TIS1/NGF-IB	Nuclear protein
JE/MIP1	Cytokine
KC/MGSA	Cytokine
TIS11	Not known
COX2/TIS10	Inducible prostaglandin synthase
i-NOS	Inducible nitric oxide synthase

either cellular proliferation to produce new daughter cells or the hypertrophy of preexisting cells without an increase in cell number. One might expect these two forms of cellular growth to be different at a molecular level. In this review, we will focus mainly on renal regeneration following injury, compensatory renal hypertrophy following uninephrectomy, and obstructive nephropathy. An examination of early response gene expression will undoubtedly be applied to other conditions of renal growth, including diabetic hypertrophy, hormone-induced growth, and protein loading in the future.

RENAL REGENERATION FOLLOWING INJURY

Following renal injury due to ischemia or exposure to nephrotoxic compounds, renal cells proliferate to restore tissue integrity (6). The proliferative response proceeds until the denuded basement membrane is repopulated by epithelial cells. Regeneration may involve a dedifferentation of existing cells, proliferation, and, finally, differentiation to regenerate lost functions (7). The proliferative response is the in vivo equivalent of growth following monolayer wounding in cell culture. As such, early response gene expression following renal injury may parallel what has been seen following mitogen stimulation in cultured cells.

Following renal ischemia and reperfusion, several groups have observed the rapid and transient induction of several early response genes (8). As in the case of mitogen-stimulated cells in culture, the early response gene c-*fos*, which encodes half of the AP-1 transcriptional activator complex, and *egr*-1, which encodes a zinc-finger containing transcription factor (9), are reproducibly induced in the kidney following ischemia-reperfusion injury (10,11). The pattern of induction is both rapid and transient; peak levels of mRNA are seen 1 hr after reflow for both c-*fos* and *egr*-1. Reperfusion is required for gene expression to be observed. Two other early response genes, KC and JE, which encode secreted cytokines are also expressed following ischemic injury (12). Ischemia-reperfusion injury does not induce all genes nonspecifically, since epidermal growth factor (EGF) and superoxide dismutase mRNA levels are decreased rather than increased following ischemia (11,13). Like ischemia-reperfusion injury, administration of folic acid—a tubular cell toxin—induces cell necrosis followed by a proliferative hyperplastic response (14). The early response genes, TIS1, *egr*-1, and TIS11 are all rapidly and transiently induced in response to folic acid (15). In short, the patterns of early response gene expression following tubular injury parallel that seen following mitogen stimulation in cultured cells. One might speculate that tubular injury and necrosis initiate a proliferative regenerative program corresponding in vivo to that stimulated by mitogens in vitro.

To define which cells in the kidney express *egr*-1 following ischemia-reperfusion injury in the rat, Bonventre et al. examined kidney tissue by immunohistochemical techniques using a specific antibody (16). They observed maximal expression of *egr*-1 protein in the thick ascending limb and principal cells of the cortical and medullary collecting ducts. Curiously, other cells known to be exquisitely sensitive to ischemic injury, such as those of the S1 segment of the proximal tubule, did not express *egr*-1 protein in response to ischemia-reperfusion injury. *Egr*-1 expression in cells, therefore, cannot be solely attributed to the degree of ischemic injury; its role in the kidney following ischemia-reperfusion injury is more complex than simply the regenerative response following injury. This study underscores the importance of defining which cells in the tissue express the gene product of interest.

COMPENSATORY RENAL HYPERTROPHY

Triggered by unilateral nephrectomy, compensatory renal hypertrophy in the adult animal is a unique form of cell growth that is associated neither with significant cell proliferation nor with differentiation (5). Instead, proximal tubular cells enlarge in size, with little or no increase in cellular DNA content, while retaining their differentiated phenotype. To distinguish how this form of renal cell growth differs from a proliferative response, several investigators have studied the differences in early response gene expression by comparing the two processes. Being the first nuclear events to occur following an extracellular stimulus, early response gene expression might be able to distinguish hypertrophy from hyperplasia and to identify the molecular basis for the hypertrophic stimulus.

One of the first studies using early response genes in studying compensatory renal hypertrophy was performed by Beer et al. (17). They compared patterns of gene expression following uninephrectomy, which results in hypertrophy, with partial hepatectomy, which results in regenerative hyperplasia. They observed that the patterns of expression for c-*myc*, c-*fos*, and other genes were different in the hypertrophic kidney compared to the regenerating liver. Bailey et al. observed that mRNA for c-*myc* and c-*Ha-ras* were increased within hours following nephrectomy in both the contralateral kidney and in the undisturbed liver (18). This pattern of gene expression was not seen following sham laparotomy. Probing with a series of cell-cycle-regulated genes, Norman et al. observed that the patterns of gene expression seen following unilateral nephrectomy differed qualitatively from that seen after folic acid administration in that there was no significant induction of the genes that were induced by nephrotoxic injury (14). These studies were extended by others to study the expression of early response genes following these two renal growth stimuli. Ouellette et al. observed that although *egr*-1 mRNA was expressed following uninephrectomy, its mRNA level was much lower than that seen following ischemia-reperfusion injury (10). Moreover, in their study, c-*fos* mRNA was not detectable following unilateral nephrectomy. Kujubu et al. observed that while TIS1, *egr*-1, and TIS11 were highly inducible following folic acid stimulation, they were expressed at a much lower level after unilateral nephrectomy, similar to that seen following sham operation (15). Unlike Ouellette et al., Nakamura, et al. observed c-*fos*, c-*jun*, and c-*myc* expression following unilateral nephrectomy; however, they did not compare their results to those seen following a hyperplastic stimulus (19). Recently, Terzi et al. observed that while c-*fos* and c-*jun* mRNA was not detected following either sham operation or uninephrectomy, both were detectable following $1^5/_6$ nephrectomy (20). Their expression correlated with an increase in renal function without any significant change in protein/DNA ratio. They concluded that $1^5/_6$ nephrectomy is followed primarily by a hyperplastic rather than a hypertrophic response in pubertal rats. The same observation has been made in adult animals; i.e., the more extensive the ablation, the more proliferation contributes to the growth response.

One particularly interesting early response gene is COX-2/TIS10, which encodes for a newly described inducible form of prostaglandin endoperoxide synthase, the rate-limiting enzyme in prostaglandin biosynthesis (21). Pelayo and Shanley observed that in response to unilateral nephrectomy, the remaining kidney demonstrates an increase in prostaglandin biosynthesis (22). Logan et al. suggest that compensatory hypertrophy can be inhibited by indomethacin, implicating a role for prostaglandin biosynthesis in compensatory renal growth (23). Recently, Harris et al. observed induction of COX-2/TIS10 in the juxtaglomerular apparatus of the remaining kidney following contralateral nephrectomy (24). Further elucidation of the role of COX-2/TIS10 in renal hypertrophy is undoubtedly forthcoming.

In summary, these studies suggest that compensatory renal hypertrophy following unilateral nephrectomy is a form of cellular growth that, from the earliest nuclear events, differs from cell proliferation. This suggests that the stimuli and signaling events involved in these two processes are distinct. It is likely that unilateral nephrectomy induces a particular collection of early response genes characteristic of compensatory hypertrophy. These genes remain to be identified. Identification of such genes will help to define the molecular basis for the hypertrophic signal. Therapeutic modulation of such signals may either enhance compromised renal function or prevent the deleterious consequences of prolonged hyperfunction.

UNILATERAL URETERAL OBSTRUCTION

Complete unilateral ureteral obstruction results in a number of complex pathophysiological changes in both the obstructed and unobstructed kidneys. In addition to rapid vasoconstrictive changes associated with acute ureteral obstruction, the obstructed kidney, over time, demonstrates interstitial fibrosis and tubular atrophy due to the triggering of an apoptotic program (25). In contrast, the unobstructed kidney undergoes compensatory hypertrophy akin to that seen following unilateral nephrectomy. With this model one can make direct comparisons between hyperplasia of the interstitial fibroblasts and hypertrophy of the proximal tubular epithelial cells within the same animal.

Sawczuk et al. examined the expression of several genes following unilateral ureteral obstruction (26). They observed that the early response genes, c-*fos* and c-*myc* mRNAs, were induced within minutes following unilateral ureteral obstruction in both the obstructed and unobstructed kidneys but not in sham operated kidneys. Expression of the early response genes, therefore, could not distinguish between the two processes. Interestingly, mRNA for SGP-2 (sulfated glycoprotein-2), a gene associated with apoptosis in androgen-deprived prostatic cells, was detectable only in the obstructed kidney within 30 min after ureteral ligation (27). The authors speculate that expression of these genes regulates the expression of growth factors in obstructive nephropathy. They observed that mRNA for EGF decreases in the obstructed kidney but increases for transforming growth factor (TGF)-beta (28).

Ureteral obstruction acutely results in an increase in eicosanoid production (29). Yanagisawa et al. demonstrated that increases in glomerular eicosanoid production in rats following bilateral ureteral obstruction are mediated by increased enzymatic activities of cyclooxygenase and 5-lipoxygenase (30). One wonders if COX2/TIS10 may also be induced in this system as it is in compensatory renal hypertrophy following unilateral nephrectomy.

The fact that c-*fos* and c-*myc* mRNA were expressed early in both cell death and cell hypertrophy following ureteral obstruction underscores limitations in the approach of examining early response gene expression alone. Many early response genes can be induced by a wide variety of stimuli and represent the initial steps in many distinct biological processes. Including a carefully performed sham procedure is essential in these types of studies, since even sham operation can induce early response gene expression.

OTHER FORMS OF RENAL GROWTH

An examination of early response genes and other forms of renal growth—including diabetes mellitus, growth hormone, pregnancy, and protein loading—has not been performed. Future studies using early response genes may prove interesting in delineating specific molecular mechanisms involved in these forms of renal growth and in showing how they differ from regenerative hyperplasia or compensatory hypertrophy.

CONCLUSIONS AND FUTURE DIRECTIONS

The molecular basis for the regulation of renal growth remains elusive. As an approach to uncover the first steps in genetic program regulating renal growth, the study of early response genes has proven valuable. However, since early response genes are often induced in response to nonspecific stimuli and cells not involved in the growth response may express these genes, early response gene expression provides only a first glimpse of a markedly complex genetic program. Future work will involve the discovery of later genes specific for the growth process of interest and the identification of kidney-specific transcription factors. Once this is accomplished, our understanding of the regulation of renal growth will be significantly enhanced.

ACKNOWLEDGMENTS

D.A.K. was supported by NIH Physician Scientist Award USPHS 1K11 01815, NIH Renal Training Grant DK-07006, Penn Center for Molecular Studies of Kidney Diseases DK-45191, and the University of Pennsylvania Research Foundation. L.G.F was supported by grants from the Medical Research Council and the Wellcome Trust, UK

REFERENCES

1. Herschman HR. Primary response genes induced by growth factors and tumor promoters. Annu Rev Biochem 1993; 60:281–319.
2. Altin JG, Kujubu DA, Raffione S, et al. Differential induction of primary response (TIS) genes in PC-12 pheochromocytoma cells and the unresponsive variant PC12nnr5. J Biol Chem 1991; 266:5401–5406.
3. Kujubu DA, Stimmel JB, Law RE, et al. Early responses of PC-12 cells to NGF and EGF: effect of K252a and 5′-methylthioadenosine on gene expression and membrane protein methylation. J Neurosci Res 1993; 36:58–65.
4. Kujubu DA, Lim RW, Varnum BC, Herschman HR. Induction of transiently expressed genes in PC-12 pheochromocytoma cells. Oncogene 1987; 1:257–262.
5. Fine L. The biology of renal hypertrophy. Kidney Int 1986; 29:619–634.
6. Bonventre JV. Mechanisms of ischemic acute renal failure. Kidney Int 1993; 43:1160–1178.
7. Bacallao R, Fine LG. Molecular events in the organization of renal tubular epithelium: From nephrogenesis to regeneration. Am J Physiol 1989; 257:F913–F924.
8. Safirstein R. Gene expression in nephrotoxic and ischemic acute renal failure. J Am Soc Nephrol 1994; 4:1387–1395.
9. Sukhatme VP, Cao X, Chang LC, et al. A zinc finger-encoding gene coregulated with c-fos during growth and differentiation, and after cellular depolarization. Cell 1988; 53:37–43.
10. Ouellette AJ, Malt RA, Sukhatme VP, Bonventre JV. Expression of two "immediate early" genes, egf-1 and c-fos, in response to renal ischemia and during compensatory renal hypertrophy in mice. J Clin Invest 1990; 85:766–771.
11. Rosenberg ME, Paller MS. Differential gene expression in the recovery from ischemic renal injury. Kidney Int 1991; 39:1156–1161.
12. Safirstein R, Megyesi J, Saggi SJ, et al. Expression of cytokine-like genes JE and KC is increased during renal ischemia. Am J Physiol 1991; 261:F1095–F1101.
13. Safirstein R, Price PM, Saggi SJ, Harris RC. Changes in gene expression after temporary renal ischemia. Kidney Int 1990; 37:1515–1521.
14. Norman JT, Bohman RE, Fischman G, et al. Patterns of mRNA expression during early cell growth differ in kidney epithelial cells destinged to undergo compensatory hypertrophy versus regenerative hyperplasia. Proc Natl Acad Sci USA 1988; 85:6768–6772.
15. Kujubu DA, Norman JT, Herschman HR, Fine LG. Primary response gene expression in renal hypertrophy and hyperplasia: Evidence for different growth initiation processes. Am J Physiol 1991; 260:F823–F827.
16. Bonventre JV, Sukhatme VP, Bamberger M, et al. Localization of the protein product of the immediate early growth response gene, Egr-1, in the kidney after ischemia and reperfusion. Cell Reg 1991; 2:251–260.
17. Beer DG, Zweifel KA, Simpson DP, Pitot HC. Specific gene expression during compensatory renal hypertrophy in the rat. J Cell Physiol 1987; 131:29–35.
18. Bailey A, Sanchez JD, Rigby D, et al. Stimulation of renal and hepatic c-myc and c-Ha-ras expression by unilateral nephrectomy. Oncogene Res 1990; 5:287–293.
19. Nakamura T, Ebihara I, Tomino Y, et al. Gene expression of growth-related proteins and ECM constituents in response to unilateral nephrectomy. Am J Physiol 1992; 262:F389–F396.
20. Terzi F, Ticozzi C, Burtin M, et al. Subtotal and unilateral nephrectomy: Two different mechanisms for renal compensatory growth. J Am Soc Nephrol 1993; 4:478.
21. Kujubu DA, Fletcher BS, Varnum BC, et al. TIS10, a phorbol ester tumor promoter inducible mRNA from Swiss 3T3 cells, encodes a novel prostaglandin syunthase/cyclooxygenase homologue. J Biol Chem 1991; 266:12866–12872.
22. Pelayo JC, Shanley PF. Glomerular and tubular adaptive responses to acute nephron loss in the rat. J Clin Invest 1990; 85:1761–1769.

23. Logan JL, Lee SM, Benson B, Michael UF. Inhibition of compensatory renal growth by indomethacin. Prostaglandins 1986; 31:253–262.
24. Harris RC, Akai Y, Homma T, et al. Mitogen-activated cyclooxygenase (COX-2) is expressed in cultured mesangial cells and in the juxtaglomerular apparatus in vivo and increases following uninephrectomy. J Am Soc Nephrol 1993; 4:454.
25. Gobe GC, Axelsen RA. Genesis of renal tubular atrophy in experimental hydronephrosis in the rat: Role of apoptosis. Lab Invest 1987; 56:273–281.
26. Sawczuk IS, Hoke G, Olsson CA, et al. Gene expression in response to acute unilateral ureteral obstruction. Kidney Int 1989; 35:1315–1319.
27. Connor J, Buttyan R, Olsson CA, et al. SGP-2 expression as a genetic marker of progressive cellular pathology in experimental hydronephrosis. Kidney Int 1991; 39:1098–1103.
28. Walton G, Buttyan R, Garcia-Montes E, et al. Renal growth factor expression during the early phase of experimental hydronephrosis. J Urol 1992; 148:510–514.
29. Yanagisawa H, Morrissey J, Morrison AR, Klahr S. Eicosanoid production by isolated glomeruli of rat with unilateral obstruction. Kidney Int 1990; 37:1528–1535.
30. Yanagisawa H, Jin Z, Kurihara N, et al. Increases in glomerular eicosanoid production in rats with bilateral ureteral obstruction are mediated by enhanced enzyme activities of both the cyclooxygenase and 5-lipoxygenase pathways. Proc Soc Exp Biol Med 1993; 203:291–296.

3

Epithelial Cell Polarity: Molecular Mechanisms

Dennis Brown
Massachusetts General Hospital and Harvard Medical School, Boston, Massachusetts

INTRODUCTION

Epithelial cells are characterized by the establishment and maintenance of distinct plasma membrane domains that contain different proteins and lipids (1,2). This characteristic apical and basolateral membrane identity depends upon the correct targeting and insertion of membrane components by the intracellular sorting machinery. It must be retained in the face of a high level of membrane fusion and fission that, if allowed to proceed in an uncontrolled fashion, would tend to cause an eventual randomization of all cellular membranes. Kidney epithelial cells have been extensively used in cell biological and physiological studies on cell polarity (3) because they are able to modulate their plasma membrane structure and function in response to a wide variety of stimuli, including hormones, growth factors, nutrients, ionic conditions, and extracellular matrix. Such responses involve the precise and regulated insertion of functionally important membrane components that are both newly synthesized, and are recycling back and forth between the plasma membrane and intracellular vesicles (4).

The intracellular sorting machinery that allows epithelial cells to maintain their functional polarity is highly complex and involves the coordinated interaction of many cellular components at different points of the trafficking pathway. Signals that are encoded within the sorted molecules themselves play a major role in determining the final destination of each protein, but these signals must be recognized by other components of the pathway in order to ensure packaging into the correct transport vesicles as the proteins exit the Golgi apparatus. These vesicles must then be moved within the cell to their destination, and they must fuse and deliver their cargo to a predetermined docking site—not to any random membrane they encounter on the way. Once incorporated into a selected membrane domain, many proteins are anchored in that domain via interaction with cytoskeletal elements. Finally, other proteins that are endocytosed or transcytosed must be able to recognize and insert sequentially into more than one type of intracellular membrane.

This review concentrates on selected aspects of protein sorting and, where applicable, draws on examples that are relevant to kidney epithelial cell function.

SORTING SIGNALS ON PROTEINS

It is well established that many, if not all, membrane proteins contain information that is used by the intracellular sorting machinery to direct the protein to its correct location (1,2). In addition, secreted proteins and some proteins produced on free ribosomes also contain sorting information. This information takes different forms; it includes short, well-conserved amino acid sequences usually in the cytoplasmic tail of the protein; longer, less conserved sequences that impart specific characteristics (e.g., hydrophobicity) to a segment of the protein; posttranslational modifications to the protein, including phosphorylation of sugar residues, proteolytic cleavage, or the addition of a glycosyl-phosphatidyinositol lipid anchor; and correct folding and oligomerization of the protein.

The GPI Anchor—An Apical Targeting Signal

Many proteins of eukaryotic cells are anchored in the plasma membrane, as well as to the membrane of intracellular organelles, by covalent linkage to glycosyl-phosphatidylinositol (GPI) (5–7). Proteins anchored by GPI have none of their sequence embedded in the lipid bilayer, and they lack the cytoplasmic tail that is of functional significance to many conventional transmembrane proteins, such as hormone and growth factor receptors and ion channels. Such GPI-linked proteins are, therefore, located exclusively on the extracellular leaflet of the plasma membrane and are oriented facing the lumenal side of intracellular compartments. The structure of a typical GPI anchor is shown in Fig. 1. Proteins linked by GPI are a diverse family of molecules with no evident shared functional characteristics (8). They include membrane-bound enzymes, adhesion molecules, activation antigens, differentiation markers, protozoan coat components, and other miscellaneous glycoproteins. Over a hundred GPI-anchored proteins have now been identified.

By comparing GPI-anchored proteins with their membrane localization pattern, it was discovered that these proteins appear to be targeted almost exclusively to the apical plasma membrane domain in polarized epithelial cells. Several endogenous GPI-anchored proteins are restricted to the apical surface of a variety of cultured epithelial cells (9,10), including MDCK, LLC-PK$_1$, Caco-2 and SK-CO15 cells. Conversion to a GPI-anchored form of a viral glycoprotein (herpes simplex glycoprotein gD-1) that is normally targeted to the basolateral membrane resulted in its delivery to the apical plasma membrane of MDCK cells (11). Conversely, when GPI-anchored proteins (such as alkaline phosphatase) are given a transmembrane anchor, they can be inserted into the basolateral plasma membrane (12).

It has been proposed, therefore, that the GPI anchor is a strong targeting signal that directs proteins to the apical plasma membrane in epithelial cells. The extracellular domain of these molecules may, therefore, be a major factor in determining their membrane targeting properties. This is supported by experiments in which a truncated form of Thy-1 (a GPI-anchored protein identified first on the plasma membrane of murine thymocytes), lacking a COOH-terminal sequence

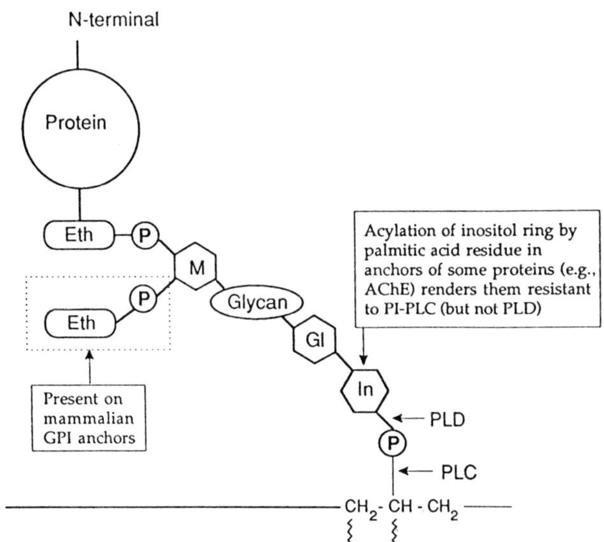

Figure 1 Diagram showing structure of a phosphatidylinositol-glycan anchor used to attach GPI-linked proteins to the membrane. Sites of cleavage by phospholipase C (PLC) and phospholipase D (PLD) are indicated. Abbreviations: In = inositol; Eth = ethanolamine; M = mannose; P = phosphate; GI = glucosamine. (From Ref. 8.)

that is required for attachment of the GPI anchor, was constructed and expressed in MDCK cells. This truncated molecule was secreted at the apical pole of these cells, indicating that the protein ectodomain contains apical targeting information (13).

Some evidence also suggests that GPI-anchored proteins may be segregated into specific regions of the membrane bilayer that are rich in cholesterol (14); they may, therefore, be subject to the same factors that regulate the flow of specific lipids to the apical plasma membrane in epithelial cells (15). These GPI-anchored proteins appear to be concentrated in specific membrane specializations known as caveoli that are cholesterol-rich, but some GPI-linked proteins can also be found to a lesser extent in clathrin-coated vesicles. While GPI-anchored proteins have no coated pit retention signal (see below), they are probably retained in coated pits by interaction of their ectodomain with adjacent transmembrane proteins. Caveoli have been identified as compartments that are involved in the internalization of folate, and these structures also internalize other ligands, including cholera toxin, that bind to lipidic receptors (15a). Previously referred to as "smooth" or "uncoated" invaginations on the cell surface, it has now been established that these structures have a characteristic striated coating material on their cytoplasmic surface (16). One component of this coating material is recognized and labeled by antibodies raised against a 22-kDa substrate for v-*src* tyrosine kinase in Rous sarcoma virus–transformed chick embryo fibroblasts. Immunogold labeling shows that this antibody binds to the filaments that form the coat. The protein present in the filaments has been named caveolin (16).

In addition to its role as an apical targeting signal, the GPI anchor may be involved in aspects of the cellular signal transduction mechanism. A common property of many GPI-anchored proteins expressed on resting T lymphocytes is their ability to activate cell proliferation when they bind monoclonal antibodies that are subsequently cross-linked with secondary antibodies, in the presence of phorbol esters (17–19).

GPI-Anchored Proteins in the Kidney

Several GPI-anchored proteins are present in the kidney. A partial list is presented below. Interestingly, Tamm-Horsfall glycoprotein and carbonic anhydrase type IV, both GPI-linked proteins, are expressed apically and basolaterally in the kidney. However, it is not yet clear whether both apical and basolateral forms of the protein are in fact GPI-linked or whether alternative RNA splicing leads to a GPI-linked apical form and a transmembrane-anchored basolateral form of these proteins.

1. *Alkaline Phosphatase*. Alkaline phosphatase was one of the first ectoenzymes identified as having a GPI linkage. It is abundant on the apical brush-border microvilli of proximal tubules but is also found on apical membranes of other cells in the urinary tubule, including collecting duct epithelial cells (20).
2. *Aminopeptidases*. Two aminopeptidases of the proximal tubule brush border are known to be GPI-anchored; aminopeptidase P (21) and renal dipeptidase (22).
3. *5′Nucleotidase*. This GPI-anchored ectoenzyme is located in the brush border of the proximal tubule as well as other tubule segments. It is one of a number of ectonucleotidases found on the plasma membrane of many epithelial cell types and may work in concert with brush-border ecto-ATPase (23), which has a conventional transmembrane anchor, to hydrolyze various adenine nucleotides to adenosine and inorganic phosphate.
4. *Uromucoid* (*Tamm-Horsfall glycoprotein*). Tamm-Horsfall glycoprotein is present in distal convoluted tubules and thick ascending limbs of Henle. It is identical to uromucoid, an immunosuppressive glycoprotein originally described in the urine of pregnant women. It was believed to be a typical secretory protein, but it is now known that uromucoid can be anchored to the plasma membrane by a GPI anchor, as shown by expressing cDNA encoding this protein in HeLa, Caco-2, MDCK, COS, and AT-20 cells (24). The appearance of soluble uromucoid in the urine might then be the result of the action of endogenous phospholipases in the kidney or of protease action. By immunocytochemistry, uromucoid can also be detected on the basolateral plasma membranes of thick ascending limb cells (25). It is unknown whether this basolateral form of the protein is also GPI-anchored or whether an alternative splicing event produces a conventionally membrane-linked form in thick ascending limb cells.
5. *Membrane-associated carbonic anhydrase type IV*. The presence of a membrane-associated form

of carbonic anhydrase in some nephron segments has been recognized for many years (26). Immunocytochemical data using antibodies against carbonic anhydrase type IV (CAIV) have localized this enzyme in rat kidney to the S2 segment of the proximal convoluted tubule and the thick ascending limbs of Henle (27). Staining is strongest in the apical plasma membrane in both tubule segments, but there is significant reactivity of the antibodies with the basolateral membranes also. In human kidney, it has been shown that a large portion of CAIV exists as a GPI-anchored protein, because the enzyme can be released from kidney membranes by PI-specific phospholipase C (28). These membranes presumably derive from apical membranes of the urinary tubule epithelial cells. However, a transmembrane-linked form of the enzyme is also detectable in human kidney, indicating that an alternative splicing event may occur. Thus, the intriguing possibility exists that the apical or basolateral targeting of kidney CAIV may be directed by a modification of the anchor used to attach this protein to the plasma membrane.

6. *Thy-1*. Thy-1 was originally described on the plasma membrane of murine thymocytes but is present on glomerular mesangial cells and neurons. Anti–Thy-1 antibodies induce mesangial cell damage in the rat, resulting in a mesangial proliferative nephritis (29). In these diseased animals as well as in cultured mesangial cells, antibody interaction with the mesangial cells results in increased extracellular matrix production (30) and glomerular accumulation of macrophages and platelets.

Basolateral and Endocytotic Sorting Signals on Proteins

Until relatively recently, it was thought that basolateral proteins were delivered to their destination via a default pathway—i.e., that no specific sorting information was required. In the past three or four years, however, sorting signals have been identified on proteins destined for delivery to the basolateral plasma membrane of epithelial cells, indicating that basolateral protein targeting is a highly specific and controlled process. Furthermore, many cell surface proteins, particularly receptors, contain small sequences of amino acids on their cytoplasmic tails that enables these proteins to be recognized and internalized via clathrin-coated pits. Interestingly, the same signals that govern receptor-mediated endocytosis also determine basolateral targeting in some proteins. These signals are discussed together below. In addition, a second category of basolateral sorting signal exists, which appears to be independent of the signal for endocytosis.

Signals That Overlap with Endocytotic Motifs

Several receptor molecules that are internalized from the cell surface by clustering in clathrin-coated pits contain a four–amino acid motif in their cytoplasmic tails. The first one to be identified was the NPXY motif of the LDL receptor and the related proximal tubule glycoprotein gp330 (31). Other similar sequences have been identified, which all contain a tyrosine residue that is critical for endocytosis—for example, the YXRF sequence in the transferrin receptor (32). The selective concentration of molecules containing such sequences in clathrin-coated pits is shown for the CR3 complement receptor in Fig. 2 (33). It is now recognized that there is a correlation between the ability of many (but not all) proteins to cluster in coated pits and their delivery to the basolateral plasma membrane of epithelial cells. This implies that the same domain of the cytoplasmic tail may be involved in both processes. For example, wild-type mouse IgG Fc receptor and nerve growth factor receptor are both basolaterally targeted in transfected cells, and both undergo active endocytosis. However, mutated receptors were targeted apically and showed a lower rate of endocytosis (34,35).

The role of a critical tyrosine residue in this process was shown in mutagenesis experiments on a lysosomal membrane glycoprotein, LGP120, and influenza virus hemagglutinin, both of which are initially targeted to the basolateral membrane (36,37). The LGP120 is then rapidly internalized and delivered to its final lysosomal destination. A role of this residue in clathrin-mediated endocytosis was shown by elegant studies on natural mutations in the LDL receptor, in which a single amino acid change from tyrosine to cysteine results in failure of the receptor to be internalized and the appearance of the phenotype of familial hypercholesterolemia (38). This defect was subsequently duplicated in an oocyte expression system and resulted in a sevenfold decrease in the rate of internalization of the altered LDL receptor (39).

The NPXY or related sequence in the cytoplasmic tail of these proteins allows them to take up

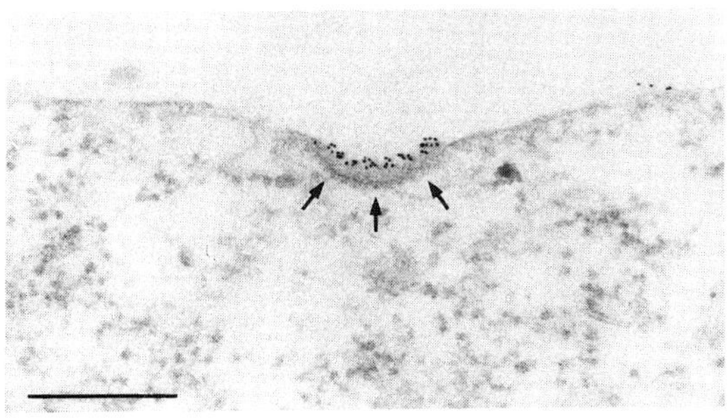

Figure 2 Cell surface localization, using the immunogold procedure, of the human CR3 complement receptor, a protein with NPXF motifs in its cytoplasmic domain. Gold particle labeling for CR3 is concentrated in a clathrin coated pit (arrows) and is sparse on the rest of the membrane. Bar = 0.5 μm. (From Ref. 33.)

a conformation known as a β-turn (40). It is possible that this protein conformation can be recognized by both the coated-pit retention mechanism and by the basolateral targeting mechanism of epithelial cells. In the case of the coated-pit mechanism, this recognition is believed to occur via specific adaptor proteins that are located in coated pits (41). These proteins recognize signals in the tails of some transmembrane proteins and cause their retention in coated pits. Interestingly, adaptors found in cell surface coated pits are distinct from those found in coated pits in the Golgi region of cells. It is possible, therefore, that adaptor-like molecules may also be involved in basolateral sorting by specifically binding to those proteins that bear this type of basolateral sorting signal.

Signals That Are Independent of Endocytotic Determinants

The polymeric immunoglobulin receptor is delivered from the Golgi to the basolateral plasma membrane of epithelial cells, where it binds extracellular polymeric IgA and IgM and then transports them by transcytosis to the apical plasma membrane. This process is physiologically important in intestinal absorptive epithelial cells, where it is involved in the development of mucosal immunity. Casanova et al. (42) reported that a mutant receptor lacking the 14 amino acids of the cytoplasmic tail adjacent to the transmembrane region was delivered directly to the apical cell membrane. Furthermore, when placental alkaline phosphatase was engineered to contain this 14–amino acid sequence, this normally apical protein was delivered to the basolateral plasma membrane. The 14–amino acid sequence had no homology to sequences in other basolateral proteins, suggesting that it confers some general structural feature that is required for basolateral targeting.

How does this type of sorting sequence function? One hypothesis is that the signal is a positive signal that actively directs the protein into the basolateral pathway by interacting with a specific "receptor," for example. The second possibility is that the sequence acts as a negative sorting signal that denies the protein access to the specific apical pathway; thus, the basolateral pathway would still be a modified default pathway for any protein that could not be recognized by the apical sorting mechanism. This issue remains unresolved.

As discussed earlier, the LDL receptor contains a classic clathrin-coated pit retention sequence that also is involved in the basolateral targeting of this protein. However, the situation is more complex, because mutation of the tyrosine to an alanine in this domain resulted in a large decrease in endocytosis but had little effect on basolateral targeting. It was found that a second, more distal region containing two tyrosine residues was also present toward the C terminal of the cytoplasmic tail of the LDL-receptor (43). This region was competent to direct basolateral targeting, even in the absence of the more proximal NPXY motif. Mutation of one of the distal tyrosine motifs (tyrosine 35) to an alanine resulted in a reduced efficiency of basolateral targeting but had no effect on endocytosis. Mutation or deletion of both proximal and distal motifs was required to completely abolish basolateral targeting. In such double mutants, the LDL receptor was found only at the apical plasma membrane of transfected MDCK cells. Thus, the structural requirements for endocytosis and basolateral targeting can be different, but both depend upon critical tyrosine residues for their function.

Gp 330—the Heymann Nephritis Antigen—in the Kidney

A clear example that the NPXY coated-pit retention sequence need not necessarily function as a basolateral targeting signal is provided by gp330, a glycoprotein that is located on the apical plasma membrane of renal proximal tubules as well as in several other cell types (44). This is the protein implicated in the pathogenesis of Heymann nephritis, a rat model of human membranous glomerulonephritis (45). It was originally described as being restricted to clathrin-coated pits in proximal tubule epithelial cells as well as glomerular podocytes (46). Subsequent studies have shown unequivocally that it is also present on the microvillar brush border in the proximal tubule (47,48), although the microvillar form may have a modified cytoplasmic domain that is not recognized by antibodies reacting with the coated-pit form (49). Partial cDNA sequences encoding gp330 revealed considerable homology to the LDL receptor, including the presence of two NPXY sequences in the cytoplasmic tail (50), and it is also homologous to the LDL-receptor–related proteins. Nevertheless, this protein is exclusively located on the apical plasma membrane of proximal tubule cells. Thus, in this case, a strong coated-pit retention sequence is present in a protein that also has a powerful but as yet undefined apical targeting signal.

Sorting of Lysosomal Hydrolases

One of the best-established sorting signals is present on soluble lysosomal hydrolases. Posttranslational modification of these hydrolases in the *cis*-Golgi results in the addition of phosphate groups to one or more N-linked oligosaccharide mannose residues on these glycoproteins. The resulting mannose-6-phosphate residues are recognized by a specific receptor, the mannose-6-phosphate receptor, which is present in the Golgi cisternae, probably in the *trans*-Golgi region (51–53). Following this interaction, the receptor-hydrolase complex buds off from the trans-Golgi network in clathrin-coated vesicles, which deliver the complex to a low-pH compartment, in which the hydrolase dissociates from the receptor. The receptor is recycled back to the Golgi, whereas the vesicles containing the soluble hydrolases fuse with lysosomes, thus delivering the hydrolases to their correct destination.

ROLE OF MICROTUBULES IN PROTEIN TARGETING

Microtubules and Epithelial Cell Polarity

Microtubule disruption interferes severely with intracellular membrane traffic, secretory processes, lysosomal distribution, and the processing and packaging of proteins at the level of the Golgi apparatus (54–58). Colchicine severely disrupts the structure of the Golgi apparatus (57), and following Golgi disruption by nocodazole, the reclustering of scattered Golgi elements occurs along microtubules (59). Despite these dramatic effects on intracellular organization, the role of microtubules in the generation and maintenance of epithelial cell polarity is controversial. Conflicting results have been obtained concerning microtubule involvement in the polarized insertion of viral proteins in epithelial cells (60,61). Much less work has been performed using endogenous proteins, but nocodazole inhibits the normal insertion of an endogenous apical membrane protein in cultured cells (62), and microtubule disruption has a dramatic effect on cell polarity in intestinal epithelial cells (54,58). We have also shown that colchicine inhibits the apical targeting of gp330 (63) and proton pumps (64) in the proximal tubule, but that it does not cause their mistargeting to the basolateral plasma membrane (see below). The effect of colchicine on gp330 targeting in proximal tubules is illustrated in Fig. 3.

Microtubules influence the intracellular movement of organelles and transporting vesicles via so-called microtubule motors (kinesin and cytoplasmic dyneins); these cytosolic proteins can induce ATP-dependent organelle movement along isolated microtubules in either an anterograde or retrograde direction (65,66). The pH-dependence of lysosomal distribution in fibroblasts may result from the selective switching on or off of different microtubule motors at different cytoplasmic pH values (55). Microtubules are involved in the movement of transporting vesicles to the apical pole

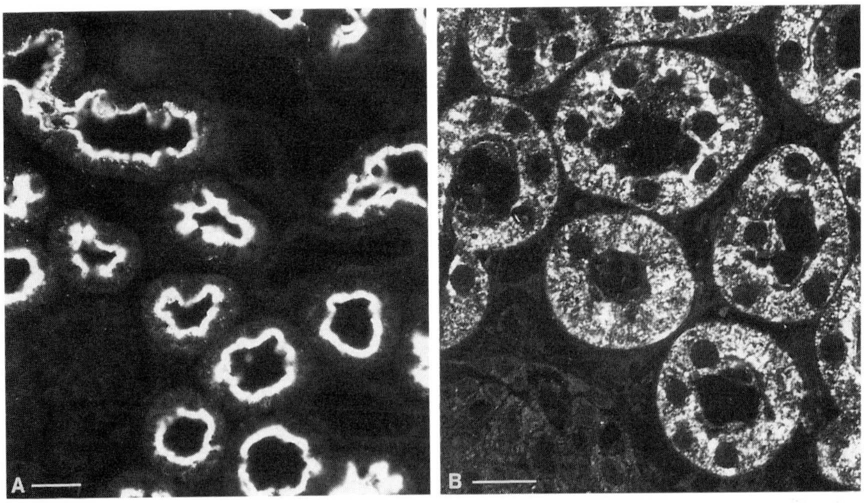

Figure 3 Immunofluorescence micrographs showing effect of microtubule disruption on localization of the apical membrane protein, gp330, in rat renal epithelial cells. Panels A and B show gp330 before (A) and after (B) colchicine treatment of rats for 8 hr. The normal apical location is absent in (B), and vesicles containing gp300 are instead scattered throughout the cytoplasm. Bar = 20 μm. (From Ref. 63.)

of epithelial cells, and that this movement may be pH-dependent is of clear relevance to the physiological response of collecting duct intercalated cells to different acid-base conditions. Indeed, in turtle bladder, acidification in response to CO_2 is inhibited by colchicine (67), and in the kidney collecting duct, nocodazole inhibits the antidiuretic response to vasopressin in isolated perfused tubules (68) as well as in intact animals (69).

Microtubules and Protein Targeting in the Kidney

Gp330 Targeting

GP330 is a highly glycosylated protein restricted to the apical plasma membrane of proximal tubule epithelial cells. As discussed above, it is the major antigen involved in the pathology of Heymann nephritis in rats, and it is homologous to the LDL receptor and to LRP (the α_2-macroglobulin receptor). In control rats, gp330 is located on the brush border, in apical invaginations (clathrin-coated pits) and in apical vesicles. It is also located in coated pits on glomerular podocytes. Six hours after injection of colchicine, however, vesicles containing gp330 were dispersed throughout the entire cytoplasm of the cell (63). Many vesicles were packed into basolateral infoldings, close to the plasma membrane, but there was no significant insertion of gp330 into the basolateral membrane (Fig. 3). When rabbit anti-gp330 antiserum was injected intravenously into colchicine-treated rats, immune complexes appeared in the glomerular basement membrane but could not be detected in peritubular basement membranes. This supports the conclusion that colchicine treatment does not result in the insertion of gp330 into the basolateral plasma membrane of proximal tubule cells. The results indicate that while microtubules are involved in the accumulation of gp330-containing vesicles at the apical pole of the cell, other factors must be required for fusion with the plasma membrane to occur.

However, not all brush border proteins are affected in the same way by colchicine, because another brush border enzyme, dipeptidyl peptidase IV, is retained on microvilli even after extended periods of microtubule disruption. In contrast to gp330, immunogold labeling shows that DPPIV is not concentrated in clathrin-coated pits in normal rat proximal tubule (70).

H^+ATPase Targeting

Distinct subtypes of intercalated cells are present in cortical collecting ducts (71–73). These so-called A and B cells are acid-secreting and bicarbonate-secreting cells, respectively (74,75). A cells have proton pumps on the apical plasma membrane and a band-3–like chloride bicarbonate exchanger on their basolateral plasma membrane, whereas B cells can insert proton pumps into their basolateral membrane but immunocytochemical detection of an apical anion exchanger in B cells has been elusive (76–78). The fact that intercalated cell subpopulations, illustrated in Fig. 4, can maintain an opposite polarity with respect to proton pumps is a finding of great cell biological interest, since most proteins have specific targeting signals that address them to one pole only of epithelial cells.

One possibility that might explain differential targeting of proton pumps is that the apical and basolateral versions of the proton ATPase may not be identical in subunit composition; this difference could confer domain specificity on the targeting process. Indeed, subunit isoforms that confer cell and organelle specificity (but not differential plasma membrane polarity) to proton pumps have been identified (79–81). Alternatively, the microtubular network could be different in cells with apical or basolateral proton pumps, so that vesicles containing the pumps move selectively to only one pole of the cell. It has been proposed that microtubule tracks are important for the delivery of apical but not basolateral proteins. Microtubule depolymerization might, therefore, result in basolateral rather than apical insertion of proton pumps. This prediction assumes that vesicles carrying proton pumps are competent to fuse with either apical or basolateral plasma membranes and that the specificity of the process lies exclusively in the delivery of the vesicles to the appropriate membrane domain. However, this is clearly not the case with another apical membrance protein, gp330, which is present in vesicles that do not fuse with the wrong (i.e., the basolateral) plasma membrane (see above and Fig. 3).

In rats treated for up to 24 hr with colchicine to induce microtubule depolymerization, proton pumps were no longer polarized to one pole of the cell but were concentrated in numerous vesicles scattered throughout the cytoplasm (64). A similar scattered distribution was seen in A and B intercalated cells as well as in epithelial cells of the proximal tubule. The A-type cells in the inner stripe of the outer medulla did not concentrate proton pumps in their basolateral plasma membranes, indicating that microtubule depolymerization alone is not sufficient to account for the final differences in the membrane distribution of proton pumps seen in A and B intercalated cells.

Taken together, these results suggest that (a) microtubules can be involved in the targeting of intracellular vesicles to both the apical and basolateral pole of epithelial cells; (b) microtubules are not involved in the final fusion event, since "misdirected" apical vesicles do not fuse with the basolateral plasma membrane; and (c) the effect of microtubule disruption on membrane protein distribution is protein-specific rather than membrane-specific.

THE FUSION MACHINE

The evidence discussed above indicates that proteins contain specific signals that ultimately direct them to precise membrane destinations. The trafficking vesicles that contain these proteins are, at least partially, directed by the microtubule network of the cell. The remaining missing link is the elucidation of the recognition and fusion proteins that enable only certain vesicles to dock with predetermined membrane domains. A considerable amount of work is now being performed to isolate

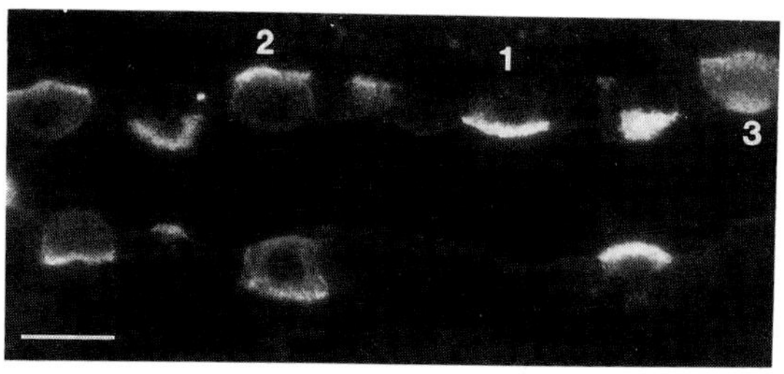

Figure 4 Immunofluorescence localization of H^+ ATPase in rat kidney cortical collecting duct. Intercalated cells are heavily stained and show different patterns of staining. Apical staining is present in A cells (cell 1), whereas B cells have either a predominantly basolateral staining (cell 2) or a diffuse pattern of staining (cell 3). Bar = 10 μm.

the multitude of soluble and membrane-associated proteins that appear to be involved in this process. This is rapidly and briefly reviewed in the final part of this chapter as an illustration of the growing complexity of protein-targeting pathways.

Among the first category of proteins found to be involved in vesicle trafficking was a family of low-molecular-weight *ras*-like GTP-binding proteins known as *rab* proteins (82). There are at least 30 known members of this group, and they are involved in all aspects of vesicle transport, from the RER to the Golgi, intra-Golgi transport, endosome fusion, exocytosis, and endocytosis. Different *rab* proteins have been located on different intracellular compartments by organelle fractionation and immunocytochemistry. However, while these proteins have been implicated in GTP-dependent vesicle transport and fusion processes in cell-free assay systems and permeabilized cells, the precise mode of action of these proteins is not clear.

One low-molecular-weight G protein, ARF (ADP-ribosylation factor), is present in the cytoplasmic coating material that is associated with specialized transport vesicles in the Golgi (83). It is believed to be important in coat assembly, but other proteins are also involved (84). In addition to the small GTP-binding proteins, roles in intracellular trafficking for the large heterotrimeric G proteins are also being discovered. One of these, $G\alpha_{i3}$, is present on Golgi cisternae; it controls the rate of constitutive secretion of a heparan sulfate proteoglycan (85) and perhaps other proteins also. Heterotrimeric G proteins have also been implicated in RER to Golgi transport (86) and exocytosis (87); they also participate in clathrin-coated vesicle-mediated endocytosis (88).

Finally, transmembrane proteins that are homologous to the synaptic vesicle protein synaptobrevin/VAMP (vesicle-associated membrane protein) are present on some transport vesicles. These SNARE proteins are receptors for a complex of two soluble proteins called NSF (n-ethylmaleimide sensitive fusion protein) and SNAP (a soluble NSF binding protein), which together may somehow form a cross link between vesicle-associated SNARE proteins and a plasma membrane receptor (89). Again by homology with the synaptic vesicle/presynaptic membrane system, a second category of NSF-SNAP receptors that are homologous to syntaxin have been identified. These proteins, may be the plasma membrane receptor for vesicles and are called t-SNARES (target membrane SNARES) to distinguish them from v-SNARES (vesicle membrane SNARES) (89).

While the components of the fusion machine are now being identified, it will require further effort to learn how they function to determine specificity. Already, interactions between the various components of the fusion machine are being elucidated, including interactions between the *rab* GTP-binding proteins and the SNARE transmembrane "receptor" proteins.

SUMMARY

This review has dealt with some important aspects of protein and vesicle targeting in eukaryotic cells. The process involves signals within individual proteins, vesicle transport by cytoskeletal elements including microtubules, and a complex fusion machinery that includes both membrane-associated and soluble components. These processes are of critical importance to the establishment and maintenance of the polarized epithelial cell phenotype and therefore to normal kidney function. It is likely that a breakdown of one or more of these pathways would result in renal tubule pathology; indeed, defects in protein targeting have been described in both renal ischemia (90) and polycystic kidney disease (91,92).

REFERENCES

1. Rodriguez-Boulan E, Powell S. Polarity of epithelial and neuronal cells. Annu Rev Cell Biol 1992; 8:395–427.
2. Caplan M, Matlin KS. Sorting of membrane and secretory proteins in polarized epithelial cells. In: Matlin KS, Valentich JD eds. Functional Epithelial Cells in Culture. New York: Alan R Liss, 1989:71–127.
3. Simons K. Membrane traffic in an epithelial cell line derived from the dog kidney. Kidney Int 1987; 32 (suppl 23):201–207.
4. Brown D. Membrane recycling and epithelial cell function. Am J Physiol 1989; 256:F1–F12.
5. Low M. The glycosyl-phosphatidylinositol anchor of membrane proteins. Bicohim Biophys Acta 1989; 988:427–454.

6. Ferguson MA, Williams AF. Cell-surface anchoring of proteins via glycosyl-phosphatidylinositol structures. Annu Rev Biochem 1988; 57:285–320.
7. Cross GA. Glycolipid anchoring of plasma membrane proteins. Annu Rev Cell Biol 1990; 6:1–39.
8. Brown D, Waneck GL. Glycosyl-phosphatidylinositol-anchored membrane proteins. J Am Soc Nephrol 1992; 3:895–906.
9. Lisanti MP, Sargiacomo M, Graeve L, et al. Polarized apical distribution of glycosyl-phosphatidylinositol-anchored proteins in a renal epithelial cell line. Proc Natl Acad Sci USA 1988; 85:9557–9561.
10. Lisanti MP, Le-Bivec A, Saltiel AR, Rodriguez-Boulan E. Preferred apical distribution of glycosyl-phosphatidyinositol (GPI) anchored proteins: A highly conserved feature of the polarized epithelial cell phenotype. J Membr Biol 1990; 113:155–167.
11. Lisanti MP, Caras IW, Gilbert T, et al. Vectorial apical delivery and slow endocytosis of a glycolipid-anchored fusion protein in transfected MDCK cells. Proc Natl Acad Sci USA 1990; 87:7419–7423.
12. Brown DA, Crise B, Rose JK. Mechanism of membrane anchoring affects polarized expression of two proteins in MDCK cells. Science 1989; 245:1499–1501.
13. Powell SK, Lisanti MP, Rodriguez-Boulan EJ. Thy-1 expresses two signals for apical localization in epithelial cells. Am J Physiol 1991; 260:C715–C720.
14. Rothberg KG, Ying Y-S, Kamen BA, Anderson RGW. Cholesterol controls the clustering of the glycophospholipid-anchored membrane receptor for 5-methyltetrahydrofolate. J Cell Biol 1990; 111:2931–2938.
15. Simons K, Van Meer G. Lipid sorting in epithelial cells. Biochemistry 1988; 27:6197–6202.
15a. Montesano R, Roth J, Robert A, Orci L. Non-coated membrane invaginations are involved in binding and internalization of cholera and tetanus toxin. Nature 1982; 296:651–653.
16. Rothberg KG, Heuser JE, Donzell WC, et al. Caveolin, a protein component of caveolae membrane coats. Cell 1992; 68:673–682.
17. Robinson PJ. Phosphatidylinositol membrane anchors and T-cell activation. Immunol Today 1991; 12:35–41.
18. Presky DH, Low MG, Shevach EM. Role of phosphatidylinositol-anchored proteins in T cell activation. J Immunol 1990; 144:860–868.
19. Rock KL, Reiser H, Bamezai A, et al. The LY-6 locus: A multigene family encoding phosphatidylinositol-anchored membrane proteins concerned with T-cell activation. Immunol Rev 1989; 111:195–224.
20. Verpooten GF, Nouwen EJ, Hoylaerts MF, et al. Segment-specific localization of intestinal-type alkaline phosphatase in human kidney. Kidney Int 1989; 36:617–625.
21. Hooper NM, Hryszko J, Turner HJ. Purification and characterization of pig kidney aminopeptidase P: A glycosyl-phosphatidylinositol-anchored ectoenzyme. Biochem J 1990; 267:509–515.
22. Hooper NM, Keen JN, Turner AJ. Characterization of the glycosyl-phosphatidylinositol-anchored human renal dipeptidase reveals that it is more extensively glycosylated that the pig enzyme. Biochem J 1990; 265:429–433.
23. Sabolic I, Culic O, Lin S-H, Brown D. Localization of ecto-ATPase in the rat kidney and isolated renal cortical vesicles. Am J Physiol 1992; 262:F217–F228.
24. Rindler MJ, Naik SS, Li N, et al. Uromodulin (Tamm-Horsfall glycoprotein/uromucoid) is a phosphatidyinositol-linked membrane protein. J Biol Chem 1990; 265:20784–20789.
25. Friedman J, Hoyer JR, Seiler MW. Formation and clearance of tubulointerstitial immune complexes in kidneys of rats immunized with heterologous sera to Tamm-Horsfall protein. Kidney Int 1982; 21:575–582.
26. Wistrand PJ. Properties of membrane-bound carbonic anhydrase. Ann NY Acad Sci 1984; 429:195–206.
27. Brown D, Zhu X-L, Sly WS. Localization of membrane-associated carbonic anhydrase type IV in kidney epithelial cells. Proc Natl Acad Sci USA 1990; 87:7457–7461.
28. Zhu XL, Sly WS. Carbonic anhydrase IV from human lung: Purification, characterization, and comparison with membrane carbonic anhydrase from human kidney. J Biol Chem 1990; 265:8795–8801.
29. Yamamoto T, Wilson CB. Quantitative and qualitative studies of antibody-induced mesangial cell damage in the rat. Kidney Int 1987; 32:514–525.
30. Floege J, Johnson RJ, Gordon K, et al. Increased synthesis of extracellular matrix in mesangial proliferative nephritis. Kidney Int 1992; 40:477–488.
31. Chen WJ, Goldstein JL, Brown MS. NPXY, a sequence often found in cytoplasmic tails, is required for coated pit-mediated internalization of the low density lipoprotein receptor. J Biol Chem 1990; 265:3116–3123.
32. Collawn JF, Stangel M. Kuhn LA, et al. Transferrin receptor internalization sequence YXRF implicates a tight turn as the structural recognition motif for endocytosis. Cell 1990; 63:1061–1072.
33. Rabb H, Michishita M, Sharma P, et al. Cytoplasmic tails of human complement receptor type 3 (CR3, CD11b/CD18) regulate ligand avidity and the internalization of occupied receptors. J Immunol 1993; 151:990–1002.
34. Hunziker W, Mellman I. Expression of macrophage-lymphocyte Fc receptors in MDCK cells: Polarity and

trancytosis differ for isoforms with or without coated pit localization domains. J Cell Biol 1991; 109:3291–3302.
35. Le Bivic A, Sambuy Y, Patzak A, et al. An internal deletion in the cytoplasmic tail reverses the apical localization of human NGF receptor in transfected MDCK cells. J Cell Biol 1991; 115:607–618.
36. Brewer CB, Roth MG. A single amino acid change in the cytoplasmic domain alters the polarized delivery of influenza virus hemagglutinin. J Cell Biol 1991; 114:413–421.
37. Hunziker W, Harter C, Matter K, Mellman I. Basolateral sorting in MDCK cells requires a distinct cytoplasmic domain determinant. Cell 1991; 66:907–920.
38. Davis CG, Lehrman MA, Russell DW, et al. The J.D. mutation in familial hypercholesterolemia: Amino acid substitution in cytoplasmic domain impedes internalization of LDL receptors. Cell 1986; 45:15–24.
39. Peacock SL, Bates MP, Russell DW, et al. Human low density lipoprotein receptor expressed in Xenopus oocytes. Conserved signals for O-linked glycosylation and receptor-mediated endocytosis. J Biol Chem 1988; 263:7838–7845.
40. Trowbridge IS. Endocytosis and signals for internalization. Curr Opin Cell Biol 1991; 3:634–641.
41. Robinson MS. Adaptins. Trends Cell Biol 1992; 2:293–297.
42. Casanova JE, Apodaca G, Mostov KE. An autonomous signal for basolateral sorting in the cytoplasmic domain of the polymeric immunoglobulin receptor. Cell 1991; 66:65–75.
43. Matter K, Hunziker W, Mellman I. Basolateral sorting of LDL receptor in MDCK cells: The cytoplasmic domain contains two tyrosine-dependent targeting determinants. Cell 1992; 71:741–753.
44. Zheng G, Bachinsky DR, Stamenkovic I, et al. Organ distribution in rats of gp330, LRP/α_2MR, RAP and RAP binding sites. J Histochem Cytochem 1994; 42:531–542.
45. Kerjaschki D, Farquhar MG. The pathogenic antigen of Heymann nephritis is a membrane glycoprotein of the renal proximal tubule brush border. Proc Natl Acad Sci USA 1982; 79:5557–5561.
46. Kerjaschki D, Farquhar MG. Immunocytochemical localization of the Heymann nephritis antigen (gp330) in glomerular cells of normal Lewis rats. J Exp Med 1983; 157:667–686.
47. Chatelet F, Brianti E, Ronco P, et al. Ultrastructural localization by monoclonal antibodies of brush border antigens expressed by glomeruli: I. Renal distribution. Am J Pathol 1986; 122:500–511.
48. Abbate M, Bachinsky D, Zheng G, et al. Location of gp330/α_2-m receptor-associated protein (α_2-MRAP) and its binding sites in kidney; Distribution of endogenous α_2-MRAP is modified by tissue processing. Eur J Cell Biol 1993; 61:139–149.
49. Bachinsky DR, Zheng G, Niles JL, et al. Detection of two forms of gp330: Their role in Heymann nephritis. Am J Pathol 1993; 143:598–611.
50. Raychowdhury R, Niles JN, McCluskey RT, Smith JA. Autoimmune target in Heymann nephritis is a glycoprotein with homology to the LDL-receptor. Science 1989; 244:1163–1165.
51. Brown WJ, Goodhouse J, Farquhar MG. Mannose-6-phosphate receptors for lysosomal enzymes cycle between the Golgi complex and endosomes. J Cell Biol 1986; 103:1235–1247.
52. Griffiths G, Hoflack B, Simons K, et al. The mannose-6-phosphate receptor and the biogenesis of lysosomes. Cell 1988; 52:329–341.
53. Sly WS, Fisher HD. The phosphomannosyl recognition system for intracellular and intercellular transport of lysosomal enzymes. J Cell Biochem 1982; 18:319–347.
54. Achler C, Filmer D, Merte C, Drenckhahn D. Role of microtubules in polarized delivery of apical membrane proteins to the brush border of the intestinal epithelium. J Cell Biol 1989; 109:179–189.
55. Heuser J. Changes in lysosome shape and distribution correlated with changes in cytoplasmic pH. J Cell Biol 1989; 108:855–864.
56. Matteoni R, Kreis TE. Translocation and clustering of endosomes and lysosomes depends on microtubules. J Cell Biol 1987; 105:1253–1265.
57. Patzelt C, Brown D, Jeanrenaud B. Inhibitory effect of colchicine on amylase secretion by rat parotid glands: Possible localization in the Golgi area. J Cell Biol 1977; 73:578–593.
58. Pavelka M, Ellinger A, Gangl A. Effect of colchicine on rat small intestinal adsorptive cells: I. Formation of basolateral microvillus borders. J Ultrastruct Res 1983; 85:249–259.
59. Kreis T. Reclustering of scattered Golgi elements occurs along microtubules. Eur J Cell Biol 1989; 48:250–263.
60. Salas P, Misek D, Vega-Salas D, et al. Microtubules are not critically involved in the biogenesis of epithelial cell surface polarity. J Cell Biol 1986; 102:1853–1867.
61. Rindler MJ, Ivanov IE, Sabatini DD. Microtubule-acting drugs lead to the nonpolarized delivery of the influenza hemagglutinin to the cell surface of polarized Madin-Darby canine kidney cells. J Cell Biol 1987; 104:231–241.
62. Eilers U, Klumperman J, Hauri HP. Nocodazole, a microtubule-active drug, interferes with apical protein delivery in cultured intestinal epithelial cells. J Cell Biol 1989; 108:13–22.
63. Gutmann EJ, Niles JL, McCluskey RT, Brown D. Colchicine-induced redistribution of an endogenous

apical membrane glycoprotein (gp 330) in kidney proximal tubule epithelium. Am J Physiol 1989; 257:C397–C407.
64. Brown D, Sabolic I, Gluck S. Colchicine-induced redistribution of proton pumps in the proximal tubule. Kidney Int 1991; 40 (suppl 33):S79–S83.
65. Schroer TA, Sheetz MP. Functions of microtubule-based motors. Annu Rev Physiol 1991; 53:629–652.
66. Vale RD. Intracellular transport using microtubule-based motors. Annu Rev Cell Biol 1987; 3:347–378.
67. Stetson DL, Steinmetz PR. Role of membrane fusion in CO_2 stimulation of proton secretion by turtle bladder. Am J Physiol 1983; 245:C113–C120.
68. Phillips ME, Taylor A. Effect of nocodazole on the water permeability response to vasopressin in rabbit collecting tubules in vitro. J Physiol (Lond) 1989; 411:529–544.
69. Dousa TP, Barnes LD. Effects of colchicine and vinblastine on the cellular action of vasopressin in the mammalian kidney: A possible role of microtubules. J Clin Invest 1974; 54:252–262.
70. Brown D, Sabolic I. Specialized endosomal pathways for water channel and proton pump recycling in kidney epithelial cells. J Cell Sci 1993; 17(suppl):49–59.
71. Madsen KM, Tisher CC. Structure-function relationships along the distal nephron. Am J Physiol 1986; 250:F1–F15.
72. Schwartz GJ, Barasch J, Al-Awqati Q. Plasticity of functional epithelial polarity. Nature 1985; 318:368–371.
73. Brown D, Hirsch S, Gluck S. An H^+ ATPase is present in opposite plasma membrane domains in subpopulations of kidney epithelial cells. Nature 1988; 331:622–624.
74. Muto S, Yasoshima K, Yoshitomi K, et al. Electrophysiological identification of α and β intercalated cells and their distribution along the rabbit distal nephron segments. J Clin Invest 1990; 86:1829–1839.
75. Furuya H, Breyer MD, Jacobson HR. Functional characterization of α and β intercalated cells in rabbit cortical collecting duct. Am J Physiol 1991; 261:F377–F385.
76. Alper SL, Natale J, Gluck S, et al. Subtypes of intercalated cells in rat kidney collecting duct defined by antibodies against erythroid band 3 and renal vacuolar H^+-ATPase. Proc Natl Acad Sci USA 1989; 86:5429–5433.
77. Schuster VL, Fejes-Toth G, Naray-Fejes-Toth A, Gluck S. Colocalization of H^+ ATPase and band 3 anion exchanger in rabbit collecting duct intercalated cells. Am J Physiol 1991; 260:F506–F517.
78. Drenckhahn D, Schluter K, Allen DP, Bennett V. Co-localization of band 3 with ankyrin and spectrin at the basal membrane of intercalated cells in the rat kidney. Science 1985; 230:1287–1289.
79. Hemken P, Guo XL, Wang ZQ, et al. Immunologic evidence that vacuolar H+ ATPases with heterogeneous forms of Mr 31,000 subunit have different membrane distributions in mammalian kidney. J Biol Chem 1992; 267:9948–9957.
80. Nelson RD, Guo X-L, Masood K, et al. Selectively amplified expression of an isoform of the vacuolar H+ATPase Mr 56,000 subunit in renal intercalated cells. Proc Natl Acad Sci USA 1992; 89:3541–3545.
81. Puopolo K, Kumamoto I, Adachi I, et al. Differential expression of the "B" subunit of the vacuolar H^+ ATPase in bovine tissues. J Biol Chem 1992; 267:3696–3706.
82. Zerial M, Stenmark H. Rab GTPases in vesicular transport. Curr Opin Cell Biol 1993; 5:613–620.
83. Serafini T, Orci L, Amherdt M, et al. ADP-ribosylation factor is a subunit of the coat of Golgi-derived COP-coated vesicles: A novel role for a GTP-binding protein. Cell 1991; 67:239–253.
84. Serafini T, Stenbeck G, Brecht A, et al. A coat of Golgi-derived non-clathrin-coated vesicles with homology to the clathrin coated vesicle coat protein β-adaptin. Nature 1991; 349:215–220.
85. Stow JL, de Almeida JB, Narula N, et al. A heterotrimeric G protein, $G\alpha_{i3}$, on Golgi membranes regulates the secretion of a heparan sulfate proteoglycan in LLC-PK_1 epithelial cells. J Cell Biol 1991; 114:1113–1124.
86. Schwaninger E, Plutner H, Bokoch G, Balch W. Multiple GTP-binding proteins regulate vesicular transport from the ER to Golgi membranes. J Cell Biol 1992; 119:1077–1095.
87. Aridor M, Rajmilevich G, Beaven MA, Sagi-Eisenberg R. Activation of exocytosis by the heterotrimeric G-protein G_{i3}. Science 1993; 262:1569–1572.
88. Carter L, Redelmeier T, Woollenweber L, Schmidt S. Multiple GTP-binding proteins participate in clathrin-coated vesicle-mediated endocytosis. J Cell Biol 1993; 120:37–45.
89. Söllner T, Whiteheart SW, Brunner M, et al. SNAP receptors implicated in vesicle targeting and fusion. Nature 1993; 362:318–324.
90. Molitoris BA. The potential role of ischemia in renal disease progression. Kidney Int Suppl 1992; 36.
91. Avner ED, Sweeney WEJ, Nelson WJ. Abnormal sodium pump distribution during renal tubulogenesis in congenital murine polycystic kidney disease. Proc Natl Acad Sci USA 1992; 89:7447–7451.
92. Wilson PD, Sherwood AC, Palla K, et al. Reversed polarity of Na(+) -K(+)-ATPase: Mislocation to apical plasma membranes in polycystic kidney disease epithelia. Am J Physiol 1991; 260:F420–F430.

4

Regulation of Coordinately Expressed Collagen Genes

Yutaka Inagaki, Shizuko Tanaka, Sharada Truter, and Francesco Ramirez
Brookdale Center for Molecular Biology, Mount Sinai School of Medicine, New York, New York

INTRODUCTION

The collagens represent a family of proteins commonly characterized by one or more domains made of repeated Gly-X-Y triplets (1). These macromolecules are responsible for maintaining the structural integrity of the body organs, and for influencing a variety of cellular activities (1,2). Production of different collagen types during development and in adulthood is therefore critical for cell-matrix interactions and for tissue integrity. The biosynthesis and degradation of collagen molecules represent the opposite ends of the balance that regulates extracellular matrix remodeling and thus the physiology of tissue repair. This balance is, in turn, the product of a dynamic interplay between mesenchyme-specific genes and the cytokines released by inflammatory cells (2). Environmental insults interfering with this delicate equilibrium result in either decreased tissue integrity or excessive collagen deposition (2). The latter is the central hallmark of fibrosis, a pathological process that irreversibly damages organ function (2). Thus, fibrosis can be generalized as a chronic and uncontrolled inflammatory/repair process that alters the normal interplay between cellular stimuli and matrix proteins coding genes (2).

Diabetic nephropathy is one example of the consequences of deregulated collagen gene expression and excessive collagen protein production (3). During the early phase of the disease, there is substantial accumulation of matrix components, with the consequential increase in the relative surface/volume area of the globular and tubular basement membranes. This pathology is in turn reflected in the chronicization of the tubuloepithelial and glomerulal hypertrophy which characterizes the early phase of diabetes (3). In the latter phase, excessive deposition of matrix components is accompanied by decreased metalloproteases activity. This combination ultimately leads to substantial thickening of the globular and tubular basement membranes, a feature readily noticeable in the diabetic kidney about 3 years after the appearance of insulin deficiency (3). Immunohistopathological examination of diabetic lesions in human patients and in experimentally induced animals has often pointed to a causal involvement of type I and type IV collagens in the progression of diabetic nephropathy (4). Unfortunately, the phenomenological nature of these studies has significantly hindered our understanding of how this causal association is first established and through which mechanisms is subsequently developed. As a result, the cause(s) of sustained collagen elevation during diabetic nephropathy remains obscure.

There are also several practical reasons why our understanding of deregulated collagen production in kidney disease has not progressed as fast as in other systems. First, there is the lack of a reliable cellular system in which to analyze systematically the onset and development of the metabolic alteration. Second, a problem is posed by the wide variety of experimental means that have been used by different groups to investigate the same phenomenon. Last, the significant variability in the histopathology of the animal models utilized to recreate the human condition is also problematic. The insulin-dependent streptozoticin-diabetic rat is a case in point, for it has often yielded conflicting results. Some studies have indicated that the diabetic kidneys of these animals express substantially high levels of $\alpha1$(IV) collagen mRNA (5). Others have denied this finding and shown a decrease in steady-state levels of $\alpha1$(IV) collagen mRNA, which parallels that normally occurring in aging rats (6). Another unclarified point is the role of inflammatory cytokines, particularly transforming growth factor (TGF)-β, in triggering and sustaining collagen upregulation in diseased kidney cells. Preliminary findings have recently shown that anti-TGF-β antibodies reverse the high-glucose–mediated induction of collagen production in cultured mesangial cells (7). This result is also consistent with the noted elevation of TGF-β in the kidney glomeruli of diabetic patients and experimentally stimulated rats (8).

This review is intended to give a brief review of our current understanding of collagen gene regulation by discussing control of type I and IV collagen production. The latter is critical to the formation of the functional architecture of the kidney, while the former is an extensively studied paradigm for cytokine modulation. It is our hope that this review will be read with the idea in mind that this information will eventually be instrumental in deciphering the pathology of the diseased kidney.

COLLAGEN GENE REGULATION

Collagen synthesis relies upon the utilization of diversified regulatory programs that employ time- and cell-type–specific promoters and enhancers (8). As a result, collagen gene transcription appears to be orchestrated by complex interactions between a variety of *cis*-acting regulatory elements and *trans*-acting nuclear factors (8).

Analysis of collagen gene expression has mostly relied on the utilization of an experimental protocol that is, in turn, composed of two distinct techniques. In the first approach, chimeric genes are transfected into cultured cells in order to examine the ability of a given promoter sequence to direct tissue-specific transcription of a reporter gene. This functional test can be carried out transiently, using stably integrated transfectants, or in transgenic mice. In the second approach, various DNA-binding assays are used to identify specific sites of interaction with nuclear proteins within a given promoter sequence. Once identified, the consequences of specific nucleotide substitutions on binding affinity and transcriptional activity are tested by the same two experimental approaches. A good correlation between the functional and binding results is ultimately interpreted as inferring a physiological role for these DNA/protein interactions. We now briefly discuss the results of these kind of studies performed on the coordinately regulated type I and IV collagen genes.

TYPE I COLLAGEN GENES

Type I collagen is the most prominent member of the fibrillar class of collagen molecules which, in addition, includes types II, III, V, and XI (1). Type I collagen is virtually present in every tissue with significant prevalence in bone, skin, tooth, tendon, and ligaments (1). The most common molecular form of type I collagen consists of two $\alpha1$ chains and one $\alpha2$ chain. Like all the other fibrillar collagens, they are initially synthesized as precursor procollagens that assemble intracellularly into procollagen trimers (1). Following secretion, the trimers undergo maturation with the proteolytic loss of the terminal propeptides (1).

The type I procollagens are encoded by two distinct genes (COL1A1 and COL1A2), which are located on different chromosomes (9). The coding sequences of the type I collagen genes are distributed among more than 50 exons in a remarkably similar manner (9). This, in turn, implies that COL1A1 and COL1A2 probably arose from a common progenitor that already possessed a multiexon structure (9). The large triple-helical domains of the type I procollagen chains are encoded by 42 exons. The majority of these coding units are 54 bp or a multiple of this in length. Thus, the core of the progenitor collagen gene might have evolved through a variety of recombinant events from an ancestral 54-bp exon coding for six Gly-X-Y triplets (9). The C-terminal propeptide coding domains of the COL1A1 and COL1A2 genes are also divided into the same four exons. This indirectly suggests that this protein domain, too, developed under strict evolutionary pressure (9). Indeed, there is ample evidence indicating that the C-terminal propeptide plays a critical role in the assembly and formation of the trimeric precursor molecule. The structurally heterogeneous N-terminal propeptides are also encoded by the same number of exons in both genes; however, the significance of this intriguing observation is obscure (9).

Transcription of COL1A1 and COL1A2 is tightly controlled, in that steady-state mRNA levels parallel the relative ratio of the protein chains (9). Altered production of type I collagen constitutes a focal problem in numerous fibrotic disorders that affect the function of several organs, including the kidney. These biosynthetic changes are believed to be elicited by cytokines released by the cells in response to as yet unidentified stimuli (10,11). To gain some insight into the modulation of type I collagen synthesis, several investigators have examined the factors that participate in the formation of active transcriptional complexes.

COL1A1 Gene Regulation

The COL1A1 promoter region between nucleotides –222 to +16 of the mouse gene contains sufficient sequence information to direct high reporter gene expression in NIH-3T3 fibroblasts (12). Several nuclear protein binding sites have been mapped within this basal COL1A1 promoter, including the recognition sequences for inhibitory factors 1 and 2 (IF1 and IF2) (12). Inhibitory factor 1 binds to two adjacent sites located between –190 to –170 and between –160 to –130; there is also an IF1-binding counterpart in the proximal segment of the COL1A2 promoter (13). Inhibitory factor 2 is a metalloprotein interacting with one of the two GC boxes located within a segment (–130 to –80) that also contains two CCAAT motifs (1). The initial suggestion that IF2 may be the ubiquitous transcription factor Sp1 was subsequently confirmed by additional studies (14,15). The proximal of the aforementioned CCAAT motifs is the site of binding of a transcriptional activator, CBF, which was originally identified in the COL1A2 promoter (see below).

A negative regulator of transcription binds to a sequence upstream of the basal promoter region (–339 to –361) of the COL1A1 gene; this factor is exclusively expressed in type I collagen-producing cells (16). Interestingly, the recognition sequence for this repressor shows a high degree of homology to the tissue-specific negative regulator of the COL1A2 promoter (see below). Further upstream, at about –1600, is a *cis*-acting element (TAE) that mediates the stimulation of TGF-β on collagen synthesis by cultured fibroblasts (17). Despite the presence of potential NF-1 and AP-2 binding sites, neither of the two transcription factors interacts with the TAE (17).

Tissue-specific expression of COL1A1 gene is governed by interactions between promoter and intron-1 sequences (8). Although there is still some controversy about the nature of the intron contribution to transcriptional regulation, several lines of evidence indicate that this genomic region plays some important role in COL1A1 gene expression (18). One of these examples is the so-called Mov13 mouse transgenic line. Generated by insertional mutagenesis, Mov 13 mice harbor a provirus sequence integrated in the first intron of COL1A1 and, as a result, the gene is transcriptionally inactive (19). The proviral integration is associated with changes in chromatin conformation, and with de novo methylation of the sequences bordering the site of integration (20,21). Thus, the transcriptional block of COL1A1 is believed to be caused by the provirus disruption of the interactions between *cis*-acting elements residing upstream and downstream of the initiation site of transcription (18). However, tooth rudiments from 13-day homozygous Mov 13 embryos express COL1A1 and develop normally (22). Hence, odontoblasts seem to utilize a different regulatory program than other type I collagen producing cells, such as fibroblasts. Although their identity is obscure, the *cis*-acting elements of the odontoblasts' program must be located sufficiently distant from intron 1 to remain unaffected by the change in chromatin configuration (8).

Additional examples of diversified COL1A1 regulatory programs have recently been reported in the rat system. Functional assays in stably transfected cells and transgenic mice have indicated that COL1A1 chimeric constructs utilize differential regulatory domains of the –3.6-kb promoter in osseous and fibroblastic cells (23). Similarly, COL1A1 promoter activity is downregulated in transfected primary bone cells compared to transgenic calvarial cells (24). Presumably, this difference reflects the architectural and/or environmental signals to which bone cells are normally exposed within the bone tridimensional context.

COL1A2 Gene Regulation

The COL1A2 gene displays a more compact promoter anatomy than the COL1A1 gene in that the sequence from –346 to +1 is sufficient to sustain high and cell-type-specific gene expression and to respond to cytokine treatment (25–29). An early report of an enhancer activity within the gene's first intron has been subsequently refuted (29,30). Two major areas of DNA-protein interactions are present in the basal COL1A2 promoter.

The first site of binding maps between nucleotides –84 and –80 and displays a characteristic CCAAT motif (31). Mutations introduced in the CCAAT sequence abrogate protein binding in vitro, and reduce substantially promoter activity in vivo (31). The *trans*-acting factor that binds at this site, CBF, consists of three distinct components: subunit A (CBF-A, Mr 39 kDa), subunit B (CBF-B, Mr 41 kDa) and subunit C (CBF-C, Mr 40 kDa) (32). The A and B subunits are structurally homologous to the yeast Hap3 and Hap2 transcription factors that regulate the respiratory function of this organism (33,34). Interestingly, the yeast subunits can be functionally interchanged with various other mammalian CCAAT-binding proteins (35). Although the structure of the CBF-C is unknown, available evidence suggests that this subunit is tightly associated with CBF-A (32).

The CBF complex is believed to be involved in the coordinated regulation of the type I collagen genes. This conclusion is based on results in a reconstituted in vitro assay showing that CBF stimulates accurate initiation of transcription of the COL1A1 promoter (36). It should, however, be noted that CBP proteins have multiple and overlapping recognition specificities and that the CCAAT-motif can interact with functionally diverse regulatory factors (37).

The second regulatory area of the COL1A2 promoter was originally linked to an NF-1-mediated response to TGF-β induction (38). More recent work has refuted this early observation and provided some new insights on the mechanisms of cytokine action on collagen gene expression (see below). The cytokine-responsive area of the COL1A2 promoter extends from –330 to –255 and includes two nuclear factor–bound regions: Box A and Box B (28). The 5′ half of the former is the site of binding of a transcriptional repressor, while Sp1 binds to its 3′ half (28). As already mentioned, the repressor binding site is somewhat similar to the upstream recognition sequence for the COL1A1 repressor and, additionally, both repressors are found in collagen-expressing cells (28). The factor(s) interacting with Box B has not yet been characterized.

Cytokines and Fibrosis

Irrespective of the initial stimuli, activation of a fibrotic process is caused by the deregulated action of several biological signals, collectively referred to as cytokines, released by the cells of the inflammatory/repair system (39). One of these, TGF-β, is a potent stimulator of fibroblast proliferation and of type I collagen production (40). Tumor necrosis factor (TNF)-α, on the other hand, exerts an antagonistic action on TGF-β stimulation, for it inhibits fibroblast type I collagen synthesis (41). The TGF-β responsive element (TbRE) of the COL1A2 gene includes the 3′ half of Box A (Box 3A) and the neighboring Box B (28).

In TGF-β activated fibroblasts, there is a rapid increase in the binding affinity of TbRE protein complex (TbRC) which parallels the stimulation of the endogenous COL1A2 gene (28). The increase includes Sp1, but only as an indirect effect of another interacting factor of the TbRC. This conclusion is based on the observation that the Sp1 site of Box 3A alone does not exhibit the same protein-binding increases as a probe containing Box 3A and Box B (28). The proposed model of TGF-β stimulation can also be extended to explain the inhibitory effect of TNF-α. This cytokine induces similar but not identical changes in the binding pattern of the TbRC; it also stimulates the interaction of the repressor at the Box 5A site (28).

The antagonistic stimuli of the cytokines at the TbRE site are therefore elaborated by changing either the identity of the Sp1-interacting factors, the nature of their modifications, or by a combination of both (28). In addition to reducing the positive action of the TbRC by one of the above mechanisms, TNF-α increases the effectiveness of the negative factor, with the overall result of a substantial downregulation in COL1A2 gene transcription (28). Finally, the presence of an Sp1-like sequence in the upstream TAE of COL1A1 reiterates that common regulatory programs might be shared by these coordinately expressed genes (28).

TYPE IV COLLAGEN GENE REGULATION

Type IV collagen forms a two-dimensional poligonal mesh that serves as the basic scaffold upon which the complex basement membrane network is built (1). The most common form of type IV collagen trimer is composed of two $\alpha1$ chains and one $\alpha2$ chain (1). The type IV collagen molecules consist of the following structurally distinct regions: a central triple helix with numerous noncollagenous interruptions, a large C-terminal globular domain (NC1), and a small N-terminal globular domain (2). Like type I collagen, type IV collagen is also assembled intracellularly into a heterotrimer but, unlike type I collagen, this is not followed by its extracellular processing (1).

The type IV polypeptides are encoded by two closely linked genes (COL4A1 and COL4A2) located on human chromosome 13 (42). The type IV coding genes are relatively large and fragmented into numerous exons (43). Unlike the fibrillar collagen genes, they do not display the characteristic 54-bp coding unit, nor do they have an identical exon/intron organization (43). Recent work has identified four additional chains ($\alpha3$, $\alpha4$, $\alpha5$, and $\alpha6$) of type IV collagen, encoded by genes that are similarly arranged in a head-to-head configuration on human chromosomes 2 (COL4A3 and COL4A4) and X (COL4A5 and COL4A6) (44,45). Genomic and sequence comparisons indicate a closer evolutionarily kinship between COL4A1, COL4A3, and COL4A5 than between them and COL4A2, COL4A4, and COL4A6. This is consistent with the hypothesis that the duplication of the three clusters followed rather than preceded the formation of the ancestral $\alpha1/\alpha2$ gene pair (43).

As it is discussed more extensively elsewhere in this book, the gene clusters on chromosomes 2 and X are also of great relevance to kidney physiopathology. They are, in fact, the diseased loci of the autosomal and sex-linked forms of Alport's syndrome (43,46). In addition, the noncollagenous (NC1) domain of the $\alpha3$(IV) chain is the primary target of autoantibodies produced in Goodpasture's syndrome (43,46).

Aside from illustrating a common evolutionary origin, the identical arrangement of the type IV collagen pairs implies that coexpression of these genes is under the control of similar regulatory mechanisms. Below, we discuss some of these mechanisms by using the most extensively studied system, namely the COL4A1-COL4A2 gene cluster. Because of the remarkable sequence conservation, results from the human and mouse systems are combined together. In closing, however, we point to unresolved differences in the regulation of these two genes in the mammalian species.

The region that separates the COL4A1 and COL4A2 genes is approximately 130 bp long. At its center and within an interrupted dyad of symmetry is a sequence rich in GC boxes to which apparently binds the transcription activator Sp1 (42,47). The common promoter works bidirectionally, for it directs transcription irrespective of its orientation to the reporter gene. But high reporter gene activity by the bidirectional promoter requires the presence of an enhancer element located in the first intron of COL4A1 (42,47). The enhancer contains potential cAMP and serum-responsive elements in addition to a novel nuclear protein-binding sequence that is also present in the common promoter sequence (42,47,48). Finally, a negative *cis*-acting regulatory sequence is present in the third intron of COL4A2 (42). Thus, coordinated transcription of COL4A1 and COL4A2 genes is a complex process that involves an interacting network of both positive and negative *cis*-acting sequences residing within a common chromosomal domain.

Teratocarcinoma cells treated with retinoic acid and cAMP mimic the phenotypic and biosynthetic changes that characterize the differentiation of parietal endoderm cells from the inner cell mass of the developing mouse embryo (50). Thickening of basement membranes and increased type IV collagen deposition is also the hallmark of numerous clinical conditions whose etiopathology is yet to be defined. Promoter-enhancer plasmids transiently expressed in differentiated teratocarcinoma cells and fibroblasts stimulate high reporter gene activity in the former but not in the latter (43,50). This finding is consistent with the level of endogenous gene activity in these two cell lines. Surprisingly, however, the plasmids are also transcriptionally active in undifferentiated teratocarcinoma cells that express very little type IV collagen (50). In contrast, stably integrated constructs are transcriptionally inactive in undifferentiated teratocarcinoma cells (47). One explanation for this apparent discrepancy is that the promoter elements of the stably integrated construct are inaccesible to the cognate *trans*-acting factors because of chromosome-associate changes, like methylation (43,48). Alternatively, additional cell type–specific elements in the proximity of but distinct from the intron-1 enhancer may be responsible for mediating retinoic acid and cAMP induction in differentiating teratocarcinoma cells (51).

As previously stated, some differences have been noted in transfection experiments using either the human or mouse gene constructs; they may reflect true species-specific differences or they may be the result of experimental discrepancies. The most important of these differences is the presence in the human system of an enhancer activity in the first intron of the COL4A2 rather than the COL4A1 gene (42). Unlike the mouse COL4A1 enhancer, the human COL4A2 element exerts its action only on its own gene. Another minor difference is the yet to be identified mouse counterpart of the silencer residing in the third intron of the human COL4A2 gene (42). Finally, the precise role of the mouse intron 1 in specifying the differentiation program of type IV producing cells remains somewhat controversial (47,51).

SUMMARY

In conclusion, the analysis of the regulation of collagen gene expression is adding an additional layer of complexity to an already intricate biological system. The examples discussed in this review exemplify this point. They illustrate how coordinately expressed genes exploit both common and unique DNA-protein interactions in order to amplify regulatory potentials, irrespective of their physical relationships. This and related work on other aspects of collagen regulation will eventually provide a full account of collagen function in normal and diseased conditions. This process will also benefit from a better understanding of the role played by the cytokines in modulating collagen biosynthesis during development, organogenesis, and differentiation as well as in the progression of pathological conditions.

ACKNOWLEDGMENTS

The authors wish to thank Dr. Gerard Karsenty for many stimulating discussions and Ms. Mary Sozomenu for the preparation of the manuscript. This is article 150 from the Brookdale Center for Molecular Biology.

REFERENCES

1. van der Rest M, Garrone R. Collagen family of proteins. FASEB J 1991; 5:2814–2823.
2. Hay ED. Collagen and other matrix glycoproteins in embryogenesis. In: Hay ED, ed. Cell Biology of Extracellular Matrix, 2nd ed. New York: Plenum Press, 1991:419–462.
3. Myers BD. Diabetes and the kidney. In: Wingaarden JB, Smith LH, eds. Cecil Textbook of Medicine, 18th ed. Philadelphia: WB Saunders, 1988:624–627.
4. Ziyadeh FN. The extracellular matrix in diabetic nephropathy. Am J Kidney Dis 1993; 22:736–744.
5. Ihm CG, Lee GSL, Nast CC, et al. Early increased renal procollagen $\alpha1$(IV) mRNA levels in streptozotocin induced diabetes. Kidney Int 1992; 41:768–777.
6. Poulsom R, Kurkinen M, Prockop DJ, Boot-Hanford RP. Increased steady-state levels of laminin $\beta1$ mRNA in kidneys of long-term streptozotocin-diabetic rats: No effect of aldose reductase inhibitor. J Biol Chem 1988; 263:10072–10076.
7. Yamamoto T, Nakamura T, Noble NA, et al. Expression of transforming growth factor β is elevated in human and experimental diabetic nephropathy. Proc Natl Acad Sci USA 1993; 90:1814–1818.
8. Ramirez F, Di Liberto M. Complex and diversified regulatory programs control the expression of vertebrate collagen genes. FASEB J 1990; 4:1616–1623.
9. Ramirez F. In: Olsen BR, Nimni EM, eds. Molecular Biology, Vol. 4. Organization and Evolution of Fibrillar Collagen Genes in Collagen. Boca Raton, FL: CRC Press, 1989:21–30.
10. Sporn MB, Harris ED. Proliferative diseases. Am J Med 1981; 70:1231–1236.
11. Seyer JM. Mediators of increased collagen synthesis in fibrosing organs. Fundam Appl Toxicol 1985; 5:228–239.
12. Karsenty G, de Crombrugghe B. Two different negative and one positive regulatory factors interact with a short promoter segment of the alpha 1(I) collagen gene. J Biol Chem 1988; 265:9934–9942.
13. Karsenty G, de Crombrugghe B. Conservation of binding sites for regulatory factors in the coordinately expressed $\alpha1$(I) and $\alpha2$(I) collagen promoters. Biochem Biophys Res Commun 1991; 177:538–544.
14. Karsenty G, Ravazzolo R, de Crombrugghe B. Purification and functional characterization of a DNA-binding protein that interacts with a negative element in the mouse $\alpha1$(I) collagen promoter. J Biol Chem 1991; 266:24842–24848.
15. Nehls MC, Rippe RA, Veloz L, Brenner DA. Transcription factors nuclear factor I and Sp1 interact with the murine collagen $\alpha1$(I) promoter. Mol Cell Biol 1991; 11:4065–4073.
16. Ritzenthaler JD, Goldstein RH, Fine A, Smith BD. Regulation of the $\alpha1$(I) collagen promoter via a transforming growth factor-β activation element. J Biol Chem 1993; 268:13625–13631.

17. Slack JL, Liska D, Bornstein P. Regulation of expression of the type I collagen genes. Am J Med Genet 1993; 45:140–151.
18. Ravazzolo R, Karsenty G, de Crombrugghe B. A fibroblast-specific factor binds to an upstream negative control element in the promoter of the mouse α1(I) collagen gene. J Biol Chem 1991; 266:7382–7387.
19. Schnieke A, Harbers K, Jaenisch R. Embryonic lethal mutation in mice induced by retrovirus insertion in the alpha (1) collagen gene. Nature 1983; 304:315–320.
20. Breindl M, Harbers K, Jaenisch R. Retrovirus-induced lethal mutation in collagen I gene of mice is associated with an altered chromatin structure. Cell 1984; 38:9–16.
21. Sander D, Jaenisch R. Retrovirus-induced de novo methylation of flanking host sequences correlates with gene inactivity. Nature 1985; 315:594–597.
22. Kratochwil K, von der Mark K, Kollar EJ, et al. Retrovirus-induced insertional mutation in Mov13 mice affects collagen I expression in a tissue-specific manner. Cell 1988; 57:807–816.
23. Pavlin D, Lichtler AC, Bedalov A, et al. Differential utilization of regulatory domains within the α1(I) collagen promoter in osseous and fibroblastic cells. J Cell Biol 1992; 116:227–236.
24. Krebsbach PH, Harrison JR, Lichtler AC, et al. Transgenic expression of COL1A1-chloramphenicol acetyltransferase fusion genes in bone: Differential utilization of promoter elements in vivo and in cultured cells. Mol Cell Biol 1993; 13:5168–5174.
25. Schmidt A, Rossi P, de Crombrugghe B. Transcriptional control of the mouse α2(I) collagen gene: Functional deletion analysis of the promoter and evidence for cell-specific expression. Mol Cell Biol 1986; 6:347–354.
26. Boast S, Su MW, Ramirez F, Sanchez M, Avvedimento EV. Functional analysis of cis-acting DNA sequences controlling transcription of human type I collagen genes. J Biol Chem 1990; 265:13351–13356.
27. Kähäri VM, Chen YQ, Su MW, et al. Tumor necrosis factor-α and interferon-γ suppress the activation of human type I collagen gene expression by transforming growth factor-β1. J Clin Invest 1990; 86:1489–1495.
28. Inagaki Y, Truter S, Tanaka S, DiLiberto M, Ramirez F. TGF-β stimulates α2(I) collagen gene expression through a cis-acting element that contains an Sp1 binding site. J Biol Chem 1995, in press.
29. Rossi P, de Crombrugghe B. Identification of a cell-specific transcriptional enhancer in the first intron of the mouse α2 (type I) collagen gene. Proc Natl Acad Sci USA 1987; 84:5590–5594.
30. Goldberg H, Helaakoski T, Garrett LA, et al. Tissue-specific expression of the mouse α2(I) collagen promoter. J Biol Chem 1992; 267:19622–19630.
31. Karsenty G, Golumbek PT, de Crombrugghe B. Point mutations and small substitution mutations in three different upstream elements inhibit the activity of the mouse α2(I) collagen promoter. J Biol Chem 1988; 263:13909–13915.
32. Maity SN, Sinha S, Ruteshouser CE, de Crombrugghe B. Three different polypeptides are necessary for DNA binding of the mammalian heteromeric CCAAT binding factor. J Biol Chem 1992; 267:16574–16580.
33. Maity SN, Vuorio T, de Crombrugghe B. The B subunit of a rat heteromeric CCAAT-binding transcription factor shows a striking sequence identity with the yeast Hap2 transcription factor. Proc Natl Acad Sci USA 1990; 87:5378–5382.
34. Vuorio T, Maity SN, de Crombrugghe B. Purification and molecular cloning of the "A" chain of a rat heteromeric CCAAT-binding protein. J Biol Chem 1990; 265:22480–22486.
35. Chodosh LA, Baldwin AS, Carthew RW, Sharp, PA. Human CCAAT-binding proteins have heterologous subunits. Cell 1988; 53:11–24.
36. Maity SN, Golumbek PT, Karsenty G, de Crombrugghe B. Selective activation of transcription by a novel CCAAT binding factor. Science 1988; 241:582–585.
37. Johnson PF, McKnight SL. Eukaryotic transcriptional regulatory proteins. Annu Rev Biochem 1989; 58:799–839.
38. Rossi P, Karsenty G, Roberts AB, et al. A nuclear factor 1 binding site mediates the transcriptional activation of a type I collagen promoter by transforming growth factor-β. Cell 1988; 52:405–414.
39. Diegelmann RF, Lindblad WJ, Cohen I. Fibrogenic processes during tissue repair. In: Nimni, EM, ed. Collagen: Biochemistry and Biomechanics. Boca Raton, FL: CRC Press, 1988:113–131.
40. Rizzino A. Transforming growth factor-β: Multiple effects on cell differentiation and extracellular matrices. Dev Biol 1988; 130:411–422.
41. Solis-Herruzo J, Brenner DA, Chojkier M. Tumor necrosis factor α inhibits collagen gene transcription and collagen synthesis in cultured human fibroblasts. J Biol Chem 1988; 263:5841–5845.
42. Poschl E, Pollner R, Kuhn K. The genes for the α1(IV) and α2(IV) chains of human basement membrane collagen type IV are arranged head-to-head and separated by a bidirectional promoter of unique structure. EMBO J 1988; 7:2687–2695.
43. Hudson BG, Reeders ST, Tryggvason K. Type IV collagen: Structure, gene organization, and role in human diseases. J Biol Chem 1993; 268:26033–26036.
44. Mariyama M, Zhang K, Yang-Feng TL, Reeders ST. Colocalization of the genes for the α3(IV) and α4(IV) chains of type IV collagen to chromosome 2 bands q35–q37. Genomics 1992; 13:809–813.

45. Zhou J, Mochizuki T, Smeets H, et al. Deletion of the paired $\alpha5$(IV) and $\alpha6$(IV) collagen genes in inherited smooth muscle tumors. Science 1993; 261:1167–1169.
46. Tryggvason K, Zhou J, Hostikka SL, Sariola H. Type IV collagen in normal and diseased glomerular basement membrane. Adv Nephrol 1993; 22:1–14.
47. Burbelo P, Martin G, Yamada Y. $\alpha1$(IV) and $\alpha2$(IV) collagen genes regulated by a bidirectional promoter and a shared enhancer. Proc Natl Acad Sci USA 1988; 85:9674–9682.
48. Burbelo PD, Horikoshi S, Yamada Y. DNA methylation and collagen IV gene expression in F9 teratocarcinoma cells. J Biol Chem 1990; 265:4839–4843.
49. Fischer G, Schmidt C, Opitz J, et al. Identification of a novel sequence element in the common promoter region of the human type IV genes involved in the regulation of divergent transcription. Biochem J 1993; 292:687–695.
50. Killen PD, Burbelo PD, Martin GR, Yamada Y. Characterization of the promoter for the $\alpha1$(IV) collagen gene: DNA sequences within the first intron enhance transcription. J Biol Chem 1988; 263:8706–8709.
51. Tanaka S, Kaytes P, Kurkinen M. An enhancer for transcription of collagen IV genes is activated by FS cell differentiation. J Biol Chem 1993; 268:7196–7204.

5
Laminin

Rainer Deutzmann
University of Regensburg, Regensburg, Germany

INTRODUCTION

Laminin is a high-molecular-weight multidomain protein of the extracellular matrix. It is composed of three polypeptide chains that form a dilulfide-linked complex with a unique cruciform structure. In the adult organism, laminin is restricted to basement membranes, whereas during embryogenesis it is also found in punctate pattern in the mesenchyme. In addition to being a major structural component of basement membranes, laminin is important in mediating cell matrix interactions (for review, see Refs. 1–5). It has been implicated in a variety of biological processes, including cell adhesion and spreading, migration, and neurite outgrowth. Laminin is already expressed in the preimplantation embryo (6) and has been shown to be essential for development of kidney epithelia (7); recently, mutations in *Drosophila* were described that could be lethal in development or give rise to adults with reduced viability and defects in a number of tissues (8). These few examples already indicate its diverse functions in embryogenesis.

A major progress toward understanding the various biological effects of laminin at the molecular level was allocation of several activities to distinct sites of the molecule and identification of receptors involved in these interactions. One of the most important findings in the last few years was the discovery that laminin is a family of related molecules that differ by substitution of constituent polypeptide chains for corresponding isoforms (9–11). This might modify or change biological activities, and tissue- and stage-specific expression of the various isoforms might play a role in morphogenesis and maintenance of organ function.

Apart from being essential in tubulogenesis, the role of laminins in kidney development and function is largely unknown, but several conclusions can be drawn from related studies. Therefore the present review first summarizes structural and functional data on laminins that are probably of general importance for all tissues; with that background, kidney-specific aspects are discussed.

STRUCTURE OF LAMININ AND ITS ISOFORMS

Classic Laminin

Laminin was originally discovered in the matrix of the transplantable mouse Engelbreth-Holm-Swarm (EHS) tumor (12) and in cell cultures of murine parietal yolk sac carcinoma cells (13). Such tumor lines produce relatively large amounts of basement membrane–like material from which individual compounds can easily be isolated. The EHS tumor turned out to be the best source of laminin; by simple extraction with nondenaturing buffers in the presence of EDTA, quantities in the order of 100 mg from 50 g of tissue can be obtained (14). This allowed detailed structural and functional studies, leading to a rapid development of laminin research. Laminin from EHS tumor became the prototypic laminin, even though it is realized now that it is just a member of a large family. To avoid confusion, the type of laminin originally isolated from the mouse tumor will be referred to here as EHS laminin.

EHS laminin consists of three genetically distinct polypeptide chains—one A chain of about 400 kDa and two smaller B chains of about 200 kDa each. Following a recently introduced systematic nomenclature, these polypeptides will be designated B1e, B2e, and Ae (15).

Rotary shadowing electron microscopy revealed a cruciform structure with three short arms and one long arm. Two of the short arms have the same length of 34 nm and contain a central and a terminal globule separated by rodlike domains, whereas the third short arm is considerably longer (48 nm) and exhibits an additional globular domain. The long arm has a length of 77 nm and forms a flexible rod with a large terminal globular domain (1,2).

The constituent Ae, B1e, and B2e chains have been sequenced from mouse (16–19), human (20–23), and *Drosophila* (8,24–28). The sequence data, together with biochemical and biophysical data of EHS-laminin and protein sequencing of proteolytic fragments, allowed the construction of the molecular model shown in Fig. 1. (For details, see Refs. 1 and 2).

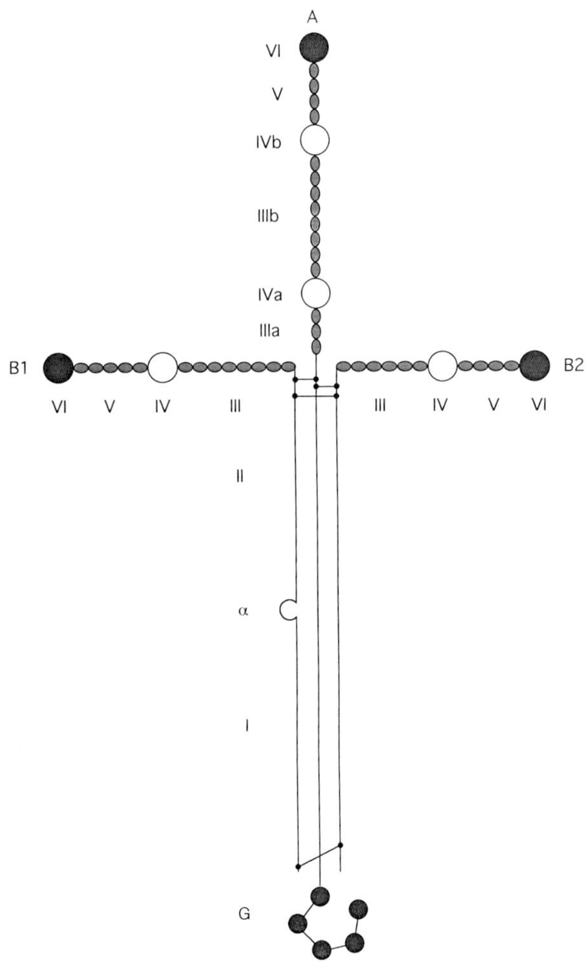

Figure 1 Structural model of laminin. The cruciform structure is formed by three polypeptide chains of the type A, B1, and B2. The N termini of the chains are at the distal ends of the short arms; the C termini are at the end of domain I (B chains) and domain G (A chain). Domains I and II are α-helical and interrupted in the B1 chain by a short domain α. Domains III and V are formed by numerous EGF-like repeats, the number of which is different in the three chains. Domains IV and VI form globular structures; domain G consists of five homologous repeats. The B chains are linked by an established disulfide bond in domain I and by further not yet localized bonds at the center of the cross.

In summary, the C-terminal ends of all three chains are located at the distal end of the long arm. The chains run in parallel orientation through the long arm and diverge at the center of the cross. The B chains and the N-terminal two-thirds of the A chain are homologous to each other. Domains I and II of the long arm are α-helical and show numerous heptad repeats in their amino acid sequence, typical for coiled coil α-helices. In laminin, the three chains probably form a triple-coiled coil α-helix in the stalk of the long arm. Domains I and II of the B1e chain are interrupted by a short, cysteine-rich domain α, which is lacking in the other two chains. The short-arm domains II and IV are formed by a great number of short cysteine-rich repeats about 40 to 50 amino acids in length which show homology to epidermal growth factor (EGF). These EGF-like repeats have been observed in a number of different proteins and have been suggested to be signals for cellular growth and differentiation (29,30). The inner globular domains IVa and IVb of the Ae chain and domain IV of the B2e chain are homologous to each other as well as the three N-terminal domains VI. A distinct feature of the Ae chain is the C-terminal domain G, which forms the terminal globular domain of the long arm of EHS laminin. This domain, which is missing in the B chains, contains five internal homologous repeats (G1 to G5), each consisting of about 200 residues. They exhibit homology with a sex hormone–binding globulin and the *Drosophila* gene product "crumbs" (31). From the latter homology, a role in epithelial polarization was speculated about (32).

EHS laminin contains 74 potential glycosylation sites. They are concentrated in the long arm and more than half of these are located in the Ae chain. Two studies reported a 12–15% glycosylation (33,34), but after fractionation by lectin affinity chromatography, molecules containing up to 25–30% carbohydrates were obtained (35,36). Most of the carbohydrates analyzed are complex-type asparagine-linked oligosaccharides encompassing many different structures (33–35). Carbohydrates have been implicated in a variety of cellular interactions (37), some of which are addressed below, under "Functions of Laminin."

Laminin Isoforms

Early indications for the existence of laminin isoforms came from immunochemical and biochemical investigations of laminin isolated from human placenta either as pepsin fragments or in intact form; furthermore, monoclonal antibodies revealed antigenic differences between laminins isolated from tumor cells and normal tissues (5). During mouse embryogenesis, the B chains were detected at the 2- to 4-cell stage, but the Ae chain was not found until the 16-cell stage (6). The mRNAs for the laminin chains were expressed in a disproportionate manner in many organs and cells (38–42); in particular, expression of the Ae chain was generally very low (22,39–42). The existence of isoforms was evident when structural data became available. In the meantime, more than ten novel laminin chains have been described, and the majority of them have already been cloned. In the past, various isoforms were designated in a nonsystematic manner, which caused some confusion even among insiders. Sometimes the same name refers to a particular chain or to the complete laminin molecule. A listing of recommended names for the polypeptide chains (according to Ref. 15) is given in Table 1; included also is a new nomenclature based on Greek letters followed by arabic numerals, which will probably be introduced in the near future (15a). Assembly of the chains to functional laminin molecules is discussed in the next chapter (see Fig. 2).

The first variant that had been sequenced was the B1s chain (s-laminin), which is highly homologous to the B1e chain (43,44). This laminin subunit is concentrated at synaptic sites in muscle, but it is also abundant in some nonmuscle basement membranes, such as perineurial basement membranes.

The best-known laminin isoform is the Am chain (merosin). Merosin was initially identified as an 80-kDa protein from human placenta (45), but subsequent studies showed that it is a carboxyterminal fragment of an A-chain variant (46). The complete sequence of the human Am chain was finished in 1994 and the gene was localized to 6q22→23 (47). It has the same domain structure as the Ae chain, and the sequences are 47% identical. The Am chain undergoes proteolytic cleavage yielding a 300-kDa chain, which remains bound to the B chains, and an 80-kDa fragment, which remains noncovalently associated (45,46). Human merosin heavy chain is most probably identical to the mouse heart laminin recently described (48). Antibodies against the Am chain typically stain the basement membranes of striated muscle, trophoblasts, and Schwann cells.

Two laminin isoforms have been characterized in skin epithelial basement membranes. One

Table 1 Nomenclature of Laminin Subunits

Ae	(α1):	A chain of EHS laminin
Am	(α2):	Merosin, M chain (A chain variant of muscle laminin)
At	(α3):	Truncated A-chain variant of kalinin (and K laminin ?)
Ble	(β1):	B1 chain of EHS laminin
Bls	(β2):	s Laminin, B1 chain variant (synapse, glomerulus)
Blt	(β3):	Truncated B1 chain variant of kalinin
B2e	(γ1):	B2 chain of EHS laminin
B2t	(γ2):	Truncated B2-chain variant of kalinin

Source: From Refs. 15 and 15a.

variant, kalinin, was shown to be a component of basement membranes from stratified epithelia (49). Immunoelectron microscopy localized it to the anchoring filaments of the skin. Kalinin is very similar or even identical to the proteins BM600/nicein (50,51) or epiligrin (52), discovered in other laboratories. In cultures of keratinocytes, kalinin is synthesized and secreted as a high-molecular-weight precursor formed by disulfide-bonded peptides with molecular weights of 200, 155, and 140 kDa, respectively. The molecule is then processed to its final tissue form by cleavage of the 200- and 155-kDa peptides to the mature 165- and 105-kDa chains (53). The molecule has a rod-like structure terminating in globular regions, indicating that the short arms are almost completely missing. Therefore all three chains must be different from EHS laminin; they are named At-B1t-B2t (t = truncated). The human B2t chain was sequenced recently; it lacks the globular domain VI (54). Another laminin variant in the dermal-epidermal basement membrane was termed K laminin (55). This Y-shaped variant contains normal B1e and B2e chains but a novel 190-kDa isoform of the A chain, which is at least closely related to the 200/165-kDa At chain of kalinin. The occurrence of

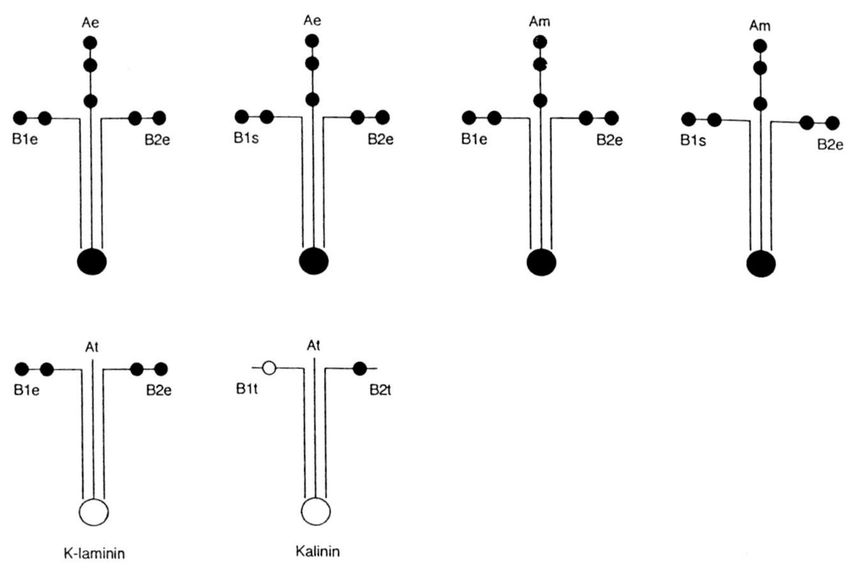

Figure 2 Schematic representation of six laminin variants. The isoforms containing Ae and Am chains have been identified in tissue; for kalinin and K laminin putative models are shown, since At and B1t chains have not yet been sequenced.

kalinin and K laminin is not restricted to skin; it has been observed in some other epithelial basement membranes as well.

Laminin variants containing smaller A-chain variants have been described from cultured 3T3 cells (56), from bovine aorta endothelial cells (57), and from RN22 schwannoma cells (58,59). The relationship of these A-chain variants to each other and to the At chain of kalinin is not known.

Recently two novel A-chain variants with the size of the normal Ae chains have been observed. One of these chains has been isolated from bovine kidneys and mainly identified on the basis of immunological differences from the Ae chain (60). The other 400-kDa chain variant is produced by several normal and transformed endothelial cells (Sorokin L., Girg W., Goepfert T., Deutzmann R.; unpublished results). Even though this novel A chain has a molecular weight of 400 kDa, it is not immunoprecipitated or detected in immunoblots by monoclonal antibodies raised against the Ae chain; furthermore it was not detected by polymerase chain reaction (PCR) techniques and by Northern blotting using various cDNA clones and specific oligonucleotides from the tumor A chain. The relation of this A chain to the kidney isoform (60) is not yet known. Interestingly, additional expression of the short A chain reported in Ref. 57 was also observed in most of the endothelial cells investigated, so that endothelial cells are obviously capable of synthesizing several laminin isoforms. Using sensitive PCR methods, even low levels of the Ae chain were detected in primary endothelial cells from bovine aorta but not in other endothelial cells (Deutzmann et al.; unpublished results).

Clones encoding a B1-chain–like peptide were recently isolated from an eye library (61), but the sequence has not yet been completed.

LAMININ GENE EXPRESSION AND CHAIN ASSEMBLY

Laminin gene expression is regulated spatially and temporally during embryonic development. The earliest models were F9 teratocarcinoma cells which, after treatment with retinoic acid, developed into endoderm-like cells accompanied by increased production of laminin and other basement proteins (62–64). The steady-state levels of the RNAs for the Ae, B1e, and B2e chains increased in a coordinate manner (39,65). Uncoordinated expression of laminin chains in other systems is presumably due to the existence of isoforms (38–42). Studies on the promotor regions will allow the regulatory mechanisms to be analyzed more precisely.

The gene structures of human laminin B1e and B2e chains (66,67) and *Drosophila* A, B1, and B2 chains (27,68,69) have been determined. The genes for the mouse B chains have been characterized (70), and sequence data from their 5′-flanking regions have been reported (71–73).

The human B1e gene has a length of 90 kb and contains 34 exons (66); the gene for the human B2e chain spans 58 kb and comprises 28 exons (67). The two genes were shown to be located on chromosomes 7 and 1, respectively. Even though the laminin B1e and B2e chains are very similar in structure, with highly conserved patterns of domains, the exon-intron structures are remarkably different; only three introns are in the same locations on the two genes. It is noteworthy that in general the exon-intron structure does not correlate with the domain structures.

The 5′-flanking regions of the B chains have been analyzed in some detail (66,67,71–73; see Ref. 70 for review). One feature is the absence of TATA and CAAT boxes in the promoter regions of both human and murine B1e and B2e chain genes. Lack of TATA boxes is common for most housekeeping genes. Both human and murine B1e and B2e chains contain several GC boxes and one (mouse B1 and B2) or more AP2 sites. In addition, both B1e-chain genes contain a retinoic acid response element (RARE), and a glucocorticoid response element–like sequence has been observed in the gene for the human B1e chain. The mouse B2e-chain gene contains nine nearly identical repeats of eleven nucleotides and a cAMP response–like sequence (71). Computer analysis revealed four highly homologous sequences of 14 to 42 bp between the human and mouse B2e-chain genes (67), which might therefore be important for the regulation of the B2 chain expression.

First attempts have been made to analyze the regulation of promoter activity. Best studied is induction of mouse laminin B1e gene transcription by retinoic acid. When transfected into F9 cells, B1e chain promoter–CAT constructs were inefficient in activating transcription, even after treatment with retinoic acid, but cotransfection with vectors expressing either h-retinoic acid receptors (RARs)-α, $-\beta$, or $-\gamma$ induced transcription (72). Mutation/deletion analysis identified the region from

–471 to –432 of the B1e-chain gene as important for promoter activity. Three stereo-aligned TGACC-like motifs were found to be crucial for binding of the RARs (73). A strong correlation was obtained between retinoic acid inducibility in vivo and efficiency of RAR binding in vitro, but RARs bound to the retinoic acid–responsive element of the laminin B1e chain gene with much weaker affinity than to that of the RAR-β gene. These results demonstrated that the retinoic acid induction of the laminin B1e gene is mediated by direct binding of RARs to the LamB1 promoter. Yet transcription starts only 24 hr after addition of retinoic acid and is cyclohexamide-sensitive. This might be due to the weakness of binding or might reflect additional regulation by retinoic acid–dependent processes and/or retinoic acid–inducible factors (73).

The promoter of the mouse B2e-chain gene was found to be considerably more active than the promoter of the mouse B1e-chain gene (70). Deletion analysis showed that a fragment of –94 to +106 was sufficient for promoter activity. Footprint analysis revealed that several sequence motifs between –94 and –30 interact with nuclear factors from astrocytes. Interestingly, in astrocytes which do not express B1e chains, B1e-chain promoter CAT constructs had very little activity.

The processing and assembly of the laminin Ae, B1e, and B2e chains to a ternary complex has been the subject of several biosynthetic studies (74–76). The chains are glycosylated with N-linked high-mannose oligosaccharides and are further processed in the Golgi apparatus before secretion; the combination of the subunits occurs before trimming of the subunits; glycosylation is not necessary for subunit assembly (75,76). Disulfide-linked B1e-B2e chain dimers were reported as intermediates in laminin biosynthesis, and addition of the Ae chain was considered as the rate-limiting step (75,76), even though, in another study, initial random association of the polypeptide chains was suggested (77).

Since a number of novel laminin chains have been identified, which chains can combine with each other is an important question. Recent studies on the reassociation of separated chains and theoretical calculations that included the Ae, Am, B1e, B1s, and B2e chains predict that none of the laminin chains appears to be designed for the formation of homodimers (78,79). Probably the chains can be divided into three groups defined by the Ae, B1e, and B2e chains. For assembly of a heterotrimeric molecule, one member of each group should be required, but assembly from two members of the same group and one member of another is unfavorable. For example, combination of two Ae chains, one Ae with one Am chain, or B1e with B1s should not occur. This problem was experimentally approached in studies using monoclonal antibodies against the Ae, Am, B1e, B1s, and B2 chains: immunfluorescence of tissue sections detected no more than one chain of each group in the same region of a basement membrane, and in large pepsin fragments of laminins from placenta the Ae and Am chains as well as the B1e and B1s peptides were never found in the same molecule (80). Similarly, using subunit-specific antibodies, it was shown for muscle and glia-like cell lines that B1s is complexed with A and B2 but not with B1 (81). A summary of various laminin isoforms is shown in Fig. 2. Up to now, nothing is known on the existence of heterodimeric molecules, even though they could exist theoretically (78).

FUNCTIONS OF LAMININ

Self-Assembly and Interaction with Other Basement Membrane Proteins

In the last few years, considerable progress was made in understanding the supramolecular architecture of basement membranes from its constituent molecules such as type IV collagen and laminin (for review, see Refs. 82 and 83). It is well established that type IV collagen forms a highly cross-linked network to which other basement membrane proteins are bound. But surprisingly, laminin is also able to form a major network polymer that is largely independent and freestanding (84). In fact, two intermeshed networks exist. Laminin polymerizes in a concentration- and temperature-dependent manner (85). This process is divalent-cation (especially calcium)–dependent (86). Laminin self-assembly is mainly mediated by interactions of the terminal globules of the short arms (87), even though long-arm interactions could contribute to supramolecular organization. Almost the same polymer observed in the collagen-rich basement membranes of the EHS tumor has been identified in collagen-free basement membranes of embryonic carcinoma cells (84).

Many basement membranes contain isoforms of laminin. Very little is known about their potential to aggregate. Yet the ability to isolate merosin using chelating agents indicates a Ca-dependent aggregation for this isoform too. In general, one might expect those laminins with a structure similar to that of EHS laminin to polymerize, whereas isoforms like kalinin would be unlikely to polymerize if not complexed to other molecules.

The best-characterized interaction of laminin with other basement membrane molecules is the binding of nidogen/entactin (88). Laminin and nidogen form a stable 1:1 complex, which can be extracted under nondenaturing conditions from mouse EHS tumor (14). The binding site on laminin has recently been mapped to a single EGF-repeat in domain III of the B2 chain (89). Therefore all laminin variants having the B2 chain should be able to bind nidogen. Nidogen has been demonstrated to bind to type IV collagen and has been proposed to mediate binding of laminin to the collagen network (90). Direct interaction of laminin with type IV collagen has also been reported (91,92).

Laminin and the laminin-nidogen complex additionally have the potential to cross-link by transglutamination to other proteins (93,94), thus stabilizing interactions by forming covalent bonds.

In addition, laminin has binding potential for heparin and heparan sulfate proteoglycan. Even though interactions with short-arm structures might exist (83,95–97), the major binding site is certainly located at the end of the long arm (83,98,99). Heparin was able to alter laminin polymerization, which could be important in the deposition and dissociation of basement membranes (83). When isolated from cell culture media, laminin was often found to be complexed to proteoglycans, and the stability of the complex against high salt concentrations indicated that protein-protein interactions should also be possible in addition to protein–heparan sulfate binding (5).

Cellular Interactions

The major functions of laminin involve its ability to interact with cells and to modulate cell behavior. These functions include cell adhesion, spreading, migration, differentiation, and stimulation of neurite outgrowth. Far more than a hundred articles have been published on the biological role of laminin; it is impossible to cover all aspects in this short survey. The reader is referred to several recent reviews (1–5). Effects on nerve cells are summarized in Refs. 100 and 101; the role of laminin and other extracellular matrix proteins in cell migration and invasion is discussed in Ref. 102.

Most of the studies on cellular interactions of laminin have been carried out in in vitro cell and organ culture systems using EHS laminin and its fragments, which is often not the natural substrate. Therefore the relevance for the in vivo situation must be carefully considered. Nevertheless, these investigations have certainly been very successful in elucidating the fundamental molecular interaction mechanisms.

Since laminin is a huge multidomain molecule, it has been of interest to assign the various functions to individual domains and to establish which cellular receptors are involved. Two major approaches were based on proteolytic fragments and synthetic peptides, respectively. Synthetic peptides designed according to distinct sequence regions certainly have the advantage of permitting an accurate localization of binding sites. Mapping of the RGDS sequence is the most famous example (103). However, in the absence of a definite approach, it is necessary to use as many techniques as possible to validate the identification of an adhesive sequence. Stringent criteria that should be fulfilled have recently been evaluated (103,104). A summary of various laminin peptides reported to be biologically active is given in Refs. 2 and 103.

Functional studies with fragments are limited in their ability to map exact binding sequences, but they certainly have the advantage that the proteolytic fragments are usually in their native conformation and correctly glycosylated. With this approach, it has been possible to unambigously identify two major cell-binding regions in EHS laminin: one of these is located at the center of the cross, the other one at the end of the long arm (see Fig. 3). Initial studies revealed that the proteolytic fragment 1, comprising central short-arm structures, acts as an effective substrate for cell adhesion and is able to bind to cells and to displace laminin from its cellular receptors (3,4); additionally, fragment 1 has been shown to decrease the metastatic potential of tumor cells (105). Recent studies (106–108) demonstrated that many cells can bind to the center of the cross only after proteolytic activation: they did not bind to fragments containing intact short arms (E1-4, E1x) but did bind to fragment P1 obtained by drastic pepsin cleavage (see Ref. 2 for a detailed description of the fragments

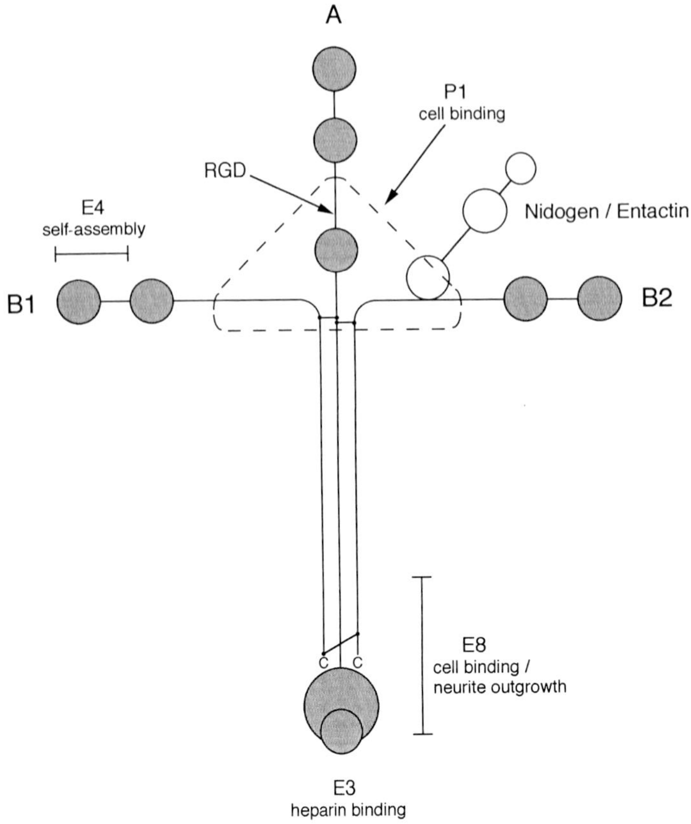

Figure 3 Schematic representation of laminin structure and localization of some important biologically active fragments and binding sites. Nidogen binds to an EGF repeat of the B2 chain, RGD denotes the localization of the RGD (Arg-Gly-Asp) cell-binding sequence.

and their nomenclature). Binding could be inhibited with rather low concentrations of RGD-containing peptides, in agreement with the occurrence of a single RGD sequence in that region of the Ae chain (108). This site seems to be cryptic and might be activated during tissue remodeling and tumor invasion. It is noteworthy that this RGD sequence is not conserved in the human Ae chain, so it remains to be seen whether similar adhesion mechanisms will work in the human system as well. In contrast, some other cells were found to bind in an RGD-independent manner to fragment E1-X, and the binding activity was stable over a wide temperature range (109,110). These results indicate that at least two different recognition mechanisms exist for the central part of the molecule.

Two cell-binding sites have been postulated in studies using synthetic peptides (96,111,112). One of these, containing the sequence YIGSR, was active in mediating cell adhesion, chemotaxis, and receptor binding (111); it also inhibited formation of tumor metastases (112). This is in contrast to findings that recombinant B1 chain, containing this sequence, did not stimulate cell binding (113) and that the peptide did not inhibit cell binding to fragment P1 (108).

In addition to stimulating cell adhesion, regions in the center of the cross seem to possess growth-promoting activity (114,115). Fragment P1 had a mitogenic effect which, in dose response and time dependence, was similar to that of EGF, even though it did not compete with EGF for binding to the EGF receptor (115). It is tempting to speculate that this function is mediated by one of the numerous EGF repeats in fragment P1, since growth-promoting activities had been observed with a large number of proteins carrying such EGF-like domains (29,30).

The major cell-binding site of laminin is obviously located at the end of the long arm and has been mapped to a proteolytic fragment E8 (106,107,109); see Fig. 3. Fragment E8 competitively inhibits the high-affinity binding of laminin to cells, and antibodies against fragment E8 block neurite growth, cell adhesion, and spreading on laminin substrates. In addition, fragment E8 stimulates neurite outgrowth (116), promotes cell locomotion (117), and is involved in establishing epithelial cell polarity (see below). Fragment E8 was shown to comprise domains G1 to G3 and the adjacent part of a rod-like domain (118). The missing domains G4 and G5 of the large terminal globule of the A chain are lost in the production of fragment E8 by limited proteolysis and can be recovered as the well-known heparin binding fragment E3, which has cell-binding activity only for a very limited number of cells (119,120). The various effects of fragment E8 depend on native structure; denaturation or separation of the chains under native conditions abolished its biological activity (121). In attempts to narrow down the binding sites, at least eight different peptides from various regions have been suggested to be active (2,122,123), including the sequence IKVAV from just above the carboxyl globule of the A chain (124), which was also claimed to be active for cell growth and for inducing c-*fos* and c-*jun* expression and DNA binding activity (125). On the other hand, strong support for the findings from proteolytic fragments that a native structure formed by all three polypeptide chains is essential for biological activity (121) has recently been provided by a study using hybrids of recombinant Ae-chain peptides and the corresponding B-chain peptides from fragment E8 (126). Further studies are certainly needed to establish precisely which regions are relevant for the in vivo effects.

At present only very limited information is available on the biological activities of laminin isoforms. Merosin has been reported to stimulate cell adhesion and neurite outgrowth in a manner similar to that of EHS laminin (127), and epiligrin/kalinin has been shown to support cell adhesion with different receptors involved (52). This indicates that some isoforms can have similar biological activities, at least in in vitro assays, but subtle differences might exist that could elicit distinct in vivo effects.

Identification of the cellular receptors that recognize the various sites on laminin is of key importance in understanding the cellular activities (reviewed in Ref. 128). Receptors of the integrin family (129) certainly play a major role. At least six members have been reported to interact with laminin: $\alpha1\beta1$, $\alpha2\beta1$, $\alpha3\beta1$, $\alpha6\beta1$, $\alpha7\beta1$, $\alpha v\beta3$ (128). The binding sites on laminin are in many cases not known, and some integrins bind more than one ligand. The most specific integrin receptor seems to be $\alpha6\beta1$; fragment E8 is the only ligand known today (119,130,131). This interaction has been well documented. Its implications for kidney development are discussed below. In some cells like myoblasts, $\alpha6$ is replaced by $\alpha7$ ($=\alpha'$), with the same binding specificity for fragment E8 (132,133). Another integrin capable of binding to the long arm of human laminin seems to be $\alpha3\beta1$. The nature of integrins binding to the cell adhesion site located at the center of the cross is more controversial. Binding to the cryptic site is probably mediated by $\beta3$ integrins such as the vitronectin receptor (108,119), whereas an RGDS-independent site in fragment E1-X might be recognized by $\alpha1\beta1$ (110, 130).

Apart from integrins, a variety of other receptors have been reported to bind to laminin. The longest known and still the most controversial receptor is the 67-kDa laminin receptor, which might be identical to a 67-kDa elastin/laminin receptor (see Ref. 128 for review). This receptor was considered to be crucial for laminin binding and tumor metastasis (for recent reports, see Refs. 134 and 135). Interestingly, full-length clones for this receptor encoded a 33-kDa protein (not a 67-kDa protein) lacking a signal peptide and a transmembrane domain. Recently this 33-kDa protein has been reported to be part of the translation machinery (136). A variety of other proteins with molecular weights between 30 and about 110-kDa have been described (128) but not yet thoroughly characterized. Recently the structure of dystroglycan has been determined (137); it is a transmembrane protein that links dystrophin, the product of the Duchenne muscular dystrophy gene, to the extracellular matrix. It has been shown to bind to laminin. Dystroglycan is not homologous to integrin subunits and may be a proteoglycan.

In addition to protein-protein interactions, sugar residues can also serve as recognition sites in cell binding to laminin. Since EHS laminin is highly glycosylated, it is not surprising that some lectins have been found to bind to laminin (37,128). A role of laminin carbohydrates in cell matrix interaction is also evident from the observation that unglycosylated laminin did not induce cell spreading and that glycosylation influenced interaction of laminin with an $\alpha6$ integrin subunit (37).

Another class of cell surface molecules that can act as receptor for poly-N-acetyllactosamin glycoconjugate on laminin are cell surface glycosyltransferases (see Ref. 138 and references therein).

These proteins were implicated in cell-cell adhesion, cell migration, and neurite outgrowth. A carbohydrate structure, identified as 3′-sulfoglucuronic acid attached to a lactosamin core, has been found to be important in the adhesion of neuronal cells (139,140). Whether this mechanism is operative in nonneural cells as well is not yet known.

More work will be required to elucidate the relative importance of these nonintegrin receptors and carbohydrates and how they act in concert with integrin receptors in signal transduction.

LAMININ IN ADULT KIDNEY

Laminin is a major component of all renal basement membranes; however, numerous immunohistochemical studies were in some disagreement on their ultrastructural localization. Some immunoelectron microscopic investigations indicated the presence of laminin in the lamina rara, others showed a distribution throughout the lamina rara and lamina densa (141–144). But now there is general agreement that laminin is distributed throughout all layers. The different results can probably be explained by differences in experimental methods and antibodies used. Since laminin forms a complicated network within the basement membrane (83) on the one side and interacts with cells on the other side, epitopes should be present in all layers. But molecular orientation in the meshwork might differ at various locations. As shown originally for cornea (145), short arms involved in aggregation can be concentrated in the central layers, with the long arms oriented to the surface and thus available for cellular interactions. In kidney, a monoclonal antibody directed against the long arm of EHS laminin stained the lamina rara of Bowman's capsule; whereas in distal tubules, both the lamina rara and densa were heavily labeled (146). The glomerular basement membrane is formed by fusion of epithelial and endothelial basement membranes. Molecular mechanisms are unclear, but basement membrane parts synthesized by one cell are apparently spliced into previously formed basement membrane (142). This would result in a very complicated distribution of laminin and its variants.

The cells lining the continuous basement membrane along the nephron have different functions in urine production and homeostasis of the internal milieu. Therefore differences in composition and/or organization of the underlying basement membrane should be expected if they are actively involved in the regulation of these processes. In agreement with this idea, different proportions of laminin, other noncollagenous proteins, and collagen Type IV have been observed (143,147–150), and investigations with monoclonal antibodies clearly showed heterogeneity of laminin distribution in kidney (146,151–155). In one of the first studies, a monoclonal antibody raised against light chains of laminin isolated from a mouse parietal yolk sac cell line recognized all tubular and glomerular basement membranes but not those of blood vessels or smooth muscle, whereas a second one stained predominantly the basement membrane of the convoluted portion of proximal tubule segments and the thin and thick ascending limb of Henle's loop (151).

Those studies could not strictly distinguish between the different accessibility/location of epitopes and compositional heterogeneity with respect to various laminin chains. This question was addressed systematically in recent work. The most surprising result was that laminin, containing the classic Ae chain, has a very restricted distribution in adult kidney. Specific polyclonal antibodies against the E3 fragment comprising the carboxyterminal 400 amino acids of the Ae chain (118) stained proximal tubules only; all other epithelial and endothelial basement membranes were negative. Moreover, the Ae chain was not detected by immunoblotting and immunoprecipitation (156,157). This is in marked contrast to the abundant staining of epithelial basement membranes in embryonic mouse kidneys (see below). Restricted expression of the Ae chain is further indicated by finding low mRNA levels for the Ae chain in comparison to the B chains (39,40,157). These results suggest that the Ae chain is replaced by other isoforms, the identity of which remains to be established. Possible candidates could be the recently described 400-kDa chain from kidney and the long and short A chains from endothelial cells (see "Laminin Isoforms," above). Even though evidence for the lack of laminins with a classic A chain is quite convincing, in one study a mAb (4C7) for the human Ae chain stained both glomerular and tubular basement membranes even though staining was fainter than that of blood vessels (158). The discrepancy is not yet clear. A possible explanation would be that this antibody recognizes a novel A chain.

In contrast to the Ae chain, the B2e chain has a broad distribution and could be localized within glomerular and tubular basement membranes. Antibodies to laminin B1 stained tubular but not glomerular basement membranes, whereas antibodies to s laminin stained glomerular basement membranes far more intensely than tubular basement membranes (43,158). This is consistent with the idea that B1 and s laminin are mutually exclusive. Recently it has been shown that the truncated B2t chain is expressed by epithelial cells in collecting tubules (54). It should be expected, therefore, that other constituent chains of kalinin will be found as well.

LAMININ IN KIDNEY DEVELOPMENT

Basement membranes are of fundamental importance in the development of epithelia (7,159,160), and the roles played by the individual components is the topic of many investigations. In kidney, only the role of laminin in the formation of tubular epithelium from mesenchyme has been studied in detail.

Differentiation starts with an interaction between the ureter bud and the nephrogenic mesenchyme. (161,162). The mesenchyme stimulates ingrowth and branching of the ureter to form the collecting ducts. In turn, signals from the ureter induce differentiation of mesenchymal cells to interstitium and tubular epithelium. This conversion is also observed in vitro in transfilter culture systems (163). Metanephric mesenchyme from mouse embryos is dissected free of the uretric bud and cultered on top of a filter. Inducer tissue is placed on the other side and cocultured for a certain period of time. In these assays, the ureter can be replaced by a variety of other epithelial tissues such as spinal cord. Even though inducing and responding tissues remain separated, morphological differentiation into epithelium starts at day 2 and clearly polarized cells can be observed on day 3.

Expression of the A and B chains of laminin has been studied extensively in both in vivo and in vitro development using organ culture and transfilter assays. In the kidney mesenchyme induced for 24 hr, the B1e and B2e chains were detected by immunofluorescence and by Western and Northern blotting, but only trace amounts of Ae-chain message were found (156,157). With the onset of epithelial development, Ae-chain mRNA levels increased dramatically. In situ hybridization revealed that the Ae chain was locally expressed in those areas where new tubules formed (157). Tubule formation could be inhibited with polyclonal antibodies against fragments E8 and E3 (156) and partially with monoclonal antibodies against E3 (164). Antibodies against short-arm structures had no effect. The start of laminin Ae chain expression with the onset of tubular differentiation was also observed in another study, using chimeric kidneys, between mouse and chicken and mouse-specific antibodies (165).

These results demonstrate that a laminin variant, containing the classic A chain, is important for the development of the kidney epithelia and that the terminal part of the long arm of the molecule is involved in these processes. That is, the same region is implicated that had already been shown to contain the major cell-binding- and neurite-outgrowth-promoting sites, which had both been mapped to fragment E8. Consistent with these findings, the integrin $\alpha6$ subunit, identified as a specific receptor for fragment E8, colocalized with the Ae chain and appeared at the same time in the developing kidney, and a monoclonal antibody directed against the $\alpha6$ subunit significantly interfered with kidney tubulogenesis (166). Taken together, these results clearly indicate that interaction of fragment E8 with an $\alpha6$ integrin, probably $\alpha6\beta1$, plays a major role in tubule development.

It is tempting to speculate that after establishing epithelial polarity, the Ae chain is no longer needed and is largely replaced by other isoforms more suited to fulfill the requirements of adult epithelial cells. Loss of laminin epitopes during glomerular basement assembly in developing mouse kidneys was also reported in another study, but the laminin chain involved was not further identified (167).

Tubulogenesis involves conversion of mesenchymal cells to epithelial cells, whereas the principal mode of epithelial cell development is branching morphogenesis, and the roles of laminin in these processes might be different. The Ae chain of laminin, even though it is not widely expressed by cells of adult kidney epithelium, has been observed in the embryonic basement membranes of cells of the ureter lineage, indicating a possible role in development. Information on how this isoform influences cell differentiation is still lacking, but the mechanism might be similar to that working in other branching epithelia such as lung. Polyclonal antibodies against laminin inhibited murine lung morphogenesis when added to organ cultures of embryonic lung (168). When a series of monoclonal antibodies were tested, two antibodies inhibited branching activity, which bound near the center of the cross and at the globular end regions of the B chains in the short arms, respectively. Antibodies against long-arm structures did not alter lung morphogenesis (169). This would indicate a crucial role for the center of the cross, containing the second cell-binding site and potentially mitogenic regions (see "Cellular Interactions," above). During intestinal development, laminin A chain was present in the basement membrane underlying embryonic or crypt epithelial cells, which might indicate a role in establishment of cell polarity or in cell growth (170). The domains involved are not known.

By immunofluorescence, the endothelial basement membranes were shown to lack the Ae chain at all developmental stages in mouse kidney and also in other organs (164,171); only basement membranes of large vessels and heart could be stained (171). Therefore final elucidation of the role of laminins in the modulation of endothelial cell behavior will not be possible until specific probes for the isoforms involved are available. Some in vitro investigations have already been performed using laminin from EHS tumors. Endothelial cells are capable of adhering to EHS laminin (172,173), the center of the cross being more effective for nontransformed cells (172). More interestingly, laminin was reported to influence endothelial cell development. It mediated formation of tubelike structures (174,175), and several distinct sites involved in these processes were postulated from work with synthetic peptides (176). How this work fits with lack of Ae chain in endothelial basement membranes and the presence of other isoforms remains to be seen. It could be that endothelial laminins have biological activities similar to those of EHS laminin. It has also been suggested that the Ae chain might be only transiently expressed at the leading edge of growing capillaries, thus escaping detection by immunological methods (7). Angiostatic steroids were reported to stimulate the synthesis of the 400-kDa chain in preference over the short variant (57). Similar switches might occur in vivo.

CONCLUSIONS

Investigations of the last few years have collected conclusive evidence for the importance of extracellular matrix and especially laminin in tissue function and development, but we are far from a comprehensive understanding. One of the most important tasks in the near future will certainly be to identify and localize the laminin variants involved and their interactions with the respective receptors. This will be essential for understanding their roles, in cooperation with other extracellular matrix molecules, for normal kidney function and pathological disorders. At present this understanding is very limited (177). In this respect our knowledge on integrin receptors (178,179) and type IV collagen, the second major basement membrane protein, is much more advanced. The identification of new polypeptide chains has allowed us to investigate disorders like Goodpasture's syndrome and Alport's syndrome, discussed in another chapter of this book. It seems conceivable that absent or aberrant expression of laminin chains and altered receptor interactions might have severe consequences for kidney function. But at the moment that is rather speculative.

NOTE ADDED IN PROOF

The paper referred to in the text as "Sorokin L, Girg W, Goepfert T, Deutzmann R, unpublished results" has now been published (180).

REFERENCES

1. Engel J. Structure and function of laminin. In: Rohrbach DH, Timpl R, eds. Molecular and Cellular Aspects of Basement Membranes. Academic Press, 1993:147–176.
2. Beck K, Hunter I, Engel J. Structure and function of laminin: Anatomy of a multidomain glycoprotein. FASEB J 1990; 4:148–160.

3. Timpl R. Structure and biological activity of basement membrane proteins. Eur J Biochem 1989; 180:487–502.
4. Timpl R, Dziadek M. Structure, development, and molecular pathology of basement membranes. Int Rev Exp Pathol 1986; 29:1–112.
5. Paulsson M. Basement membrane proteins: Structure, assembly, and cellular interactions. Crit Rev Biochem Mol Biol 1992; 27:93–127.
6. Cooper AR, MacQueen HA. Subunits of laminin are differentially synthesized on mouse eggs and early embryos. Dev Biol 1983; 96:467–471.
7. Ekblom P. Basement membranes in development. In: Rohrbach DH, Timpl R, eds. Molecular and Cellular Aspects of Basement Membranes. Academic Press, 1993:359–383.
8. Henchcliffe C, Garcia-Alonso L, Tang J, Goodman CS. Genetic analysis of laminin A reveals diverse functions during morphogenesis in Drosophila. Development 1993; 118:325–337.
9. Tryggvason K. The laminin family. Curr Opin Cell Biol 1993; 5:877–882.
10. Paulsson M. Laminin and collagen IV variants and heterogeneity in basement membrane composition. In: Rohrbach DH, Timpl R, eds. Molecular and Cellular Aspects of Basement Membranes. Academic Press, 1993:177–187.
11. Engvall E. Laminin variants: Why, where and when? Kidney Int 1993; 43:2–6.
12. Timpl R, Rohde H, Gehron Robey P, et al. Laminin—A glycoprotein from basement membranes. J Biol Chem 1979; 254:9933–9937.
13. Chung AE, Jaffe R, Freeman IL, et al. Properties of a basement membrane related glycoprotein synthesized in culture by a mouse embryonal carcinoma-derived cell line. Cell 1979; 16:277–287.
14. Paulsson M, Aumailley M, Deutzmann R, et al. Laminin-nidogen complex: Extraction with chelating agents and structural characterization. Eur J Biochem 1987; 166:11–19.
15. Engel J, Hunter I, Schulthess T, et al. Assembly of laminin isoforms by triple and double stranded coiled-coil structures. Biochem Soc Trans 1991; 19:839–843.
15a. Burgeson RE, Chiquet M, Deutzmann R, et al. A new nomenclature for the laminins. Matrix Biol 1994; 14:209–211.
16. Sasaki M, Kato S, Kohno K, et al. Sequence of the cDNA encoding the laminin B1 chain reveals a multidomain protein containing cysteine-rich repeats. Proc Natl Acad Sci USA 1987; 84:935–939.
17. Sasaki M, Yamada Y. The laminin B2 chain has a multidomain structure homologous to the B1 chain. J Biol Chem 1987; 262:17111–17117.
18. Sasaki M, Kleinman HK, Huber H. Laminin, a multidomain protein: The A chain has a unique globular domain and homology with the basement membrane proteoglycan and the laminin B chains. J Biol Chem 1988; 263:16536–16544.
19. Durkin ME, Bartos BB, Liu SH. Primary structure of the mouse laminin B2 chain and comparison with laminin B1. Biochemistry 1988; 27:5198–5204.
20. Pikkarainen T, Eddy R, Fukushima Y, et al. Human laminin B1 chain. A multidomain protein with gene (LAMB1) locus in the q22 region of chromosome 7. J Biol Chem 1987; 262:10454–10462.
21. Pikkarainen T, Kallunki T, Tryggvason K. Human laminin B2 chain: Comparison of the complete amino acid sequence with the B1 chain reveals variability in sequence homology between different structural domains. J Biol Chem 1988; 263:6751–6758.
22. Nissinen M, Vuolteenaho R, Boot-Hanford R, et al. Primary structure of the human laminin A chain: Limited expression in human tissues. Biochem J 1991; 276:369–379.
23. Haaparanta T, Uitto J, Ruoshlahti E, Engvall E. Molecular cloning of the cDNA encoding human laminin A chain. Matrix 1991; 11:151–160.
24. Montell DJ, Goodman CS. Drosophila substrate adhesion molecule: Sequence of laminin B1 chain reveals domains of homology with mouse. Cell 1988; 53:463–473.
25. Chi HC, Hui CF. Primary structure of the Drosophila laminin B2 chain and comparison with human, mouse, and Drosophila laminin B1 and B2 chains. J Biol Chem 1989; 264:1543–1550.
26. Montell DJ, Goodman CS. Drosophila laminin: Sequence of B2 subunit and expression of all three subunits during embryogenesis, J Cell Biol 1989; 109:2441–2453.
27. Kusche-Gullberg M, Garrison K, MacKrell AJ, et al. Laminin A chain: Expression during Drosophila development and genomic sequence. EMBO J 1992; 11:4519–4527.
28. Mackrell AJ, Kusche-Gullberg M, Garrison K, Fessler JH. Novel Drosophila laminin A chain reveals structural relationships between laminin subunits. FASEB J 1993; 7:375–381.
29. Appella E, Weber IT, Blasi F. Structure and function of epidermal growth factor-like regions in proteins. FEBS Lett 1988; 231:1–4.
30. Engel J. EGF-like domains in extracellular matrix proteins: Localized signals for growth and differentiation? FEBS Lett 1989; 251:1–7.
31. Joseph DR, Baker ME. Sex hormone-binding globulin, androgen-binding protein, and vitamin K-dependent

protein S are homologous to laminin A, merosin and Drosophila crumbs protein. FASEB J 1992; 6:2477–2481.
32. Patthy L. Laminin A-related domains in crb protein of Drosophila and their possible role in epithelial polarization. FEBS Lett 1991; 289:99–101.
33. Arumugham RG, Hsieh TCY, Tanzer ML, Laine RA. Structures of the asparagine-linked sugar chains of laminin. Biochem Biophys Acta 1986; 883:112–126.
34. Fujiwara S, Shinkai H, Deutzmann R, et al. Structure and distribution of N-linked oligosaccharide chains on various domains of mouse tumor laminin. Biochem J 1988; 252:453–461.
35. Knibbs RN, Perini F, Goldstein IJ. Structure of the major concanavalin A reactive oligosaccharides of the extracellular matrix component laminin. Biochemistry 1989; 28:6379–6392.
36. Chandrasekaran S, Dean JW, Grininger MS, Tanzer ML. Laminin carbohydrates are implicated in cell signalling. J Cell Biochem 1991; 46:115–124.
37. Tanzer ML, Chandrasekaran S, Dean JW, Giniger MS. Role of laminin carbohydrates on cellular interactions. Kidney Int 1993; 43:66–72.
38. Boot-Handford RP, Kurkinen M, Prockop DJ. Steady state levels of MRNAs coding for the type IV collagen and laminin polypeptide chains of basement membranes exhibit marked tissue specific stoichiometric variations in the rat. J Biol Chem 1987; 262:12475–12478.
39. Kleinman HK, Ehihara I, Killen PD, et al. Genes for basement membrane proteins are coordinately expressed in differentiating F9 cells but not in normal adult murine tissues. Dev Biol 1987; 122:373–378.
40. Laurie GW, Horikoshi S, Killen PD, et al. In situ hybridization reveals temporal and spatial changes in cellular expression of mRNA for a laminin receptor, laminin, and basement membrane (type IV) collagen in the developing kidney. J Cell Biol 1989; 109:1351–1362.
41. Olsen D, Nagayoshi T, Fazio M, et al. Human laminin: Cloning and sequence analysis of cDNAs encoding A, B1 and B2 chains, and expression of the corresponding genes in human skin and cultured cells. Lab Invest 1989; 60:772–782.
42. Kücherer-Ehret A, Pottgiesser J, Kreutzberg GW, et al. Developmental loss of laminin from the interstitial extracellular matrix correlates with decreased laminin expression. Development 1990; 110:1285–1293.
43. Hunter DD, Shah V, Merlie JP, Sanes JR. A laminin-like adhesive protein concentrated in the synaptic cleft of the neuromuscular junction. Nature 1989; 338:229–234.
44. Porter, BE, Justice MJ, Copeland NG, et al. S-Laminin: Mapping to mouse chromosome 9 and expression in the linked mutants tippy and ducky. Genomics 1993; 16:278–281.
45. Leivo I, Engvall E. Merosin, a protein specific for basement membranes of Schwann cells, striated muscle, and trophoblast, is expressed late in nerve and muscle development. Proc Natl Acad Sci USA 1988; 5:1544–1548.
46. Ehrig K, Leivo I, Argraves WS, et al. Merosin, a tissue specific basement membrane protein, is a laminin-like protein. Proc Natl Acad Sci USA 1990; 87:3264–3268.
47. Vuolteenaho R, Nissinen M, Sainio K, et al. Complete primary structure, chromosomal assignment and expression of the M and A chains in human fetal tissues. J Cell Biol 1994; 124:381–394.
48. Paulsson M, Saladin K, Engvall E. Structure of laminin variants: The 300-kDa chains of murine and bovine heart laminin are related to the human placenta merosin heavy chain and replace the A chain in some laminin variants. J Biol Chem 1991; 266:17545–17551.
49. Rousselle P, Lunstrom GP, Keene DR, Burgeson RE. Kalinin: An epithelium-specific basement membrane adhesion molecule that is a component of anchoring filaments. J Cell Biol 1991; 114:567–576.
50. Verrando P, Hsi BL, Yeh CJ. Monoclonal antibody GB3, a new probe for the study of human basement membranes and hemidesmosomes. Exp Cell Res 1987; 170:116–128.
51. Marchisio PC, Cremona O, Savoia P, et al. The basement membrane protein BM-600/nicein codistributes with kalinin and the integrin $\alpha 6\beta 4$ in human cultures keratinocytes. Exp Cell Res 1993; 205:205–212.
52. Carter WG, Ryan MC, Gahr PJ. Epiligrin, a new cell adhesion ligand for integrin $\alpha 31\beta 1$ in epithelial basement membranes. Cell 1991; 65:599–610.
53. Marinkovich MP, Lunstrum GP, Burgeson RE. The anchoring filament protein kalinin is synthesized as a high molecular weight precursor. J Biol Chem 1992; 267:17900–17906.
54. Kallunki P, Sainio K, Eddy R, et al. A truncated laminin chain homologous to the B2 chain: Structure, spatial expression, and chromosomal assignment. J Cell Biol 1992; 119:679–693.
55. Marinkovich MP, Lunstrom GP, Keene DR, Burgeson RE. The dermal-epidermal junction of human skin contains a novel laminin variant. J Cell Biol 1992; 119:695–703.
56. Aratani Y, Kitagawa Y. Enhanced synthesis and secretion of type IV collagen and entactin during adipose conversion of 3T3-L1 cells and production of unorthodox laminin complex. J Biol Chem 1988; 263:16163–16169.
57. Tokida Y, Aratani Y, Morita A, Kitagawa Y. Production of two variant laminin forms by endothelial cells and shift of their relative levels by angiostatic steroids. J Biol Chem 1990; 265:18123–18129.

58. Davies GE, Manthorpe M, Engvall E, Varon S. Isolation and characterization of rat Schwannoma neurite-promoting factor: Evidence that the factor contains laminin. J Neurosci 1985; 5:2662–2671.
59. Edgar D, Timpl R, Thoenen H. Structural requirements for the stimulation of neurite outgrowth by two variants of laminin and their inhibition by antibodies. J Cell Biol 1988; 106:1299–1306.
60. Lindblom A, Engel J, Paulsson M. Characterization of native laminin from bovine kidney and comparison with other laminin variants. Eur J Biochem 1994; 219:383–392.
61. O'Rear J. A novel laminin B1 chain variant in avian eye. J Biol Chem 1992; 267:20555–205557.
62. Strickland S, Smith KK, Marotti KR. Hormonal induction of differentiation in teratocarcinoma stem cells: Generation of parietal endoderm by retinoic acid and dibutyryl cyclic AMP. Cell 1980; 21:347–355.
63. Carlin B, Durkin ME, Bender B, et al. Synthesis of laminin and entactin by F9 cells induced with retinoic acid and dibutyryl cyclic AMP. J Biol Chem 1983; 258:7729–7737.
64. Morita A, Kitagawa Y, Sugimota E. Reversible effects of dibutyryl cAMP on laminin and type IV collagen secretion from retinoic acid treated F9 cells. J Cell Physiol 1985; 125:263–272.
65. Durkin ME, Philips SL, Chung AE. Control of laminin synthesis during differentiation of F9 embryonal carcinoma cells: A study using cDNA clones complementary to the mRNA species for the A, B1 and B2 subunits. Differentiation 1986; 32:260–266.
66. Vuolteenaho R, Chow LT, Tryggvason K. Structure of the human laminin B1 chain gene. J Biol Chem 1990; 265:15611–15616.
67. Kallunki T, Ikonen J, Chow LT, et al. Structure of the human laminin B2 chain gene reveals extensive divergence from the B1 chain gene. J Biol Chem 1991; 266:221–228.
68. Chi HC, Juminaga D, Wang SY, Hui CF. Structure of Drosophila gene for thc laminin B2 chain. DNA Cell Biol 1991; 10:451–466.
69. Gow CH, Chang HY, Lih CJ, et al. Analysis of the Drosophila gene for the laminin B1 chain. DNA Cell Biol 1993; 12:573–587.
70. Yamada Y, Kühn K. Genes and regulation of basement membrane collagen and laminin synthesis. In: Rohrbach DH, Timpl R, eds. Molecular and Cellular Aspects of Basement Membranes. Academic Press, 1993:121–146.
71. Ogawa K, Burbelo PD, Sasaki M, Yamada Y. The laminin B2 chain promotor contains unique repeat sequences and is active in transient transfection. J Biol Chem 1988; 263:8384–8389.
72. Vasios GW, Gold JD, Petkovich M, et al. A retinoic acid-responsive element is present in the 5′-flanking region of the laminin B1 gene. Proc Natl Acad Sci USA 1989; 86:9099–9103.
73. Vasios GW, Mader S, Gold JD, et al. The late retinoic acid induction of laminin B1 gene transcription involve RAR binding to the responsive element. EMBO J 1991; 10:1149–1158.
74. Cooper AR, Kurkinen M, Taylor A, Hogan BLM. Studies on the biosynthesis of laminin by murine parietal endoderm cells. Eur J Biochem 1981; 119:189–197.
75. Morita A, Sugimoto E, Kitagawa Y. Post-translational assembly and glycosylation of laminin subunits in parietal endoderm-like F9 cells. Biochem J 1985; 229:259–264.
75a. Morita A, Kitagawa Y, Dugimoto E. Abnormal laminin secretion from parietal endoderm-like F9 cells in the presence of monensin. J Biochem 1985; 98:561–568.
76. Peters BP, Hartle RJ, Krzesicki F, et al. The biosynthesis, processing, and secretion of laminin by human choriocarcinoma cells. J Biol Chem 1985; 260:14732–14742.
77. Wu C, Friedman R, Chung AE. Analysis of the assembly of laminin and the laminin entactin complex with laminin chain specific monoclonal and polyclonal antibodies. Biochemistry 1988; 27:8780–8787.
78. Hunter I, Schulthess T, Engel J. Laminin chain assembly by triple and double stranded coiled-coil structures. J Biol Chem 1992; 267:6006–6011.
79. Beck K, Dixon TW, Engel J, Parry DAD. Ionic interactions in the coiled-coil domain of laminin determine the specificity of chain assembly. J Mol Biol 1993; 231:311–323.
80. Engvall E, Earwicker D, Haaparanta T, et al. Distribution and isolation of four laminin variants: Tissue restricted distribution of heterodimers assembled from five different subunits. Cell Reg 1990; 1:731–740.
81. Green TL, Hunter DD, Wing CH, et al. Synthesis and assembly of the synaptic cleft protein s-laminin by cultured cells. J Biol Chem 1992; 267:2014–2022.
82. Yurchenco PD, Schittny JC. Molecular architecture of basement membranes. FASEB J 1990; 4:1477–1590.
83. Yurchenco PD, O'Rear J. Supramolecular organization of basement membranes. In: Rohrbach DH, Timpl R, eds. Molecular and Cellular Aspects of Basement Membranes. Academic Press, 1993:20–47.
84. Yurchenco PD, Cheng YS, Colognato H. Laminin forms an independent network in basement membranes. J Cell Biol 1992; 117:1119–1133.
85. Yurchenco PD, Tsilibary EC, Charonis AS, Furthmayr H. Laminin polymerization in vitro: Evidence for a two step assembly with domain specificity. J Biol Chem 1985; 260:7636–7644.
86. Paulsson M. The role of Ca^{2+} binding in the self-aggregation of laminin-nidogen complexes. J Biol Chem 1988; 263:5424–5430.

87. Yurchenco PD, Cheng YS. Self-assembly and calcium-binding sites in laminin. J Biol Chem 1993; 268:17286–17299.
88. Timpl R, Aumailley M. Other basement membrane proteins and their calcium-binding potential. In: Rohrbach DH, Timpl R, eds. Molecular and Cellular Aspects of Basement Membranes. Academic Press, 1993:211–235.
89. Mayer U, Nischt R, Pöschl E, et al. A single EGF-like motif of laminin is responsible for high affinity nidogen binding. EMBO J 1993; 12:1879–1885.
90. Aumailley M, Battaglia C, Mayer U, et al. Nidogen mediates the formation of ternary complexes of basement membrane components. Kidney Int 1993; 43:7–12.
91. Charonis AS, Tsilibary EC, Yurchenco PD, Furthmayr H. Binding of laminin to type IV collagen: A morphological study. J Cell Biol 1985; 100:1848–1853.
92. Laurie GW, Bing JT, Kleinman HK, et al. Localization of binding sites for laminin, heparansulfate proteoglycan and fibronectin on basement membrane (type IV) collagen. J Mol Biol 1986; 189:205–216.
93. Aeschlimann D, Paulsson M. Cross-linking of laminin-nidogen complexes by tissue transglutaminase: A novel mechanism for basement membrane stabilization. J Biol Chem 1991; 266:15308–15317.
94. Usui T, Takagi J, Saito Y. Propolypeptide of von Willebrand factor serves as a substrate for factor XIIIa and is cross-linked to laminin. J Biol Chem 1993; 268:12311–12316.
95. Kousi-Koliakos K, Koliakos GG, Tsilibary EC, et al. Mapping of three major heparin-binding sites on laminin and identification of a novel heparin-binding site on the B1 chain. J Biol Chem 1989; 264:17971–17978.
96. Charonis AS, Skubitz APN, Koliakos GG, et al. A novel synthetic peptide from the B1 chain of laminin with heparin-binding and cell adhesion-promoting activities. J Cell Biol 1988; 107:1253–1260.
97. Skubitz APN, McCarthy JB, Charonis AS, Furcht LT. Localization of three distinct heparin-binding domains of laminin by monoclonal antibodies. J Biol Chem 1988; 263:4861–4868.
98. Ott U, Odermatt E, Engel J, et al. Protease resistance and conformation of laminin. Eur J Biochem 1982; 123:63–72.
99. Battaglia C, Mayer U, Aumailley M, Timpl R. Basement membrane heparan sulfate proteoglycan binds to laminin by its heparan sulfate chains and to nidogen by sites in the protein core. Eur J Biochem 1992; 208:359–366.
100. Venstrom KA, Reichardt LF. Extracellular matrix 2: Role of extracellular matrix molecules and their receptors in the nervous system. FASEB J 1993:996–1003.
101. Reichardt LF, Tomaselli KJ. Extracellular matrix molecules and their receptors: Functions in neural development. Annu Rev Neurosci 1991; 14:531–570.
102. Goodman SL. Role of extracellular matrix in cell migration and invasion. In: Rohrbach DH, Timpl R, eds. Molecular and Cellular Aspects of Basement Membranes. New York: Academic Press, 1993:345–358.
103. Humphries MJ. Peptide sequences in matrix proteins recognized by adhesion receptors. In: Rohrbach DH, Timpl R, eds. Molecular and Cellular Aspects of Basement Membranes. New York: Academic Press, 1993:289–308.
104. Yamada KM. Adhesive recognition sequences. J Biol Chem 1991; 266:12809–12812.
105. Barsky SH, Rao CN, Williams JE, Liotta LA. Domains of laminin which alter metastasis in a murine model. J Clin Invest 1984; 74:843–848.
106. Aumailley M, Nurcombe V, Edgar D, et al. The cellular interactions of laminin fragments. J Biol Chem 1987; 262:11532–11538.
107. Nurcombe V, Aumailley M, Timpl R, Edgar D. The high affinity binding of laminin to cells: Assignation of a major cell-binding site to its short arms. Eur J Biochem 1989; 180:9–14.
108. Aumailley M, Gerl M, Sonnenberg A, et al. Identification of the Arg-Gly-Asp sequence in laminin A chain as a latent cell-binding site being exposed in fragment P1. FEBS Lett 1990; 262:82–86.
109. Goodman SL, Deutzmann R, von der Mark K. Two independent cell binding domains in laminin react with differentially expressed cell surface receptors. J Cell Biol 1987; 105:589–598.
110. Goodman SL, Aumailley M, von der Mark H. Multiple cell surface receptors for the short arms of laminin: $\alpha 1\beta 1$ integrin and RGD-dependent proteins mediate cell attachment only to domains III in murine tumor laminin. J Cell Biol 1991; 113:931–941.
111. Graf J, Iwamoto Y, Sasaki M, et al. Identification of an amino acid sequence in laminin mediating cell attachment, chemotaxis, and receptor binding. Cell 1987; 48:989–996.
112. Iwamoto Y, Robey FA, Graf J, et al. YIGSR, a synthetic laminin pentapeptide, inhibits experimental metastasis formation. Science 1987; 238:1132–1134.
113. Pikkarainen T, Schulthess T, Engel J, Tryggvason K. Recombinant laminin B1 chains exhibit intact short-arm domains but do not form oligomeric molecules. Eur J Biochem 1992; 209:571–582.
114. Terranova VP, Aumailley M, Sultan LH, et al. Regulation of cell attachment and cell number by fibronectin and laminin. J Cell Physiol 1986; 127:473–479.
115. Panayotou G, End P, Aumailley M, et al. Domains of laminin with growth-factor activity. Cell 1989; 56:93–101.

116. Edgar D, Timpl R, Thoenen H. The heparin-binding domain of laminin is responsible for its effects on neurite outgrowth and neuronal survival. EMBO J 1984; 3:1463–1468.
117. Goodman SL, Deutzmann R, Nurcombe V. Locomotory competence and laminin-specific cell surface binding-sites are lost during myoblast differentiation. Development 1989; 106:795–802.
118. Deutzmann R, Huber J, Schmetz K, et al. Structural study of long arm fragments of laminin: Evidence for repetitive C-terminal sequences in the A chain, not present in the B chains. Eur J Biochem 1988; 177:35–45.
119. Sonnenberg A, Linders CJT, Modderman PW, et al. Integrin recognition of different cell-binding fragments of laminin (P1,E3,E8) and evidence that $\alpha 6\beta 1$ but not $\alpha 6\beta 4$ functions as a major receptor for fragment E8. J Cell Biol 1990; 110:2145–2155.
120. Taraboletti G, Rao CN, Krutzsch HC, et al. Sulfatide-binding domain of the laminin A chain. J Biol Chem 1990; 265:12253–12258.
121. Deutzmann R, Aumailley M, Wiedemann H, et al. Cell adhesion, spreading and neurite stimulation by laminin fragment E8 depends on maintenance of secondary and tertiary structure in its rod and globular domain. Eur J Biochem 1990; 191:513–522.
122. Skubitz APN, Letourneau PC, Wayner E, Furcht LT. Synthetic peptides from the carboxy-terminal globular domain of the A chain of laminin: Their ability to promote cell adhesion and neurite outgrowth, and interact with heparin and the $\beta 1$ integrin subunit. J Cell Biol 1991; 115:1137–1148.
123. Gehlsen KR, Sriramarao P, Furcht LT, Skubitz APN. A synthetic peptide derived from the carboxy terminus of the laminin A chain represents a binding site for the $\alpha 3\beta 1$ integrin. J Cell Biol 1992; 117:449–459.
124. Tashiro K, Sephel GC, Weeks B, et al. A synthetic peptide containing the IKVAV sequence from the A chain of laminin mediates cell attachment, migration, and neurite outgrowth. J Biol Chem 1989; 264:16174–16182.
125. Kubota S, Tashiro K, Yamada Y. Signaling site of laminin with mitogenic activity. J Biol Chem 1992; 267:4285–4288.
126. Sung U, O'Rear JJ, Yurchenco PD. Cell and heparin binding in the distal long arm of laminin: Identification of active and cryptic sites with recombinant and hybrid glycoprotein. J Cell Biol 1993; 123:1255–1268.
127. Engvall E, Earwicker D, Day A, et al. Merosin promotes cell attachment and neurite outgrowth and is a component of the neurite-promoting factor of RN22 Schwannoma cells. Exp Cell Res 1992; 198:115–123.
128. Mecham RP. Laminin receptors. Annu Rev Cell Biol 1991; 7:71–91.
128a. Mecham RP. Receptors for laminin on mammalian cells. FASEB J 1991; 5:2538–2546.
129. Hynes RO. Integrins: Versatility, modulation, and signaling in cell adhesion. Cell 1992; 69:11–25.
130. Hall DE, Reichardt LF, Crowley E, et al. The $\alpha 1/\beta 1$ and $\alpha 6/\beta 1$ integrin heterodimers mediate cell attachment to distinct sites on laminin. J Cell Biol 1990; 110:2175–2184.
131. Aumailley M, Timpl R, Sonnenberg A. Antibody to integrin $\alpha 6$ subunit specifically inhibits cell-binding to laminin fragment E8. Exp Cell Res 1990; 188:55–60.
132. Kramer RH, Vu MP, Cheng YF, et al. The laminin-binding integrin $\alpha 7\beta 1$: Functional characterization and expression in normal and malignant melanocytes. Cell Reg 1991; 2:805–817.
133. von der Mark H, Dürr J, Sonnenberg A, et al. Skeletal myoblasts utilize a novel $\beta 1$-series integrin and not $\alpha 6\beta 1$ for binding to the E8 and T8 fragments of laminin. J Biol Chem 1991; 266:23593–23601.
134. Cioce V, Margulies IMK, Sobel ME, Castronovo V. Interaction between the 67 kilodalton metastasis-associated laminin receptor and laminin. Kidney Int 1993; 43:30–37.
135. Campo E, Monteagudo C, Castronovo V, et al. Detection of laminin receptor mRNA in human cancer cell lines and colorectal tissues by in situ hybridization. Am J Pathol 1992; 141:1073–1083.
136. Auth D, Brawermann G. A 33-kDa polypeptide with homology to the laminin receptor: Component of translation machinery. Proc Natl Acad Sci USA 1992; 89:4368–4372.
137. Ibraghimov-Beskrovnajya O, Ervasti JM, Leville CJ, et al. Primary structure of dystrophin-associated glycoproteins linking dystrophin to the extracellular matrix. Nature 1992; 355:696–702.
138. Evans SC, Lopez LC, Shur BD. Dominant negative mutation in cell surface $\beta 1$,4-galactosyltransferase inhibits cell-cell and cell-matrix interactions. J Cell Biol 1993; 120:1045–1057.
139. Hall H, Liu L, Schachner M, Schmitz B. The L2/HNK-1 carbohydrate mediates adhesion of neural cells to laminin. Eur J Neurosci 1993; 5:34–42.
140. Bronner-Frazer M. Perturbation of cranial neural crest migration by the HNK-1 antibody. Dev Biol 1987; 123:321–331.
141. Abrahamson DR. Recent studies on the structure and pathology of basement membranes. J Pathol 1986; 149:257–278.
142. Abrahamson DR. Structure and development of the glomerular capillary wall and basement membrane. Am J Physiol 1987; 253:F783–F794.
143. Kerjaschki D, Sawada H, Farquhar MG. Immunoelectron microscopy in kidney research: Some contributions and limitations. Kidney Int 1986; 30:229–245.

144. Farquhar MG. The glomerular basement membrane: A selective macromolecular filter. In: Hay ED, ed. Cell Biology of Extracellular Matrix. New York: Plenum Press, 1991:365–418.
145. Schittny JC, Timpl R, Engel J. High resolution immunoelectron microscopic localization of laminin, nidogen, and heparan sulfate proteoglycan in epithelial basement membrane of mouse cornea reveals different topological orientations. J Cell Biol 1988; 107:1599–1610.
146. Abrahamson DR, Irwin MH, St. John PL, et al. Selective immunoreactivities of kidney basement membranes to monoclonal antibodies against laminin: Localization of the end of the long arm and the short arms to discrete microdomains. J Cell Biol 1989; 109:3477–3491.
147. Desjardins M, Bendayan M. Heterogenous distribution of type IV collagen, entactin, heparan sulfate proteoglycan, and laminin among renal basement membranes as demonstrated by quantitative immunocytochemistry. J Histochem Cytochem 1989; 37:885–897.
148. Grant DS, Leblond CP. Immunogold quantitation of laminin, type IV collagen and heparansulfate proteoglycan in a variety of basement membranes. J Histochem Cytochem 1988; 36:271–283.
149. Kefalides NA, Howard P, Ohno N. Heterogeneity in basement membranes determines their structure and function. In: Shibata S, ed. Basement Membranes. New York: Elsevier Science Publishers, 1985:73–87.
150. Martinez-Hernandez A, Chung AE. The ultrastructural localization of two basement membrane components: Entactin and laminin in rat tissues. J Histochem Cytochem 1984; 32:289–298.
151. Jaffe R, Bender B, Santamaria M, Chung AE. Segmental staining of the murine nephron by monoclonal antibodies directed against the GP-2 subunit of laminin. Lab Invest 1984:51:88–96.
152. Wan YJ, Wu TC, Chung AE, Damjanov I. Monoclonal antibodies to laminin reveal the heterogeneity of basement membranes in the developing and adult mouse tissues. J Cell Biol 1984; 98:971–979.
153. Hessle H, Sakai LY, Hollister DW, et al. Basement membrane diversity detected by monoclonal antibodies. Differentiation 1984; 26:49–54.
154. Leu FJ, Engvall E, Damjanov I. Heterogeneity of basement membranes of the human genitourinary tract revealed by sequential immunofluorescence staining with monoclonal antibodies to laminin. J Histochem Cytochem 1986; 34:483–489.
155. Horikoshi S, Koide H, Shirai T. Monoclonal antibodies against laminin A chain and B chain in the human and mouse kidneys. Lab Invest 1988; 58:532–538.
156. Klein G, Langegger M, Timpl R, Ekblom P. Role of laminin A chain in the development of epithelial cell polarity. Cell 1988; 55:331–341.
157. Ekblom M, Klein G, Mugrauer G, et al. Transient and locally restricted expression of laminin A chain mRNA by developing epithelial cells during kidney organogenesis. Cell 1990; 60:337–346.
158. Sanes JR, Engvall E, Butkowski R, Hunter D. Molecular heterogeneity of basal laminae: Isoforms of laminin and collagen IV at the neuromuscular junction and elsewhere. J Cell Biol 1990; 111:1685–1699.
159. Bernfield M, Banerjee S, Koda JE, Rapraeger AC. Remodeling of basement membrane: Morphogenesis and maturation. Ciba Found Symp 1984; 108:179–196.
160. Grobstein C. Mechanisms of organogenetic tissue interaction. Natl Cancer Inst Monogr 1967; 26:279–299.
161. Ekblom P. Renal development. In: Seldin DW, ed. The Kidney: Physiology and Pathophysiology. New York: Raven Press, 1992:475–501.
162. Saxen L. Organogenesis of the Kidney. Cambridge: Cambridge University Press, 1987.
163. Grobstein C. Trans-filter induction of tubules in mouse metanephrogenic mesenchyme. Exp Cell Res 1956; 10:424–440.
164. Sorokin LM, Conzelmann S, Ekblom P, et al. Monoclonal antibodies against laminin A chain fragment E3 and their effects on binding to cells and proteoglycan and on kidney development. Exp Cell Res 1992; 201:137–144.
165. Holm K, Ristelli L, Sariola H. Differential expression of the laminin A and B chains in chimeric kidneys. Cell Diff 1988; 24:223–228.
166. Sorokin LM, Sonnenberg A, Aumailley M, et al. Recognition of the laminin E8 cell-binding site by an integrin possessing the $\alpha 6$ subunit is essential for epithelial polarization in developing kidney tubules. J Cell Biol 1990; 111:1265–1273.
167. Abrahamson DR, St John PL. Loss of laminin epitopes during glomerular basement membrane assembly in developing mouse kidneys. J Histochem Cytochem 1992; 40:1943–1953.
168. Schuger L, O'Shea S, Rheinheimer J, Varani J. Laminin in lung development: Effects of anti-laminin antibody in murine lung morphogenesis. Dev Biol 1990; 137:26–32.
169. Schuger L, Skubitz AMP, O'Shea KS, et al. Identification of laminin domains involved in branching morphogenesis: Effects of anti-laminin monoclonal antibodies on mouse embryonic lung development. Dev Biol 1991; 146:531–541.
170. Simo P, Simon-Assmann P, Bouziges F, et al. Changes in the expression of laminin during intestinal development. Development 1991; 112:477–487.
171. Klein G, Ekblom M, Fecker L, et al. Differential expression of laminin A and B chains during development of embryonic mouse organs. Development 1990; 110:823–837.

172. Aumailley M, Timpl R, Risau W. Differences in laminin fragment interactions of normal and transformed endothelial cells. Exp Cell Res 1991; 196:177–183.
173. Tashiro KI, Sephel GC, Greatorex D, et al. The RGD containing site of the mouse laminin A chain is active for cell attachment, spreading, migration and neurite outgrowth. J Cell Physiol 1991; 146:451–459.
174. Kubota Y, Kleinman HK, Martin GR, Lawley TJ. Role of laminin and basement membrane in the morphological differentiation of human endothelial cells into capillary-like structures. J Cell Biol 1988; 107:1589–1598.
175. Grant DS, Tashiro KI, Segui-Real B. Two different laminin domains mediate the differentiation of human endothelial cells into capillary-like structures. Cell 1989; 58:933–943.
176. Schnaper HW, Kleinman HK, Grant DS. Role of laminin in endothelial cell recognition and differentiation. Kidney Int 1993; 43:20–25.
177. Rohrbach DH, Murrah VA. Molecular aspects of basement membrane pathology. In: Rohrbach DH, Timpl R, eds. Molecular and Cellular Aspects of Basement Membranes. Academic Press, 1993:396–419.
178. Korhonen M, Laitinen L, Ylänne J, et al. Integrins in developing, normal and malignant human kidney. Kidney Int 1992; 41:641–644.
179. Goligorsky MS, Lieberthal W, Racusen L, Simon EE. Integrin receptors in renal tubular epithelium: New insights into pathophysiology of acute renal failure. Am J Physiol 1993; 33:F1–F8.
180. Sorokin L, Girg W. Göpfert T, Hallmann R, Deutzmann R. Expression of novel 400 kDa laminin chains by mouse and bovine endothelial cells. Eur J Biochem 1994; 223:603–610.

6
Metalloproteinases

Malcolm Davies
University of Wales College of Medicine, Royal Infirmary, Cardiff, Wales, United Kingdom

David H. Lovett
San Francisco Veterans Affairs Medical Center and University of California at San Francisco, San Francisco, California

INTRODUCTION

The mammalian matrix metalloproteinases (MMPs) constitute a family of structurally related enzymes which are the products of related genes (1–3). These proteinases, which are involved in the turnover of the extracellular matrix, share the following characteristics: (a) they have the potential to degrade at least one component of the ECM, (b) they are optimally active at neutral pH, (c) they have an absolute requirement for Zn^{2+} and are inhibited by metal chelating agents such as EDTA and 1,10-phenanthroline, (d) they are secreted in an inactive proform and undergo proteolytic cleavage of an amino-terminal domain during activation, and (e) the active forms are all inhibited by specific tissue inhibitors of metalloproteinases (TIMPs).

Domain Sequences

The analysis of cDNA sequences of cloned MMPs as well as biochemical and immunological data have shown that this family of proteinases can be divided into three subgroups: the interstitial collagenases, the gelatinases (formally referred to as type IV collagenases), and the stromelysins (Table 1). Consideration of the predicted amino acid sequence data of each enzyme has demonstrated a number of distinctive domains that are conserved in all the MMPs (Fig. 1). The first is a leader sequence or predomain sequence that targets the enzymes for secretion. The second represents a propeptide sequence of approximately 80 amino acids that contains the highly conserved sequence PRCGVPDV, critical to activation of the proenzyme, which is situated just upstream, N terminal to the catalytic domain. This prodomain is removed when the enzyme becomes permanently active. The third or catalytic domain contains a conserved zinc-chelating motif (VAAHEXGHXXGXXH), thought to be the Zn^{2+}-binding site. The fourth domain is the disulfide-bonded C-terminal domain of about 250 amino acids with sequence similarities to hemopexin. This domain is not essential for proteolytic activity, as demonstrated by matrilysin (Fig. 1), a truncated MMP lacking the C-terminal domain. This domain, however, is important to a number of interactions central to the function of the MMPs. First, it is involved in the substrate specificity of collagenase (4) and the binding of pro- and active stromelysin-1 to collagen fibrils (5). Second, this domain represents a region that interacts with a putative cell surface receptor for gelatinase A (72-kDa type IV gelatinase), an event that is likely to be important in the activation of this MMP (6,7). Finally, there is compelling evidence that TIMP-1 binds to the C-terminal domain of gelatinase B (92-kDA type IV gelatinase), whereas gelatinase A preferentially binds with TIMP-2 (8–11). The two gelatinases have larger Mr values due to the insertion into the catalytic domain of a unique region immediately adjacent to the putative binding region composed of three 58-residue head-to-head repeats with extensive homology to the

Table 1 Matrix-Degrading Metalloproteinases and Their Substrate Specificity[a]

	Native collagen					Gelatin type				Noncollagenous molecules			
Enzyme (Mr)	I	III	IV	V	VII	I	III	IV	V	PG	FN	LM	GBM
PMN collagenase (75 K)	+	+	–	–	+	(+)	(+)	(+)	–	–	–	–	–
Collagenase (52 K)	+	+	–	–	+	(+)	(+)	(+)	–	–	–	–	–
Gelatinase B (92 K)	–	–	+	+	–	+	+	+	+	–	+	–	+
Gelatinase A (72 K)	–	–	+	(+)	–	+	+	+	+	–	+	–	+
Stromelysin-1 (53 K)	–	+	+	+	nd	+	+	+	+	+	+	+	+
Stromelysin-2 (53 K)	–	+	+	+	nd	+	+	(+)	+	+	+	+	nd
Stromelysin-3 (54 K)[b]	–	nd	+	nd	nd	+	nd	nd	nd	+	+	+	nd
Matrilysin (28 K)	–	–	–	–	nd	+	+	+	+	+	+	+	nd

[a]The list is incomplete and lists mainly substrates relevant to the glomerular ECM. Abbreviations: Lack of activity by an enzyme against a substrate = –; good activity = +; slight activity = (+); not determined = nd; FN = fibronectin; PG = proteoglycan; LM = laminin; GGBM =glomerular basement membrane.

[b]Based on the properties of a 28-kDa protein produced by expressing stromelysin-3 in a mouse myeloma cell system. However, it has been questioned whether this proteinase is a true member of the MMP family (19).

collagen-binding domain of fibronectin (12,13). Gelatinase B possesses a further insert with sequence similarities to the α2-chain of type V collagen and thus represents the largest member of the MMP group. The full genomic structure of interstitial collagenase, stromelysin-1, the gelatinases, and martrilysin has been determined (14,15). Collagenase and stromelysin consist of 10 exons of similar length that are both mapped to the long arm human chromosome 11. In the gelatinases, there are three additional exons to provide for the gelatin-binding domain. The first five exons of matrilysin are highly homologous to those of the stromelysin group; however the C-terminal sixth exon is unique (15).

Substrate Specificity

The MMP family of proteinases have the combined ability to degrade all the normally occurring components of connective tissue matrices including basement membranes (BMs) (see Table 1). Gelatinase A and gelatinase B have similar substrate specificities. They degrade native type IV collagen, the major component of BMs, and thus were initially referred to as type IV collagenases. However, these enzymes can also degrade collagen types V, VII, and X and fibronectin. In addition, they have considerable activity against denatured interstitial collagens (gelatin), and for this reason are now referred to as gelatinases. The third group of MMPs, the stromelysins, are distinguished from the other MMPs by their ability to degrade the core protein of proteoglycans (stromelysin-I was originally named proteoglycanase). These enzymes have a broad range of proteinase activity and degrade type IV and IX collagens, fibronectin, laminin, and elastin. While these enzymes have a similar domain structure to collagenase, they do not cleave interstitial collagens. Also included in this group of MMPs is matrilysin (formally called PUMP-1). Matrilysin lacks the C-terminal hemopexin-like domain and thus represents the smallest member of the MMP gene family. It also exhibits a broad spectrum of substrate specificity similar to that of stromelysin-1. This includes the ability to hydrolyze casein, gelatin, fibronectin, and proteoglycans (16–19). In contrast to stromelysin-1, matrilysin does not degrade type IV collagen or elastin.

As opposed to the MMPs mentioned above, the interstitial collagenases exhibit a relatively restricted substrate specificity in that they uniquely cleave collagen I, II, and III at a single locus within the helical region approximately three-quarters the distance from the N terminal. The collagen fragments released by these enzymes are rapidly denatured at physiological temperatures and thus become substrates for other proteinases, particularly the gelatinases. The involvement of two MMPs in the degradation of interstitial collagen is further emphasized by recent findings that interstitial

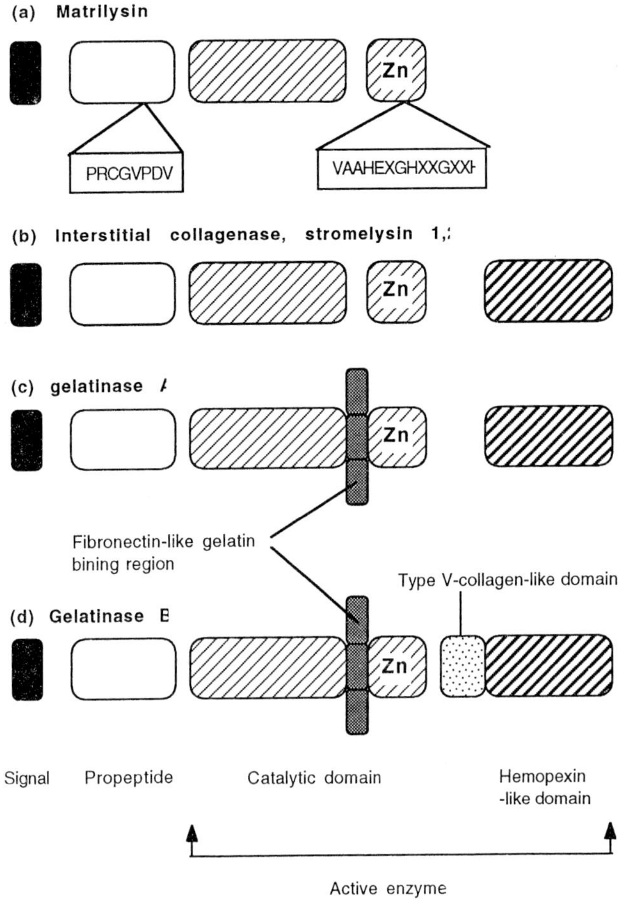

Figure 1 Domain structure of matrix metalloproteinases.

collagenase can form a complex with gelatinase B (10). Such an interaction in vivo would favor the rapid and efficient degradation of the collagen fibrils to small peptides.

Activation of Latent Metalloproteinases

In vitro, the latent forms of MMPs are activated by physical forces (i.e., heat) or chemical compounds (i.e., organomercurials, alkylating agents) as well as by limited proteolysis (i.e., trypsin). The precise role of these different agents is not clear, but it is likely to involve modification by the so-called cysteine switch mechanism of Cys_{73} present in the highly conserved $PRC_{73}GXPX$ region of the propeptide domain (Fig. 1) (20,21). The essential feature is that the propeptide domain is folded in such a manner that the Cys_{73} residue can interact with the active site Zn^{2+} (see Fig. 2), thus preventing the accessibility of the water molecule required in the cleavage mechanism. Disruption of the coordination between the Zn^{2+}-cysteine molecules results in conformational changes and the rapid attainment of protease activity. This initial step is followed by autoproteolysis (Fig. 1C) of the C-terminal side of the conserved PRCGXPD site with loss of Cys_{73} and the generation of a stable active enzyme. As a consequence of this rearrangement, the N terminal domain is lost and the active enzyme is considerably smaller than its latent form.

The mechanisms by which the latent form of MMPs are activated in vivo are unclear. Biochemical studies with purified or recombinant latent forms of stromelysin, collagenase, and gelatinase B and a streptokinase-plasminogen system to generate plasmin show that activation can

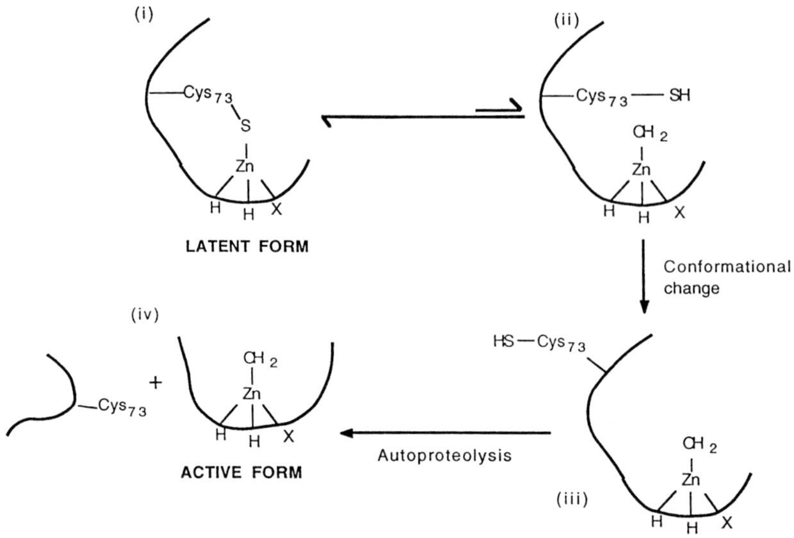

Figure 2 The "cysteine switch" mechanism for the activation of matrix metalloproteinases.

be achieved by the serine proteinase (22,23). Studies with cell monolayers plated on collagen and gelatin films also implicate plasmin as a potential physiological activator (24). In these studies, the activation of stromelysin occurred rapidly, whereas that of interstitial collagenase required the concerted action of plasmin and stromelysin. In addition, stromelysin can considerably enhance the trypsin and chemical activation of collagenase by as much as five- to eightfold. This suggests that the activation mechanism of the MMPs in vivo probably involves a proteolytic cascade system from plasminogen activator, through plasmin and stromelysin to collagenase and gelatinase B and subsequent autoactivation (see Fig. 3).

Although several in vivo studies have identified gelatinase activities of 58 to 62 kDa that correspond to the active form of gelatinase A, this MMP is resistant to proteolytic cleavage by plasmin (and trypsin), indicating that an alternative mechanism to the plasminogen cascade system must exist. It is now generally believed that the activation of gelatinase A does not occur in the soluble phase but rather involves an interaction between an activator located on the surface and the C-terminal domain of the enzyme (7,25,26). The expression of this activator is dependent on the stimulation of these cells with agents such as concanavalin A, phorbol ester, or extracellular matrix. In addition, immunological and ligand-binding studies indicate that progelatinase A binds to high-affinity plasma membrane receptors on fibroblast and tumor cells (27). Since these receptors are present on nonstimulated cells as well, they are presumably distinct entities to the membrane activator. A truncated form of gelatinase lacking the C-terminal domain cannot bind to the receptor or be activated by the membrane activator, indicating an important role for the C domain in the regulation of gelatinase A (26). Based on the above, the following mechanism has been proposed for the in vivo activation of progelatinase A and for its proform/ TIMP-2 complex (see Ref. 6). The proform through the C-terminal domain first binds to a specific cell surface receptor for gelatinase A, occupancy of which also allows the membrane activator to interact with the same domain. The result of these events is the formation of a multiprotein complex within which a conformational change of the proenzyme allows the intermolecular autolytic reactions to proceed and establish full enzymatic activity. Little is known about the nature of the membrane activator other than that it is extractable by detergents from plasma membrane and that trypsin pretreatment inactivates the capacity of membrane preparations to process gelatinase A. In vitro, the activation is sensitive to metal ion chelators and excess TIMP-2 but not to cysteine or serine inhibitors. The effect of EDTA is probably due to inhibition of the proenzyme autolytic cleavage step rather than inhibition of the membrane activator or active MMP. The initial binding process probably involves an interaction between the cell membrane receptor and the C-terminal domain of the proenzyme. Since TIMP-2 also binds to

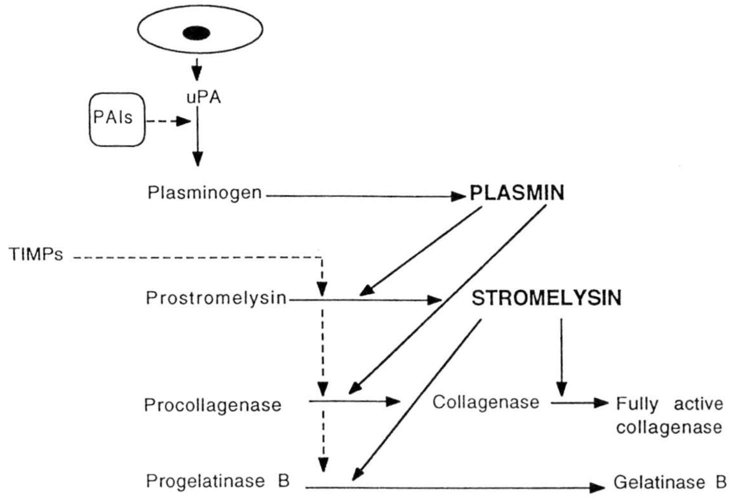

Figure 3 The putative plasminogen/plasmin cascade for the activation of matrix metalloproteinases. This mechanism does not include the activation of gelatinase A (see text).

this domain and inhibits the activation process, it is likely that the balance between TIMP-2, progelatinase A, and active gelatinase is a key factor in the regulation of the cell-mediated activation and function of this enzyme. Given that the location of these molecules is restricted to the cell membrane, the ability of active gelatinase A to remodel the extracellular matrix (ECM) is also restricted to the immediate environment of cells, a feature that is likely to be significant for migration and proliferation of cells. In this respect, recent findings indicate that antiproteolytic agents such as TIMPs and synthetic MMP inhibitors inhibit tumor cell invasion and vascular smooth muscle proliferation and migration in vitro and in vivo (28,29).

Tissue Inhibitors of Metalloproteinases

The activity of the MMPs is modulated by the presence of the tissue inhibitors of metalloproteinases (TIMPs). Several different TIMPs have been identified, among which three have been cloned and sequenced; they are TIMP-1, a glycoprotein of molecular mass 28.5 kDa (30–32); TIMP-2, a nonglycosylated protein (21 kDa) (33,34); and TIMP-3 (21 kDa) (35). TIMP-1 and TIMP-2 share about 40% homology, in which the locations of all 12 cysteines are conserved. These cysteine residues form disulfide bonds, giving rise to a protein structure of six loops shared equally between two domains.

Both TIMP-1 and TIMP-2 inhibit all MMPs, interacting with each active enzyme with a 1:1 stoichiometry to form tight enzyme-inhibitor complexes. The inhibitors are not modified by this interaction and, following dissociation of the complexes, the free inhibitor is available to recomplex with active MMPs (36). Recent experiments with truncated forms of TIMP-1 and TIMP-2 that retain the anti-MMP activity indicate that the N-amino domain is the major structural feature involved in the formation of the enzyme/inhibitor complex (37). The role of the C-terminal region of TIMPs has not been elucidated, but it is possible that this domain binds to the C-terminal regions of latent gelatinases. Of particular interest is the observation that TIMP-1 binds preferentially to progelatinase B, whereas TIMP-2 complexes with progelatinase A (8–11). The physiological significance of such specific interactions is as yet unknown, but one proposed role is that they serve to regulate the in vivo activation of progelatinase A and progelatinase B (10,25).

GLOMERULAR METALLOPROTEINASES

The characterization of the matrix-degrading enzymes secreted by the intrinsic cells of the glomerulus has been the focus of investigation of several laboratories for over a decade. The primary reasons for this extensive interest relate to our current limited understanding of the mechanisms involved in the basal turnover of the glomerular extracellular matrix as well as the concept that excessive synthesis of such activities could participate in the development of glomerular injury. Studies in this area may be divided into two general categories, including those utilizing tissue culture of glomerular cells and those examining the expression of matrix-degrading enzymes in vivo. Due to the relative ease of culture, virtually all reports in this area have involved mesangial cells, primarily of either rat or human origin. Initial reports partially defined an enzymatic activity present in the culture supernates of rat mesangial cells with properties consistent with the MMP family, including function at neutral pH, zinc dependence, and secretion in latent, proenzyme form (38). This study also indicated that the activity was capable of extensively degrading insoluble glomerular BM type IV collagen. Subsequent purification of this activity to apparent homogeneity, using rat and human mesangial cell sources, provided convincing evidence for identification as the 72-kDa type IV collagenase (39,40). Additionally, protein sequencing of tryptic peptides derived from purified human mesangial-cell enzyme demonstrated identity at the amino acid level with the 72-kDa type IV collagenase (gelatinase A) expressed by H-*ras*–transformed tracheobronchial epithelial cells (12).

Investigation into the mesangial-cell–specific features of 72-kDa type IV collagenase synthesis has revealed several unusual aspects. In most studied cell lines, the synthesis of this particular enzyme is constitutive and demonstrates little if any responsiveness to inflammatory cytokines. In contrast, the synthesis of gelatinase A by early passage rat mesangial cells is greatly stimulated by exposure to interleukin-1, tumor necrosis factor, phorbol ester, and second-messenger analogues (41). As detailed below, the 72-kDa type IV collagenase is also induced by transforming growth factor (TGF)-β1. These observations initially raised the question as to whether the mesangial cell product represented a previously unrecognized second isoform of the enzyme. Homology cloning of the rat 72-kDa type IV collagenase cDNA, which exploited the conserved PRCCV and zinc-binding loci, definitively identified this enzyme as the homologue of the human enzyme cloned from H-*ras* epithelial cells. Recent efforts from our laboratory have focused on the 5′ regulatory regions involved in the distinctive patterns of mesangial cell regulation of 72-kDa type IV collagenase synthesis. Sequencing of nearly 2000 bp of the upstream regulatory region has identified several AP-2–like consensus sequences as well as one AP-1 site located within the first exon (D.H.L.; unpublished observations). To extend these findings, a series of deletion constructs were directionally cloned into promoterless luciferase expression vectors and transiently transfected into cultured rat mesangial cells. The initial series of constructs has permitted the identification of a basal proximal promoter located between -57 and 3 bp relative to the transcriptional start site. A major increment in transcriptional activity was observed following addition of 1200 bp of upstream sequence, which appeared to be specific for expression in mesangial cells. Further fine mapping of this construct has defined an 80-bp region with strong position- and orientation-independent enhancer activity. Gel shift analysis demonstrates interaction of this sequence with two nuclear proteins, and the molecular characterization of these transcription factors is currently in progress.

While the predominant MMP secreted by mesangial cells appears to be the 72-kDa type IV collagenase, others have presented preliminary evidence for the secretion of a stromelysin-like activity (42). Earlier studies from our laboratories had indicated the presence of a casein-degrading activity in mesangial cell supernates, also suggestive of a stromelysin-like activity. This activity was subsequently purified from both rat and human sources and characterized at the functional and molecular levels. The purified enzyme readily degrades fibronectin, proteoglycans, and denatured collagens and was noted on casein substrate gels to have an approximate molecular mass of 31 and 26 kDa. Definitive identification of this enzyme was obtained with a homology cloning strategy similar to that discussed for gelatinase A and led to the surprising result that the activity represented matrilysin (PUMP-1) (43). While matrilysin mRNA had previously been identified as a transcript within certain tumor cells, this represented the first report of matrilysin synthesis by a nontransformed cell. The mesangial matrilysin transcript is processed in a tissue-specific manner, yielding a transcript with repeated 3′-untranslated region ATTA motifs commonly found in cytokines with limited mRNA stability. Mesangial cell synthesis of this enzyme was greatly enhanced by incubation with inflammatory cytokines, with a synergistic effect observed with interleukin-1 and tumor necrosis factor. A polyclonal antibody to the C-terminal region of the matrilysin protein was prepared and demonstrated the enhanced mesangial cell synthesis of this enzyme in several forms of acute inflammatory glomerulonephritis.

Metalloproteinases in Renal Disease

The preparation of highly specific antibodies to the mesangial-cell matrix metalloproteinases has permitted the evaluation of enzyme expression within normal glomeruli and during the course of experimental immune complex–mediated glomerulonephritis (44). Histochemical studies at the light and electron microscopic levels indicated that there is a low but consistent level of gelatinase A expression by approximately 10% of the intrinsic mesangial cells. Notably, the enzyme protein was localized almost exclusively at sites adjacent to the basement membrane, suggesting that the normal function of this enzyme is the basal turnover of the GBM. Induction of the Thy-1.1 model of immune complex–mediated glomerulonephritis led to a massive increment in gelatinase A expression, particularly within foci of actively proliferating mesangial cells. In addition, heavy concentrations of the enzyme were detected by immunogold technique within regions of evolving mesangiolysis and at sites of specific basement membrane discontinuity. Thus, enhanced expression of gelatinase A in this model of glomerular disease may be directly associated with the evolution of matrix and BM injury. These observations have recently been extended (45) to a consideration of the potential role of TGF-β1 in the induction of gelatinase A synthesis in this model. Invitro studies clearly demonstrate a stimulatory effect of TGF-β1 on gelatinase A synthesis by cultured human mesangial cells, such that the net effect is on the accumulation of this MMP in excess of TIMP inhibitor protein. The effects of TGF-β1 on gelatinase A synthesis are complex and appear to be mediated at both the transcriptional and translational levels, resulting in prolonged synthesis of the enzyme. These observations were extended to an analysis of gelatinase A and TGF-β1 mRNA expression in vivo during the course of the Thy-1.1 model of nephritis. Remarkably, induction of acute nephritis was associated with a synchronous increase of mRNA expression for both factors, which occurred exclusively within the proliferating mesangial cells. These in vivo findings suggest that there is a direct linkage between augmented TGF-β1 expression and synthesis of the gelatinase A enzyme.

FUTURE DIRECTIONS

Future efforts in this field should focus on the extension of purely in vitro observations to either clinical biopsy material or experimental models of glomerular disease. The current activities of this laboratory are focused on the direct analysis of the function(s) of the 72-kDa type IV collagenase enzyme in vivo. These efforts involve the specific targeting of glomerular mesangial cells in vivo using cationic immunoliposomes as DNA delivery modules. Two forms of genetic constructs are currently under evaluation for the specific inhibition of mesangial-cell gelatinase A synthesis. These include episomally replicating vectors expressing antisense gelatinase A transcripts as well as retroviral constructs expressing specific gelatinase A mRNA-degrading ribozyme sequences. Hopefully, such studies will offer further insights into the mechanisms of glomerular disease and provide the basis for future attempts at specific therapeutic modalities.

REFERENCES

1. Docherty AJP, Murphy G. The tissue metalloproteinase family and the inhibitor TIMP: A study using cDNAs and recombinant proteins. Ann Rheum Dis 1990; 49:469–479.
2. Woessner JF. Matrix metalloproteinases and their inhibitors in connective tissue remodelling. FASEB J 1991; 5:2145–2154.
3. Matrisian LM. The matrix-degrading metalloproteinases. Bioessays 1992; 14:455–463.
4. Clark IM, Cawston TE. Fragments of human fibroblast collagenase: Purification and characterization. Biochem J 1989; 263:201–206.
5. Allan JA, Hembry RM, Angal S, et al. Binding of latent and high active Mr forms of stromelysin to collagen is mediated by the C-terminal domain. J Cell Sci 1991; 99:789–795.
6. Kleiner DE, Stetler-Stevensen WG. Structural biochemistry and activation of matrix metalloproteinases. Curr Opin Cell Biol 1993; 5:891–897.
7. Brown PD, Kleiner DE, Unsworth EJ, Stetler-Stevenson WG. Cellular activation of the 72 kDa type-IV procollagenase/TIMP-2 complex. Kidney Int 1993; 43:163–170.
8. Goldberg GI, Marmer BL, Grant GA, et al. Human 72 kDa type IV collagenase forms a complex with a tissue inhibitor of metalloproteinase designated TIMP-2. Proc Natl Acad Sci USA 1989; 86:8207–8211.

9. Stetler-Stevenson WG, Krutzsch HC, Liotta LA. Tissue inhibitor of metalloproteinase (TIMP-2). J Biol Chem 1989; 264:17374–17378.
10. Goldberg GI, Strongin A, Collier IE, et al. Interaction of 92-kDa type IV collagenase with the tissue inhibitor of metalloproteinases prevents dimerization, complex formation with interstitial collagenase, and activation of the proenzyme with stromelysin. J Biol Chem 1992; 267:4583–4591.
11. Kleiner DE, Unsworth EJ, Krutzsch HC, Stetler-Stevenson WG. Higher-order complex formation between the 72-kilodalton type-IV collagenase and tissue inhibitor of metalloproteinases-2. Biochemistry 1992; 31:1665–1672.
12. Collier IE, Wilhelm SM, Eisen AZ, et al. H-ras oncogene-transformed human bronchial epihelial cells (TBE-1) secrete a single metalloproteinase capable of degrading basement membrane collagen. J Biol Chem 1988; 263:6579–6587.
13. Wilhelm SM, Collier IE, Marmer BL, et al. SV40 transformed human lung fibroblasts secrete a 92 kDa type IV collagenase which is identical to that secreted by human macrophages. J Biol Chem 1989; 264:17213–17221.
14. Collier IE, Bruns GAP, Goldberg GI, Gerhard DS. On the structure and chromosome location of the 72- and 92-kDa human type IV collagenase gene. Genomics 1991; 9:429–434.
15. Gaire M, Magbanua Z, McDonnell S, et al. Structure and expression of the human gene for the matrix metalloproteinase matrilysin. J Biol Chem 1994; 269:2032–2040.
16. Wilhelm SM, Collier IE, Kronerberger AZ, et al. Human skin fibroblast stromelysin: Structure, glycosylation, substrate specificity, and differential expression in normal and tumorigenic cells. Proc Natl Acad Sci USA 1987; 84:6725–6729.
17. Murphy G, Cockett ML, Ward RV, Docherty AJP. Matrix degradation of elastin, type IV collagen and proteoglycan: A quantitative comparison of the activities of 95 kDa and 72 kDa gelatinases, stromelysin-1 and -2 and punctuated metalloproteinase (PUMP). Biochem J 1991; 279:277–279.
18. Chin JR, Murphy G, Werb Z. Stromelysin, a connective tissue degrading metalloproteinase secreted by stimulated rabbit synovial fibroblasts in parallel with collagenase. J Biol Chem 1985; 260:12367–12376.
19. Murphy G, Segain J-P, O'Shea M, et al. The 28-kDa N-terminal domain of mouse stromelysin-3 has the general properties of a weak metalloproteinase. J Biol Chem 1993; 268:15435–15441.
20. Springman EB, Angleton EL, Birkedal-Hansen H, et al. Multiple modes of activation of latent human fibroblast collagenase: Evidence for the role of CYS^{73} active-site zinc complex in latency and a "cysteine switch" mechanism for activation. Proc Natl Acad Sci USA 1990; 87:364–368.
21. Salowe SP, Marcy AI, Cuca GC, et al. Characterization of zinc-binding sites in human stromelysin-1: Stoichiometry of the catalytic domain and identification of a cysteine ligand in the proenzyme. Biochemistry 1992; 31:4535–4540.
22. He C, Wilhelm SM, Pentland AP, et al. Tissue cooperation in a proteolytic cascade activating human interstitial collagenase. Proc Natl Acad Sci USA 1989; 86:2632–2636.
23. Murphy G, Ward RV, Gavrilovic J, Atkinson S. Physiological mechanisms for metalloproteinase activation. Matrix 1992; (Suppl 1):224–230.
24. Atkinson SJ, Ward AV, Reynolds JJ, Murphy G. Cell-mediated degradation of type IV collagen and gelatin film is dependent on the activation of matrix metalloproteinases. Biochem J 1992; 288:605–611.
25. Ward RV, Atkinson SJ, Slocombe PM, et al. Tissue inhibitor of metalloproteinase-2 inhibits the activation of 72 kDa gelatinase by fibroblast membranes. Biochem Biophys Acta 1991; 1079:242–246.
26. Murphy G, Wilenbrock F, Ward RV, et al. The C-terminal domain of the 72 kDa gelatinase is not required for catalysis, but is essential for membrane activation and modulates interactions with tissue inhibitors of metalloproteinases. Biochem J 1992; 283:637–641.
27. Enonard HP, Remacle AG, Noel AC, et al. Tumor cell surface-associated binding site for the Mr 72,000K type IV collagenase. Cancer Res 1992; 52:5845–5848.
28. Mignatti P, Rifkin DB. Biology and biochemistry of proteinases in tumor invasion. Physiol Rev 1993; 73:161–195.
29. Southgate KM, Davies M, Booth RFG, Newby AC. Involvement of Extracellular-matrix-degrading metalloproteinases in rabbit aortic smooth-muscle cell proliferation. Biochem J 1992; 288:93–99.
30. Carmichael DF, Sommer A, Thompson RC, et al. Primary structure and cDNA cloning of human fibroblast collagenase inhibitor. Proc Natl Acad Sci USA 1986; 83:2407–2411.
31. Cawston TE, Galloway WA, Mercer E, et al. Purification of rabbit bone inhibitor of collagenase. Biochem J 1981; 195:159–165.
32. Welgus HG, Stricklin GP. Human skin fibroblast inhibitor: Comparative studies in human connective tissues, serum and amniotic fluid. J Biol Chem 1983; 258:12259–12264.
33. Boone TC, Johnson MJ, DeClerk YA, Langley KE. cDNA cloning and expression of a metalloproteinase inhibitor related to tissue inhibitor of metalloproteinases. Proc Natl Acad Sci USA 1990; 87:587–594.
34. DeClerk YA, Yean T-D, Ratkin BJ, et al. Purification and characterization of two related but distinct metalloproteinase inhibitors secreted by bovine endothelial cells. J Biol Chem 1989; 264:17445–17453.

35. Pavloff N, Staskus PW, Kishnani NS, Hawkes SP. A new inhibitor of metalloproteinases from chicken—CHIMP-3—a 3rd member of the TIMP family. J Biol Chem 1992; 267:17321–17326.
36. Murphy G, Koklitis P, Carne AF. Dissociation of tissue inhibitor of metalloproteinase (TIMP) from enzyme complexes yields fully active inhibitor. Biochem J 1989; 261:1031–1034.
37. Murphy G, Houbrechts A, Cockett MI, et al. The N-terminal domain of tissue inhibitor of metalloproteinase retains metalloproteinase inhibitory activity. Biochemistry 1991; 30:8097–8102.
38. Lovett DH, Sterzel RB, Kashgarian M. Neutral proteinase activity produced in vitro by cells of the glomerular mesangium. Kidney Int 1986; 23:342–340.
39. Davies M, Thomas GJ, Martin J, Lovett DH. The purification and characterisation of a glomerular basement membrane-degrading neutral proteinase from rat mesangial cells. Biochem J 1988; 251:419–425.
40. Martin J, Davies M, Thomas GJ, Lovett DH. Human mesangial cells secrete a GBM-degrading neutral proteinase and a specific inhibitor. Kidney Int 1989; 36:790–801.
41. Marti HP, McNeil L, Davies M, et al. Homology cloning of rat 72 kDa type IV collagenase: Cytokine and second-messenger inducibility in glomerular mesangial cells. Biochem J 1993; 291:441–446.
42. Kawanishi S, Imai E, Moriiyama T, et al. Differential regulation of tissue inhibitors of metalloproteinases (TIMP)-1, TIMP-2, and stromelysin gene by interleukin-1 (IL)1) and TGF-β in cultured rat mesangial cells (abstr). J Am Soc Nephrol 1991; 2:577.
43. Marti HP, McNeil L, Thomas GJ, et al. Molecular characterization of a low-molecular-mass matrix metalloproteinase secreted by glomerular mesangial cells as PUMP-1. Biochem J 1992; 285:899–905.
44. Lovett DH, Johnson RJ, Marti HP, et al. Structural characterisation of the mesangial cell type IV collagenase and enhanced expression in a model of complex-mediated glomerulonephritis. Am J Pathol 1992; 141:85–98.
45. Marti H-P, Lee L, Kashgarian M, Lovett DH. Transforming growth factor-β1 stimulates glomerular mesangial cell synthesis of the 72 kDa type IV collagenase. Am J Pathol 1994; 144:82–94.

7
Molecular Biology of Renin

Timothy L. Reudelhuber
Clinical Research Institute of Montreal, Montreal, Canada

INTRODUCTION

The Circulating and Tissue Renin-Angiotensin System

The renin-angiotensin system (RAS) plays a critical role in the maintenance and modulation of blood pressure in mammals and has been implicated in the pathophysiology associated with several diseases including hypertension, cardiac hypertrophy, and myocardial infarction as well as retinopathies and nephropathies (1–4). For this reason, there has been a major effort in the past several years to understand the molecular mechanisms governing the biosynthesis of the components of the RAS, so that novel means might be developed to control their activities. In the classic view of the RAS (Fig. 1), the glycoprotein angiotensinogen (Aogen) is secreted into the circulation by the liver, where it is cleaved by renin, an aspartyl protease secreted by the kidney, to release the decapeptide angiotensin I (AI). Angiotensin-converting enzyme (ACE), a metalloprotease produced by and anchored to the surface of endothelial cells, then cleaves two amino acids from the carboxyl terminus of AI to release the octapeptide angiotensin II (AII). Angiotensin II exerts its action by binding to specific high-affinity receptors on target cells, resulting in vasoconstriction, increased aldosterone secretion from the adrenal gland, and possibly the proliferation of smooth muscle cells. Aldosterone, in turn, regulates sodium resorption from the proximal tubule and consequently fluid and electrolyte balance.

The concentration of Aogen in human blood is 1.3 μM (5), very close to the Km (1.15 μM) (6) of purified human renin for human Aogen. Under these conditions, the overall activity of the circulating RAS would be dependent on the concentrations of both renin and Aogen. Renin itself is first synthesized as an inactive precursor, or zymogen, called prorenin. Evidence to date suggests that prorenin is analogous to the circulating "big" or "inactive" renin and can be present at three to five times the level of "active" renin in the circulation of humans (7). It is unlikely that prorenin is activated once it is in the circulation; injection of monkeys with large excesses of recombinant human prorenin does not result in a detectable increase in either blood pressure or AII (8,9). Thus, the concentration of circulating active renin is a major determinant of the activity of the RAS and the conversion of prorenin to renin occurs by proteolysis before secretion into the circulation.

Protein and/or messenger RNA (mRNA) encoding all of the components of the RAS including angiotensin receptors have been colocalized within several additional tissues, including brain, kidney, adrenal and pituitary glands, heart and vasculature, and reproductive tissues (2,10–13), leading to the suggestion that tissue renin-angiotensin systems (tRAS) might function in a locally restricted manner. It should be noted, however, that for a given tRAS to be functionally active, a tissue would presumably need not only to express the renin gene but also to activate the resulting prorenin. In humans, circulating active renin drops to undetectable levels within 2 days after nephrectomy (14). In contrast, while prorenin also drops acutely, it continues to be detected even years after nephrectomy (5,7,15). In rats, the case seems a bit different: although several extrarenal tissues contain prorenin mRNA and/or protein (16), nephrectomy results in the disappearance of both renin and prorenin

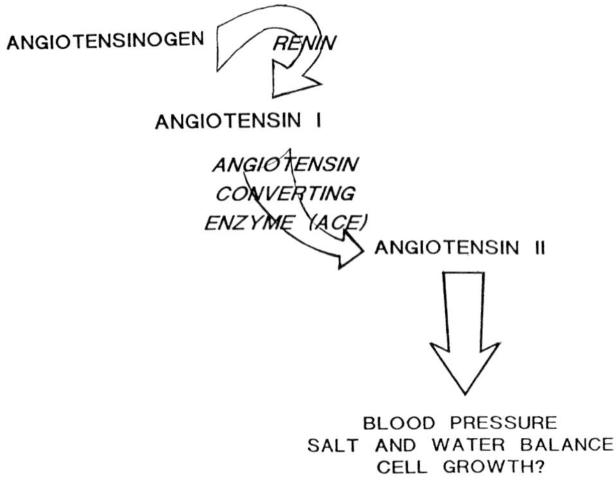

Figure 1 Schematic representation of the renin-angiotensin system.

from the circulation (17). In anephric patients, circulating AI and AII concentrations fall to less than 7% of levels in control subjects (5), while in rats, circulating angiotensins are undetectable within 48 hr after nephrectomy (18). Taken together, these results strongly suggest that while the kidney can release both prorenin and renin, it is the predominant (if not exclusive) source of circulating active renin, while nonrenal sources secrete predominantly (if not exclusively) prorenin.

Isolated, perfused rat hindlimbs are also capable of generating angiotensin peptides (19–22), suggesting that they too contain a source of active renin. However, peripheral generation of angiotensin peptides is eliminated if the animal is nephrectomized prior to limb isolation and perfusion. Similarly, renin activity present in cardiovascular tissues disappears with nephrectomy (23). Thus, renin of renal origin not only plays a key role in the activity of the circulating RAS but may also be taken up by some tissues and used to generate angiotensin peptides peripherally (21,22,24).

Local synthesis of all of the components of the RAS has been demonstrated within the kidney. Angiotensinogen mRNA is present in the proximal tubule (25). Renin is readily detected by immunocytochemistry in the juxtaglomerular (JG) cells of the afferent arteriole (Fig. 2) and to a much lesser extent in proximal connecting and cortical collecting tubules of the adult kidney (26,27). Using in situ hybridization, however, only the JG apparatus is found to contain renin mRNA (28), suggesting that renin found in the proximal tubule may be taken up from the circulation. The AII receptors of the AT_1 subtype are found in the efferent and afferent arterioles of the glomerulus as well as in mesangial cells (29–31). Multiple functions have been proposed for the intrarenal RAS (32,33); AII constriction of the afferent arteriole would have the effect of reducing glomerular flow and glomerular capillary pressure, with a corresponding decrease in glomerular filtration rate (GFR). Conversely, constriction of the efferent arteriole, while also reducing flow, would increase glomerular pressure and GRF. The action of AII on mesangial cells results in a morphological appearance of contraction with a corresponding decrease in the glomerular capillary ultrafiltration coefficient (K_f). In the proximal tubule, AII is thought to regulate sodium and pH balance through modulation of the activity of the Na/H antiporter. Thus, there is much compelling evidence that locally produced components of the RAS may play an important role in both the physiology and the pathophysiology of renal function.

Modulation of Renin Release

Renin release from the kidney is modulated by a number of factors (34,35). It is increased in response to low blood pressure or a drop in sodium chloride concentrations in the distal tubule; it is increased by sympathetic nerve activity. Renin secretion from the kidney is decreased in response to elevations

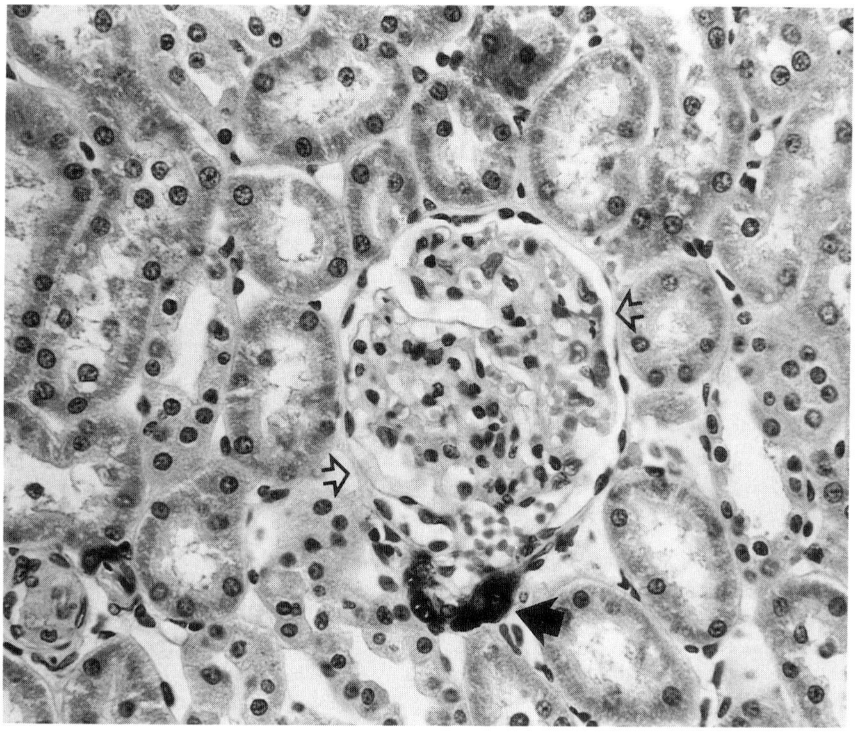

Figure 2 Immunohistochemical staining of a mouse renal cortex with an antibody to renin. The juxtaglomerular apparatus of the afferent arteriole (solid arrowheads) at the base of the glomerulus (open arrowheads) is heavily stained. (Courtesy of D. Ramla, IRCM, Montreal, Canada.)

in blood pressure and elevations in the concentrations of a number of humoral factors including AII, vasopressin, endothelin, adenosine, and atrial natriuretic factor. Expression of the renin gene in the kidney is also developmentally regulated (36,37). Both renin protein and renin mRNA are detected in cells surrounding the lumen of developing intrarenal arteries. As renal development proceeds, renin expression colocalizes most strongly with the newer portions of elongating arteries and gradually disappears in the more mature vessels. By 1 week of age, renin expression is primarily restricted to the JG apparatus in much the same pattern seen in adult mammals. Treatment of rats with either a low-salt diet, diuretics, ACE inhibitors, or a selective AT_1 receptor antagonist causes renin immunostaining to reappear along the afferent arteriole in a pattern of decreasing intensity as the distance from the glomerulus increases (38). Taken together, these results are consistent with a model in which smooth muscle cells in the kidney are generally capable of expressing renin during embryogenesis and lose this ability in the adult. Some specialized cells near the JG apparatus apparently retain the ability to "switch on" renin gene expression, possibly in response to expression of a locally produced factor which may itself be under tonic control by AII.

DETERMINANTS OF RENIN GENE EXPRESSION

Organization and Species Variation

The genes encoding mouse, rat, and human renins have been cloned and characterized (39–43). Their genomic organization and the deduced amino acid sequence of their encoded renins confirm the close relatedness of renin to other aspartyl proteinases. Human and rat genomes contain only one renin gene (41–44). In humans, the renin gene is located on the short arm of chromosome 1 at the q32 band (45), while in rats it is located on chromosome 13 at the q13 band (46). Mice must be subdivided into two categories (47); some strains have a single renin gene locus. In this case, the allele is referred to as Ren-1^{c} and is located on chromosome 1. Other strains of mice initially characterized as having high levels of renin in the submandibular gland (SMG) were subsequently found to have a duplicated renin gene locus adjacent to the *Ren-1* gene. In this case, the two loci are called *Ren-1*^{d} and *Ren-2*^{d}. *Ren-1*^{c}, *Ren-1*^{d}, and *Ren-2*^{d} are all expressed to approximately the same level in the kidney (48,49), while *Ren-2*^{d} is expressed at perhaps a hundred times the level of the *Ren-1* genes in the SMG (50). The differential pattern of expression of the mouse renin genes may be due to insertional elements in the DNA flanking their coding sequences (51,52).

Molecular Determinants of Renin Expression

The ability to generate transgenic animals expressing renin genes from various species has provided the most clear-cut information regarding the DNA sequences necessary for the tissue-specific expression of the renin genes. A gene fragment containing 2.5 kb of 5′-flanking DNA, all of the natural exons and introns, as well as 3 kb of 3′-flanking DNA of the mouse *Ren-2* gene has been reported to be appropriately expressed in the kidney of transgenic mice (53). Likewise, a *Ren-1*^{d} genomic DNA fragment including approximately 5 kb of 5′-flanking and 4 kb of 3′-flanking DNA also gives cell-type–specific expression in transgenic mice and contains DNA sequences that determine the minor differences in the tissue-distribution of expression of *Ren-1*^{c} and *Ren-1*^{d} (54). A human renin genomic DNA fragment containing as little as 900 bp of 5′-flanking and 400 bp of 3′-flanking DNA is also capable of driving JG cell-specific expression in mice (55). These experiments suggest that DNA sequences contained within the injected genomic DNA fragments are sufficient for directing tissue-specific expression of the renin genes. Experiments to more precisely define DNA sequences required for this expression have been limited: Sola et al. (56) have generated transgenic mice with a hybrid gene containing approximately 2.5 kb of mouse *Ren-2* 5′-flanking DNA linked to the coding sequences for the simian virus 40 large T antigen (an oncogene). However, in spite of the fact that a genomic DNA fragment containing the identical 5′-flanking DNA drives correct tissue-specific expression transgenic mice (53), the hybrid gene caused the appearance of tumors with a tissue distribution that did not match the expected pattern for renin (56). When a similar approach is used including approximately 4.6 kb of *Ren-2* 5′-flanking DNA, tumors are detected specifically in renin-expressing tissues (57). Why does tissue-specific expression of the genomic *Ren-2* gene only require 2.5 kb of flanking DNA while correct expression of the hybrid gene requires a much longer DNA fragment? One possible explanation for these results is that DNA sequences within 2.5 kb of the transcription start site of the mouse *Ren-2* gene participate in directing the expression of this gene but have to act in concert with additional DNA sequences (perhaps redundant) either farther upstream in 5′-flanking DNA or within the gene or 3′-flanking DNA to direct expression of *Ren-2* in the appropriate tissues.

Several groups have used the approach of introducing hybrid genes containing various portions of renin gene 5′-flanking DNA into tissue culture cells as a method to further define important gene control elements (47,58). While this approach has the advantage of being more rapid and less costly than generating transgenic animals, the conclusions to be drawn regarding the determinants of basal expression of the renin gene are also more limited. Such analyses carried out with relatively short DNA fragments of the mouse renin 5′-flanking DNAs (within 500 bp of the transcription start site) have led to the identification of putative stimulatory as well as inhibitory sequences (59–61). Evidence has also been presented for the interaction of tissue-specific (62) and species-specific (63) transcription factors with this region of the mouse gene 5′-flanking DNA. Nevertheless, it should be noted that the cells used to carry out these analyses do not express their endogenous renin genes and that a 2.5-kb fragment *Ren-2* 5′-flanking DNA is insufficient to drive tissue-specific expression in transgenic mice (56). Thus, the current studies regarding putative control elements in the mouse renin gene will need to be confirmed in transgenic animals.

A hybrid gene containing only 100 bp of human renin 5′-flanking DNA is accurately transcribed in prorenin-expressing human primary chorion cells (64), suggesting that at least some of the elements necessary for the tissue-specific expression of human renin are located very near the start site of transcription. Catanzaro and colleagues (65) have recently reported that this region of the human renin 5′-flanking DNA contains a short DNA sequence which is highly conserved in the analogous regions of the mouse and rat renin genes and binds a member of the POU family of homeotic transcription factors. They suggest that binding of different members of this transcription factor family might drive expression of the renin genes at different levels in different tissues and may also account for the observed modulation of renin gene expression during development. As with the mouse renin genes, however, it will be important to demonstrate that this region of the 5′-flanking DNA is sufficient to account for the observed tissue specificity in human renin gene expression using transgenic animals.

POSTTRANSLATIONAL MODIFICATION OF PRORENIN

Translation and Covalent Modification

In mice, rats, and humans, renin is synthesized as a protein precursor of 400 to 406 amino acids (44,66,67). A signal peptide encoded at the amino terminus directs the nascent polypeptides to the rough endoplasmic reticulum (RER). Upon insertion into the RER, the signal peptide is removed to generate prorenin, and posttranslational modification begins. There are two consensus sequences for N-glycosylation in human renin and three such sites in rat and mouse (*Ren-1*) renal renins (44,67,68). Curiously, mouse SMG renin (*Ren-2*) is devoid of potential glycosylation sites. The glycosylation sites on renin may be modified to different extents within the RER and Golgi lamellae, resulting in multiple species of renin and prorenin that can be separated by either isoelectric focusing or lectin affinity chromatography (69,70). In human renin, mannose residues on the carbohydrate side chains may also be partially phosphorylated (71), creating a classic lysosomal targeting signal. The importance of the glycosylation of prorenin and renin is most obvious in clearance of the protein from the circulation (72,73), although some evidence has accumulated that glycosylation may also affect intracellular transit time (74), efficiency of intracellular sorting (75), and stability (76) (protease sensitivity?) of prorenin. Rat prorenin can be fractionated into multiple isoelectric species even after enzymatic deglycosylation (77). In contrast, recombinant human prorenin in which the glycosylation sites have been eliminated by protein engineering migrates as a single isoelectric species (78), suggesting that human prorenin does not undergo covalent modifications other than *N*-glycosylation.

"Variant" Renins

Several "variant" renins have also been proposed: There have been several reports of intracellular generation of angiotensins (79). In the kidney, AII is abundant in the secretory granules of renin-expressing cells in the afferent arterioles (Fig. 3), suggesting that renin (and by inference ACE) can express its activity prior to secretion from the cell (80). In addition to intragranular renin, there have been occasional reports of cytoplasmic and membrane-bound renin activity (81,82), although the actual biochemical mechanism that would lead to their generation is still unclear. More striking is the finding that many cells produce what may be a specific renin-binding protein (RnBP). This protein was first demonstrated in whole kidney lysates, where a portion of the active renin is found in complex with a protein of roughly 40,000 molecular weight. Subsequently, cloning of the cDNAs encoding RnBP from pigs, rats, and humans has revealed some interesting features (83–86). First, the interaction of RnBP with active renin is species-specific and of high affinity (0.2 n*M* with porcine RnBP and renin) and results in the inactivation of renin. Second, the genes for RnBP do not encode an obvious signal peptide, suggesting that RnBP is a cytoplasmic protein. How this protein would interact with the renin generated within the secretory pathway remains a mystery. Finally, mRNA encoding RnBP is widely distributed in rat tissues, although the actual cellular site of production in the kidney and other tissues has not yet been reported. It is still possible, therefore, that RnBP plays a role in the tissue uptake or metabolism of active renin.

Intracellular Sorting of Prorenin

In Vivo Studies

Much of what we understand about the secretion of renin has been derived from ultrastructural studies on the JG cells of the kidney. These cells are modified smooth muscle cells that make up approximately 0.1% of the cellular mass of the adult kidney (87). Whike JG cells resemble other neuroendocrine cells in their rich cytoplasmic content of dense-core secretory granules, they are

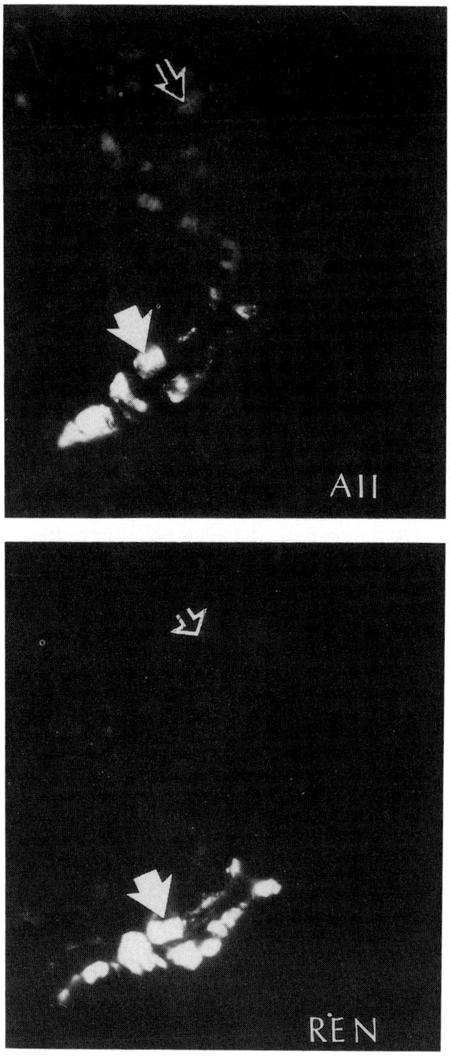

(A)

(B)

Figure 3 Colocalization of angiotensin II and renin in the juxtaglomerular cells of the kidney. Rat kidney cortex was stained using the fluorescein-labeled second antibody method with a specific antiserum for angiotensin II (A). Antibody conjugates were subsequently removed by a low pH wash and the section was restained with an antirenin antibody (B). Note that all AII-containing cells also contain renin immunoreactivity (solid arrowheads), while mesangial cells stain for angiotensin II but not renin (open arrowheads). (Courtesy of D. Ramla, IRCM, Montreal, Canada.)

distinguished from these other cell types by two rather striking characteristics. First, rhomboid, paracrystalline structures can be sometimes be seen budding off from the trans-Golgi network (TGN) and in membrane-bound structures within the cytoplasm. These structures are seen most frequently at times of high renin synthesis and may play a role in the overall mechanism of renin biosynthesis. Second, the secretory granules of JG cells are atypical and display many similarities to lysosomes. At the ultrastructural level, the electron-dense matrix of these granules is sometimes seen to contain multiple vesicular inclusions and membrane fragments; some micrographs suggest that these granules are capable of micropinocytosis and autophagy of other cellular organelles (88,89). The JG cell granules are also immunoreactive to antibodies against a number of lysosomal enzymes, including acid phosphatase, β-glucuronidase, arylsulfatase, *N*-acetyl-β-glucosaminidase, and cathepsins B, D, H, and L (89,90). These results, combined with the apparent lack of any recognizable, classic lysosomal structures, have led some investigators to suggest that JG cells do not contain the type of secretory granules seen in many endocrine cell types but rather have adapted lysosomes for the processing, storage, and secretion of prorenin (89).

Using antibodies to various portions of the human prorenin prosegment, Taugner and colleagues have demonstrated that the paracrystalline structures budding off from the TGN of JG cells contain prorenin (91). These structures, which have been called protogranules, subsequently fuse together to form a membrane-bound structure containing multiple protogranules, among which small round vesicles can be seen. The protogranules eventually lose their individual structures and fuse to form a relatively amorphous, low-density, membrane-bound vesicle, they have been termed the "immature" or "juvenile" secretory granules. It is within the immature granules that prorenin activation is thought to begin (see below). In some micrographs, these immature granules can be seen to fuse directly with the plasma membrane (89), which would presumably result in the release of partially activated prorenin and would correspond, therefore, to a "basal" pathway of secretion of both prorenin and active renin. Immature granules that are not released from the cell become progressively more electron-dense, possibly due to a second stage of aggregation which radiates from a central focal point. These structures have been referred to as "intermediate" granules. These most dense granules are referred to as "mature" granules and are frequently seen to contain inclusions which resemble bits of membrane or cellular organelles. Mature secretory granules contain only active renin. Taken together, these results suggest that the proteolytic activation of prorenin in the JG cells of the kidney occurs within maturing secretory granules and that JG cells are capable of releasing both prorenin and renin constitutively and active renin via the regulated release of mature secretory granules (Fig. 4).

In Vitro Studies

All mammalian cells possess the ability to secrete proteins via the constitutive secretory pathway in which proteins are directly exported to the cell surface from the TGN. Some specialized endocrine and neuroendocrine cells may also export proteins by the regulated secretory pathway. Proteins secreted in this manner are sorted at the TGN to dense-core secretory granules, and they are stored there until the cell receives a signal triggering their release. Little is known about the precise molecular signals that target proteins to dense-core secretory granules. However, the ability to direct the expression of heterologous proteins in cultured cells of various origins has enabled the definition of

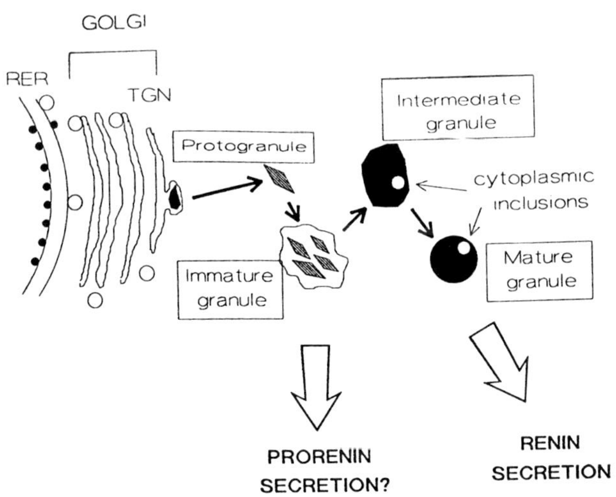

Figure 4 Proposed pathways of biosynthesis and secretion of prorenin and renin in the juxtaglomerular cells of the kidney. RER, rough endoplasmic reticulum; GOLGI, golgi lamellae; TGN, trans-Golgi network.

certain characteristics of the constitutive and regulated secretory pathways (92–94): (a) The constitutive secretory pathway is the "default" route for protein secretion from cells (i.e., there is no targeting signal other than the signal peptide necessary for secretion from this pathway). (b) Targeting information for the regulated secretory pathway (via secretory granules) is contained within the targeted protein. (c) Secretory granule targeting information is universal (i.e., recognized across species and tissue barriers) and dominant (i.e., fusion of a granule-targeted protein to one secreted constitutively will result in granule targeting of the hybrid). In spite of this apparent universal nature of the sorting machinery, there is no extended sequence homology between proteins sorted to granules. There is, in fact, no consensus regarding the actual mechanism of sorting, although models proposing a specific receptor in the TGN and selective aggregation of targeted proteins have been proposed (92,94,95).

In an effort to define the protein sequences responsible for targeting prorenin to secretory granules, recombinant expression vectors encoding prorenins from various species have been introduced into cell-culture models containing constitutive and regulated secretory pathways. Expression of either human prorenin (96,97), mouse *Ren-1* (98), mouse *Ren-2* (99), or rat prorenin (99) in mouse pituitary AtT-20 cells (which contain secretory granules and process endogenous POMC to ACTH and other peptides) leads to secretory-granule targeting of a portion of the expressed prorenin. In the case of the mouse *Ren-2* and human prorenins, activation also appears to occur in the granules. Human prorenin is also sorted to the regulated secretory pathway in PC12 rat pheochromocytoma cells (100) and rat somatomammotrophic GH4 cells (101), although in these two cases prorenin is not activated in granules. These results imply that prorenin must contain primary or higher-order structural information directing it to the regulated secretory pathway (secretory granules).

The finding that cells in tissue culture faithfully direct human prorenin to dense-core secretory granules has made it possible to study this intracellular event by modifying the expressed prorenins by site-directed mutagenesis. Neither the replacement of the native signal peptide of human prorenin with a signal peptide from a constitutively secreted immunoglobulin M (IgM) nor the elimination of the two glycosylation sites on human prorenin prevented its targeting to secretory granules in transfected AtT-20 cells (102). The dispensability of the carbohydrate residues for granule sorting is also evidenced by the fact that mouse *Ren-2* prorenin (which is naturally nonglycosylated) is sorted to granules in AtT-20 cells (98). The processing of prorenin to renin is also not required; prorenin molecules containing mutations in the paired basic amino acids at the native processing site cannot be activated in AtT-20 cells but are nevertheless sorted to the regulated pathway and released as prorenin in response to secretagogues (103). In addition, regulated secretion of prorenin is seen in transfected PC12 and GH4 cells, which contain granules but apparently lack a processing enzyme capable of activating prorenin (100,101). Finally, the prosegment can also be deleted from human prorenin, and the resulting "prerenin" is secreted in a regulated manner in both PC12 and AtT-20 cells (100,102,104). By deduction, a sorting signal would appear to be located within the protein domain corresponding to active renin.

As previously mentioned, there is no obvious linear homology between the putative sorting peptide in the human prorenin prosegment and peptide sequences contained within other proteins destined for the secretory granule, such as POMC, growth hormone, insulin and atrial natriuretic factor (T. L. Reudelhuber; unpublished results). This result suggests that potential homologies in secretory granule sorting peptides may either be in secondary or tertiary structure rather than the linear amino acid sequence. Alternatively, multiple sorting receptors may exist or a given sorting receptor may have the capacity to interact with a wide spectrum of binding sequences, thereby restricting homologies to subsets of secretory granule sorted proteins. Discrimination between these possibilities will likely have to await the further characterization of minimal sorting peptides in both prorenin and other proteins secreted by the regulated pathway.

In summary, results to date suggest the following regarding the secretory granule targeting machinery for renin: First, the sorting of prorenin to granules and/or its retention in the maturing granules is not quantitative, either in the JG cells of the kidney or in tissue culture models. In both cases, as much as 80% of the prorenin may be secreted in the inactive form by either the constitutive or basal pathway. Second, since the targeting of prorenin to secretory granules can occur in the absence of its proteolytic processing, these two intracellular events appear to be independent. Moreover, since intracellular cleavage of prorenin has not been reported in the absence of targeting to secretory granules, it is likely that targeting precedes processing. This latter conclusion is also supported by immunoelectron microscopic studies of JG cells, in which prorenin disappears (is cleaved to renin) in the maturing granule. Third, the signal(s) responsible for directing prorenin to secretory granules appears to be functional in cultured endocrine cell types from a variety of tissues and species, suggesting that it shares some homology (not yet evident) to secretory granule targeting sequences with other granule resident proteins.

Proteolytic Processing of Prorenin

In Vivo Studies

Antibodies specific for the prosegment of human prorenin stain predominantly protogranules and immature granules and show little or no staining of intermediate and mature granules (91). In contrast, an antibody that reacts with both prorenin and renin stains all of these granular structures (91). These results suggest that the proteolytic activation of prorenin occurs after secretory granule targeting, at early stage of granule maturation. Release of immature granules may account for "constitutive-like" or "basal" release not only of prorenin but also of small amounts of active renin. The role of the secretory granule in processing prorenin is further supported by biochemical studies: granule fractions purified from kidney homogenates contain predominantly active renin (105). In addition, renin is secreted more slowly than prorenin from human renal cortical slices and with kinetics that are consistent with its storage in secretory granules (106), and pharmacological stimuli that cause a release of secretory granules result in an acute and preferential release of active renin into the circulation (107).

Amino-terminal sequencing of renin isolated from human kidney lysates suggests that activation occurs by the proteolytic removal of a 43–amino acid prosegment from the amino terminus of prorenin (108). This processing site follows a pair of basic amino acids in human renin. Processing of prorenin in the mouse SMG gland occurs at the analogous position (109), but processing of rat renal renin seems to occur after a threonine residue located 7 amino acids toward the carboxyl terminus relative to the analogous position in human renin (77,110). The proteolytic cleavage site of mouse renal prorenin is currently unknown. Rat renal and mouse SMG renins subsequently undergo an additional internal processing event, converting "one-chain" active renin to a "two-chain" molecule (77,109,110) in which the two halves are held together by a disulfide bridge. It is not known whether mouse renal renin also undergoes a similar secondary cleavage. Notably, while renal renins appear to be processed within secretory granules, mouse SMG renin may be processed to one-chain renin within the Golgi apparatus and only a portion of the protein is further processed in granules to yield the two-chain protein (111). Thus, while renins from mice, rats, and humans share many similarities in protein structure and function, differences exist in the way these proteins are modified within the secretory apparatus.

In Vitro Studies

Activation of prorenin may occurr by a variety of means. In vitro, acidification (112) or prolonged storage in the cold (113) of purified prorenin can result in its partial and reversible activation in the absence of proteolysis, presumably due to an unfolding of the prosegment and exposure of the active site of the enzyme. Prorenin can also be irreversibly activated by the proteolytic removal of its prosegment. Studies carried out with purified recombinant human prorenin suggest that proteolytic removal of the complete prosegment is not necessary to derive active renin (114,115).

In the human kidney, cleavage of prorenin is highly specific and occurs at a pair of basic amino acids (Lys-Arg), resulting in removal of a 43–amino acid prosegment from the amino terminus of prorenin (6). There are six additional pairs of basic amino acids in human prorenin (68)—including Lys-Lys, Arg-Arg, and Arg-Lys within the body of renin; two Lys-Arg pairs in the prosegment; and the Lys-Lys-Arg triplet in the body of renin; none of these appear to be cleaved in the kidney. AtT-20 cells transfected with a human preprorenin expression vector also cleave prorenin at the same site as that reported for renin purified from human kidney lysates (96). Many proteases are capable of activating human prorenin in vitro, including trypsin, plasmin, tissue and plasma kallikreins, and cathepsin B (7,116,117). While most of these enzymes are likely to be physiologically irrelevant due to their tissue distribution, nevertheless some cleave prorenin with the correct site specificity (114). One hypothesis to explain the cleavage-site selectivity displayed by enzymes in vitro, AtT-20 cells, and the kidney is that primary and/or higher-order structural determinants on prorenin render the native processing site uniquely sensitive to proteolytic cleavage. This hypothesis was directly tested by introducing single amino acid mutations in human preprorenin surrounding the natural cleavage site and expressing the resultant recombinant proteins to proteolytic activation either by trypsin or by the endogenous processing enzyme in AtT-20 cells (118). The results suggest that amino acids, in addition to the pair of basic amino acids surrounding the cleavage site, affect the ability of both trypsin and the AtT-20 processing enzyme to cleave prorenin. Notably, while a proline at position -4 is essential for processing of human prorenin in AtT-20 cells and is correlated with predicted formation of a β-turn at this position, other site-directed mutations suggest that this structural feature in addition to a pair of basic amino acids is not sufficient to lead to proteolytic activation of prorenin (118). In contrast to the case with human prorenin, neither mouse renal prorenin (99) nor rat prorenin (99,119) are processed at the analogous positions in transfected AtT-20 cells. In both cases, mutagenesis of the natural substrates has demonstrated that this is also due to the particular arrangement of amino acids immediately adjacent to the native processing site (96,99,118,120).

Although many of the enzymes which activate human prorenin in vitro may be physiologically irrelevant, there are some notable exceptions: Do et al. recently characterized an enzyme from human whole-kidney lysates which correctly processes human prorenin to active renin (121). Subsequent purification and partial amino acid sequencing of this putative prorenin processing enzyme (PPE) revealed that it is cathepsin B (117). While cathepsin B is a lysosomal enzyme expressed in a broad variety of cell types (122), it appears to colocalize with renin not only in the lysosome-like granules of JG cells (89,90) but also in the more classic secretory granules of prorenin-containing human pituitary lactotrophs (123). In vitro, cathepsin B cleaves human prorenin with the correct specificity and with a Km in the nanomolar range (117). For these reasons, cathepsin B has been proposed as the renal PPE. In a similar effort, an enzyme capable of processing mouse SMG prorenin (the product of the *Ren-2* gene) has been isolated from submaxillary glands (124). This enzyme, which has been called PRECE, was subsequently revealed to be identical to the mGK-13 gene product (125) (also known as the epidermal growth factor–binding protein type B), a member of the kallikrein gene family. While PRECE can activate mouse SMG prorenin to generate one-chain renin, it is unable to carry out the second cleavage to yield the two-chain form (124). In addition, kidney glandular kallikrein cannot activate mouse SMG prorenin, and PRECE is unable to activate mouse renal or human prorenins (124). Recently, a second enzyme capable of converting moused SMG prorenin to one-chain renin has also been isolated from mouse submaxillary gland (126).

As an alternative approach to biochemical purification and in vitro testing of candidate PPEs, cell culture transfection assays have been developed to directly test for the ability of candidate processing enzymes to cleave prorenin within the appropriate intracellular environment. When human prorenin is cotransfected into rat pituitary GH4C1 cells (which contain secretory granules but are normally unable to activate human prorenin) with an expression vector encoding the mouse subtilisin-like endoprotease PC1, the cells are rendered capable of selectively processing prorenin at the identical site as that reported for the human kidney. Interestingly, this processing event does not occur in cells devoid of secretory granules (CHO and BSC-40) and is not due to any apparent differences in processing of PC1 in these cell types (119). When tested in a similar assay, neither furin (101), PC2 (119), nor human cathepsin B (C. Mercure and T. Reudelhuber; unpublished) are able to process human prorenin. In a similar assay, mouse SMG prorenin is correctly processed by mouse PC1 (127), and mouse PC6 (also called PC5) (128); it is not processed by furin (129). As of this date, there have been no published reports of enzymes capable of activating either mouse renal prorenin (*Ren-1*) or rat prorenin.

Transgenic Studies

As mentioned above, rat renal renin does not have the same amino terminus as human renal renin (77,110), and the amino terminus of active mouse renal renin is still unknown. This, combined with the species specificity of some of the PPEs described above, raises the possibility that species-specific differences exist in the processing enzymes that activate prorenins. In contrast to these findings is the experience of expressing prorenins from various species in transgenic animals. Ohkubo et al. have expressed rat renin in ectopic tissues of transgenic mice by placing the prorenin coding sequences under the control of a mouse metallothionein gene promoter (130). Mating of the rat prorenin-expressing mouse strain with another strain which had been rendered transgenic for rat angiotensinogen resulted in a "double transgenic" strain with elevated blood pressure (130). As only mice containing both of the rat transgenes had elevated pressures, the implication is that the rat prorenin had been activated in the mouse tissues, although the tissue site of activation was not determined. In similar approaches, injection of either mouse (55,131) or rat (132) embryos with the intact human prorenin gene resulted in the generation of transgenic animals with active human renin in their circulation. Thus, in spite of the apparent species selectivity of PPE activities reported in vitro, the rodent kidney probably expresses an enzyme(s) capable of activating prorenins from rats, mice, and humans.

Some experiments suggest that tissues in addition to the kidney may be able to activate prorenin and use it to generate AII locally. Mullins et al. have generated transgenic rats with a genomic mouse Ren-2 gene (133). These rats, which express both the endogenous rat renin as well as mouse SMG renin, are severely hypertensive even though expression of the mouse transgene is virtually undetectable in their kidneys. Active mouse renin was also undetectable in the circulation of the transgenic rats, although mouse prorenin was present. Notably, the mouse transgene was expressed at high levels in the adrenals and was detectable in other tissues such as brain. Could renin be generated within tissues such as the adrenal and act locally to produce AI? In support of this possibility is the finding that explants of normal human adrenal and various adrenal tumors secrete small but detectable amounts of active renin when placed in organ culture (134,135).

GENES OF THE RAS AND THE GENETICS OF CARDIOVASCULAR DISEASE

Linkage of the Renin Gene with Hypertension in Animal Models and Humans

Because of the obvious involvement of the RAS in the pathophysiology of hypertension and other cardiovascular diseases, several groups have undertaken studies to determine whether mutations in the renin gene might be causally related to the etiology of some of these diseases. Genetic analysis in both humans and laboratory animals suggests that blood pressure modulation is a polygenic trait involving at least four to five genes in addition to numerous environmental factors (136–138). Several strains of laboratory rats and mice have been developed that display inheritable hypertension, lending support to the implication of a genetic element. Dahl and colleagues (136) have used selective breeding to derive rats that develop hypertension when maintained on a high-sodium diet (Dahl S or salt-sensitive rats), while their "control" counterparts, the salt-resistant rats (R), remain normotensive on the same diet. Rapp and colleagues have inbred the original stocks of Dahl S and R rats (139) and have used selective cross-breeding of these inbred strains to examine the role of the renin gene locus in this form of hypertension (140). The renin gene alleles in the inbred S and R strains can be distinguished by a restriction fragment length polymorphism (RFLP) detected by the enzyme BglII. Naturally, all of the progeny of a cross between the S and R strains are heterozygous for the S and R renin alleles (Fig. 5; F_1 generation). Interbreeding of the F_1 generation yields a second generation (the F_2 generation), which now displays the expected Mendelian distribution for the S and R renin gene alleles. Blood pressure measurements performed on lightly anesthetized rats using a tail cuff revealed that those rats homozygous for the S renin gene allele have a mean blood pressure that is 20 mmHg higher than that of rats homozygous for the R renin gene allele (Fig. 5), while those heterozygous for the two alleles have an intermediate blood pressure. It is notable that the blood pressures seen in the ren^S/ren^S rats of the F_2 generation did not attain the levels seen in the original inbred S strain (171 mmHg vs. 210 mmHg, respectively). Moreover, the cross-bred rats required maintenance on a high-sodium diet for longer periods of time than the inbred strain to achieve maximal blood pressure increases (12 vs. 8 weeks, respectively). As it has been previously estimated that two to four independent loci account for the blood pressure differences between the S and R strains (141), these differences may reflect the obviously mixed genetic backgrounds in the F_2 generation.

The important contribution of genetic background on the cosegregation of renin gene alleles with blood pressure in inbred Dahl rats has been supported by other breeding experiments. When F_1 progeny of a cross between the inbred S and the R strains are crossed with the parental inbred R strain (back-crossed), there is no correlation between the segregation of the renin alleles and

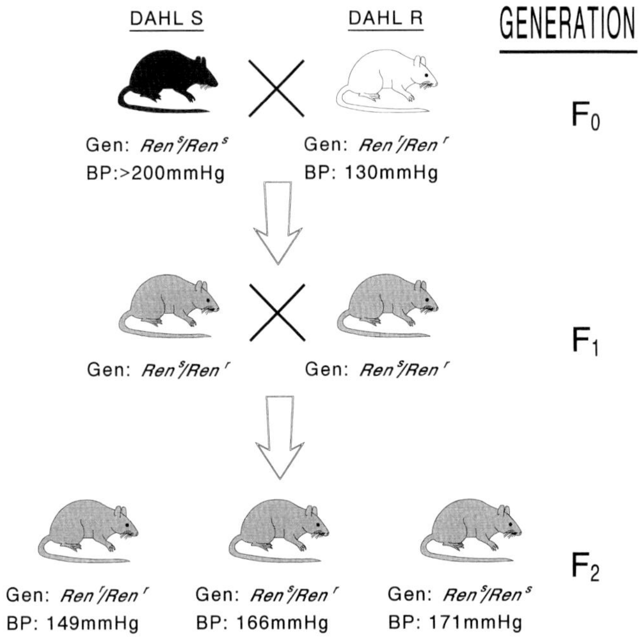

Figure 5 Strategy used to test for association of the renin gene with elevations in blood pressure in inbred laboratory rat strains. BP, the systolic blood pressure in male rats as determined by the tail cuff method; Gen, genotype; *Ren*^{r} and *Ren*^{s}, the renin alleles of the Dahl salt-resistant (S) and salt-sensitive (R) rats, respectively. (From Ref. 140.)

salt-induced hypertension (142). In contrast, crossing of the F_1 generation with the inbred S parental strain yields the previously mentioned correlation. While all of the aforementioned studies have been carried out using inbred strains of Dahl rats, the renin allele distribution in the original outbred Dahl rats show a less obvious linkage to blood pressure. The outbred salt-resistant rat is indeed homozygous for the same R renin allele as the inbred strain, but the salt-sensitive rats display a random distribution of the S and R alleles as well as an additional renin gene allele named Z (143). Molecular analysis of the cloned S and R renin genes alleles has shown that the BglII polymorphism is due to an insertion/deletion in the first intron of the gene (144). More recently, Rapp and coworkers have identified at least seven different alleles of the renin gene in laboratory strains of rats based on insertion/deletions in intron 1 (145). However, no obvious differences have yet been found between the two renin gene alleles or their encoded proteins that might explain the salt-induced blood pressure differences between the S and R strains of Dahl rats (146).

Using an approach similar to that use in the analysis with Dahl rats, Kurtz and colleagues have determined that the renin gene allele of the spontaneously hypertensive rats (SHR) co-segregates with an increase in catheter-measured mean arterial pressure (MAP) in the F_2 generation of crosses with the normotensive Lewis rat strain (147). As in the study of the Dahl/Rapp rats, the RFLP used in this study was also a BglII polymorphism which is due to a varying repeat in the first intron of the renin gene, suggesting that such a polymorphism can be linked to hypertension even in the absence of a high-salt diet. Perhaps surprisingly, the SHR-linked renin allele most closely resembles the R renin allele in Dahl rats, which in the aforementioned studies was correlated with normal blood pressure. In further contrast to the case with the inbred Dahl rats, the greatest increase in blood pressure was seen in rats of the F_2 generation, which were heterozygous for the SHR renin gene allele (147). Using a similar approach, Lindpaintner et al. (148) have analyzed the segregation of the renin allele from stroke-prone spontaneously hypertensive rat (SPSHR) in cross-breeding experiments with the normotensive WKY strain. Analysis of rats in the F_2 generation showed no correlation between transmission of the SPSHR renin allele and either systolic or diastolic pressure, heart rate, responses of blood pressure to either stress or dietary sodium, plasma renin activity, ventricular hypertrophy, or tissue water content. In cross-breeding experiments using the Lyon hypertensive (LH) rat strain, a microsatellite marker in the LH renin gene allele cosegregates with an increment in diastolic pressure in the F_2 generation of crosses with the normotensive (LN) rat strain (149).

In humans, there is also strong evidence of familial predisposition to hypertension (138,150). Numerous studies have tested for cosegregation of polymorphisms in the human renin gene with hypertension in the general population. To date, however, population studies have not established linkage of the renin gene with human hypertension (151–153). In an effort to overcome some of the inherent complications of population studies, Jeunemaitre et al. (154) have undertaken a study of renin gene linkage to hypertension among siblings with hypertensive parents. In this approach, the frequency of various polymorphisms within the general population is determined and the probability that two siblings will share a given allele is then calculated. If the observed frequency of allele sharing between affected siblings is significantly higher than the calculated value, linkage is predicted to be positive. This approach, termed sib-pair linkage, is more likely to uncover a genetic linkage in a complex multifactorial disease due to a reduction in the randomization of the gene pool. Jeunemaitre et al. (154) used combinations of three RFLPs (TaqI, HinfI, and HindIII) to define eight allelic variants of the human renin gene. Sib-pair linkage analysis was performed on siblings from 57 families in which subjects displayed sustained hypertension of early onset. However, sharing of alleles among the hypertensive siblings did not occur at a frequency higher than that predicted to occur by random segregation (154).

In conclusion, there is evidence for renin gene linkage in some animal models of genetically determined hypertension, but this linkage is extremely sensitive to the genetic background of the host animal and may be manifest in different ways (systolic, diastolic, mean arterial, or pulse pressure). In humans, linkage has not been established, although studies using restricted ethnic groups and families to reduce the complexity of the gene pool have perhaps not been adequately pursued. In addition, the use techniques for detection of polymorphic variations that are more sensitive than RFLP analysis (155,156) may significantly refine current analyses.

Other RAS Genes and Cardiovascular Disease

While it has been difficult to establish linkage of the human renin gene to hypertension, analysis of the genes encoding other components of the RAS (Fig. 1) has yielded more positive results. In a sib-pair linkage study similar to that described above for renin, a significant association was established between a polymorphism in the human angiotensinogen gene and hypertension (157). In addition, while studies have not established linkage of polymorphisms in the genes encoding either human ACE or the human At1 AII receptor with hypertension (158,159), a polymorphism in the human ACE gene is linked to increased risk for myocardial infarction (160). In contrast, in some genetic animal models of hypertension, a microsatellite marker near the ACE gene appears to cosegregate with increased blood pressure (161–163). These results confirm the role of the RAS as an inheritable component of cardiovascular pathologies and reinforce the possibility that mutations within or near the renin gene may play a role in more restricted subtypes of cardiovascular disease.

FUTURE PERSPECTIVES

Although it will soon be 100 years since Tigerstedt and Bergman reported that a saline extract of rabbit kidney could raise blood pressure (164), renin and the components of the RAS have not yet finished revealing their secrets. While there is an indisputable role of the circulating RAS in the modulation of blood pressure, the interaction of this system with the components of the various tissue RAS remains largely a matter of conjecture. In particular, the components of the RAS within the kidney have been suggested to play a key role not only in blood pressure modulation but also in the microvascular pathology associated with chronic renal disease (165). Perhaps even more perplexing, however, is the role of the RAS in various nonrenal tissues. This question is rendered all the more fascinating in light of the fact that, to date, no one has reported a case of mutations that would eliminate expression of renin in mammals. It is interesting to speculate that the RAS plays some important role in gestational development of mammals which is no longer evident in adults. For example, activation of any given tRAS might only require transient expression of a prorenin processing enzyme and the generated angiotensin peptides might function not only in regulating local circulation but also perhaps in acting as chemoattractants for cell migration or as angiogenic or generalized growth factors. Such a model might serve to explain the high levels of renin gene expression seen in early gestational sacs in humans (166) and the fluctuating levels of renin gene expression seen in tissues of the developing mouse (37). The ability to selectively "knock out" specific genes in the mouse genome (167) should enable the testing of such a hypothesis in the near future.

ACKNOWLEDGMENTS

The author would like to thank Dr. Djamel Ramla for the provision of immunohistochemical data presented in this publication and Dr. K. W. Gross for his reading of the manuscript and insightful comments. This work was supported by a grant from the Medical Research Council of Canada to the Multidisciplinary Research Group on Hypertension. T.L.R. is the recipient of the Merck-Frosst Chair in Clinical and Molecular Pharmacology.

REFERENCES

1. Lindpaintner K, Ganten D. Tissue renin-angiotensin systems and their modulation: The heart as a paradigm for new aspects of converting enzyme inhibition. Cardiology 1991; 79(suppl 1):32–44.
2. Griendling KK, Murphy TJ, Alexander RW. Molecular biology of the renin-angiotensin system. Circulation 1993; 87:1816–1828.
3. Danser AH, van den Dorpel MA, Deinum J, et al. Renin, prorenin, and immunoreactive renin in vitreous fluid from eyes with and without diabetic retinopathy. J Clin Endocrinol Metab 1989; 68:160–167.
4. Neuringer JR, Brenner BM. Hemodynamic theory of progressive renal disease: A 10-year update in brief review. Am J Kidney Dis 1993; 22:98–104.
5. Campbell DJ, Kladis A, Skinner SL, Whitworth JA. Characterization of angiotensin peptides in plasma of anephric man. J Hypertens 1991; 9:265–274.
6. Do YS, Shinegawa T, Tam S, et al. Characterization of pure human renal renin: Evidence for a subunit structure. J Biol Chem 1987; 262:1037–1043.
7. Hsueh WA, Baxter JD. Human prorenin. Hypertension 1991; 17:469–479.
8. Lenz T, Sealy JE, Lappe RW, et al. Infusion of recombinant human prorenin into rhesus monkeys: Effects on hemodynamics, renin-angiotensin-aldosterone axis and plasma testosterone. Am J Hypertens 1990; 3:257–261.
9. Lenz T, Sealey JE, Maack T, et al. Half-life, hemodynamic, renal, and hormonal effects of prorenin in cynomolgus monkeys. Am J Physiol 1991; 260:R804–R810.
10. Paul M, Wagner J, Dzau VJ. Gene expression of the renin-angiotensin system in human tissues: Quantitative analysis by the polymerase chain reaction. J Clin Invest 1993; 91:2058–2064.
11. Mulrow PJ. Adrenal renin: A possible local regulator of aldosterone production. Yale J Biol Med 1989; 62:503–510.
12. Ganong WF, Deschepper CF, Steele MK, Intebi A. Renin-angiotensin system in the anterior pituitary of the rat. Am J Hypertens 1989; 2:320–322.
13. Ganong WF. Angiotensin II in the brain and pituitary: Contrasting roles in the regulation of adenohypophyseal secretion. Horm Res 1989; 31:24–31.
14. Sealey JE, Rubattu S. Prorenin and renin as separate mediators of tissue and circulating systems. Am J Hypertens 1989; 2:358–366.
15. Hosoi M, Kim S, Tabata T, et al. Evidence for the presence of differently glycosylated forms of prorenin in the plasma of anephric man. J Clin Endocrinol Metab 1992; 74:680–684.
16. Suzuki F, Ludwig G, Hellmann W, et al. Renin gene expression in rat tissues: a new quantitative assay method for rat renin mRNA using synthetic cRNA. Clin Exp Hypertens 1988; 10:345–359.
17. Kim S, Hosoi M, Nakajima K, Yamamoto K. Immunological evidence that kidney is primary source of circulating inactive prorenin in rats. Am J Physiol 1991; 260:E526–536.
18. Nussberger J, Flückiger J-P, Hui KY, et al. Angiotensin I and II disappear completely from circulating blood within 48 hours after binephrectomy: Improved measurement of angiotensins in rat plasma. J Hypertens 1991; 9(suppl 6):S230–S231.
19. Campbell DJ, Ziogas J, Kladis A. Metabolism of tetradecapeptide, angiotensinogen and angiotensin I and II by isolated perfused rat hindlimbs. Clin Exp Pharmacol Physiol 1990; 17:335–350.

20. Kuczera M, Hilgers KF, Lisson C, et al. Local angiotensin formation in hindlimbs of uremic hypertensive and renovascular hypertensive rats.J Hypertens 1991; 9:41–48.
21. Hilgers KF, Hilgenfeldt U, Veelken R, et al. Angiotensinogen is cleaved to angiotensin in isolated rat blood vessels. Hypertension 1993; 21:1030–1034.
22. Kato H, Iwai N, Inui H, et al. Regulation of vascular angiotensin release. Hypertension 1993; 21:446–454.
23. von Lutterotti N, Catanzaro DF, Sealey JE, Laragh JH. Renin is not synthesized by cardiac and extrarenal vascular tissues: A review of experimental evidence (see comments). Circulation 1994; 89:458–470.
24. Danser AHJ, Sassen LMA, Admiraal PJJ, et al. Regional production of angiotensins I and II: Contribution of vascular kidney-derived renin. J Hypertens 1991; 9(suppl 6):S234–S235.
25. Ingelfinger JR, Zuo WM, Fon EA, et al. In situ hybridization evidence for angiotensinogen messenger RNA in the rat proximal tubule: An hypothesis for the intrarenal renin angiotensin system. J Clin Invest 1990; 85:417–423.
26. Hackenthal E, Metz R, Bührle CP, and Taugner R. Intrarenal and intracellular distribution of renin and angiotensin. Kidney Int 1987; 20(suppl):S4–S17.
27. Gomez RA, Lynch KR, Chevalier RL, et al. Renin and angiotensinogen gene expression and intrarenal renin distribution during ACE inhibition. Am J Physiol 1988; 254:F900–F906.
28. Deschepper CF, Mellon SH, Cumin F, et al. Analysis by immunocytochemistry and in situ hybridization of renin and its mRNA in kidney, testis, adrenal, and pituitary of the rat. Proc Natl Acad Sci USA 1986; 83:7552–7556.
29. Gasc JM, Monnot C, Clauser E, Corvol P. Co-expression of Type 1 angiotensin II receptor (AT1R) and renin mRNAs in juxtaglomerular cells of the rat kidney. Endocrinology 1993; 132:2723–2725.
30. Kakinuma Y, Fogo A, Inagami T, Ichikawa I. Intrarenal localization of angiotensin II type 1 receptor mRNA in the rat. Kidney Int 1993; 43:1229–1235.
31. Paxton WG, Runge M, Horaist C, et al. Immunohistochemical localization of rat angiotensin II AT1 receptor. Am J Physiol 1993; 264:F989–F995.
32. Dzau VJ, Ingelfinger JR. Molecular biology and pathophysiology of the intrarenal renin-angiotensin system. J Hypertens 1989; 7:S3–S8.
33. Ichikawi I, Harris RC. Angiotensin actions in the kidney: Renewed insight into the old hormone (review). Kidney Int 1991; 40:583–596.
34. Gomez RA, Chevalier RL, Carey RM, Peach MJ. Molecular biology of the renal renin-angiotensin system (review). Kidney Int 1990; 30(suppl):S18–S23.
35. Burns KD, Homma T, Harris RC. The intrarenal renin-angiotensin system (review). Semin Nephrol 1993; 13:13–30.
36. Gomez RA, Lynch KR, Sturgill BC, et al. Distribution of renin mRNA and its protein in the developing kidney. Am J Physiol 1989; 257:F850–F858.
37. Jones CA, Sigmund CD, McGowan RA, et al. Expression of murine renin genes during fetal development. Mol Endocrinol 1990; 4:375–383.
38. Gomez RA, Chevalier RL, Everett AD, et al. Recruitment of renin gene-expressing cells in adult rat kidneys. Am J Physiol 1990; 259:F660–F665.
39. Holm I, Ollo R, Panthier J, Rougeon F. Evolution of aspartyl proteases by gene duplication: The mouse renin gene is organized in two homologous clusters of four exons. EMBO J 1984; 3:557–562.
40. Fukamizu A, Nishi K, Cho T, et al. Structure of the rat renin gene. J Mol Biol 1988; 201:443–450.
41. Hobart PM, Fogliano M, O'Connor BA, et al. Human renin gene: Structure and sequence analysis. Proc Natl Acad Sci USA 1984; 81:5026–5030.
42. Miyazaki H, Fukamizu A, Hirose S, et al. Structure of the human renin gene. Proc Natl Acad Sci USA 1984; 81:5999–6003.
43. Hardman JA, Hort YJ, Catanzaro DF, et al. Primary structure of the human renin gene. DNA 1984; 3:457–468.
44. Burnham CE, Hawelu-Johnson CL, Frank BM, Lynch KR. Molecular cloning of rat renin cDNA and its gene. Proc Natl Acad Sci USA 1987; 84:5605–5609.
45. Cohen-Haguenauer O, Soubrier F, Van Cong N, et al. Regional mapping of the human renin gene to 1q32 by in situ hybridization. Ann Genet 1989; 32:16–20.
46. Mori M, Ishizaki K, Serikawa T, Yamada J. Instability of the minisatellite sequence in the first intron of the rat renin gene and localization of the gene to chromosome 13q13 between FH and PEPC loci. J Hered 1992; 83:204–207.
47. Sigmund CD, Gross KW. Structure, expression, and regulation of the murine renin genes (review). Hypertension 1991; 18:446–457.
48. Field LJ, Gross KW. Ren-1 and Ren-2 loci are expressed in mouse kidney. Proc Natl Acad Sci USA 1985; 82;6196–6200.
49. Fabian JR, Field LJ, McGowan RA, et al. Allele-specific expression of the murine Ren-1 genes. J Biol Chem 1989; 264:17589–17594.

50. Field LJ, McGowan RA, Dickinson DP, Gross KW. Tissue and gene specificity of mouse renin expression. Hypertension 1984; 6:597–603.
51. Panthier JJ, Dreyfus M, Roux TL, Rougeon F. Mouse kidney and submaxillary gland renin genes differ in their 5′ putative regulatory sequences. Proc Natl Acad Aci USA 1984; 81:5489–5493.
52. Field LJ, Philbrick WM, Howles PN, et al. Expression of tissue-specific Ren-1 and Ren-2 genes of mice: Comparative analysis of 5′-proximal flanking regions. Mol Cell Biol 1984; 4:2321–2331.
53. Tronik D, Dreyfus M, Babinet C, Rougeon F. Regulated expression of the Ren-2 gene in transgenic mice derived from parental strains carrying only the Ren-1 gene. EMBO J 1987; 6:983–987.
54. Mullins JJ, Sigmund CD, Kane-Haas C, et al. Expression of the DBA/2J Ren-2 gene in the adrenal gland of transgenic mice. (Erratum appears in EMBO J 1990; 9:972.) EMBO J 1989; 8:4065–4072.
55. Sigmund CD, Jones CA, Kane CM, et al. Regulated tissue- and cell-specific expression of the human renin gene in transgenic mice. Circ Res 1992; 70:1070–1079.
56. Sola C, Tronik D, Dreyfus M, et al. Renin-promoter SV40 large T-antigen transgenes induce tumors irrespective of normal cellular expression of renin genes. Oncogene Res 1989; 5:149–153.
57. Sigmund CD, Jones CA, Fabian JR, et al. Tissue and cell specific expression of a renin promoter-reporter gene construct in transgenic mice. Biochem Biophys Res Commun 1990; 170:344–350.
58. Morris BJ. Molecular biology of renin. II: Gene control by messenger RNA, transfection and transgenic studies (review). J Hypertens 1992; 10:337–342.
59. Paul M, Burt DW, Krieger JE, et al. Tissue specificity of renin promoter activity and regulation in mice. Am J Physiol 1992; 262:E644–E650.
60. Horiuchi M, Pratt RE, Nakamura N, Dzau VJ. Distinct nuclear proteins competing for an overlapping sequence of cyclic adenosine monophosphate and negative regulatory elements regulate tissue-specific mouse renin gene expression. J Clin Invest 1993; 92:1805–1811.
61. Barrett G, Horiuchi M, Paul M, et al. Identification of a negative regulatory element involved in tissue-specific expression of mouse renin genes. Proc Natl Acad Sci USA 1992; 89:885–889.
62. Horiuchi M, Nakamura N, Tang SS, et al. Molecular mechanism of tissue-specific regulation of mouse renin gene expression by cAMP: Identification of an inhibitory protein that binds nuclear transcriptional factor. J Biol Chem 1991; 266:16247–16254.
63. Loudon JA, Fukamizu A, Murakami K, Morris BJ. Species differences in binding of submandibular nuclear proteins to renin promoter DNA. Clin Exp Pharmacol Physiol 1993; 20:283–288.
64. Duncan KG, Haidar MA, Baxter JD, Reudelhuber TI. Regulation of human renin expression in chorion cell primary cultures. Proc Natl Acad Sci USA 1990; 87:7588–7592.
65. Sun J, Oddoux C, Lazarus A, et al. Promoter activity of human renin 5′-flanking DNA sequences is activated by the pituitary-specific transcription factor Pit-1. J Biol Chem 1993; 268:1505–1508.
66. Murakami K, Hirose S, Miyazaki H, et al. Complementary DNA sequences of renin: State-of-the-art review. Hypertension 1984; 6:95–100.
67. Panthier JJ, Rougeon F. Kidney and submaxillary gland renins are encoded by two non-allelic genes in Swiss mice. EMBO J 1983; 2:675–678.
68. Imai T, Miyazaki H, Hirose S, et al. Cloning and sequence analysis of cDNA for human renin precursor. Proc Natl Acad Sci USA 1983; 80:7405–409.
69. Katz SA, Marvin RL, Lee J, et al. Analysis of active renin heterogeneity. Proc Soc Exp Biol Med 1991; 197:387–392.
70. Hosoi M, Kim S, Yamamoto K. Evidence for heterogeneity of glycosylation of human renin obtained by using lectins. Clin Sci 1991; 81:393–399.
71. Faust PL, Chirgwin JM, Kornfeld S. Renin, a secretory glycoprotein, acquires phosphomannosyl residues. J Cell Biol 1987; 105:1947–1955.
72. Shier DN, Malvin RL. Differential secretion and removal of multiple renin forms. Am J Physiol 1985; 249:R79–R84.
73. Kim S, Hiruma M, Ikemoto F, Yamamoto K. Importance of glycosylation for hepatic clearance of renal renin. Am J Physiol 1988; 255:E642–E651.
74. Paul M, Nakamura N, Pratt RE, Dzau VJ. Glycosylation influences intracellular transit time and secretion rate of human prorenin in transfected cells. J Hypertens 1988; 6:S487–S489.
75. Baxter JD, James MN, Chu WN, et al. The molecular biology of human renin and its gene. Yale J Biol Med 1989; 62:493–501.
76. Hori H, Yoshino T, Ishizuka Y, et al. Role of N-linked oligosaccharides attached to human renin expressed in COS cells. FEBS Lett 1988; 232:391–394.
77. Kim S, Hosoi M, Kikuchi N, Yamamoto K. Amino-terminal amino acid sequence and heterogeneity in glycosylation of rat renal renin. J Biol Chem 1991; 266:7044–7050.
78. Su Y and Reudelhuber TL. Molecular characterization of human prorenin isoelectric forms. J Hypertens 1993; 11:141–146.
79. Ganong WF. Origin of the angiotensin II secreted by cells. Proc Soc Exp Biol Med 1994; 205:213–219.

80. Inagami T, Mizuno K, Naruse K, et al. Intracellular formation and release of angiotensins from juxtaglomerular cells. Kidney Int 1990; 30(suppl):S33–S37.
81. Okamura T, Clemens DL, Inagami T. Renin, angiotensins and angiotensin-converting enzyme in neuroblasotoma cells: Evidence for intracellular generation of angiotensins. Proc Natl Acad Sci USA 1981; 78:6940–6943.
82. Nishimura K, Wand P, Erdos EG. Kallikrein and renin in the membrane fractions of the rat kidney. Hypertension 1980; 2:538–545.
83. Inoue H, Fukui K, Takahashi S, Miyake Y. Molecular cloning and sequence analysis of a cDNA encoding a porcine kidney renin-binding protein. J Biol Chem 1990; 265:6556–6561.
84. Tada M, Takahashi S, Miyano M, Miyake Y. Tissue-specific regulation of renin-binding protein gene expression in rats. J Biochem 1992; 112:175–182.
85. Inoue H, Takahashi S, Fukui K, Miyake Y. Leucine zipper motif in porcine renin-binding protein (RnBP) and its relationship to the formation of an RnBP-renin heterodimer and an RnBP homodimer. J Biol Chem 1991; 266:11896–11900.
86. Takahashi S, Inoue H, Miyake Y. The human gene for renin-binding protein. J Biol Chem 1992; 267:13007–13013.
87. Taugner R, Bührle CP, Nobiling R. Ultrastructural changes associated with renin secretion from the juxtaglomerular apparatus of mice. Cell Tiss Res 1984; 237:459–472.
88. Taugner R, Metz R, Rosivall L. Macroautophagic phenomena in renin granules. Cell Tissue Res 1988; 251:229–231.
89. Taugner R, Hackenthal E. On the character of the secretory granules in juxtaglomerular epithelioid cells. Int Rev Cytol 1988; 110:93–131.
90. Matsuba H, Watanabe T, Watanabe M, et al. Immunocytochemical localization of prorenin, renin, and cathepsins B, H, and L in juxtaglomerular cells of rat kidney. J Histochem Cytochem 1989; 37:1689–1697.
91. Taugner R, Kim SJ, Murakami K, Waldherr R. The fate of prorenin during granulopoiesis in epithelioid cells: Immunocytochemical experiments with antisera against renin and different portions of the renin prosegment. Histochemistry 1987; 86:249–253.
92. Miller SG, Moore H. Regulated secretion. Curr Opin Cell Biol 1990; 2:642–647.
93. Rothman JE, Orci L. Molecular dissection of the secretory pathway. Nature 1992; 355:409–415.
94. Kelly RB. Secretory granule and synaptic vesicle formation. Curr Opin Cell Biol 1991; 3:654–660.
95. Reaves BJ, Dannies PS. Is a sorting signal necessary to package proteins into secretory granules? Mol Cell Endocrinol 1991; 79:C141–C145.
96. Fritz LC, Haidar MA, Arfsten AE, et al. Human renin is correctly processed and targeted to the regulated secretory pathway in mouse pituitary AtT-20 cells. J Biol Chem 1987; 262:12409–12412.
97. Pratt RE, Flynn JA, Hobart PM, et al. Different secretory pathways of renin from mouse cells transfected with the human renin gene. J Biol Chem 1988; 263:3137–3141.
98. Landenheim, Seidah N, Lutfalla G, Rougeon F. Stable and transient expression of mouse submaxillary gland renin cDNA in AtT20 cells: Proteolytic processing and secretory pathways. FEBS Lett 1989; 245:70–74.
99. Nagahama M, Nakayama K, Murakami K. Sequence requirements for prohormone processing in mouse pituitary AtT-20 cells: Analysis of prorenins as model substrates. Eur J Biochem 1991; 197:135–140.
100. Chidgey MA, Harrison TM. Renin is sorted to the regulated secretory pathway in transfected PC12 cells by a mechanism which does not require expression of the propeptide. Eur J Biochem 1990; 190:139–144.
101. Hatsuzawa K, Hosaka M, Nakagawa T, et al. Structure and expression of mouse furin, a yeast Kex2-related protease: Lack of processing of coexpressed prorenin in GH4C1 cells. J Biol Chem 1990; 265:22075–22078.
102. Chu WN, Baxter JD, Reudelhuber TL. A targeting sequence for dense core secretory granules resides in the protein moiety of human prorenin. Mol Endocrinol 1990; 4:1905–1913.
103. Nakayama K, Nagahama M, Kim WS, et al. Prorenin is sorted into the regulated secretory pathway independent of its processing to renin in mouse pituitary AtT-20 cells. FEBS Lett 1989; 257:89–92.
104. Nagahama M, Nakayama K, Murakami K. Effects of propeptide deletion on human renin secretion from mouse pituitary AtT-20 cells. FEBS Lett 1990; 264:67–70.
105. Kawamura M, McKenzie JC, Hoffman LH, et al. The storage form of renin in renin granules from rat kidney cortex. Hypertension 1986; 8:706–711.
106. Pratt RE, Carleton JE, Richie JP, et al. Human renin biosynthesis and secretion in normal and ischemic kidneys. Proc Natl Acad Sci USA 1987; 84:7837–7840.
107. Toffelmire EB, Slater K, Corvol P, et al. Response of plasma prorenin and active renin to chronic and acute alterations of renin secretion in normal humans: Studies using a direct immunoradiometric assay. J Clin Invest 1989; 83:679–687.
108. Do YS, Shinagawa T, Tam H, et al. Characterization of pure human renal renin. J Biol Chem 1987; 262:1037–1043.
109. Misono KS, Chang J, Inagami T. Amino acid sequence of mouse submaxillary gland renin. Proc Natl Acad Sci USA 1982; 79:4858–4862.

110. Campbell DJ, Valentijn AJ, Condron R. Purification and amino-terminal sequence of rat kidney renin: Evidence for a two-chain structure. J Hypertens 1991; 9:29–33.
111. Pratt RE, Ouellette AJ, Dzau VJ. Biosynthesis of renin: Multiplicity of active and intermediate forms. Proc Natl Acad Sci USA 1983; 80:6809–6813.
112. Derkx FH, Schalekamp MP, and Schalekamp MA. Two-step prorenin-renin conversion: Isolation of an intermediary form of activated prorenin. J Biol Chem 1987; 262:2472–2477.
113. Pitarresi TM, Rubattu S, Heinrikson R, Sealey JE. Reversible cryoactivation of recombinant human prorenin. J Biol Chem 1992; 267:11753–11759.
114. Heinrikson RL, Hui J, Zürcher-Neely H, Poorman RA. A structural model to explain the partial catalytic activity of human prorenin. Am J Hypertens 1989; 2:367–380.
115. Shinagawa T, Do YS, Baxter J, Hsueh WA. Purification and characterization of human truncated prorenin. Biochemistry 1992; 31:2758–2764.
116. Frohlich ED, Iwata T, Sasaki O. Clinical and physiologic significance of local tissue renin-angiotensin systems. Am J Med 1990; 87(suppl 6B):6B-19S–6B-23S.
117. Wang PH, Do YS, Macaulay L, et al. Identification of renal cathepsin B as a human prorenin-processing enzyme. J Biol Chem 1991; 266:12633–12638.
118. Chu WN, Mercure C, Baxter JD, Reudelhuber TL. Molecular determinants of human prorenin processing. Hypertension 1992; 20:782–787.
119. Benjannet S, Reudelhuber T, Mercure C, et al. Pro-protein conversion is determined by a multiplicity of factors including convertase processing, substrate specificity and intracellular environment. J Biol Chem 1992; 267:11417–11423.
120. Hosaka M, Nagahama M, Kim W-S, et al. Arg-X-Lys/Arg-Arg Motif as a signal for precursor cleavage catalyzed by furin within the constitutive secretory pathway. J Biol Chem 1991; 266:12127–12130.
121. Shinagawa T, Do YS, Baxter JD, et al. Identification of an enzyme in human kidney that correctly processes prorenin. Proc Natl Acad Sci USA 1990; 87:1927–1931.
122. San Segundo B, Chan SJ, Steiner DF. Differences in cathepsin B mRNA levels in rat tissues suggest specialized functions. FEBS Lett 1986; 201:251–256.
123. Saint-Andrë JP, Rohmer V, Pinet F, et al. Renin and cathepsin B in human pituitary lactotroph cells: An ultrastructural study. Histochemistry 1989; 91:291–297.
124. Nakayama K, Kim W-S, Nakagawa T, et al. Substrate specificity of prerenin converting enzyme of mouse submandibular gland. J Biol Chem 1990; 265:21027–21031.
125. Kim WS, Nakayama K, Nakagawa T, et al. Mouse submandibular gland prorenin-converting enzyme is a member of glandular kallikrein family. J Biol Chem 1991; 266:19283–19287.
126. Kim WS, Nakayama K, Murakami K. The presence of two types of prorenin converting enzymes in the mouse submandibular gland. FEBS Lett 1991; 293:142–144.
127. Nakayama K, Hosaka M, Hatsuzawa K, Murakami K. Cloning and functional expression of a novel endoprotease involved in prohormone processing at dibasic sites. J Biochem 1991; 109:803–806.
128. Nakagawa T, Hosaka M, Torii S, et al. Identification and functional expression of a new member of the mammalian Kex2-like processing endoprotease family: Its striking structural similarity to PACE-4. J Biochem 1993; 113:132–135.
129. Hatsuzawa K, Nagahama M, Takahashi S, et al. Purification and characterization of furin, a kex2-like processing endoprotease, produced in Chinese hamster ovary cells. J Biol Chem 1992; 267:16094–16099.
130. Ohkubo H, Kawakami H, Kakehi Y, et al. Generation of transgenic mice with elevated blood pressure by introduction of the rat renin and angiotensinogen genes. Proc Natl Acad Sci USA 1990; 87:5153–5157.
131. Fukamizu A, Sugimura K, Takimoto E, et al. Chimeric renin-angiotensin system demonstrates sustained increase in blood pressure of transgenic mice carrying both human renin and human angiotensinogen genes. J Biol Chem 1993; 268:11617–11621.
132. Ganten D, Wagner J, Zeh K, et al. Species specificity of renin kinetics in transgenic rats harboring the human renin and angiotensinogen genes. Proc Natl Acad Sci USA 1992; 89:7806–7810.
133. Mullins JJ, Peters J, Ganten D. Fulminant hypertension in transgenic rats harbouring the mouse Ren-2 gene. Nature 1990; 344:541–544.
134. Sarzani R, Fallo F, Dessi-Fulgheri P, et al. Local renin-angiotensin system in human adrenals and aldosteronomas. Hypertension 1992; 19:702–707.
135. Racz K, Pinet F, Gasc JM, et al. Coexpression of renin, angiotensinogen, and their messenger ribonucleic acids in adrenal tissues. J Clin Endocrinol Metab 1992; 75:730–737.
136. Dahl LK, Heine M, Tassinari L. Role of genetic factors in susceptibility to experimental hypertension due to chronic excess salt ingestion. Nature 1962; 194:480–482.
137. Creager MA, Roddy MA, Holland KM, et al. Sodium depresses arterial baroreceptor reflex function in normotensive humans. Hypertension 1991; 17:989–996.
138. Williams RR. Will gene markers predict hypertension? Hypertension 1989; 14:610–613.

139. Rapp JP, Dene H. Development and characteristics of inbred strains of Dahl salt-sensitive and salt-resistant rats. Hypertension 1985; 7:340–349.
140. Rapp JP, Wang SM, Dene H. A genetic polymorphism in the renin gene of Dahl rats cosegregates with blood pressure. Science 1989; 243:542–544.
141. Knudsen KD, Dahl LK, Thompson K, et al. Effects of chronic excess salt ingestion. Inheritance of hypertension in the rat. J Exp Med 1970; 132:976–1000.
142. Rapp JP, Wang SM, Dene H. Effect of genetic background on cosegregation of renin alleles and blood pressure in Dahl rats. Am J Hypertens 1990; 3:391–396.
143. O'Dowd BF, Rapp JP. Heterogeneity of renin alleles in outbred Dahl salt-sensitive (Brookhaven) rats. Hypertension 1991; 18:9–11.
144. Wang SM, Rapp JP. Structural differences in the renin gene of Dahl salt-sensitive and salt-resistant rats. Mol Endocrinol 1989; 3:288–294.
145. Rapp JP, Dene H, Deng AY. Seven renin alleles in rats and their effects on blood pressure. Kidney Int 1994; 12:348–355.
146. Alam KY, Wang Y, Dene H, Rapp JP. Renin gene nucleotide sequence of coding and regulatory regions in Dahl rats. Clin Exp Hypertens 1993; 15:599–614.
147. Kurtz TW, Simonet L, Kabra PM, et al. Cosegregation of the renin allele of the spontaneously hypertensive rat with an increase in blood pressure. J Clin Invest 1990; 85:1328–1332.
148. Lindpaintner K, Takahashi S, Ganten D. Structural alterations of the renin gene in stroke-prone spontaneously hypertensive rats: Examination of genotype-phenotype correlations. J Hypertens 1990; 8:763–773.
149. Dubay C, Vincent M, Samani N, et al. Genetic determinants of diastolic and pulse pressure map to different loci in Lyon hypertensive rats. Nature Genet 1993; 3:354–357.
150. Ward R. Familial aggregation and genetic epidemiology of blood pressure. In: Laragh JH, Brenner BM, eds. Hypertension: Pathophysiology, Diagnosis and Treatment. New York: Raven Press, 1990: 81–100.
151. Naftilan AJ, Williams R, Burt D, et al. A lack of genetic linkage of renin gene restriction fragment length polymorphisms with human hypertension. Hypertension 1989; 14:614–618.
152. Zee RY, Ying LH, Morris BJ, Griffiths LR. Association and linkage analyses of restriction fragment length polymorphisms for the human renin and antithrombin III genes in essential hypertension. J Hypertens 1991; 9:825–830.
153. Soubrier F, Jeunemaitre X, Rigat B, et al. Similar frequencies of renin gene restriction fragment length polymorphisms in hypertensive and normotensive subjects. Hypertension 1990; 16:712–717.
154. Jeunemaitre X, Rigat B, Charru et al. Sib pair linkage analysis of renin gene haplotypes in human essential hypertension. Hum Genet 1992; 88:301–306.
155. Morris BJ. Identification of essential hypertension genes. J Hypertens 1993; 11:115–120.
156. Soubrier F, Cambien F. Renin-angiotensin system genes as candidate genes in cardiovascular diseases. Trends Endocrinol Metab 1993; 3:250–258.
157. Jeunemaitre X, Soubrier F, Kotelevtsev YV, et al. Molecular basis of human hypertension: Role of angiotensinogen. Cell 1992; 71:169–180.
158. Harrap SB, Davidson HR, Connor JM, et al. The angiotensin I converting enzyme gene and predisposition to high blood pressure. Hypertension 1993; 21:455–460.
159. Jeunemaitre X, Lifton RP, Hunt SC, et al. Absence of linkage between the angiotensin converting enzyme locus and human essential hypertension. Nature Genet 1992; 1:72–75.
160. Cambien F, Poirier O, Lecerf L, et al. Deletion polymorphism in the gene for angiotensin-converting enzyme is a potent risk factor for myocardial infarction. Nature 1992; 359:641–644.
161. Deng Y, Rapp JP. Cosegregation of blood pressure with angiotensin converting enzyme and atrial natriuretic peptide receptor genes using Dahl salt-sensitive rats. Nature Genet 1992; 1:267–272.
162. Hilbert P, Lindpaintner K, Bedckmann JS, et al. Chromosomal mapping of two genetic loci associated with blood-pressure regulation in hereditary hypertensive rats. Nature 1991; 353:521–529.
163. Jacob HJ, Lindpaintner K, Lincoln SE, et al. Genetic mapping of a gene causing hypertension in the stroke-prone spontaneously hypertensive rat. Cell 1991; 67:213–224.
164. Tigerstedt R, Bergman PG. Niere and Kreislauf. Skand Arch Physiol 1898; 8:223–271.
165. Rosenberg ME, Smith LJ, Correa-Rotter R, Hostetter TH. The paradox of the renin-angiotensin system in chronic renal disease. Kidney Int 1994; 45:403–410.
166. Itskovitz J, Rubattu S, Levron J, Sealey JE. Highest concentrations of prorenin and human chorionic gonadotropin in gestational sacs during early human pregnancy. J Clin Endocrinol Metab 1992; 75:906–910.
167. Capecchi MR. Altering the genome by homologous recombination. Science 1989; 244:1288–1292.

8
Angiotensin II and the Renin-Angiotensin System

Kenneth E. Bernstein
Emory University, Atlanta, Georgia

Eric Clauser
College de France, Paris, France

Marÿke Brink
Ciba-Geigy Ltd., Basel, Switzerland

INTRODUCTION

A basic description of the renin-angiotensin system is that renin, produced by the juxtaglomerular cells of the kidney, enzymatically cleaves the amino terminal ten amino acids of the serum glycoprotein angiotensinogen to release the peptide angiotensin I (Fig. 1). This peptide is an inactive intermediate and it is further processed by angiotensin-converting enzyme (ACE) into the eight–amino acid peptide angiotensin II. Angiotensin II binds to high-affinity cell surface receptors and causes a remarkable diversity of physiological effects designed to elevate blood pressure (1). Angiotensin II induces vascular smooth muscle constriction and raises peripheral vascular resistance. In response to angiotensin II, both renal proximal tubular epithelium and cells of the gut increase absorption of salt and water. Within the adrenal, glomerulosa cells are stimulated to produce aldosterone. Angiotensin II elevates the resistance of both efferent and afferent arterioles and increases filtration fraction. Mesangial cells are thought to contract in response to angiotensin II and to regulate the hemodynamics of individual glomeruli (2). In the heart, angiotensin II is associated with positive inotrophy. In the brain, angiotensin II induces a variety of responses, including the onset of thirst and increased vasopressin release (3). These and other actions of angiotensin II act to increase intracellular volume, peripheral vascular resistance, and blood pressure.

Given the physiological diversity of angiotensin II, it is not surprising that pharmaceutical companies sought inhibitors of angiotensin II synthesis and actions. Three strategies are readily apparent: inhibit the enzymatic action of renin, inhibit the enzymatic action of ACE, or competitively inhibit the binding of angiotensin II to cell surface receptors. While pharmaceuticals directed against renin have been synthesized, none have yet achieved wide clinical use (4). By comparison, inhibitors of ACE are now widely prescribed for the treatment of hypertension and heart failure. Research to develop ACE inhibitors was stimulated by the discovery that the venom of the South American pit viper *Bothrops jararaca* contains natural ACE inhibitors (5). This and the functional characterization of ACE as a zinc peptidase similar to carboxypeptidase A served as the basis for an elegant series of pharmacological constructions that succeeded in developing the sulfhydryl ACE inhibitor captopril (6). Now many different compound such as enalapril, ramipril, benazepril, and cilazapril are available for the treatment of human disease (7). The ACE inhibitors have demonstrated a clinical effectiveness far beyond that originally envisioned by pharmaceutical investigators. For the patient suffering from heart failure, these drugs reduce afterload and decrease patient mortality (8,9). They are not only

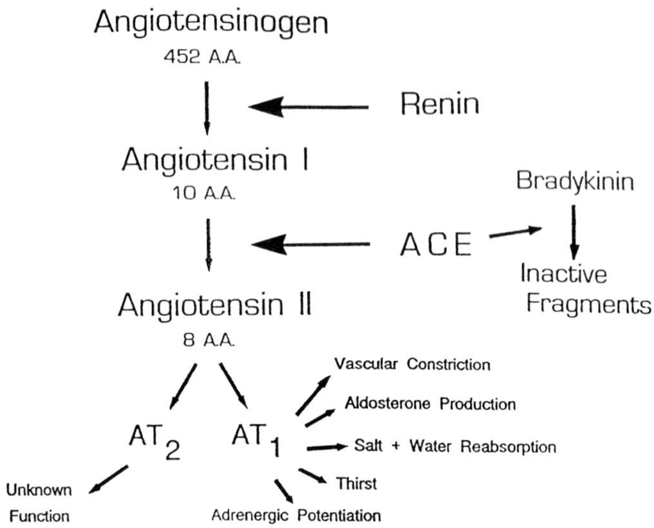

Figure 1 Angiotensin II is an eight–amino acid peptide produced by the sequential cleavage of angiotensinogen by renin and angiotensin-converting enzyme (ACE). Renin is very specific in its substrate specificity and only cleaves angiotensinogen, releasing the amino terminal 10 amino acids. Angiotensin-converting enzyme is a less selective enzyme and cleaves many small peptides including angiotensin I and bradykinin. The two major types of angiotensin II receptors are called AT_1 and AT_2. All of the hemodynamic and cardiovascular function associated with angiotensin II are a result of its interaction with the AT_1 receptor. The exact function of the AT_2 receptor is not known.

effective in treating the hypertension associated with high serum renin levels but are also efficacious for the majority of hypertensive patients presenting with normal or even low serum renin levels (7). Experimental animal models also suggest that ACE inhibitors may ameliorate certain forms of progressive renal disease (10,11). In the rat, ACE inhibitors prevent the neointimal formation observed after balloon angiography (12). In summary, the full clinical spectrum of this class of drugs is still being investigated.

A third locus for interruption of the renin-angiotensin system is angiotensin II receptor inhibitors. During the development of these compounds, peptidic and nonpeptidic inhibitors were developed that discriminate between two major classes of angiotensin II receptors (13,14). These receptor subtypes are now termed AT_1 (blocked by the pharmaceutical DuP753) and AT_2 (blocked by the compound PD123177 or CGP42112). The use of these specific inhibitors has allowed assignment of function to the individual receptor subtypes, and many experiments have demonstrated that virtually all the hemodynamic and cardiovascular effects associated with angiotensin II are mediated by the AT_1 receptor subtype (15). The specific AT_1 receptor inhibitor, DuP753, is now called losartan and is in the final phases of clinical trials.

While the focus of this chapter is on the structure of ACE and the AT_1 receptor subtype, we first present a brief summary of angiotensinogen and renin to emphasize the interaction among the individual components of the renin-angiotensin system. This collection of enzymes is highly integrated and operates in a coordinate fashion to maintain physiological homeostasis of blood pressure, volume, and electrolyte composition.

ANGIOTENSINOGEN

Human angiotensinogen is a glycoprotein of 452 amino acids produced predominantly by the liver and secreted into the blood (16,17). Physical isolation of this protein has shown that it is heterogeneous in molecular weight. For instance, within the human, two major species of 61.4 and

65.4 kDa have been identified. Angiotensinogen is a member of the serpin superfamily of proteins, which are thought to have been derived from an ancestral gene encoding a serine protease inhibitor. Other members of this family include α1-antitrypsin and antithrombin III. Like α1-antitrypsin, angiotensinogen is an acute-phase reactant and production by the liver is markedly elevated in response to stresses such as bacterial infection. High serum levels of angiotensinogen are observed during pregnancy. Liver production of this protein is also stimulated by glucocorticoids, thyroid hormones, and sex steroids. Nephrectomy, with the resultant decrease of serum renin, also leads to a marked elevation of liver angiotensinogen mRNA. Finally, angiotensin II, the final active product of the renin-angiotensin system, participates in a positive feedback loop that stimulates the hepatic production of angiotensinogen. This feedback loop would have the effect that during periods of high angiotensin II production, the peptide stimulates production of its own precursor protein to ensure constant availability of renin substrate. There is no known function of angiotensinogen other than as the precursor of angiotensin II. Recent work has suggested that genetic polymorphisms in the angiotensinogen gene play an important causitive role in some instances of hypertension and preeclampsia (18,19).

RENIN

Renin production by the kidney is one of the central mechanisms regulating blood pressure. The existence of this protein was first suggested in 1898 when Robert Tigerstedt demonstrated that a saline extract of rabbit kidney was capable of elevating the blood pressure of rabbits when injected intravenously. Renin is produced by the juxtaglomerular apparatus located at the base of each glomerulus. Critical to the production of renin are (a) specialized baroreceptor cells located in the glomerular afferent arteriole and (b) the macula densa, a portion of the distal tubule anatomically in juxtaposition to the afferent arteriole. The juxtaglomerular apparatus senses both the afferent arterial pressure and the amount of sodium chloride delivered to the distal tubule. A decrease in blood pressure, hypovolemia, or decreased sodium chloride presentation to the distal tubule all trigger increased renin release. In contrast, high serum levels of angiotensin II inhibit renin secretion, a classic inhibitory pathway in which the final product of the renin-angiotensin system leads to a feedback inhibition of its own formation (20,21).

Renin is an aspartyl proteinase distantly related to pepsin. It is produced as a preproprotein that in the human has a molecular weight of approximately 45,000 Da. In the human, the renin signal peptide (the presegment) is 23 amino acids (22). An additional 43 amino acids (the prosegment) is eventually removed to produce the active enzyme, which contains 340 amino acids. It is often stated that renin production of angiotensin I is the rate-limiting step in the generation of angiotensin II. One of the first models of hypertension in animals was developed by Harry Goldblatt in the early 1930s, when he demonstrated that constriction of one renal artery and removal of the second kidney resulted in persistent hypertension. It is now known that disease in this model is triggered by a marked elevation in the production of renin by the remaining kidney after sensing a reduced renal blood flow.

ANGIOTENSIN-CONVERTING ENZYME

Angiotensin-converting enzyme (ACE) is a zinc-containing dipeptidyl carboxypeptidase that is responsible for the release of the dipeptide His-Leu from the carboxyl end of angiotensin I. While renin is extraordinarily precise in its substrate specificity, ACE is enzymatically far more promiscuous, and many other small peptides (enkephalines, substance P, luteinizing hormone–releasing hormone etc.) can be cleaved by this enzyme (23). Angiotensin-converting enzyme converts bradykinin into inactive fragments and thus functionally degrades this potent vasodilator. It is perhaps because of the wide diversity of substrates that inhibitors of ACE are so effective in the treatment of hypertension and other cardiovascular diseases.

Many different tissues produce ACE, but it is the production of the enzyme by vascular endothelium that is thought most important to the regulation of blood pressure. Nascent ACE protein contains a 29–amino acid signal sequence, and its amino terminus is extruded from the cell. A carboxyl terminal hydrophobic anchor sequence secures the protein to the luminal face of the endothelial cell membrane. Thus angiotensin II is formed at the luminal surface of endothelial cells in close proximity to vascular smooth muscle, a critical target organ for this vasoconstrictor. Studies have examined the ACE levels in human sera, and while levels vary by up to fourfold among individuals, no significant association with clinical hypertension has been identified (24,25). The isozyme of ACE produced by endothelium and other somatic tissues is called somatic ACE.

Primary Structure of Somatic ACE

The primary structure of human somatic ACE was first elucidated by cloning and sequencing the corresponding cDNA (26). The cloning strategy included purification of somatic ACE protein from human kidney and the determination of amino acid sequence from the amino terminus and internal regions of the protein. Mixtures of oligonucleotides were then synthesized and used to screen human endothelial cDNA libraries. Analysis of cDNA showed that somatic ACE is 1306 amino acids.

A striking feature of the ACE sequence is the presence of two internal homologous domains, each of which is now known to be catalytic (Fig. 2). Each domain is composed of 357 amino acids, and overall the two domains are 68% identical in amino acid sequence. Higher conservation of sequence (89%) is present in the centers of the domains, where residues potentially involved in catalysis have been identified by comparison with the active sites of other metallopeptidases, such as thermolysin and neutral endopeptidase. The finding that somatic ACE contains two potentially independent catalytic domains was very unexpected, since previous biochemical studies had strongly implied only a single catalytic site per molecule (27,28). However, the cloning of mouse and rabbit somatic ACE cDNA confirmed that all mammalian ACE molecules contain this peculiar structure and include two potential catalytic domains (29,30).

Human ACE is encoded by a single gene located on chromosome 17 (31). It spans 21 kilobases and is made up of 25 exons (32). Each of the two homologous domains of the enzyme are encoded by a cluster of eight exons (exons 4 to 11 and exons 16 to 23). Corresponding exons are similar in size and in the codon phase at the exon-intron boundaries. The similarity of the exon-intron organization of the two clusters strongly suggests that the mammalian ACE gene is the result of an ancestral gene duplication event.

Structure-Function Analysis of Human Somatic ACE

The elucidation of the primary structure of somatic ACE raised the question of the functional significance of two potential catalytic sites. Are both sites truly catalytic? And if so, do they differ in substrate specificity and kinetics? These questions were solved for human somatic ACE using the technique of site-directed mutagenesis. This powerful technique allows selective change of a protein's amino acid sequence. The development of this technology by Michael Smith resulted in his being awarded the 1993 Nobel Prize in Chemistry. Modification of the protein sequence is performed at the level of the DNA encoding the protein (Fig. 3). The DNA is first cloned into a vector to produce single-stranded DNA. This is then hybridized in vitro with a synthetic oligonucleotide that, while complementary to a specific region of the sequence, also contains a *mutated* codon. Using DNA polymerase, the oligonucleotide containing the mutation is extended into a DNA strand complementary to the original single-stranded DNA template. The replication in bacteria of a double-stranded DNA, one strand of which corresponds to wild-type sequence while the other strand corresponds to

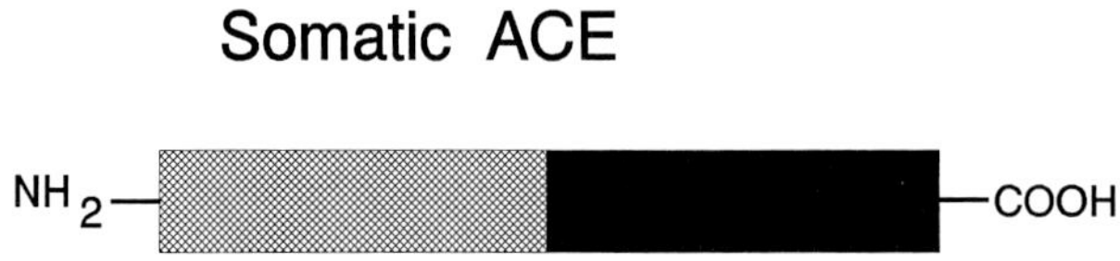

Figure 2 The isozyme of angiotensin-converting enzyme (ACE) made by endothelium and other somatic tissues is called somatic ACE. Though it is a single polypeptide chain, somatic ACE is functionally composed of two homologous amino acid domains, each of which is independently catalytic. The amino acid homology of these two domains and their similar exonic structure suggest that the modern ACE gene is the result of a gene duplication event.

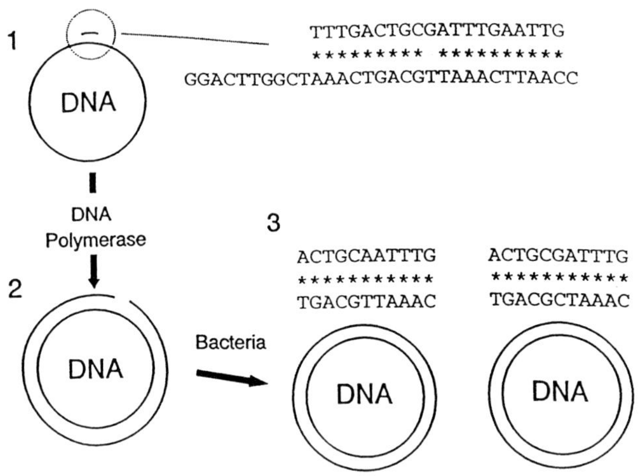

Figure 3 Site-directed mutagenesis. The DNA of interest is cloned into a vector to produce single-stranded DNA (panel 1). This is then hybridized in vitro with an oligonucleotide containing the desired mutation. The enzyme DNA polymerase is used to extend the oligonucleotide (panel 2). Once transfected into bacteria, each of the two DNA strands will be duplicated, resulting in two populations of DNA. One population contains wild-type DNA while the other incorporates the mutation into both DNA strands (panel 3). By recloning into bacteria, one can easily select for and prepare pure DNA containing the desired mutation.

the complementary sequence with the exception of the introduced mutation, eventually results in two different populations of DNA molecules. One population is double-stranded DNA bearing the mutated codon on both DNA strands, and this new gene can be introduced into eucaryotic cells to express the mutated protein.

Site-directed mutagenesis was used to analyze each of the potential catalytic sites of the human somatic ACE gene (33–35). Eight different mutated enzymes were produced in Chinese hamster ovary cells (CHO). Two of these were truncated enzymes containing either the amino or the carboxyl terminal catalytic domains. The six other enzymes contained point mutations of the ACE sequence, changing selected histidines to lysine or glutamic acids to aspartic acid. Analysis of these mutated ACE molecules demonstrated that both catalytic sites are active, have an absolute zinc requirement, and appear to function independently. However, the two active sites present differences in their substrate-specificity. Both sites bind angiotensin I with the same affinity (K_m = 16 μM), but the carboxyl terminal domain hydrolyzed this peptide three times faster than the amino terminal domain (k_{cat} = 35 s^{-1} and 12 s^{-1} respectively). Similar results were observed for the hydrolysis of substance P. Bradykinin, though, was cleaved with similar kinetics by each of the catalytic domains of ACE (K_m = 0.24 and 0.54 μM and k_{cat} = 8 and 5 s^{-1} for the carboxyl and amino terminal domains respectively). Finally, LHRH was hydrolyzed 10 times faster by the amino terminal domain than by the carboxyl terminal domain, despite a similar affinity for this substrate (K_m = 235 and 160 μM, k_{cat} = 8.5 and 0.8s^{-1} respectively). Another difference between the two catalytic sites is the modulating effect of chloride, the presence of which is important for the catalytic activity of the carboxyl terminal domain but not of the amino terminal domain. These data indicate that both active sites of somatic ACE possess dipeptidyl carboxypeptidase activity, but under physiologic conditions the carboxyl terminal domain is more active. Moreover the amino terminal domain exhibits an unusual amino terminal endoproteolytic activity, suggesting that the two catalytic domains of ACE may have different physiological functions.

Testis ACE

As early as 1971, researchers were surprised to find that testis contains large amounts of ACE and that the protein found in this tissue is biochemically distinct from the ACE enzyme produced by endothelium (36). Subsequent analysis has demonstrated that developing male germ cells (developing sperm) produce large amounts of ACE mRNA encoding a protein approximately half as large as that observed in somatic tissues. For example, in the mouse, the ACE enzyme produced by somatic tissues is composed of 1312 amino acids, while the testis isozyme contains only 732 (37). Despite the smaller size, testis ACE is fully catalytic with K_m and K_{cat} values, similar to the protein produced by somatic tissues (38). Analysis of cDNA encoding testis ACE established two significant features of this enzyme (Fig. 4). First, the amino terminal 66 amino acids of testis ACE is sequence-unique to the testis isozyme. Second, the remainder of the testis ACE protein, 666 amino acids, is identical to the carboxyl terminal catalytic domain of somatic ACE. Within all mammals studied to date, the ACE gene is encoded within a single genetic locus. Developing germ cells are unique in that they begin mRNA transcription of ACE within the 12th intron of the somatic ACE gene. The result is a protein in which the first exon of testis ACE, encoding the amino terminal 66 amino acids, is sequence-treated as intronic by all somatic tissues. Due to the start of mRNA transcription in the middle of the ACE gene, testis ACE contains only one catalytic domain.

While the function of ACE in the development of male germ cells is not at present understood, substantial progress has been made in understanding the unique transcriptional initiation site recognized by male germ cells. Transgenic mouse studies have demonstrated that, located within the 12th intron of the somatic ACE gene, is a DNA sequence that serves as a male germ cell–specific promoter for testis ACE transcription (39,40). This was proven by taking a small portion of the 12th intron of the mouse gene (the putative promoter) and linking it to a reporter gene encoding *E. coli* β-galactosidase. The hybrid DNA construct was then microinjected into the pronuclei of fertilized mouse ova, which were reimplanted into surrogate mothers (Fig. 5). In approximately one-third of the offspring, the injected DNA was integrated into the genomic DNA of the fertilized ovum and thus was present in every cell of the progeny mice. If the injected DNA contains a tissue-specific promoter, the reporter gene will be expressed only in those tissues recognizing the promoter region.

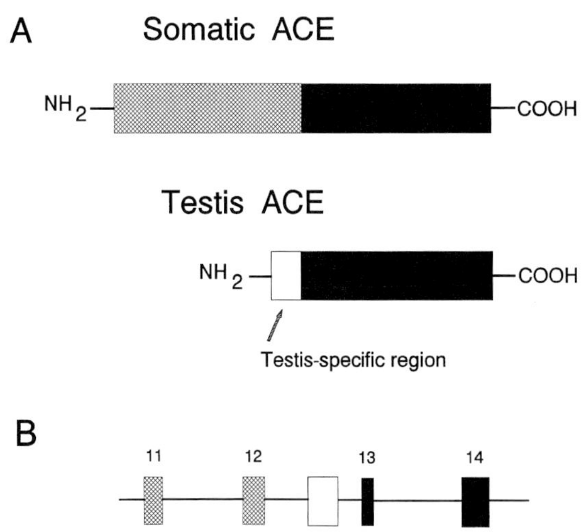

Figure 4 (A) Testis angiotensin-converting enzyme (testis ACE) is an isozyme of ACE produced by developing male germ cells. It contains only one catalytic domain. The amino terminal 66 amino acids of testis ACE is not found in somatic ACE. The remainder of the testis ACE protein is identical in sequence to the carboxyl terminal catalytic domain of somatic ACE. (B) A portion of the genomic organization of the ACE gene. The 11th, 12th, 13th and 14th exons of somatic ACE are indicated with boxes. Somatic tissues eliminate the information between the 12th and the 13th exons, treating it as intronic. In contrast male germ cells begin transcription of testis ACE within this identical portion of DNA, and thus DNA considered intronic by somatic tissues encodes the 1st exon of testis ACE including the 66 amino acids of the testis specific region. The second exon of testis ACE is the 13th exon of somatic ACE, the 3rd exon of testis ACE is the 14th exon of somatic ACE etc.

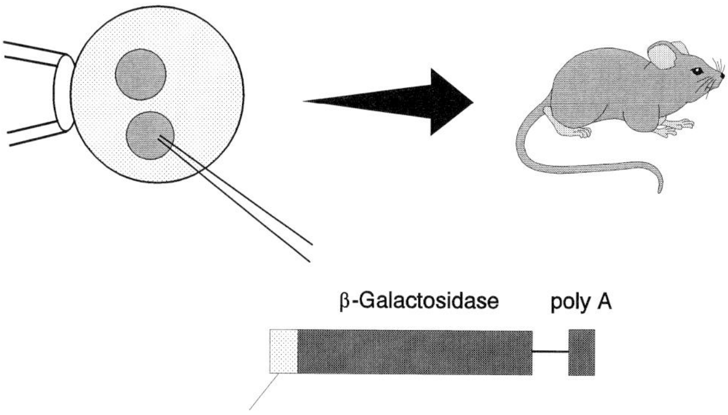

Figure 5 The testis ACE promoter region was linked to a reporter gene encoding *E. coli* β-galactosidase. Fertilized mouse ova were collected before pronuclei fusion and microinjected with the DNA construct. In some ova the injected construct was integrated into the genomic DNA. After reimplantation of the ova into surrogate mothers, the progeny mice were examined for the tissue-specific expression of β-galactosidase. The testis ACE promoter contruct resulted in transgenic mice expressing high levels of β-galactosidase within developing male germ cells.

When mice were made transgenic for the testis ACE construct, high levels of β-galactosidase expression were observed only in developing male germ cells. It is clear from this and other experimental data that the unique biochemistry within developing male germ cells results in the recognition of a tissue-specific testis ACE promoter, the initiation of RNA transcription within the 12th intron of the somatic gene, and the production of an enzyme with only one catalytic domain.

ANGIOTENSIN II RECEPTORS

Early indications for a heterogeneity of angiotensin II receptors came from studies with substituted peptide analogues of angiotensin II. For example, in the intestinal tract and the adrenal medulla, substitution of phenylalanine in position 8 of the octapeptide chain did not affect the activity of angiotensin II, whereas in the majority of tissues, this phenylalanine is absolutely required (41). Other biochemical studies showed that certain ions, sulfhydryl reducing agents, and guanyl nucleotides affected angiotensin II binding in different ways, depending on the tissue (42–44). Great progress in understanding angiotensin II receptors followed the development of peptidic and nonpeptidic receptor antagonists (13,14,45). Analogues such as losartan (DuP753) are highly selective for the AT_1 receptor. In contrast, analogues like CGP42112, PD123177, and PD123319 have a high affinity only for the AT_2 receptor. Studies using these analogues have demonstrated that virtually all of the cardiovascular manifestations of angiotensin II are a direct result of ligand binding to the AT_1 receptor subtype (15,46). The AT_1 receptor is a member of the large superfamily of G protein–associated receptors. This large group of molecules contains seven discrete hydrophobic regions that are thought to form α-helices and to traverse the cell membrane seven times. Other G protein–coupled receptors include rhodopsin as well as receptors for adrenergic, muscarinic, dopaminergic, and a host of other peptide ligands such as bradykinin and vasopressin. The elucidation of the general structure of this superfamily of receptors and their mechanisms for intracellular signaling has been one of the major achievements of the 1980s (47).

The Type 1 Angiotensin II Receptor

The structure of the type 1 angiotensin II (AT_1) recpetor was elucidated in 1992 by expression cloning (48,49). Expression cloning is a methodology in which cDNA is prepared within a vector capable of transcriptional initiation once placed within a permissive cell type. To clone the AT_1 receptor, mRNA was isolated from cultured rat aortic smooth muscle cells and cDNA was then prepared and inserted into the vector pCDM8. This vector contains a strong viral promoter immediately upstream of the cDNA cloning site (50). It also contains sequence encoding the SV40 origin of replication. When pCDM8 is transfected into COS-7 cells, a monkey cell line that constitutively expresses the SV40 large T antigen protein, the vector is replicated to a high copy number. Both the high copy number and the strong viral promoter combine to drive COS-7 transcription of the cloned cDNA. The COS-7 cells contain a very low level of endogenous angiotensin II binding activity. Pools of cDNA cloned into pCDM8 were transfected into COS-7 cells, and the cells were then screened for the acquisition of angiotensin II binding capacity. Positive pools were subdivided until a unique cDNA encoding the AT_1 receptor was identified. Several independent experimental criteria were used to verify that this procedure indeed encoded the true AT_1 receptor. Perhaps most convincing was a pharmacological potency series in which analogues of angiotensin II were assessed for their relative ability to inhibit the binding of $[^{125}I]$Sar1, Ile8-angiotensin II to COS-7 cells transfected with the putative AT_1 receptor cDNA. These studies demonstrated that the cDNA encoded a receptor with binding characteristics indistinguishable from those of the endogenous AT_1 receptor (48). For instance, the cloned cDNA encoded a receptor with an inhibition constant (K_i) for DuP753 of 6.3 n*M*; the inhibition constant for the AT_2-specific ligand PD123177 was > 1 m*M*.

The AT_1 receptor is composed of 359 amino acids and is readily identifiable as a member of the G protein–coupled receptor superfamily. By analogy with other G protein–coupled receptors, it is postulated that the amino terminus of the AT_1 receptor lies outside the plasma membrane. The protein then traverses the plasma membrane seven discrete times, giving rise to three extracellular loops, three intracellular protein loops, and a carboxyl terminal intracellular tail (Fig. 6). Based on this model, the AT_1 receptor has four extracellular cysteine residues. Those positioned in the second and third extracellular domains are at positions conserved among many different G protein–coupled receptors and are thought to form a disulfide bridge. The two additional cysteines in the first and fourth extracellular domains may also form a disulfide bridge and may account for the known sensitivity of the AT_1 receptor to such reducing agents as dithiothreitol (DTT).

Concomitant with our description of the rat AT_1 receptor, Sasaki et al. described the cloning

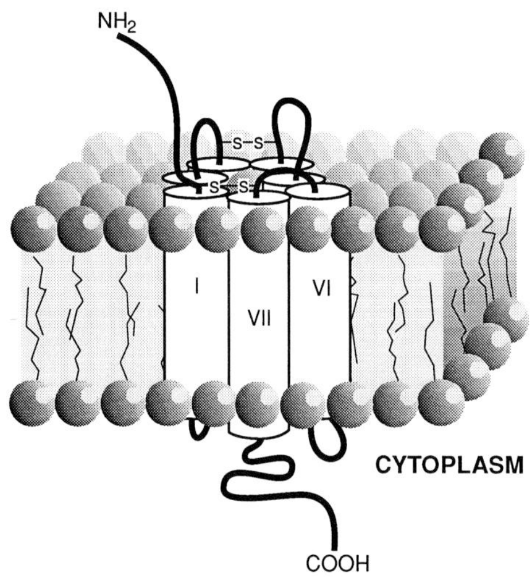

Figure 6 A schematic representation of the AT_1 receptor. In this drawing, cylinders represent the seven hydrophobic regions thought to transverse the plasma cell membrane. The amino terminus is thought to be outside the cell, while the carboxyl terminus is intracellular. Disulfide bonds link the first extracellular domain to the fourth and the second extracellular domain to the third. This drawing is meant to emphasize that the AT_1 receptor protein forms a three-dimensional structure within the cell membrane. (From Ref. 51.)

of the equivalent molecule from bovine adrenal (49). The AT_1 receptor has subsequently been cloned from the human, mouse, rabbit, and turkey (51–53). Rodents appear unique in containing two AT_1 receptor genes. These are now referred to as the AT_{1a} and AT_{1b} receptor subtypes (our original cDNA description is AT_{1a}) and share 95% amino acid homology (Fig. 7). In contrast to the coding regions, the 5′ and 3′ untranslated regions are only about 60% identical in nucleic acid sequence. A significant structural difference between the AT_{1a} and AT_{1b} receptors is the absence of cysteine

```
                                                        1
RAT AT1A      MALNSSAEDGIKRIQDDCPKAGRHSYIFVMIPTLYSIIFVVGIFGNSLVV   50
RAT AT1B      -T----T-----------------N--------------M----------
MOUSE AT1A    ------T------------R------------------------------
MOUSE AT1B    ------I-----------------N-------------------------
BOVINE        -I----T-----------------N---I---------------------
HUMAN         -I----T-----------------N-------------------------

                                     2
RAT AT1A      IVIYFYMKLKTVASVFLLNLALADLCFLLTLPLWAVYTAMEYRWPFGNHL   100
RAT AT1B      --------------------------------------------------
MOUSE AT1A    --------------------------------------------------
MOUSE AT1B    ------------------------------------------Q-------
BOVINE        ------------------------------------------------Y-
HUMAN         ------------------------------------------------Y-

                        3                                 4
RAT AT1A      CKIASASVSFNLYASVFLLTCLSIDRYLAIVHPMKSRLRRTMLVAKVTCI   150
RAT AT1B      --------------------------------------------------
MOUSE AT1A    --------------------------------------------------
MOUSE AT1B    --------------------------------------------------
BOVINE        --------------------------------------------------
HUMAN         --------------------------------------------------

RAT AT1A      IIWLMAGLASLPAVIHRNVYFIENTNITVCAFHYESRNSTLPIGLGLTKN   200
RAT AT1B      ---------------Y--------------------Q-------------
MOUSE AT1A    --------------------------------------------------
MOUSE AT1B    ------------------------------------Q-------------
BOVINE        ----L-------TI-----F----------------Q-----V-------
HUMAN         ----L--------I-----F----------------Q-------------

                     5                                  6
RAT AT1A      ILGFLFPFLIILTSYTLIWKALKKAYEIQKNKPRNDDIFRIIMAIVLFFF   250
RAT AT1B      ----V---------------------K----T------------------
MOUSE AT1A    --------------------------------------------------
MOUSE AT1B    ----V---V-----------------K----T------------------
BOVINE        --------------------T-------------K----K--L-------
HUMAN         ---------------------------------------K----------

                                                     7
RAT AT1A      FSWVPHQIFTFLDVLIQLGVIHDCKISDIVDTAMPITICIAYFNNCLNP    300
RAT AT1B      -------------------I-R--E-A----------------------
MOUSE AT1A    --------------------------A----------------------
MOUSE AT1B    ---------S--------------E-A-V--------------------
BOVINE        -----------M-------L-R----E------------L---------
HUMAN         ---I---------------I-R--R-A----------------------

RAT AT1A      FYGFLGKKFKKYFLQLLKYIPPKAKSHSSLSTKMSTLSYRPSDNMSSSAKKPASCFEVE   359
RAT AT1B      ----------------------T----AG----------------------S--F----
MOUSE AT1A    -----------------------------------------------A-------S---
MOUSE AT1B    ----------R-------------R--AG--------------------R-S-Y-----
BOVINE        ----------------------------N-------------E-GN--T----P-I---
HUMAN         ----------R-----------------N---------------V---T----P-----
```

Figure 7 Comparison of several AT_1 receptors. The amino acid sequence of the rat AT_{1A} receptor is presented in its entirety (48). Identity with this sequence is indicated by a dash. The seven predicted regions of membrane-associated helices are indicated. (From Ref. 51.)

residue 355 in the AT_{1b} receptor (54). In the AT_{1a} receptor, this residue is found and may serve as a site for palmitoylation, a posttranslational modification that would anchor the carboxyl terminal tail of the receptor to the plasma membrane. In the rat, the AT_{1a} receptor is the primary isoform expressed by vascular smooth muscle cells and is predominant in liver, kidney, heart, aorta, lung, and testis (55). The AT_{1b} receptor subtype is the predominant molecule found in the adrenal cortex, uterus, and pituitary. Expression of AT_{1b} in the pituitary is modified by estrogen levels. Both AT_1 receptors bind angiotensin II with a similar affinity. The functional significance of two highly related AT_1 receptor proteins in rodents is not understood.

In an effort to localize the AT_1 receptor in rat tissues, an affinity-purified polyclonal antiserum was prepared against the peptide QDDCPKAGRHC (56). This corresponds to amino acids 15 to 24 of the rat AT_{1a} and AT_{1b} receptors, a region located in the extracellular amino terminus. The antiserum can immunochemically detect AT_1 receptor protein within paraffin-imbedded tissues. Survey of rat tissues showed AT_1 receptors in liver, vascular smooth muscle, and the granulosa cells of the adrenal. In addition, smooth muscle in the bronchi and gut as well as in the ureter and epididymis reacted positively with the antisera. Within the kidney, all vascular smooth muscle stained intensely positive. This included the smooth muscle of both afferent and efferent arterials. Staining was observed in the thick ascending limb within the inner stripe of the outer medulla. Proximal tubular epithelium demonstrated AT_1 receptors and glomerular staining was observed within the mesangium.

Structure of the Type 1 Angiotensin II Receptor Ligand Binding Site

Elucidation of the primary structure of the AT_1 receptor indicates that it belongs to the family of G protein–associated receptors. The function of these receptors is to bind an extracellular ligand and then to transduce a signal activating an intracellular effector such as phospholipase C. The precise amino acids of the AT_1 receptor that participate in these functions can be identified by the technique of site-directed mutagenesis. Consider the nature of the AT_1 binding site. Studies of other G protein–coupled receptors showed that the ligand-binding domain of the bioamine receptors clearly involves the polar residues of the transmembrane domains and not the extracellular sequences of these receptors. This surprising conclusion resulted from extensive site-directed mutagenesis of adrenergic receptors and from three-dimensional molecular computer modeling of these proteins (47). In contrast, the receptors for the pituitary glycoprotein hormones such as TSH and LH bind ligand in an extracellular binding site encoded by a large amino terminal domain (57). While study of the AT_1 receptor is not yet complete, what is known is that mutations of the potential N-glycosylation sites located on the amino terminal segment and the second extracellular loop do not modify the expression or the pharmacology of the receptor (58). In contrast, mutation of any of the four cysteines located on the extracellular segments destroys the ability of the AT_1 receptor to bind angiotensin II, either by impairing expression at the cell surface or by modifying the structure of the binding site. A conserved aspartate residue (Asp74) located in the second transmembrane domain was recently mutated in the rat AT_1 receptor (59). This Asp is known to influence ligand affinity in other G protein–coupled receptors and is the target of regulation by sodium for the α_2-adrenergic receptor (60). Mutation of this residue in the AT_1 receptor does not change the affinity for angiotensin II but does strongly modify the specificity of this mutated receptor for AT_1 and AT_2 antagonists. Finally, we recently mutated several polar residues of the third and fifth transmembrane domains and identified Lys102, and Lys199, located close to the extracellular loops, as essential in the binding of both angiotensin II and nonpeptidic AT_1 antagonists. In contrast, Asn111 seems involved in the binding of nonpeptidic AT_1 antagonists only (C. Monnot et al.; in preparation). While these data are as yet unable to give the precise structure of the AT_1 ligand binding site, the emerging picture indicates that polar residues of the transmembrane domains and the correct disulfide bridge formation are necessary components. Moreover, these results suggest that the binding sites for angiotensin II and nonpeptidic antagonists are not strictly overlapping; the binding site for angiotensin II appears to be at the junction of the extracellular space and the cell membrane, while that for nonpeptidic antagonists appears to be deeper in the cell membrane and formed by polar residues of the transmembrane domains.

Intracellular Signaling Mediated by the Type 1 Angiotensin II Receptor

When angiotensin II binds to the AT_1 receptor, it triggers a complex series of intracellular, diffusible second messengers. While there are substantial experimental data to indicate that the AT_1 receptor activates heterotrimeric G proteins known to bind and hydrolyze GTP, it is also possible that a second class of monomeric 20- to 25-kDa G proteins such as $p21^{ras}$ are involved in signaling (51). It is known that the AT_1 receptor can both inhibit adenylate cyclase and stimulate phospholipase C. Modification of adelynate cyclase activity is associated with coupling to the G protein subclass G_i, while stimulation of phospholipase C is typical of G_q. Ohnishi et al. have examined whether cloned AT_1 receptors will couple to several different signal transduction pathways (61). Using Chinese hamster ovary cell lines which were stably transfected with the AT_1 receptor construct, they demonstrated that angiotensin II will activate phospholipase C, stimulate dihydropyridine-sensitive voltage-dependent calcium channels, and inhibit adenylate cyclase activity. These data are in sharp contrast to those for adrenergic receptors which appear linked to only a single signaling mechanism. A recent review has summarized the current state of understanding of angiotensin II signaling (62).

The sequences of the AT_1 receptor that interact with the α subunit of G proteins are not known. However, by analogy with other G protein–coupled receptors, one suspects that amino acids in the second and third intracellular loops and the proximal segment of the carboxyl terminal domain are important for this function. One recent study supported this hypothesis when it showed that mutations in the second intracellular loop and the distal part of the third intracellular loop suppressed angiotensin II–induced second-messenger production, presumably by preventing AT_1 coupling to a G protein (63). Other residues of the AT_1 receptor are certainly essential for the receptor to adopt the correct conformation after ligand binding to allow activation of the G protein. As an example, mutation of Asp74 in the second transmembrane domain does not change the affinity of angiotensin II for this receptor but completely abolished its coupling to the G protein (59). This residue cannot be in contact to the G protein but is certainly essential for the activation of the receptor. The structure-function analysis of the AT_1 receptor is just beginning and should provide important information on how a receptor for a peptide such as angiotensin II differs from the bioamine receptors.

The Type 2 Angiotensin II Receptor

As previously indicated, a second class of angiotensin II receptors, termed AT_2, has been defined. The AT_2 binding sites have been reported in the pancreas, distinct areas of the brain, the adrenal, the kidney, the renal arteries, the heart, the aorta, the uterine myometrium, the ovary, and the intestine (64). Both the number and the tissue localization of the AT_2 subtype differ between species. For example, in the rat and rabbit kidney cortex, more than 90% of the angiotensin II binding sites are the AT_1 subtype (65). In contrast, the kidney cortex of the monkey contains equal amounts of both AT_1 and AT_2 receptors. Interestingly, AT_2 receptor antagonists have no effect on plasma renin activity in either the rat or the monkey (66). Grone et al. identified both receptor subtypes in the cortex and medulla of fetal and adult human renal tissue (67).

A major unanswered question is the functional role of the AT_2 receptor. Both AT_1 and AT_2 subtype antagonists have been shown to inhibit proximal tubule sodium reabsorption in the microperfused rat kidney (68). Results obtained by Keiser et al. suggest that the AT_2 receptor may be related to water handling in the dog kidney (69). Functional responses associated with the AT_2 receptor have been reported in the brain and in cultured cells. Unfortunately, the number of studies on this topic remains limited, and an increasing number of studies describe negative data with AT_2-selective antagonists. At present, no functional response has been definitively linked to the AT_2 receptor in adults.

In the fetus, abundant expression of the AT_2 receptor is found in the dermis and in tissues derived from embryonic mesoblasts such as skeletal muscle (70). Surprisingly, these receptors rapidly disappear within days after birth. The AT_2 receptor has also been identified in immature brain and during development of the aorta. Its expression is upregulated in skin wounds and perhaps during neointimal formation following vascular injury. The distribution of the AT_2 receptor points to a role in growth and development, and it has been suggested that angiotensin II in fetal life may modulate the effects of growth factors (64). Lu et al., however, reported no effects of a 7-day infusion of either PD123319 or losartan in 14-day pregnant rats except for a downregulation of angiotensin II binding sites in fetal skin (71).

The AT_2 receptor has recently been cloned using an expression-cloning strategy. It was found to share the seven-transmembrane-domain topology and some key amino acid residues found in many G protein–coupled receptors and to be 34% identical in amino acid sequence to the AT_1 receptor (72). The AT_2 receptor, however, is not affected by GTPγS (73) and thus seems to have a unique intracellular signaling pathway. Mukoyama et al. speculate that the AT_2 receptor belongs to a class of receptors for which G protein coupling has not been demonstrated. A conserved motif in the third intracellular loop distinguishes this class from the classic G protein–coupled receptors. Interestingly, other members of this class—like somatostatin SSTR1, dopamine D3, and frizzled protein Fz—all exhibit fetal and developmental or neuronal-specific expression. In conclusion, cloning of the AT_2 receptor has provided further support for the hypothesis that the AT_2 receptor is involved in growth and development. The availability of the sequence for the AT_2 receptor allows the development of specific tools like antibodies and probes for in situ hybridization. Future studies will probably give more insight into the function of the AT_2 receptor.

DIVERSITY OF ANGIOTENSIN II FUNCTION

The renin-angiotensin system has been implicated in many physiological and pathological processes besides abnormalities in blood pressure. Central to this is the concept that components of the renin-angiotensin system may be synthesized locally within individual tissues (74). This local generation of angiotensin II is apart from and under different control mechanisms than the systemic generation of angiotensin II. Take, for example, the heart. The mRNA encoding each of the components of the renin-angiotensin system has been identified in cardiac tissue. Evidence exists that protein is synthesized and that this results in the local production of angiotensin II. It has been suggested that within cardiac tissue, angiotensin II may act as a growth factor (75). Other studies have suggested that angiotensin II plays a role in the cardiac fibrosis observed during chronic heart failure (76). Additional local renin-angiotensin systems have been studied in the brain, pituitary, blood vessels, fat and testes. Not surprisingly, components of the renin-angiotensin system have been identified in lower organisms including birds, amphibians, and fish.

Several recent studies have implicated angiotensin II in diseases apart from high blood pressure. Cambien et al. have recently demonstrated linkage between a locus in the ACE gene and some cases of myocardial infarction (77). A similar analysis has implicated the renin-angiotensin system in the origins of preeclampsia (19). Powell et al. have demonstrated that ACE inhibitors prevent the neointimal proliferation that has been observed after balloon angiography in animals (12). Unfortunately, while a similar disease process is observed in humans, ACE inhibitors appear far less efficacious in them. If the past is any guide to the future, the understanding of the renin-angiotensin system in human disease will continue to expand.

REFERENCES

1. Smith JB. Angiotensin-receptor signaling in cultured vascular smooth muscle cells. Am J Physiol 1986; 250:F759–F769.
2. Blantz RC, Konnen KS, Tucker BJ. Angiotensin II effects upon the glomerular microcirculation and ultrafiltration coefficient of the rat. J Clin Invest 1976; 57:419–434.
3. Saavedra J. Brain and pituitary angiotensin. Endocr Rev 1991; 13:329–380.
4. Brunner HR, Nussberger J, Waeber B. Angiotensin II blockade compared with other pharmacological methods of inhibiting the renin-angiotensin system. J Hypertens 1993; 11:S53–S58.
5. Ondetti MA, Williams NJ, Sabo EF, et al. Angiotensin-converting enzyme inhibitors from the venom of Bothrops jararaca: Isolation, elucidation of structure, and synthesis. Biochemistry 1971; 10:4033–4039.
6. Skeggs LT, Dorer FE, Kahn JR, et al. Experimental renal hypertension: The discovery of the renin-angiotensin system. In: Soffer RL, ed. Biochemical Regulation of Blood Pressure. New York: Wiley Interscience, 1981:3–38.
7. Berecek KH, King SJ, Wu JN. Angiotensin-converting enzyme and converting enzyme inhibitors. In: Raizada MK, Phillips MI, Sumners C, eds. Cellular and Molecular Biology of the Renin-Angiotensin System. Boca Raton, FL: CRC Press, 1993:183–220.

8. The CONSENSUS Trial Study Group. Effects of enalapril on mortality in severe congestive heart failure: Results of the Cooperative North Scandinavian Enalapril Survival Study (CONSENSUS). N Engl J Med 1987; 316:1429–1435.
9. The SOLVD Investigators. Effect of enalapril on survival in patients with reduced left ventricular ejection fractions and congestive heart failure. N Engl J Med 1991; 325:293–302.
10. Zatz R, Dunn BR, Meyer TW, et al. Prevention of diabetic glomerulopathy by pharmacological amelioration of glomerular capillary hypertension. J Clin Invest 1986; 77:1925–1930.
11. Lafferty HM, Brenner BM. Are glomerular hypertension and "hypertrophy" independent risk factors for progression of renal disease? Semin Nephrol 1990; 10:294–304.
12. Powell JS, Clozel J-P, Müller RKM, et al. Inhibitors of angiotensin-converting enzyme prevent myointimal proliferation after vascular injury. Science 1989; 245:186–188.
13. Timmermans PBMWM, Wong PC, Chiu AT, Herblin WF. Nonpeptide angiotensin II receptor antagonists. Trends Pharmacol Sci 1991; 12:55–62.
14. Whitebread S, Mele M, Kamber B, De Gasparo M. Preliminary biochemical characterization of two angiotensin II receptor subtypes. Biochem Biophys Res Commun 1989; 163:284–291.
15. Wong PC, Hart SD, Zaspel AM, et al. Functional studies of nonpeptide angiotensin II receptor subtype-specific ligands: DuP753 (AII-1) and PD123177 (AII-2). J Pharmacol Exp Therp 1990; 255:584–592.
16. Tewksbury DA. Angiotensinogen: Biochemistry and molecular biology. In: Laragh JH, Brenner BM, eds. Hypertension: Pathophysiology, Diagnosis, and Management. New York: Raven Press, 1990:1197–1216.
17. Lynch KR, O'Connell DP. Molecular, biochemical and functional biology of angiotensinogen. In: Raizada MK, Phillips MI, Sumners C, eds. Cellular and Molecular Biology of the Renin-Angiotensin System. Boca Raton, FL: CRC Press, 1993:131–148.
18. Jeunemaitre X, Soubrier F, Kotelevtsev Y, et al. Molecular basis of human hypertension: Role of angiotensinogen. Cell 1992; 71:169–180.
19. Ward K, Hata A, Juenemaitre X, et al. A molecular variant of angiotensinogen associated with preeclampsia. Nature Genet 1993; 4:59–61.
20. Krieger JE, Dzau VJ. Molecular biology of hypertension. Hypertension 1991; 18:I3–I17.
21. Baxter JD, Duncan K, Chu W, et al. Molecular biology of human renin and its gene. Rec Prog Horm Res 1991; 47:211–257.
22. Heinrikson RL, Poorman RA. The biochemistry and molecular biology of recombinant human renin and prorenin. In: Laragh JH, Brenner BM, eds. Hypertension: Pathophysiology, Diagnosis, and Management. New York: Raven Press, 1990:1179–1196.
23. Skidgel RA, Erdös EG. Novel activity of human angiotensin I converting enzyme: Release of the NH2- and COOH-terminal dipeptides from the luteinizing hormone-releasing hormone. Proc Natl Acad Sci USA 1985; 82:1025–1029.
24. Rigat B, Hubert C, Alhenc-Gelas F, et al. An insertion/deletion polymorphism in the angiotensin I–converting enzyme gene accounting for half the variance of serum enzyme levels. J Clin Invest 1990; 86:1343–1346.
25. Jeunemaitre X, Lifton RL, Hunt SC, et al. Absence of linkage between the angiotensin converting enzyme locus and human essential hypertension. Nature Genet 1992; 1:72–75.
26. Soubrier F, Alhenc-Gelas F, Hubert C, et al. Two putative active centers in human angiotensin I–converting enzyme revealed by molecular cloning. Proc Natl Acad Sci USA 1988; 85:9386–9390.
27. Bunning P, Riordan JF. The functional role of zinc in angiotensin converting enzymes: Implications for the enzyme mechanism. J Inorg Biochem 1985; 24:183–198.
28. Bull HG, Thornberry NA, Cordes MHJ, et al. Inhibition of rabbit lung angiotensin converting enzyme by *N*-alpha-((S)-1-carboxy-3-phenyl propyl)-L-alanyl-L-proline and *N*-alpha-((S)-1-carboxy-3-phenyl propyl-L-lysyl-L-proline. J Biol Chem 1985; 260:2952–2963.
29. Bernstein KE, Martin BM, Edwards AS, Berstein EA. Mouse angiotensin I–converting enzyme is a protein composed of two homologous domains. J Biol Chem 1989; 264:11945–11951.
30. Kumar RS, Kusari J, Roy SN, et al. Structure of testicular angiotensin-converting enzyme: A segmental mosaic isozyme. J Biol Chem 1989; 264:16754–16758.
31. Mattei MG, Hubert C, Alhenc-Gelas F, et al. Angiotensin 1 converting enzyme gene is on chromosome 17. Cytogenet Cell Genet 1989; 51:1041.
32. Hubert C, Houot AM, Corvol P, Soubrier F. Structure of the angiotensin 1–converting enzyme gene. J Biol Chem 1991; 266:15377–15383.
33. Wei L, Alhenc-Gelas F, Corvol P, Clauser E. The two homologous domains of the human angiotensin I converting enzyme are both catalytically active. J. Biol Chem 1991; 266:9002–9008.
34. Jaspard E, Wei L, Alhenc-Gelas. Differences in the properties and enzymatic specificities of the two active sites of angiotensin I-converting enzyme (kininase II). J Biol Chem 1993; 268:9496–9503.
35. Wei L, Clauser E, Alhenc-Gelas F, Corvol P. The two homologous domains of human angiotensin I converting enzyme interact differently with competitive inhibitors. J Biol Chem 1992; 267:13398–13405.

36. Cushman DW, Cheung HS. Concentrations of angiotensin-converting enzyme in tissues of the rat. Biochim Biophys Acta 1971; 250:261–265.
37. Howard TE, Shai S-Y, Langford KG, et al. Transcription of testicular angiotensin-converting enzyme (ACE) is initiated within the 12th intron of the somatic ACE gene. Mol Cell Biol 1990; 10:4294–4302.
38. El-Dorry HA, Bull HG, Iwata K, et al. Molecular and catalytic properties of rabbit testicular dipeptidyl carboxypeptidase. J Biol Chem 1982; 257:14128–14133.
39. Langford KG, Shai S-Y, Howard TE, et al. Transgenic mice demonstrate a testis specific promoter for angiotensin converting enzyme (ACE). J Biol Chem 1991; 266:15559–15562.
40. Howard TE, Balogh R, Overbeek P, Bernstein KE. Sperm specific expression of angiotensin-converting enzyme (ACE) is mediated by a 91 base pair promoter encoding a CRE-like element. Mol Cell Biol 1992; 13:18–27.
41. Peach MJ, Levens NR. Molecular approaches to the study of angiotensin receptors. Adv Exp Med 1980; 130:171–194.
42. Birabeau MA, Capponi AM, Vallotton MB. Solubilized adrenal angiotensin II receptors: Studies on the site of action of sodium and calcium ions, and on the role of disulfide bridges. Mol Cell Endocrinol 1984; 37:181–189.
43. Gunther S. Characterization of angiotensin receptor subtypes in rat liver. J Biol Chem 1984; 259:7622–7629.
44. Bouscarel B, Blackmore PF, Exton JH. Characterization of the angiotensin II receptor in primary cultures of rat hepatocytes: Evidence that a single population is coupled to two different responses. J Biol Chem 1988; 263:14913–14919.
45. De Gasparo M, Whitebread S, Mele M, et al. Biochemical characterization of two angiotensin II receptor subtypes in the rat. J Cardiovasc Pharmacol 1990; 16:s31–s35.
46. Chiu AT, Leung KH, Smith RD, Timmermans PBMWM. Defining angiotensin receptor subtypes. In: Raizada MK, Phillips MI, Sumners C, eds. Cellular and Molecular Biology of the Renin-Angiotensin System. Boca Raton, FL: CRC Press 1993:245–271.
47. Caron MG, Lefkowitz RJ. Catecholamine receptors: structure, function and regulation. Rec Prog Horm Res 1993; 48:277–291.
48. Murphy TJ, Alexander RW, Griendling KK, et al. Isolation of a cDNA encoding the vascular type-1 angiotensin II receptor. Nature 1991; 351:233–236.
49. Sasaki K, Yamano Y, Bardham S, et al. Cloning and expression of a complementary DNA encoding a bovine adrenal angiotensin II type-1 receptor. Nature 1991; 351:230–233.
50. Afuffo A, Seed B. Molecular cloning of a CD28 cDNA by a high-efficiency COS cell expression system. Proc Natl Acad Sci USA 1984; 84:8573–8577.
51. Bernstein KE, Berk BC. The biology of angiotensin II receptors. Am J Kidney Dis 1993; 22:745–754.
52. Burns KD, Inagami T, Harris RC. Cloning of a rabbit kidney cortex angiotensin receptor that is present in proximal tubule epithelium. Am J Physiol 1993; 264:F645–F654.
53. Murphy TJ, Nakamura Y, Takeuchi K, Alexander RW. A cloned angiotensin receptor isoform from turkey adrenal gland is pharmacologically distinct from mammalian angiotensin receptors. Mol Pharmacol 1993; 44:1–7.
54. Kakar SS, Neill JD. Angiotensin receptor subtypes (AT_{1a} and AT_{1b}): Cloning and expression. In: Raizada MK, Phillips MI, Sumners C, eds. Cellular and Molecular Biology of the Renin-Angiotensin System. Boca Raton, FL: CRC Press, 1993:293–306.
55. Kitami Y, Okura T, Marumoto K, et al. Differential gene expression and regulation of type-1 angiotensin II receptor subtypes in the rat. Biochem Biophys Res Commun 1992; 188:446–452.
56. Paxton WG, Runge M, Horaist C, et al. Immunohistochemical localization of the rat AT_1 receptor. Am J Physiol 1993; 264:F989–F995.
57. Xie YB, Wang H, Segaloff DL. Extracellular domain of lutropin/choriogonadotropin receptor expressed in transfected cells binds choriogonadotropin with high affinity. J Biol Chem 1990; 265:21411–21414.
58. Yamano Y, Ohyama K, Chaki S, et al. Identification of amino acid residues of rat angiotensin II receptor for ligand binding by site directed mutagenesis. Biochem Biophys Res Comm 1992; 187:1426–1431.
59. Bihoreau C, Monnot C, Davies E, et al. Asp 74 mutations of the rat angiotensin II receptor (AT_{1a}) confer changes in antagonist affinities and abolish G protein coupling. Proc Natl Acad Sci USA 1993; 90:5133–5137.
60. Horstman DA, Brandon S, Wilson AL, et al. An aspartate conserved among G-protein receptors confers alloteric regulation of alpha-2-adrenergic receptors by sodium. J Biol Chem 1990; 265:21590–21595.
61. Ohnishi J, Ishido M, Shibata T, et al. The rat angiotensin II AT_{1a} receptor couples with three different signal transduction pathways. Biochem Biophys Res Commun 1992; 186:1094–1101.
62. Catt KJ, Sandberg K, Balla T. Angiotensin II receptors and signal transduction mechanisms. In: Raizada MK, Phillips MI, Sumners C, eds. Cellular and Molecular Biology of the Renin-Angiotensin System. Boca Raton, FL: CRC Press 1993:307–356.

63. Ohyama K, Yamano Y, Chaki S, et al. Domains for G-protein coupling in angiotensin II receptor type 1: Studies by site-directed mutagenesis. Biochem Biophys Res Commun 1992; 189:677–683.
64. Bottari SP, De Gasparo M, Steckelings UM, Levens NR. Angiotensin II receptor subtypes: Characterization, signalling mechanisms, and possible physiological implications. Frontiers Neuroendocrinol 1993; 14:123–171.
65. Chang RSL, Lotti VJ. Angiotensin receptor subtypes in rat, rabbit, and monkey tissues: Relative distribution and species dependency. Life Sci 1991; 49:1485–1490.
66. Gibson RE, Thorpe HH, Cartwright ME, et al. Angiotensin II receptor subtypes in renal cortex of rats and rhesus monkeys. Am J Physiol 1991; 261:F512–F518.
67. Grone HJ, Simon M, Fuchs E. Autoradiographic characterization of angiotensin receptor subtypes in fetal and adult human kidney. Am J Physiol 1992; 262:F326–F331.
68. Cogan MG, Liu FY, Wong PC. Comparison of inhibitory potency by nonpeptide angiotensin II receptor antagonists PD123177 and DuP753 on proximal nephron and renal transport. J Pharmacol Exp Ther 1991; 259:687–691.
69. Keiser JA, Bjork FA, Hodges JC, Taylor DG. Renal hemodynamic and excretory responses to PD 123319 and losartan, nonpeptide AT_1 and AT_2 subtype-specific angiotensin II ligands. J Pharmacol Exp Ther 1992; 262:1154–1160.
70. Aguilera G, Johnson MC, Feuillan P, Millan M. Developmental expression of angiotensin II receptors: Distribution, characterization, and coupling mechanisms. In: Raizada MK, Phillips MI, Sumners C, eds. Cellular and Molecular Biology of the Renin-Angiotensin System. Boca Raton, FL: CRC Press, 1993:413–431.
71. Lu GH, Overhiser RW, Keiser JA, Panek RL. Characterization of angiotensin II receptors in the rat fetus following 7 day administration of PD123319 and DuP753. FASEB J 1992; 6:A1017.
72. Mukoyama M, Nakajima M, Horiuchi M, et al. Expression cloning of type-2 angiotensin receptor reveals a unique class of seven-transmembrane receptors. J Biol Chem. In press.
73. Bottari SP, Taylor V, King IN, et al. Angiotensin II AT_2 receptors do not interact with guanine nucleotide binding proteins. Eur J Pharmacol 1991; 207:157–163.
74. Phillips MI, Speakman EA, Kimura B. Tissue renin-angiotensin systems. In: Raizada MK, Phillips MI, Sumners C, eds. Cellular and Molecular Biology of the Renin-Angiotensin System. Boca Raton, FL: CRC Press, 1993:97–130.
75. Pratt RE, Dzau VJ. Molecular and cellular biology of angiotensin-mediated growth of the cardiovascular system. In: Raizada MK, Phillips MI, Sumners C, eds. Cellular and Molecular Biology of the Renin-Angiotensin System. Boca Raton, FL: CRC Press, 1993:471–883.
76. Weber KT, Brilla CG, Campbell SE, et al. Myocardial fibrosis: Role of angiotensin II and aldosterone. Basic Res Cardiol 1993; 88(suppl 1):107–124.
77. Cambien F, Poirier O, Lecerf L, et al. Deletion polymorphism in the gene for angiotensin-converting enzyme is a potent risk factor for myocardial infarction. Nature 1992; 359:641–644.

9

Mineralocorticoid Receptors and Specificity-Conferring Mechanisms

John W. Funder
Baker Medical Research Institute, Melbourne, Australia

INTRODUCTION

In 1987 the human mineralocorticoid receptor (hMR) was cloned and sequenced (1), establishing it as a member of what is now recognized as a steroid/thyroid/retinoid/orphan receptor family of nuclear transactivating factors. The hMR was shown to be the longest member (984aa) of the superfamily cloned to date and to share the domain structure characteristic of family members. Within this family, the N-terminal domain varies enormously in length (from 24 amino acids in vitamin D_3 receptors to 602 in hMR), and in sequence, with no significant homologies between even closely related family members. The central DNA binding domain is the area of maximally conserved identity (≥40%) over a stretch of 66 to 68 amino acids, with a total of 9 invariant cysteines, 8 of which complex two zinc ions to form two "zinc fingers." The C-terminal ligand (signal) binding domain is an area of moderately conserved identity between family members, ranging from ~25–57%. Mineralocorticoid receptors form part of a more closely related subfamily within the superfamily, sharing ≥90% amino acid identity in the DNA-binding domain, and ≥50% identity in the ligand-binding domain, with glucocorticoid receptors (GR) (2), progesterone receptors (PR) (3) and androgen receptors (AR) (4).

The hMR cloning studies also allowed two experiments with results that appear counterintuitive. First, Northern blot analyses of various tissue extracts showed that in the rat, MR were expressed at much higher levels in the hippocampus than in the kidney. Second, the same authors showed that whereas expressed hMR-bound aldosterone with relatively high affinity (K_d 1.7 n*M*), the receptors were unable to distinguish between aldosterone and the physiological glucocorticoid cortisol or corticosterone (in the rat and mouse). In fact, neither of these findings was unexpected, as it had been demonstrated some years previously that renal mineralocorticoid receptors and the hippocampal "corticosterone-preferring sites" (5) appeared indistinguishable on a variety of criteria, including trypsin fragmentation patterns (6) and high equivalent affinity for aldosterone and corticosterone when transcortin-free cytosols were compared in vitro (7).

Although hippocampal and renal MR—recombinant or in cytosol extracts—show equivalent binding of aldosterone and corticosterone in vitro, in in vivo studies major differences were seen. When adrenalectomized rats are injected with [^{3}H]aldosterone or [^{3}H]corticosterone under conditions to produce similar plasma-free levels of both tracer, uptake and retention of the two steroids into hippocampal "MR" was equivalent; tracer binding to tissue glucocorticoid receptors was blocked by concurrent injection of excess RU28362, a highly selective GR agonist. In the kidney and colon, however, a very different pattern was seen, with uptake and retention ≥ 10 times lower for corticosterone than for aldosterone (8,9).

Two inferences can be drawn from these in vivo data. First, given that the circulating levels of glucocorticoids are orders of magnitude higher than those of aldosterone, under physiological conditions the hippocampal MR are presumably overwhelmingly occupied by glucocorticoids rather than by aldosterone. The physiological role(s) of such high-affinity glucocorticoid receptors and the mechanism(s) of their action are the subject of very active inquiry, but largely outside the ambit of this chapter. Second, given the difference in specificity in the kidney and colon between in vivo and in vitro studies, there must exist prereceptor mechanisms excluding corticosterone and thus conferring in vivo aldosterone selectivity on what are intrinsically nonselective MR.

The nature of the in vivo mechanism conferring such specificity on epithelial MR was suggested by studies on patients with the syndrome of apparent mineralocorticoid excess (AME). Such patients have the stigmata of marked mineralocorticoid excess, including salt sensitivity and severe hypertension, but with suppressed renin and low aldosterone levels (10). They have, however, a very abnormal profile of urinary cortisol metabolites consistent with a range of enzyme defects, most notably that of 11β-hydroxysteroid dehydrogenase (11βHSD), which in the kidney predominantly acts to convert cortisol to cortisone (11,12). Subsequently, licorice was shown to block 11βHSD and to cause a very mild forme fruste of AME (13).

These studies were interpreted as evidence of the high intrarenal cortisol levels consequent upon low renal 11βHSD activity overcoming the normal prereceptor specificity-conferring mechanisms (13). In vivo studies using carbenoxolone to block 11βHSD in the rat, however, showed that 11βHSD itself appears to be the prereceptor specificity-conferring mechanism by converting corticosterone to its receptor-inactive 11-keto congener, 11-dehydrocorticosterone (14); aldosterone, in contrast, is not so metabolized, as its uniquely reactive 18-aldehyde group cyclizes with the 11-OH to form a hemiketal bridge and thus protect it from enzymatic attack. Parallel studies on kidney slices using glycyrrhizic acid to inhibit 11βHSD were similarly interpreted in support of a key role for 11βHSD in aldosterone action (15).

In the studies on the index case of AME, it had been found that the patient was more sensitive to administered cortisol than to aldosterone in terms of sodium retention and blood pressure elevation. This seemed difficult to explain if the action of cortisol in the syndrome was merely via normally protected MR, at which aldosterone is equivalently active, but consistent with an additional cortisol effect through GR in the same cells, for which aldosterone has very low affinity. To test this possibility, carbenoxolone was administered to patients with pseudohypoaldosteronism (PHA), a syndrome characterized by the absence or low levels of mineralocorticoid receptors (16). Given carbenoxolone to inhibit renal 11βHSD, such patients respond by a decrease in urinary Na^+/K^+ and a prompt increase in plasma HCO_3^-, hallmarks of mineralocorticoid action on the kidney and consistent with a classic mineralocorticoid effect via glucocorticoid receptors (17).

In studies to further explore this possibility, adrenalectomized rats were given the selective GR agonist RU28362; in the presence of carbenoxolone, their urinary electrolyte response was equivalent to that of aldosterone. In the presence of carbenoxolone, corticosterone had a similar effect on urinary electrolytes, an effect which was blocked by the MR antagonist RU28318 and the glucocorticoid antagonist RU38486 given together but not by either given alone (17). Finally, in a series of elegant studies on cultured cortical collecting tubule cells grown to confluence on a grid between two chambers, aldosterone, dexamethasone, and RU28362 were shown to have indistinguishable effects on Na^+ and K^+ flux, and the resultant potential difference between the chambers measured as a short-circuit current (18).

Taken together, these studies underline the crucial specificity-conferring role of 11βHSD in excluding glucocorticoids not only from MR in aldosterone target tissues but equally from GR. Reflecting the ≥90% homology in the DNA-binding domain in the MR/GR/PR/AR subfamily, all four receptors appear able to initiate transcription from classic hormone response elements (HRE), which are imperfect palindromes with a consensus sequence GGAAGAnnnTGTTCT. There may indeed be variations on this basic HRE theme, which may bind one or other member of the subfamily with higher or lower affinity, as has been suggested by very recent studies on Na-K ATPase α_1 subunit gene expression (19). In addition, a clear distinction between MR and GR action has been found at composite response elements (CoRE), which contain not only a nonconsensus sequence binding motif for MR and GR but also an AP-1 binding site for *jun*/*fos* dimers. At such CoRE, activated GR can block transcription induced via the AP-1 site, whereas activated MR cannot (20), although they can bind to the CoRE and thus potentially act as an antagonist of the GR effect (21). While MR-specific actions at the genomic level via any or all of these mechanisms cannot be excluded as components of physiological aldosterone action, there would appear to be very considerable overlap between MR and GR in aldosterone target cells, providing, of course, that glucocorticoids can access these cells. Given this degree of overlap, and the intrinsic inability of MR to distinguish between mineralocorticoids and physiological glucocorticoids, the role of 11βHSD in excluding glucocorticoids from aldosterone target tissues becomes doubly important.

To date, the role of "protection" of MR (and GR) in aldosterone target tissues has been ascribed to 11βHSD activity in the generic sense. One species of 11βHSD has been purified from rat liver (22), and the corresponding rat (23), human (24), and sheep (25) cDNA sequences have been established. This species (11βHSD1) is expressed at highest levels in liver, lung, testis, and renal proximal convoluted tubule, none of which are classic sites of aldosterone action; it is NADP-preferring and has a relatively high (1 to 2 μM) K_m for corticosterone and cortisol. Given its tissue localization and its very low affinity for physiological glucocorticoids, it appeared highly unlikely to be the species of 11βHSD protecting aldosterone target tissues. On this basis the necessity to search for a second species (11β HSD) was proposed (26). Such activity has been shown histochemically in distal tubular cells, distinguished from 11βHSD1 by its NAD-dependence (27), and in cultured cortical tubule preparations by its NAD-dependence, its low K_m for corticosterone (~15 nM), and its apparent unidirectionality (28). Very recently, the cDNA coding for human (29) and ovine (30) 11βHSD2 has been cloned and sequenced and the expressed enzyme shown to be operationally unidirectional with a very low (nanomolar) K_m for corticosterone and cortisol.

There are three recent series of studies related to MR which may prove of relevance to aldosterone action and/or extend our current concepts of specificity-conferring mechanisms in mineralocorticoid action. First, in studies contransfecting MR and/or GR into a human neuroblastoma cell line with an MMTV-luciferase reporter, Trapp et al. (31) have shown that at low (1 to 2 nM) cortisol concentrations, transcriptional activation in the presence of both MR and GR was very much higher than the sum of the activities in the presence of either receptor alone. In gel supershift assays, both MR and GR bound the radiolabeled 27-nucleotide MMTV-LTR fragment and were supershifted by the appropriate antibody only (HRE-MR by anti-MR, HRE-GR by anti-GR). When the labeled HRE-containing sequence was incubated with MR plus GR, the resultant complex was totally supershifted by either anti-GR or anti-MR. Finally, these authors have established, again by binding to labeled HRE-containing fragments, that mixtures of MR and GR bind with higher affinity than equivalent overall amounts of MR or GR alone. These studies constitute very strong evidence for the formation of MR:GR heterodimers, both in broken-cell and whole-cell systems, and that such heterodimers may be more potent transactivating factors than homodimers of MR or GR. The extent to which these processes contribute to aldosterone action via classic MR and the physiological circumstances under which such mechanisms might be operant remains to be determined.

Second, MR in the guinea pig have been shown to have affinity for aldosterone, corticosterone, and cortisol indistinguishable from that of rat MR (32). The guinea pig has a very different pituitary-adrenal axis from that in other species—superagonist ACTH (33) reflecting an Ala24Pro substitution (33,34), very high circulating cortisol levels, low affinity/capacity transcortin, and low affinity GR, estimated to have ~one-twentieth the affinity of those in the mouse (35), and recently shown to reflect in large part a point mutation in the ligand binding domain substituting Trp for an otherwise invariant Cys (36). That the MR appear not to share this drive toward a lower affinity may be interpreted in several ways. In non-epithelial tissues, where MR are unprotected by 11βHSD, it would appear that such receptors may operate as always occupied in the guinea-pig and thus probably in other species, albeit to a lesser degree. For epithelial tissues, the very high circulating cortisol levels pose an even more acute problem for aldosterone occupancy than in other species; whether guinea-pig 11βHSD2 shows increases in affinity and/or capacity commensurate with the elevated cortisol levels or whether there exist additional cortisol-excluding mechanisms in guinea-pig epithelia remains to be explored.

Third, some such additional specificity-conferring mechanisms have been proposed to exclude deoxycorticosterone and progesterone from epithelial MR, given that although such steroids will bind to 11βHSD1, they are not substrates for the enzyme. On theoretical grounds and on the basis of the known patterns of corticosterone metabolism by the rat kidney (37), a likely candidate would appear to be the enzyme 3α,20β steroid reductase (38). Recent observations from this laboratory underline the necessity to explore such mechanisms for excluding progesterone (Funder and Myles; in preparation). Historically, progesterone was considered to have 10–15% the affinity of aldosterone and cortisol for human MR (1), still a level to be reckoned with in the luteal phase and pregnancy.

More recently, progesterone has been claimed to have an affinity for hMR more than a hundredfold higher than aldosterone (39), an extraordinarily high figure and derived from internally inconsistent observations.

Given this three orders of magnitude discrepancy in reported values and the notoriously stickiness of progesterone, we have determined the affinity of progesterone for MR in epithelial (colon) and nonepithelial (hippocampus) tissues, controlling for nonspecific sequestration of progesterone by parallel studies with [^{3}H]progesterone and [^{3}H]aldosterone, in the absence and presence of RU38486 to exclude tracer from GR and any PR present, and at 4°C to minimize the possibility of steroid metabolism. Under these conditions, progesterone has equivalent affinity for MR as aldosterone and cortisol in the guinea pig, and ~threefold higher affinity in the rat. The implications of such a high affinity for MR occupancy by progesterone in nonepithelial tissues (presuming that they are unprotected against progesterone occupancy, just as they are unprotected against glucocorticoids) appears profound, if beyond the scope of this chapter; the implications for epithelial tissues are similarly profound and provide a challenge for the immediate future in terms of their elucidation.

CONCLUSION

In summary, mineralocorticoid receptors are found in both epithelial and nonepithelial tissues and appear to have equivalent high affinity for aldosterone, the physiological glucocorticoids cortisol and corticosterone, and progesterone. In nonepithelial tissues, these receptors—in contrast with classic GR—are of such affinity that they will be largely occupied over the range of circadian glucocorticoid concentrations. In epithelial tissues, these receptors are protected against glucocorticoid occupancy by the operation of an enzyme 11βHSD2, clearly distinct from the species (11βHSD1), both of which have been cloned and sequenced. The role of progesterone in the operation of MR in nonepithelial tissues and the mechanisms which may operate to exclude high luteal and pregnancy levels from MR in epithelial tissues remain to be explored.

REFERENCES

1. Arriza JL, Weinberger C, Cerelli G, et al. Cloning of human mineralocorticoid receptor complementary DNA: Structural and functional kinship with the glucocorticoid receptor. Science 1987; 237:268–275.
2. Hollenberg SM, Weinberger C, Ong ES, et al. Primary structure and expression of a functional human glucocorticoid receptor cDNA. Nature 1985; 318:635–641.
3. Jeltsch JM, Krozowski Z, Quirin-Stricker C, et al. Cloning of the chicken progesterone receptor. Proc Natl Acad Sci USA 1986; 83:5424–5428.
4. Chang C, Kokontis J, Liao S. Molecular cloning of human and rat complementary DNA encoding androgen receptors. Science 1988; 240:324–326.
5. de Kloet ER, Wallach G, McEwen BS. Differences in corticosterone and dexamethasone binding to rat brain and pituitary. Endocrinology 1975; 96:598–609.
6. Wrang O, Yu Z-Y. Mineralocorticoid receptor in rat kidney and hippocampus: Characterization and quantitation by isoelectric focusing. Endocrinology 1983; 113:243–250.
7. Krozowski ZS, Funder JW. Renal mineralocorticoid receptors and hippocampal corticosterone binding species have identical intrinsic steroid specificity. Proc Natl Acad Sci USA 1983; 80:6056–6060.
8. Sheppard K, Funder JW. Mineralocorticoid specificity of renal type I receptors: In vivo binding studies. Am J Physiol 1987; 252:E224–E229.
9. Sheppard K, Funder JW. Type I receptors in parotid, colon and pituitary are aldosterone-selective in vivo. Am J Physiol 1987; 253:E467–E471.
10. Ulick S, Ramirez LC, New M. An abnormality in reductive metabolism in a hypertensive syndrome. J Clin Endocrinol Metab 1977; 44:799–802.
11. Ulick S, Levine LS, Gunczler P, et al. A syndrome of apparent mineralocorticoid excess associated with defects in the peripheral metabolism of cortisol. J Clin Endocrinol Metab 1979; 49:757–764.
12. Stewart PM, Shackleton CHL, Edwards CRW. The cortisol-cortisone shuttle and the genesis of hypertension. In Mantero F, Vecsei P, eds. Corticosteroids and Peptide Hormones in Hypertension, Serono Symposia Publications. New York: Raven Press, 1987:163–177.
13. Stewart PM, Wallace AM, Valentino R, et al. Mineralocorticoid activity of liquorice: 11-beta-hydroxysteroid dehydrogenase deficiency comes of age. Lancet 1987; 2:821–824.

14. Funder JW, Pearce PT, Smith R, Smith AI. Mineralocorticoid action: Target-tissue specificity is enzyme, not receptor, mediated. Science 1988; 242:583–585.
15. Edwards CRW, Stewart PM, Burt D, et al. Localization of 11β-hydroxysteroid dehydrogenase—Tissue specific protector of the mineralocorticoid receptor. Lancet 1988; 2:986–989.
16. Armanini D, Kuhnle U, Strasser T, et al. Aldosterone-receptor deficiency in pseudohypoaldosteronism. N Engl J Med 1985; 313:1178–1181.
17. Funder JW, Pearce P, Myles K, Roy LP. Apparent mineralocorticoid excess, pseudohypoaldosteronism and urinary electrolyte excretion: Towards a redefinition of "mineralocorticoid" action. FASEB J 1990; 4:3234–3238.
18. Naray-Fejes-Toth A, Fejes-Toth G. Glucocorticoid receptors mediate mineralocorticoid-like effects in cultured collecting duct cells. Am J Physiol 1990; 259:F672–F678.
19. Stewart PM, Whorwood C. The effect of 11β-OHSD on mineralocorticoid and glucocorticoid gene transcription. Steroids 1994; 59:90–95.
20. Pearce D, Yamamoto KR. Mineralocorticoid and glucocorticoid receptor activities distinguished by nonreceptor factors at a composite response element. Science 1993; 259:1661–1665.
21. Funder JW. Mineralocorticoids, glucocorticoids, receptors and response elements. Science 1994; 259:1132–1133.
22. Lakshmi V, Monder C. Purification and characterization of the corticosteroid 11β-dehydrogenase component of the rat liver 11β-hydroxysteroid dehydrogenase complex. Endocrinology 1989; 123:2390–2398.
23. Agarwal AK, Monder C, Eckstein B, White PC. Cloning and expression of rat cDNA encoding corticosteroid 11β-dehydrogenase. J Biol Chem 1989; 264:18939–18943.
24. Tannin GM, Agarwal AK, Monder C, et al. The human gene for 11 beta-hydroxysteroid dehydrogenase: Structure, tissue distribution, and chromosomal localization. J Biol Chem 1991; 266:16653–16658.
25. Yang K, Smith CL, Dales D, et al. Cloning of an ovine 11β-hydroxysteroid dehydrogenase complementary deoxyribonucleic acid: Tissue and temporal distribution of its messenger ribonucleic acid during fetal and neonatal development. Endocrinology 1992; 131:2120–2126.
26. Funder JW. 11β-hydroxysteroid dehydrogenase and the meaning of life. Mol Cell Endocrinol 1990; 68:C3–C5.
27. Mercer WR, Krozowski ZS. Localization of an 11β-hydroxysteroid dehydrogenase activity to the distal nephron of the rat kidney: Evidence for the existence of two species of dehydrogenase in the rat kidney. Endocrinology 1992; 130:540–542.
28. Rusvai E, Naray-Fejes-Toth A. A new isoform of 11 beta-hydroxysteroid dehydrogenase in aldosterone target cells. J Biol Chem 1993; 268:10717–10720.
29. Albiston A, Obeyesekere V, Smith R, et al. Cloning and tissue distribution of the human 11-beta hydroxysteroid dehydrogenase type II enzyme. Mol Cell Endocrinol 1994; 105:R11–R17.
30. Agarwal AK, Mune T, Monder C, et al. NAD^+-dependent isoform of 11β-hydroxysteroid dehydrogenase: Cloning and characterization of cDNA from sheep kidney. J Biol Chem 1994; 269:25959–25962.
31. Trapp T, Rupprecht R, Castren M, et al. Heterodimerization between mineralocorticoid and glucocorticoid receptor: A new principle of glucocorticoid action in the CNS. Neuron 1994; 13:1–20.
32. Myles K, Funder JW. Type I (mineralocorticoid) receptors in the guinea-pig. Am J Physiol. In press.
33. Smith AI, Wallach CA, Moritz RL, et al. Isolation, amino acid sequence and superagonist steroidogenic activity of guinea-pig ACTH. J Endocrinol 1987; 15:R5–R8.
34. Keightley M-C, Funder JW, Fuller PJ. Molecular cloning and sequencing of a guinea-pig pro-opiomelanocortin cDNA. Mol Cell Endocrinol 1991; 82:89–98.
35. Kraft N, Hodgson AJ, Funder JW. Glucocorticoid receptor and effector mechanisms: A comparison of the corticosensitive mouse with the corticoresistant guinea-pig. Endocrinology 1979; 104:344–349.
36. Keightley M-C, Fuller PJ. Unique sequences in the guinea-pig glucocorticoid receptor induce constitutive transactivation and decrease steroid sensitivity. Mol Endocrinol. In press.
37. Hoyer GA, Tsiakiras D, Siebe H, Hierholzer K. Corticosteroid metabolism in isolated rat kidney in vitro: III. Structure analysis of lipid soluble metabolites of corticosterone. Pflugers Arch 1984; 400:377–380.
38. Funder JW. A la recherche du temps perdu. In: Bonvalet J-P, Farman N, Lombes M, Rafestin-Oblin M-E, eds. Aldosterone: Fundamental Aspects. France: John Libbey Eurotext, 1991:77–83.
39. Rupprecht R, Reul JMHM, van Steensel B, et al. Pharmacological and functional characterization of human mineralocorticoid and glucocorticoid receptor ligands. Eur J Pharmacol 1993; 247:145–154.

10
Endothelin Generation, Receptors, and Cellular Signaling

Barbara J. Ballermann
Johns Hopkins School of Medicine, Baltimore, Maryland

INTRODUCTION

Endothelins are secreted 21–amino acid peptides first discovered as potent vasoconstrictor activity in supernatants of cultured vascular endothelial cells. There are three known members of the mammalian endothelin family, and homologous peptides exist in snake venoms. The endothelins are powerful vasoconstrictors with long-lasting effects on vascular smooth muscle contractility. Exogenous endothelin administration in experimental animals results in sustained hypertension and reduced renal perfusion, suggesting a role in systemic blood pressure control and possibly in hypertensive disorders. However, recent findings in transgenic mice with a heterozygous deletion of the endothelin-1 gene suggest that the actions of endothelin-1 are more complicated than that, given that such mice are hypertensive even though circulating endothelin-1 levels are suppressed.

In the kidney and elsewhere, endothelins are produced not only by endothelial cells, as the name would imply, but also by a number of other cell types. Furthermore, endothelins have diverse functional effects in various cells. Whereas the molecular mechanisms of activation of endothelin synthesis and their cellular signaling mechanisms are reasonably well known at this time, their role in physiology and pathophysiology remains incompletely understood.

THE ENDOTHELINS

The endothelins-1, -2, -3 (ET-1, -2 and -3) are three structurally similar mammalian peptides that bear striking structural homology to sarafotoxin S6b, found in the venom of the snake *Atractaspis engaddensis* (1). ET-1 was first isolated from endothelial cells (2), hence the name "endothelin." The mature endothelins and sarafotoxin S6b are 21 amino acid peptides, each with two internal disulfide bonds that create a hairpin loop structure. Sequence variability between the mammalian peptides is restricted to the hairpin loop, while the carboxyl terminus with a terminal tryptophan residue is highly conserved (Figure 1).

Endothelins are products of three distinct genes, with chromosomal localizations in humans at 6p23-p24 for ET-1, 1p34 for ET-2, and 20q13.2-q13.3 for ET-3 (3). Structurally, the ET-1 and ET-3 genes are very similar, each consisting of five exons and four introns (4–6). Although it has not been fully examined, the ET-2 gene likely has a similar structural arrangement. Exon 1 of ET-1 and -3 genes contains a 5′ untranslated region and encodes the first 22 amino acids of preproET, including a signal peptide sequence. The sequence encoding the mature ET peptides is located in exon 2, and a highly homologous ET-like sequence is found in exon 3. Since exons 2 and 3 encode a string of similar amino acids, it is probable that exon 3 arose through an exon duplication event (4). Further, since ET-3 shows greater sequence homology with sarafotoxin S6b than with ET-1, it is also likely that the ET-3 sequence represents a more direct evolutionary descendant of the

Endothelin-1: Cys-Ser-Cys-Ser-Ser-Leu-Met-Asp-Lys-Glu-Cys-Val-Tyr-Phe-Cys-His-Leu-Asp-Ile-Ile-Trp

Endothelin-2: Cys-Ser-Cys-Ser-Ser-Trp-Leu-Asp-Lys-Glu-Cys-Val-Tyr-Phe-Cys-His-Leu-Asp-Ile-Ile-Trp

Endothelin-3: Cys-Thr-Cys-Phe-Thr-Tyr-Lys-Asp-Lys-Glu-Cys-Val-Tyr-Tyr-Cys-His-Leu-Asp-Ile-Ile-Trp

Sarafotoxin S6b: Cys-Thr-Cys-Lys-Asp-Met-Thr-Asp-Lys-Glu-Cys-Leu-Tyr-Phe-Cys-His-Gln-Asp-Val-Ile-Trp

Figure 1 Amino acid sequences of the endothelins and sarafotoxin S6b. Disulfide bridges are indicated by the dark lines. Stippled boxes indicate nonconserved residues.

sarafotoxin S6b gene or a common ancestor (7). Given the high degree of variation in untranslated sequences between the different ET genes and their location on different chromosomes but the high degree of sequence conservation for each ET gene between species, the duplication events that gave rise to the three mammalian ETs must have occurred prior to the emergence of mammals. Furthermore, since the ET-like sequence (in exon 3) is contained in ET-1 and ET-3 genes (and presumably also in the ET-2 gene), the exon duplication must have occurred prior to the gene duplication events that generated ET-2 and ET-1 (7). Though the biological roles for each of the ET peptides are as yet incompletely understood, conservation of the three genes between mammalian species suggests that they have critical functions.

The promoter sequences and transcriptional regulation have been studied most extensively for the ET-1 gene. A typical TATA sequence is present 26 bp upstream of the exon 1 cap site (4). The 5′ flanking region contains an AP-1 element at -110 to -102, predicted to interact with the FOS•JUN complex. This region is necessary for ET-1 expression in endothelial cells, binds and is *trans*-activated by the products of the *fos* and *jun* genes (4,6,8). Consistent with the effects of AP-1 binding proteins, ET-1 transcription is transiently activated by phorbol esters, though prolonged exposure of cells to phorbol esters leads to suppression of ET-1 transcription (9,10). Another region necessary for ET-1 expression in endothelial cells, TTATCT, corresponds to bp-136 through -131 and binds the zinc-finger protein GATA-2 (11). A 119-bp region of the ET-1 promoter containing the AP-1 and GATA-2 binding sites is necessary to direct endothelial cell–specific expression (12). Because another GATA protein, GATA-1, is restricted to cells of erythroid lineage, it was reasoned that the GATA-2 site in ET-1 might be responsible for endothelium-restricted expression (11). However, the finding that GATA-2 is widely expressed in a number of cell lines that also express ET-1 is consistent only with the view that this sequence is necessary but not sufficient for endothelium-specific expression (11). It has also been noted that the GATA motif and AP-1 sites are often found together. Further, erythroid-specific expression of the β-globin gene requires activation of a GATA-associated AP-1 site by a tissue-specific factor, NFE-2 (11). Activation of endothelial cells by phorbol esters alone does not lead to sustained transcriptional activation of the ET-1 gene, but the AP-1 site in the ET-1 promoter is required for basal expression in these cells. Also, GATA-2 alone cannot explain tissue-restricted expression of the ET-1 gene. Nevertheless, the promoter element containing AP-1 and GATA-2 sites does direct endothelium-specific expression of ET-1 (11,12). It therefore is tempting to speculate that, like NFE-2 for erythroid cells, an as yet unidentified endothelium-specific AP-1 binding factor could be necessary for endothelium-directed expression of ET-1.

By contrast to endothelial cells, the GATA-2 binding domain is neither necessary nor sufficient to drive ET-1 promoter activity in Cos-1 cells (13). In these cells, promoter activity between bp -647 and -127 was found when expressed without the bp -127 to 0 region, but the full sequence bp -647 through 0 had repressor activity in Cos-1 cells. In addition, Benatti et al. (13) reported expression of two distinct ET-1 mRNA species in placenta, which suggested transcription of the ET-1 gene from two different start sites in that tissue, one similar to and one dissimilar from the endothelial cell start site. Taken together with the findings that GATA-2 was an effective and necessary *trans*-activator in endothelial but not in COS-1 cells, it has been proposed that preproET-1 can be transcribed from two independent promoters in different tissues (13).

In addition to tissue-restricted expression of ET-1, transcriptional regulation by hormones and mediators has also been extensively examined. ET-1 release is regulated by a number of calcium-activating mediators, inflammatory mediators, mediators stimulating cAMP and cGMP production, and physical factors (14). Several consensus motifs for nuclear factor 1 and hexanucleotide sequences thought to represent acute-phase reactant response elements were identified throughout the ET-1 gene (6). It is of interest that transforming growth factor β, thought to activate gene transcription through nuclear factor 1, induces preproET-1 transcription in several cell types (14). Endotoxin, interleukin-1, and tumor necrosis factor-α can also induce preproET-1 expression; the precise DNA element mediating induction by these mediators is not known, though at least some participation of factors binding to the AP-1 site have been postulated (15–17). Whereas shear stress reduces ET-1 expression by endothelial cells (10,18), cyclical strain, which results in stretching of the cells, significantly increased ET-1 expression by cultured human umbilical vein endothelial cells, an effect that was inhibited by a PKC blocker (19). Since activation of PKC alone is not an effective stimulus for sustained ET-1 transcription, it is possible that cyclical strain signals ET-1 transcription through an additional mechanism. Exposure of endothelial cells to fluid shear stress represses ET-1 expression by the cells (18). This effect is seen as a response to pulsatile and steady laminar shear but not to cyclical stretching of the cells or reversing shear. Further, the shear-stress effect required a region in the ET-1 promoter between -2.9 and -2.5 kb, whereas the region containing the GATA-2 and AP-1 sites was not sufficient for transcriptional downregulation. In this regard, prolonged exposure to phorbol esters leads to transcriptional repression of the ET-1 gene and cAMP (10) and cGMP (20,21) reduce ET-1 gene expression. However, neither PKC activation, cAMP generation, nor GATA-2 expression could explain regulation of preproET expression by shear stress, but an element far upstream from this area seemed to be required (10).

Finally, it is of interest that the 3′ untranslated regions of the ET-1 and ET-3 genes contain AU-rich regions that are thought to confer RNA instability (6). The half-life of ET-1 mRNA has been estimated to be 30 min or less (9), consistent with the view that the message for this mediator is unstable and therefore also subject to potential regulation.

ENDOTHELIN-1–CONVERTING ENZYME

Mature ETs are produced from the ~203-aa preproETs through at least four proteolytic cleavage events. As with most secreted peptides, the preproET signal peptide is first cleaved to produce proET (2). Within the proET sequences, sites for cleavage by ubiquitous dibasic pair–specific peptidases cleave the prosequence at amino acids 53 and 92 for proET-1 (2). Intracellular processing of proET-1 therefore results in a 46-aa peptide, larger than the mature 21-aa bioactive form. This precursor, named "big ET-1," is at least two orders of magnitude less potent than the mature 21-aa peptide in eliciting smooth muscle cell contraction (22). Cleavage of big ET-1 and ET-2 occurs at an unusual Trp-Val site, cleavage of ET-3 at Trp-Ile. Conversion of big ET-1 to mature ET-1 by cathepsin-D has been documented (23), though it is doubtful that this enzyme is the physiological ET-1–converting enzyme, since it is expressed in lysosomes, has an acidic pH optimum for big ET-1, and degrades the carboxyl terminus of ET-1 at higher pH. Recently, evidence from several studies converged in the purification to apparent homogeneity of a metalloproteinase from endothelial cell plasma membranes that represents the endothelial ET-1 converting enzyme (24). This enzyme functions best at neutral pH and is inhibited by phosphoramidon but not thiorphan. Inhibition is also achieved by EDTA, with Zn^{2+} restoring activity more effectively than other divalent cations. It is therefore likely that the endothelial ET-1 converting enzyme is a zinc-containing metalloproteinase. The K_m and V_{max} of the enzyme were ~3.3 μM and ~410 nmol/min/mg protein when big ET-1 served as substrate. The relatively high K_m would be consistent with the view that substrate concentration is rate-limiting under most circumstances. Structure-activity studies showed that this big ET-1–converting enzyme cleaves big ET-2 with a potency approximately one order of magnitude less than big ET-1 and has almost no activity against big ET-3. It is therefore likely that at least one additional ET-converting enzyme exists. Of interest, big ET–converting enzyme activity in vascular smooth muscle cell membranes (25) acts on both big ET-3 and big ET-1, and these substrates compete with each other for cleavage. Thus, VSMC may well express the alternate ET-converting enzyme. Given the degree of specificity of endothelial-cell big ET-1-converting enzyme for big ET-1, it seems likely that tissue specificity for the various ETs is not dependent only on the specific ET gene product or on the specific ET receptor genes expressed but also on the specificity of the converting enzyme.

ENDOTHELIN RECEPTORS

Pharmacological and genetic evidence points to the existence of at least three ET receptors. Conventional binding studies have shown several distinct ET binding sites in crude tissue and membrane preparations which bind the ETs and related toxins with characteristic potency orders (26). Such studies suggested the presence of binding sites with high and low affinities, sites that preferred ET-1 and ET-2 over ET-3, others which preferred ET-3 over ET-1 and ET-2, and a third subtype that bound all three ETs with the same affinity (27–29). Three distinct cDNAs encoding ET-A, -B, and -C (ET_AR, ET_BR, and ET_CR) receptors with ET isopeptide binding preferences similar to those found by pharmacological means were subsequently cloned (30–32).

Expression cloning strategies in *Xenopus* oocytes and in Cos-1 cells resulted in the isolation of cDNAs for the ET_AR and ET_BR, respectively (30,31). The proteins predicted from the respective nuleotide sequences are monomers and, like others in the G protein–coupled receptor superfamily, contain seven membrane-spanning domains, each with an extracellular N terminal and an intracellular C terminal domain. For the human ET_AR and ET_BR consisting of 427 and 442 amino acids, respectively, there is an overall sequence homology of 55%. The highly conserved regions correspond to transmembrane-spanning domains and intracellular loops, whereas divergence was noted in the sequence and length of the extracellular N terminus. Putative glycosylation sites were identified for both in the extracellular domain and sequences consistent with a G protein–binding site were present on the third intracellular loop. The ET_AR exhibits selectivity for ET-1 and -2 and binds ET-3 and sarafotoxin S6b with an exceedingly low affinity (30). By contrast, the ET_BR binds all three peptides with nearly equal affinity and, when ET_BR is expressed in Cos-1 cells, all three peptides stimulate intracellular Ca^{2+} mobilization and inositol trisphosphate generation (31). Expression of ET_AR was found greatest in heart and lung, followed by brain, kidney, and small and large intestine. Relatively little expression was found in adrenal and liver (30,33). ET_BR was strongly expressed in heart, kidney, and brain and somewhat less in heart, uterus, stomach, and adrenal; but expression was also clearly present in liver (31,34). Arterial smooth muscle as well as the smooth muscle cell line A10 express ET_AR and not ET_BR (30).

Pigment dispersion in dermal melanophores of *Xenopus laevis* is stimulated by ET-3 with a potency nearly three orders of magnitude greater than ET-1 and ET-2. This functional potency order predicted expression of an ET receptor subtype distinct from ET_AR and ET_BR. An ET C receptor (ET_CR) was consequently cloned from these cells, using a PCR approach with degenerate oligonucleotide primers corresponding to the conserved transmembrane domains of ET-AR and -BR (32). The ET_CR nucleotide sequence is 47% and 52% homologous with ET_AR and ET_BR, respectively. The predicted amino acid sequence of this ET-3–selective receptor also places it into the seven-transmembrane-domain G protein–coupled receptor superfamily (32). Tissue-specific expression of ET_CR in mammals has not been reported to date.

The genes for human ET_AR and ET_BR have been cloned and their structures have been explored (33,34). The human ET_AR gene is a single-copy gene that localizes to human chromosome 4. It spans over 40 kb and contains eight exons with seven introns. The 5′ flanking region contains a putative SP-1 binding site 27 bp upstream of the transcription initiation site but no TATA box. In addition, a CArG box, four GATA domains, an octanucleotide sequence representing an inverted MyoD-E2A binding site, and a hexanucleotide sequence representing an inverted "acute-phase reactant element" were identified. All of these elements presumably function to regulate receptor expression. The ET_AR mRNA was highly expressed in aorta. In cultured cells, message was found in mesangial cells but not in human umbilical vein endothelial cells. The gene for human ET_BR similarly exists as a single-copy gene located on human chromosome 13. It spans approximately 24 kb and contains seven exons with six introns. The 5′ flanking region lacks TATA and CCAAT boxes but contains putative SP-1 sites just upstream of the transcription initiation sequence. The promoter region also contains a GATA motif, a hexanucleotide "acute-phase reactant" sequence, and four "E" box sequences. Two distinct mRNA species, 4.3 and 1.7 kb in size, arise from the ET_BR gene and are due to different lengths of the 3′ polyadenylated tail.

Examination of domain homology with other receptors has placed the receptors into the G protein–coupled receptor superfamily and suggested that the putative G protein–binding site is located in the third cytoplasmic loop. Further, all three ET receptors contain proline residues in transmembrane-spanning domains 4 to 7, which are conserved in this superfamily. Several cysteines, which may be palmitoylated, are located in the carboxyl terminus near the seventh transmembrane-spanning domain. A number of serine residues, sites for potenial phosphorylation, are also present in the carboxyl terminal cytoplasmic tail. In ET_AR, sequence similarity with domain 9 of serine/threonine protein kinase family was observed near transmembrane domain 5, but the significance of this region is not known.

A number of synthetic ET_AR- and ET_BR-selective ligands have been produced (26) and some of these have been used to probe the location of ligand binding sites in $ET_{A/B}R$ chimeric receptors produced by mutagenesis (35) (Table 1). Ligand binding and function were then examined in transiently transfected cells. Each of a large number of different chimeric proteins bound ET-1, whereas transmembrane helices 4 to 6, with their adjacent loops, conferred specificity for ET-3 and synthetic ET_BR-selective agonists. By contrast, specificity for BQ 123, an ET_AR-selective antagonist, was conferred by transmembrane regions 1 to 3 and 7 with adjacent loops. These data can be interpreted to indicate that the carboxyl terminal tail region of the ETs interacts with a different receptor domain than the ET loop region, the former likely requiring the N terminus and last extracellular loop of the receptor and the latter the second extracellular loop (Figure 2). Specificity for ET-3 seems to be conferred by the last extracellular loop. Point mutations of two residues that differed by charge between ET_AR and ET_BR did not result in alterations of binding affinities.

One of the remarkable aspects of ET-receptor binding is the nearly irreversible nature of receptor-ligand interaction and the prolonged desensitization of the receptor. These phenomena are as yet unexplained. The affinity of many G protein–coupled receptors for agonist ligands is profoundly decreased with G protein activation. No decrease in ET receptor affinity for agonist ligands has been reported with G protein activation. Given the exceedingly slow dissociation rates of ETs from these receptors, an intruiging possibility, which may need to be explored, is that G protein activation in the case of ET receptors could lead to an increase in ligand affinity. Effects of carboxyl terminal mutations on the ET_AR rate of resensitization have been examined (36). Deletion of 51 carboxyl-terminal amino acids rendered ET_AR nonfunctional, whereas deletion of up to 36 carboxyl-terminal residues gave a fully functional receptor. No changes were observed in duration of the desensitized state of the receptor.

MOLECULAR SIGNALING MECHANISMS

As noted above, all three ET receptors cloned so far are members of the G protein–coupled receptor superfamily. Receptor-coupled G proteins represent a large superfamily of heterotrimeric proteins that consist of α, β, and γ subunits (37). They are divided into several subgroups ($G\alpha_i$, $G\alpha_{s/o}$, $G\alpha q$, and $G\alpha_{12}$), based principally on the structure of the α subunit, which determines the receptor association, target substrate, and toxin sensitivity (38). The various G protein α subunits furthermore

Table 1 Potency Orders for Natural Ligands of the Three Known Endothelin Receptors and Specificities of Some Antagonists and Agonists

Receptor	Ligand potency orders	Antagonists	Agonists
ET_AR	ET-1 = ET-2 >> ET-3 = S6b	BQ-123 FR139317 Ro 46-2005[a]	
ET_BR	ET-1 = ET-2 = ET-3 = S6b	Ro 46-2005	BQ3020 IRL1620
ET_CR	ET-3 = S6b >> ET-1 = ET-2	Unknown	Unknown

[a]Ro46-2005 is the first orally active endothelin receptor antagonist (126).
Source: Ref. 26.

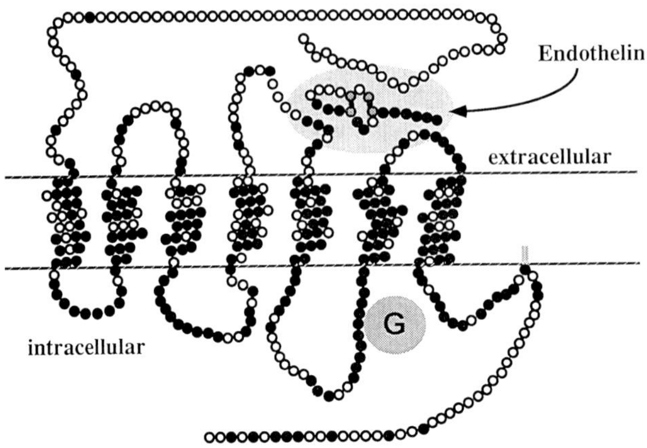

Figure 2 Schematic representation of ET_AR (35) and ET-1. A two-dimensional representation of a plausible location for the endothelin-binding pocket is shown by the stippled area between the ET_AR N terminus and the second and third extracellular loops. Each circle represents one amino acid residue. For the receptor, the open circles are not conserved between ET_AR and ET_BR. For ET-1, the open circles are not conserved between the endothelin peptides. For ET_AR, the stippled lines anchoring the carboxyl terminus in the membrane represents a potentially palmitoylated residue. The putative location of the G protein binding site is also shown. (From Ref. 35.)

differ by their affinity for GTP, their intrinsic GTPase activity, and their affinities for $\beta\gamma$ subunits. Receptor-ligand binding results in exchange of GDP for GTP on the α subunit, dissociation of α from the $\beta\gamma$ subunits, and interaction of the GTP-activated α subunit with a target effector protein. Inactivation of $G\alpha$ occurs through the intrinsic GTPase activity of the α subunit, which returns it to the GDP-bound $\beta\gamma$-associated state. The well-known cholera toxin–sensitive $G\alpha_s$ subgroup of G proteins is associated with receptors that stimulate adenylyl cyclase activity, and members of this group are irreversibly activated by cholera toxin through ADP ribosylation on an internal arginine residue of the α_s subunit. By contrast, the subgroup of $G\alpha_i$s is inhibitory to adenylyl cyclase and is inactivated by pertussis toxin through α_i subunit ADP-ribosylation on a carboxyl-terminal cysteine residue. That ET-receptor signaling is mediated by G proteins has been concluded from the finding that the three cloned ET receptors show strong structural homology with the G protein–coupled receptor superfamily (30–32). Also, cell signaling by ETs is augmented by nonhydrolyzable analogues of GTP, which, after receptor-ligand–stimulated binding to the α subunit, cannot be inactivated by α subunit GTPase activity (26). Further, a number of studies suggest that at least some of the actions of the ETs on cells can be inhibited by pertussis toxin (14,26).

That ET receptors can be coupled to pertussis-toxin–sensitive G proteins is strongly suggested by reports that ET has a strongly inhibitory effect on adenylyl cyclase (26). For example, Kohan et al. (39) found that ET-1 profoundly inhibits cAMP accumulation in response to vasopressin in inner medullary collecting duct (IMCD) cells. This response was equally elicited by ET-1 and ET-3 and was not inhibited by BQ123, an ET_AR antagonist. Pertussis toxin and PKC inhibition both blocked the effect on cAMP accumulation. Indomethacin did not block the ET effect on cAMP accumulation. These findings therefore suggest a direct inhibition of adenylyl cyclase through ET_BR in IMCD, not involving prostaglandin actions. In C6 glioma cells (40), ET-1 also inhibited adenylyl cyclase activity. The effect was completely eliminated by pertussis toxin pretreatment. Acute PKC activation by phorbol esters did not alter adenylyl cyclase activity, but the inhibitory effect of ET-1 on adenylyl cyclase was blunted by PKC activation. This study also supports the view that ET-1 can activate a pertussis toxin–sensitive G_i inhibitory to adenylyl cyclase and independent of PKC activation.

In all cells studied so far, including vascular smooth muscle (41,42) glomerular mesangial cells (43,44), renal medullary interstitial cells (45), and endothelial cells (46,47), ET receptor stimulation by agonists has been found to activate the phospholipase C signaling cascade, with the consequent hydrolysis of phosphatidylinositol 4,5 bisphosphate to release water-soluble inositol 1,4,5 trisphosphate (IP3) and diacylglycerol, which remains membrane-associated. The IP3 is metabolized further to yield several inositol phosphate products, some of which can act as intracellular mediators (48,49). Transfection of CHO cells with both ET_AR and ET_BR confers ET-sensitive PLC activity (50). The phosphatidylinositol-specific phosholipases C (PLC) fall into three distinct groups, phospholipases C-β, -γ, and -δ (38). PLC-β are activated by G protein–coupled receptors, whereas PLC-γ are stimulated by receptor tyrosine kinases. The mechanism of PLC-δ activation is not understood. A G protein subfamily, Gq, which consists of four members with distinct α subunits (αq, α11, α14, and α16), none of them with a pertussis toxin–sensitive domain, has been shown to interact with PLC-β1 and -2 in a highly specific manner (51,52). Reconstituted PLCs-β were activated only by G protein α subunits in the Gq family (53,54), and the activation was Ca^{2+}-insensitive (38). Further, cotransfection of Gαq cDNAs and PLC-β1 cDNAs resulted in a large stimulation of phosphatidyl 4,5 inositol hydrolysis, whereas other classes of Gα subunits were without effect (55). It is known that members of the Gαq and Gα11 mediate thromboxane A2, bradykinin, angiotensin, histamine, vasopressin, and muscarinic acetylcholine receptor signaling via PLC (38). When the liberation of IP3 in response to ET-1 was examined, responses were either not inhibited by pertussis toxin (56,57), or were partially inhibited (58,59). Taken together with the studies of PLC-β specificity for Gαqs, such findings are consistent with the view that pertussis toxin–insensitive members of the Gαq subgroup are involved in mediating PLC activation by ET. Direct evidence of ET_BR coupling to $G_{\alpha q}$ comes from studies in rat liver, where ET-stimulated PLC activity was selectively inhibited by antibodies directed against $C\alpha_q$ but not by antibodies against $G\alpha_s$ (60). In the same study, ET inhibited a plasma membrane Ca^{2+} extrusion pump. That effect was inhibited only by antibodies to $G\alpha_s$ but not to $G\alpha_q$. However, ET-stimulated PLC activation by a pertussis toxin–sensitive G protein (G_i or G_o) is strongly suggested by findings in mesangial cells, where pertussis toxin treatment led to partial inhibition of ET responses, including IP_3 generation. Furthermore, there was inhibition of pertussis toxin–mediated ADP ribosylation in ET-pretreated but not vehicle-treated cells (58). Hence, association of ETs with their respective receptors activates at least one common signaling pathway in all cells so far investigated, namely activation of phospholipase C, likely of the β subgroup, via a G protein, likely in the $G\alpha_q$ subfamily. How pertussis toxin–sensitive PLC activity can be explained awaits further studies.

Stimulation of cells with ETs results in a rapid rise of intracellular Ca^{2+} concentration (42–46). The large but transient Ca^{2+} peak is then followed by a sustained elevation in intracellular Ca^{2+} concentrations (48). It has been conclusively shown by a number of investigators that the initial and transient Ca^{2+} peak in response to ET results from mobilization of Ca^{2+} from intracellular stores, and that it coincides with the rise in IP_3 generation. It is also well known that IP_3 releases Ca^{2+} from intracellular, membrane-bound Ca^{2+} storage sites by interacting with specific receptors. The details of studies showing IP_3-mediated Ca^{2+} release (14) by the ETs is therefore not reiterated here.

The molecular mechanisms of the sustained phase of cytosolic Ca^{2+} elevations in response to the ETs are less well understood. The universal finding of the dependence of this phase of cytosolic Ca^{2+} elevation on the presence of extracellular Ca^{2+} together with studies reporting ET-stimulated Ca^{2+} uptake by cells support the view that Ca^{2+} enters cells from the extracellular space (42–46). Further, the entry of Ca^{2+} into cells in response to stimulation with ET-1 has been dissociated from the initial peak response in that modest but sustained elevations of intracellular Ca^{2+}, dependent on Ca^{2+} influx, were observed at concentrations of extracellular ET below the threshold for PLC activation (61). There are a large number of studies reporting that vasoconstrictor effects of the ETs are inhibited by antagonists of voltage-sensitive dihyropyridine Ca^{2+} channels, although others find no effect (14). Inhibitors of dihydropyridine Ca^{2+} channels furthermore tend not to inhibit the sustained phase of Ca^{2+} entry into cells stimulated by ET (45), though inhibition of the sustained elevation in intracellular Ca^{2+} by diltiazem has been reported (62). Treatment of vascular smooth muscle cells with ET-1 did increase the open probability of voltage-sensitive Ca^{2+} channels when the cells were depolarized in a stepwise fashion (63). This effect was seen in patch-clamp experiments only when cells remained intact, suggesting that the alteration in voltage sensitivity of this channel was dependent on ET-induced intracellular signals. In patch-clamp studies of guinea-pig portal vein smooth muscle cells (64), activation of two voltage-sensitive Ca^{2+} currents by ET was found in whole cell and cell-attached studies. This report suggest that ET augments both the nifedipine-sensitive and resistant Ca^{2+} channels in the smooth muscle cell membranes of the guinea pig portal vein and that ET acts indirectly on the voltage-dependent Ca^{2+} channel. An indirect, G protein–dependent action on voltage-dependent

Table 2 Renal Sites of Action

Cell type	Endothelin peptide	Stimulatory signals	Inhibitory signals	Receptor subtypes
Glomerulus				
Endothelial cells	ET-1	Bradykinin Thrombin TNF α Interferon γ	Shear stress	? ET_BR
Mesangial cells	ET-1	TGF-β1 Thrombin Thromboxane A2 Vasopressin	Atrial peptide Nitric oxide	ET_AR ET_BR
Epithelial cells	ET-1	TGF-β1 Thrombin Complement C5b-9		
Medulla				
Inner medullary collecting duct cells	ET-1	Hypertonicity	Nitric oxide Atrial peptide TNF α Interferon γ	ET_BR
Medullary interstitial cells	ET-3			ET_AR
Vasa recta	ET-1			ET_AR

Ca^{2+}-channel activity was also noted by Lauer et al. (65), who found an effect of ET-1 on the activity of a voltage sensitive Ca^{2+} current in cell-attached ventricular myocytes in the presence but not in the absence of GTP. This action of ET on the transmembrane Ca^{2+} current was inhibited by GDP beta S but could not be blocked by pertussis toxin. In cardiac myocytes, ET-1 also inhibited a delayed rectifying K^+ current, a response that was abolished by the PKC inhibitor staurosporine (66). The authors conclude that these effects of ET on K^+ conductances would prolong the action potential and increase Ca^{2+} influx across the sarcolemma (66). In freshly isolated smooth muscle cells from arcuate and interlobar rat renal arteries, Gordienko et al. (67) also reported activation of both L- and T-type Ca^{2+} conductances by ET-1. However, they suggested that the initial event of intracellular Ca^{2+} mobilization triggers activation of a Ca^{2+}-dependent chloride conductance, which leads to cell depolarization with consequent activation of the voltage-dependent Ca^{2+} channels. Earlier studies by the same group (68) had also provided evidence for a similar mechanism of action in primary cultures of mesangial and vascular smooth muscle cells. Taking the patch-clamp studies and in vivo findings together, it is likely that the ETs regulate the sensitivity of voltage-dependent Ca^{2+} channels in smooth muscle cells and cardiac myocytes, though the effect is not a direct one. The initial event may involve a G protein and K^+ and/or Cl^- channel activation.

Evidence for Ca^{2+} influx via receptor-operated Ca^{2+} channels has also been obtained. Wilkes et al. (45) found that the sustained phase of intracellular Ca^{2+} elevation in ET-treated medullary interstitial cells was returned to baseline in cells treated with Ni^{2+}, while dihydropyridine Ca^{2+}-channel blockade had no effect. Similarly, Simonson and Dunn reported Mn^{2+}-sensitive Ca^{2+} influx in ET-treated mesangial cells, whereas inhibitors of voltage sensitive Ca^{2+} channels were without effect (61). In A10 vascular smooth muscle cells known to express only ET_AR, Ca^{2+} entry also appeared to be best explained via a receptor-operated channel (69). Chan and Greenberg (70) reported inhibition of ET-stimulated Ca^{2+} entry into a neural cell line by an apparently selective inhibitor of receptor-gated Ca^{2+} channels. Thus, the increase in intracellular Ca^{2+} concentration in response to ET stimulation results from at least three separate effects, liberation of Ca^{2+} from intracellular stores through the action of IP_3, an effect on the sensitivity of voltage-dependent Ca^{2+} channels, and possibly an effect on receptor-operated Ca^{2+} channels.

Another common effect of ET-receptor activation is the stimulation of protein kinase C (PKC) activity. PKC activation requires diacylglycerol generation and is accompanied by mobilization of the enzyme from the cytosol to the plasma membrane (48). It seems clear that the initial stimulation of PKC involves PLC-mediated diacylglycerol generation, whereas a second, sustained phase of diacylglycerol release is responsible for the prolonged activation of PKC by ET as well as other mediators, including the phorbol esters (48). PCK activation plays a central role in many of the ET-mediated effects on cells, some of which are discussed below. As with other members of these signaling cascades, a family of enzymes with PKC activity is known. There are at least four Ca^{2+}-dependent (alpha, beta I, beta II, and gamma) and four Ca^{2+}-independent (delta, epsilon, zeta, and eta) isoenzymes (71). Both classes of PKC isoenzymes have been implicated in smooth muscle contraction, though only the PKC alpha, beta, epsilon, and zeta isoenzymes have been identified in smooth muscle (71). In neonatal cardiac myocytes, ET-1–mediated actions were only partly inhibited after phorbol ester–induced downregulation of PKC alpha, delta, and epsilon. Since PKC zeta was present but not downregulated, the authors hypothesized that the ET-1 effect in PKC downregulated cells was mediated through PKC zeta (72). The same authors (73) probed adult rat heart myocytes with specific antibodies to PKC isotypes and found the Ca^{2+}-independent PKC zeta—but not alpha, beta-1, gamma, or delta. In unstimulated cells, the PKC zeta was present in the cytosol and rapidly and completely shifted to the plasma membrane on activation with phorbol ester. In these cells, translocation of the PKC zeta was also observed with ET-1. In contrast, studies by Chen (74) suggest that ET-1 translocated PKC alpha and delta but not epsilon and zeta in the C6 glioma cell line. Which PKC isoenzymes are involved in mediating ET action in smooth muscle, mesangial, endothelial, and renal epithelial cells remains to be shown. Nevertheless, it is noteworthy that ET activated a Ca^{2+}-independent PKC in the cardiac myocytes, suggesting that not all actions of ET in these cells require Ca^{2+}

Another critical component of the ET-generated cellular signal is the activation of phospholipase D, responsible for the sustained release of diacylglycerol (75). This enzyme uses primarily phosphatidylcholine as substrate, generating phosphatidic acid, which is then metabolized further to diacylglycerol through the action of phosphatidic acid phosphomonoesterase (48). The generation of diacylglycerol by PLD may well explain the sustained activation of PKC in response to ET (48), although PKC is also involved in activating PLD. In this regard, the activation of PLD by ET-1 in rat fibroblasts was found to be additive with PLD activation by phorbol esters, suggesting that both PKC-dependent and -independent pathways stimulate PLD in response to ET in these cells (76). Studies in fibroblasts, mesangial cells, and renal medullary interstitial cells all demonstrate that ET-stimulated PLD activity is partially inhibited by PKC inhibitors, though downregulation of PKC by prolonged incubation with phorbol ester completely abolishes ET-sensitive PLD activity (76–80). That PKC regulates PLD activity was also suggested from findings in fibroblasts overexpressing PKC β-1. In these cells, ET-stimulated PLD activity was activated to a much greater extent than in controls (81). However, overexpression of PKC markedly increases ET-receptor expression in fibroblasts, which could explain the enhanced PLD activation (82). Though PLD is thought to require Ca^{2+} for activation, chelation of intracellular Ca^{2+} did not alter PLD activity in cultured mesangial cells (78). In contrast, the contractile response of rat aorta to ET-1 was markedly inhibited by removal of extracellular Ca^{2+} (83). PLD activation was also observed in response to ET, but unlike the findings in cultured cells, the response was not sensitive to inhibition of PKC, though it was blocked by removal of extracellular Ca^{2+}. The PLD response to ET-1 was, furthermore, additive with the activation of PKC by phorbol ester. The authors of this study (83) therefore concluded that not all responses to ET-1 are mediated by PKC and that the PLD response can be seen in the absence of PKC activation and can be sensitive to cytosolic Ca^{2+}. Similarly, in smooth muscle of rabbit iris sphincters, ET-1–stimulated PLD activity was independent of PKC (84). It is therefore attractive to hypothesize that ET-receptor activation results in direct activation of PLD and that PKC positively regulates this response. Whether this involves G protein–mediated signaling is unclear. It is also known that phosphatidylinositol 4,5 bisphosphate hydrolysis by PLC is negatively regulated by protein kinase C (48). In this regard, Challiss et al. (85) reported that ET-1 stimulates PLC and PLD in human neuroblastoma/epithelioma cells. The activation of PLC was inhibited when PKC was stimulated and enhanced when PKC was inhibited. When the PLD products were diverted from phosphatidic acid to phosphatidyl butanol or phosphatidate phosphohydrolase, PLC activity increased. It was therefore concluded that diacylglycerol produced from phosphatidylcholine by PLD would activate PKC and would concomitantly downregulate ET-stimulated PLC. As with other Ca^{2+}-mobilizing agonists, ET-receptor activation therefore seems to trigger PKC activity first through the PLC, while the sustained response involves PLD activation and inhibition of PLC.

Phospholipase A_2 is the third phospholipase activated by ET-receptor stimulation (86–88). Both ET_AR and ET_BR mediate this effect (50). In vascular smooth muscle cells, the predominant cyclooxygenase product formed is thromboxane A_2; in brain microvessel endothelial cells prostaglandin F_2 alpha; and in mesangial as well as medullary interstitial cells and inner medullary collecting duct cells, prostaglandin E_2 (86–90). Findings suggesting direct stimulation of adenylyl cyclase activity by the ETs can be explained by autocrine stimulation of the cells with prostaglandins (89,91). As with PLD, the question of whether activation occurs via a direct or indirect mechanism has been addressed. In rat mesangial cells, sustained activation of PLA_2 was observed after ET-receptor activation, whereas acute responses were desensititzed (90). Furthermore, in vascular smooth muscle cells, PKC activation was dissociated from the activation of PLA_2 (92). In cultured rat renal medullary interstitial cells (RMIC), stimulation with ET resulted in PGE_2 production—but from phosphatidylethanolamine, not phosphatidylinositol 4,5, bisphosphate—arguing against PI-PLC–mediated mechanism (93). This study suggests that in RMIC, there is either a direct coupling of PLA_2 to the ET receptor or that phospholipase A_2 stimulation is secondary to ET-stimulated Ca^{2+} influx (93).

In addition to the pathways described above, ET receptors also activate tyrosine kinase cascades. Such responses are partially though not uniformly PKC-dependent. For instance, in neonatal cardiac myocytes, ET-1 stimulated MAP kinase and MAP kinase phosphorylation, similar to the response elicited by phorbol ester. Whereas PKC downregulation abolished the phorbol ester response, that to ET-1 was only partially inhibited (72), suggesting that a portion of the response was PKC independent. Similarly, Sugimoto et al. (94) reported that ET-1 and phorbol esters stimulated MAP kinase activity in rat glomerular mesangial cells, an effect inhibited by atrial natriuretic peptide (ANP). Since ANP also inhibited ET-1–stimulated translocation of PKC in these cells, it was concluded that MAP kinase activation in mesangial cells was mediated by PKC (94).

In fibroblasts, proteins associated with focal adhesion plaques, namely paxillin and the focal adhesion kinase p125FAK, are tyrosine-phosphorylated in response to ET (95,96). The phosphorylation of paxillin by ET-1 was dissociated from both PKC activation and mobilization of intracellular Ca^{2+}. Similarly, tyrosine phosphorylation of p125FAK in quiescent Swiss 3T3 cells by ET-1 was dissociated from activation of PKC in that the time course of phosphorylation for p125FAK differed, while phosphorylation of 80k/MARKS (a specific PKC substrate) coincided with PKC activation. Also, depletion or inhibition of PKC eliminated 80K/MARKS but not p125FAK phosphorylation, and the concentration of ET-1 required for PKC activation was greater than for p125FAK phosphorylation (96). The tyrosine phosphorylation of p125FAK was furthermore dissociated from the agonist-induced Ca^{2+} response. However, cytochalasin D, an agent that selectively disrupts actin microfilaments, inhibited the p125FAK tyrosine phosphorylation in response to ET-1, while Ca^{2+} signaling and PKC activation were not disturbed. These observations led the authors to conclude that the p125FAK tyrosine phosphorylation is dependent on an intact actin cytoskeleton and that it is activated in response to ET-1 by mechanisms that do not require PKC or mobilization of intracellular Ca^{2+} (96).

In mesangial cells, the mitogenic response to ET-1 may also involve a tyrosine phosphorylation cascade. Simonson et al. (97) found that ET-1 induced tyrosine phosphorylation of several proteins in the quiescent mesangial cells, an effect that was inhibited by herbimycin A and genistein. One of these was the nonreceptor protein tyrosine kinase pp60csrc, which was autophosphorylated and activated by ET-1. Since phosphorylation of p125FAK by constitutively activated pp60src was previously demonstrated (96), it is tempting to speculate that pp60src is one of the central players in the ET-1–mediated tyrosine phosphorylation cascade. Simonson et al. (97) also reported that ET-1–stimulated c-fos induction and AP-1 binding and thymidine incorporation in the mesangial cells; these responses were abolished in the presence of either tyrosine kinase inhibitor. The effect on tyrosine phosphorylation and on cell proliferation was shown to be mediated by ET_AR in mesangial cells and was not linked to a pertussis-toxin–sensitive G protein. PKC activation was necessary but not sufficient in eliciting the mitogenic effect. This study therefore suggests that ET_AR activation in mesangial cells stimulates a mitogenic response and that this response is mediated, in part, through tyrosine phosphorylation events.

Activation of Na^+/H^+ exchange is another response elicited by ET receptor activation. The Na^+/H^+ exchanger is activated by a large number of stimuli, among them PKC, reductions in intracellular pH, and cell shrinkage. In vascular smooth muscle cells, Koh et al. (98) found transient acidification in response to ET-1, followed by a Na^+ and amiloride-sensitive intracellular alkalinization indicating activation of Na^+/H^+ exchange. Since this effect was inhibited by PKC inhibitors and by the Ca^{2+}-channel antagonist nicardipine, they concluded that ET-1–stimulated Na^+/H^+ exchange is linked to Ca^{2+} influx and activation of PKC. However, Winkel et al. (99) showed that an antibody directed against amino acids 658 to 815 in the cytoplasmic tail of the Na^+/H^+ exchanger abolished activation by Et-1 and thrombin, but not phorbol ester, cell acidification, or cell shrinkage. Also, PKC depletion did not affect Na^+/H^+ exchange activation by Et-1. These findings indicate that PKC activation and Na^+/H^+ activation by ET-1 can be dissociated.

RENAL EXPRESSION AND FUNCTIONS

All cultured endothelial cells examined to date express ET-1 mRNA in abundance and secrete the mature peptide. In keeping with these observations, glomerular capillary endothelial cells in culture express ET-1 mRNA and secrete the mature ET-1 peptide (9). In these cells, ET-1 expression was stimulated by a number of agonists that also serve to activate the PLC signaling cascade, though prolonged stimulation of protein kinase C with phorbol ester inhibited ET-1 transcription (9). Inflammatory mediators, among them TNFα and interferon γ, also augmented ET-1 expression and secretion by these cells (17,100). Whereas expression of ET-1 mRNA can be shown by PCR in microdissected renal glomeruli (101), in situ hybridization studies have suggested, that the level of ET-1 expression in the renal microvasculature is low (2) compared with expression in larger vessels. Since cultured endothelial cells exhibit a less differentiated phenotype than those in vivo, it is possible that high levels of ET-1 expression in vitro do not reflect the in vivo situation. In keeping with this view are the findings that exposure to chronic shear stress, a condition under which glomerular endothelial cells differentiate (102), markedly downregulates ET-1 mRNA expression in cultured cells (10,18).

Expression of ET-1 mRNA in most other renal vessels with the exception of outer medullary vasa recta bundles, also tends to be low under normal conditions (2,103). Glomerular mesangial cells (104) and epithelial cells (105) also express ET-1 mRNA and can secrete the mature protein under culture conditions, suggesting that they have the potential of producing this protein in vivo. However, secretion of ET-1 by these cells was markedly less than that observed for cultured endothelial cells in vitro (104,105). In cultured mesangial cells, transforming growth factor β, thrombin, and a thromboxane A_2 analogue all stimulated ET-1 expression and secretion (104). In mesangial cells, ET-1 secretion was also stimulated by vasopressin and markedly inhibited by atrial peptides through a cGMP-mediated effect (106). The cGMP-mediated inhibition of ET-1 production by these cells suggests that nitric oxide could mimic these effects. In cultured glomerular epithelial cells, transforming growth factor-β, complement C5b-9, and thrombin stimulated ET-1 release, whereas EGF was without effect (105). Given that all three resident glomerular cells can express and release ET-1 and that a number of inflammatory and platelet-derived mediators can augment ET-1 expression, it has been proposed that ET-1 may play a significant pathophysiological role in glomerular inflammation (107).

Both ET_AR and ET_BR are expressed in abundance by cultured glomerular mesangial cells, and a large number of studies have shown the mitogenic and contractile actions of the ETs in these cells (14,27,44,107). The contractile and mitogenic response to ET-1 is accompanied by a marked increase in mesangial cell PGE_2 production, presumably on the basis of PLA_2 activation (90). ET receptors are observed in glomeruli under normal conditions (29,103,108,109). Further, a lowering in the glomerular capillary ultrafiltration coefficient and an increase in filtration fraction are in keeping with the physiological responsiveness of glomerular mesangial cells to ETs (44,110). Nevertheless, whereas acute studies show that ET-1 is a potent and long-lived renal vasoconstrictor, it is also known that the cellular response to ET rapidly desensitizes. In this regard, a profound downregulation of ET receptors and desensitization of the cells to acute stimulation with ET were observed when mesangial cells were chronically exposed to glomerular endothelial cell–derived ET-1 (90). Contraction of isolated afferent and efferent arterioles in response to ET application (111) and the marked increase in overall renal vascular resistance observed in response to ET infusion (44,110,112) supports the view that small resistance vessels in the kidney are also responsive to ET.

In the kidney, ET-1 is most abundantly expressed in the renal medulla, and in that site the predominant localization is in the outer medulla (103). In this location, both vasa recta and tubules express mRNA for the peptide. Of the tubule segments devoid of vascular elements, the inner medullary collecting duct (IMCD) epithelial cells express ET-1 and ET-3 in greatest abundance (110,113,114). Localization of large amounts of immunoreactive ET-1 and ET-3 to the inner medulla has also been shown by radioimmunoassay of tissue extracts (115). In IMCD cells, the ETs are expressed under basal, unstimulated conditions in vivo. In contrast to endothelium, ET-1 synthesis by IMCD cells is not augmented by vasopressin, thrombin, or bradykinin, but freshly isolated IMCD segments were observed to increase ET-1 mRNA expression and ET-1 release when exposed to a hypertonic environment (116). Isolated glomeruli also expressed high levels of ET-1 under basal conditions, but they did not respond to alterations in extracellular tonicity (116). In IMCD, ET-1 synthesis is also inhibited by nitric oxide and atrial peptides, effects mediated through cGMP as a second messenger (20). ET-1 synthesis was more profoundly inhibited by interferon γ and tumor necrosis factor α through as yet undefined mechanisms (20).

Binding sites for ET are also expressed in large amounts in the inner medulla of the kidney, as shown by autoradiographic techniques on tissue slices (103,108) and in membranes prepared from the renal medulla (29). Indeed, the highest abundance of ET binding sites in mammals is the inner medulla of the kidney. It is furthermore of interest that expression of ET-1 mRNA appears to be localized to the outer medulla, whereas the greatest abundance of ET receptors is in the inner medulla (103). In microdissected nephron segments devoid of vascular elements, ET receptors were most abundant in IMCD. PCR techniques have shown that ET_BR is expressed predominantly in the IMCD, whereas ET_AR seems to be confined to vascular elements, including glomeruli, arcuate artery, and vasa recta (109,117). Though IMCD expresses the greatest abundance of ET receptors, the cortical collecting duct and outer medullary collecting duct also express ET receptors, with a significant preponderance of the ET_BR subtype (109,118). Rat medullary interstitial cells (RMIC) express ET receptors of the ET_AR subtype based on the findings that ET-3 does not bind to receptors on their surface (45).

In the IMCD, ET-1 inhibits vasopressin-stimulated cAMP generation and water permeability via a mechanism that requires PKC activation and is not dependent on ET-stimulated prostaglandin synthesis (119,120). Conversely, AVP-stimulated cAMP accumulation in IMCD increases in the presence of neutralizing ET-1 antibodies (121). Taken together, the findings of ET-1 and -3 synthesis by IMCD, expression of ET_BR, and reduction of vasopressin-mediated intracellular events by ET-1 antibodies provide evidence that the ET system acts in an autocrine fashion to modulate water permeability in the collecting duct. In IMCD, ET-1 also stimulates phospholipase A_2 and consequently prostaglandin E_2 (PGE_2) synthesis, PGE_2 antagonizes vasopressin-mediated water permeability in cortical and inner medullary collecting ducts, providing an additional mechanism of ET-1–mediated inhibition of vasopressin action. In IMCD, ET-1 also inhibits solute transport through a PGE_2-mediated inhibition of Na^+, K^+ATPase activity (91). In keeping with these observations, Oishi et al. (120) reported inhibition of both vasopressin-stimulated water and solute reabsorption by rat cortical collecting ducts. Furthermore, ET-1 markedly stimulates PGE_2 synthesis by RMIC (45). It is therefore plausible to propose that ET-1 secreted by IMCD cells could act on RMIC to generate PGE_2, which then inhibits vasopressin action in IMCD in a paracrine fashion.

PATHOPHYSIOLOGY

Given the vasoconstrictor actions of the endothelins (122), a number of studies have examined the possibility that ET-1 plays a role in pathophysiological states where renal or systemic vasoconstriction predominates, among them hypertensive states, acute renal failure induced by renal artery clamping, administration of cyclosporine, congestive heart failure, hepatorenal syndrome, and sepsis (123). In most of these studies, involvement of endothelin was inferred through measurements either of circulating or tissue endothelin levels, endothelin mRNA expression, and/or receptor expression. Interruption of ET-1 action with specific neutralizing antibodies or, more recently, with specific receptor antagonists is providing more direct information regarding the possible involvement of the endothelins in pathophysiology and the likely therapeutic potential of endothelin inhibitors in clinical medicine.

A role for ET-1 in hypertensive states has been sought. Circulating levels of the peptide are not elevated in patients with essential hypertension and normal renal function (124,125). In hypertensive patients with renal insufficiency, circulating ET-1 levels are elevated (126,127), presumably due to diminished ET-1 clearance (128). Blood vessel constrictor responses to ET-1 are reported as diminished (129) and elevated (130) as compared with nonhypertensive individuals. In rat models of hypertension, diminished and enhanced blood vessel reactivity to ET-1 has also been reported (131,132) and, similar to the findings in humans, circulating ET-1 levels are elevated only if hypertension is severe enough to result in renal insufficiency (133). Recent studies in mice made deficient in ET-1 by disruption of the ET-1 gene (ET-1^-) surprisingly showed that circulating ET-1 levels were lower in heterozygous ET-1^-/ET-1^+ mice than in wild-type controls, but blood pressure was consistently higher (134). Hence, contrary to what might be predicted from the known pharmacological effects of ET-1, reduced ET-1 expression due the absence of one ET-1 allele appears to be associated with higher, not lower, blood pressures in mice. This, and the generally negative studies in humans with essential hypertension and in rat models of hypertension would argue against a causal role for ET-1 overexpression in essential hypertension.

Chronic hypoxia is known to produce pulmonary hypertension in experimental animals and in humans. In experimental animals, chronic hypoxia, achieved by exposing rats to reduced oxygen tension in inspired air, results in increased ET-1 expression by pulmonary endothelium, while ET-1 expression in other organs remains unchanged (135,136). The pulmonary hypertension observed under these conditions can be reversed with endothelin-receptor antagonists (137). It therefore seems likely that endothelin produced locally in the lung, in response to hypoxia, contributes significantly to pulmonary hypertension, at least early in the disease.

Renal ischemia induced by renal artery clamping in rats is associated with a prolonged decrement in renal blood flow and GFR after the obstruction is relieved. Administration of ETA-(138,139) and ETB-(140) receptor antagonists prior to renal artery clamping is protective against renal vasoconstriction and decrements in GFR as well as tubular injury (138). Such studies strongly suggest that ET-1–mediated mechanisms participate in the renal vasoconstrictor response to renal artery occlusion and reflow. However, it has also been noted that the receptor antagonists must be administered prior to renal artery occlusion and that they are ineffective if given only during the reflow period. Whether ET-1 plays a role only in the initiation phase or whether delivery of the antagonists is hindered in the postocclusion period is as yet not known. Nevertheless, the finding that preadministration of the receptor antagonist is necessary implies that administration of endothelin-receptor antagonists in humans with established postischemic acute renal failure may not be of benefit.

Renal vasoconstriction and decrements in GFR are also commonly observed in patients treated with cyclosporine. Cyclosporine stimulates ET-1 synthesis by endothelial cells in vitro (141), and Kon et al. (142) reported a rapid increase in circulating ET-1 levels after acute cyclosporine administration in rats. In glomeruli of rats given cyclosporine but perfused with anti ET-1 antibody, blood flow was maintained, whereas a marked decrement in single glomerular plasma flow rate was observed in those not perfused with ET antibody (142). Similarly, in isolated, perfused kidneys, Perico et al. (143) found a dose-dependent decrease in GFR and renal blood flow in response to cyclosporine, an effect that was prevented by pretreatment with neutralizing ET-1 antibodies. Administration of ETA receptor antagonist in rats prior to cyclosporine administration also resulted in protection against renal vasoconstriction, but the receptor antagonist did not reverse cyclosporine-induced vasoconstriction once established (144). In patients with kidney transplants, renal hypoperfusion was observed within 2 to 4 hr after cyclosporine administration and was found to be associated with a significant increase in ET-1 excretion (145). Interestingly, in renal biopsy specimens from patients with renal transplants, immunoreactive ET-1 in renal vessles appeared diminished in association with acute vascular rejection and with cyclosporine toxicity, while no changes were observed with interstitial/tubular rejection (146). The mechanism of cyclosporine-induced, endothelin-dependent renal vasoconstriction is not entirely clear at this point. There appears to be enhanced ET-1 synthesis by endothelial cells (141), though the rapidity of increase in ET-1 concentrations after cyclosporine administration and the reduction in ET-1 immunoreactivity in tissues (142,146) suggests that there must also be release of ET-1 from a preformed pool. In addition, an increase in rat glomerular ET receptor density has also been reported with cyclosporine administration (147). Such findings suggest that the cyclosporine effect might be mediated, in part, by upregulation of receptors cell surface receptors. FK506 also stimulates ET-1 synthesis by endothelial cells in vitro, with a concentration-response relationship similar to that of cyclosporine (148). It has been postulated that the reduced renal toxicity of FK506, when compared with cyclosporine, might be explained by the fact that lower doses of FK506 are necessary for the same therapeutic effect.

Endothelin-mediated effects on the renal vasculature have also been implicated in radiocontrast-induced nephrotoxicity. In rats (149,150) and in dogs (151), iodinated radiocontrast agents increase plasma ET-1 concentrations. As with cyclosporine administration, the increase in ET-1 release occurs rapidly, within 15 min after administration (149), again implying release of preformed ET-1. However, the ET_AR antagonist CP170687 did not protect against radiocontrast-induced renal vasoconstriction except when the radiocontrast material was administered together with a prostaglandin synthesis inhibitor (152). These findings are consistent with the view that endothelin is released by radiocontrast but that its vasoconstrictor effect can be offset markedly by vasodilatory prostaglandins.

Endothelin levels have also been found elevated in patients with the hepatorenal syndrome (153), cirrhosis (154), sepsis (155), congestive heart failure (156), chronic renal failure (157), and preeclampsia (158). In experimental animals, reduction in renal mass is associated with increased circulating ET-1 levels (159). In each of these conditions, diminished renal clearance, and/or increased endothelin production could be implicated. Furthermore, it has been postulated that increments in plasma ET-1 concentrations merely reflect endothelial cell damage (160). To what degree the high circulating levels of endothelin alter systemic and renal hemodynamics in these pathophysiological states will need further clarification with specific endothelin receptor antagonists (161).

SUMMARY

Rapid progress is being made in defining the molecules of the ET system and its signaling cascades. There is very strong evidence that the ETs regulate renal vascular and inner medullary functions. A large literature has also explored the physiological effects of the ETs (14). Among these, the potential pathophysiological consequences of ET-mediated vasoconstrictor effects have led to the speculation that ET may have a role to play in the pathogenesis of hypertension, renal ischemia, and cyclosporine toxicity. Studies using transgenic mice furthermore suggest that ET-1 expression is necessary for normal embryonic development (134). Nevertheless, the precise functional roles of the endothelins in development, physiology, and pathophysiology as well as many of the details of gene regulation and intracellular signaling are as yet incompletely understood. There is much to be done.

REFERENCES

1. Inoue A, Yanagisawa M, Kimura S, et al. The human endothelin family: Three structurally and pharmacologically distinct isopeptides predicted by three separate genes. Proc Natl Acad Sci USA 1989; 86:2863–2867.
2. Yanagisawa M, Kurihara H, Kimura S, et al. A novel potent vasoconstrictor peptide produced by vascular endothelial cells. Nature (London) 1988; 332:411–415.
3. Arinami T, Ishikawa M, Inoue A, et al. Chromosomal assignments of the human endothelin family genes: The endothelin-1 gene (EDN1) to 6p23-p24, the endothelin-2 gene (EDN2) to 1p34, and the endothelin-3 gene (EDN3) to 20q13.2-q13.3. Am J Hum Genet 1991; 48:990–996.
4. Bloch KD, Friedrich SP, Lee M-E, et al. Structural organization and chromosomal assignment of the gene encoding endothelin. J Biol Chem 1989; 264:10851–10857.
5. Bloch KD, Eddy RL, Shows TB, Quertermous T. cDNA cloning and chromosomal assignment of the gene encoding endothelin-3. J Biol Chem 1989; 264:18156–18161.
6. Inoue A, Yanagisawa M, Takuwa Y, et al. The human preproendothelin-1 gene. J Biol Chem 1989; 264:14954–14959.
7. Landan G, Bdolah A, Wollberg Z, et al. Evolution of the sarafotoxin/endothelin superfamily of proteins. Toxicon 1991; 29:237–244.

8. Lee M-E, Dhaly MS, Temizer DH, et al. Regulation of endothelin-1 gene expression by Fos and Jun. J Biol Chem 1991; 266:19034–19039.
9. Marsden PA, Dorfman DM, Collins T, et al. Regulated expression of endothelin 1 in glomerular capillary endothelial cells. Am J Physiol 1991; 261:F117–F125.
10. Malek AM, Greene AL, Izumo S. Regulation of endothelin 1 gene by fluid shear stress is transcriptionally mediated and independent of protein kinase C and cAMP. Proc Natl Acad Sci USA 1993; 90:5999–6003.
11. Lee M-E, Temizer DH, Clifford JA, Quertermous T. Cloning of the GATA-binding protein that regulates endothelin-1 gene expression in endothelial cells. J Biol Chem 1991; 266:16188–16192.
12. Lee M-E, Bloch KD, Clifford JA, Quertermous T. Functional analysis of the endothelin-1 gene promoter: Evidence for an endothelial cell-specific cis-acting sequence. J Biol Chem 1990; 265:10446–10450.
13. Benatti L, Bonecchi L, Cozzi L, Sarmientos P. Two preproendothelin 1 mRNAs transcribed by alternative promoters. J Clin Invest 1993; 91:1149–1156.
14. Simonson MS. Endothelins: Multifunctional renal peptides. Physiol Rev 1993; 73:375–411.
15. Sugiura M, Inagami T, Kon V. Endotoxin stimulates endothelin-release in vivo and in vitro as determined by radioimmunoassay. Biochem Biophys Res Commun 1989; 161:1220–1227.
16. Yoshiqumi M, Kurihara H, Moriat T, et al. Interleukin 1 increases the production of endothelin-1 by cultured endothelial cells. Biochem Biophys Res Commun 1990; 166:324–329.
17. Marsden PA, Brenner BM. Transcriptional regulation of the endothelin-1 gene by TNF-α. Am J Physiol 1992; 262:C854–C861.
18. Malek A, Izumo S. Physiological fluid shear stress causes downregulation of endothelin-1 mRNA in bovine aortic endothelium. Am J Physiol 1992; 263:C389–C396.
19. Wang DL, Tang CC, Wung BS, et al. Cyclical strain increases endothelin-1 secretion and gene expression in human endothelial cells. Biochem Biophys Res Commun 1993; 195:1050–1056.
20. Kohan DE, Padilla E. Endothelin-1 production by rat inner medullary collecting duct: Effect of nitric oxide, cGMP and immune cytokines. Am J Physiol 1994; 266:F291–F297.
21. Kohno M, Yasunari K, Yokokawa K, et al. Inhibition by atrial and brain natriuretic peptides of endothelin-1 secretion after stimulation with angiotensin II and thrombin in cultured human endothelial cells. J Clin Invest 1991; 87:1999–2994.
22. Kashiwabara T, Inagaki Y, Ohta H, et al. Putative precursors of endothelin have less vasoconstrictor activity in vitro but a potent pressor effect in vivo. FEBS Lett 1989; 247:73–76.
23. Takaoka M, Hukumori Y, Shiragami K, et al. Proteolytic processing of porcine big endothelin-1 catalyzed by cathepsin D. Biochem Biophys Res Commun 1990; 173:1218–1223.
24. Ohnaka K, Takayanagi R, Nishikawa M, et al. Purification and characterization of a phosphoramidon-sensitive endothelin-converting enzyme in porcine aortic endothelium. J Biol Chem 1993; 268:26759–26766.
25. Tsukahara Y, Matsumura Y, Kuninobu K, et al. Phosphoramidon-sensitive endothelin converting enzyme in cultured vascular smooth muscle cells converts big endothelin-3 to endothelin-3. Life Sci 1993; 53:465–471.
26. Huggins JP, Pelton JT, Miller RC. The structure and specificity of endothelin receptors: Their importance in physiology and medicine. Pharmacol Ther 1993; 59:55–123.
27. Martin ER, Brenner BM, Ballermann BJ. Heterogeneity of cell-surface endothelin receptors. J Biol Chem 1990; 265:14044–14049.
28. Badr KF, Munger KA, Sugiura M, et al. High and low affinity binding sites for endothelin on cultured rat glomerular mesangial cells. Biochem Biophys Res Commun 1989; 161:776–781.
29. Martin ER, Marsden PA, Brenner BM, Ballermann BJ. Identification and characterization of endothelin binding sites in rat renal papillary and glomerular membranes. Biochem Biophys Res Commun 1989; 162:130–137.
30. Arai H, Hori S, Aramori I, et al. Cloning and expression of a cDNA encoding an endothelin receptor. Nature 1990; 318:730–732.
31. Sakurai T, Yanagisawa M, Takuwa Y, et al. Cloning of a cDNA encoding a non-isopeptide-selective subtype of the endothelin receptor. Nature 1990; 318:732–735.
32. Karne S, Jayawickreme CK, Lerner MR. Cloning and characterization of an endothelin-3 specific receptor (ET_CReceptor) from Xenopus laevis dermal melanophores. J Biol Chem 1993; 268:19126–19133.
33. Hosoda K, Nakao K, Tamura N, et al. Organization, structure, chromosomal assignment, and expression of the gene encoding the human endothelin-A receptor. J Biol Chem 1992; 267:18797–18804.
34. Arai H, Nakao K, Takaya K, et al. The human endothelin-B receptor gene: Structural organization and chromosomal assignment. J Biol Chem 1993; 268:3463–3470.
35. Sakamoto A, Yanagisawa M, Sawamura T, et al. Distinct subdomains of human endothelin receptors determine their selectivity to $endothelin_A$-selective antagonist and $endothelin_B$-selective agonists. J Biol Chem 1993; 268:8547–8553.
36. Cyr CR, Rudy B, Kirs RM. Prolonged desensitization of the human endothelin A receptor in Xenopus oocytes. J Biol Chem 1993; 268:26071–26074.

37. Exton JH. Role of G proteins in activation of phosphoinositide phospholipase C. Adv Sec Mess Phosphopro Res 1993; 28:65–72.
38. Rhee SG, Choi KD. Regulation of inositol phospholipid-specific phospholipase C Isozymes. J Biol Chem 1992; 267:12393–12396.
39. Kohan DE, Padilla E, Hughes AK. Endothelin B receptor mediates ET-1 effects on cAMP and PGE2 accumulation in rat IMCD. Am J Physiol 1993; 265:F670–F676.
40. Lin WW, Chuang DM. Endothelin- and ATP-induced inhibition of adenylyl cyclase activity in C6 glioma cells: Role of G_i and calcium. Mol Pharmacol 1993; 44:158–165.
41. Resink TJ, Scott-Burden T, Buhler FR. Endothelin stimulates phospholipase C in cultured vascular smooth muscle cells. Biochem Biophys Res Commun 1988; 157:1360–1368.
42. Marsden PA, Danthuluri NR, Brenner BM, et al. Endothelin action on vascular smooth muscle involves inositol trisphosphate and calcium mobilization. Biochem Biophys Res Commun 1989; 158:86–93.
43. Simonson MS, Wann S, Mene P, et al. Endothelin stimulates phospholipase C, Na^+/H^+ exchange, c-fos expression, and mitogenesis in rat mesangial cells. J Clin Invest 1989; 83:708–712.
44. Badr KF, Murray JJ, Breyer MD, et al. Mesangial cell, glomerular, and renal vascular responses to endothelin in the kidney. J Clin Invest 1989; 83:336–342.
45. Wilkes BM, Ruston AS, Mento P, et al. Characterization of endothelin 1 receptor and signal transduction mechanisms in rat medullary interstitial cells. Am J Physiol 1991; 260:F579–F589.
46. Stanimirovic DB, Yamamoto T, Uematsu S, Spatz M. Endothelin-1 receptor binding and cellular signal transduction in cultured human brain endothelial cells. J Neurochem 1994; 62:592–601.
47. Hirata Y, Emori T, Eguchi S, et al. Endothelin receptor subtype B mediates synthesis of nitric oxide by cultured bovine endothelial cells. J Clin Invest 1993; 91:1367–1373.
48. Nishizuka Y. Intracellular signaling by hydrolysis of phospholipids and activation of protein kinase C. Science 1992; 258:607–614.
49. Sasakawa N, Nakaki T, Kato R. Stimulus-responsive and rapid formation of inositol pentakisphosphate in cultured adrenal chromaffin cells. J Biol Chem 1990; 265:17700–17705.
50. Aramori I, Nakanishi S. Coupling of two endothelin receptor subtypes to differing signal transduction in transfected Chinese hamster ovary cells. J Biol Chem 1992; 267:12468–12474.
51. Simon MI, Strathmann MP, Gautam N. Diversity of G proteins in signal transduction. Science 1991; 252:802–808.
52. Smrcka AV, Hepler JR, Brown KO, Sternweis PO. Regulation of polyphosphoinositide-specific phospholipase C activity by purified Gq. Science 1991; 250:804–807.
53. Taylor SJ, Chae HZ, Rhee SG, Exton JH. Activation of the beta 1 isozyme of phospholipase C by alpha subunits of the Gq class of G proteins. Nature 1991; 350:516–518.
54. Waldo GL, Boyer JL, Morris AJ, Harden TK. Purification of an AlF4- and G-protein beta gamma-subunit-regulated phospholipase C-activating protein. J Biol Chem 1991; 266:14217–14225.
55. Wu DQ, Lee CH, Rhee SG, Simon MI. Activation of phospholipase C by the alpha subunits of the Gq and G11 proteins in transfected Cos-7 cells. J Biol Chem 1992; 267:1811–1817.
56. Takuwa Y, Kasuya Y, Takuwa N, et al. Endothelin receptor is coupled to phospholipase C via a petussis toxin-insensitive guanine nucleotide-binding regulatory protein in vascular smooth muscle cells. J Clin Invest 1990; 85:653–658.
57. Muldoon L, Rodland KD, Forsythe ML, Magun BE. Stimulation of phosphatidylinositol hydrolysis, diacylglycerol release, and gene expression in response to endothelin, a potent new agonist for fibroblasts and smooth muscle cells. J Biol Chem 1989; 264:8529–8536.
58. Thomas, CP, Kester, M. Dunn MJ. A pertussis toxin–sensitive GTP-binding protein couples endothelin to phospholipase C in rat mesangial cells. Am J Physiol 1991; 260:F347–F352.
59. Marsault R, Vigne P, Frelin C. The effect of extracellular calcium on the contractile action of endothelin. Biochem Biophys Res Commun 1990; 171:301–305.
60. Jouneaux C, Mallat A, Serradeil-Le Gal C, et al. Coupling of endothelin B receptors to the calcium pump and phopholipase C via Gs and Gq in rat liver. J Biol Chem 1994; 269:1845–1851.
61. Simonson MS, Dunn MJ. Ca^{2+} signaling by distinct endothelin peptides in glomerular mesangial cells. Exp Cell Res 1991; 192:148–156.
62. Kai H, Kanaide H, Nakamura M. Endothelin-sensitive intracellular Ca^{2+} store overlaps with caffeine-sensitive one in rat aortic smooth muscle cells in primary culture. Biochem Biophys Res Commun 1989; 158:235–243.
63. Silberberg SD, Poder TC, Lacerda AE. Endothelin increases single-channel calcium currents in coronary arterial smooth muscle cells. FEBS Lett 1989; 247:68–72.
64. Inoue Y, Oike M, Nakao K, et al. Endothelin augments unitary calcium channel currents on the smooth muscle cell membrane of guinea-pig portal vein. J Physiol (Lond) 1990; 423:171–91.
65. Lauer MR, Gunn MD, Clusin WT. Endothelin activates voltage-dependent Ca^{2+} current by a G protein-dependent mechanism in rabbit cardiac myocytes. J Physiol 1992; 448:729–747.

66. Damron DS, Van Wagoner DR, Moravec CS, Bond M. Arachidonic acid and endothelin potentiate Ca^{2+} transients in rat cardiac myocytes via inhibition of distinct K^+ channels. J Biol Chem 1993; 268:27335–27344.
67. Gordienko DV, Clausen C, Goligorsky MS. Ionic currents and endothelin signaling in smooth muscle from rat renal resistance arteries. Am J Physiol 1994; 266:F325–F341.
68. IIjima K, Lin L, Nasjletti A, Goligorsky MS. Intracellular ramification of endothelin signal. Am J Physiol 1991; 260:C982–C992.
69. Simpson AW, Stampfl A, Ashley CC. Evidence for receptor-mediated bivalent-cation entry in A10 vascular smooth-muscle cells. Biochem J 1990; 267:277–280.
70. Chan J, Greenburg DA. SK&F96365, a receptor-mediated calcium entry inhibitor, inhibits calcium responses to endothelin-1 in NG108-15 cells. Biochem Biophys Res Commun 1991; 177:1141–1146.
71. Andrea JE, Walsh MP. Protein kinase C of smooth muscle. Hypertension 1992; 20:585–595.
72. Bogoyevitch MA, Glennon PE, Andersson MB, et al. Endothelin-1 and fibroblast growth factors stimulate the mitogen-activated protein kinase signaling cascade in cardiac myocytes: The potential role of the cascade in the integration of two signaling pathways leading to myocyte hypertrophy. J Biol Chem 1994; 269:1110–1119.
73. Bogoyevitch MA, Parker PJ, Sugden PH. Characterization of protein kinase C isotype expression in adult rat heart: Protein kinase C-epsilon is a major isotype present, and it is activated by phorbol esters, epinephrine, and endothelin. Circ Res 1993; 72:757–767.
74. Chen CC. Protein kinase C alpha, delta, epsilon and zeta in C6 glioma cells: TPA induces translocation and down-regulation of conventional and new PKC isoforms but not atypical PKC zeta. FEBS Lett 1993; 332:169–173.
75. Rando RR, Kishi Y. Structural basis of protein kinase C activation by diacylglycerols and tumor promoters. Biochemistry 1992; 31:2211–2218.
76. MacNulty EE, Plevin R, Wakelam MJ. Stimulation of the hydrolysis of phosphatidylinositol 4,5-bisphosphate and phosphatidylcholine by endothelin, a complete mitogen for Rat-1 fibroblasts. Biochem J 1990; 272:761–766.
77. Moolenaar WH, van Blitterswijk WJ. The biologically active phospholipid, lysophosphatidic acid, induces phosphatidylcholine breakdown in fibroblasts via activation of phospholipase D: Comparison with the response to endothelin. Biochem J 1992; 285:235–240.
78. van der Bend RL, de Widt J, van Corven EJ, et al. Endothelin stimulates phosphatidic acid formation in cultured rat mesangial cells: Role of a protein kinase C-regulated phospholipase D. J Cell Physiol 1992; 150:578–585.
79. Ambar I, Sokolovsky M. Endothelin receptors stimulate both phospholipase C and phospholipase D activities in different cell lines. Eur J Pharmacol 1993; 245:31–41.
80. Friedlaender MM, Jain D, Ahmed Z, et al. Endothelin activation of phospholipase D: Dual modulation by protein kinase C and Ca^{2+}. Am J Physiol 1993; 264:F845–F853.
81. Pai JK, Dobek EA, Bishop WR. Endothelin-1 activates phospholipase D and thymidine incorporation in fibroblasts overexpressing protein kinase C beta 1. Cell Reg 1991; 2:897–903.
82. Pachter JA, Mayer-Ezell R, Cleven RM, Fawzi AB. Endothelin (ETA) receptor number and calcium signalling are up-regulated by protein kinase C-beta 1 overexpression. Biochem J 1993; 294:153–158.
83. Liu Y, Geisbuhler B, Jones AW. Activation of multiple mechanisms including phospholipase D by endothelin-1 in rat aorta. Am J Physiol 1992; 262:C941–C949.
84. Zhang Y, Abdel-Latif AA. Activation of phospholipase D by endothelin-1 and other pharmacological agents in rabbit iris sphincter smooth muscle. Cell Signal 1992; 4:777–786.
85. Challiss RA, Wilkes LC, Patel V, et al. Phospholipase D activation regulates endothelin-1 stimulation of phosphoinositide-specific phospholipase C in SK-N-MC cells. FEBS Lett 1993; 327:157–160.
86. Resink TJ, Scott-Burden T, Buhler FR. Activation of phospholipase A_2 by endothelin in cultured vascular smooth muscle cells. Biochem Biophys Res Commun 1989; 158:279–286.
87. Reynolds EE, Mok LL. Role of thromboxane A_2/prostaglandin H_2 receptor in the vasoconstrictor response of rat aorta to endothelin. J Pharmacol Exp Ther 1990; 252:915–921.
88. Zoya C, Benigni A, Renzi D, et al. Endothelin and eicosanoid synthesis in cultured mesangial cells. Kidney Int 1990; 37:927–933.
89. Stanimirovic DB, Yamamoto T, Uematsu S, Spatz M. Endothelin-1 receptor binding and cellular signal transduction in cultured human brain endothelial cells. J Neurochem 1994; 62:592–601.
90. Uchida K, Ballermann BJ. Sustained activation of PGE2 synthesis in mesangial cells cocultured with glomerular endothelial cells. Am J Physiol 1992; 263:C200–C209.
91. Zeidel ML, Brady HR, Kone BC, et al. Endothelin, a peptide inhibitor of Na^+K^+ATPase in intact renal tubular cells. Am J Physiol 1989; 257:C1101–C1107.
92. Reynolds EE, Mok LL, Kurokawa S. Phorbol ester dissociates endothelin-stimulated phosphoinositide hydrolysis and arachidonic acid release in vascular smooth muscle cells. Biochem Biophys Res Commun 1989; 160:868–873.

93. Barnett RL, Ruffini L, Hart D, et al. Mechanism of endothelin activation of phospholipase A2 in rat renal medullary interstitial cells. Am J Physiol 1994; 266:F46–56.
94. Sugimoto T, Kikkawa R, Haneda M, Shigeta Y. Atrial natriuretic peptide inhibits endothelin-1-induced activation of mitogen-activated protein kinase in cultured rat mesangial cells. Biochem Biophys Res Commun 1993; 195:72–78.
95. Zachary I, Sinnett-Smith J, Turner CE, Rozengurt E. Bombesin, vasopressin, and endothelin rapidly stimulate tyrosine phosphorylation of the focal adhesion-associated protein paxillin in Swiss 3T3 cells. J Biol Chem 1993; 268:22060–22065.
96. Sinnett-Smith J, Zachary I, Valverde AM, Rozengurt E. Bombesin stimulation of p125 focal adhesion kinase tyrosine phosphorylation: Role of protein kinase C, Ca^{2+} mobilization, and the actin cytoskeleton. J Biol Chem 1993; 268:14261–14268.
97. Simonson MS, Herman WH. Protein kinase C and protein tyrosine kinase activity contribute to mitogenic signaling by endothelin-1: Cross-talk between G protein-coupled receptors and pp60c-src. J Biol Chem 1993; 268:9347–9357.
98. Koh E, Morimoto S, Kim S, et al. Endothelin stimulates Na+/H+ exchange in vascular smooth muscle cells. Biochem Int 20:375–380.
99. Winkel GK, Sardet C, Pouyssegur J, Ives HE. Role of cytoplasmic domain of the Na^+/H^+ exchanger in hormonal activation. J Biol Chem 1993; 268:3396–3400.
100. Lamas S, Michel T, Collins T, et al. Effects of interferon γ on nitric oxide synthase activity and endothelin-1 production by vascular endothelial cells. J Clin Invest 1992; 90:879–887.
101. Ujiie K, Terada Y, Nonoguchi H, et al. Messenger RNA expression and synthesis of endothelin-1 along rat nephron segments. J Clin Invest 1992; 90:1043–1048.
102. Ott MJ, Olson JL, Ballermann BJ. Chronic in vitro flow promotes ultrastructural differentiation of endothelial cells. Endothelium. In press.
103. MacCumber MW, Ross CA, Glaser BM, Snyder SH. Endothelin: Visualization of mRNAs by in situ hybridization provides evidence for local action. Proc Natl Acad Sci USA 1989; 86:7285–7289.
104. Zoya C, Orisio S, Perico N, et al. Constitutive expression of endothelin gene in cultured human mesangial cells and its modulation by transforming growth factor-β, thrombin, and a thromboxane A_2 analogue. Lab Invest 1991; 64:16–19.
105. Cybulsky AV, Stewart DJ, Cybulsky MI. Glomerular epithelial cells produce endothelin-1. J Am Soc Nephrol 1993; 3:1398–1404.
106. Kohno M, Horio T, Ikeda M, et al. Natriuretic peptides inhibit mesangial cell production of endothelin induced by arginine vasopressin. Am J Physiol 1993; 264:F678–F683.
107. Simonson MS, Dunn MJ. Endothelin peptides: A possible role in glomerular inflammation. Lab Invest 1991; 64:1–4.
108. Kohzuki M, Johnston CI, Chai SY, et al. Localization of endothelin receptors in rat kidney. Eur J Pharmacol 1989; 160:193–194.
109. Terada Y, Tomita K, Nonoguchi H, Marumo F. Different localization of two types of endothelin receptor mRNA in microdissected rat nephron segments using reverse transcription and polymerase chain reaction assay. J Clin Invest 1992; 90:107–112.
110. Kon V, Yoshioka T, Fogo A, Ichikawa I. Glomerular actions of endothelin in vivo. J Clin Invest 1989; 83:1762–1767.
111. Edwards RM, Trizna WT, Ohlstein EH. Renal microvascular effects of endothelin. Am J Physiol 1990; 259:F217–F221.
112. King AJ, Brenner BM, Anderson S. Endothelin: A potent renal and systemic vasoconstrictor peptide. Am J Physiol 1989; 256:F1951–F1058.
113. Kohan DE, Fiedoreck FT, Jr. Endothelin synthesis by rat inner medullary collecting duct cells. J Am Soc Nephrol 1991; 2:150–155.
114. Kohan DE. Endothelin synthesis by rabbit renal tubule cells. Am J Physiol 1991; 261:F221–F226.
115. Kitamura K, Tanaka T, Kato J, et al. Immunoreactive endothelin in rat kidney inner medulla: Marked decrease in spontaneously hypertensive rats. Biochem Biophys Res Commun 1989; 162:38–44.
116. Yang T, Terada Y, Nonoguchi H, et al. Effect of hyperosmolality on production and mRNA expression of ET-1 in inner medullary collecting duct. Am J Physiol 1993; 264:F684–F689.
117. Kohan DE, Hughes AK, Perkins SL. Characterization of endothelin receptors in the inner medullary collecting duct of the rat. J Biol Chem 1992; 267:12336–12340.
118. Takemoto F, Uchida S, Ogata E, Kurokawa K. Endothelin-1 and endothelin-3 binding to rat nephrons. Am J Physiol 1993; 264:F827–F832.
119. Tomita K, Nonoguchi H, Marumo F. Effect of endothelin on peptide-dependent cyclic adenosine monophosphate accumulation along the nephron segments of the rat. J Clin Invest 1990; 85:2014–2018.
120. Oishi R, Nonoguchi H, Tomita K, Marumo F. Endothelin-1 inhibits vasopressin-stimulated osmotic water permeability in inner medullary collecting duct of rat. Am J Physiol 1991; 261:F951–F956.

121. Kohan DE, Hughes AK. Autocrine role of endothelin-1 in inner medullary collecting duct: Inhibition of AVP-induced cAMP accumulation. Am J Physiol 1993; 265:F126–F129.
122. Sorensen SS, Madsen JK, Pedersen EB. Systemic and renal effect of intravenous infusion of endothelin-1 in healthy human volunteers. Am J Physiol 1992; 263:F649–F655.
123. Kon V, Badr KF. Biological actions and pathophysiologic significance of endothelin in the kidney. Kidney Int 1991; 40:1–12.
124. Schiffrin EL, Thibault G. Plasma endothelin in human essential hypertension. Am J Hypertens 1991; 4:303–308.
125. Davenport AP, Ashby MJ, Easton P, et al. A sensitive radioimmunoassay measuring endothelin-like immunoreactivity in human plasma: Comparison of levels in patients with essential hypertension and normotensive control subjects. Clin Sci 1990; 78:261–264.
126. Shichiri M, Hirata Y, Ando K, et al. Plasma endothelin levels in hypertension and chronic renal failure. Hypertension 1990; 15:493–496.
127. Kohno M, Yasunari K, Murakawa KI, et al. Plasma immunoreactive endothelin in essential hypertension. Am J Med 1990; 88:614–618.
128. Kohno MK, Murakawa K, Yasunari K, et al. Prolonged blood pressure elevation after endothelin administration in bilaterally nephrectomized rats. Metabolism 1989; 38:712–713.
129. Schiffrin El, Deng LY, Larochelle P. Blunted effects of endothelin upon small subcutaneous resistance arteries of mild essential hypertensive patients. J Hypertens 1992; 10:437–444.
130. Haynes WG, Hand MF, Johnstone HA, et al. Direct and sympathetically mediated venoconstriction in essential hypertension: Enhanced responses to endothelin-1. J Clin Invest 1994; 94:1359–1364.
131. Dohi Y, Luscher TF. Endothelin-1 in hypertensive resistance arteries: Intraluminal and extraluminal dysfunction. Hypertension 1991; 18:543–549.
132. Miyauchi T, Ishikawa T, Tomobe Y, et al. Characteristics of pressor response to endothelin in spontaneously hypertensive and Wistar-Kyoto rats. Hypertension 1989; 14:427–434.
133. Kohno M, Murakawa K, Horio T, et al. Plasma immunoreactive endothelin-1 in experimental malignant hypertension. Hypertension 1991; 18:93–100.
134. Kurihara Y, Kurihara H, Suzuki H, et al. Elevated blood pressure and craniofacial abnormalities in mice deficient in endothelin-1. Nature 1994; 368:703–710.
135. Elton TS, Oparil S, Taylor GR, et al. Normobaric hypoxia stimulates endothelin-1 gene expression in the rat. Am J Physiol 1992; 263:R1260–R1264.
136. Li H, Elton TS, Chen YF, Oparil S. Increased endothelin receptor expression in hypoxic rat lung. Am J Physiol 1994; 266:L553–L560.
137. Bonvallet ST, Zamora MR, Hasunuma K, et al. BQ 123, an ETA-receptor anatgonist attenuates hypoxic pulmonary hypertension in rats. Am J Physiol 1994; 266:H1327–H1331.
138. Kusumoto K, Kubo K, Kandori H, et al. Effects of a new endothelin antagonist, TAK-044, on postischemic acute renal failure in rats. Life Sci 1994; 55:301–310.
139. Chan L, Chittinandana A, Shapiro JI, et al. Effect of an endothelin-receptor antagonist on ischemic acute renal failure. Am J Physiol 1994; 266:F135–F138.
140. Mino N, Kobayashi M, Nakajima A, et al. Protective effect of a selective endothelin receptor antagonist, BQ-123, in ischemic acute renal failure in rats. Eur J Pharmacol 1992; 221:77–83.
141. Bunchman TE, Brookshire CA. Cyclosporine-induced synthesis of endothelin by cultured human endothelial cells. J Clin Invest 1991; 88:310–314.
142. Kon V, Sugiura M, Inagami T, et al. Role of endothelin in cyclosporine-induced glomerular dysfunction. Kidney Int 1990; 37:1487–1491.
143. Perico N, Dadan J, Remuzzi G. Endothelin mediates the renal vasoconstriction induced by cyclosporine in the rat. J Am Soc Nephrol 1990; 1:76–83.
144. Fogo A, Hellings SE, Inagami T, Kon V. Endothelin receptor antagonism is protective in in vivo acute cyclosporine toxicity. Kidney Int 1992; 42:770–774.
145. Perico N, Ruggenenti P, Gaspari F, et al. Daily renal hypoperfusion induced by clyclosporine in patients with renal transplantation. Transplantation 1992; 54:56–60.
146. Watschinger B, Vychytil A, Attar M, et al. Pattern of endothelin immunostaining during rejection episodes after kidney transplantation. Clin Nephrol 1994; 41:86–93.
147. Awazu M, Sugiura, Inagami T, et al. Cyclosporine promotes glomerular endothelin binding in vivo. J Am Soc Nephrol 1991; 1:1253–1258.
148. Takeda Y, Yoneda T, Ito Y, et al. Stimulation of endothelin mRNA and secretion in human endothelial cells by FK 506. J Cardiovasc Pharmacol 1993; 22(suppl 8)S310–S312.
149. Heyman SN, Clark BA, Kaiser N, et al. Radiocontrast agents induce endothelin release in vivo and in vitro. J Am Soc Nephrol 1992; 3:58–65.
150. Heyman SN, Clark BA, Cantley L, et al. Effects of ioversol versus iothalamate on endothelin release and radioconstrast nephropathy. Invest Radiol 1993; 28:313–318.

151. Margulies KB, Hildebrand FL, Heublein DM, Burnett JC Jr. Radiocontrast increases plasma and urinary endothelin. J Am Soc Nephrol 1991; 2:1041–1045.
152. Cantley LG, Spokes K, Clark B, et al. Role of endothelin and prostaglandins in radiocontrast-induced renal artery constriction. Kidney Int 1993; 44:1217–1223.
153. Moore K, Wendon J, Frazer M, et al. Plasma endothelin immunoreactivity in lever disease and the hepatorenal syndrome. N Engl J Med 1992; 327:1774–1778.
154. Uchihara M, Izumi N, Sato C, Marumo F. Clinical significance of elevated plasma endothelin concentration in patients with cirrhosis. Hepatology 1992; 16:95–99.
155. Badr KF. Sepsis-associated renal vasoconstriction: Potential targets for future therapy. Am J Kidney Dis 1992; 20:207–213.
156. Loffler BM, Roux S, Kalina B, et al. Influence of congestive heart failure on endothelin levels and receptors in rabbits. J Mol Cell Cardiol 1993; 25:407–416.
157. Saito Y, Kazuwa N, Shirakami G, et al. Endothelin in patients with chronic renal failure. J Cardiovasc Pharmacol 1991; 17(suppl 7):S437–S439.
158. Barden A, Beilin LJ, Ritchie J, et al. Plasma and urinary endothelin 1, prostacyclin metabolites and platelet consumption in pre-eclampsia and essential hypertensive pregnancy. Blood Press 1994; 3:38–46.
159. Benigni A, Perico N, Gaspari F, et al. Increased renal endothelin production in rats with reduced renal mass. Am J Physiol 1991; 260:F331–F339.
160. Neild GH. Endothelin plasma levels in hypertensive patients with vascular disease. J Hypertens Suppl 1994; 12:S17–S20.
161. Clozel M, Breu V, Burri K, et al. Pathophysiological role of endothelin revealed by the first orally active endothelin receptor antagonist. Nature 1993; 365:759–761.

11
The Nitric Oxide Synthase Gene Family

Kenneth D. Bloch
Harvard Medical School and Massachusetts General Hospital, Boston, Massachusetts

INTRODUCTION

In the past, vascular endothelium was viewed as a passive boundary layer between the vessel lumen and the smooth muscle cells controlling its diameter. In recent years, it has become increasingly evident that the endothelium is an active tissue regulating the thrombotic/thrombolytic balance of the luminal contents as well as the state of contraction and proliferation of the underlying smooth muscle. In 1980, Furchgott and Zawadski (1) observed that the ability of acetylcholine to relax vascular rings was critically dependent on the presence of intact endothelium. Subsequent research demonstrated that the labile substance released by acetylcholine-stimulated endothelial cells, referred to as endothelium-derived relaxing factor (EDRF), was identical to or contained nitric oxide (NO) (2–4).

Nitric oxide is a cell membrane–permeable free radical gas with a very short half-life in biological fluids. The half-life of NO is shortened in the presence of other free radicals and is lengthened in the presence of superoxide dismutase. Clinicians have long used pharmacological agents that release NO, including nitroglycerin and sodium nitroprusside, to treat elevated blood pressure and angina pectoris. Outside the vasculature, NO is an important signal transduction molecule in the central and peripheral nervous systems (5), where it serves as a neurotransmitter, and in the immune system (6), where it participates in macrophage cytotoxic activity and is a potent antiviral agent (7,8).

Formed by photochemical reactions (9), NO is likely to have been present in the primordial soup from which the first unicellular organisms arose (10). It is produced by soil bacteria during nitrification or denitrification (11) and has been found to be an important biological mediator in nonmammalian species including teleosts (12), insects (13), and the limulus crab (14). Nitric oxide may represent one of the first molecules to be involved in signal transduction.

Nitric oxide interacts with several intracellular molecular targets (reviewed in Ref. 15). It stimulates ADP-ribosyltransferase activity and inhibits several enzymes of the mitochondrial respiratory chain. It also blocks translation of mRNAs encoding proteins involved in cellular iron metabolism (16,17). Interaction of NO with the heme group in soluble guanylate cyclase stimulates the conversion of guanosine triphosphate (GTP) to cyclic guanosine monophosphate (cGMP), resulting in increased concentration of cGMP. Through its action on cGMP-dependent protein kinase, cGMP induces relaxation of smooth muscle, inhibition of proliferation of vascular smooth muscle cells, and inhibition of platelet aggregation and adhesion. Cyclic guanosine monophosphate is metabolized by a family of phosphodiesterase enzymes, some of which are cGMP-specific. The NO/cGMP signal transduction system (reviewed in Ref. 18) is illustrated in Fig. 1.

Nitric oxide is synthesized from L-arginine and oxygen by a family of enzymes called nitric oxide synthases (NOSs). These are divided into functional classes designated constitutive and inducible (19). Constitutive enzymes (cNOS) are present in unstimulated cells, including neurons and endothelial cells, and their enzyme activity is dependent on intracellular calcium concentration. The second class of enzymes is present in cells exposed to one or more cytokines. Activity of most,

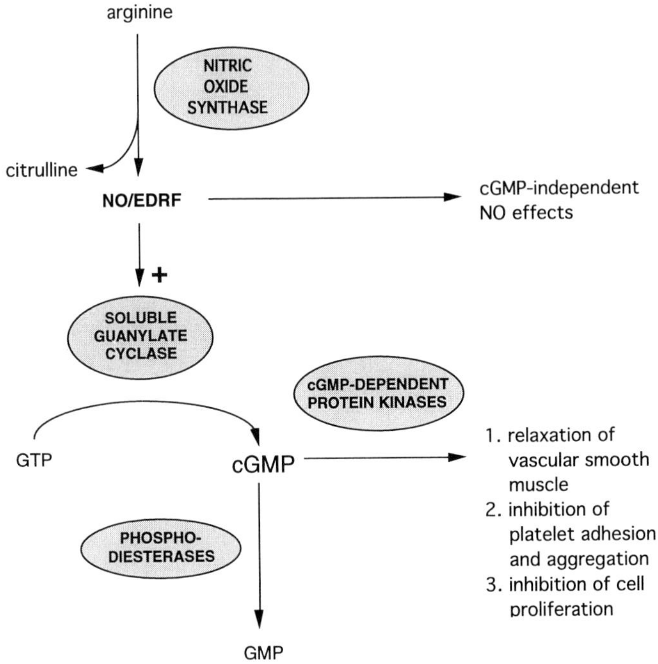

Figure 1 The nitric oxide/cGMP signal transduction system.

but not all, of the inducible enzymes is independent of intracellular calcium concentration. Inducible NOS (iNOS) isoforms have been detected in many cell types, including macrophages, endothelial cells, and smooth muscle cells. Both classes of enzymes are dependent on several cofactors including heme, FMN, FAD, NADPH, and tetrahydrobiopterin.

The biology, biochemistry, and biosynthesis of NO have been extensively reviewed (20–22). This chapter focuses on the molecular biology of the NOS gene family, including the isolation and characterization of NOS cDNA clones and genes and the regulation of NOS gene expression. Insights gained from knowledge of the predicted structure of these enzymes are also highlighted.

BRAIN NITRIC OXIDE SYNTHASE

The first NOS isoform for which a cDNA was isolated was the constitutive rat cerebellar enzyme described by Snyder and colleagues in 1991 (23). These investigators isolated NOS from rat cerebellum using classic enzyme purification techniques. Early purification attempts were unsuccessful because enzyme activity was lost during the initial stages of purification. The problem was circumvented after it was discovered that NOS enzyme activity was dependent upon calmodulin present in crude extracts: activity was detectable during the purification process only after inclusion of calmodulin in the reaction mixture (24). Purified enzyme was digested with trypsin, and the amino acid sequence of tryptic peptides was determined. Oligonucleotides corresponding to these amino acid sequences were synthesized and used in polymerase chain reactions to isolate partial cDNAs encoding brain NOS. These partial cDNAs were used to isolate a full-length cDNA. The enzyme encoded by the cDNA is a 160-kDa protein and contains regions binding enzyme cofactors, including NADPH, FAD, and FMN (Fig. 2). There is also a calmodulin binding site which is involved in rendering the enzyme sensitive to calcium. Upon searching the appropriate computer databases, Snyder's group found a protein sharing sequence homology with brain NOS called cytochrome P-450 reductase (CPR), an enzyme which transfers electrons to microsomal P-450 enzymes. Brain NOS

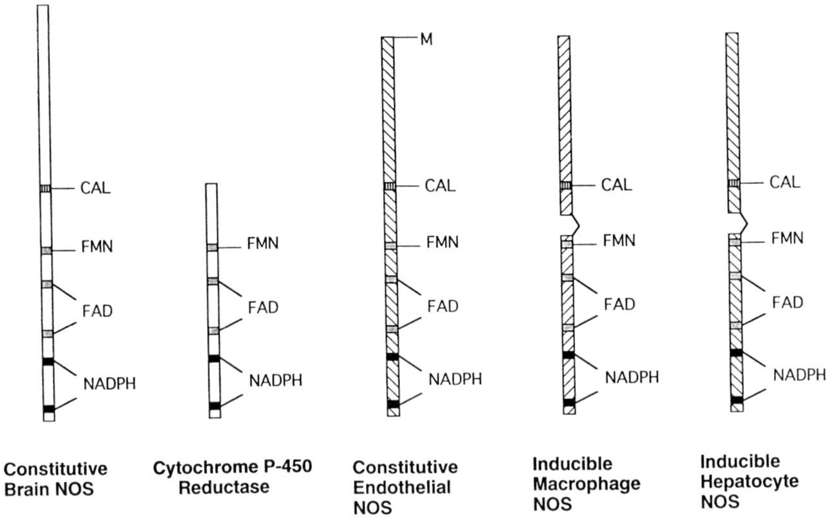

Figure 2 The nitric oxide synthase family. Calmodulin and cofactor binding sites (FMN, FAD, and NADPH) are indicated. The endothelial NOS is N-terminal myristolated (M).

and CPR are most closely related at the cofactor binding sites (Fig. 2), where there are regions of amino acid identity.

The cDNA was ligated into a eukaryotic expression vector and transfected into a human kidney cell line. Transfected cells contained calcium-dependent NOS enzyme activity as measured by the ability of cell extracts to stimulate soluble guanylate cyclase and to convert arginine to citrulline and NO_2^- (a stable metabolite of NO). The cDNA was also used to study the tissue distribution of brain NOS gene expression: RNA blot hybridization revealed brain NOS mRNA in cerebellum and other brain regions. Sessa et al. (25) detected brain NOS mRNA in poly-A^+ RNA extracted from spinal cord, stomach, large intestine, aorta, adrenal, seminal vesicle, and vas deferens. Of note, a smaller mRNA hybridizing with a brain NOS cDNA probe was detected in rat testis. The significance of this smaller mRNA is unknown.

ENDOTHELIAL NITRIC OXIDE SYNTHASE

Immunohistochemical studies using an antiserum directed against brain NOS detected immunoreactivity in vascular endothelial cells, suggesting that the constitutive NOS isoforms in brain and endothelium were identical (26). In fact, however, the two tissues contained different enzymes. Concurrently, three laboratories, including ours, described the isolation and characterization of cDNAs encoding endothelial NOS, the enzyme responsible for EDRF synthesis (27–29). Our approach was to take advantage of the homology between brain NOS and CPR. We hypothesized that amino acids conserved between two distantly related enzymes, CPR and brain NOS, are important for NOS enzyme function and are therefore likely to be present in other NOS isoforms. Degenerate oligonucleotides were synthesized corresponding to amino acid sequences shared by the two enzymes. A partial cDNA encoding a bovine endothelial NOS-related cDNA was amplified using the polymerase chain reaction. This partial cDNA was used to isolate a cDNA encoding a human vascular endothelial NOS: the translated protein is approximately 135 kDa in size and contains cofactor-binding sequences similar to those found in brain NOS (Fig. 2). Abundant endothelial NOS mRNA was detected in unstimulated human umbilical vein endothelial cells. To confirm that the encoded protein had NOS enzyme activity, the cDNA was ligated into an expression vector and transfected into NIH3T3 cells. In coculture assays, NO production by transfected cells stimulated guanylate cyclase activity in RFL-6 cells. The conversion of arginine to citrulline catalyzed by NOS in transfected cells was significantly increased by A23187, a calcium ionophore. These observations demonstrated that the endothelial cDNA encoded a calcium-regulated, constitutively expressed NOS.

Endothelial NOS shares approximately 50% of its amino acid sequence with brain NOS. Southern blot techniques revealed that endothelial and brain NOS cDNA probes hybridized to differing DNA restriction fragments, demonstrating that the two constitutive NOS isoforms were encoded by independent genes. Endothelial NOS gene expression was found in human lung, kidney, and spleen (27). In the rat, abundant endothelial NOS mRNA was detected in aorta, heart, lung, kidney, adrenal gland, spinal cord, and urogenital tissue (25). Lower concentrations of mRNA were present in all tissues tested, reflecting the ubiquitous presence of vascular endothelium (25). Regulation of endothelial NOS gene expression has been investigated in endothelial cells. Incubation of endothelial cells with tumor necrosis factor–α (TNF-α), an agent that increases NOS enzyme activity in this cell type (32,33), decreased endothelial NOS mRNA levels (30,31). This apparent discrepancy is possibly due to the presence of an inducible NOS isoform in TNF-α–treated endothelial cells. Yoshizumi et al. (34) found that TNF-α decreases endothelial NOS mRNA levels by altering transcript stability. Nishida et al. (31) observed that exposure of endothelial cells to fluid shear stress (15 dyn/cm^2 for 24 hr) increased endothelial NOS mRNA and immunoreactivity. This observation may explain the finding that chronic exposure of blood vessels to shear stress increases EDRF release (35).

Endothelial NOS is predominantly associated with the membrane fraction of cell extracts (36), while the brain isoform is located in the cytosol (24). Examination of the predicted amino acid of the endothelial enzyme did not reveal a transmembrane spanning region. However, a consensus motif for N-terminal myristolation was identified (28,29). Myristolization has a role in the regulation of several proteins involved in intracellular signaling, including the α subunits of G proteins and the pp60^{src} oncogene. Two groups of investigators (37,38) used oligonucleotide-directed mutagenesis of the consensus motif to demonstrate that endothelial NOS is myristolated and that localization of the enzyme to the membrane fraction was determined by this posttranslational modification. Michel and colleagues investigated another posttranslational modification of endothelial NOS, phosphorylation (39). They observed that activation of endothelial NOS led to phosphorylation of the enzyme and that enzyme phosphorylation was associated with translocation of the protein from the membrane to the cytoplasm. Because NO is labile once formed, these investigators suggested that location of the enzyme may determine whether NO is released from the cell.

Recently, Marsden and colleagues described the isolation and characterization of the endothelial NOS gene (40). The gene spans approximately 21 kb and contains 26 exons. Examination of the sequences flanking the 5′ end of the gene revealed multiple consensus regulatory sequences. Some of these consensus sequences may be involved in endothelial cell–specific gene expression and in the regulation of gene transcription in response to shear stress. The functional significance of these putative regulatory elements remains to be determined. Of note, 5′ flanking sequences did not contain a TATA sequence, typically present in gene promoters. These investigators also localized the endothelial NOS gene to the 7q35 to 7q36 region of human chromosome 7 and confirmed the findings of Xu et al. (41) that the brain NOS gene was localized to the 12q24.2 region of chromosome 12.

INDUCIBLE NITRIC OXIDE SYNTHASES

The second class of NOS enzymes, the inducible isoforms, are not present in unstimulated cells. After exposure for several hours to cytokines and lipopolysaccharide (LPS), either individually or in combination, cells produce large quantities of NO by a process that is, in general, calcium-calmodulin–independent. Several groups described cDNAs encoding the interferon-γ-(IFN-γ) and LPS-inducible NOS in RAW 264.7 mouse macrophages (42–44). Lyons et al. (42) and Lowenstein et al. (44) cloned a mouse macrophage iNOS cDNA using a PCR-based approach similar to that described above for cloning the endothelial NOS cDNA. Nathan and colleagues employed a different approach to isolate a macrophage iNOS cDNA (43). Using a polyclonal antiserum directed against purified macrophage iNOS, they screened a cDNA library prepared from an IFN-γ-and LPS-treated RAW 264.7 cells. This group identified two isoforms of the mouse macrophage iNOS. The two isoforms differed most at the carboxyl terminus, with one isoform being 22 amino acids shorter than the other. The shorter protein was not detected in RAW 264.7 cells and is reported to be catalytically inactive (7). The longer macrophage iNOS is 131 kDa in size and is approximately 50% homologous to the brain and endothelial constitutive NOSs (Fig. 2). When the cDNA was expressed in eukaryotic cells, abundant NOS enzyme activity, which was insensitive to calcium concentration, was detected. Despite the fact that enzyme activity is calcium-independent, the enzyme has a calmodulin binding site. Cho et al. (45) demonstrated that the enzyme has a high affinity for calmodulin even in the absence of calcium.

Lorsbach et al. (46) investigated the regulation of iNOS gene expression in RAW 264.7 cells. They found that induction of iNOS gene expression was closely correlated with NO_2^- production and cell cytotoxicity, and that LPS and IFN-γ had a synergistic effect on iNOS gene transcription. In contrast, dexamethasone (32), cyclosporine (47), and transforming growth factor-β1 (TGF-β1) (48) inhibited cytokine-induced iNOS gene expression. Vodovotz et al. (48) observed that TGF-β1 decreased iNOS enzyme levels in RAW 264.7 cells by decreasing the stability of iNOS mRNA transcripts and by increasing degradation of iNOS enzyme once synthesized. Xie et al. (49) and Lowenstein et al. (50) characterized the 5′ flanking sequences of the mouse iNOS gene. They found that the promoter contained a typical TATA sequence and a variety of putative *cis*-acting regulatory sequences Two areas within these flanking sequences were responsible for mediating induction by LPS and IFN-γ: one region appeared most important for LPS induction, while a second region mediated the response to IFN-γ.

The mouse macrophage iNOS cDNA has been used as a probe to identify iNOS mRNA in a variety of tissues and cell types including rat vascular endothelial (51) and smooth muscle cells (52,53) as well as hepatocytes (54). Geller et al. (54) investigated the expression of iNOS gene expression in rat hepatocytes. They observed that a combination of LPS with three cytokines, TNF-α, IFN-γ, and interleukin-1β (IL-1β), dramatically increased inducible NOS mRNA levels in hepatocytes. They found that iNOS gene expression in hepatocytes was inhibited by dexamethasone. More recently, these investigators (55) used the mouse macrophage cDNA to screen a cDNA library prepared from primary human hepatocytes exposed to the mixture of cytokines and LPS. They isolated a cDNA which encoded a protein sharing approximately 80% of its amino acids with the macrophage isoform, including the cofactor binding sites (Fig. 2). The hepatic cDNA was transfected into a kidney cell line, which was then assayed for NOS enzyme activity. Extracts of transfected cells converted arginine to citrulline, but this activity was sensitive to calcium-chelators and a calmodulin inhibitor. The latter observation suggested that, in contrast to macrophage iNOS, hepatic iNOS enzyme activity was calcium-sensitive.

An unresolved question is whether the hepatic and macrophage iNOS isoforms are encoded by the same gene with amino acid sequence differences attributable to species variation or whether the two iNOSs are encoded by distinct genes. The apparent calcium-sensitivity of the hepatic isoform and calcium-insensitivity of the macrophage enzyme suggested that the two iNOSs are products of distinct genes. On the other hand, Wood et al. (56) identified an iNOS isoform in cytokine-treated rat hepatocytes which shared 94% of its amino acids with the mouse macrophage enzyme and was identical to the enzyme present in cytokine-treated rat vascular smooth muscle cells (57). These investigators suggested that isoforms present in hepatocytes and macrophages are the product of the same gene.

NITRIC OXIDE SYNTHASE IN THE KIDNEY

Nitric oxide participates in many aspects of renal function. It modulates glomerular hemodynamics (58) as well as renal medullary oxygenation (59). Localized in the macula densa, the brain NOS isoform appears to participate in the regulation of afferent arteriolar tone, and thereby glomerular filtration, in response to renal tubular fluid delivery and reabsorption (60,61). Nitric oxide also appears to modulate natriuresis and diuresis via cGMP (62). Recent evidence suggests that NO also regulates renal endocrine function through cGMP: Ohigashi et al. (63) observed that nitroprusside administration increased serum erythopoeitin levels in ex-hypoxic polycythemic mice and that a cell-permeable cGMP analogue increased erythropoetin production (in a liver cell line). The modulation of renal function by NO is mediated in part by its effect on systemic blood pressure. Chronic blockade of NO synthesis (using a L-arginine analogue that inhibits all known NOS isoforms) induced systemic hypertension as well as proteinuria and glomerular sclerosis (64).

Inducible nitric oxide synthase was identified in LPS- (65) or TNF-α–treated (66) glomerular mesangial cells, and iNOS mRNA was detected in TNF-α–and IFN-γ–treated renal epithelial cells (67). The role of iNOS in the kidney is unknown, but it is conceivable that induction of NO synthesis may contribute to injury associated with glomerular inflammation.

FUTURE DIRECTIONS

Abnormalities of EDRF/NO production are likely to participate in the pathogenesis of several renal and cardiovascular diseases. Insufficient NO production may contribute to systemic and pulmonary hypertension. Excessive NO production may participate in the pathogenesis of septic shock, a condition associated with increased concentrations of cytokines in the circulation. Very high levels of NO, as might be produced by an iNOS, are cytotoxic. Nitric oxide–induced cytotoxicity may participate in the pathogeneses of some forms of vasculitis and glomeronephritis. Several studies have demonstrated that NOS inhibitors ameliorate the hemodynamic sequelae of sepsis (68,69), but these benefits are associated with important toxicities possibly attributable to inhibition of constitutive NOS isoforms.

Development of NOS enzyme inhibitors that are selective for brain, endothelial, or inducible isoforms is under way in many research centers. Critical to identification of these drugs is knowledge of the number of NOS isoforms, their enzyme characteristics, and the cellular mechanisms regulating their function. In the future, another approach to inhibiting NOS activity, for example in sepsis, may be to employ intravenous antisense oligonucleotides directed against specific iNOS isoforms. Antisense oligonucleotides have been used in culture to inhibit iNOS production by rat pulmonary artery smooth muscle cells (70). This antisense approach would require knowledge of the mRNA nucleotide sequences for each iNOS isoform.

In some clinical situations, such as systemic hypertension, it may be desirable to increase NO production. Future antihypertensive medications may augment endothelial or renal tubular NO synthesis and/or NOS gene expression, thereby causing vasodilatation and natriuresis/diuresis. Further characterization of the NOS genes and identification of their chromosomal locations may provide important insights into the causes of some forms of hypertension. Ultimately, DNA screening tests may permit identification of those individuals who are predisposed to cardiovascular and/or renal disease.

CONCLUSION

In summary, NO signal transduction, present in organisms from horseshoe crab to human beings, has important roles in regulating cardiovascular and renal function. The enzymes responsible for NO synthesis, the nitric oxide synthases, are present in many, if not all, cell types under appropriate conditions. Nitric oxide synthases are regulated at the level of gene transcription, mRNA stability, and enzyme stability. Further investigations of the NOS gene family will provide important insights into the cause and treatment of renal and vascular diseases.

REFERENCES

1. Furchgott RF, Zawadzki JV. The obligatory role of endothelial cells in the relaxation of arterial smooth muscle by acetylcholine. Nature 1980; 288:373–376.
2. Ignarro LJ, Buga GM, Wood KS, et al. Endothelium-derived relaxing factor produced and released from artery and vein is nitric oxide. Proc Natl Acad Sci USA 1987; 84:9265–9269.
3. Myers PR, Minor RL, Guerra R, et al. Vasorelaxant properties of the endothelium-derived relaxing factor more closely resemble S-nitrosocysteine than nitric oxide. Nature 1990; 345:161–163.
4. Palmer RMJ, Ferrige AG, Moncada S. Nitric oxide release accounts for the biological activity of endothelium-derived relaxing factor. Nature 1987; 327:524–526.
5. Dawson TM, Dawson VL, Synder SH. A novel neuronal messenger molecule in brain: The free radical, nitric oxide. Ann Neurol 1992; 32:297–311.
6. Nussler AK, Billiar TR. Inflammation, immunoregulation, and inducible nitric oxide synthase. J Leuk Biol 1993; 54:171–178.

7. Karupiah G, Xie QW, Buller RM, et al. Inhibition of viral replication by interferon-gamma-induced nitric oxide synthase. Science 1993; 261:1445–1448.
8. Croen KD. Evidence for antiviral effect of nitric oxide: Inhibition of herpes simplex virus type 1 replication. J Clin Invest 1993; 91:2446–2452.
9. Levine JS, Rogowski RS, Gregory GL, et al. Simultaneous measurements of NO_x, NO, and O_3 production in a laboratory discharge: Atmospheric implications. Geophys Res Lett 1981; 8:357–360.
10. Moncada S, Martin JF. Vasodilation: Evolution of nitric oxide. Lancet 1993; 341:1511.
11. Anderson IA, Levine JS. Relative rates of nitric oxide and nitrous oxide production by nitrifiers, denitrifiers, and nitrate respirers. Appl Environ Microbiol 1986; 51:938–945.
12. Li ZS, Furness JB. Nitric oxide synthase in the enteric nervous system of the rainbow trout, Salmo gairdneri. Arch Histol Cytol 1993; 56:185–193.
13. Ribeiro JM, Nussenzveig RH. Nitric oxide synthase activity from a hematophagous insect salivary gland. FEBS Lett 1993; 330:165–168.
14. Radomski MW, Martin JF, Moncada S. Synthesis of nitric oxide by the hemeocytes of the American horseshoe crab (Limulus polyphemus). Phil Trans R Soc Lond B 1991; 334:129–133.
15. Henry Y, LePoivre M, Drapier JC, et al. EPR characterization of molecular targets for NO in mammalian cells and organelles. FASEB J 1993; 7:1124–1134.
16. Drapier JC, Hirling H, Wietzerbin J, et al. Biosynthesis of nitric oxide activates iron regulatory factor in macrophages. EMBO J 1993; 12:3643–3649.
17. Weiss G, Goossen B, Doppler W, et al. Translational regulation via iron-responsive elements by the nitric oxide/NO-synthase pathway. EMBO J 1993; 12:3651–3657.
18. Schmidt HHHW, Lohmann SM, Walter U. The nitric oxide and cGMP signal transduction system: Regulation and mechanism of action. Biochim Biophys Acta 1993; 1178:153–175.
19. Moncada S, Palmer RMJ, Higgs EA. Nitric oxide: Physiology, pathophysiology, and pharmacology. Pharmacol Rev 1991; 43:109–142.
20. Nathan C. Nitric oxide as a secretory product of mammalian cells. FASEB J 1992; 6:3051–3064.
21. Marletta MA. Nitric oxide synthase structure and mechanism. J Biol Chem 1993; 268:12231–12234.
22. Snyder SH, Bredt DS. Biological roles of nitric oxide. Sci Am 1992; 266:68–77.
23. Bredt DS, Hwang PM, Glatt CE, et al. Cloned and expressed nitric oxide synthase structurally resembles cytochrome P-450 reductase. Nature 1991; 351:714–718.
24. Bredt DS, Snyder SH. Isolation of nitric oxide synthetase, a calmodulin-requiring enzyme. Proc Natl Acad Sci USA 1990; 87:682–685.
25. Sessa WC, Harrison JK, Luthin DR et al. Genomic analysis and expression patterns reveal distinct genes for endothelial and brain nitric oxide synthase. Hypertension 1993; 21:934–938.
26. Bredt DS, Hwang PM, Snyder SH. Localization of nitric oxide synthase indicating a neural role for nitric oxide. Nature 1990; 347:768–770.
27. Janssens SP, Shimouchi A, Quertermous T, et al. Cloning and expression of a cDNA encoding human endothelium-derived relaxing factor/nitric oxide synthase. J Biol Chem 1992; 267:14519–14522.
28. Lamas S, Marsden PA, Li GK, et al. Endothelial nitric oxide synthase: Molecular cloning and characterization of a distinct constitutive enzyme isoform. Proc Natl Acad Sci USA 1992; 89:6348–6352.
29. Sessa WC, Harrison JK, Barber, CM, et al. Molecular cloning and expression of a cDNA encoding endothelial cell nitric oxide synthase. J Biol Chem 1992; 267:15274–15276.
30. Marsden PA, Schappert KT, Chen HS, et al. Molecular cloning and characterization of human endothelial nitric oxide synthase. FEBS Lett 1992; 307:287–293.
31. Nishida K, Harrison DG, Navas JP, et al. Molecular cloning and characterization of the constitutive bovine aortic endothelial cell nitric oxide synthase. J Clin Invest 1992; 90:2092–2096.
32. Radomski MW, Palmer RMJ, Moncada S. Glucocorticoids inhibit the expression of an inducible, but not the constitutive, nitric oxide synthase in vascular endothelial cells. Proc Natl Acad Sci USA 1990; 87:10043–10047.
33. Lamas S, Michel T, Brenner BM, Marsden PA. Nitric oxide synthesis in endothelial cells: Evidence for a pathway inducible by TNF-α. Am J Physiol 1991; 261:C634–C641.
34. Yoshizumi M, Perrella MA, Burnett JC, Lee ME. Tumor necrosis factor downregulates an endothelial nitric oxide synthase mRNA by shortening its half-life. Circ Res 1993; 73:205–209.
35. Miller VM, Vanhoutte PM. Enhanced release of endothelium-derived factor(s) by chronic increases in blood flow. Am J Physiol 1988; 255:H446–H451.
36. Pollock JS, Forstermann U, Mitchell JA, et al. Purification and characterization of particulate endothelium-derived relaxing factor synthase from cultured and native bovine aortic endothelial cells. Proc Natl Acad Sci USA 1991; 88:10480–10484.
37. Michel T, Li GK, Busconi L. Phosphorylation and subcellular translocation of endothelial nitric oxide synthase. Proc Natl Acad Sci USA 1993; 90:6252–6256.

38. Sessa WC, Barber CM, Lynch KR. Mutation of N-myristolation site converts endothelial cell nitric oxide synthase from a membrane to a cytosolic protein. Circ Res 1993; 72:921–924.
39. Busconi L, Michel T. Endothelial nitric oxide synthase: N-terminal myristolation determines subcellular localization. J Biol Chem 1993; 268:8410–8413.
40. Marsden PA, Heng HHQ, Scherer SW, et al. Structure and chromosomal localization of the human endothelial nitric oxide synthase gene. J Biol Chem 1993; 268:17478–17488.
41. Xu W, Gorman P, Sheer D, et al. Regional localization of the gene coding for human brain nitric oxide synthase (NOS1) to 12q24.2 →24.31 by fluorescent in situ hybridization. Cytogenet Cell Genet 1993; 64:62–63.
42. Lyons CR, Orloff GJ, Cunningham JM. Molecular cloning and functional expression of an inducible nitric oxide synthase from a murine macrophage cell line. J Biol Chem 1992; 267:6370–6374.
43. Xie QW, Cho HJ, Calaycay J, et al. Cloning and characterization of inducible nitric oxide synthase from mouse macrophages. Science 1992; 256:225–228.
44. Lowenstein CJ, Glatt CG, Bredt DS, Snyder SH. Cloned and expressed macrophage nitric oxide synthase contrasts with the brain enzyme. Proc Natl Acad Sci USA 1992; 89:6711–6715.
45. Cho HJ, Xie QW, Calaycay J, et al. Calmodulin is a subunit of nitric oxide synthase from macrophages. J Exp Med 1992; 176:599–604.
46. Lorsbach RB, Murphy WJ, Lowenstein CJ, et al. Expression of the nitric oxide synthase gene in mouse macrophages activated for tumor cell killing: Molecular basis for the synergy between interferon-gamma and lipopolysaccharide. J Biol Chem 1993; 268:1908–1913.
47. Fast DJ, Lynch RC, Leu RW. Cyclosporin A inhibits nitric oxide production by L929 cells in response to tumor necrosis factor and interferon-gamma. J Interferon Res 1993; 13:235–240.
48. Vodovotz Y, Bogdan C, Paik J, et al. Mechanisms of suppression of macrophage nitric oxide release by transforming growth factor β. J Exp Med 1993; 178:605–613.
49. Xie QW, Whisnant R, Nathan C. Promoter of the mouse gene encoding calcium-independent nitric oxide synthase confers inducibility by interferon gamma and bacterial lipopolysaccharide. J Exp Med 1993; 177:1779–1784.
50. Lowenstein CJ, Alley EW, Raval P, et al. Macrophage nitric oxide synthase gene: Two upstream regions mediate induction by interferon γ and lipopolysaccharide. Proc Natl Acad Sci USA 1993; 90:9730–9734.
51. Suschek C, Rothe H, Fehsel K, et al. Induction of a macrophage-like nitric oxide synthase in cultured rat aortic endothelial cells: IL-1 beta-mediated induction regulated by tumor necrosis factor-alpha and IFN-gamma. J Immunol 1993: 151:3283–3291.
52. Nakayama DK, Geller DA, Lowenstein CJ, et al. Cytokines and lipopolysaccharide induce nitric oxide synthase in cultured rat pulmonary artery smooth muscle. Am J Respir Cell Mol Biol 1992; 7:471–476.
53. Koide M, Kawahara Y, Tsuda T, and Yokoyama M. Cytokine-induced expression of an inducible type of nitric oxide synthase gene in cultured vascular smooth muscle cells. FEBS Lett 1993; 318:213–217.
54. Geller DA, Nussler AK, DiSilvio M, et al. Cytokines, endotoxin, and glucocorticoids regulate the expression of inducible nitric oxide synthase in hepatocytes. Proc Natl Acad Sci USA 1993; 90:522–526.
55. Geller DA, Lowenstein CJ, Shapiro RA, et al. Molecular cloning and expression of inducible nitric oxide synthase from human hepatocytes. Proc Natl Acad Sci USA 1993; 90:3491–3495.
56. Wood ER, Berger H, Sherman PA, Lapetina EG. Hepatocytes and macrophages express an identical cytokine inducible nitric oxide synthase gene. Biochem Biophys Res Commun 1993; 191:767–774.
57. Nunokawa Y, Ishida N, Tanaka S. Cloning of inducible nitric oxide synthase in rat vascular smooth muscle cells. Biochem Biophys Res Commun 1993; 191:89–94.
58. Zatz R, de Nucci G. Effects of acute nitric oxide inhibition on rat glomerular microcirculation. Am J Physiol 1991; 261:F360–F363.
59. Brezis M, Heyman SN, Dinour D, et al. Role of nitric oxide in renal medullary oxygenation: Studies in isolated and intact rat kidneys. J Clin Invest 1991; 88:390–395.
60. Wilcox CS, Welch WJ, Murad F, et al. Nitric oxide synthase in macular densa regulates glomerular capillary pressure. Proc Natl Acad Sci USA 1992; 89:11993–11997.
61. Mundel P, Bachmann S, Bader M, et al. Expression of nitric oxide synthase in kidney macula densa cells. Kidney Int 1992; 42:1017–1019.
62. Lahera V, Salom MG, Mirand-Guardiola F, et al. Effects of N^G-nitro-L-arginine methyl ester on renal function and blood pressure. Am J Physiol 1991; 261:F1033–F1037.
63. Ohigashi T, Brookins J, Fisher JW. Interaction of nitric oxide and cyclic guanosine 3′,5′-monophosphate in erythropoetin production. J Clin Invest 1993; 92:1587–1591.
64. Baylis C, Mitruka B, Deng A. Chronic blockade of nitric oxide synthesis in the rat produces systemic hypertension and glomerular damage. J Clin Invest 1992; 90:278–281.
65. Shultz PJ, Tayeh MA, Marletta MA, Raji L. Synthesis and action of nitric oxide in rat glomerular cells. Am J Physiol 1991; 261:F600–F606.

66. Marsden PA, Ballerman BJ. Tumor necrosis factor activates soluble guanylate cyclase in bovine glomerular mesangial cells via an L-arginine-dependent mechanism. J Exp Med 1990; 172:1843–1852.
67. Markewitz BA, Michael JR, Kohan DE. Cytokine-induced expression of a nitric oxide synthase in rat renal tubule cells. J Clin Invest 1993; 91:2138–2143.
68. Kilbourn RG, Jubran A, Gross SS, et al. Reversal of endotoxin-mediated shock by N^G-methyl-L-arginine, an inhibitor of nitric oxide synthesis. Biochem Biophys Res Commun 1990; 172:1132–1138.
69. Petros A, Bennett D, Vallance P. Effect of nitric oxide synthase inhibitors on hypotension in patients with septic shock. Lancet 1991; 338:1557–1558.
70. Thomae KR, Geller DA, Billiar TR, et al. Antisense oligodeoxynucleotide to inducible nitric oxide synthase inhibits nitric oxide synthesis in rat pulmonary artery smooth muscle cells in culture. Surgery 1993; 114:272–277.

12
Adrenergic and Dopamine Receptors

Robert M. Graham, R. Peter Riek, S. Iismaa, and S. Chen
The Victor Chang Cardiac Research Institute, St. Vincent's Hospital, Sydney, Australia

INTRODUCTION

The kidney is richly innervated by postganglionic sympathetic fibers originating from sympathetic celiac and aortorenal plexi that receive inputs from the sixth thoracic through the second lumbar spinal nerves (1). These noradrenergic nerves extend not only to the afferent and efferent arterioles and juxtaglomerular cells but also to all portions of the nephron, including the collecting duct (2–4). Renal sympathetic nerve stimulation produces a variety of effects, including alterations in renal hemodynamics and in renin release as well as changes in renal tubular sodium and water reabsorption via actions on the proximal tubule, the ascending thick limb of the loop of Henle, and the collecting duct (3). These effects are all mediated by adrenergic receptors—integral membrane proteins that bind and are selectively activated by the catecholamines norepinephrine and epinephrine. These adrenergic receptors have been identified throughout the kidney in a distribution commensurate with the effects of renal sympathetic nerve stimulations.

Dopamine, a sympathomimetic amine precursor of norepinephrine, is postulated to be another neurotransmitter capable of regulating renal hemodynamics, renin secretion, and sodium excretion (5–7). Thus, dopaminergic innervation of the cortical vessels, particularly the glomerular vascular poles, has been demonstrated; dopamine receptor binding sites have been identified in renal tissue, including glomeruli and both presynaptic and postsynaptic sites, and low concentrations of dopamine have been shown to cause renal vasodilatation and natriuresis (7,8).

With the advent of molecular cloning, a variety of adrenergic and dopaminergic receptors have been identified, including many previously unrecognized subtypes. Availability of clones for these receptors has also resulted in significant advances in our understanding of their structure, function, and signal transduction mechanisms (9,10). In this article, these recent insights are reviewed, after a brief consideration of the renal effects mediated by adrenergic and dopaminergic receptors.

ADRENERGIC RECEPTOR–MEDIATED RESPONSES

Activation of renal sympathetics, the greater splanchnic or renal afferent nerve, or administration of catecholamines or other α-adrenergic agonists produces frequency- or dose-dependent renal vasoconstriction that is abolished by α-adrenergic receptor antagonists (11–15). In the cortex, this increased vascular resistance is due to constriction of preglomerular and efferent arteriolar segments—low levels of stimulation causing equivalent constriction of both afferent and efferent arterioles such that glomerular pressure is unchanged, while higher frequencies produce predominant preglomerular constriction and thus reduced glomerular capillary pressure. In the rat (16,17), cat (18), and dog (19), these vasoconstrictor responses are mediated by α_1-adrenergic receptors, and, more specifically, as recently demonstrated (20), by the α_{1A}-adrenergic receptor or its cloned equivalent the rat (α_{1c}- or $\alpha_{1A/c}$-adrenergic receptor; see below). Although significant renal vasoconstrictor responses can also be observed with activation of postjunctional α_2-adrenergic receptors, postjunctional α_1-adrenergic vasoconstrictor responses predominate and are of much greater magnitude than those of α_2-receptors. In the rabbit, however, α_2-adrenergic receptors may mediate neurogenic vasoconstrictor responses (21).

In addition to these direct renal sympathetic effects, activation of renal vascular adrenergic receptors produces indirect hemodynamic effects, resulting from α_1-adrenergic receptor–mediated formation of vasodilatory prostaglandins and from β-receptor stimulation of renin release (22). The former response buffers direct vasoconstrictor effects of nerve stimulation, while the increase in angiotensin II formation that results from enhanced renin release accounts, in part, for the sympathetically mediated vasoconstrictor response. This β-adrenergic receptor–mediated release of renin from the juxtaglomerular apparatus is probably the most important effect of renal β-receptor activation. In humans and the rat, this effect is attributable entirely to the β_1-subtype, although in the cat, β_2-receptors may be involved (23–25).

β-Adrenergic receptor vasodilatation has also been demonstrated for the renal vascular bed but appears to be less marked than in other vascular beds due to a low complement of vascular β-receptors in the kidney. Both glomerular and tubular β-adrenergic receptors have been identified, and activation of β-receptors has been reported to increase sodium reabsorption (26,27). However, antinatriuretic effects of renal nerve stimulation appear to be mediated predominantly by α_1-receptors (3).

In addition to the rich innervation of the renal vasculature by postganglionic sympathetic fibers, almost all tubular segments are also innervated, with the highest densities of nerve terminals in the thick ascending limb of the loop of Henle (3). Importantly, renal nerve stimulation leads to a hierarchy of adrenergic receptor–mediated responses. With low-frequency nerve stimulation, renin release increases via β_1-receptor activation. With increased nerve stimulation, sodium excretion decreases due to enhanced sodium reabsorption in the proximal tubule, ascending limb, and collecting tubules. This response can be observed in the absence of changes in hemodynamics, indicating a direct tubular effect. Despite the twofold greater density of α_2- over α_1-adrenergic receptors in the rat kidney, this antinatriuretic response appears to be α_1-receptor–mediated in dogs (28) and rabbits (29). By contrast, α_2-receptor activation in the rat may increase sodium and water excretion via a mechanism consistent with antagonism of vasopressin's actions on the cortical collecting tubule. Finally, with high-frequency nerve stimulation—as observed with dehydration, blood-volume contraction, hemorrhage, and congestive heart failure—renal α_1-adrenergic receptor–mediated vasoconstriction is observed, which may be intense (30,31).

DOPAMINERGIC RECEPTOR–MEDIATED RESPONSES

The kidney is also innervated by dopaminergic fibers (32,33), and renal dopamine is either released from these nerves or may arise from intrarenal synthesis by proximal convoluted tubules (34). This latter source accounts for up to 50% of the free dopamine excreted in the urine, but its physiological role remains uncertain (35). Renal dopaminergic nerves have been implicated in the physiological control of renal blood flow as well as water and sodium handling, and in the control of renin secretion (5–7). Also, alterations in renal dopaminergic mechanisms have been suggested to play a pathophysiological role in disease states, such as hypertension and congestive heart failure (36,37). However, the precise role of the renal dopaminergic system in the reflex regulation of renal function or in disease states still remains unclear (38). Nonetheless, dopamine receptors of both the DA_1 and DA_2 subfamilies have been identified in glomeruli, proximal tubules, medulla, and renal microvessels, and administration of dopamine or dopaminergic agonists is widely used therapeutically to maintain renal perfusion and sodium excretion in shock states and in congestive heart failure (39). Infusion of low concentrations of dopamine dilates the renal vasculature, increases renal blood flow, and reduces filtration fraction (40,41). However, high doses produce α-adrenergically mediated renal vasoconstriction. In rat and rabbit renal arteries, activation of DA_1-receptors stimulates adenylyl cyclase, although this effect is less than that observed with β-receptor activation (39). By contrast, DA_2-receptor activation inhibits adenylyl cyclase in rabbit renal arteries. However, there is little evidence for functional DA_2-receptors in the canine renal vasculature (42). Similarly, prejunctional stimulation of dopamine (DA_2) receptors during moderate levels of renal efferent nerve activity has little influence on renal vascular resistance (43).

In addition to an action of dopamine at the level of the renal vasculature, which may indirectly promote sodium excretion as a result of renal vasodilatation, dopamine may also influence sodium excretion as a result of a direct inhibition of tubular sodium reabsorption (44), by activation of the kallikrein-kinin system (45), by stimulating renin release at the level of the juxtaglomerular apparatus (46,47), and by a direct tonic inhibitory action on the secretion of aldosterone from the adrenal cortex (48).

ADRENERGIC RECEPTOR SUBTYPES AND SIGNALING

Based on pharmacological studies, receptors that mediate the actions of catecholamines were initially classified into two major types, α and β (49). Subsequently, α_1, α_2, β_1, and β_2 subtypes were identified as a result of functional and biochemical studies (50–52). Each subtype could be distinguished by its ability to selectively bind ligands (agonists and antagonists) and to activate or inhibit distinct effectors, such as adenylyl cyclase and phospholipase C, as well as phospholipases A_2 and D and various ion channels and exchangers (50,51). With the isolation, purification, and subsequent molecular cloning of these receptors, novel, previously unrecognized subtypes have been identified so that the adrenergic receptor family has now grown to nine discrete subtypes: α_{1A}, α_{1B}, α_{1D}; α_{2A}, α_{2B}, α_{2C}, and β_1, β_2, and β_3 (Table 1).

Classification of adrenergic receptors, particularly α_1-adrenergic receptors, has been problematic for several reasons. First, few drugs are available that show marked subtype selectivity (i.e., recognition by one subtype versus another with at least a 10 to 100-fold difference in affinity). Thus, the ability of pharmacological studies to discriminate between subtypes is limited. Moreover, this problem is compounded by the fact that tissues and even cell lines express more than one subtype. For example, no tissue or cell line has been found that expresses only the α_{1A}-receptor. Second, molecular cloning has revealed the existence of previous uncharacterized subtypes (e.g., the α_{1D}-adrenergic) (51,53). Third, each subtype couples similarly to multiple effector pathways. Finally, the mRNA for adrenergic receptors are frequently expressed at very low levels. Thus, the absence of mRNA by Northern blot analysis does not mean that a particular subtype is not expressed in a particular tissue. For example, a major reason for classifying the cloned α_{1c}-adrenergic receptor as a novel subtype, despite the fact that it displayed an α_{1A}-receptor pharmacology, was the inability to demonstrate expression of an mRNA for this receptor in the rat (54), the major species in which an α_{1A}-receptor had initially been described on the basis of biochemical and pharmacological studies (51).

With the more recent cloning of a rat homologue for this subtype, it is clear that the previously designated α_{1c}-receptor clone actually encodes the "classic," tissue-expressed α_{1A}-receptor (55–57). With these recent insights, it is likely that the classification of α_1-adrenergic receptor subtypes, as indicated in Table 1, will be generally adopted. Moreover, it is likely that the availability of the cloned receptors for the evaluation of each individual expressed subtype will soon allow highly subtype-selective drugs to be developed. At present the most selective compounds for the α_{1A}-receptor are oxymetazoline, 5-methylurapidil, (+)niguldipine, A-61603, and SNAP-5150; for the α_{1B}-receptor, spiperone, respiridone, and chloroethylclonidine; and for the α_{1D}-receptor, (+)norepinephrine and BMY7378. Importantly, it should be noted that WB4101, phentolamine, and benoxathian do not adequately discriminate between the various subtypes.

The classification of α_2- and β-receptors has been less problematic, although, as indicated in Table 1, a species difference is observed in the binding profile of the cloned human (α_2-C10) and rat (RG-20) receptors—the former displaying higher affinity for rauwolscine, yohimbine, and oxymetazoline and lower affinity for imiloxan than the latter (58).

A variety of subtype-selective compounds are available for discriminating β-receptor subtypes, although few have yet been simultaneously evaluated at all three subtypes using pure preparations of the cloned expressed proteins. Selective agonists include xamoterol and denopamine for β_1-receptors; salbutamol, salmeterol, and terbutaline for β_2-receptors; and BRL 37344 for β_3-receptors. Isoproterenol is nonselective (58). Selective antagonists are betaxolol, atenolol, metoprolol, bisoprolol, and CGP20712 for β_1-receptors and ICI118551 for β_2-receptors, with propranolol and CGP122177 being nonselective (58).

Molecular characterization of adrenergic receptors has also revealed that, like dopaminergic receptors, they are members of a large and functionally diverse superfamily (9,50,51). This

Table 1 Molecular Characteristics of the Cloned Adrenergic Receptors[a]

Receptor subtype	Previous/Other names	Mr (kDa)	Amino acids	Glycosylation sites (N-terminus)	Phosphorylation sites	Introns	Chromosomal location
α_{1A}	α_{1c}; $\alpha_{1A/c}$	—	466	3	PKA	1	8
α_{1B}	—	80	515	4	PKA	1	5
α_{1D}	α_{1a}; α_{1d}; $\alpha_{1a/d}$	~65	560	2	—	1	20 p13
$\alpha_{2A}(\alpha_{2D})$	α_2(C-10) (human); RG-20 (rat); Mα_2-10H (mouse)	64	450	2	PKA, βARK	0	10
α_{2B}	α_2(C-2) (human); RNG (rat); Mα_2-2H (mouse)	44	450	0	—	0	4 p16
α_{2C}	α_2(C-4) human; RG-10 (pA2d, RBα_{2B}) (rat); Mα_2-4H (mouse)	75	461	2	—	0	2
β_1	—	64	477	2	PKA, βARK	0	10 q24-q26
β_2	—	64	413	2	PKA, βARK	0	5 q31-q33
β_3	—	—	402	2	0	1	8p11-p12

[a]Lowercase subscripts in the designation of the subtypes refer to the cloned receptors; uppercase to the IUPHAR designation or corresponding pharmacologically characterized receptor (58). The apparent molecular weights (Mr) on SDS-PAGE are shown; that for the α_{2B}-receptor is based on the Mr of the tissue equivalent of this receptor found in rat neonatal lung (67). A single intron interrupting the coding sequence, at the region of the gene corresponding approximately to the end of the sixth transmembrane segment is found in an identical location in all α_1-receptor genes (84,85). It is now clear that the cloned α_{1c}-receptor corresponds to the "classical" or endogenously expressed α_{1A}-receptor; hence, this receptor is now being designated as the α_{1A}- or $\alpha_{1A/c}$-receptor. The prototypic tissues expressing this receptor are the rat submaxillary gland and rat kidney. Additionally, it is now clear that the cloned receptor previously designated as the α_{1a}- (86), α_{1d}- (53), $\alpha_{1a/d}$-receptor (87) does not correspond to the "classic" or endogenously expressed α_{1A}-receptor but to a previously unidentified subtype now termed the α_{1D}-receptor. The prototypic tissue expressing this α_{1D}-receptor, as defined from functional studies, is the rat aorta (88). The chromosomal locations refer to the human genome. More than one copy of the α_{2C}-receptor has been found in the human genome (89). The α_{1D}- (previously referred to as the α_{1a}-receptor) was initially reported to be localized to chromosome 5 (86), but more recently has been found to actually be localized to chromosome 20 (90). The pharmacological characteristics of the cloned α_{2A}-receptors show species differences. The ligand binding profile of the cloned human (α_2-C10) and pig α_2-receptors is similar to that observed for the prototypic tissues, human platelet or HT29 cells, and is designated as an α_{2A} pharmacology, whereas the profile of the cloned rat (RG-20), mouse (Mα_2-4H) and bovine α_2-receptors is similar to that observed in bovine pineal gland, rat sublingual gland or RINm5F cell line, and is designated as an α_{2D} pharmacology. The ligand binding profiles of the α_{2B}- and α_{2C}-receptors do not show species differences. Abbreviations: PKA = protein kinase A; βARK = β-adrenergic receptor kinase.

superfamily of integral-membrane cell surface proteins responds not only to sympathomimetic amines but also to a variety of neurotransmitters and hormones as well as to sensory signals, such as light, taste, and smell (Table 2). Indeed, it has been estimated that 80% of neurotransmitters, hormones, etc., utilize receptors of this superfamily for transmembrane signaling (59) and that approximately 1% of all mammalian genes encode these receptor proteins.

Despite the wide structural array of activators for the heptatopic receptors, it is of interest that the receptor proteins per se share considerable structural homology. This reflects their common mechanism of action, which involves initial recognition and binding of agonist—or, in the case of

Table 2 The Heptatopic Receptor Superfamily

Small ligand family
- Adrenergic ($\alpha_{1A,B,D}$; $\alpha_{2A\text{-}C}$; $\beta_{1\text{-}3}$)
- Dopamine (D_1, $D_{2A\text{-}B}$, $D_{3\text{-}5}$)
- Serotonin ($5HT_{1A\text{-}B}$, $5HT1D_{\alpha,\beta}$ $5HT_{1E,F}$; $5HT_{2A\text{-}C}$, $5HT_{5A,B}$, $5HT_6$, $5HT_{7A,B}$)
- Adenosine (A_1, $A_{2A,B}$, A_3)
- Histamine (H1, 2)
- Melatonin
- Acetylcholine (muscarinic, M1-5)
- Tyramine (octopamine)

Sensory family
- Opsins (rhodopsin, bacterial opsins, sensory and halorhodopsin)
- Colour vision pigments (blue, green, red)
- Odorant
- Gustatory

Peptide hormone family
- Angiotensin ($AT_{1A\text{-}C}$, AT_2, AT_3)
- Bombesin/gastrin-releasing peptide (BB_2, BB_3)
- Bombesin/neuromedin B (BB_1)
- Bradykinin (B2)
- Cholecystokinin/gastrin (CCK_A, $CCK_{B1,\ 2}$)
- Complement C5a
- Endothelin (ET_A, ET_B, ET_C)
- Follicle-stimulating hormone
- Interleukin-8 (2)
- Luteinizing hormone/chorionic gonadotropin
- Macrophage inflammatory protein 1α/RANTES
- Monocyte chemoattractant protein 1 (MCP-1A, B)
- Neurokinins (NK1-3)
- Neuropeptide Y/peptide YY (Y_1, Y_2)
- Neurotensin
- N-formyl peptide (2)
- Opioid (δ, κ, μ)
- Oxytocin
- Somatostatin ($SRIF_{1A\text{-}C}$, 2A, 2B)
- Thrombin
- Thyroid stimulating hormone
- Thyrotropin-releasing hormone
- Vasopressin (V_1, V_2)

Lipid/fatty acid family
- PGE_2 ($EP_{1,2}$, $EP_{3A\text{-}D}$)
- $PGF_{2\alpha}$
- PGI_2
- TXA_2/PGH_2
- Platelet activating factor
- Cannabinoid (anandamide)

Secretion receptor family
- Secretin
- Calcitonin ($C_{1a,\ B}$)
- Corticotropin releasing factor ($CRF_{1,\ 2}$)
- Gastric inhibitory polypeptide
- Glucagon
- Glucagon-like peptide 1

Table 2 *(Continued)*

Growth hormone releasing hormone (G_nRH_{1-3})
Parathyroid hormone / PTH-related peptide
Pituitary adenylyl cyclase activating peptide (I; I-hip; I-hop1,2; I-hip-hop1)
Vasointestinal Polypeptide ($VIP_{1,2}$)
Metabotropic family
Glutamate ($mGluR1_{a-c}$, $mGluR_{2-7}$)
Calcium sensor (BoPCaR)
Other
ATP (P_{2Y1}, P_{2U})
Orphan (15)
Viral

rhodopsin, activation of its bound ligand as a result of light-induced isomerization (60). As a consequence of these processes, the receptor protein undergoes a complex conformational change that allows it to interact specifically with one or more guanine nucleotide–binding regulator protein(s) (G protein). This interaction promotes the exchange of GTP for GDP by the α-subunit of the heterotrimeric G proteins and dissociation of α- and $\beta\gamma$-subunits of the G protein complex. In most cases, the GTP-activated α subunit is then able to activate the receptor-linked effector, although in some instances the dissociated $\beta\gamma$-subunits are involved primarily in effector activation. Signaling is then terminated by the reassociation of the $\alpha\beta\gamma$–G protein complex following hydrolysis of GTP by the GTPase activity intrinsic to the α-subunit (59). Interestingly, dissociation of the GTP-bound form of the G protein from its receptor results in a reciprocal conformational change in the receptor protein, such that its affinity for agonists is now reduced. Thus, the proportion of receptors in the high-affinity state for agonists provides important information on the degree of receptor–G-protein coupling.

The G proteins coupling receptors and effectors are generally identified on the basis of the "signature" α-subunit, although diversity among β- and γ-subunits is also apparent. At least 15 different α-subunits, 5 β-subunits and 5 γ-subunits have now been identified (61). In addition, G proteins that are not members of the heterotrimeric family can mediate adrenergic receptor signaling (62). The G proteins involved in adrenergic receptor signaling include G_s and G_{13}, which couple β-receptors to adenylyl cyclase stimulation and Na^+-H^+ antiport activation, respectively, and G_i and G_o, which couple α_2-receptors to adenylyl cyclase inhibition and calcium channel activation, respectively. For α_1-adrenergic receptors, both the G_q and G_h families can mediate receptor-coupled phospholipase-C activation (62).

ADRENERGIC RECEPTOR STRUCTURE

Cloning, sequence determination, and structure-function studies, particularly using site-directed mutagenesis approaches but also biochemical and biophysical techniques, have revealed the following insights into adrenergic receptor structure and function. Like other members of this superfamily, adrenergic receptors are composed of single polypeptide chains ranging in length from 402 to 561 amino acids (50). Each receptor contains seven stretches of 20 to 28 relatively hydrophobic amino acids that are predicted to form seven transmembrane α-helices connected by alternating extracellular and intracellular loops. Based on this structural arrangement, these receptors have been descriptively characterized as heptatopic (63) or heptahelical (64) membrane-spanning receptors, although the less accurate descriptor* G protein–coupled receptor, is now widely used.

*This descriptor is less accurate, since at least one important subgroup of this family of receptor proteins, the bacterial rhodopsins, do not couple to G proteins. Moreover, the involvement of G proteins in transmembrane signaling is not confined to the hepatopic receptors but is also observed with several single membrane-spanning receptors (65,66).

The amino terminus of each receptor is located extracellularly and in most but not all instances (67) contains several sites at which the proteins are glycosylated with N-linked oligosaccharides. Prevention of glycosylation either by the use of inhibitors of glycosylation enzymes or by site-directed mutagenesis of the oligosaccharide-linked asparagine residue(s) does not alter the ligand-binding properties or functional activity of the receptors but decreases their level of cell surface expression (10). The carboxyl terminus is located intracellularly and contains sites at which the proteins may be phosphorylated by serine/threonine kinases involved in receptor desensitization (68). The connecting intracellular and extracellular loops are generally short (~10 to 20 amino acids) except for the third intracellular loop, which is generally much longer but varies considerably between the various receptor subfamilies. This loop as well as the second intracellular loop are involved in the binding and specificity of interaction with the receptor-coupled G proteins. In most instances the carboxyl terminus also contains one or more cysteine residues in the juxtamembranous region is thioesterified with palmitic acid (10). This fatty acid modification anchors the receptor tail to the membrane and thus results in the formation of a "pseudo" fourth intracellular loop. Whether this loop is also involved in G protein coupling is presently unclear. Thus, substitution of the palmitoylated C-terminal cysteine residue in the β-receptor with a glycine prevented receptor activation of G_s (68). However, substitution of this cysteine with a leucine in the β-receptor (69), or with serine in rhodopsin (70) or alanine in the α_{2A} receptor (71) did not affect overall receptor structure or function.

In addition to the conserved C-terminal cysteine residue mentioned above, adrenergic receptors and other members of this receptor superfamily contain two highly conserved cysteine residues in the second and third extracellular loops that are critical for receptor folding, cell surface expression, and glycosylation (60,72). In rhodopsin and in the muscarinic receptor, these cysteine resisues are involved in the formation of a disulfide bridge that stabilizes receptor structure and allows maturational folding and membrane expression. In the β-adrenergic receptor, however, these conserved extracellular cysteines are not linked. Rather, this receptor probably contains two disulfide linkages involving coupling of each of the conserved cysteines with one or other of two vicinal cysteines in the third extracellular loop that are unique to the β-receptor (Fig. 1). The correct formation of these two unique disulfide bonds is required for high-affinity ligand binding and for effector activation (72). α_1-Adrenergic receptors also contain a structurally important extracellular disulfide bond that is solvent-inaccessible (73).

The seven α-helical transmembrane regions are most likely arranged in a cluster to exclude the surrounding membrane phospholipids and to form a binding pocket that allows the binding of the hydrophilic catecholamines. Like other members of this receptor superfamily, the residues in the transmembrane domains are more highly conserved than those in the intra- and extracellular loop regions (63). Within a subfamily (e.g., α_1-receptors) this transmembrane homology is 70–80%, whereas this figure is significantly lower (30–40%) when an α_1-receptor is compared with an α_2- or β- receptor, for example.

Binding of catecholamines and related synthetic ligands to adrenergic and dopaminergic receptors probably involves the formation of an ion pair interaction between the carboxylate side chain of an aspartic acid (Asp^{113} in the hamster β_2-receptor) in the upper half of the third transmembrane helix and the protonated amine of the ligands (9). This Asp residue is conserved in all biogenic amine–binding receptors including histamine and muscarinic receptors. Interestingly, in rhodopsin, the side chain of Glu^{113}, located one helix turn above the position corresponding to Asp^{113} in the β-receptor, serves as the counter ion for the Schiff base that is involved in the covalent binding of retinal to a lysine (Lys^{296}) in the seventh transmembrane helix (60). Additional interactions between adrenergic ligands and their receptors involve serine residues (Ser^{204} and Ser^{207} in the hamster β_2-receptor) in the fifth transmembrane segment, which probably form hydrogen bonds with the catecholamine aromatic ring hydroxyl groups; a phenylalanine (Phe^{290} in the hamster β_2-receptor) in the sixth transmembrane segment, which may form a hydrophobic interaction with the aromatic ring (9); and a serine in the second (Ser^{90}) or the fourth (Ser^{165}) transmembrane helix that interacts with the β-hydroxyl of catecholamines and thus is responsible for the stereoselective binding by adrenergic receptors of agonist and antagonists with a chiral center, such as the phenylethylamines (74). Interestingly, a serine equivalent to the Ser^{90} in α_2-receptors is not present in β-adrenergic receptors, suggesting that catecholamines may interact in a different manner with α_2- and β-adrenergic receptors.

Little is currently known about the amino acid determinants of subtype selectivity. Studies in

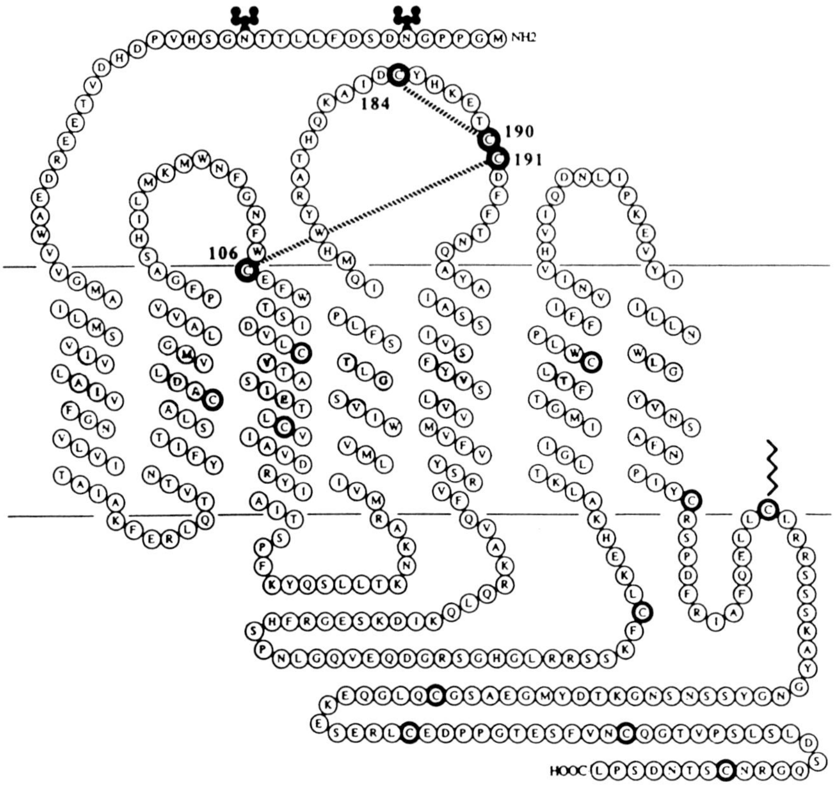

Figure 1 A secondary structure model of the hamster β_2-adrenergic receptor. The amino terminus (NH_2) is located extracellularly and the carboxyl terminus (HOOC) is located intracellularly. Horizontal lines indicate the boundaries of the plasma membrane lipid bilayer. Hatched lines show the unique disulfide bond connectivity between the conserved cysteine residues (Cys^{106}, Cys^{184}) and the vicinal cysteines (Cys^{190}, Cys^{191}) that are only found in β-adrenergic receptors. Other cysteine residues throughout the molecule are indicated by the heavy circles, including one in the C-terminal tail that is thioesterified with palmitic acid (wavy line), thus creating a fourth intracellular loop. (From Ref. 70.)

which chimeric receptors are constructed containing part of one subtype and the corresponding domains of another subtype indicate that the fourth or fourth and fifth (9) transmembrane helices are involved in determining β_1 vs. β_2 specificity of ligand binding. However, as no single amino acid has been identified that can cause this subtype switch, it is likely that multiple residues are involved in subtype selectivity. With the human α_{2A}-adrenergic receptor, a single amino acid (Cys^{201} in the fifth transmembrane domain) has been suggested to account entirely for a species difference in antagonist binding (75). However, a more recent study indicates that this species difference in ligand binding cannot be due only to this one amino acid difference (76).

The residues involved in antagonist binding also remain largely undefined. For the β-adrenergic receptor, an asparagine (Asn^{312}) appears to be required for the binding of phenoxypropanolamine antagonists (9). Also, substitution of Asp^{113} with a glutamic acid (which has a longer side chain than aspartic acid), while decreasing the affinity of the receptor for adrenergic ligands, results in antagonists now demonstrating partial agonist activity (9). Based on this observation, it has been suggested that compounds with an ability to bind simultaneously the carboxylate side chain at position 113 and the catechol binding nucleus in helices 5 and 6 will function as agonists (9). Although this postulate holds true for catecholamines, it is still unclear how the catechol nucleus of β-antagonists bind to the receptor, since these compounds lack hydroxyl substituents on the aromatic ring. Other residues that appear to be important in determining differences in the antagonist binding specificity between the β_2- and α_2-adrenergic receptors are in the seventh transmembrane helix, (e.g., Phe^{412} in the α_2-receptor) (77).

DOPAMINE RECEPTOR SUBTYPES, STRUCTURE AND SIGNALING

Like adrenergic receptors, pharmacological, biochemical, and molecular cloning studies have revealed that the dopamine receptor family is composed of a number of distinct but related proteins (Table 3). Two distinct subtypes of dopamine receptors were initially identified in the brain on the basis of pharmacological and functional studies. The D1-receptor subtype activated adenylyl cyclase, whereas the D2-receptors inhibited this effector enzyme (78,79). With the molecular cloning of dopamine receptors, many more subtypes have now been identified. Several of the receptors cloned from brain correspond to the classically described D1- and D2-receptors. Among the D1 subfamily, variants include the D_{1A}- and D_{1B}-(or D5-) receptors, that each couple to stimulation of adenylyl cyclase and to inhibition of Na^+, K^+-ATPase (10,80). These receptors share the same high level of amino acid identity (75–80%) within their transmembrane domains, as is characteristic of the adrenergic receptor subtypes of the same subfamily. In addition, the genes for these two receptors, like those of the β_1-, β_2- and α_2-receptors, are intronless. The D2-receptor subfamily, on the other hand, couple to inhibition of adenylyl cyclase and activation of K^+ channels through pertussis toxin–sensitive G proteins and are encoded by intron-containing genes. This subfamily has four members, two D_2 isoforms that result from alternative splicing as well as the closely related D_3 and D_4 receptors (10). The two isoforms of the D_2 receptor arise by the insertion of an alternatively spliced exon that encodes a 29–amino acid segment within the third intracellular loop. Therefore the short form of this receptor, D_{2A} (rat) is composed of 415 amino acids, while the long form, D_{2B}, contains 444 residues. These two isoforms, although pharmacologically identical with respect to their ligand-binding characteristics, can be distinguished functionally (81). Thus, the D_{2B} receptor inhibits cAMP production more potently than the D_{2A} isoform.

Although the structural determinants of dopamine receptor binding and signaling have not been evaluated as extensively as those of adrenergic receptors, it is likely that very similar considerations will apply for these biogenic amine–activated receptors. An important distinction, however, is that dopamine, unlike epinephrine and norepinephrine, lacks a chiral center. Not surprisingly therefore, these receptors lack one or both of the analogous serine residues thought to be involved in the stereoselectivity of ligand binding to α_2- or β-adrenergic receptors.

Interestingly, the expression of the various dopamine receptors in different tissues is very region-specific, both in the central nervous system and in the kidney. For example, the D_{1A} receptor is expressed abundantly in the basal ganglia, whereas the D_{1B} receptor is expressed exclusively in the limbic system (82). Similarly, the D_{2A} and D_3 receptors are expressed in specific regions of the kidney, including the glomeruli (83).

Table 3 Molecular Characteristics of the Cloned Dopamine Receptors

Receptor subtype	Species	Amino acid	Gycosylation site (N-terminus)	Exons	Introns	Chromosomal location[a]
D_{1A}	Human, rat	446	2	1	0	5 q35.1
D_{1B} (D5)	Rat	475	1	—	—	
	Human	477	1	1	0	4 p15.1–16.1
D_{2A}	Human, rat	415	3	6	5	11 q22 23
D_{2B}	Bovine, *Xenopus*, human	444	3	7	6	11 q22–23
D_3	Rat	446	2	6	5	
	Human	400	2	—	—	3 p13.3
D_4	Human	387	1	5	4	11 p

[a]Chromosomal locations refer to the human genome.

ACKNOWLEDGMENTS

The expert secretarial assistance of Ms. Elaine Martin is gratefully acknowledged. Studies from the authors' laboratory were supported in part by a National Institutes of Health grant (NS 19583) and by an Eccles Award from the National Health and Medical Research Council, Australia.

REFERENCES

1. Mitchell GAG. The nerve supply of the kidney. Acta Anat 1950; 10:1–9.
2. Insel PA, Snavely MD. Catecholamines and the kidney: Receptors and renal function. Annu Rev Physiol 1981; 43:625–636.
3. DiBona GF. Neural regulation of renal tubular sodium reabsorption and renin secretion. Fed Proc 1985; 44:2816–2822.
4. Barajas L, Powers K, Wang P. Innervation of the renal cortical tubules: A quantitative study. Am J Physiol 1984; 274:F50.
5. Bell C. Regulation of renal function by endogenous dopamine. In: Imbs JL, Schwartz J, eds. Peripheral Dopamine Receptors. New York: Pergamon, 1979.
6. Goldberg LI. The dopamine vascular receptor. In: Imbs JL, Schwartz J, eds. Peripheral Dopaminergic Receptors. New York: Pergamon, 1979.
7. McDonald RH, Goldberg LI, McNay JL, Tuttle EP. Effect of dopamine in man: Augmentation of sodium excretion, glomerular filtration rate and renal blood flow. J Clin Invest 1964; 43:116–120.
8. Baer PG, Navar LG. Renal vasodilation and uncoupling of blood flow and filtration rate autoregulation. Kidney Int 1973; 4:12–21.
9. Strader CD, Fong TM, Tota MR, Underwood D. Structure and function of G protein–coupled receptors. Annu Rev Biochem 1994; 63:101–132.
10. Iismaa T, Biden TJ, Shine J. G Protein–Coupled Receptors. Boca Raton, FL: CRC Press, 1994.
11. Hermansson K, Larson M, Kallskog O, Wolgast M. Influence of renal nerve activity on arteriolar resistance, ultrafiltration dynamics and fluid reabsorption. Pflugers Arch 1981; 389:85–90.
12. Kon V, Ichikawa I. Effector loci for renal nerve control of cortical microcirculation. Am J Physiol 1983; 245:F545–F553.
13. Pelayo JC, Zeigler MG, Blantz RC. Angiotensin II in adrenergic-induced alterations in glomerular hemodynamics. Am J Physiol 1984; 247:F799–F807.
14. Cooke JH, Johns EJ, MacLeod JH, Singer B. The effect of renal nerve stimulation, renal blood flow and adrenergic blockade on plasma renin activity in the cat. J Physiol 1972; 226:15–36.
15. Myers BD, Deen WM, Brenner BM. Effects of norepinephrine and angiotensin II on the determinants of glomerular ultrafiltration and proximal tubule fluid reabsorption in the rat. Circ Res 1975; 37:101–110.
16. Schmitz JM, Graham RM, Sagalowsky AI, Pettinger WA. Renal alpha$_1$- and alpha$_2$-adrenergic receptors: Biochemical and pharmacological correlations. J Pharmacol Exp Ther 1981; 219:400–406.
17. Campbell WB, Graham RM, Jackson EK. The role of renal prostaglandins in sympathetically mediated renin release in the rat. J Clin Invest 1979; 64:448–456.
18. Drew GM, Whiting SB. Evidence for two distinct types of postsynaptic alpha-adrenoceptor in vascular smooth muscle. Br J Pharmacol 1979; 67:207–215.
19. Horn PT, Kohli JD, Listinsky JJ, Goldberg LI. Regional variation in the alpha-adrenergic receptors in the canine resistance vessels. Naunyn-Schmiedeberg's Arch Pharmacol 1982; 318:166–172.
20. Clarke DE. Does the rat kidney express an α_{1C}-adrenoceptor? Evidence from operational and binding studies. Pharmacology of Adrenoceptors Satellite Symposium of the XIIth IUPHAR Congress, King of Prussia, PA, July 21–23, 1994.
21. Hesse IFA, Johns EJ. An in vivo study of the alpha-adrenoceptor subtypes on the renal vasculature in the anesthetized rabbit. J Auton Pharmacol 1984; 4:145–152.
22. Keeton TK, Campbell WB. The pharmacological alteration of renin release. Pharmacol Rev 1980; 32:81–27.
23. Buhler FR, Burkart F, Lutold BE, et al. Antihypertensive beta-blocking action as related to renin and age: A pharmacologic tool to identify pathogenic mechanisms in essential hypertension. Am J Cardiol 1975; 36:653–669.
24. Milavec-Krizman M, Evenou JP, Wagner H, et al. Characterisation of β-adrenoceptor subtypes in rat kidney with new highly selective β_1-blockers and their role in renin release. Biochem Pharmacol 1985; 34:3951–3957.
25. Johns EJ, Singer B. Comparison of the effects of propranolol and ICI 66082 in blocking the renin releasing effects of renal nerve stimulation in the cat. Br J Pharmacol 1974; 53:315–318.

26. Munzel PA, Healy DP, Insel PA. Autoradiographic localisation of β-adrenoceptors in rat kidney slices using [^{125}I] iodocyanopindolol. Am J Physiol 1984; 246:F240–F245.
27. Moss NG. Renal function and renal afferent and efferent nerve activity. Am J Physiol 1982; 243:F425–F433.
28. Osborn JL, Holdaas H, Thames MD, DiBona GF. Renal adrenoceptor mediation of antinatriuretic and renin secretion responses to low frequency renal nerve stimulation in the dog. Circ Res 1983; 53:298–305.
29. Hesse IFA, Johns EJ. The subtype of alpha-adrenoceptor involved in the neural control of renal tubular sodium reabsorption in the rabbit. J Physiol 1984; 352:527–538.
30. DiBona GF. The functions of the renal nerves. Rev Physiol Biochem Pharmacol 1982; 94:76–81.
31. Gottschalk CW, Moss NG, Colindres RE. Neural control of renal function in health and disease. In: Seldin DW, Giebisch G, eds. The Kidney: Physiology and Pathophysiology. New York: Raven Press, 1985.
32. Bell C. Regulation of renal function by endogenous dopamine. In Imbs JL, Schwartz J. eds. Peripheral Dopamine Receptors. New York: Pergamon Press, 1979.
33. Harris PJ, Navar LG. Tubular transport responses to angiotensin. Am J Physiol 1985; 248:F621–F630.
34. Hagege J, Richet G. Proximal tubule dopamine histofluorescence in renal slices incubated with L-dopa. Kidney Int 1985; 27:3–8.
35. Stevenson RK, Sole MJ, Baines AD. Neural and extraneural catecholamine production by rat kidneys. Am J Physiol 1982; 242:F261–F266.
36. Jose PA, Eisner GM, Felder RA. Dopaminergic defect in hypertension. Pediatr Nephrol 1993; 7:859–864.
37. Ganguly PK, Mukherjee K, Chen Y. Altered renal dopamine receptors during development of cardiac hypertrophy. Am J Physiol 1992; 262:E569–E573.
38. Di Bona GF. Renal dopamine containing nerves: What is their functional significance? Am J Hypertens 1990; 3:64S–67S.
39. Ruffolo Jr, RR, Hieble JP, Brooks DP, et al. Drug receptors and control of the cardiovascular system. Progr Drug Res 1991; 36:117–360.
40. Baer PG, Navar LG. Renal vasodilation and uncoupling of blood flow and filtration rate autoregulation. Kidney Int 1973; 4:12–21.
41. McDonald RH, Goldberg LI, McNay JL, Tuttle EP. Effect of dopamine in man, augmentation of sodium excretion, glomerular filtration rate and renal blood flow. J Clin Invest 1964; 43:1116–1121.
42. Horn PT, Kohli JD. Absence of postsynaptic DA2 dopamine receptors in the dog renal vasculature. Eur J Pharmacol 1991; 197:125–130.
43. Lokhandwala MF, Buckley JP. Presynaptic dopamine receptors as mediators of dopamine-induced inhibition of neurogenic vasoconstriction. Eur J Pharmacol 1977; 45:305–309.
44. Felder RA, Belcher M, Calcagno PL, Jose PA. Dopamine receptors in the proximal tubule of the rabbit. Am J Physiol 1984; 247:F499–F505.
45. Mills IH. The renal kallikrein-kinin system and sodium excretion. Q J Exp Physiol 1982; 67:393–399.
46. Kurtz A, Della Bruna R, Pratz J, Cavero I. Rat juxtaglomerular cells are endowed with DA-1 dopamine receptors mediating renin release. J Cardiovasc Pharmacol 1988; 12:658–663.
47. Antonipillai I, Broers MI, Lang D. Evidence that specific dopamine-1 receptor activation is involved in dopamine-induced renin release. Hypertension 1989; 13:463–468.
48. McCarty R, Kirby RF, Carey RM. Dopamine may be a neurohormone in the rat adrenal cortex. Am J Physiol 1984; 247:E709–E713.
49. Ahlquist RP. A study of adrenotropic receptors. Am J Physiol 1948; 153:586–600.
50. Graham RM. Adrenergic receptors: Structure and function. Cleve Clin J Med 1990; 57:481–491.
51. Hwa J, De Young MB, Perez DM, Graham RM. Autonomic control of myocardium: Alpha-adrenoceptor mechanisms. In: Burnstock G, ed. The Autonomic Nervous System. Volume VIII: The Nervous Control of the Heart. Volume eds. Shepherd J, Vatner SF. Cambridge, MA: Harvard Academic Press, 1995 (in press).
52. Homcy CJ, Graham RM. Molecular characterisation of adrenergic receptors. Circ Res 1985; 56:635–650.
53. Perez DM, Piascik MT, Graham RM. Solution-phase library screening for the identification of rare clones: Isolation of an α_{1D}-adrenergic receptor cDNA. Mol Pharmacol 1991; 40:876–883.
54. Schwinn DA, Lomasney JN, Loreng W, et al. Molecular cloning and expression of the cDNA for a novel α_1-adrenergic receptor subtype. J Biol Chem 1990; 265:8183–8189.
55. Perez DM, Chen JL, Piasick MT, et al. Is the α_{1c}-adrenergic receptor the α_{1A}-subtype? FASEB J 1994; A353:2041.
56. Rokosh DG, Bailey BA, Stewart AFR, et al. Distribution of α_{1c}-adrenergic receptor mRNA in adult rat tissue by RNase protection assay and comparison with α_{1b}, α_{1d}. Biochem Biophys Res Commun 1994; 200:1177–1184.
57. Ford APDW, William TJ, Blue DR, Clarke DE. α_1-Adrenoceptor classification: Sharpening Occam's razor. Trends Pharmacol Sci 1994; 15:167–169.
58. Bylund DB, Eikenberg DC, Hieble JP, et al. IV International Union of Pharmacology Nomenclature of Adrenoceptors. Pharmacol Rev 1994; 46:121–136.

59. Birnbaumer L, Abramowitz J, Brown AM. Receptor-effector coupling by G-proteins. Biochem Biophys Acta 1990; 1031:163–224.
60. Khorana HG. Rhodopsin photoreceptor of the rod cell: An emerging pattern for structure and function. J Biol Chem 1992; 267:1–4.
61. Conklin BR, Bourne HR. Structural elements of G_α subunits that interact with $G_{\beta\gamma}$, receptors, and effectors. Cell 1993; 73:631–641.
62. Nakaoka H, Perez DM, Baek KJ, et al. A GTP-binding protein with transglutaminase activity and receptor signalling function. Science 1994; 264:1593–1596.
63. Riek RP, Hanschumacher MK, Sung S-S, et al. Evolutionary conservation of both the hydrophilic and hydrophobic nature of transmembrane residues. J Theoret Biol. In press.
64. Yanagisawa M. The endothelin system: A new target for therapeutic intervention. Circulation 1994; 89:1320–1322.
65. Teitelbaun I, Strasheim A, Berl T. Epidermal growth factor-stimulated phosphoinositide hydrolysis in cultured rat inner medullary collecting tubule cells: Regulation by G-protein, calcium and protein kinase C. J Clin Invest 1990; 85:1044–1050.
66. Luttrell L, Kilgour E, Larner J, Romero G. A pertussis toxin–sensitive G-protein mediates some aspects of insulin action in BC3H-1 murine myocytes. J Biol Chem 1990; 265:16873–16879.
67. Lanier SM, Homcy CJ, Patenaude C, Graham RM. Identification of structurally distinct alpha $_2$-adrenergic receptors. J Biol Chem 1988; 263:14491–14496.
68. O'Dowd BF, Hnatowich M, Caron MG, et al. Palmitoylation of the human β_2-adrenergic receptor: Mutation of Cys 341 in the carboxyl tail leads to an uncoupled nonpalmitoylated form of receptor. J Biol Chem 1989; 264:7564–7569.
69. Dixon RAF, Sigal TS, Candelore MR, et al. Structural features required for ligand binding to the beta-adrenergic receptor. EMBO J 1987; 11:3269–3275.
70. Karnik SS, Ridge KD, Bhattacharya S, Khorana HG. Palmitoylation of bovine opsin and its cysteine mutations in COS-1 cells. Proc Natl Acad Sci USA 1993; 90:40–44.
71. Kennedy ME, Limbind LE. Mutations of the α_{2A}-adrenergic receptor that eliminate detectable palmitoylation do not perturb receptor-G-protein coupling. J Biol Chem 1993; 268:8003–8011.
72. Noda K, Saad Y, Graham RM, Karnik SS. The high affinity state of the β_2-adrenergic receptor requires unique interaction between conserved and non-conserved extracellular loop cysteines. J Biol Chem 1994; 269:6743–6752.
73. Parini A, Homcy CJ, Graham RM. Structural properties of the alpha $_1$-adrenergic receptor: Studies with membrane and purified receptor preparations. Circ Res 1987; 61:I-100–I-104.
74. Li Y-O, Bergsma D, Ganguly S, et al. The β-hydroxyl group of catecholamines may interact with the second transmembrane helix of the α_{2A}-adrenoceptor. Pharmacology of Adrenoceptors. Satellite Symposium of the XIIth IUPHAR Congress. King of Prussia, PA. July 21–23, 1994.
75. Link R, Daunt D, Barsh G, et al. Cloning of two mouse genes encoding alpha$_2$-adrenergic receptor subtypes and identification of a single amino acid in the mouse alpha$_2$-C10 homolog responsible for an interspecies variation in antagonist binding. Mol Pharmacol 1992; 42:16–27.
76. Blaxall HS, Heck DA, Bylund DB. Molecular determinants of the alpha $_{2D}$-adrenergic receptor subtype. Life Sci 1993; 52:255–259.
77. Suryanaryana S, Daunt DA, von Zastrow M, Kobilka BK. A point mutation in the seventh hydrophobic domain of the α_2-adrenergic receptor increases its affinity for a family of β-receptor antagonists. J Biol Chem 1992; 266:15488–15492.
78. Kebabian JW, Calne DB. Multiple receptors for dopamine. Nature 1979; 277:93–96.
79. Anderson PH, Gingrich JA, Bates MD, et al. Dopamine receptor subtypes: Beyond the D1/D2 classification. Trends Pharmacol Sci 1990; 11:231–236.
80. Caron MG, Lefkowitz RJ. Catecholamine receptors: Structure, function, and regulation. Rec Prog Horm Res 1993; 48:277–290.
81. Hayes G, Biden TJ, Selbie LA, Shine J. Structural subtypes of the dopamine D2 receptor are functionally distinct: Expression of the cloned D_{2A} and D_{2B} subtypes in a heterologous cell line. Mol Endocrinol 1992; 6:920–926.
82. Tiberi M, Jarvie KR, Silvia C, et al. Cloning, molecular characterisation, and chromosomal assignment of a gene encoding a second D1 dopamine receptor subtype: Differential expression pattern in rat brain compared with the D_{1A} receptor. Proc Natl Acad Sci USA 1991; 88:7491–7495.
83. Gao DG, Canessa LM, Mouradian MM, Jose PA. Expression of the D2 subfamily of dopamine receptor genes in kidney. Am J Physiol 1994; 266:F646–F650.
84. Ramarao CS, Kincade JM, Perez DM, et al. Genomic organisation and expression of the human α_{1B}-adrenergic receptor. J Biol Chem 1992; 267:21936–21945.
85. Weinberg DH, Trivedi P, Tan CP, et al. Cloning, expression and characterisation of human α-adrenergic receptors α_{1a}, α_{1b}, α_{1c}. Biochem Biophys Res Commun 1994; 201:1296–1304.

86. Lomasney JW, Cotecchia S, Lorenz W, et al. Molecular cloning and expression of the cDNA for the α_{1A}-adrenergic receptor. J Biol Chem 1991; 266:6365–6369.
87. Schwinn DA, Lomasney JW. Pharmacological characterisation of cloned α_1-adrenoceptor subtypes: Selective antagonists suggest the existence of a fourth subtype. Eur J Pharmacol 1992; 227:433–436.
88. Saussy D. Personal communication.
89. Chhajlani V, Rangel N, Uhlen S, Wikberg JE. Identification of an additional gene belonging to the α_2-adrenergic receptor family in the human genome by PCR. FEBS Lett 1991; 280:241–244.
90. Yang-Feng TL, Han H, Lomasney JW and Caron MG. Localisation of the cDNA for an alpha$_1$-adrenergic receptor subtype (ADR α_{1D}) to chromosome band 20p13. Cytogenet Cell Genet 1994; 66:170–171.

13

Molecular Biology of Atrial Natriuretic Peptide in the Kidney

Mark L. Zeidel
University of Pittsburgh Medical Center, Pittsburgh, Pennsylvania

INTRODUCTION

Atrial natriuretic peptide was originally discovered as an extract of cardiac atria that exhibited striking natriuretic, diuretic, and vasodilatory effects (1,2). Since this initial discovery, atrial natriuretic peptide (ANP) and several related peptides such as C-natriuretic peptide (CNP), brain natriuretic peptide (BNP), and urodilatin (URO) have been characterized. Atrial natriuretic peptide stimulates excretion of salt and water by coordinate renal and endocrine actions (3,4). In the kidney, ANP at high concentrations augments the glomerular filtration rate (GFR), reduces angiotensin-stimulated proximal tubular Na^+ reabsorption, and reduces net Na^+ reabsorption by the collecting duct. In addition, ANP inhibits vasopressin-stimulated collecting duct water reabsorption. It also directly inhibits renin secretion by the macula densa and reduces aldosterone synthesis and release by the adrenal glomerulosa cells. This peptide stimulates relaxation of vascular smooth muscle and reduces the sympathetic compensatory response to vasorelaxation, resulting in profound reductions in blood pressure. This chapter examines the different forms of ANP and related peptides, the molecular biology of ANP receptors, and the cellular mechanisms by which ANP regulates renal Na^+ excretion.

MOLECULAR BIOLOGY OF ANP AND RELATED PEPTIDES

The presence of numerous electron-dense granules in atrial myocytes and their resemblance to secretory granules in endocrine organs led Debold and colleagues to the discovery of the natriuretic, diuretic, and vasodilatory properties of atrial extracts (1,2). Several peptides of similar core structure but varying amino acid length were soon isolated, and cDNA encoding ANP was cloned (3,4).

The ANP gene is located on the short arm of chromosome 1 in humans and chromosome 4 in mice (5,6). The human gene contains 3 exons and 2 introns (see Fig. 1). In humans, the full-length mRNA is initially translated into a 150–amino acid pre pro ANP, from which a 25–amino acid amino-terminal signal peptide is cleaved, leaving a 126–amino acid pro-ANP for storage in atrial myocyte granules (4). Upon stimulation of the atrial myocyte, pro-ANP is released and rapidly cleaved by a specific serine protease (atrioactivase), releasing the carboxyl-terminal 28 amino acids (residues 99 to 126), which is termed $ANP_{1\text{-}28}$ or ANP (7,8). The fragment containing residues 1 to 99 is further degraded into several peptides, including a fragment, $ANP_{31\text{-}67}$ which has been shown to mediate natriuretic but not vasodilatory effects (see below). The posttranslational processing of ANP is similar in rodents, except that the signal peptide is 25 amino acids in length and an additional two carboxyl-terminal arginine residues are removed to yield $ANP_{1\text{-}28}$ (9–12).

The regulation of ANP secretion from cardiac myocytes has been examined in vivo (13–15)

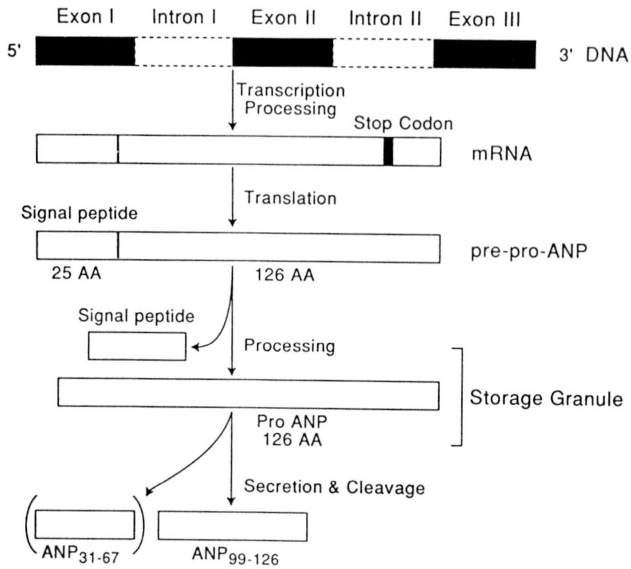

Figure 1 Model of ANP generation and release in atrial myocytes. See text for details.

and in primary cutlures of neonatal cardiocytes (12,13,16). Stretching of the atria by increased extracellular volume (13), atrial tachyarrhythmias (13,17), and congestive heart failure (14,15) markedly increases ANP secretion, tissue levels, and tissue mRNA. In primary cultures, stretch increases ANP release and mRNA levels by a calmodulin-dependent mechanism (16). Additional stimuli of ANP generation and release include $PGF_{2\alpha}$, PGE_2, and endothelin (18–20). Moreover, several tissue-specific ANP regulatory domains have been identified in or near the ANP gene (21–24). By placing putative regulatory sequences into constructs containing the chloramphenicol acetyl-transferase (CAT) reporter gene, the ability of sequences flanking the ANP gene to induce synthesis of CAT was examined. Sequences that bind c-*fos* and c-*jun* have been identified (24,25). Moreover, transient overexpression of c-*fos* and c-*jun* in cardiac myocytes can stimulate ANP release (24,25). Since expression of c-*fos* and c-*jun* is increased in hypertrophic states, it is possible that increased expression of these protooncogenes helps stimulate ANP release in cardiac hypertrophy (24).

Figure 2 shows additional peptides closely related to ANP, which are synthesized in noncardiac tissues. Several ANP analogues are formed by different posttranslational processing of the pro-ANP molecule. Thus, URO (ANP_{95-126}), which was first discovered in urine and is now known to be synthesized in renal cortex, has an amino-terminal extension (26–29). Other forms of ANP with various amino termini have been found in the brain (e.g., $ANP_{102-126}$) (30) and testis (ANP_{96-126}) (31). Two additional peptides, brain natriuretic peptide (BNP) (32) and C-type natriuretic peptide (CNP) (33), were identified in porcine brain extracts by assaying for the ability to relax chick rectum. All of these peptides share a disulfide bridge between cysteines 105 and 121 and identity of several amino acids within this disulfide ring (see Fig. 2). C-type natriuretic peptide has no carboxyl-terminal extension beyond the ring because of a stop codon just after the final CYS codon in the mRNA (34). The ANP and CNP sequences are highly conserved among species, with a single amino acid substitution in rat as compared with human ANP (4,35). By contrast, the sequences for BNP vary widely, with only 50% amino acid identity between pig, human, and rat BNPs and a range of length of the final hormone from 26 to 45 residues (35,36).

Both ANP and BNP are synthesized predominantly in the heart, with ANP levels 45-fold higher than BNP levels. Atrial ANP and BNP peptide generation is several orders of magnitude higher than ventricular synthesis, and these differences are also reflected in the mRNA levels of the respective peptides (37). In congestive heart failure (CHF), the levels of both ANP and BNP rise, with BNP rising more than ANP and ventricular BNP synthesis outstripping that of the atria (37). In addition,

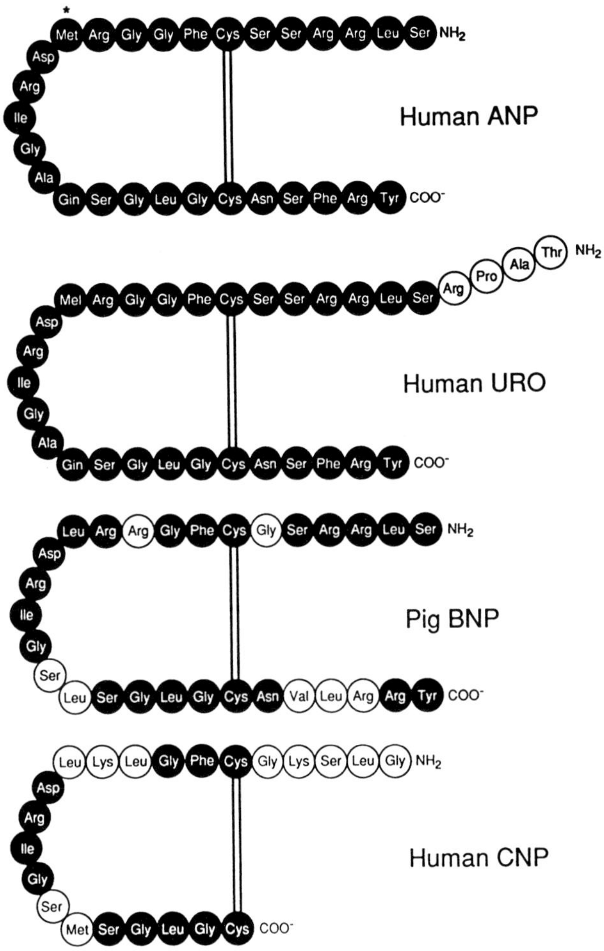

Figure 2 Amino acid sequences of human ANP, URO, and CNP and pig BNP. Identical residues are shaded. The methionine residue in ANP is replaced by an isoleucine residue in mouse, rat, bovine, and porcine ANP.

administration of BNP to patients with CHF results in a longer duration of action and more pronounced natriuretic effect than administration of ANP (38). These results suggest that BNP plays a role distinct from that of ANP in the pathophysiology of CHF (37,38).

Synthesis of URO has been localized to the renal cortical connecting tubule by autoradiography and studies in cell suspensions (26). Cortical collecting duct cells in culture can synthesize URO (26,27). At present, the renal tissue levels of URO are unknown. In addition, it is not known what factors regulate the URO synthesis and release. However, the availability of cultured renal epithelial cells that can synthesize URO may help clarify the regulation of URO secretion.

Both BNP and ANP have also been localized to the brain, although at levels below those of the heart. In brain, BNP levels are 10-fold higher than those of ANP (35). Injcctions of ANP or BNP into brain have a number of effects to regulate volume homeostasis, modifying responses such as hypothalamic vasopressin secretion, diuresis, salt appetite, heart rate, blood pressure, and water intake in response to angiotensin II (35). These activities suggest that ANP and BNP may function as neurotransmitters. C-type natriuretic peptide appears to be localized exclusively to brain, at concentrations severalfold higher than those of ANP and BNP (39). The function of CNP remains unexplored.

MOLECULAR BIOLOGY OF ANP RECEPTORS

As would be expected from ANP's physiological effects, studies of ligand binding in isolated membranes and by autoradiography to tissues in situ have identified specific ANP binding sites of high affinity in the kidney, adrenal, and vasculature. Moreover, abundant binding has also been localized to the central nervous system, eye, hepatocytes, the smooth muscle of the colon and gallbladder, and the lung parenchyma (40,41). In the kidney, binding localizes to glomeruli (42), larger renal vessels, and the inner medulla (43,44). Isolated glomeruli and medullary collecting ducts exhibit high levels of specific ANP binding as well as generation of cGMP in response to ANP (45–48). Cultured renal cell types exhibiting specific ANP binding include glomerular mesangial cells (49), vascular smooth muscle (50,51) and endothelial cells, renomedullary interstitial cells (52), and inner medullary collecting duct (IMCD) cells (45).

Early studies distinguished two classes of renal ANP receptors by their locations, ligand affinities, and ability to stimulate cGMP accumulation. One class was tightly linked to guanylate cyclase (45,49), and the other appeared to serve a clearance function, since no second-messenger response could be identified following binding of ANP (53,54). This clearance receptor, termed NPR-C (natriuretic peptide receptor-C) was purified to homogeneity from vascular smooth muscle cells and amino terminal sequence obtained (55,56). From this sequence, synthetic oligonucoeltides permitted isolation of clones encoding NPR-C (56).

By homology with other forms of particulate guanylate cyclases, two guanylate cyclase–linked ANP receptors, NPR-A and NPR-B, were cloned (57–59). Analysis of the primary structures of these three receptors (see Fig. 3) reveals four domains: an extracellular ligand binding domain, a membrane spanning domain, a kinase-like domain, and a guanylate cyclase domain (35,60). As is evident, NPR-C shares only the first two domains with NPR-A and NPR-B. The kinase-like domains contain more than 80% of the key conserved residues present in all protein kinases and share 30% identity to them. The guanylate cyclase domains of NPR-A and NPR-B share 40% homology with soluble guanylate cyclases and 88% identity with each other (35,59,60).

The differences in amino acid sequence among the three NPRs thus far identified is reflected in striking differences in ligand specificity. Thus, NPR-A binds tightly with ANP and BNP but does not interact with CNP (61); only ANP and BNP stimulate cGMP accumulation in cells in which NPR-A is transiently expressed (62). Also, BNP binds to NPR-A and stimulates cGMP accumulation in NPR-A–transfected cells with 10-fold lower potency than ANP. By contrast, NPR-B does not bind ANP or BNP (61) and does not respond to either peptide with increased guanylate cyclase activity (62). However, CNP binds to NPR-B with high affinity and stimulates cGMP generation effectively (63). Finally, NPR-C binds ANP, BNP, and CNP at roughly similar affinities and also binds to a wide variety of ANP analogues (63). This apparent lack of specificity of binding of NPR-C is consistent with a role for this receptor in buffering a variety of natriuretic hormones (35,53,54,64).

Detailed localization studies of renal NPR have been hindered by the lack of antisera specific for each of the NPR types. However, differential ligand affinities and measurements of mRNA

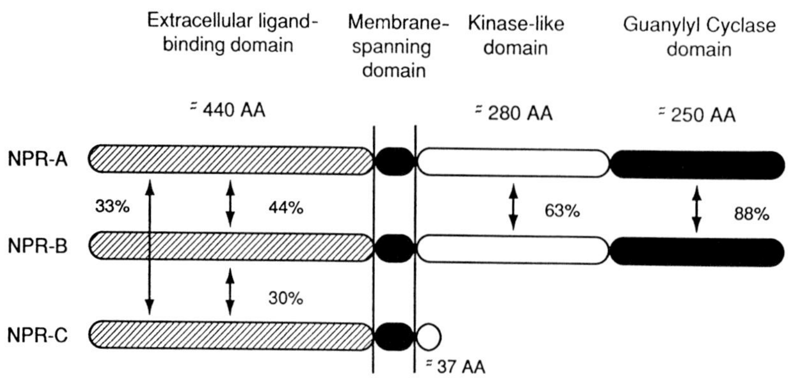

Figure 3 Structural domains of natriuretic peptide receptors (NPR). The different domains, their relative homologies to each other (percentages with arrows), and amino acid lengths are shown.

expression have allowed overall localization of NPR types. In the kidney, mRNA for NPR-A is located in glomeruli and medulla (64,65), while mRNA for NPR-C is abundant in glomeruli and large renal vessels and absent in medulla (64). Apparently, mRNA for NPR-B is absent in the kidney and appears to be localized to neural tissue, as is its principal ligand, CNP (65). In agreement with these results, glomeruli bind ANP and CNP analogues (64) but increase cGMP generation in response only to ANP (45,47,48). By contrast, IMCD cells bind only ANP and not CNP and make cGMP in response to ANP but not CNP (45).

Binding studies that take advantage of the differential ligand selectivity of NPR subtypes indicate that over 70% of glomerular and 95% of cortical NPR are NPR-C (53,54). Glomerular binding sites are predominantly located in epithelial cells and podocytes and also in mesangial cells (40,42). In the inner medulla, NPR-A are localized most prominently to renomedullary interstitial cells (52) and IMCD cells (45). Other sites of detectable NPR-A mRNA and/or ANP-induced cGMP accumulation include the cortical collecting duct and, to a lesser extent, the proximal tubule (66,67).

The molecular mechanisms underlying NPR-A and NPR-B function are only now being defined. Thus far, it has been impossible to purify NPR-A or NPR-B to homogeneity and reconstitute ANP-stimulated guanylate cyclase function (60). Therefore, the role of other membrane proteins or of membrane lipids in NPR function remains undefined. However, expression of NPR-A or NPR-B in a variety of cell types leads to induction of ligand-stimulated cGMP accumulation. The assignment of guanylate cyclase function to the carboxyl-terminal domain of NPR-A shown in Fig. 3 is supported by the homology of this region to other guanylate cyclases (59,68). Moreover, expression of the carboxyl-terminal 293 amino acid sequence in bacteria results in the appearance of guanylate cyclase activity, demonstrating that this region is sufficient to encode guanylate cyclase function (69).

The kinase-like domain of NPR-A appears to be necessary for coupling of ANP binding to guanylate cyclase function, because expression of mutant NPR-A in which this domain has been deleted results in the appearance of guanylate cyclase activity that is not stimulated by ANP (70). These results suggest that, in the wild-type NPR-A, the kinase-like domain functions to repress guanylate kinase activity, and that binding of ANP to the extracellular ligand-binding domain releases this repression, permitting guanylate cyclase activity (70).

Phosphorylation and binding of adenine nucleotides also play important regulatory roles in NPR-A function. When NPR-A is expressed in Sf9 insect cells using a recombinant baculovirus, the NPR-A present in the plasma membrane exhibits an absolute dependence on adenine nucleotides for its activity (71). Moreover, since nonhydrolyzable ATP analogues also permit ANP-stimulated guanylate cyclase activity, the role of ATP is to bind to the receptor and not to undergo hydrolysis (71). Atrial natriuretic hormone is effective in the millimolar range, the level present within the cytoplasm (71).

The role of phosphorylation in NPR-A function has been examined in mammalian cell lines with transient expression of NPR-A. Labeling transfected cells with ^{32}P demonstrated phosphorylation of serine and, to a lesser extent, threonine residues of NPR-A. Exposure of the cells to ANP led to a time-dependent dephosphorylation of NPR-A, with concomitant desensitization of cellular guanylate cyclase activity to ANP without a reduction in the level of enzyme protein (72). Moreoever, dephosphorylation of the protein with protein phosphatase A also reduced ANP-stimulated guanylate cyclase activity (72). Finally, site-directed mutagenesis of the kinase-like domain to remove phosphorylation sites reduced ANP-stimulated guanylate cyclase activity (73).

Taken together, these results support the following model for MPR-A function: Atrial natriuretic hormone binds to the ligand-binding domain of phosphorylated NPR-A in the presence of intracellular ATP, causing a shift in the three-dimensional structure of the protein, which is transmitted through the cell membrane to the kinase-like domain. This shift in structure releases the inhibitory effect of the kinase-like domain on the guanylate cyclase domain, resulting in increased cGMP generation. Continued binding of ANP to the ligand binding domain stimulates dephosphorylation of several sites, probably in the kinase-like domain, leading to inhibition of guanylate cyclase function and desensitization of the NPR-A molecule to further stimulation by ANP (35,60).

The function of NPR-C has been examined by determining the effects on ANP kinetics of infusions of CNP analogues into rats and isolated perfused rat kidneys. Thus, infusions of CNP have no natriuretic effect in isolated perfused rat kidney but potentiate the response to ANP. In the rat, infusions of CNP raise circulating ANP levels, with concomitant decrease in blood pressure and increase in salt excretion (53,54). It appears that NPR-C are continuously endocytosed from the cell surface into lysosomes and are reshuttled to the cell surface continuously, and that the rate of this recycling is not affected by the presence or absence of ligand (74). Because NPR-C carries bound ANP into the lysosomal compartment for prompt degradation (74), it serves as a buffer system for ANP and related peptides, regulating both circulating and tissue levels of these ligands.

CELLULAR MECHANISMS BY WHICH ANP REGULATES RENAL Na^+ EXCRETION

Atrial natriuretic peptide stimulates salt and water excretion by a coordinate series of actions along the nephron and at extrarenal sites (3,4,75). It reduces renin production in the macula densa and aldosterone synthesis and release in the adrenal medulla, reducing renal exposure to two potent antinatriuretic substances, angiotensin II and aldosterone. Moreover, ANP reduces the activity of renal sympathetic nerves (4). In addition to reducing the levels of these antinatriuretic influences, ANP directly increases GFR, antagonizes angiotensin II–stimulated proximal tubule volume reabsorption, inhibits collecting duct sodium reabsorption, and blunts the antidiuretic response of the collecting duct to vasopressin (see below).

Atrial natriuretic peptide increases GFR by increasing the glomerular capillary pressure, P_{GC}, (76–78) and the ultrafiltration coefficient, K_f. (79–81) The P_{GC} rises because ANP dilates arcuate, interlobular, and afferent arterioles while constricting efferent arterioles (76,78,82). This rise in P_{GC} increases the mean transcapillary hydraulic pressure gradient, increasing GFR. The K_f can also rise in response to ANP (79–81). The ultrafiltration coefficient is thought to be regulated by the contractility of mesangial cels, so that when mesangial cells contract, adjacent capillary loops are closed to filtration, so that the surface area for filtration is decreased, reducing K_f. Interestingly, cultured mesangial cells express NPR-A and release cGMP in response to ANP (46).

The increase in P_{GC} is probably due to ANP effects on the vascular smooth muscle of the preglomerular arterioles. In vascular smooth muscle, ANP binds to NPR-A, resulting in increased intracellular cGMP. This increase in cGMP causes vasodilatation by reducing intracellular calcium levels, as occurs when cGMP accumulation is stimulated by nitric oxide (NO) and its analogues (3,4). In the glomerulus, ANP may act directly on mesangial cells. However, the bulk of NPR-C and NPR-A in glomeruli appear to be located in glomerular epithelial cells (42,64). While these cells may also exhibit a contractile function, it is also possible that they cells release cGMP or a stimulant of mesangial cell–soluble guanylate cyclase, which enters adjacent mesangial cells, leading to reduced contractility. A similar mechanism probably occurs in resistance arterioles, where the endothelium releases endothelium-derived relaxing factor (EDRF), which, in turn, stimulates cGMP accumulation in adjacent vascular smooth muscle cells.

There is strong evidence that ANP reduces proximal tubule salt reabsorption. Early micropuncture studies showed no effect of ANP on basal proximal tubule function (83). However, ANP abolished the stimulatory effects of angiotensin II and norepinephrine on proximal tubule Na^+ reabsorption both in micropuncture studies and in studies of isolated perfused proximal tubules (84–86). In the studies involving isolated perfused tubules, cGMP mimicked the response to ANP (85,86). Although the density of NPR-A in proximal tubules appears low when compared with that of the IMCD (66,67), this level of receptors appears adequate to mediate the response.

Although there are modest levels of NPR-A mRNA and ANP-stimulated cGMP accumulation in the thick ascending limb and distal convoluted tubule (66,67), there is no evidence for inhibition of Na^+ reabsorption in these segments by ANP. Micropuncture studies have shown an increase in salt and water delivery out of the distal convoluted tubule in response to ANP, but this increase can be accounted for by increased GFR and reduced proximal tubule reabsorption (2,87). ANP does not alter salt and reabsorption in isolated perfused thin descending limb or in cortical and medullary thick ascending limbs of Henle (88,89).

ANP inhibits net Na^+ and water reabsorption in the cortical and medullary collecting ducts. Early studies involving retrograde microcatheterization of IMCD demonstrated that ANP increased salt and water delivery to the IMCD, consistent with inhibition of cortical collecting duct reabsorption, and that ANP abolished net salt and water reabsorption in the IMCD (2,90). These studies were confirmed by micropuncture of the terminal IMCD, demonstrating that ANP increased delivery to the site along the IMCD where the initial pipette was inserted and inhibited reabsorption between the initial pipette and the final urine (87,91). Examination of the effects of ANP in tubule segments in vitro have demonstrated direct inhibition of Na^+ and water transport. In the isolated perfused cortical collecting duct, ANP inhibits net Na^+ reabsorption and vasopressin-stimulated water reabsorption (92,93). In the isolated perfused IMCD, ANP also inhibited vasopressin-stimulated water flow (94). Moreover, some (95,96), but not all (97) laboratories have shown that ANP inhibits net Na^+ reabsorption. In freshly prepared suspensions of IMCD cells, ANP inhibits entry of Na^+ across the cell membrane, indicating a direct transport effect (98,99).

The mechanisms involved in ANP inhibition of collecting duct Na^+ transport have been examined in some detail. Studies in cell suspensions and primary cultures have demonstrated that ANP inhibits Na^+ flux via the apical amiloride-sensitive cation channel in the IMCD as follows: (a) ANP blocks amiloride-sensitive oxygen consumption of IMCD cell suspensions, and the ANP effect is abolished by the cation ionophore amphotericin (98); (b) ANP inhibits voltage-dependent, amiloride-sensitive conductive Na^+ uptake in IMCD cells (99); and (c) in primary cultures of rat IMCD cells, ANP reduces the open time of amiloride-sensitive cation channels, as measured in cell-attatched patches (100).

As discussed above, collecting duct expresses high levels of NPR-A (45). Studies of isolated collecting ducts have demonstrated that ANP stimulates cGMP accumulation with a time course and concentration response that mimics closely its inhibition of Na^+ and water transport (66,94,101). Moreover, these results were confirmed in measurements of ANP activation of NPR-A guanylate cyclase activity in IMCD cell membranes (45,102). Na^+ channel blockade is mediated by cGMP because cGMP mimics the actions of ANP in perfused tubules and cell suspensions (92,95,99,101). Moreover, addition of cGMP to patches of cell membrane detached from cultured IMCD cells reduces the open time of the amiloride-sensitive cation channel (100,103). Whether cGMP acts by binding to the channel or by stimulating a channel-associated protein kinase remains unclear. However, recent patch-clamp data support both mechanisms. G proteins have been found to be associated with amiloride-sensitive Na^+ channels in a number of epithelia, where they increase open probability (104–106). In cell detached patches, activation of G proteins with GTPγS blocked the component of channel inhibition mediated by cGMP-dependent protein kinase but did not alter the inhibition effected by cGMP itself (103,104). These results indicate that cGMP reduces the open time of the amiloride-sensitive Na^+ channel both by binding to the channel and by stimulating a GTP-dependent protein kinase which, in turn may modulate the stimulatory activity of G proteins associated with the channel A model of ANP action in IMCD is presented in Fig. 4.

Early microcatheterization studies suggested that ANP not only inhibited Na^+ reabsorption in this segment but also stimulated net Na^+ secretion (2,90). In support of this view, studies from some laboratories have shown that ANP inhibits lumen-to-bath flux of isotopic Na^+ and stimulates bath-to-lumen Na^+ flux in isolated perfused rat IMCD (95,96). The bath-to-lumen flux appears to be furosemide-sensitive (96,107). In support of these results, studies in fresh suspensions of rat IMCD cells have identified a furosemide-sensitive Na/K/2Cl cotransporter (108). The mechanisms by which ANP might regulate this cotransporter remain unclear but likely involve cGMP (95,96).

ANP inhibits vasopressin-stimulated water reabsorption in cortical and inner medullary collecting ducts. In the isolated perfused rabbit cortical collecting duct, ANP inhibited the hydroosmotic response to vasopressin but not to forskolin, which directly stimulates cAMP accumulation, or to exogenous cAMP (93). These results suggest that ANP blunts the vasopressin response by blocking vasopressin-stimulated cAMP accumulation (93). By contrast, ANP inhibited the hydroosmotic response to both vasopressin and exogenous cAMP in isolated perfused rat cortical and inner medullary collecting ducts (92,94), suggesting that ANP acts at a step in the hydroosmotic response beyond the generation of cAMP. Indeed, ANP did not inhibit vasopressin-stimulated cAMP generation in microdissected rat or rabbit cortical and medullary collecting duct segments (66).

An additional issue related to the mechanism of ANP action is the location of NPR-A on either the apical or basolateral membrane domain. Studies performed in cell suspensions or in cell cultures grown on plastic cannot distinguish the sidedness of hormone action. However, in isolated perfused inner medullary and cortical collecting ducts, ANP regulation of Na^+ or water transport occurred when the hormone was applied to the basolateral and not the apical surface (92–95). These findings were confirmed in studies using rabbit IMCD cells grown on filter-bottom supports, because basolateral but not apical ANP inhibited apical amiloride-sensitive Na^+ uptake (109). By contrast, Sonnenberg has perfused the apical surface of IMCDs in situ with ANP using microcatheterization and shown that luminal ANP reduces net Na^+ reabsorption as well as does luminal amiloride; both agents in the lumen did not give additive effects (110).

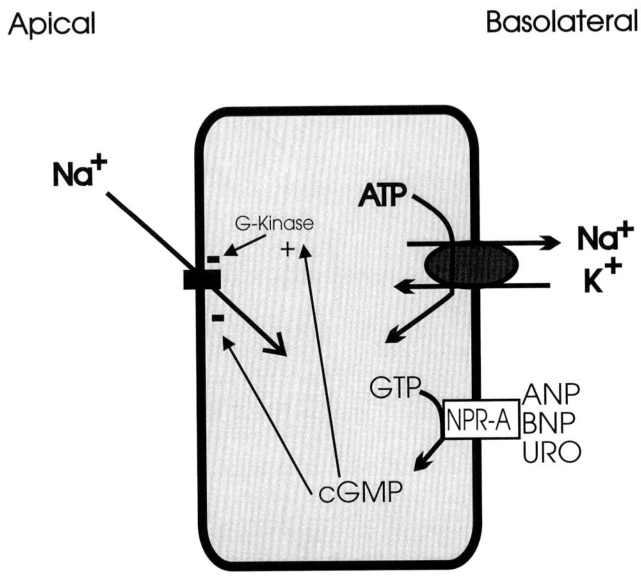

Figure 4 Model of action of ANP to inhibit Na^+ reabsorption in the IMCD. See text for details.

A potential luminal action of ANP in the collecting duct has two important physiological consequences: (a) The neutral endopeptidase of the renal brush border represents a major site of ANP degradation. Indeed, inhibitors of this enzyme have been shown to stimulate salt excretion without necessarily raising plasma levels of the peptide. This natriuretic effect may be due to an increase in the levels of intraluminal ANP, leading to enhanced inhibition of collecting duct Na^+ reabsorption (105,111). (b) Clearly, URO is synthesized in the connecting segment of the cortex, and, as expected from its similar structure and ability to bind to NPR-A, has been shown to inhibit IMCD Na^+ transport in vivo and in cell suspensions in a manner identical to that of ANP. However, it is not clear how URO might reach the IMCD. If URO were active from the luminal side, then it could be secreted into the lumen at the connecting segment and reach luminal NPR-A in the IMCD via the urine (105,111).

As noted above, processing of the ANP prohormone leads to release of an additional prohormone fragment, ANP_{31-67}. This peptide has been shown to circulate (112) and to stimulate diuresis and natriuresis without altering GFR in intact animals (113). In IMCD cell suspensions, this peptide inhibited Na^+ transport at concentrations above 1 p*M* via a mechanism distinct from that of ANP involving stimulation of PGE_2 generation and inhibition of Na, K-ATPase (114). Whether circulating or renally generated ANP_{31-67} inhibits Na^+ reabsorption in the IMCD or other tubular segments in vivo remains unclear, although this peptide may represent an additional mechanism by which the cardiac atria may regulate renal Na^+ excretion.

FUTURE DIRECTIONS

As specific antisera directed against selective epitopes of the different NPR types become available, definitive localization of these receptors in health and disease should become possible. These results will help resolve the glomerular localization of receptors and allow determination of whether receptors are present on luminal as well as basolateral collecting duct membranes. The mechanisms regulating URO production remain unclear, as do the pathways by which it reaches target epithelial cells. Studies in cultured cells that produce URO should reveal important regulatory mechanisms. Correlation of these measurements in cultured cells with urine and tissue levels will help define the physiological role of URO. The physiological role of ANP_{31-67} in regulating Na^+ excretion also remains to be defined. Finally, the development of atrial peptide analogues that bind to specific receptor subtypes may result in agents which lower blood pressure and increase Na^+ excretion in salt-retentive states. Potential examples include CNP analogues, which, by binding to clearance receptors, may increase levels of functional ANP.

REFERENCES

1. Debold AJ, Borrenstein HB, Veress AT, Sonnenberg H. A rapid and potent natriuretic response to intravenous injection of atrial myocardial extract in rats. Life Sci 1981; 28:89–94.
2. Sonnenberg H, Cupples WA, De Bold AJ, Veress AT. Intrarenal localization of the natriuretic effects of cardiac atrial extract. Can J Physiol Pharmacol 1982; 60:1149–1152.
3. Brenner BM, Ballermann BJ, Gunning ME, Zeidel ML. The diverse actions of atrial natriuretic peptide. Physiol Rev 1990; 70:665–688.
4. Ballermann BJ, Zeidel ML. Atrial Natriuretic Peptide. In: Seldin DW, Giebisch G, eds. The Kidney, Physiology and Pathophysiology. New York: Raven Press, 1992.
5. Nemer M, Chamberland M, Sirois D, et al. Gene structure of human cardiac hormone precursor, pronatriodilatin. Nature 1984; 312:654–656.
6. Yang-Feng TL, Floyd-Smith G, Nemer M, et al. The pronatriodilatin gene is located on the distal short arm of human chromosome 1 and on mouse chromosome 4. Am J Hum Genet 1985; 37:1117–1124.
7. Imada T, Takayanaki R, Inagami T. Identification of a peptidase which processes atrial natriuretic factor precursor to its active form with 28 amino acid residues in particulate fractions of rat atrial homogenate. Biochem Biophys Res Comm 1987; 143:587–592.
8. Imada T, Takayanagi R, Inagami T. Atrioactivase: Specific peptidase in bovine atria for processing of proatrial natriuretic factor: Purification and characterization. J Biol Chem 1988; 263:9515–9523.
9. Maki M, Takayanagi R, Misono KS, et al. Strucure of rat atrial natriuretic factor precursor deduced from cDNA sequence. Nature 1984; 309:722–724.
10. Oikawa S, Imai M, Ueno A, et al. Cloning and sequence analysis of cDNA encoding a precursor of human atrial natriuretic polypeptide. Nature 1984; 309:724–726.
11. Seidman CE, Duby AD, Choi E, et al. The structure of rat preproatrial natriuretic factor by a complementary DNA clone. Science 1984; 225:324–326.
12. Bloch KD, Scott JA, Zisfein JB, et al. Biosynthesis and secretion of pro atrial natriuretic factor by cultured rat cardiocytes. Science 1985; 230:1168–1171.
13. Lang RE, Tholken H, Ganten D, et al. Atrial natriuretic factor—A circulating hormone stimulated by volume loading. Nature 1985; 314:364–367.
14. Burnett JC, Kao PC, Hu DC, et al. Atrial natriuretic peptide in congestive heart failure in the human. Science 1986; 231:1145–1147.
15. Cody RJ, Atlas SA, Laragh JH, et al. Atrial natriuretic factor in normal subjects and heart failure patients: Plasma levels and renal, hormonal, and hemodynamic responses to peptide infusion. J Clin Invest 1986; 78:1362–1374.
16. Gardner DG, Wirtz H, Dobbs LG. Stretch-dependent regulation of atrial peptide synthesis and secretion in cultured atrial cardiocytes. Am J Physiol 1992; 263:E239–E244.
17. Williams TDM, Walsh KP, Canepa-Anson R, et al. Atrial natriuretic peptide response to rapid atrial pacing in cardiac-denervated dogs. Am J Physiol 1989; 257:R162–R167.
18. Gardner DG, Schultz HD. Prostaglandins regulate the synthesis and secretion of the atrial natriuretic peptide. J Clin Invest 1990; 86:52–59.
19. Kovacic-Milivojevic B, Schultz HD, Gardner DG. Arachidonic acid metabolites regulate the secretion of atrial natriuretic peptide in cultured rat atrial cardiocytes. Can J Physiol Pharmacol 1991; 69:1493–1499.
20. Gardner DG, Newman ED, Nakamura KK, Nguyen KP. Endothelin increases the synthesis and secretion of atrial natriuretic peptide in neonatal rat cardiocytes. Am J Physiol 1991; 261:E177–E182.
21. Wu JP, Kovacic-Milivojevic B, Lapointe MC, et al. Cis-active determinants of cardiac-specific expression in the human atrial natriuretic peptide gene. Mol Endocrinol 1991; 5:1311–1322.
22. Seidman CE, Bloch KD, Zisfein J, et al. Molecular studies of the atrial natriuretic factor gene. Hypertension 1985; 7(suppl 1):I31–I34.
23. Rosenzweig A, Seidman CE. Atrial natriuretic factor and related peptide hormones. Annu Rev Biochem 1991; 60:229–255.
24. Rosenzweig A, Halazonetis TD, Seidman JG, Seidman CE. Proximal regulatory domains of rat atrial natriuretic factor gene. Circulation 1991; 84:1256–1265.
25. Kovacic-Milivojevic B, Gardner DG. Divergent regulation of the human atrial natriuretic peptide gene by c-jun and c-fos. Mol Cell Biol 1992; 12:292–301.
26. Ritter D, Needleman P, Greenwald JE. Synthesis and secretion of an atriopeptin-like protein in rat kidney cell culture. J Clin Invest 1991; 87:208–212.
27. Ritter D, Chao J, Needleman P, et al. Localization, synthetic regulation, and biology of renal atriopeptin-like prohormone. Am J Physiol 1992; 263:F503–F509.

28. Saxenhofer H, Raselli A, Weidmann P, et al: Urodilatin, a natriuretic factor from kidneys, can modify renal and cardiovascular function in men. Am J Physiol 1990; 259:F832–F838.
29. Schulz-Knappe P, Honrath U, Forssmann WG, Sonnenberg H. Endogenous natriuretic peptides: Effect on collecting duct function in rat kidney. Am J Physiol 1990; 259:F415–F418.
30. Shiono S, Nakao K, Morii N, et al. Nature of atrial natriuretic polypeptide in rat brain. Biochem Biophys Res Comm 1986; 135:728–736.
31. Pandey KN, Orgebin-Crist M. Atrial natriuretic factor in mammalian testis: Immunological detection in spermatozoa. Biochem Biophys Res Comm 1991; 180:437–444.
32. Sudoh T, Kangawa K, Minamino N, Matsuo H. A new natriuretic peptide in porcine brain. Nature 1988; 332:78–81.
33. Sudoh T, Minamino N, Kangawa K, Matsuo H. C-type natriuretic peptide (CNP): A new member of natriuretic peptide family identified in porcine brain. Biochem Biophys Res Commun 1990; 168:863–870.
34. Tawaragi Y, Fuchimara K, Tanaka S, et al. Gene precursor structures of human C-type natriuretic peptide. Biochem Biophys Res Commun 1991; 175:645–651.
35. Koller KJ, Goeddel DV. Molecular biology of the natriuretic peptides and their receptors. Circulation 1992; 86:1081–1088.
36. Sudoh T, Maekawa K, Kojima M, et al. Cloning and sequence analysis of cDNA encoding a precursor for rat brain natriuretic peptide. Biochem Biophys Res Commun 1989; 159:1427–1434.
37. Mukoyama M, Nakao K, Hosoda K, et al. Brain natriuretic peptide as a novel cardiac hormone in humans: Evidence for an exquisite dual natriuretic peptide system, ANP and BNP. J Clin Invest 1991; 87:1402–1412.
38. Yoshimura M, Yasue H, Morita E, et al. Hemodynamic, renal and hormonal responses to brain natriuretic peptide infusion in patients with congestive heart failure. Circulation 1991; 84:1581–1588.
39. Minamino N, Makino Y, Tateyam H, et al. Characterization of immunoreactive human C-type natriuretic peptide in brain and heart. BBRC 1991; 179:535–542.
40. Bianchi C, Gutkowska J, Thibault G, et al. Radioautographic localization of atrial natriuretic factor in rat tissues. Histochemistry 1985; 82:441–450.
41. Bianchi C, Anand-Srivastava MB, deLean A, et al. Localization and characterization of specific receptors for atrial natriuretic factor in the ciliary processes of the eye. Curr Eye Res 1986; 5:283–287.
42. Bianchi C, Gutkowska J, Thibault G, et al. Distinct localization of atrial natriuretic factor and angiotensin II binding sites in the glomerulus. Am J Physiol 1986; 251:F594–F602.
43. Mendelsohn FA, Allen AM, Chai SY, et al. Overlapping distribution of receptors for atrial natriuetic peptide and angiotensin II visualized by in vitro autoradiography: Morphological basis of physiological antagonism. Can J Physiol Pharmacol 1987; 65:1517–1522.
44. Chai SY, Sexton PM, Allen AM, et al. In vitro autoradiographic localization of ANP receptors in rat kidney and adrenal gland. Am J Physiol 1986; 250:F753–F760.
45. Gunning ME, Ballermann BJ, Silva P, et al. Characterization of ANP receptors in rabbit inner medullary collecting duct cells. Am J Physiol 1988; 255:F324–F330.
46. Ballermann BJ, Hoover RL, Karnovsky MJ, Brenner BM. Physiologic regulation of atrial natriuretic peptide receptors in rat renal glomeruli. J Clin Invest 1985; 76:2049–2056.
47. Martin ER, Ballermann BJ. Atrial natriuretic peptide receptors. In: Stein J, Brenner BM, eds. Contemporary Issues in Nephrology: Recent Advances in Atrial Natriuretic Peptides. New York: Churchill Livingstone, 1989. In press.
48. Martin ER, Lewicki JA, Scarborough RM, Ballermann BJ. Expression and regulation of ANP receptor subtypes in rat renal glomeruli and papillae. Am J Physiol 1989; 257:F649–F657.
49. Ballermann BJ, Hoover RL, Karnovsky MJ, Brenner BM. Physiologic regulation atrial natriuretic peptide receptors in rat renal glomeruli. JCI 1985; 76:2049–2056.
50. Schenk DB, Phelps MN, Porter JG, et al. Identification of the receptor for atrial natriuretic factor on cultured vascular cells. J Biol Chem 1985; 260:14887–14890.
51. Scarborough RM, Schenk DB, McEnroe GA, et al. Truncated atrial natriuretic peptide analogs: Comparison between receptor binding and stimulation of cyclic GMP accumulation in cultured vascular smooth muscle cells. J Biol Chem 1986; 261:12960–12964.
52. Fontoura BM, Nussenzveig DR, Pelton KM, Maack T. Atrial natriuretic factor receptors in cultured renomedullary interstitial cells. Am J Physiol 1990; 258:C692–C699.
53. Maack T, Suzuki M, Almeida FA, et al. Physiological role of silent receptors to atrial natriuretic factor. Science 1987; 238:675–678.
54. Almeida FA, Suzuki M, Scarborough RM, et al. Clearance function of type C receptors of atrial natriuretic factor in rats. Am J Physiol 1989; 256:R469–R476.
55. Schenk DB, Phelps MN, Porter JG, et al. Purification and subunit composition of atrial natriuretic peptide receptor. Proc Natl Acad Sci USA 1987; 84:1521–1525.
56. Fuller F, Porter JG, Arfsten AE, et al. Atrial natriuretic peptide clearance receptor: Complete sequence and functional expression of cDNA clones. J Biol Chem 1988; 263:9395–9401.

57. Chinkers M, Garbers DL, Chang MS, et al. A membrane form of guanylate cyclase is an atrial natriuretic peptide receptor. Nature 1989; 338:78–83.
58. Singh S, Garbers DL. Molecular cloning of membrane forms of guanylyl cyclase. Methods Enzymol 1991; 195:414–423.
59. Schulz S, Singh S, Bellet RA, et al. The primary structure of a plasma membrane guanylate cyclase demonstrates diversity within this new receptor family. Cell 1989; 58:1155–1162.
60. Wong SK, Garbers DL. Receptor guanylyl cyclases. J Clin Invest 1992; 90:299–305.
61. Bennett BD, Bennett GL, Vitangcol RV, et al. Extracellular domain-IgG fusion proteins for three natriuretic peptide receptors. J Biol Chem 1991; 266:23060–23067.
62. Koller KJ, Lowe DG, Minamino N, et al. Differential activation of the human natriuretic peptide guanylate cyclases. In: Imura H, Matsuo H, Masaki T, eds. Peptide Regulation of Cardiovascular Function. Osaka: Takeda Science Foundation, 1991:91–99.
63. Koller KJ, Lowe DG, Bennett GL, et al. Selective activation of the B natriuretic peptide receptor by C-type natriuretic peptide (CNP). Science 1991; 252:120–123.
64. Maack T, Okolicany J, Koh GY, Price DA. Functional properties of atrial natriuretic factor receptors. Semin Nephrol 1993; 13:50–60.
65. Wilcox JN, Augustine A, Goeddel DV, Lowe DG. Differential regional expression of three natriuretic peptide recpetor genes within primate tissues. Mol Cell Biol 1991; 11:3454–3462.
66. Nonoguchi H, Knepper MA, Manganiello VC. Effects of atrial natriuretic factor on cyclic guanosine monophosphate and cyclic adenosine monophosphate accumulation in microdissected nephron segments from rats. J Clin Invest 1987; 79:500–507.
67. Terada Y, Moriyama T, Martin BM, et al. RT-PCR microlocalization of mRNA for guanylyl cyclase-coupled ANF receptor in the kidney. Am J Physiol 1991; 261:F1080–F1087.
68. Thorpe DS, Garbers DL. The membrane form of guanylate cyclase: Homology with a subunit of the cytoplasmic form of the enzyme. J Biol Chem 1989; 264:6545–6549.
69. Thorpe D, Morkin E. The carboxyl region contains the catalytic domain of the membrane form of guanylyl cylcase. J Biol Chem 1990; 265:14717–14720.
70. Chinkers M, Garbers DL. The protein kinase domain of the ANP receptor is required for signaling. Science 1989; 245:1392–1394.
71. Chinkers M, Singh S, Garbers DL. Adenine nucleotides are required for activation of rat atrial natriuretic peptide receptor/guanylyl cyclase expressed in a baculovirus system. J Biol Chem 1991; 266:4088–4093.
72. Potter LR, Garbers DL. Dephosphorylation of the guanylyl cyclase—A receptor causes desensitization. J Biol Chem 1992; 267:14531–14534.
73. Koller KJ, Lipari MT, Goeddel DV. Proper glycosylation and phosphorylation of the type A natriuretic peptide receptor are required for hormone-stimulated guanylyl cyclase activity. J Biol Chem 1993; 268:5997–6003.
74. Koh GY, Nussenzveig DR, Okolicany J, et al. Dynamics of atrial natriuretic factor-guanylate cyclase receptors and receptor-ligand complexes in cultured glomerular mesangial and renomedullary interstitial cells. J Biol Chem 1992; 267:11987–11994.
75. Zeidel ML, Brenner BM. Actions of atrial natriuretic peptides on the kidney. Semin Nephrol 1987;7:91–97.
76. Dunn BR, Ichikawa I, Pfeffer JM, et al. Renal and systemic hemodynamic effects of synthetic atrial natriuretic peptide in the anesthetized rat. Circ Res 1986; 59:237–246.
77. Marin-Grez M, Fleming JT, Steinhausen M. Atrial natriuretic peptide causes preglomerular vasodilatation and postglomerular vasoconstriction in rat kidney. Nature 1986; 324:473–476.
78. Veldkamp PJ, Carmines PK, Inscho EW, Navar LG. Direct evaluation of the microvascular actions of ANP in juxtamedullary nephrons. Am J Physiol 1988; 254:F440–F444.
79. Appel RG, Wang J, Simonson MS, Dunn MJ. A mechanism by which atrial natriuretic factor mediates its gomerular actions. Am J Physiol 1986; 251:F1036–F1042.
80. Singhal PC, Decandido S, Satriano JA, et al. Atrial natriuretic peptide and nitroprusside cause relaxation of cultured rat mesangial cells. Am J Physiol 1989; 257:C86–C93.
81. Fried TA, McCoy RN, Osgood RW, Stein JH. Effect of atriopeptin II on determinants of glomerular filtration rate in the in vitro perfused dog glomerulus. Am J Physiol 1986; 250:F1119–F1122.
82. Murray RD, Itoh S, Inagami T, et al. Effects of synthetic atrial natriuretic factor in the isolated perfused rat kidney. Am J Physiol 1985; 249:F603–F609.
83. Cogan MG. Atrial natriuretic factor can increase renal solute excretion primarily by raising glomerular filtration. Am J Physiol 1986; 250:F710–F714.
84. Harris PJ, Thomas D, Morgan TO. Atrial natriuretic peptide inhibits angiotensin-stimulated proximal tubular sodium and water reabsorption. Nature 1987; 326:697–698.
85. Garvin JL. Inhibition of Jv by ANF in rat proximal straight tubules requires angiotensin. Am J Physiol 1989; 257:F907–F911.

86. Garvin JL. ANF inhibits norepinephrine-stimulated fluid absorption in rat proximal straight tubules. Am J Physiol 1992; 263:F581–F585.
87. Briggs JP, Steipe B, Schubert G, Schnermann J. Micropuncture studies of the renal effects of atrial natriuretic substance. Pflugers Arch 1982; 395:271–276.
88. Kondo Y, Imai M, Kangawa K, Matsuo H. Lack of direct action of human atrial natriuretic polypeptide on the in vitro perfused segments of Henle's loop isolated from rabbit kidney. Pflugers Arch 1986; 406:273–278.
89. Peterson LN, De Rouffignac C, Sonnenberg H, Levine DZ. Thick ascending limb response to dDAVP and atrial natriuretic factor in vivo. Am J Physiol 1987; 252:F374–F381.
90. Sonnenberg H, Honrath U, Chong CK, Wilson DR. Atrial natriuretic factor inhibits sodium transport in medullary collecting duct. Am J Physiol 1986; 250:F963–F966.
91. Van de Stolpe A, Jamison RL. Micropuncture study of the effect of ANP on papillary collecting duct in the rat. Am J Physiol 1988; 254:F477–F483.
92. Nonoguchi H, Sands JM, Knepper MA. ANF inhibits NaCl and fluid absorption in cortical collecting duct of rat kidney. Am J Physiol 1989; 256:F179–F186.
93. Dillingham MA, Anderson RJ. Inhibition of vasopressin action by atrial natriuretic factor. Science 1986; 231:1572–1573.
94. Nonoguchi H, Sands JM, Knepper MA. Atrial natriuretic factor inhibits vasopressin-stimulated osmotic water permeability in rat inner medullary collecting duct. J Clin Invest 1988; 82:1383–1390.
95. Rocha AS, Kudo LH. Atrial peptide and cGMP effects on NaCl transport in inner medullary collecting duct. Am J Physiol 1990; 259:F258–F268.
96. Rocha AS, Kudo LH. Factors governing sodium and chloride transport across the inner medullary collecting duct. Kidney Int 1990; 38:654–667.
97. Sands JM, Nonoguchi H, Knepper MA. Hormone effects on NaCl permeability of rat inner medullary collecting duct. Am J Physiol 1988; 255:F421–F428.
98. Zeidel ML, Seifter JL, Lear S, et al. Atrial peptides inhibit oxygen consumption in kidney medullary collecting duct cells. Am J Physiol 1986; 251:F379–F383.
99. Zeidel ML, Kikeri D, Silva P, et al. Atrial natriuretic peptides inhibit conductive sodium uptake by rabbit inner medullary collecting duct cells. J Clin Invest 1988; 82:1067–1074.
100. Light DB, Schwiebert EM, Karlson KH, Stanton BA. Atrial natriuretic peptide inhibits a cation channel in renal inner medullary collecting duct cells. Science 1989; 243:383–385.
101. Zeidel ML, Silva P, Brenner BM, Seifter JL. Cyclic GMP mediates effects of atrial peptides on medullary collecting duct cells. Am J Physiol 1987; 252:F551–F559.
102. Gunning ME, Silva P, Brenner BM, Zeidel ML. Characteristics of ANP-sensitive guanylate cyclase in inner medullary collecting duct cells. Am J Physiol 1989; 256:F766–F775.
103. Light DB, Corbin J, Stanton BA. Dial ion-channel regulation by cyclic GMP and cyclic GMP-dependent protein kinase. Nature 1990; 344:336–339.
104. Light DB, Ausiello DA, Stanton BA. Guanine nucleotide binding protein alpha-i-3, directly activates a cation channel in rat inner medullary collecting duct cells. JCI 1990; 84:352–356.
105. Zeidel ML. Hormonal regulation of inner medullary collecting duct sodium transport. Am J Physiol. In press.
106. Schafer JA, Hawk CT. Regulation of Na^+ channels in the cortical collecting duct by AVP and mineralocorticoids (editorial). Kidney Int 1992; 41:255–268.
107. Kudo LH, van Baak AA, Rocha AS. Effect of vasopressin on sodium transport across inner medullary collecting duct. Am J Physiol 1990; 258:F1438–F1447.
108. Grupp C, Pavenstadt-Grupp I, Grunewald RW, et al. A Na-K-Cl cotransporter in isolated rat papillary collecting duct cells. Kidney Int 1989; 36:201–209.
109. Zeidel ML: Renal actions of atrial natriuretic peptide: Regulation of collecting duct sodium and water transport. Annu Rev Physiol 1990; 52:747–759.
110. Sonnenberg H, Honrath U, Wilson DR. In vivo microperfusion of inner medullary collecting duct in rats: Effect of amiloride and ANF. Am J Physiol 1990; 259:F222–F226.
111. Goetz K. Renal natriuretic peptide (urodilatin?) and atriopeptin: Evolving concepts. Am J Physiol 1991; 261:F921–F932.
112. Winters CJ, Sallman AL, Baker BJ, et al. The N-terminus and a 4000-MW peptide from the midportion for the N-terminus of the atrial natriuretic factor prohormone each circulate in humans and increase in congestive heart failure. Circulation 1989; 80:438–449.
113. Martin DR, Pevahouse JB, Trigg DJ, et al. Three peptides from the ANP prohormone amino terminus are natriuretic and/or kaliuretic. Am J Physiol 1990; 258:F1401–F1408.
114. Gunning ME, Brady HR, Otuechere G, et al. Atrial natriuretic peptide (31–67) inhibits Na^+ transport in rabbit inner medullary collecting duct cells: Role of prostaglandin E2. J Clin Invest 1992; 89:1411–1417.

14
Kinins and Kidney Function

Harry S. Margolius
Medical University of South Carolina, Charleston, South Carolina

INTRODUCTION

It is now clear that tissue kallikreins and their kinin products are important regulators of renal function and participate in the actions of drugs affecting the kidney. These phylogenetically ancient enzymes and peptides have responsibilities for the regulation of renal hemodynamics and for handling electrolyte and water movements across renal epithelial cells. These conclusions are the result of important discoveries concerning the molecular characterization of system components, including the substrate kininogens, the formative and destructive proteases and peptidases, and the kinin receptors; the localization of system components in the kidney; the regulation of their gene expression; interrelations among system components and other renal regulatory hormones and mechanisms; and finally, new data describing system aberrancies during or prior to the appearance of systemic diseases or renal manifestations of diseases, including hypertension and diabetes mellitus. This chapter summarizes these findings with particular emphasis upon the molecular biology of the renal kallikrein-kinin system and also upon important questions raised by recent discoveries but not yet answered.

COMPONENT CHARACTERIZATION, LOCALIZATION, AND REGULATION

Kininogens

The single human kininogen gene is localized to chromosome 3q26 $\rightarrow$ qter, close to two other related genes, the α-2-HS-glycoprotein and the histidine-rich glycoprotein. It codes for the production of both high-molecular-weight (HMW, 626aa, 88 to 120 kDa) and low-molecular-weight (LMW, 409aa, 50 to 68 kDa) kininogens via alternative splicing from 11 exons spread over a 27-kb pair span. Figure 1 (1) illustrates the relationships between the human kininogen gene and the mRNAs for HMW and LMW kininogens. The nine exons upstream of the kinin sequence code for the same amino acids in both kininogens, the portion of exon 10 downstream of the kinin is unique to HMW kininogen mRNA, whereas exon 11 is uniquely expressed in LMW kininogen mRNA. There is an interesting gene duplication in the rat that results in the K gene coding for HMW and LMW kininogens and a so-called T gene coding for T kininogens. Although these rat genes are highly homologous (>90%), the production of T kininogens and K kininogens, and hence T kinin (ile-ser-bradykinin) and K kinins (lys-bradykinin and bradykinin), are regulated differently in the rat by hormones or stress (2).

All kininogens are single-chain glycoproteins with an amino-terminal heavy chain and smaller but variable carboxyl-terminal light chains with the kinin moiety intervening. Multiple disulfide bridges are present in each form, with the heavy and light chains connected by a single bridge. Separate functions are resident in each section of the molecules, including the inhibition of cysteine

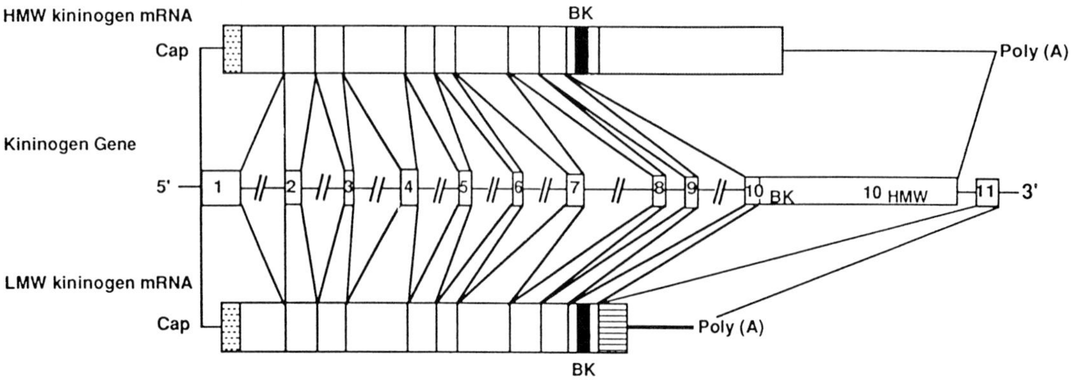

Figure 1 Schematic representation of the human kininogen gene and mRNAs for HMW and LMW kininogens. The protein-coding regions are indicated by the open boxes, cap sites are stippled, and the bradykinin (BK) sequences are indicated by the black bars. Note that only short segments of exon 10 and exon 11 are transcribed in LMW kininogen mRNA, whereas all of exon 10 but not exon 11 is transcribed in HMW kininogen mRNA. (From Ref. 1.)

proteinases such as the cathepsins and calpain (heavy chains), binding regions for endothelial surfaces and promotion of contact activation of clotting factors (light chain of HMW), and, of course, the binding to kinin receptors by kinin released from the molecules by the proteolytic kallikreins.

The kidney is presented with kininogens that are synthesized elsewhere, primarily in the liver (3), then secreted and transported in plasma (HMW kininogen concentration, 80 μg/ml; LMW kininogen concentration, 160 μg/ml) as well as on platelet and neutrophil plasma membranes (4,5). The HMW kininogen also exists in platelet granules and is secreted after platelet activation. Both HMW and LMW kininogens also occupy binding sites upon the unstimulated platelet, forming a ready reservoir for kinin release after proteolysis. In addition, human vascular endothelial cells contain mRNA for HMW kininogen (6), and kininogen is found in rat vascular smooth muscle cells grown in defined media containing no serum. In addition, mRNA for LMW kininogen, the preferred substrate for tissue (renal) kallikrein, is detectable in human kidney cortex and medulla (7). A unique rodent model for the study of kininogens is available in the Brown Norway Katholiek rat. These animals express all kininogen mRNAs but do not export synthesized kininogens, thus demonstrating nondetectable levels of HMW (8) and very low levels of LMW kininogen in plasma. Urinary kinin excretion in these rats is about 5% of normal (9). The usefulness of these rats for studies of kinin function is discussed below.

Using antibodies specific for human LMW kininogen and tissue kallikrein and immunohistochemistry, Figueroa and colleagues (10) described the spatial relationships of kininogen and kallikrein in the human kidney (Fig. 2). The work demonstrates kallikrein in connecting tubule cells and kininogen in principal cells of the same tubule just preceding the collecting duct. The site is juxtaposed to the afferent arteriole, where synthesized kallikrein (known to traffic to basolateral membranes of these epithelial cells) might affect interstitial cell or vascular wall function via local kinin formation. Alternatively, known kallikrein trafficking to the apical membranes of these epithelial cells, with subsequent tubular secretion, might find kininogen in the adjacent principal cells to generate kinin locally so as to affect tubular ion and water transport. Some recent reviews survey the likelihood of each of these rational possibilities (2).

Kallikreins and Kallikrein Inhibitors

Renal kallikrein is the so-called "true" tissue kallikrein, a serine proteinase product of a gene in a small gene family of three in the human but much larger families of up to 20 in the rat, of which 13 are identified, and 25 genes in the mouse. The human genes are clustered on chromosome 19 at q13.2-13.4. The analogous locus in the mouse is on chromosome 7, but the locus is not yet determined

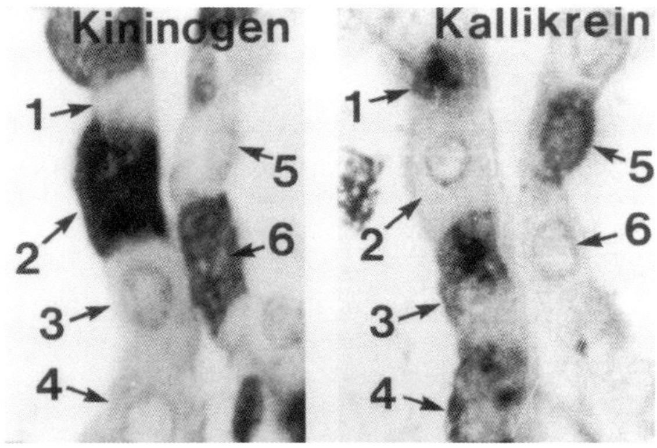

Figure 2 Serial sections of human renal connecting tubule immunostained for kininogen and kallikrein. Cells 2 and 6 show immunoreactive kininogen but not kallikrein. Cells 1, 3, 4, and 5 contain immunoreactive kallikrein but not kininogen. X3000. (From Ref. 10.)

in the rat. As noted in Table 1, the human gene is called *KLK1* and is expressed in pancreatic and salivary duct cells as well as kidney and intestine (11). The human neutrophil contains tissue kallikrein mRNA showing that expression also occurs here. The closely related human *KLK3* gene is of interest because it is expressed only in prostate and codes for the prostate-specific antigen (PSA). Prostate-specific antigen has high (60%) sequence homology to tissue kallikrein, is also a serine proteinase, and is, of course, important in the detection of prostatic carcinoma. The *KLK2* gene is also expressed only in prostate, but the product has no known function.

In the rat kidney, three kallikrein genes are expressed in addition to rat *KLK1*, the "true" tissue kallikrein gene. All of these genes (Table 2) regardless of species consist of five exons and four introns. Both the regulatory elements in flanking sequences of the rat genes and their protein products are highly homologous (>74%). *KLK7*, producing a proteinase also known as esterase B, is actually expressed at a 10-fold higher level in the rat kidney than *KLK1*, but its functional importance, cellular localization, and substrate are unknown (12). Other kallikrein genes of unknown function, *KLK4* and *KLK9*, are also expressed in rat kidney. Some studies suggest that renal kallikrein mRNA is also detectable by in situ hybridization at the glomerular vascular pole using a kallikrein cDNA as the probe. However, more specific oligonucleotide probes for true kallikrein failed to detect rK1 at this site, raising the possibility of another gene family member being expressed here. The true tissue kallikreins of human and rodent (hK1 and rK1) are acidic glycoproteins of 24 to 45 kDa. Most of the molecular-weight variation is due to variable glycosylation; for example, human urinary kallikrein is about 20% carbohydrate. The purified human renal enzyme is synthesized as a zymogen called prokallikrein, with an attached 17–amino acid signal peptide preceding a 7–amino acid activation

Table 1 The Human Tissue Kallikrein Genes (Species Designation: HSA)

Gene designation	Previous gene designations	mRNA/cDNA	Protein	Protein designation
KLK1	KLK1, hRKALL	λHK1 & phKK25 cDNAs	Tissue kallikrein (renal/pancreas/ salivary/intestine)	hK1
KLK2	KLK2, hGK-1, hKK-3			hK2
KLK3	PSA, PA, APS	λHPSA-1 & PSA cDNAs	PSA (prostate-specific antigen)	hK3

Source: Ref. 1.

Table 2 The Rat Tissue Kallikrein Genes (Species Designation: RNO)

Gene designation	Previous gene designations	mRNA/cDNA	Protein	Protein designation
KLK1	rGK-1 true tissue kallikrein	PS RSK1105 cDNA	Tissue kallikrein, renal kallikrein	rK1
KLK2	rGK-2 RSKG-5	S2	Tonin	rK2
KLK3	rGK-3 RSKG-50	S1		rK3
KLK4	rGK-4			rK4
KLK5	rGK-5	pseudogene?		
KLK6	rGK-6			rK6
KLK7	RSKG-7	K1	k7, esterase B, proteinase A	rK7
KLK8	rGK-8	P1	k8	rK8
KLK9		S3	SEV, KLP-S3, prostate K	rK9
KLK10		rKLK10 mRNA	Endopeptidase k, antigen gamma, proteinase B & t-kininogenase	rK10
KLK11	rGK-7	pseudogene?		
KLK12	RSKG-3			rK12
KLK13	RSKG-9	pseudogene		

Source: Ref. 1.

sequence, which must be cleaved to activate the enzyme. Several proteinases are capable of activating prokallikrein, including a human renal thiol proteinase; but the enzymes responsible for the regulation of kallikrein activation in situ are still unknown.

Once activated, renal kallikrein cleaves LMW kininogen at a met-lys N-terminal bond and an arg-ser C-terminal bond to release lys-bradykinin (kallidin). In most mammals including humans, tissue kallikrein cleaves lys-bradykinin from kininogens whereas plasma kallikrein releases bradykinin. Conversion of lys-bradykinin to bradykinin can occur via the action of aminopeptidases, but the peptides are generally equipotent and such conversion is not considered important. Several inhibitors of the enzymatic activity of tissue kallikreins are known, including aprotinin—the bovine basic pancreatic trypsin inhibitor—a 6.5-kDa 58-aa polypeptide; and a newly described serine proteinase inhibitor (a serpin) called kallistatin (13). Aprotinin is commercially available and is widely used experimentally as a tissue kallikrein inhibitor, although it is not specific in this regard and efficiently inhibits other serine proteinases. Kallistatin, a 58-kDA acidic protein, slowly forms heat-stable complexes with active tissue kallikrein (and other serine proteinases) that can be blocked by heparin. The protein is measurable in plasma of rats and humans. Its precise in vivo target is unknown and its role in regulating kallikrein activity locally remains to be explored.

Kinins and Kinin Receptors

Kinin formed within the kidney is detectable in urine, renal interstitial fluid, and—under some circumstances (i.e., drug-induced kininase inhibition)—even in renal venous blood. However, both the local and systemic half-life of kinins is widely considered to be very short, on the order of 10 to 30 sec. Concentrations of kinins in biological fluids are actually quite low—for example, a few picograms per milliliter in human plasma, but for years they were overestimated by assays that did not adequately inhibit kinin-generating enzymes or used nonspecific antisera which falsely elevated the estimates. On the other hand, the potency with which kinins exert a broad spectrum of effects on biological targets has, if anything, been underestimated, as an understanding of all the peptidase contributors to kinin catabolism, particularly in the kidney, is still incomplete. Clear evidence for powerful effects of kinins on renal vascular resistance, electrolyte and water excretion, as well as on renal functional modulators (such as renin and angiotensin, eicosanoids, catecholamines, nitric oxide, atriopeptin, vasopressin, and endothelin) establishes that the renal kallikrein-kinin system has important regulatory roles in the mammalian kidney (2). Further support for this notion, in addition to the localization information noted above, includes the remarkably high daily turnover rate of mammalian renal kallikrein (estimated to be 3 hr in the rat) (14), the high concentrations of renal kininases in discrete locales (e.g., proximal tubular brush borders) (15,16), and the identification of kinin receptor sites in cortical and medullary collecting tubules, interstitial cells, mesangial cells, and glomerular membranes (17,18). The effects of exogenous kinins to decrease afferent arteriolar resistance (and efferent resistance to a lesser degree) also point to the existence of kinin receptors in renal vasculature.

These receptors are presently characterized as BK1, BK2, and perhaps BK3. Receptors of the BK1 type are less prominent than BK2 and are notably present in the rabbit vasculature, especially after insult with for example, *Escherichia coli* endotoxin or lipopolysaccharide. Then the principal ligand for such entities, des-Arg^9-bradykinin, will produce a marked vasodilation and hypotension, an effect not noted in more normal vasculature, although the peptide can also produce contraction in some vascular smooth muscle preparations. These receptors have been described in several species and cell lines but are not cloned. Indeed, there are few ligand-binding and second-messenger studies of BK1 receptors. However recent work has detected their coexistence with BK2 receptors on rat mesangial cells (18), and a recent preliminary report has demonstrated physically distinct mRNA species for B1 and B2 receptors obtained from the human cell line W138 and expressed in *Xenopus* oocytes (19). Antisense oligonucleotides and the oocyte expression system were used to show sequence differences between the human B1 receptor encoding mRNA and that for B2 receptor. These data seem the strongest evidence to date, supporting the existence of separate kinin receptors.

The BK2 receptors mediate most of the actions of kinins. Both the rat and human BK2 receptor genes have been cloned and expressed (20,21). The rat BK2 receptor cDNA was obtained from a uterus library using *Xenopus* oocytes to assay for expression based upon bradykinin-induced ion currents. Six rounds of clonal selection were required to obtain the single cDNA encoding this BK2 receptor. The predicted protein sequence is for 366 aa with a MW of 41,696 Da and seven putatative transmembrane domains. Strong homology is present to the histamine H2 receptor as well as to neurotensin and tackykinin receptors. As expected, the potency of bradykinin and lys-bradykinin were equal ($EC_{50} \sim 1.9$ to 2.9 n*M*) insofar as induced ion currents in the oocyte and the BK1 receptor agonist des-Arg^9-bradykinin had no effect on oocytes expressing the BK2 receptor. Although the rat uterus has several times as much receptor message as any other tissue, the amounts in kidney are at least equivalent to that in heart, lung, testes and brain.

cDNA or DNA encoding the human BK2 receptor has also been isolated (21,22). The predicted amino acid sequence from each is 81% identical to the rat smooth muscle BK2 receptor. The encoded protein is 364 aa long with the features of a seven transmembrane domain G protein–coupled receptor. There is conservation of potential N-glycosylation sites and consensus sites for phosphorylation by protein kininases. It is interesting that the highest degree of homology between the human B2 kinin receptor and other known proteins is with the rat angiotensin receptor (32%) (21). Either the cDNA or the gene could be transfected into CHO or COS cells with resultant stable expression of high levels of kinin binding, high sensitivity to specific receptor blockade, and even coupling to the Ca^{2+}-phosphatidylinositol cascade. Interestingly, the level of human BK2 receptor mRNA density was fivefold higher in kidney than any other screened tissues, including uterus, lung, brain, heart, and testes (21). The isolation of these receptors from human and rat will be very helpful to discerning kinin roles and to therapeutic advances based upon receptor antagonism or stimulation.

A third BK receptor (BK3) is being explored in bovine aortic endothelial cells or the microvasculature of guinea-pig hindbrain. At these sites, variant responses to BK1 or BK2 agonists and antagonists suggest possible interaction with a non-BK1 or non-BK2 receptor (22).

Kininases

The half-life of kinins is a function of both formation and destruction. Peptidases that hydrolyze kinins are known as kininases, although none are known to be specific for these peptides. Both aminopeptidases and carboxypeptidases can terminate kinin biological activity, but the latter predominate; in rats, kininase II (ACE, or angiotensin I–converting enzyme) and neutral endopeptidase 24.11 (NEP 24.11, enkephalinase) each remove COOH-terminal Phe^8-Arg^9, thus inactivating kinins. Carboxypeptidases M, N, a Y-like carboxypeptidase, and another NEP (24.15) can also efficiently catabolize kinins. Both kininase II and NEP 24.11 are present in high concentrations in proximal tubular brush borders and the latter, along with the carboxypeptidase Y-like enzyme, are the major kinin-destroying enzymes of rat urine. However, the former (ACE) has been known since the early 1970s to be bifunctional, either forming angiotensin II or hydrolyzing kinins. Although also occurring as a soluble plasma enzyme, this kininase is highly concentrated on the lumenal surface of vascular endothelial cells as well as the aforementioned renal proximal tubular cell apical membranes. The human lung vasculature is rich in this enzyme but, interestingly, levels in kidney are about sixfold higher. For a considerable time, all therapeutic actions of converting enzyme inhibitors were emphatically considered to result from inhibition of angiotensin II formation. It is now clear that retardation of kinin destruction is likely to play a significant part in their efficacy, especially insofar as beneficial cardiac effects are concerned. For example, the ability of these inhibitors to reduce infarct size, left ventricular hypertrophy, or postischemic reperfusion injury is either attenuated or abolished by concomitant administration of the kinin BK2-receptor blocking agent HOE140 (23). These data, along with the corroborating changes in plasma kinin level, suggest that locally produced kinins, at least in cardiac tissue, contribute to the beneficial effects of ACE inhibition. A new kinin method assay has shown that ACE inhibition from a single dose (20 mg PO) of quinapril given to healthy volunteers produces significant elevations of plasma kinins for up to 8 hr, concomitant with significant reductions in angiotensin II levels of shorter duration (24). Such data now allow us to ask interesting questions about local kinin contributions to the function (or dysfunction) of other organs, including the kidney.

Regulation

Any questions concerning local (or systemic) roles for kallikrein-kininogen-kinin systems ultimately reach issues of system regulation in situ. The fact is that at present, there is little available information concerning the coordinate regulation of system components in response to various biochemical, physiological, or pathological stimuli. However, bits of regulatory information are appearing at an increasing rate. For example, T kininogen and HMW kininogen synthesis in cultured hepatocytes can be augmented by glucocorticoid, and maternal estrogen appears to be responsible for high circulating T kininogen in neonatal rats or at puberty. Liver kininogen mRNA levels are about fourfold higher in female rats than in male rats. Estradiol can increase while progesterone will decrease liver kininogen mRNA in ovariectomized rats. Interestingly, estradiol and progesterone both increase renal kallikrein mRNA in the same animals (2). Whether these findings have relevance to cardiovascular or renal function remains to be studied. In addition, some inflammatory stimuli, such as a carrageenan injection into the rat paw, induce a marked rise in plasma T kininogen but not K kininogen levels (3). The mediators for this response are unclear.

More information is available about possible regulatory influences on kidney kallikrein (2). Both urinary and renal tissue kallikrein levels and synthesis rate can be increased by diets low in sodium (14). In addition, diets high in potassium augment urinary kallikrein excretion or renal kallikrein levels. Chronic high levels of mineralocorticoids can increase renal kallikrein levels, and adrenalectomy reduces them. Renal kallikrein mRNA is twice as high in female rats as in male rats. Various hormones affect these renal mRNA and protein levels, including testosterone, thyroxine, and insulin. Each significantly increases kallikrein synthesis and the level of enzyme activity. Vasopressin can also increase, but norepinephrine decreases kallikrein release from rat renal cortical slices. The latter effect is accompanied by a reduction in de novo kallikrein synthesis and can be prevented by B_1-adrenergic blockade. Thus, there is now ample opportunity to examine coordinate alterations in substrate and formative enzyme levels or gene expression in relation to pharmacologically induced or pathological changes in renal function.

This conclusion is reinforced by some recent studies of renal kinin receptors. These receptors were well characterized in binding studies using ^{125}I-tyr^8-BK, a partial BK2 agonist, and mesangial cells or glomerular membranes (18,25). In addition to describing both BK1 and BK2 receptors in rat kidney and evaluating them in Goldblatt experiments, these studies showed that after 28 days of low sodium intake, there was a marked reduction in BK2 binding-site density concomitant with increased renal and urinary kallikrein. Water deprivation conversely resulted in a reduction in renal kallikrein level and an increase in BK2 receptor density. This work suggests that there is an inverse relation between presumptive renal kinin levels (inferred from augmented kallikrein activity) and BK receptor density. Most recently, these clues were augmented by a new technique allowing the direct measurement of renal interstitial kinin levels and showing that such levels change markedly in response to stimuli (26).

INTERRELATIONS OF KALLIKREINS AND KININS WITH RENAL REGULATORY HORMONES

Renin-Angiotensin-Aldosterone

The only certain in situ biochemical connection here is that angiotensin I–converting enzyme also efficiently catabolizes kinins. Increasing data now show that converting enzyme inhibition by various drugs leads to changes in circulating or local kinin levels, which have significant functional consequences. The availability of the specific and potent antagonists of BK2 receptors are now allowing collection of data showing the specific biochemical or functional consequences that are due to the actions of either administered or accumulated kinins (24). Another connection previously suggested as a result of some in vitro studies was that kallikrein could serve as a prorenin activating enzyme. This possibility in vivo is no longer considered convincing. Similarly, because a tissue kallikrein was capable of generating angiotensin II from a plasma protein fraction in vitro, suggestions of alternative pathways for formation of the pressor peptide were made. Again, no convincing evidence for such a role in vivo exists. Thus, the two systems now appear likely to function in concert to maintain renal blood flow and excretory capability. That is, while diets low in sodium (or high in potassium) or other systemic challenges (e.g., water deprivation) stimulate renin gene expression, renin synthesis, and increased systemic levels of angiotensin and aldosterone in defense of circulatory homeostasis, many of the same stimuli augment renal kallikrein and kinin production in what is probably a local defense of renal blood flow and glomerular filtration rate by vasodilator actions on renal cortical blood vessels and perhaps particularly afferent arterioles. The explanations for changes in the two systems in opposite directions—such as occurs in the 2K, 1C rat, with high renin and angiotensin levels but lowered renal kallikrein—are not yet well explained. The notion that such changes in kallikrein (among the earliest observed in the kidney enzyme) may only be some secondary response to a more important interstitial kinin level or kinin receptor change (25), especially in the nonclipped kidney, which collectively promotes a compensatory excretory response to the contralateral insult, is now an operational question, given the availability of specifc receptor blockers and other resources (e,g,m Brown-Norway rats of the Katholiek strain which produce no LMW or HMW kininogen). These and other chemical and biological tools will help unravel the related roles of these intertwined vasoactive peptide systems.

Atrial Natriuretic Peptides

Relations to other regulatory hormones are also being sought. In vitro, tissue kallikrein was found capable of forming "atriopeptin" from its precursors as well as catabolizing the active peptide (27,28). Administration of this powerful natriuretic diuretic agent affects urinary kallikrein excretion; conversely, cardiac tissue contains a kallikrein-like enzyme that colocalizes in atriopeptin-containing granules (29,30). Recent work now localizes the synthesis and secretion of an atriopeptin-like hormone from distal cortical connecting tubule cells of the mouse and rat, which also contain kallikrein (31). Because atriopeptin receptors, activation of which may modulate renal sodium reabsorption, exist downstream in the inner medullary collecting ducts, the hormone synthesized locally in the kidney may affect both tubular function and even, perhaps, renin secretion via interstitial release from the same synthetic site. The role of renal kallikrein produced in the same cells (or, perhaps, kinins) in this local atriopeptin production requires further study.

Eicosanoids

The renal kallikrein-kinin system activates eicosanoid synthesis in various renal cellular sites. Several studies show that kinins stimulate arachidonic acid release and subsequent eicosanoid synthesis in renal vasculature as well as interstitial and epithelial cells (32–34). These all seem, thus far, to occur via activation of BK2 receptors and phospholipase A_2-mediated arachadonic acid release. Stimulation of PGE_2 production is known to occur in response to kinins added to the lumenal surface of collecting duct cells (which conceivably enhances a kinin-induced natriuresis at this site) as well as in glomerular arterioles and in mesangial and renomedullary interstitial cells. Vascular PGI_2 synthesis is powerfully stimulated by kinins, but so is vascular or platelet synthesis of the vasoconstrictor thromboxane. Most studies attempting to interrupt these linkages with, for example, cyclooxygenase inhibitors or kinin receptor blockers or to modify putative relationships with converting enzyme inhibition or lipopolysaccharide-induced endotoxic shock disclose a significant connection between kinins and prostaglandins and especially their vasodilator and natriuretic properties (35). These connections may relate to some actions of vasopressin in the distal nephron (36). This peptide stimulates renal cellular kallikrein release and kinin production, but kinin inhibits vasopressin-induced water and perhaps sodium reabsorption in collecting ducts, probably via the production of PGE_2 at this site (37). Thus, it is reasonable to hypothesize that there is a local, negative feedback loop between kinins, eicosanoids, and vasopressin in the distal nephron.

Nitric oxide

Nitric oxide is another mediator now implicated in kinin-induced vasodilation and hypotension (38). Recent work has shown that in the rat and dog renal vasculature, the vasodilation produced by administered bradykinin is partially dependent upon nitric oxide synthesis and as such could be markedly attenuated by either N^G-monomethyl-L-arginine or N^{ω}-nitro-L-arginine, inhibitors of nitric oxide synthetase (39). These studies now bring consideration of nitric oxide, known from the earliest studies of Furchgott to be a responsible mediator for kinin-induced vasodilation, to the renal circulation. Questions concerning this relation are of great interest because there is a renal vascular hyperresponsiveness to bradykinin, particularly in the spontaneously hypertensive rat, in terms of both nitric oxide–dependent, and independent actions (Fig. 3).

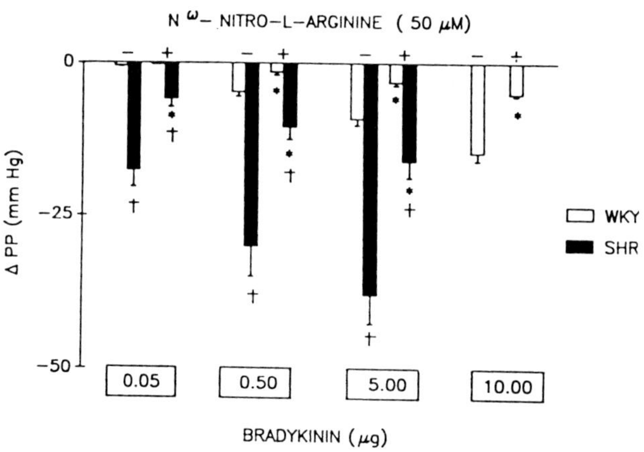

Figure 3 Bar graph shows effect on perfusion pressure (PP) of bolus injections of bradykinin in isolated kidneys of Wistar-Kyoto (WKY) rats and spontaneously hypertensive rats (SHR) perfused with (+) and without (–) N^{ω}-nitro-L-arginine-containing media. Results are mean ± SEM of eight to nine experiments. *Significant difference ($p < 0.05$) relative to data in kidneys perfused without N^{ω}-nitro-L-arginine. †Significant difference ($p < 0.01$) relative to data in WKY rats. (From Ref. 39.)

KALLIKREINS, KININS, AND RENAL FUNCTION

Hemodynamics and Excretion

Speculations about the role of this system in renal function and blood pressure regulation began in 1909, when the hypotensive property of human urine, now known to represent excreted renal kallikrein, was discovered (40). The earliest definitive studies of the effects of kinins on renal function were carried out by Webster and Gilmore (41) and Gill et al (42). They showed the natriuretic/diuretic capabilities of a kinin in dog and human and were soon followed by work showing that stimulation of water and electrolyte excretion was a function of increased renal blood flow. Indeed, the most consistently observed renal effect of kinins is to reduce renal vascular resistance. Unlike other vasodilators, bradykinin can increase blood flow without significant change in glomerular filtration rate or absolute proximal reabsorption but with a marked increase in fluid delivery to the distal nephron (43). This latter effect may contribute to the observed increased urine volume and sodium excretion seen with exogenously administered kinin into kidneys. It appears that the natriuresis and diuresis are the result of an effect of kinins on renal papillary blood flow, which inhibits sodium reabsorption distally secondary to a washout of the medullary solute gradient, rather than upon cortical blood flow, or, as mentioned above, glomerular filtration rate (44). Support for this contention is derived from several studies using either inhibitors of renal kininases such as captopril and phosphoramidon (the latter being an inhibitor of neutral endopeptidase 24.11) or chronic treatment with desoxycorticosterone (DOC), also known to raise endogenous kinin levels, followed by specific blockers of renal kinin BK2 receptors. The work generally indicates that increases in papillary blood flow, urine volume, and sodium excretion induced by kininase inhibition or with chronic DOC treatment can be either attenuated or abolished by kinin BK2 receptor blockade (45). Thus, it is now clear that *endogenously* produced kinin significantly affects renal hemodynamics and excretory function. This conclusion is supported by studies of renal function, just beginning to appear, in kininogen-deficient Brown Norway Katholiek rats. These animals exhibit a brisk hypertensive response to a 2% NaCl diet seemingly related to sodium and fluid retention (9). What is still uncertain is whether the observed natriuretic/diuretic responses are all a result of effects upon renal hemodynamics in the papilla or might include a component of distal tubular inhibition of electrolyte reabsorption (or stimulation of electrolyte secretion) (46,47). Regardless, the weight of present opinion suggests that intrarenal kinins modulate renal excretory function predominantly by effects upon renal vasculature.

Tubuloglomerular Feedback

Among the most interesting possible assignments of a role in renal function for kallikrein and kinins is that in tubuloglomerular feedback (TGF). Recent studies have established in either normal or hydronephrotic kidneys that bradykinin can differently reset TGF (48). The turning point is increased by kinin in control rats but is decreased in the hydronephrotic animals. Although concentrations of kinin used in the perfusates were extremely high, no kininase inhibitors were used concomitantly. It was suggested that endogenously produced kinin might, via effects upon prostaglandin production in the normal rats, lower TGF sensitivity, or that it might, via effects upon thromboxane synthesis in hydronephrotic rats, increase TGF sensitivity. In the hydronephrotic kidney, bradykinin is known to stimulate thromboxane synthesis. The work complements a previous study which showed that the serine proteinase inhibitor aprotinin was able to diminish or prevent the attenuation of TGF induced by the converting enzyme/kininase II inhibitor captopril (49). This work suggested that endogenous renal kinin production might be reducing TGF (lowering sensitivity and increasing turning point). Finally, a study by Ushiogi et al. (50) characterized the effects of TGF inhibition by salt loading on the salt sensitivity of blood pressure in the spontaneously hypertensive rat (SHR). The results, including crossover studies which perfused tubules of the various groups of SHR and W/Ky with previously collected tubular fluids from salt-loaded or control rats, showed that TGF was augmented in SHR and not affected by salt loading. It appeared that this resetting in SHR might be related to defective activation of a humoral feedback inhibitory substance in response to chronic salt load, resulting in a greater blood pressure increase in SHR vs. control animals. Several working hypotheses can be formulated based upon these findings and the renal kallikrein-kinin system abnormalities known to exist in SHR. Collectively, these studies compel more evaluation of endogenous renal kallikrein-kinin system behavior in relation to this important connection between tubular and glomerular function.

Vectorial Ion and Water Transport

As stated above, the specific local roles of kinin, generated from renal distal tubular kininogen by adjacent kallikrein, in ion and water transport is uncertain. However, it is clear that kinin BK2 receptors are coupled to cellular systems in polarized epithelia, which lead to marked changes in vectorial ion and water transport. Many epithelia (e.g., rat colonic, porcine papillary collecting duct, guinea pig gallbladder) have been shown to secrete anions, predominantly chloride but also bicarbonate in voltage-clamp experiments in response of kinin; these actions are partially prostaglandin-dependent and can be blocked by inhibitors of Na^+, K^+, Cl^- cotransport such as furosemide or bumetanide (2,51,52). However, the actions of locally generated renal kinins on ion and water transport are still mysterious. Some studies of isolated perfused cortical collecting ducts from rats have suggested that kinin inhibits either electroneutral NaCl absorption or stimulates NaCl secretion (46). However, that work was challenged recently by studies which found no effects whatsoever of kinin or any electrophysiological property of this tissue (47). The use of more specific system modulators such as receptor blockers, the Brown-Norway rats, or animals subject to transgenic or homologous recombination experiments will shed light on this question.

KALLIKREIN-KININ SYSTEM FUNCTION IN RENAL AND SYSTEMIC DISEASES

Hypertension

The earliest evaluations of renal kallikrein in humans with arterial hypertension were carried out in the 1930s (2). Urinary kallikrein excretion in hypertensives was found to be significantly less than in comparable normotensive subjects. Even then, the notion that this finding might represent a deficiency in an endogenous renal vasodilator system which was contributory to the hypertensive state was prominently considered. Progress in addressing this possibility has been rather slow, unlike the enormous, sustained interest provoked on behalf of the renin-angiotensin system by the Goldblatt experiment. Today, interest in possible renal kallikrein-kinin contributions to the pathogenesis of human hypertensive diseases is growing because of a series of provocative findings reaching from epidemiological surveys (see below) to gene polymorphism-cosegregation analyses (53). However, the case for involvement is still weaker than the easily demonstrable importance of vasoconstrictor influences in human hypertension.

While it is clear that patients with essential hypertension excrete less kallikrein that do normotensive subjects in general, there is much overlap in any of the population studies carried out over the past 20 years (54). That is, many hypertensive subjects show normal urinary kallikrein excretion. Black subjects, adults or children, excrete markedly less kallikrein than whites, regardless of blood pressure, with black hypertensives generally showing the lowest measured levels (55,56). In recent years, studies of kallikrein and other system components in more homogeneous human populations have begun to appear. For example, Japanese patients with low-renin forms of hypertension show significant reductions in both active urinary kallikrein and kinin (57). They also demonstrate higher levels of a kallikrein inhibitory material in urine. Reduced urinary kininogen and increased total kininase and neutral endopeptidase 24.11 are also present in such hypertensive patients (2).

Epidemiological surveys in children stimulated interest in relations between renal kallikrein and blood pressure (55,58). These studies examined blood pressures, kallikrein, and other variables repetitively over long intervals and showed that kallikrein excretion was familially aggregated and that families of children with the lowest kallikrein excretions showed significantly higher blood pressures than did families of children with the highest kallikrein excretions. These efforts have been extended in recent years. For example, urinary kallikrein and diastolic blood pressure are negatively correlated in newborn infants, 2 to 4 days old, and such correlations are detectable in infants up to 18 months of age (59). In another approach, Berry et al. (60) examined family history of hypertension in a large population (57 Utah pedigrees containing 391 youths and 405 normotensive adults) and found that individuals with a higher urinary kallikrein excretion genotype were less likely to have one or two hypertensive parents than those with a lower excretion genotype. The data suggested that the higher excretion rate represents a genotype associated with a reduced risk of essential hypertension (60). Such studies, while provocative, require extension in a variety of ways before the case for a contributory role of renal kallikrein and kinins in the origins of some human forms of hypertension is established.

Work in rodent forms of hypertension is proceeding more rapidly. Goldblatt hypertensive rats were the first animal model shown to have reduced urinary kallikrein excretion and renal level of the enzyme (2). This occurs principally in the compromised kidney, and levels in the contralateral kidney are either normal or reduced to a lesser extent. These changes are now being studied in relation to the different salt-handling properties of the two kidneys. In addition, these differences are now being elaborated upon by examination of BK2 receptor density, which is increased to a greater extent in the contralateral kidney than in the clipped one (25). These increases could signify an augmented kinin-induced PGE_2 release in compensatory response to the higher perfusion pressure this kidney faces. This contralateral kidney is already known to show higher renal blood flow, glomerular filtration rate, and sodium excretion. Experiments with specific kinin receptor blockade will be forthcoming.

All genetic models of rat hypertension—including the SHR, Dahl, Milan, New Zealand, Fawn-hooded, and Sabra strains—have been evaluated for rate of urinary kallikrein excretion and compared with their control strains; the excretion rate is reduced in each (2). It is important to point out that few of these studies had been carried out longitudinally with respect to age, and it was generally unclear whether the urine kallikrein abnormality preceded or followed the appearance of hypertension. One early study in Milan rats showed significantly lower levels in newborn animals of the hypertensive vs. the control strain (61). A more recent effort showed renal tissue active kallikrein in SHR was only 53% of values in WKY within 12 hr of birth, whereas total enzyme level (including prokallikrein) was not different between strains (62). The difference persists between SHR and SKY at 4, 8, and 12 weeks of age. This work suggested a possible defect in renal prokallikrein activation but not in synthesis rate in the SHR.

Studies in Dahl salt-sensitive (SS/Jr) vs. salt-resistant (SR/Jr) rats are providing interesting new information concerning renal kallikrein-kinin activity in these highly inbred strains. Here, renal kallikrein levels and ureteral kinin excretion are increased and kininases reduced in young SR/Jr compared with SS/Jr. Furthermore, BK2 receptor blockade markedly reduces RBF and GFR in SR/Jr but not SS/Jr. These studies suggest the possibility that an augmented renal kallikrein-kinin system activity could be associated with the resistance to hypertension displayed by SR/Jr.

The BK2 receptor blocker HOE140 was recently used to show that chronic systemic BK2 receptor blockade in rats chronically treated with DOC results in an earlier and greater rise in blood pressure than seen in rats treated with DOC alone (63). This, and other recent studies are suggesting that endogenously produced kinins are indeed participating in arterial blood pressure regulation.

Diabetes Mellitus

Rats with streptozotocin-induced diabetes mellitus have markedly altered renal kallikrein-kinin system function (64). Early in the course of the diabetic state, these animals, treated with some insulin, also show glomerular hyperfiltration along with increased renal kallikrein synthesis, levels, and urinary excretion (65,66). Treatment of such animals with aprotinin or a BK2 receptor antagonist reduces renal blood flow and glomerular filtration rate to levels equal to those in normal rats (66). These studies were recently confirmed in patients with type I (insulin-dependent) diabetes mellitus in whom filtration rate, blood flow, and renal tubular sodium reabsorption were measured (67). Patients with glomerular hyperfiltration showed greater active kallikrein and PGE_2 excretion than patients with normal glomerular filtration rate or otherwise normal subjects. Both kallikrein and PGE_2 levels correlated directly with glomerular filtration rate, and the former also correlated directly with distal tubular sodium reabsorption. These findings in diabetic rats and patients suggest that renal kallikrein, kinins, and PGE_2 contribute to the glomerular hyperfiltration of human diabetes.

Other Nephropathies

The ability of converting enzyme inhibition to reduce proteinuria in nephrotic rats is dependent on the renal kallikrein-kinin system. Recent work has shown, in confirmation of earlier studies, that urinary kallikrein excretion as well as renal levels of kallikrein mRNA are reduced in passive Heymann nephritis (68). However, converting enzyme inhibition restores kallikrein mRNA levels to normal, partially increases urinary kallikrein excretion, and reduces urinary albumin excretion. The data suggest reversal of a transcriptional suppression of renal kallikrein gene(s) without concomitant effect on renin RNA. The studies further implicate renal kallikreins and kinins in renal responses to insult.

Over the past 25 years, a large number of studies have disclosed abnormality in components of this system in renal diseases or systemic diseases with renal features, including Bartter's syndrome, primary aldosteronism, pheochromocytoma, cirrhosis, hepatorenal syndrome, heavy metal poisonings, polycystic renal disease, and others (2). Many drugs affecting renal function also affect levels of system components, including antihypertensive agents, diuretics, and cyclooxygenase inhibitors. With the significant advances in our understanding of the renal kallikrein-kinin system's component structure, localization, and regulation and the ability to manipulate components with stimuli or inhibitors, it is likely that the understood contributions of the system to normal renal function and pathology will lead to new therapeutic strategies based upon stimulation or interdiction of kinin actions.

REFERENCES

1. Müller-Esterl W, Iwanga S, Nakaniski S. Kininogens revisited. Trends Biochem Sci 1986; 11:336–339.
2. Bhoola KD, Figueroa CD, Worthy K. Bioregulation of kinins: Kallikreins, kininogens, and kininases. Pharmacol Rev 1992; 44:1–80.
3. Nakaniski S. Substance P precursor and kininogen: Their structures, gene organizations, and regulation. Physiol Rev 1987; 67:1117–1142.
4. Schmaier AH. Zuckerberg A, Silverman C, et al. High molecular weight kininogen: A secreted platelet protein. J Clin Invest 1983; 71:1477–1489.
5. Gustafson EJ, Schmaier AH, Wachtfogel YT, et al. Human neutrophils contain and bind high-molecular-weight kininogen. J Clin Invest 1989; 84:28–35.
6. Schmaier AH, Kuo A, Lundberg D, et al. The expression of high-molecular-weight kininogen on human umbilical vein endothelial cells. J Biol Chem 1988; 263:16327–16333.
7. Iwai N, Matsunaga M, Kita T, et al. Detection of low molecular kininogen messenger mRNA in human kidney. J Hypertens 1988; 6(suppl 4):S399–S400.
8. Lattion AL, Baussant T, Alhenc-Gelas F, et al. The high-molecular mass kininogen deficient rat expresses all kininogen mRNA species, but does not export the high-molecular-mass kininogen synthesized. FEBS Lett 1988; 239:59–64.
9. Majima M, Yoshida O, Mihara H, et al. High sensitivity to salt in kininogen-deficient Brown Norway Katholiek rats. Hypertension 1993; 22:705–714.
10. Figueroa CD, MacIver AG, Mackenzie JC, Bhoola KD. Localisation of immunoreactive kininogen and tissue kallikrein in the human nephron. Histochemistry 1988; 89:437–442.
11. Berg T, Bradshaw RA, Carretero OA, et al. A common nomenclature for members of the tissue (glandular) kallikrein gene families. In: Fritz H, Müller-Esterl W, Jochum M, et al., eds. Recent Progress on Kinins. Basel: Birkhauser Verlag, 1992; 38(suppl 1):19–25.
12. Brady JM, MacDonald RJ. The expression of two kallikrein gene family members in the rat kidney. Arch Biochem Biophys 1990; 278:342–349.
13. Zhou GX, Chao L, Chao J. Kallistatin: A novel human tissue kallikrein inhibitor. J Biol Chem 1992; 267:25873–25880.
14. Miller DH, Chao J, Margolius HS. Tissue kallikrein synthesis and its modification by testosterone or low dietary sodium. Biochem J 1984; 218:37–43.
15. Ward PE, Erdös EG, Gedney CD, et al. Isolation of membrane-bound renal enzymes that metabolize kinins and angiotensins. Biochem J 1976; 157:643–650.
16. Schulz WW, Hagler HK, Buja LM, Erdös EG. Ultrastructural localization of angiotensin I-converting enzyme (EC 3.4.15.1) and neutral metalloendopeptidase (EC 3.4.24.11) in the proximal tubule of the human kidney. Lab Invest 1988; 59:789–797.
17. Hall JM. Bradykinin receptors: pharmacological properties and biological roles. Pharmacol Therap 1992; 56:131–190.
18. Bascands J-L, Pecher C, Ronaud S, Emond C, Tack JL, Bastie MJ, Burch R, Regoli D, Girolami JP. Evidence for existence of two distinct bradykinin receptors on rat mesangial cells. Am J Physiol 1993; 264:F548–F556.

19. Webb M, Phillips E, Skidmore E, Brown M, McIntyre P. Molecular studies on B1 and B2 bradykinin receptors (abstr). Kinin '93, Guaruja, Brazil, Oct 17–22, 1993; L111.
20. McEachern AE, Shelton ER, Bhakta S, Obernolte R, Bach C, Zuppan P, Fujisaki J, Aldrich RW, Jarnagin K. Expression cloning of a rat B_2 bradykinin receptor. Proc Natl Acad Sci USA 1991; 88:7724–7728.
21. Hess JF, Borkowski JA, Young GS, Strader CD, Ransom RW. Cloning and pharmacological characterization of a human bradykinin (BK-2) receptor. Biochem Biophys Res Comm 1992; 184:260–268.
22. Eggerickx D, Raspe E, Bertrand D, Vassart G, Parmentier M. Molecular cloning, functional expression and pharmacological characterization of a human bradykinin B2 recepto gene. Biochem Biophys Res Comm 1992; 187:1306–1313.
23. Linz W and Schölkens BA. Role of bradykinin in the cardiac effects of angiotensin-converting enzyme inhibitors. J Cardiovasc Pharmacol 1992; 20(Suppl 9):583–590.
24. Pellaconi A, Brunner HR, Nussberger J. Plasma kinin levels during ACE-inhibition: relationships with the reinin-angiotensin system (abstr). Kinin '93, Guaruja, Brazil, Oct 17–22, 1993; P89.
25. Edmond C, Bascands J-L, Rakotoarivony J, Praddaude F, Boinpart G, Pecher C, Ader J-L, Girolami J-P. Glomerular B_2-kinin-binding sites in two-kidney, one-clip hypertensive rats. Am J Physiol 1991; 260:F626–F634.
26. Siragy HM, Jaffa AA, Margolius HS. Stimulation of renal interstitial kinins by sodium depletion. Am J Hypertens 1993; 6:863–866.
27. Briggs J, Marin-Grez M, Steipe B, Schubert G, Schnermann J. Inactivation of atrial natriuretic substance by kallikrein. Am J Physiol 1984; 247:F480–F484.
28. Currie MG, Geller DM, Chao J. Margolius HS, Needleman P. Kallikrein activation of a high molecular weight atrial peptide. Biochem Biophys Res Comm 1984; 120:461–466.
29. Lopez C, Jimenez W, Arroyo V, La Villa G, Martinez-Pardo A, Gaya J, Rivera F. Effects of atrial natriuretic peptide on urinary kallikrein excretion and renal function in rats. Eur J Pharmacol 1989; 168:1–6.
30. Simson J, Currie M, Chao L, Chao J. Co-localization of a kallikrein-like serine protease (arginine esterase A) and atrial natriuretic peptide in rat atrium. J Histochem Cytochem 1989; 37:1913–1917.
31. Ritter D, Chao J, Needleman P, Tetens E, Greenwald J. Localization, synthetic regulation, and biology of renal atriopeptin-like hormone. Am J Physiol 1992; 263:F503–F509.
32. Grenier F, Rollins T, Smith W. Kinin-induced prostaglandin synthesis by renal papillary collecting tubule cells in culture. Am J Physiol 1981: 241:F94–F104.
33. Welsh C, Dubyak G, Douglas J. Relationship between phospholipase C activation and prostaglandin E2 and cyclic adenosine monophosphate production in rabbit tubular epithelial cells. Effects of angiotensin, bradykinin, and arginine vasopressin. J Clin Invest 1988; 81:710–719.
34. Thomasson D, Zenser T, Davis B. Cortical interstitial cell interactions induce sensitivity of hydronephrotic kidney to bradykinin. Kidney Int 1988; 33:71–76.
35. Wang Y-X, Gavras I, Lammek B, Bresnahan M, Gavras H. Effects of bradykinin and prostaglandin inhibition on systemic and regional hemodynamics in conscious normotensive rats. J Hyperten 1991; 9:805–812.
36. Friedlander G, Amiel C. Protein kinase C activators and bradykinin selectively inhibit vasopressin-stimulated cAMP synthesis in MDCK cells. Biochim et Biophys Acta 1987; 929:311–317.
37. Schuster VL. Mechanism of bradykinin, ADH, and cAMP interaction in rabbit cortical collecting duct. Am J Physiol 1985; 249:F645–F653.
38. Fulton D, McGiff J, Quilley J. Contribution of NO and cytochrome P450 to the vasodilator effect of bradykinin in the rat kidney. Brit J Pharmacol 1992; 107:722–725.
39. Cachofeiro V, Nasjletti A. Increased vascular responsiveness to bradykinin in kidneys of spontaneously hypertensive rats: Effects of N^{ω}-nitro-L-arginine. Hypertension 1991; 18:683–689.
40. Abelous J, Bardier E. Les substances hypotensives de l'urine humaine normale. Compt Rend Soc Biol 1909; 66:511–512.
41. Webster M, Gilmore J. Influence of kallidin-10 on renal function. Am J Physiol 1964; 206:714–718.
42. Gill JR Jr, Melmon KL, Gillespie L Jr, Bartter FC. Bradykinin and renal function in normal man: Effects of adrenergic blockade. Am J Physiol 1965; 209:844–848.
43. Stein J, Congbalay R, Karsh D, et al. The effect of bradykinin on proximal tubular sodium reabsorption in the dog: Evidence for functional nephron heterogeneity. J Clin Invest 1972; 51:1709–1721.
44. Roman R, Kaldunski M, Scicli A, Carretero O. Influence of kinins and angiotensin II on the regulation of papillary blood flow. Am J Physiol 1988; 255:F690–F698.
45. Fenoy FJ, Roman RJ. Effect of kinin receptor antagonists on renal hemodynamic and natriuretic responses to volume expansion. Am J Physiol 1992; 263:R1136–R1140.
46. Tomita K, Pisano JJ, Burg MB, Knepper MA. Effects of vasopressin and bradykinin on anion transport by the rat cortical collecting duct. J Clin Invest 1986; 77:136–141.
47. Rouch AJ, Chen L, Troutman SL, Shafer JA. Na^+ transport in isolated rat CCD: Effects of bradykinin, ANP, clonidine and hydrochlorothiazide. Am J Physiol 1991; 260:F86–F95.

48. Morsing P, Persson EG. Kinin and tubuloglomerular feedback in normal and hydronephrotic rats. Am J Physiol 1991; 260:F868–F873.
49. Schnermann J, Briggs JP, Schubert G, Marin-Grez M. Opposing effects of captopril and aprotinin on tubuloglomerular feedback responses. Am J Physiol 1984; 247:F912–F918.
50. Ushiogi Y, Takabatake T, Häberle DA. Blood pressure and tubuloglomerular feedback mechanism in chronically salt-loaded spontaneously hypertensive rats. Kidney Int 1991; 39:1184–1192.
51. Cuthbert AW, Margolius HS. Kinins stimulate net chloride secretion by the rat colon. Br J Pharmacol 1982; 75:587–598.
52. Baird AW, Margolius HS. Bradykinin stimulates electrogenic bicarbonate secretion by the guinea pig gallbladder. J Pharmacol Exp Ther 1989; 248:268–272.
53. Pravenec M, Kren V, Kunes J, et al. Cosegregation of blood pressure with a kallikrein gene family polymorphism. Hypertension 1991; 17:242–246.
54. Margolius HS. Tissue kallikreins and kinins: Regulation and roles in hypertensive and diabetic diseases. Annu Rev Pharmacol 1989; 29:343–364.
55. Zinner SH, Margolius HS, Rosner B, et al. Familial aggregation urinary kallikrein concentration in childhood. Am J Epidemiol 1976; 104:124–132.
56. Levy S, Lilley J, Frigon R, Stone R. Urinary kallikrein and plasma renin activity as determinants of renal blood flow: The influence of race and dietary sodium intake. J Clin Invest 1977; 60:129–138.
57. Nakahashi Y, Shimamoto K, Ura N, et al. Comprehensive studies on the renal kallikrein-kinin system in essential hypertension. In: Greenbaum LM, Margolius, HS, eds. Kinins IV: Part B. Advances in Experimental Medicine & Biology. New York: Plenum Press, 1986; 198B:351–357.
58. Zinner SH, Margolius HS, Rosner BR, Kass EH. Stability of blood pressure rank and urinary kallikrein concentration in childhood. Circulation 1978; 58:908–915.
59. McGarvey ST, Zinner SH, Margolius HS. Urinary kallikrein and blood pressure in infants and children. In: Iimura O, Margolius HS, eds. Renal Function, Hypertension and Kallikrein-Kinin System. Tokyo: Hokusen-Sha, 1988:161–168.
60. Berry TD, Hasstedt SJ, Hunt SC, et al. A gene for high urinary kallikrein may protect against hypertension in Utah kindreds. Hypertension 1989; 13:3–8.
61. Favaro S, Baggio B, Antonello A, et al. Renal kallikrein content of spontaneously hypertensive rats. Clin Sci 1975; 49:69–71.
62. Praddaude F, Tran-Van T, Ader J-L. Renal kallikrein activity in rats developing spontaneous hypertension. Clin Sci 1989; 76:311–315.
63. Madeddu P, Anania V, Pargaglia PP, et al. Chronic kinin receptor blockade induces hypertension in deoxycorticosterone-treated rats. Br J Pharmacol 1993; 108:651–657.
64. Mayfield R, Namm DH, Squires J, et al. Development of hypertension in rats made diabetic with streptozotocin is associated with decreased urinary kallikrein excretion. Diabetes 1985; 34:22–28.
65. Jaffa AA, Miller DH, Bailey GS, et al. Abnormal regulation of renal kallikrein in experimental diabetes and the effects of insulin on prokallikrein synthesis, activation and excretion. J Clin Invest 1987; 80:1651–1659.
66. Harvey JN, Jaffa AA, Margolius HS, Mayfield RK. Renal kallikrein and the hemodynamic abnormalities of the diabetic kidney. Diabetes 1990; 39:299–304.
67. Harvey JN, Edmundson AW, Jaffa AA, et al. Renal excretion of kallikrein and eicosanoids in patients with type I (insulin-dependent) diabetes mellitus: Relationship to glomerular and tubular function. Diabetologia 1992; 35:857–862.
68. Hutchison FN, Webster SK, Jaffa AA. Altered renal kallikrein and renin gene expression in nephrotic rats and modulation by converting enzyme inhibition. J Clin Invest 1993; 92:1073–1079.

15

Cyclooxygenases

William L. Smith and David DeWitt
Michigan State University, East Lansing, Michigan

INTRODUCTION AND OVERVIEW

Prostanoids, which include the prostaglandins (PGs) and thromboxanes (TXs), are synthesized via the pathway shown in Fig. 1 (1). Prostanoid biosynthesis can be envisioned as occurring in three stages: (a) hormone-induced activation of phospholipase(s) leading to the hydrolysis of esterified arachidonate from precursor phospholipids; (b) conversion of arachidonate to the prostaglandin endoperoxide PGH_2 mediated by PGH synthases (cyclooxygenases); and (c) isomerization [in the cases of PGD_2, PGE_2, prostacyclin (PGI_2), and thromboxane A_2 (TXA_2)] or reduction (in the case of $PGF_{2\alpha}$) of PGH_2 by specific synthases or reductases to yield the major biologically active prostanoids (2). Following their synthesis and exit from the cell, prostanoids act on the parent cell and adjoining cells in an autocrine and paracrine fashion, respectively, activating specific G protein–linked prostanoid receptors to stimulate or inhibit changes in the levels of second messengers (3–8). Prostanoids can be viewed as local hormones that coordinate responses to circulating hormones such as arginine vasopressin, angiotensin II, and bradykinin, which elicit prostanoid synthesis (3). For example, in the case of the renal collecting tubule, PGE_2 is synthesized in response to arginine vasopressin (9) and acts on collecting tubule cells themselves to attenuate the antidiuretic effect of arginine vasopressin (AVP) and on neighboring thick limb cells to modulate NaCl reabsorption necessary for antidiureses (3,10,11).

In this review, we concentrate on one component of the prostaglandin biosynthetic pathway—the PGH synthase or cyclooxygenase. In fact, there are two closely related PGH synthase isozymes, called PGH synthase-1 and -2. The goal of this review is to summarize information on (a) the enzymology of PGH synthases, including their interactions with nonsteroidal anti-inflammatory agents, and (b) the regulation of expression of the genes for each of the two PGH synthases.

RENAL COMPARTMENTATION OF PGH SYNTHASES-1 AND -2

As discussed in more detail below, PGH synthase-1 is considered to be a "constitutive" enzyme, whereas PGH synthase-2 is "inducible." The distribution of PGH synthase-1 in kidneys has been studied using antibodies specific for this isozyme (12,13). PGH synthase-1 immunoreactivity is highly compartmentalized. Those renal cells expressing substantial levels of this constitutive form of the enzyme include collecting tubule epithelia, vascular endothelial cells, medullary interstitial cells, and epithelial cells of the thin limb of Henle's loop. Prostanoids are well established to have multiple tubular and vascular effects in the kidney (10,11,14,15). Those prostanoid responses which have been characterized most extensively at the cellular and molecular levels are the effects of PGE_2 on the collecting tubule and thick ascending limb (10,11,16) and the effects of TXA_2/PGH_2 analogs on renal mesangial cells and vascular endothelial cells (14,15). Thus, most of the known actions of

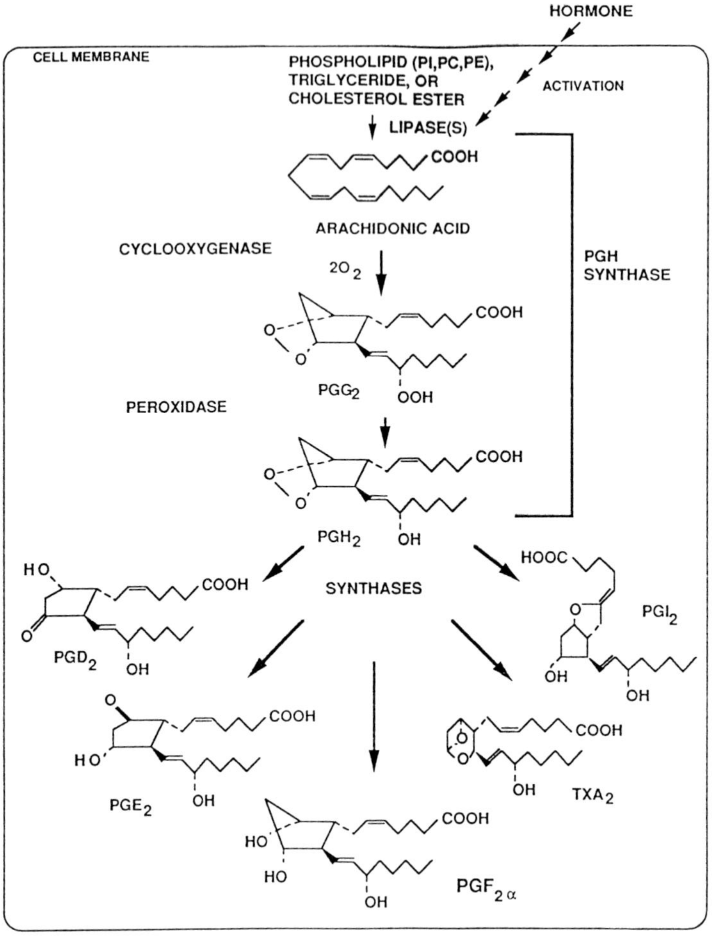

Figure 1 Biosynthetic pathway for the formation of prostanoids. All the products of the pathway are shown in this figure. However, usually only one prostanoid is formed as a major product by a given cell type; for example, platelet cells form almost exclusively TXA_2, renal collecting tubule epithelia form mainly PGE_2, and endothelial cells from large arteries form mainly PGI_2. Abbreviations: PI, PC, and PE = phosphatidylinositol, -choline, and -ethanolamine, respectively; PGH_2, PGG_2, PGD_2, PGE_2, $PGF_{2\alpha}$ = prostaglandins; H_2, G_2, D_2, E_2, and $F_{2\alpha}$ respectively; PGI_2 = prostacyclin; and TXA_2 = thromboxane A_2. (From Ref. 1.)

prostanoids in the kidney can be attributed to the production of prostanoids via pathways involving PGH synthase-1.

Staining of normal rabbit kidney with two different antipeptide antibodies generated against PGH synthase-2 has failed to reveal any positive staining (W. L. Smith and D. L. DeWitt; unpublished observations). However, in situ hybridization using murine probes for PGH synthases-1 and -2 has indicated that there are trace amounts of PGH synthase-2 in the renal cortex, although the cellular location has not been determined (C. D. Breder, D. L. DeWitt, and W. L. Smith; unpublished observations). As discussed below, PGH synthase-2 appears to be dramatically upregulated in situations associated with increased cell replication or differentiation. Thus, this isozyme might not be expected to be present in abundance in kidney except under conditions of inflammation and/or associated tissue repair such as seen with the hydronephrotic kidney model (13,17,18).

THE ENZYMOLOGY OF PGH SYNTHASES

Prostaglandin Endoperoxide (PGH) Synthase Isozymes

As noted above, the second step in prostanoid biosynthesis is the conversion of arachidonate to PGH_2, and this conversion is catalyzed by PGH synthase (Fig. 1). Historically, this enzyme has been called "cyclooxygenase." However, this term correctly refers only to the dioxygenase reaction catalyzed by PGH synthase, in which arachidonic acid is converted to PGG_2. A second activity of PGH synthase, a peroxidase activity, catalyzes the two-electron reduction of the 15-hydroperoxyl group of PGG_2 to PGH_2. During the past 2 years, it has become apparent that there are two distinct PGH synthase isozymes called PGH synthase-1 and -2. Each enzyme is encoded by a different gene. Both enzymes catalyze cyclooxygenase and peroxidase reactions with comparable efficiencies. Figure 2 compares the deduced amino acid sequences of PGH synthases-1 and -2 from several species.

PGH synthase 1 is the enzyme that was originally purified from ovine and bovine vesicular glands in the mid 1970s (19,20). cDNAs encoding PGH synthases-1 have been cloned from mouse (21), human (22,23), and sheep (24–26). PGH synthases-1 have relatively large signal peptides, which—in the case of the sheep enzyme—is cleaved between amino acid residues 24 and 25 to yield a mature enzyme having 576 amino acids and the N-terminal sequence ADPGAP. The deduced amino acid sequences of PGH synthases-1 from sheep, human, and mouse are about 90% identical. The biggest sequence differences are among the signal peptides and the ten amino acids immediately preceding the RPS(P)TEL sequences at the C terminus.

PGH synthases 2 were identified by sequence homology to PGH synthase-1 as (a) a v-*src*-inducible gene product from chicken fibroblasts (27,28) and (b) a phorbol ester-inducible immediate early gene product called TIS10 from murine 3T3 cells (29). cDNAs encoding mouse PGH synthases-2 have been expressed in vitro and shown to exhibit both cyclooxygenase and peroxidase activities (30,31). The amino acid sequences of PGH synthases-1 and -2 are about 60% identical (and about 75% homologous) for isozymes from the same species (21–23,29,32). PGH synthase-2 differs significantly from PGH synthase-1 at positions prior to amino acid residue 30; fully processed rat PGH synthase-2 has the N-terminal sequence ANPCC, corresponding to cleavage of seventeen amino acids from the N terminus of the deduced sequence of the murine enzyme (Fig. 2) (33). Notably, all PGH synthases-2 contain an 18–amino acid insert, not seen with PGH synthases-1, near the C termini.

For technical reasons, most of the enzymological studies on PGH synthase have been performed with ovine PGH synthase-1. Those residues and sequences that have been identified as being critical in the catalytic functions of ovine PGH synthase-1 are discussed below. All of these residues are conserved in the PGH synthases-2 (Fig. 2), suggesting that the mechanism of catalysis is essentially the same for both PGH synthase isozymes.

The C-terminal P(S)TEL sequence is common to all PGH synthases-1 and -2 except the chicken PGH synthase-2 (Fig. 2). This P(S)TEL sequence resembles the D(T)EL sequences involved in retaining enzymes within the endoplasmic reticulum (34). However, substantial alterations can be made in this sequence in ovine PGH synthase-1 without apparently affecting its subcellular location (M. K. Regier, J. C. Otto, and W.L. Smith; unpublished observations), thus arguing against the P(S)TEL sequence acting as an endoplasmic reticulum (ER) retention signal for PGH synthases.

PGH Synthase Catalysis

The Cyclooxygenase Reaction

The cyclooxygenase and peroxidase reactions catalyzed by PGH synthases-1 and -2 occur at two physically distinct but neighboring sites on the proteins. The best evidence for this is that indomethacin (35,36), aspirin (35,36), or fatty acid analogues (37), each of which acts as a competitive inhibitor of arachidonate binding and blocks the cyclooxygenase activity of PGH synthase-1 without affecting the peroxidase activity of the enzyme. Moreover, several mutants of PGH synthase-1 have been prepared which lack cyclooxygenase activity but express peroxidase activity (24,38). A model for the relationship between the cyclooxygenase and peroxidase active sites is presented below after these two activities are discussed individually.

```
Chick-2    MLLPCALLAALL-----------------AAGHAANPCCSLPCQNRGECMTTGFDRYECD
Human-2    MLARALLLCAVL-----------------ALSHTANPCCSHPCQNRGVCMSVGFDQYKCD
Mouse-2    MLFRAVLLCAAL-----------------GLSQAANPCCSNPCQNRGECMSTGFDQYKCD
Mouse-1    MSRRSLSLWFPLLLLLLLPPTPSVLLADPGVPSPVNPCCYYPCQNQGVCVRFGLDNYQCD
Human-1    MSR-SLLLRFLLLLLLL-PPLP-VLLADPGAPTPVNPCCYYPCQHQGICVRFGLDRYQCD
Sheep-1    MSRQSISLRFPLLLLLL-SPSP-VFSADPGAPAPVNPCCYYPCQHQGICVRFGLDRYQCD
                   10        20        30        40        50

Chick-2    CTRTGYYGENCTTPEFFTWLKLLIKPTPNTVHYILTHFKGVWNIINNSPFLRDTIMRYVL
Human-2    CTRTGFYGENCSTPEFLTRIKFLLKPTPNTVHYILTHFKGFWNVVNNIPFLRNAIMSYVL
Mouse-2    CTRTGFYGENCTTPEFLTRLKLLLKPTPNTVHYILTHFKGVWNIVNNIPFLRSLTMKYVL
Mouse-1    CTRTGYSGPNCTIPEIWTWLRNSLRPSPSFTHFLLTHGYWLWEFVNAT-FIREVLMRLVL
Human-1    CTRTGYSGPNCTIPGLWTWLRNSLRPSPSFTHFLLTHGRWFWEFVNAT-FIREMLMLLVL
Sheep-1    CTRTGYSGPNCTIPEIWTWLRTTLRPSPSFIHFLLTHGRWLWDFVNAT-FIRDTLMRLVL
           60        70        80        90        100       110

Chick-2    TSRSHLIDSPPTYNSDYSYKSWEAYSNLSYYTRSLPPVGHDCPTPMGVKGKKELPDSKLI
Human-2    TSRSHLIDSPPTYNADYGYKSWEAFSNLSYYTRALPPVPDDCPTPLGVKGKKQLPDSNEI
Mouse-2    TSRSYLIDSPPTYNVHYGYKSWEAFSNLSYYTRALPPVADDCPTPMGVKGNKELPDSKEV
Mouse-1    TVRSNLIPSPPTYNSAHDYISWESFSNVSYYTRILPSVPKDCPTPMGTKGKKQLPDVQLL
Human-1    TVRSNLIPSPPTYNSAHDYISWESFSNVSYYTRILPSVPKDCPTPMGTKGKKQLPDAQLL
Sheep-1    TVRSNLIPSPPTYNIAHDYISWESFSNVSYYTRILPSVPRDCPTPMGTKGKKQLPDAEFL
            120       130       140       150       160       170

Chick-2    VEKFLLRRKFIPDPQGTNVMFTFFAQHFTHQFFKTDHKRGPGFTKAYGHGVDLNHIYGET
Human-2    VGKLLLRRKFIPDPQGSNMMFAFFAQHFTHQFFKTDHKRGPAFTNGLGHGVDLNHIYGET
Mouse-2    LEKVLLRREFIPDPQGSNMMFAFFAQHFTHQFFKTDHKRGPGFTRGLGHGVDLNHIYGET
Mouse-1    AQQLLLRREFIPAPQGTNILFAFFAQHFTHQFFKTSGKMGPGFTKALGHGVDLGHIYGDN
Human-1    ARRFLLRRKFIPDPQGTNLMFAFFAQHFTHQFFKTSGKMGPGFTKALGHGVDLGHIYGDN
Sheep-1    SRRELLRRKFIPDPQGTNLMFAFFAQHFTHQFFKTSGKMGPGFTKALGHGVDLGHIYGDN
            180       190       200       210       220       230

Chick-2    LERQLKLRLRKDGKLKYQMIDGEMYPPTVKDTQAEMIYPPHVPEHLQFSVGQEVFGLVPG
Human-2    LARQRKIRLFKDGKMKYQIIDGEMYPPTVKDTQAEMIYPPQVPEHLRFAVGQEVFGLVPG
Mouse-2    LDRQHKLRLFKDGKLKYQVIGGEVYPPTVKDTQVEMIYPPHIPENLQFAVGQEVFGLVPG
Mouse-1    LERQYHLRLFKDGKLKYQVLDGEVYPPSVEQASVLMRYPPGVPPERQMAVGQEVFGLLPG
Human-1    LERQYQLRLFKDGKLKYQVLDGEMYPPSVEEAPVLMHYPRGIPPQSQMAVGQEVFGLLPG
Sheep-1    LERQYQLRLFKDGKLKYQMLNGEVYPPSVEEAPVLMHYPRGIPPQSQMAVGQEVFGLLPG
            240       250       260       270       280       290

Chick-2    LMMYATIWLREHNRVCDVLKQEHPEWDDEQLFQTTRLILIGETIKIVIDDYVQHLSGYHF
Human-2    LMMYATIWLREHNRVCDVLKQEHPEWGDEQLFQTSRLILIGETIKIVIDDYVQHLSGYHF
Mouse-2    LMMYATIWLREHNRVCDILKQEHPEWGDEQLFQTSRLILIGETIKIVIDDYVQHLSGYHF
Mouse-1    LMLFSTIWLREHNRVCDLLKEEHPTWDDEQLFQTTRLILIGETIKIVIEEYVQHLSGYFL
Human-1    LMLYATLWLREHNRVCDLLKAEHPTWGDEQLFQTTRLILIGETIKIVIEEYVQQLSGYFL
Sheep-1    LMLYATIWLREHNRVCDLLKAEHPTWGDEQLFQTARLILIGETIKIVIEEYVQQLSGYFL
            300       310       320       330       340       350

Chick-2    KLKFDPELLFNQRFQYQNRIAAEFNTLYHWHPLLPDTFQIHNQEYTFQQFLYNNSIMLEH
Human-2    KLKFDPELLFNKQFQYQNRIAAEFNTLYHWHPLLPDTFQINDQKYNYQQFIYNNSILLEH
Mouse-2    KLKFDPELLFNQQFQYQNRIASEFNTLYHWHPLLPDTFNIEDQEYSFKQFLYNNSILLEH
Mouse-1    QLKFDPELLFRAQFQYRNRIAMEFNHLYHWHPLMPNSFQVGSQEYSYEQFLFNTSMLVDY
Human-1    QLKFDPELLFGVQFQYRNRIATEFNHLYHWHPLMPDSFKVGSQEYSYEQFLFNTSMLVDY
Sheep-1    QLKFDPELLFGAQFQYRNRIAMEFNQLYHWHPLMPDSFRVGPQDYSYEQFLFNTSMLVDY
            360       370       380       390       400       410

Chick-2    GLSHMVKSSKRQIAGRVAGGKNVPAAVQKVAKASIDQSRQMRYQSLNEYRKRFMLKPFKS
Human-2    GITQFVESFTRQIAGRVAGGRNVPPAVQKVSQASIDQSRQMKYQSFNEYRKRFMLKPYES
Mouse-2    GLTQFVESFTRQIAGRVAGGRNVPIAVQAVAKASIDQSREMKYQSLNEYRKRFSLKPYTS
Mouse-1    GVEALVDAFSRQRAGRIGGGRNFDYHVLHVAVDVIKESREMRLQPFNEYRKRFGLKPYTS
Human-1    GVEALVDAFSRQIAGRIGGGRNMDHHILHVAVDVIRESREMRLQPFNEYRKRFGMKPYTS
Sheep-1    GVEALVDAFSRQPAGRIGGGRNIDHHILHVAVDVIKESRVLRLQPFNEYRKRFGMKPYTS
            420       430       440       450       460       470

Chick-2    FEELTGEKEMAAELEELYGDIDAMELYPGLLVEKPRPGAIFGETMVEIGAPFSLKGLMGN
Human-2    FEELTGEKEMSAELEALYGDIDAVELYPALLVEKPRPDAIFGETMVEVGAPFSLKGLMGN
Mouse-2    FEELTGEKEMAAELKALYSDIDVMELYPALLVEKPRPDAIFGETMVELGAPFSLKGLMGN
Mouse-1    FQELTGEKEMAAELEELYGDIDALEFYPGLLLEKCQPNSIFGESMIEMGAPFSLKGLLGN
Human-1    FQELVGEKEMAAELEELYGDIDALEFYPGLLLEKCHPNSIFGESMIEIGAPFSLKGLLGN
Sheep-1    FQELTGEKEMAAELEELYGDIDALEFYPGLLLEKCHPNSIFGESMIEMGAPFSLKGLLGN
            480       490       500       510       520       530

Chick-2    TICSPEYWKPSTFGGKVGFEIINTASLQSLICNNVKGSPFTAFHVLNPEPTETATINVST
Human-2    VICSPAYWKPSTFGGEVGFQIINTASIQSLICNNVKGCPFTSFSVPDPELIKTVTINASS
Mouse-2    PICSPQYWKPSTFGGEVGFKIINTASIQSLICNNVKGCPFTSFNVQDPQPTKTATINASA
Mouse-1    PICSPEYWKPSTFGGDVGFNLVNTASLKKLVCLNTKTCPYVSFRVPDYPGDDGSVIV---
Human-1    PICSPEYWKPSTFGGEVGFNIVKTATLKKLVCLNTKTCPYVSFRVPDASQDDGPAVE---
Sheep-1    PICSPEYWKASTFGGEVGFNLVKTATLKKLVCLNTKTCPYVSFHVPDPRQEDRPGVE---
            540       550       560       570       580       590

Chick-2    SNFAMEDINPTLLLKEQSAEL
Human-2    SRSGLDDINPTVLLKERSTEL
Mouse-2    SHSRLDDINPTVLIKRRSTEL
Mouse-1    ---------------RRSTEL
Human-1    ---------------RPSTEL
Sheep-1    ---------------RPPTEL
                            600
```

Mechanism of the Cyclooxygenase Reaction

The formation of PGG_2 from arachidonate and two molecules of O_2 is depicted in Fig. 3 (39). PGH synthases are believed to bind arachidonate having a kink in the carbon chain due to rotation about the bond between C-9 and C-10 (39). The enzyme then abstracts the *pro-S* hydrogen atom from C-13 in the initial step in the cyclooxygenase reaction (39–44). Hydrogen atom abstraction is followed by insertion of an O_2 molecule from the solvent side at C-11. Serial cyclization of the 11-peroxyl radical produces a bicyclic endo-peroxide having *trans* aliphatic chains. Addition of a second O_2 to the carbon radical at C-15 also occurs from the solvent side yielding PGG_2.

Kinetics of Cyclooxygenase Catalysis

The cyclooxygenase activity of PGH synthase can be continuously monitored by measuring O_2 consumption using an O_2 electrode. Typically, one observes a rapid increase in the rate of O_2 uptake which decreases to zero within about 5 min (Fig. 4). This decrease in O_2 uptake is due to "suicide inactivation" of the enzyme (45–47). On average, each enzyme molecule catalyzes the synthesis of about 1300 moles of PGG_2 before the cyclooxygenase is inactivated (48). The rate of suicide inactivation is proportional to the concentration of enzyme-substrate complex and independent of product formation. This indicates that suicide inactivation results from the decay of an unstable enzyme-substrate intermediate to a catalytically incompetent enzyme. The chemical changes that underlie suicide have not been established. However, it is known that suicide inactivation is temporally associated with the formation of singlet protein tyrosyl radical signals (49–51). This process is discussed in further detail below. Although the suicide inactivation is of interest from a mechanistic standpoint, it is not clear that the suicide reaction is important in vivo. For example, with vascular endothelial cells, it takes repeated exposure to high levels of arachidonate to inactivate the enzyme (52). One would imagine that in most cells, the amount of enzyme present far exceeds the demands for product formation. A possible exception to this generalization might be platelets, where new PGH synthase cannot be synthesized.

Although the initial rate of the cyclooxygenase reaction is usually the maximal rate, there are various experimental maneuvers that expose a lag period prior to achieving the maximal rate (45,46,49,53–55) (Fig. 4).* Studies of the kinetic lag phase have established that an alkyl hydroperoxide is required for the cyclooxygenase reaction to occur. A hydroperoxide oxidizes the cyclooxygenase to a form that is able to abstract the 13-*pro-S* hydrogen from arachidonate. As described in more detail below, hydroperoxide activation of the cyclooxygenase involves oxidation of the heme group present at the peroxidase active site of PGH synthase.

Peroxidase Reaction

Both PGH synthase-1 and -2 display peroxidase activities that can catalyze the reduction of various hydroperoxides to their corresponding alcohols with concomitant oxidation of reducing cosubstrates. The peroxidase activity of PGH synthase-1 has a preference for secondary alkyl hydroperoxides such as the 15-hydroperoxyl group of PGG_2, but it displays some activity even toward H_2O_2 (59,60). Characterization of the reduction of various hydroperoxides, including the conversion of 10-hydroperoxy-8c,12t-octadecadienoic acid (10-HpODE) to 10-HODE by PGH synthase-1, has established that hydroperoxides are reduced simultaneously by two electrons (56,58). This type of peroxide reduction reaction is found with all known heme peroxidases (40).

*For example, addition of reduced glutathione (GSH) plus GSH peroxidase to the reaction mixture will slow or prevent initiation of the cyclooxygenase reaction (56,57); inhibition by GSH peroxidase can be overcome by the addition of N-ethylmaleimide. The lag phase induced by GSH peroxidase can be eliminated by adding low concentrations of fatty acid hydroperoxides (57,58).

Figure 2 Deduced amino acid sequences of PGH synthases-1 and -2. Boldface letters are shown for the signal peptides of PGH synthases-1 and -2, for the 18–amino acid insert of PGH synthase-2 near the C terminus, for histidine (H) residues important in cyclooxygenase and peroxidase activities and heme binding, for the tyrosine (Y) residue essential for cyclooxygenase catalysis, and for the serine (S), which is acetylated by aspirin. Numbering is for ovine PGH synthase-1. Sequences are shown for chicken PGH synthase-2 (27), human PGH synthase-2 (32), murine PGH synthase-2 (29), murine PGH synthase-1 (21), human PGH synthase-1 (22,23), and ovine PGH synthase-1 (24–26).

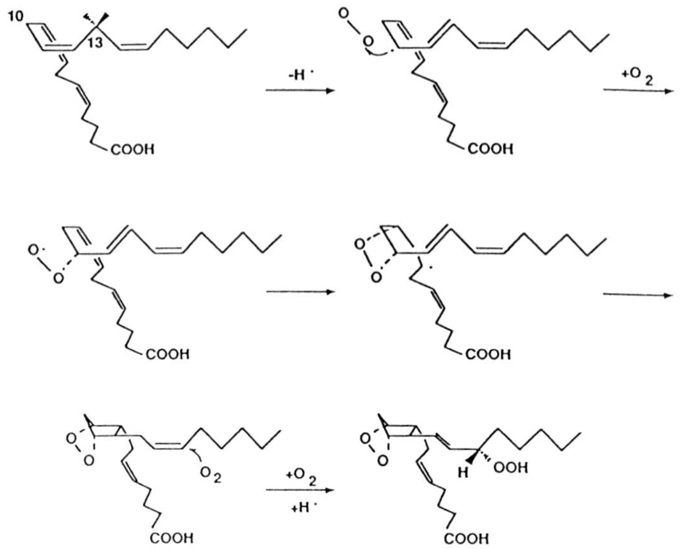

Figure 3 Mechanism for the oxygenation of arachidonic acid by PGH synthases. (From Ref. 83.)

PGH synthase contains a heme prosthetic group: Fe^{3+}- protoporphyrin IX (61). The heme group is required for peroxidase (and cyclooxygenase) activity (57,62–64). Addition of peroxides to ovine PGH synthase-1 in the absence of reducing agents causes formation of a spectral Intermediate I which is very similar to Compound I of horseradish peroxidase (61) and corresponds to a two-electron oxidized heme having an iron in the 4+ state and the porphyrin group oxidized to a radical cation (Fig. 5). Spectral Intermediate I isomerizes with time to spectral Intermediate II, which is analogous to Compound II of horseradish peroxidase and Compound ES of cytochrome *c* peroxidase (61). Compound II intermediates have iron in the 4+ state and a neutral porphyrin ring (40,41). In addition to these spectral changes, an EPR signal at $g = 2.005$ is formed at the same time as Intermediate II when ovine PGH synthase-1 is incubated with hydroperoxides (50,51,65–69). This EPR signal is due to a protein tyrosyl radical. The tyrosyl radical is formed by an intramolecular electron transfer from a tyrosine of PGH synthase to the porphyrin π cation radical of Intermediate I (65,66) (Fig. 5).

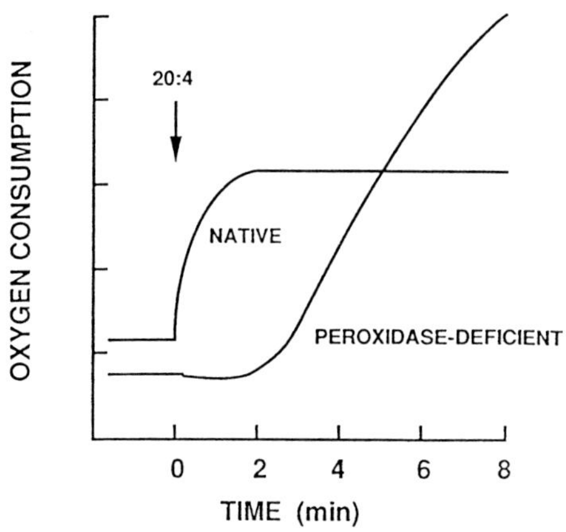

Figure 4 Comparison of O_2 consumption by cyclooxygenase activities of native PGH synthase-1 and peroxidase-deficient forms of PGH synthase-1. (From Ref. 83.)

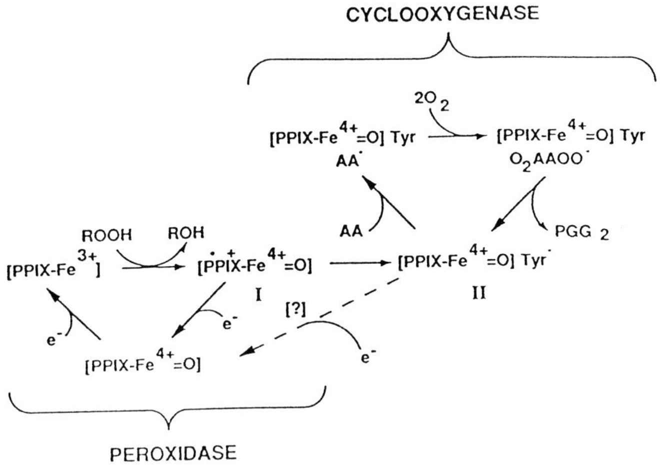

Figure 5 Model for peroxide-dependent activation of cyclooxygenase activity of ovine PGH synthase-1 via formation of an intermediate tyrosyl radical. Abbreviations: PPIX-Fe^{3+}, heme; AA, arachidonic acid. (From Ref. 83.)

In brief, the peroxidase activity of PGH synthase-1 has properties that closely resemble those of other heme peroxidases. PGH synthase-1 (a) catalyzes a two-electron hydroperoxide reduction, (b) undergoes a peroxide-dependent heme oxidation, and (c) has a very high catalytic efficiency (70).

Hydroperoxide-Dependent Activation of Cyclooxygenase Activity

The dependence of cyclooxygenase activity on hydroperoxide, the appearance of oxidized heme intermediates and a tyrosyl radical signal, and the removal of the 13-*pro-S* hydrogen atom from arachidonate as the initiating step in the cyclooxygenase reaction appear to be related. Ruf and coworkers developed the model depicted in Fig. 5 to explain these interrelationships (66). According to this model, a two-electron oxidation of the heme group at the peroxidase active site of PGH synthase by a hydroperoxide causes formation of a Compound I-like Intermediate I. Intermediate I abstracts a hydrogen atom from a neighboring tyrosine, yielding Intermediate II, which contains a Fe^{4+}, a neutral protoporphyrin IX, and a protein tyrosyl radical. The tyrosyl radical abstracts the 13-*pro-S* hydrogen from a molecule of arachidonate positioned in the cyclooxygenase active site, thereby initiating cyclooxygenase catalysis.

The tyrosine residue responsible for the EPR signal has not been established with certainty. However, Tyr385 is at the cyclooxygenase active site of PGH synthase-1 (71) (see Fig. 7 below) and replacement of Tyr385 with a phenylalanine yields a protein with an altered EPR spectrum (69).

Although the Ruf model integrates the cyclooxygenase and peroxidase functions of PGH synthases, the proposed role of a tyrosyl radical in cyclooxygenase catalysis still remains controversial. There are several different tyrosyl radical signals associated with the interaction of hydroperoxides with PGH synthase-1 (50,51,65–69). Indeed, one of these tyrosyl radical signals remains even after the enzyme has undergone suicide inactivation (50,68). Thus, an alternative (or additional) explanation for the tyrosyl radical signal(s) is that it is a marker for enzyme undergoing suicide inactivation. Tyrosyl radical signals have been observed in other systems, including one in which met-myoglobin interacts with hydrogen peroxide; in this instance, peroxide-dependent oxidation of the heme group of met-myoglobin leads to generation of tyrosyl radicals which, in turn, react with the heme (72). It is conceivable that suicide inactivation of PGH synthase involves a similar reaction.

General Chemical Properties of PGH Synthases

Including the signal peptides, PGH synthases-1 and -2 have predicted subunit molecular weights of approximately 65,500. Nevertheless, native PGH synthase-1 has an M_r = 72,000 on SDS-PAGE

(19,20) and, typically, PGH synthase-2 appears as a doublet (or triplet) with subunit molecular weights of 72 and 74 kDa (73,74). The differences between the calculated and experimentally determined molecular weights are due to the presence of asparagine-linked oligosaccharides. There are three high-mannose oligosaccharides, one $Man_7(NAcGln)_2$ and two $Man_9(NAcGln)_2$ groups (75), which are linked to ovine PGH synthase-1 at Asn68, Asn144, and Asn 410 (73); there is one additional site of N-glycosylation in PGH synthase-2 which, in the case of the murine enzyme, is at Asn580 (73). Glycosylation at Asn410 is required for PGH synthase-1 to fold into its active conformation.

Although the subunit molecular weight of PGH synthase-1 is 72,000, the enzyme is solubilized from membranes in the form of a dimer (76,77). The enzyme is also a dimer in its crystalline state (M. Garavito; personal communication). Residues 25 to 70 of PGH synthases are homologous to epidermal growth factor (EGF) (78). It appears that this region of the protein is responsible for dimer formation (M. Garavito; personal communication).

Subcellular Location of PGH Synthases

PGH synthases-1 and -2 have both been localized to the endoplasmic reticulum and the nuclear membrane using immunocytochemistry (79–81). The significance of the nuclear location is not clear. The outer membrane of the nuclear envelope is continuous with the endoplasmic reticulum (ER). However, it is possible that nuclear synthesis of prostanoids is independent of ER synthesis.

PGH synthase-1 can be solubilized only by treatment of membranes with detergents (19,20), suggesting that the enzyme is an integral membrane protein. However, the nature of the interaction of the enzyme with membranes is incompletely resolved. Asn-linked oligosaccharides are found only on the lumen side of the ER, and the finding that PGH synthases are N-glycosylated indicates that at least a portion of the protein chain is in the ER (73). Moreover, recent studies using antipeptide antibodies indicate that both the N and C termini as well as a region near the middle of the protein sequence are in the lumen of the ER (J. C. Otto and W. L. Smith; unpublished observations). These findings, along with the globular structure apparent from crystallographic studies, suggest that PGH synthase-1 is a lumenal ER protein. Ovine PGH synthase-1 may be anchored to the lumenal side of the ER via a peptide segment involving residues 70 to 140 (M. Garavito; personal communication). Figure 6 depicts a model for the orientation of PGH synthase-1 in the lumen of the ER.

Heme Binding to PGH Synthase

As noted earlier, heme is required for both the cyclooxygenase and peroxidase activities of PGH synthase-1. The consensus is that there is one heme per subunit (40,41,57,61–64). Various spectral studies have indicated that the heme group is liganded by imidazole groups at the fifth and sixth

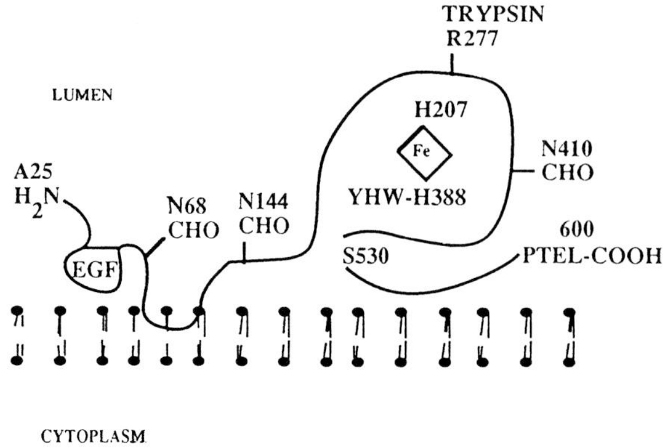

Figure 6 Orientation of ovine PGH synthase-1 in the endoplasmic reticulum. The N terminus of the mature enzyme is Ala25. The C terminus is Leu600. Abbreviation: CHO, N-glycosylation sites.

coordination positions of the iron (61,82). A combination of x-ray crystallographic studies and site-directed mutagenesis have indicated that His388 is the proximal heme ligand and His207 is the distal heme ligand (55,83); M. Garavito; personal communication).

Structure of PGH Synthase Active Sites

Figure 7 (83) depicts a dual cyclooxygenase/peroxidase active site model for ovine PGH synthase-1. The two active sites of PGH synthase-2 would be expected to be analogous. An alkyl hydroperoxide (ROOH) is shown interacting with the heme group at the peroxidase active site. Bound peroxide would undergo a two-electron reduction to its corresponding alcohol with concomitant oxidation of the heme group. The heme group would have two potential fates: (a) two sequential one-electron reductions regenerating ground state heme—the typical peroxidase reaction—or (b) abstraction of a hydrogen atom from a neighboring tyrosine—Tyr385—to produce an activated cyclooxygenase having a tyrosyl radical. Once a tyrosyl radical was formed, it would be capable of abstracting the 13-*pro-S* hydrogen from arachidonate positioned at the cyclooxygenase active site. Oxygen insertion and cyclization would follow. Also shown in the model is the residue Ser530 (Fig. 7). The hydroxyl group of the side chain of Ser530 is acetylated when PGH synthase-1 is incubated with aspirin (21,84).

Interaction of PGH Synthase Isozymes with Aspirin and Other Nonsteroidal Anti-Inflammatory Drugs

Although other nonsteroidal anti-inflammatory drugs (NSAIDs) cause apparent "irreversible" inactivation of the cyclooxygenase (85), aspirin is the only NSAID that causes covalent modification of PGH synthase (e.g., 86). In the case of ovine PGH synthase-1, replacement of Ser530 with an alanine by site-directed mutagenesis yields a functional S530A PGH synthase-1 mutant that is not acetylated by aspirin (21,38). This result establishes that Ser530 is not required for either substrate binding or catalysis. Replacements of Ser530 with amino acids which are roughly isosteric with an acetylated Ser530 (e.g., Asn or Leu) yields mutant enzyme forms which, like the aspirin-acetylated native enzyme, retain peroxidase activity but lack cyclooxygenase activity (21,38). These observations have led to the concept that acetylation of PGH synthase-1 by aspirin places a bulky group at Ser530 which interferes with the binding of arachidonate to the cyclooxygenase active site of the enzyme (without interfering with the binding of alkyl peroxides to the peroxidase active site) (Fig. 7).

Aspirin also causes the acetylation of PGH synthase-2. Acetylation occurs on Ser516 of human

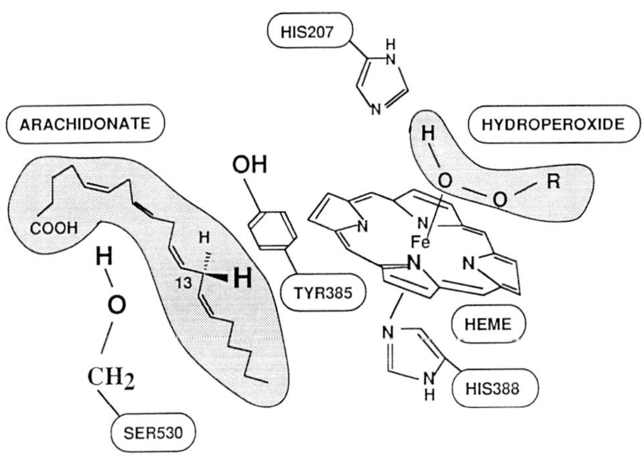

Figure 7 Model showing proposed interrelationships of the cyclooxygenase and peroxidase active sites of ovine PGH synthase-1. (From Ref. 83.)

PGH synthase-2, a residue which is homologous to Ser530 of ovine PGH synthase-1 (M. Lecomte and W. L. Smith; unpublished results). Importantly, the effect of aspirin acetylation of PGH synthase-2 is different from that of PGH synthase-1. Acetylated PGH synthase-2 is still able to catalyze the oxygenation of arachidonate; however, the product is 15*R*-HETE (15*R*-hydroxy-5c, 8c, 11c, 13t-eicosatetraenoic acid) instead of PGH_2 (31,87). It will be of interest to determine if 15*R*-HETE formation is related to the anti-inflammatory action of aspirin.

PGH synthase-1 is potently inhibited by most NSAIDs which, in turn, are competitive inhibitors of the binding of arachidonate to the cyclooxygenase active site of the enzyme (85). Although PGH synthase-1 has been assumed to be the site of action of NSAIDs, the discovery of PGH synthase-2 (and its potential association with inflammation noted below) has suggested that it is PGH synthase-2, and not PGH synthase-1, which is the principal therapeutic target of NSAIDs acting as anti-inflammatory agents. Recent studies with murine PGH synthases-1 and -2 expressed in vitro have indicated (a) that NSAIDs do inhibit PGH synthase-2 and (b) that there are significant differences among known NSAIDs to inhibit the cyclooxygenase activities of the two isozymes (31) (Table 1). Sulindac sulfide, indomethacin, and proxicam are all significantly better inhibitors of PGH synthase-1 than PGH synthase-2. Ibuprofen, flurbiprofen, and meclofenamate inhibit murine PGH synthases-1 and -2 with comparable potencies. 6-Methoxy-2-napthylacetic acid (6-MNA), the active metabolite of nabumetone (Relafen), has slight preference for inhibiting PGH synthase-2. Similar results have been observed with human PGH synthases-1 and -2 (O. Laneuville, D. L. DeWitt, and W. L. Smith; unpublished results). These studies suggest that agents can be identified or designed that will be isozyme-specific. Development of isozyme-specific inhibitors of PGH synthases could lead to a new generation of NSAIDs lacking the ulcerogenic activity of the current drugs in this group.

EXPRESSION OF PGH SYNTHASES

Tissue Distribution of PGH Synthase Isozymes

PGH synthase-1 is present in many cell lines and in extracts of virtually all mammalian tissues (28,88) (Table 2). In contrast, Northern "zoo" blots have indicated that PGH synthase-2 mRNA is detectable in prostate, brain, testis, and lung but is in very low abundance or undetectable in kidney

Table 1 Inhibition of murine PGH synthase isozymes by Non-Steroidal Anti-Inflammatory Drugs[a]

Specificity	Inhibitor	ID_{50} for PGHS-1 (μM)	ID_{50} for PGHS-2 (μM)	ID_{50} (PGHS-2)[b] / ID_{50} (PGHS-1)
Equipotent	Flurbiprofen	0.46– 0.50	2.1– 3.4	5.7
	(S)-Ibuprofen	8.9 – 14	7.2– 8.2	0.672
	Meclofenamic acid	2.0 – 2.5	13 – 18	6.92
	Docosahexaenoic acid	11	13 – 17	1.36
$PGHS_{mu}$-1	Piroxicam	9.0 – 24	70 –240	9.54
	Indomethacin	4.9 – 8.1	130 –160	22.3
	Sulindac sulfide[c]	0.3 – 0.5	11 – 14	30.9
$PGHS_{mu}$-2	6-MNA[d]	200 –280	15 – 55	0.14

[a]Values presented represent the range of values obtained from individual experiments and not the statistical variance of a single measurement.
[b]Ratio of average ID_{50} values.
[c]The active metabolite of sulindac.
[d]6-MNA; 6-methoxy-2-naphthyl acetic acid, the active metabolite of nabumetone (Relafen).
Source: Ref. 31.

Table 2 Comparison of PGH Synthase-1 and PGH Synthase-2

	PGHS-1	PGHS-2
Homology	Approximately 60% identical, 75% similar at the amino acid–sequence level. Protein regions believed to be important for enzyme function that are conserved include EGF homology domain (78), heme ligand sites (55), aspirin acetylation "active" site (38), and glycosylation sites (73). Enzymatic activities (*V*max) and affinity for arachidonate (*K*m) are essentially identical (31).	
Regulation	Constitutive (90,102).	Inducible (28,29,90–97)
Range of expression	Can increase 2- to 4-fold (90).	Can increase 10- to 80-fold (28,29,90–97)
Tissue expression	Platelets (23), endothelial cells (94,95), stomach,[a] kidney (12,13), smooth muscles, most tissues (28).	Prostate (28), brain (28), activated monocytes (91–93), or fibroblasts (28,29,90,98), synoviacytes during inflammation (96), follicles preceding ovulation (33,97). Can be expressed in most tissues but requires stimulation by growth factors, cytokines, phorbol esters, or hormones.
Effect of glucocorticoids	Little or none (90,99)	Inhibits expression (90,97–100).
Proposed role of enzyme	"Housekeeping gene," to produce prostaglandins involved in the autocrine/paracrine responses of cells to circulating hormones, and which help regulate normal renal and stomach function and vascular homeostasis.	1. "Inflammatory response gene," member of family of genes induced during inflammation (101), may produce prostaglandins involved in inflammation. 2. "Immediate early gene" member of gene family thought to control mitogenesis; may produce prostaglandins involved in cell growth (28,90). 3. Produce prostaglandins essential for signal transduction regulating ovulation (33,97).

[a]Staining of normal rabbit stomach fundus with antipeptide antibodies to PGH synthases-1 and -2 revealed positive staining for PGH synthase-1 but not PGH synthase-2.

and most other major organs (28); with the exception of Rat-1 cells and mitogen-stimulated mouse 3T3 fibroblasts, common cell lines lack appreciable PGH synthase-2 mRNA (29).

Differential Expression of PGH Synthase-1 and -2 Genes

In Swiss mouse 3T3 cells, mRNA levels of both PGH synthase genes are increased by serum and growth factors, TPA, and cAMP (28,29,89,90) (Table 2). However, PGH synthase-2 mRNA levels are upregulated much more dramatically than PGH synthase-1 mRNA levels; furthermore, the temporal order of expression of the two genes is different. In serum-stimulated quiescent 3T3 cells, PGH synthase-2 mRNA increases dramatically from undetectable levels within as little as 30 min, peaking at from 1 to 3 hr after stimulation and then rapidly declining (90). Serum-induced changes in the levels of PGH synthase-1 mRNA in 3T3 cells involve two- to threefold increases in mRNA levels which occur only 3 to 4 hr poststimulation but which remain elevated 6 to 8 hr after stimulation (29,90).

PGH synthase-2 is now known to be induced in a number of different cell types. LPS can stimulate PGH synthase-2 expression in monocytes and macrophages (91–93), and tumor necrosis factor, phorbol esters, LPS, and IL-1 can induce PGH synthase-2 in vascular endothelial cells (94,95). PGH synthase-2 is also increased in synoviacytes during inflammation (96), and there is a dramatic transient increase in PGH synthase-2 in rat follicles immediately preceding ovulation (33,97); this latter event can be viewed as a local inflammatory response. Typically PGH synthase-2 expression increases by as much as 10- to 80-fold. While only a limited number of tissues and cell types have been examined, it seems likely that PGH synthase-2 can be expressed in almost any cell or tissue with the appropriate stimuli. An important aspect of the regulated induction of PGH synthase-2 is that it can be completely inhibited by anti-inflammatory glucocorticoids such as dexamethasone (90,98–100). Thus, PGH synthase-2 appears to belong to a family of similarly regulated, glucocorticoid-sensitive inflammatory-response genes (101).

Serum treatment of rat renal mesangial cells has been shown to stimulate PGH synthase-1 gene expression, apparently via a protein kinase C–dependent mechanism (102); it is not known whether PGH synthase-2 mRNA levels are also affected in mesangial cells.

Structure of Genes for PGH Synthases-1 and -2

The intron/exon structures of the murine (103) and human (22) PGH synthase-1 genes and the murine PGH synthase-2 gene (30) are illustrated in Fig. 8. The PGH synthase-1 gene is 22 kb and consists of 11 exons. The intron/exon structure of the human and murine PGH synthase-1 genes are vitrually identical (22,103). The murine PGH synthase-2 gene is much smaller (about 8 kb) but, interestingly, the locations of the intron/exon boundaries are the same except for the first exon (30). The introns present in the gene for murine PGH synthase-2 are much smaller than those in PGH synthase-1 (Fig. 8).

The nucleotide sequences of the 5′-end of the genes for PGH synthases-1 and -2 have been determined (30,103); the transcriptional start sites for both genes have also been defined. There are numerous consensus response elements present in the 5′-flanking regions of each gene. For example, there are three AP-1–like elements (for the binding of *fos/jun* dimers) in the 5′-flanking region of the PGH synthase-1 gene; there is also a putative negative glucocorticoid response element (nGRE) neighboring an AP-1 site. There is no TATA box. The functional relevance of these putative response elements has yet to be tested. A region containing approximately 1 kb upstream of the transcriptional start site of murine PGH synthase-2 has been sequenced and shown to contain AP-1 and SP-1 sites and a putative TATA box. When this upstream regulatory region of the PGH synthase-2 gene is coupled to a luciferase reporter gene and transfected into NIH 3T3 cells, luciferase activity is induced in response to both serum and phorbol ester treatments (29). Curiously, although it has been established that serum will induce the expression of PGH synthase-2, there are no obvious serum response elements (SREs) in the 5′-end of the gene. A region containing approximately 350 bp upstream of the transcriptional start site of murein PGH synthase-2 has been shown to contain sequences involved in responses to both serum and phorbol ester (30,99). The sequence involved in the cAMP-dependent induction of the PGH synthase-2 gene is located between –192 and –54; the subregion –142/–120 contains a *cis*-acting C/EPBβ promoter element and mutations within this element decrease forskolin inducibility (97).

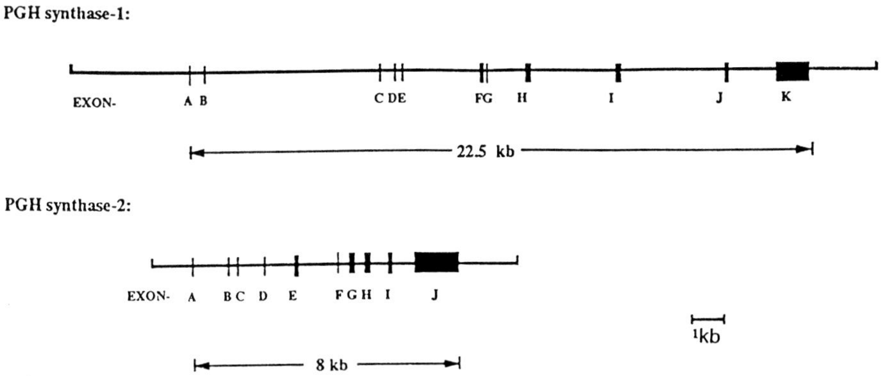

Figure 8 Structures of the two genes coding for murine PGH synthases-1 and -2. Exons are denoted with letters. (PGH synthase-1 gene structure is from Ref. 103 and PGH synthase-2 gene structure Ref. 30. Adapted from Ref. 1.)

Why Are There Two PGH Synthase Isozymes?

As discussed above, PGH synthase-1 is a constitutive enzyme present in most tissues, albeit at different levels in different cell types. PGH synthase-1 provides for prostaglandins that are required rapidly and on an ongoing basis—most commonly to modulate responses to changes in the levels of circulating hormones. For example, PGE_2 is formed in the collecting tubule via PGH synthase-1 when AVP concentrations in blood increase, and the newly formed PGE_2 modulates tubular responses to AVP (11). In contrast to PGH synthase-1, PGH synthase-2 is undetectable in most cells and tissues. PGH synthase-2 appears in cells beginning about 2 hr following mitogenic or inflammatory challenge and then disappears within 2 to 3 hr. PGH synthase-2 is an immediate early gene, and prostaglandins formed via PGH synthase-2 presumably function in replication (e.g., 104).

Many of the cells in which PGH synthase-2 is induced already contain appreciable levels of PGH synthase-1. Thus, the role of PGH synthase-2 could be to augment constitutive prostaglandin production. Alternatively, a PGH synthase-2 system could operate independent of PGH synthase-1 by producing different prostaglandin products or prostaglandins targeted to different locations than those generated through PGH synthase-1. Several experimental observations argue that PGH synthase-2 does not simply act in concert with PGH synthase-1 to augment total cellular prostaglandin synthesis. Most notably, in LPS-stimulated macrophages (91) and in IL-1-, serum-, or PDGF-stimulated fibroblasts (90,105), total cellular PGH synthase activity increases only about twofold despite dramatic increases in PGH synthase-2.

There is also an indirect argument for the existence of separate prostaglandin-forming systems involving PGH synthases-1 and -2: the apparent existence of multiple arachidonate release mechanisms, each of which appears to be temporally correlated with the expression of PGH synthase-1 and PGH synthase-2. Domin and Rozengurt (106) have documented a biphasic release of arachidonate in PDGF-stimulated 3T3 cells. The first phase occurs rapidly, is coincident with an increase in $cPLA_2$ activity, and is cycloheximide-insensitive. A second phase of arachidonate mobilization begins after 20 min, is involved in most of the total arachidonate release, is dependent on de novo protein synthesis, but is not associated with the activation of $cPLA_2$. The mechanism for the second phase of arachidonate release is not resolved, but Habenicht et al. (107) have suggested that it requires the uptake of extracellular LDL. In any event, it appears that there are both constitutive and inducible mechanisms for arachidonate release, just as there are constitutive and inducible PGH synthases.

ACKNOWLEDGMENTS

Work in the authors' laboratories has been supported by U.S.P.H.S. NIH Grants DK22042, DK42509, and GM40713 and Grants-in-Aid from the American Heart Association of Michigan.

REFERENCES

1. Smith WL. Prostanoid biosynthesis and mechanisms of action. Am J Physiol 1992; 263:F181–F191.
2. Smith WL, Marnett LJ, DeWitt DL. Prostaglandin and thromboxane biosynthesis. Pharmacol Ther 1991; 49:153–179.
3. Smith WL. The eicosanoids and their biochemical mechanisms of action. Biochem J 1989; 259:315–324.
4. Coleman RA, Kennedy I, Humphrey PPA, et al. Prostanoids and their receptors. In: Hansch C, Sammes PG, Taylor JB, eds. Comprehensive Medicinal Chemistry. Oxford: Pergamon Press, 1990:643–714.
5. Sonnenburg WK, Zhu J, Smith WL. A prostaglandin E receptor coupled to a pertussis toxin sensitive guanine nucleotide regulatory protein in rabbit cortical collecting tubule cells. J Biol Chem 1990; 265:8479–8483.
6. Hirata M, Hayashi Y, Ushikubi F, et al. Cloning and expression of cDNA for a human thromboxane A_2 receptor. Nature 1991; 389:617–620.
7. Sugimoto Y, Namba T, Honda A, et al. Cloning and expression of a cDNA for mouse prostaglandin E receptor EP3 subtype. J Biol Chem 1992; 267:6463–6466.
8. Namba T, Sugimoto Y, Negishi M, et al. Alternative splicing of C-terminal tail of prostaglandin E receptor subtype EP3 determines G-protein specificity. Nature 1993; 365:166–170.
9. Kirschenbaum MA, Lowe AG, Trizna W, Fine LG. Regulation of vasopressin action by prostaglandins. J Clin Invest 1982; 70:1193–1204.
10. Hebert RL, Jacobson HR, Breyer MD. PGE_2 inhibits AVP-induced water flow in cortical collecting ducts by protein kinase C activation. Am J Physiol 1990; 259:F318–F325.
11. Smith WL, Sonnenburg WK, Allen ML, et al. The biosynthesis and actions of prostaglandin in the renal collecting tubule and thick ascending limb. In: Dunn MJ, Patrono C, Cinotti GA, eds. Renal Eicosanoids. New York: Plenum Press, 1989:131–148.
12. Smith WL, Bell TG. Immunohistochemical localization of the prostaglandin-forming cyclooxygenase in renal cortex. Am J Physiol 1978; 235:F451–F460.
13. Smith WL, Bell TG, Needleman P. Increased renal tubular synthesis of prostaglandins in the rabbit kidney in response to urethral obstruction. Prostaglandins 1979; 18:269–276.
14. Mene P, Simonson MS, Dunn MJ. Prostaglandins, thromboxane and leukotrienes in the control of mesangial function. In: Dunn MJ, Patrono C, Cinotti GA, eds. Renal Eicosanoids. New York: Plenum Press, 1989:167–197.
15. Schlondorff D. Interactions of platelet activating factor and prostaglandins in the glomerulus and in mesangial cells. In: Dunn MJ, Patrono C, Cinotti GA, eds. Renal Eicosanoids. New York: Plenum Press, 1989:199–220.
16. Nakao A, Allen ML, Sonnenburg WK, Smith WL. Regulation of cAMP metabolism by prostaglandin E_2 in the cortical and medullary thick ascending limb of Henle's loop. Am J Physiol 1989; 256:C652–C657.
17. Morrison AR, Moritz H, Needleman P. Mechanism of enhanced renal prostaglandin biosynthesis in ureter obstruction. Role of de novo protein synthesis. J Biol Chem 1978; 253:8210–8212.
18. Nishikawa K, Morrison A, Needleman P. Exaggerated prostaglandin biosynthesis and its influence on renal resistance in the isolated hydronephrotic rabbit kidney. J Clin Invest 1977; 59:1143–1150.
19. Hemler ME, Lands WEM, Smith WL. Purification of the cyclooxygenase that forms prostaglandins: Demonstration of two forms of iron in the holoenzyme. J Biol Chem 1976; 251:5575–5579.
20. Miyamoto T, Ogino N, Yamamoto S, Hayaishi O. Purification of prostaglandin endoperoxide synthetase from ovine vesicular gland microsomes. J Biol Chem 1976; 251:2629–2636.
21. DeWitt DL, El-Harith EA, Kraemer SA, et al. The aspirin and heme-binding sites of ovine and murine prostaglandin endoperoxide synthases. J Biol Chem 1990; 265:5192–5198.
22. Yokoyama C, Tanabe T. Cloning of human gene encoding prostaglandin endoperoxide synthase and primary structure of the enzyme. Biochem Biophys Res Commun 1989; 165:888–894.
23. Funk CD, Funk LB, Kennedy ME, et al. Human platelet/erythroleukemia cell prostaglandin G/H synthase: cDNA cloning, expression, and gene chromosomal assignment. FASEB J 1991; 5:2304–2312.
24. DeWitt DL, Smith WL. Primary structure of prostaglandin G/H synthase from sheep vesicular gland determined from the complementary DNA sequence. Proc Natl Acad Sci USA 1988; 85:1412–1416.
25. Merlie JP, Fagan D, Mudd J, Needleman P. Isolation and characterization of the complementary DNA for sheep seminal vesicle prostaglandin endoperoxide synthase (cyclooxygenase). J Biol Chem 1988; 3550–3553.
26. Yokoyama C, Takai T, Tanabe T. Primary structure of sheep prostaglandin endoperoxide synthase deduced from cDNA sequence. FEBS Lett 1988; 231:347–351.
27. Xie W, Chipman JG, Robertson DL, et al. Expression of a mitogen-responsive gene encoding prostaglandin synthase is regulated by mRNA splicing. Proc Natl Acad Sci USA 1991; 88:2692–2696.
28. Simmons DL, Xie W, Chipman JG, Evett GE. Multiple cyclooxygenases: Cloning of a mitogen-inducible

form. In: Bailey JM, ed. Prostaglandins, Leukotrienes, Lipoxins, and PAF. New York: Plenum Press, 1991:67–78.
29. Kujubu DA, Fletcher BS, Varnum BC, et al. TIS10, a phorbol ester tumor promoter-inducible mRNA from Swiss 3T3 cells, encodes a novel prostaglandin synthase/cyclooxygenase homologue. J Biol Chem 1991; 266:12866–12872.
30. Fletcher BS, Kujubu DA, Perrin DM, Herschman HR. Structure of the mitogen-inducible TIS10 gene and demonstration that the TIS10-encoded protein is a functional prostaglandin G/H synthase. J Biol Chem 1992; 267:4338–4344.
31. Meade EA, DeWitt DL, Smith WL. Differential inhibition of prostaglandin endoperoxide synthase (cyclooxygenase) isozymes by aspirin and other nonsteroidal anti-inflammatory drugs. J Biol Chem 1993; 268:6610–6614.
32. Hla T, Maciag T. Cyclooxygenase gene expression is down-regulated by heparin-binding (acidic fibroblast) growth factor-1 in human endothelial cells. J Biol Chem 1991; 266:24059–24063.
33. Sirois J, Richards JS. Purification and characterization of a novel, distinct isoform of prostaglandin endoperoxide synthase induced by human chorionic gonadotropin in granulosa cells of rat preovulatory follicles. J Biol Chem 1992; 267:6382–6388.
34. Noiva R, Lennarz WJ. Protein disulfide isomerase: A multifunctional protein resident in the lumen of the endoplasmic reticulum. J Biol Chem 1992; 267:3553–3556.
35. Van der Ouderaa FJ, Buytenhek M, Nugteren DH, van Dorp DA. Acetylation of prostaglandin endoperoxide synthetase with acetylsalicylic acid. Eur J Biochem 1980; 109:1–8.
36. Mizuno K, Yamamoto S, Lands WEM. Effects of non-steroidal anti-inflammatory drugs on fatty acid cyclooxygenase and prostaglandin hydroperoxidase activities. Prostaglandins 1982; 23:743–757.
37. Marshall PJ, Kulmacz RJ. Prostaglandin H synthase: Distinct binding sites for cyclooxygenase and peroxidase substrates. Arch Biochem Biophys 1988; 266:162–170.
38. Shimokawa T, Smith WL. Prostaglandin endoperoxide synthase: The aspirin acetylation region. J Biol Chem 1992; 267:12387–12392.
39. Hamberg M, Samuelsson B. On the mechanism of the biosynthesis of prostaglandins E_1 and $F_{1\alpha}$. J Biol Chem 1967; 242:5336–5343.
40. Marnett LJ, Maddipati KR. Prostaglandin H synthase. In: Everse J, Everse K, Grisham M, eds. Peroxidases: Chemistry and Biology. Boca Raton, FL: CRC Press, 1991:293–334.
41. Smith WL, Marnett LJ. Prostaglandin endoperoxide synthase: Structure and catalysis. Biochem Biophys Acta 1991; 1083:1–17.
42. Mason RP, Kalyanaraman B, Tainer BE, Eling TE. A carbon-centered free radical intermediate in the prostaglandin synthetase oxidation of arachidonic acid. J Biol Chem 1980; 255:5019–5022.
43. Schreiber J, Eling TE, Mason RP. The oxidation of arachidonic acid by the cyclooxygenase activity of purified prostaglandin H synthase: Spin trapping of a carbon-centered free radical intermediate. Arch Biochem Biophys 1986; 249:126–135.
44. Kwok P-Y, Muellner FW, Fried J. Enzymatic conversion of 10,10-difluoro-arachidonic acid with PGH synthase and soybean lipoxidase. J Am Chem Soc 1987; 109:3692–3698.
45. Smith WL, Lands WEM. Oxygenation of polyunsaturated fatty acids during prostaglandin biosynthesis by sheep vesicular gland. Biochemistry 1972; 11:3276–3282.
46. Hemler ME, Cook HW, Lands WEM. Prostaglandin biosynthesis can be triggered by lipid peroxides. Arch Biochem Biophys 1979; 193:340–345.
47. Kulmacz RJ. Prostaglandin G_2 levels during reaction of prostaglandin H synthase with arachidonic acid. Prostaglandins 1987; 34:225–240.
48. Marshall PJ, Kulmacz RJ, Lands WEM. Constraints on prostaglandin biosynthesis in tissues. J Biol Chem 1987; 262:3510–3517.
49. Smith WL, Eling TE, Kulmacz RJ, et al. Tyrosyl radicals and their role in hydroperoxide-dependent activation and inactivation of prostaglandin endoperoxide synthase. Biochemistry 1992; 31:3–7.
50. Lassmann G, Odenwaller R, Curtis JF, et al. Electron spin resonance investigation of tyrosyl radicals to prostaglandin H synthase. J Biol Chem 1991; 266:20045–20055.
51. Tsai A-L, Palmer G, Kulmacz RJ. Prostaglandin H synthase. Kinetics of tyrosyl radical formation and of cyclooxygenase catalysis. J Biol Chem 1992; 267:17753–17759.
52. Kent RS, Diedrich SL, Whorton AR. Regulation of vascular prostaglandin synthesis by metabolites of arachidonic acid in perfused rabbit aorta. J Clin Invest 1983; 72:455–465.
53. Hemler ME, Lands WEM. Evidence for a peroxide-initiated free radical mechanism of prostaglandin biosynthesis. J Biol Chem 1980; 255:6253–6261.
54. Ogino N, Ohki S, Yamamoto S, Hayaishi O. Prostaglandin endoperoxide synthetase from bovine vesicular gland microsomes. J Biol Chem 1978; 253:5061–5065.
55. Shimokawa T, Smith WL. Essential histidines of prostaglandin endoperoxide synthase: His-309 is involved in heme binding. J Biol Chem 1991; 266:6168–6173.

56. Marnett LJ, Chen Y-NP, Maddipati KR, et al. Functional differentiation of cyclooxygenase and peroxidase activities of prostaglandin synthase by trypsin treatment: Possible location of a prosthetic heme binding site. J Biol Chem 1988; 263:16532–16535.
57. van der Ouderaa FJ, Buytenhek M, et al. On the haemoprotein character of prostaglandin endoperoxide synthetase. Biochim Biophys Acta 1979; 572:29–42.
58. Markey CM, Alward A, Weller PE, Marnett LJ. Quantitative studies of hydroperoxide reduction by prostaglandin H synthase. J Biol Chem 1987; 262:6266–6277.
59. Ohki S, Ogino N, Yamamoto S, Hayaishi O. Prostaglandin hydroperoxidase, an integral part of prostaglandin endoperoxide synthetase from bovine vesicular gland microsomes. J Biol Chem 1979; 254:829–836.
60. Kulmacz RJ, Lands WEM. Requirements for hydroperoxide by the cyclooxygenase and peroxidase activities of prostaglandin H synthase. Prostaglandins 1983; 25:531–540.
61. Lambeir AM, Markey CM, Dunford HB, Marnett LJ. Spectral properties of the higher oxidations states of prostaglandin H synthase. J Biol Chem 1985; 260:14894–14896.
62. Roth GJ, Machuga ET, Strittmatter P. The heme-binding properties of prostaglandin synthetase from sheep vesicular gland. J Biol Chem 1981; 256:10018–10022.
63. Ruf HH, Schuhn D, Nastainczyk W. EPR titration of ovine prostaglandin H synthase with hemin. FEBS Lett 1984; 165:293–295.
64. Kulmacz RJ, Lands WEM. Prostaglandin H synthase: Stoichiometry of heme cofactor. J Biol Chem 1984; 259:6358–6363.
65. Karthein R, Dietz R, Nastainczyk W, Ruf HH. Higher oxidation states of prostaglandin H synthase: EPR study of a transient tyrosyl radical in the enzyme during the peroxidase reaction. Eur J Biochem 1988; 171:313–320.
66. Dietz R, Nastainczyk W, Ruf HH. Higher oxidation states of prostaglandin H synthase: Rapid electronic spectroscopy detected two spectral intermediates during the peroxidase reaction with prostaglandin G_2. Eur J Biochem 1988; 171:321–328.
67. Kulmacz RJ, Ren Y, Tsai A-L, Palmer G. Prostaglandin H synthase: Spectroscopic studies of the interaction with hydroperoxides and with indomethacin. Biochemistry 1990; 29:8760–8771.
68. DeGray JA, Lassmann G, Curtis JF, et al. Spectral analysis of the protein-derived tyrosyl radicals from prostaglandin H synthase. J Biol Chem 1992; 267:23583–23588.
69. Tsai A-L, Hsi LC, Kulmacz RJ, Smith WL. Characterization of the tyrosyl radicals in ovine prostaglandin H synthase-1 by isotope replacement and site-directed mutagenesis. J Biol Chem. In press.
70. Ple P, Marnett LJ. Alkylaryl sulfides as peroxidase reducing substrates for prostaglandin H synthase: Probes for the reactivity and environment of the ferryl-oxo complex. J Biol Chem 1989; 264:13983–13993.
71. Shimokawa T, Kulmacz RJ, DeWitt DL, Smith WL. Tyrosine-385 of prostaglandin endoperoxide synthase is required for cyclooxygenase catalysis. J Biol Chem 1990; 265:20073–20076.
72. Catalano CE, Choe YS, Ortiz de Montellano PR. Reactions of the protein radical in peroxide-treated myoglobin. J Biol Chem 1989; 264:10534–10541.
73. Otto JC, DeWitt DL, Smith WL. N-glycosylation of prostaglandin endoperoxide synthase-1 and -2 and their orientation in the endoplasmic reticulum. J Biol Chem 1993; 268:18234–18242.
74. Sirois J, Richards JS. Purification and characterization of a novel, distinct isoform of prostaglandin endoperoxide synthase induced by human chorionic gonadotropin in granulosa cells of rat preovulatory follicles. J Biol Chem 1992; 267:6382–6388.
75. Mutsaers JHGM, van Halbeek H, Kamerling JP, Vliegenthart JFG. Determination of the structure of the carbohydrate chains of prostaglandin endoperoxide synthase from sheep. Eur J Biochem 1985; 147:569–574.
76. Roth GJ, Siok CJ, Ozols J. Structural characteristics of prostaglandin synthetase from sheep vesicular gland. J Biol Chem 1980; 255:1301–1304.
77. van der Ouderaa FJ, Buytenhek M, Nugteren DH, van Dorp DA. Purification and characterization of prostaglandin endoperoxide synthetase from sheep vesicular gland. Biochim Biophys Acta 1977; 487:315–331.
78. Toh H. Prostaglandin endoperoxide synthase contains an EGF-like domain. FEBS Lett 1989; 258:317–319.
79. Rollins TE, Smith WL. Subcellular localization of prostaglandin-forming cyclooxygenase in Swiss mouse 3T3 fibroblasts by electron microscopic immunocytochemistry. J Biol Chem 1980; 255:4872–4875.
80. Regier MK, DeWitt DL, Schindler MS, Smith WL. Subcellular localization of prostaglandin endoperoxide (PGH) synthase-2 in murine 3T3 cells. Arch Biochem Biophys 1993; 301:439–444.
81. Kujubu DA, Reddy ST, Fletcher BS, Herschman HR. Expression of the protein product of the prostaglandin synthase-1/TIS10 gene in mitogen-stimulated Swiss 3T3 cells. J Biol Chem 1993; 268:5425–5430.
82. Kulmacz RJ, Tsai A-L, Palmer G. Heme spin states and peroxide-induced radical species in prostaglandin H synthase. J Biol Chem 1987; 262:10524–10531.
83. Smith WL, Marnett LJ. Prostaglandin endoperoxide synthases. In: Sigel H, Sigel M, eds. Metal Ions in Biological Systems. Vol. 30. New York: Marcel Dekker, 1994. In press.

84. Roth GJ, Machuga ET, Ozols J. Isolation and covalent structure of the aspirin modified, active site region of prostaglandin synthetase. Biochemistry 1983; 22:4672–4675.
85. Rome LH, Lands WEM. Structural requirements for time-dependent inhibition of prostaglandin biosynthesis by anti-inflammatory drugs. Proc Natl Acad Sci USA 1975; 72:4863–4865.
86. Stanford N, Roth GJ, Shen TY, Majerus PW. Lack of covalent modification of prostaglandin synthetase (cyclooxygenase) by indomethacin. Prostaglandins 1977; 13:669–675.
87. Holtzman MJ, Turk J. Shornick LP. Identification of a pharmacologically distinct prostaglandin H synthase in cultured epithelial cells. J Biol Chem 1992; 267:21438–21445.
88. Smith WL. Prostaglandin biosynthesis and its compartmentation in vascular smooth muscle and endothelial cells. Annu Rev Physiol 1986; 48:251–262.
89. DeWitt DL, Kraemer SA, Meade EA. Serum induction and superinduction of PGG/H synthase mRNA levels in 3T3 fibroblasts. In: Samuelsson B, ed. Prostaglandins and Related Compounds II. Vol. 21. New York: Raven Press, 1991:75–90.
90. DeWitt DL, Meade EA. Serum and glucocorticoid regulation of gene transcription and expression of the prostaglandin H synthase-1 and prostaglandin H synthase-2 isozymes. Arch Biochem Biophys. In press.
91. Lee SH, Soyoola E, Chanmugam P, et al. Selective expression of mitogen-inducible cyclooxygenase in macrophages stimulated with lipopolysaccharide. J Biol Chem 1992; 267:25934–25938.
92. O'Sullivan GM, Chilton FH, Huggins EM Jr, McCall CE. Lipopolysaccharide priming of alveolar macrophages for enhanced synthesis of prostanoids involves induction of a novel prostaglandin H synthase. J Biol Chem 1992; 267:14547–14550.
93. O'Sullivan MG, Huggins EM, Meade EA, et al. Lipopolysaccharide induces prostaglandin H synthase-2 in alveolar macrophages. Biochem Biophys Res Commun 1992; 187:1123–1127.
94. Maier JAM, Hla T, Maciag T. Cyclooxygenase is an immediate-early gene induced by interleukin-1 in human endothelial cells. J Biol Chem 1990; 265:10805–10808.
95. Jones DA, Carlton DP, McIntyre TM, et al. Molecular cloning of human prostaglandin endoperoxide synthase type II and demonstration of expression in response to cytokines. J Biol Chem 1993; 268:9049–9054.
96. Sano H, Hla T, Maier JAM, et al. In vivo cyclooxygenase expression in synovial tissue of patients with rheumatoid arthritis and osteoarthritis and rats with adjuvant and streptococcal cell wall arthritis. J Clin Invest 1992; 89:97–108.
97. Sirois J, Richards JS. Transcriptional regulation of the rat prostaglandin endoperoxide synthase 2 gene in granulosa cells. J Biol Chem 1993; 268:21931–21938.
98. O'Banion MK, Winn VD, Young DA. cDNA cloning and functional activity of a glucocorticoid-regulated inflammatory cyclooxygenase. Proc Natl Acad Sci USA 1992; 89:4888–4892.
99. Kujubu DA, Herschman HR. Dexamethasone inhibits mitogen induction of the TIS10 prostaglandin synthase/cyclooxygenase gene. J Biol Chem 1992; 267:7991–7994.
100. Masferrer JL, Seibert K, Zweifel B, Needleman P. Endogenous glucocorticoids regulate an inducible cyclooxygenase enzyme. Proc Natl Acad Sci USA 1992; 89:3917–3921.
101. Jonat C, Rahmsdorf HJ, Park K, et al. Antitumor promotion and antiinflammation: down-modulation of AP-1 (fos/jun) activity by glucocorticoid hormone. Cell 1990; 62:1189–1204.
102. Simonson MS, Wolfe JA, Konieczkowski M, et al. Regulation of prostaglandin endoperoxide synthase gene expression in cultured rat mesangial cells: Induction by serum via a protein kinase C-dependent mechanism. Mol Endocrinol 1991; 5:441–451.
103. Kraemer SA, Meade EA, DeWitt DL. Prostaglandin endoperoxide synthase gene structure: Identification of the transcriptional start site and 5′-flanking regulatory sequences. Arch Biochem Biophys 1992; 293:391–400.
104. Nakao A, Watanabe T, Taniguchi S, et al. Characterization of prostaglandin $F_{2\alpha}$ receptor of mouse 3T3 fibroblasts and its functional expression in Xenopus laevis oocytes. J Cell Physiol 1993; 155:257–264.
105. Lin AL, Bienkowski MJ, Gorman RR. Regulation of prostaglandin H synthase mRNA levels and prostaglandin biosynthesis by platelet-derived growth factor. J Biol Chem 1989; 264:17379–17383.
106. Domin J, Rozengurt E. Platelet-derived growth factor stimulates a biphasic mobilization of arachidonic acid in Swiss 3T3 cells. J Biol Chem 1993; 268:8927–8934.
107. Habenicht AJR, Salbach P, Goerig M, et al. The LDL receptor pathway delivers arachidonic acid for eicosanoid formation in cells stimulated by platelet derived growth factor. Nature 1990; 345:634–636.

16

Renal Prostanoid Receptors

Richard M. Breyer and Matthew D. Breyer
Vanderbilt University, Nashville, Tennessee

INTRODUCTION

The kidney is a major site of arachidonic acid release and its subsequent enzymatic conversion to multiple bioactive eicosanoids. Arachidonic acid is metabolized via several distinct enzymatic pathways including lipoxygenase, cytochrome P-450, and the cyclooxygenase (COX) pathways. Of these pathways, the biological relevance and importance of the COX metabolites is perhaps most clearly established. Cyclooxygenase metabolizes arachidonate to multiple oxygenated derivatives, including prostaglandin E_2 (PGE_2), prostaglandin $F_{2\alpha}$($PGF_{2\alpha}$) prostaglandin D_2 (PGD_2), prostacyclin (PGI_2), and thromboxane A_2 (TxA_2), known collectively as prostanoids. While the production of these autacoids occurs in all cells and tissues, the kidney is a particularly rich source of prostanoids. Unlike classical circulating hormones, such as insulin or vasopressin, prostanoids act locally on the tissues in which they are synthesized or on tissues adjacent to those in which they are synthesized. The production of prostanoids is stimulated by several hormones—including angiotensin, vasopressin, and bradykinin—and they are thought either to mediate or modulate the many of the actions of these hormones at the level of their target tissues.

The kidney is also an important biological target for eicosanoid action. Not only do the different COX metabolites of arachidonic acid (e.g., PGE_2, $PGF_{2\alpha}$, PGI_2) each have distinct effects in their target tissues, but a given prostaglandin may also have multiple physiological effects in a given target tissue. For example PGE_2 is predominantly a vasodilator in some vascular beds, while it is a vasoconstrictor in other vascular beds (1,2). There is now excellent evidence that the diverse effects of an individual prostanoid are mediated by distinct receptor subtypes for that ligand.

Pharmacological studies using structural analogues of prostaglandins provided initial evidence that multiple receptors existed for each prostaglandin. These studies also suggested the existence of multiple receptors for individual prostanoids. For example, the PGE_2 analogue butaprost was active only in vascular beds where PGE_2 was a vasorelaxant, whereas butaprost was totally inactive in vascular beds where PGF_2 was a vasoconstrictor. Conversely, the PGE_2 analogue sulprostone was active only in vascular beds where PGE_2 was a vasoconstrictor and inactive in vascular beds where PGE_2 was a vasodilator. Based upon these studies, the existence of multiple PGE_2 receptors was proposed (2,3). The nomenclature for the prostanoid receptors has now been standardized, so that all PGE_2 receptors are referred to as E-prostanoid receptors or EP receptors; thromboxane receptors are TP receptors; $PGF_{2\alpha}$ are FP; PGD_2 receptors are designated DP receptors, and PGI_2 receptors are designated IP receptors (Table 1). Subtypes of the prostaglandin receptors are designated by subscript, so that EP_1, EP_2, and EP_3 refer to different isoforms of PGE_2 receptors. The intrarenal distribution (Fig. 1), function, and molecular biology of each of receptor is reviewed below.

Table 1 Prostanoid Receptor Pharmacology and Signaling

Eicosanoid	Receptor	Agonist	Antagonist	Signaling
Thromboxane A2	TP	I-BOP U46619 STA2	Bay U3405 AH19437	↑ IP3/DAG
PGI_2 (prostacyclin)	IP	Cicaprost AP-227 Iloprost	—	↑ cAMP
PGE	EP			
	EP_1	17-phenyl-trinor PGE2 Iloprost Sulprostone	SC19220 AH6809	↑ IP3/DAG
	EP_2	Butaprost AH13205 11-deoxy PGE1 19(R)-OH-PGE2 (?)	—	↑ cAMP
	EP_3	M&B 28767 Sulprostone 11-deoxy-PGE1	—	Gi/ ↓ cAMP
	EP_4	?	AH23848 (?)	↑ cAMP
$PGF_{2\alpha}$	FP	Fluprostenol	—	↑ IP3/DAG
PGD	DP	BW 245C	BW A868C	↑ cAMP

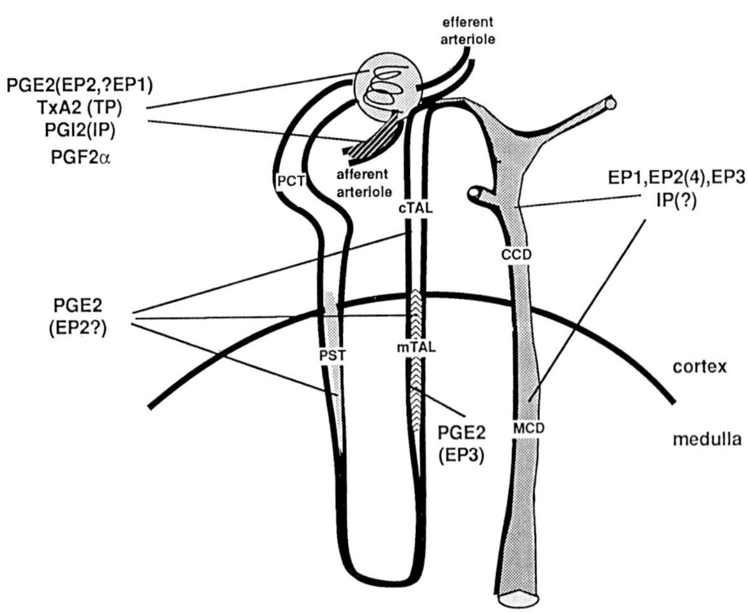

Figure 1 Segmental localization and distribution of the prostanoid receptors in the kidney. This distribution is based both on molecular studies (in the case of the EP3 receptor) and functional studies (for the other prostanoid receptors), suggesting the presence of these receptors in each nephron segment.

PROSTANOID RECEPTOR STRUCTURE

At the writing of this chapter, cDNA sequences for all the prostanoid receptors except the DP receptor have been reported. All prostanoid receptors identified thus far couple to their intracellular effectors via guanine nucleotide regulatory proteins (G proteins) (4,5,6). The primary structure of each of the cloned receptors possesses seven hydrophobic stretches of amino acids characteristic of G protein–coupled receptors. These seven hydrophobic domains are believed to represent transmembrane α-helices by analogy with the structure of bacteriorhodopsin (7,8) and rhodopsin (9). G protein–coupled receptors bind their cognate ligands with these seven transmembrane α-helices and couple to the G protein by their intracellular sequences, particularly the third intracellular loop and the proximal portion of the C-terminal tail (Fig. 2). (For review, see Refs. 10 and 11.) The distal region of the C-terminal tail of G protein–linked receptors is thought to be a target for regulatory phosphorylation by protein kinases such as protein kinase A as well as receptor-specific kinases (12–14).

THE TXA_2 RECEPTOR

Thromboxane A_2 is a labile arachidonic acid metabolite that is a potent vasoconstrictor as well as a stimulant of platelet aggregation (15). The receptor for TXA_2 (or TP receptor) was the first eicosanoid receptor cloned (16). The initial success in cloning of this prostanoid receptor depended upon the purification of the human TP receptor protein. Narumiya and coworkers purified a 57-kDa glycoprotein from human platelets using the TP receptor antagonist S-145 to develop a ligand-affinity chromatography strategy. This purified protein displayed binding properties consistent with a TP receptor (17). The purification obtained in these studies was sufficient to allow partial amino acid sequence analysis, which was used in turn to design oligonucleotide probes for screening cDNA libraries. Using this strategy, a 2.9-kb clone encoding the full-length coding region for the TP receptor was isolated from a human placenta cDNA library (16). This clone encoded a protein of 343 amino acids (37.4 kDa) containing the seven hydrophobic stretches of amino acids. The discrepancy between the deduced molecular weight of the cloned TP receptor and the observed molecular weight for the purified receptor is presumably due to glycosylation of the receptor protein.

When expressed in COS 7 cells, this clone displayed the characteristic ligand-binding properties of the human TP receptor: S-145 > ONO-3708 (TP antagonist) > STA_2 (TP agonist) >> $PGF_{2\alpha}$ PGE_2 > PGI_2 > TXB_2. Signal transduction properties of this receptor were evaluated in *Xenopus* oocytes, where agonist stimulation opened a phosphatidylinositol (PI) turnover-dependent Ca^{2+} channel, consistent with the PI turnover observed for the endogenous receptor in vivo. A limited Northern blot analysis revealed significant expression of a 2.8-kb species in both placenta and lung, the two tissue types evaluated.

Oligonucleotide primers derived from the human TP receptor were used to amplify a fragment of the mouse TP receptor, and this fragment was used to isolate a full-length murine TP receptor from a mouse lung cDNA library, 76% identical with the human TP receptor cDNA (18). Expression of this clone demonstrated similar ligand binding and signal transduction properties as compared with the human TP receptor. Extensive Northern blot analysis demonstrated a major mRNA species hybridized at 2.0 kb in a number of tissues, and a second species of 3.0 kb was evident in thymus. Overall, the highest level of expression was observed in the thymus, followed by spleen, lung, and kidney. Lower levels of expression were observed in heart, uterus, and brain. Using restriction fragment length polymorphisms in interspecific back-crossed mice, the *Tbxa2r* gene encoding the TP receptor was mapped to chromosome 10 (19). More recently, the rat homologue cDNA has also been cloned and displays properties similar to the human and mouse TP receptor cDNAs (20).

Screening a human genomic library resulted in the isolation of a single TXA_2 receptor gene comprising three exons spanning 15 kb (21). Using in situ hybridization, the gene encoding the human TXA_2 receptor was localized to chromosome 19. The first exon is in the 5′ untranslated region (UTR) while the second and third exons encode the receptor protein. Differential transcription initiation results in the incorporation of two alternate 5′UTR exons. The two coding exons are separated by a 4.3-kb intron in the region comprising the sixth transmembrane domain. No evidence for multiple isoforms of the TXA_2 receptor protein was found in the genomic structure, although there is pharmacological evidence for the existence of multiple isoforms (15,22).

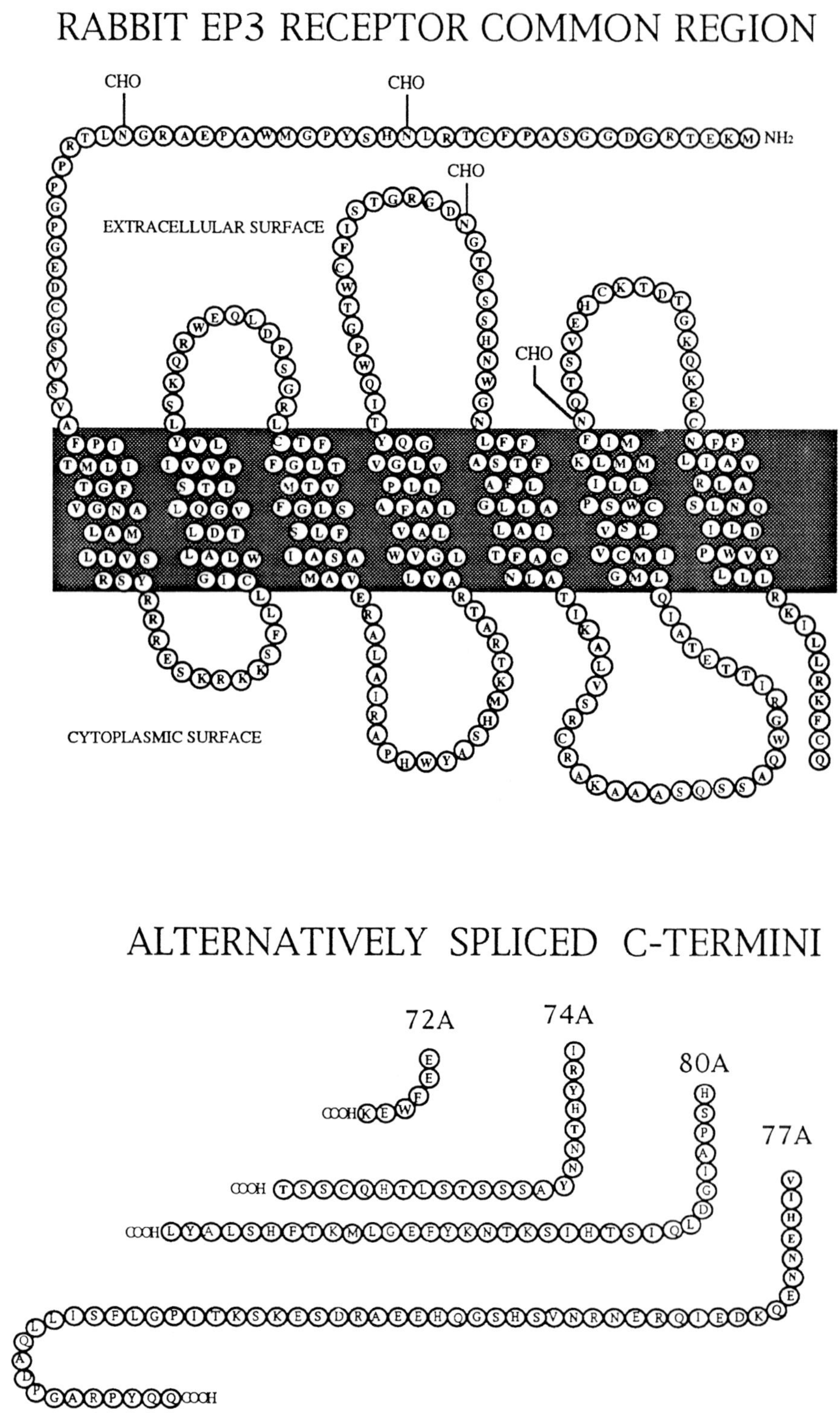

Figure 2 The deduced amino acid sequence of the rabbit EP3 receptors, showing the typical seven transmembrane structure of a G protein–coupled receptor. The four receptor isoforms are identical up until Gln355, at which point the sequences diverge. The unique sequence for each receptor is shown below. The transmembrane-spanning regions of G protein–coupled receptors largely determine the ligand-binding specificity. The intracellular third loop and the C-terminal tail have been implicated in coupling specificity and regulation.

In the kidney, TxA_2 causes intense vasoconstriction, thus decreasing glomerular filtration rate (23). These effects are mediated by glomerular TP receptors coupled to PI hydrolysis, protein kinase C activation, and glomerular mesangial cell contraction (24). Although the TP receptor has now been cloned and characterized, the intrarenal distribution of its mRNA—including the renal vasculature and glomerulus—has not been reported (e.g., using either in situ hybridization or microdissection with PCR). Thus pharmacological studies suggesting the existence of specific glomerular TP receptors have not been confirmed at the molecular level. Important pathogenic roles for TxA_2 and glomerular TP receptors in mediating renal dysfunction in glomerulonephritis, diabetes mellitus, and sepsis have also been proposed (25–27). Roles for TP receptors in modulating tubule epithelial function in the kidney are poorly substantiated (28).

PROSTAGLANDIN E_2 RECEPTORS

Prostaglandin E_2 is the major renal cyclooxygenase metabolite of arachidonate and is the major prostanoid excreted in the urine (20,30–33). The kidney also possesses abundant PGE_2 binding sites (6,34–36). At least four subtypes of PGE_2 receptor had been proposed (2,3,37–39), based upon pharmacological studies performed in smooth muscle. These E-prostanoid receptors (EP receptors) are designated EP_1, EP_2, EP_3, and EP_4. Recently cDNAs for three separate PGE_2 receptors have been cloned using strategies based upon homology with the TP receptor.

The EP_1 receptor causes smooth muscle contraction of guinea pig ileum and dog fundus and is selectively activated by 17-phenyl-trinor-PGE_2 and sulprostone and antagonized by SC19220 and AH6809 (Fig. 3). EP_2 receptors relax smooth muscle in cat trachea and guinea pig ileum; they are activated by butaprost and AY23636 but not sulprostone. The EP_3 receptors cause smooth muscle contraction in chick ileum and inhibit acid secretion in rat gastric mucosa, are activated by both sulprostone and AY23636, but are not antagonized by SC19220. Recently, a fourth receptor subtype, tentatively designated EP4, has been proposed in pig saphenous vein, where it causes EP2-like smooth muscle relaxation, but it is not activated by EP_2–selective agonists (38,39).

The existence of multiple PGE_2 receptors corresponds nicely with studies demonstrating that PGE_2 couples to multiple signaling pathways. Thus PGE_2 stimulates phosphatidylinositol turnover via a G protein–mediated mechanism as well as modifying cAMP generation and cAMP generation via G_s and Gi (40–44). To our knowledge, PGE_2 is the only prostanoid described for which multiple signaling mechanisms have been reported in vivo (45). These distinct signaling pathways are mediated by different receptors.

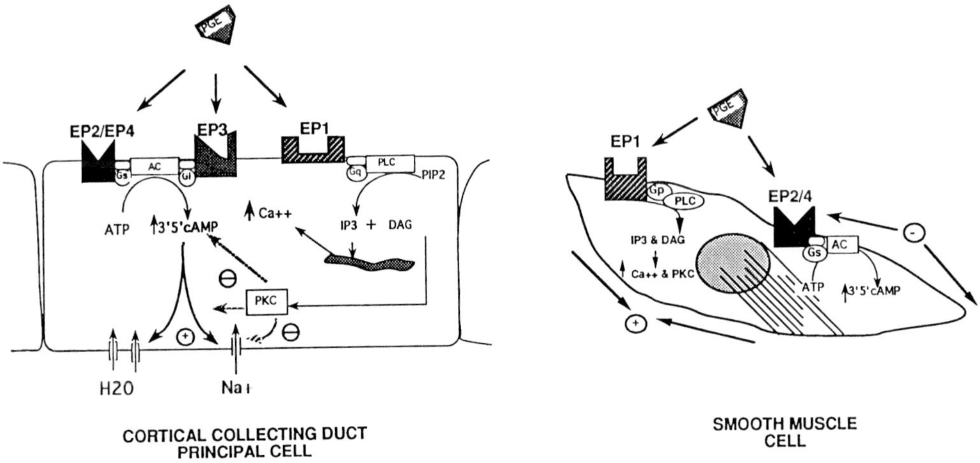

Figure 3 Distinct signaling mechanisms and functional consequences of EP receptor subtype activation. The left panel shows the effect of EP receptor activation on salt and water transport in the cortical collecting duct. The right panel shows the effect of EP receptor activation on vascular smooth muscle.

The EP_3 Receptor

The EP_3 receptor subtype is unique among the cloned prostanoid receptors in that molecular biology strategies have revealed a number of previously undetected receptor isoforms. Using homology-based cloning, a number of laboratories have cloned a large family of EP_3 receptors from the rabbit (46), mouse (47–49), cow (51), human (52,53), and rat (20,54). The multiple isoforms of the EP_3 receptor family have been shown to be derived from a single gene in rabbit (46), rat (54), and mouse (50), and the gene encoding the mouse EP_3 receptor, *Ptgepr3*, has been mapped to the distal end of chromosome 3 (19). Four alternatively spliced isoforms have been found in both the rabbit (Fig. 2) and cow, three isoforms have been found in the mouse and human, and two occur in the rat (54). Taken together, there are 15 receptor isoform cDNAs cloned from five species, which, based upon sequence homology, fall into eight classes. This suggests either that there is a large interspecies variation or, alternatively, that there is a very large number of receptor isoforms in each species of which only a small fraction have been cloned.

For each species, the receptor isoforms are identical throughout the seven-transmembrane domain and the constant portion of the receptor is about 85% homologous across species. The EP_3 receptors have essentially similar ligand-binding properties when transfected in mammalian cell lines. The rabbit EP_3 receptor transfected into COS1 cells bound $[^3H]PGE_2$ with a K_D of 320 p*M*. Competition experiments with a panel of natural and synthetic prostanoid analogues had the following order of affinity: M&B 28767 >sulprostone $\geq PGE_2 = PGE_1 > PGF_{2\alpha} > PGD_2 >$ 8-epi $PGF_{2\alpha}$, in good agreement with in vivo functional agonist order of potency of the rabbit renal G_i coupled EP_3 receptor (40,41,44).

Physiological evidence suggests that the EP_3 receptor signals via inhibition of cAMP generation, and the cloned mouse, bovine, and human receptors were shown to signal through this pathway when expressed in cell culture systems. A subset of bovine EP_3 receptor splice variants also signaled via *stimulation* of cAMP and phosphatidylinositol hydrolysis when expressed in CHO cells. These unexpected signaling effects were observed only at agonist concentrations five orders of magnitude higher than the concentration required for Gi-mediated effects, rendering the physiological significance of this observation uncertain. Nonetheless, it is of interest that different C termini of the alternative splice variants of the bovine EP_3 receptor have distinct signal transduction characteristics in vitro. The physiological significance of the multiple splice variants remains to be determined.

Renal Effects of EP_3 Receptor Activation

The intrarenal distribution of the EP_3 receptor has been mapped both by in situ hybridization in rabbit kidney (55) (Fig. 4) and polymerase chain reaction in microdissected rat nephron segments (56). These studies demonstrate high levels of EP_3 mRNA expression in medullary thick ascending limb as well as lower levels of expression in the medullary and cortical collecting duct. Interestingly, while EP_3 mRNA was detected in rat cortical thick ascending limb (TAL), no significant expression of EP_3 mRNA was detected in the rabbit cortical TAL. The differential expression of EP_3 mRNA in the medullary vs. cortical TAL of the rabbit parallels the distinct functional effects of PGE_2 on ion transport in these segments of the rabbit nephron. Stokes found that while PGE_2 markedly inhibited Cl^- absorption in the rabbit medullary TAL, it had no effect on rabbit cTAL Cl^- transport (57). The similar distribution of the EP_3 receptor and the functional effects of PGE_2 suggests that activation of the EP_3 receptor may be responsible for inhibition of NaCl absorption in the TAL.

In contrast, EP_3 receptor activation appears to have little effect on $Na+$ absorption in the isolated perfused rabbit cortical collecting duct (44). Instead, the EP_3 receptor appears to be responsible for the classic effect of PGE_2 to inhibit vasopressin-stimulated water permeability in the CCD (44) (Fig. 3). As previously discussed, multiple isoforms of the EP_3 receptor, generated by alternative splicing and differing only in their C-terminal tails, appear to exist in the kidney. While some studies suggest differences in signaling or desensitization of these EP_3 isoforms when expressed in COS or CHO cells, the physiological significance of these EP_3 isoforms in the kidney remains to be characterized (46,48,49).

The EP_1 Receptor

The EP_1 receptor was originally identified by its ability to cause smooth muscle contraction in a variety of tissues. A cDNA encoding the human EP_1 receptor was recently isolated from a human

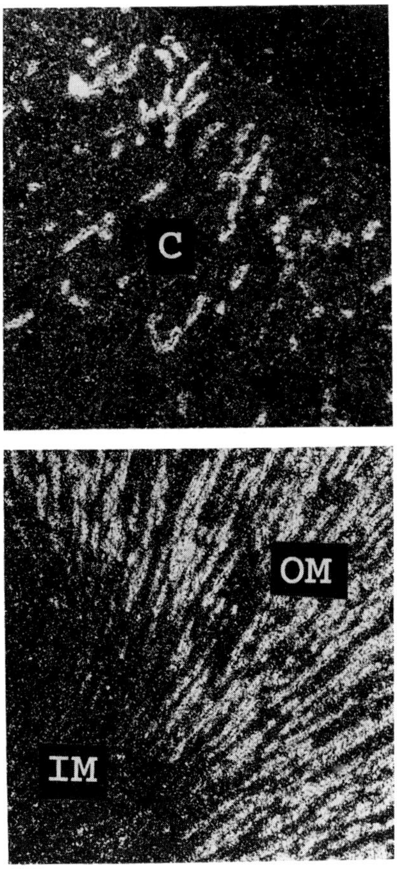

Figure 4 In situ hybridization and intrarenal localization of the rabbit EP3 receptor. Cortex (C) (upper panel); and inner (IM) and outer (OM) medulla (lower panel). Shown are dark-field exposures at ×50 magnification.

erythroleukemia cell line (58). This cDNA encoded a protein of 402 aa and conferred high-affinity $[^3H]PGE_2$ binding (Kd = 1 n*M*) when expressed in COS cells. The $[^3H]PGE_2$ binding could be displaced by a panel of natural and synthetic prostaglandins, which follow the order of potency typical of an EP1 receptor: $PGE_2 > PGE_1 > PGF_{2\alpha} >$ AH6809 > SC19220 > $PGD_2 >$ butaprost. In electrophysiological assays, oocytes expressing the EP_1 clone displayed a ligand-mediated Cl^- current characteristic of Ca^{2+}-coupled receptors.

The mouse EP_1 receptor, which was cloned from kidney, shares 85% sequence identity with the human clone (59). Ligand-binding and signal-transduction properties are essentially identical to those of the human clone with the exception that, unlike the human clone, the mouse clone did not demonstrate binding of the EP_1 antagonist AH6809. Northern blot analysis demonstrated high levels of expression of the mouse EP_1 receptor mRNA in the kidney, with lower levels of expression in the lung. No expression was observed in a variety of other tissues, including brain, thymus, heart, liver, ileum, and stomach.

The functional renal effects of EP_1 receptor activation are not fully characterized. While PGE_2 is thought of predominantly as a glomerular vasodilator (60–62), vasoconstrictor effects of PGE_2 have also been described (63). Prostaglandin E_2 has also been demonstrated to increase Ca^{2+} in cultured mesangial cells, suggesting the presence of an intraglomerular PGE_2 receptor coupled to PI hydrolysis and glomerular contraction (64). It may be that a vasoconstrictor EP_1 receptor mediates glomerular vasoconstriction.

Activation of the EP_1 receptor in the cortical collecting duct may also mediate PGE_2 inhibition of sodium transport, since PGE_2 inhibits sodium transport by a mechanism dependent on increased $[Ca^{2+}]i$ due to the release of Ca^{2+} from intracellular stores (43,44). The ability of PGE_2 to increase intracellular Ca^{2+} in the CCD is mimicked most potently by 17-phenyl trinor-PGE_2, followed by sulprostone. This action is not reproduced by either the EP_3-selective compound MB28767 or the EP_2/EP_3-active compound 11-deoxy-PGE_2 (65). This rank order of potency is consistent with the $[Ca^{2+}]i$ coupled effects of PGE_2 on Na+ transport being mediated via an EP_1 receptor.

The EP_2 (and EP_4) Receptors

The EP_2 receptors are defined by their ability to relax smooth muscle, presumably by raising intracellular cAMP concentration. Narumiya and coworkers recently isolated a cDNA clone by screening a P815 mastocytoma library with an EP_3 probe at low stringency (66). This cDNA encodes a protein of 513 aa, which has 36% homology to the mouse EP_3 receptor. The gene encoding this murine receptor, *Pgerep2*, mapped to the centromeric region of chromosome 15, a region homologous to the human *hChr5p*. When expressed in COS-1 cells this cDNA clone conferred $[^3H]PGE_2$ binding to cell membranes with a ligand order of affinity consistent with an EP receptor and caused an increase in intracellular cAMP in a dose-dependent manner. It bound misoprostol an $EP_{2/3}$ selective compound with high affinity; however, it did not bind the classic EP_2 selective ligand, butaprost. Northern analysis demonstrated high levels of expression in ileum, spleen, thymus, and lung. No expression was observed in a number of other tissues tested. Unexpectedly, the kidney was among those tissue showing no expression despite well-described EP_2-like effects. In contrast, the human homologue of the mouse EP_2 receptor, which was cloned from a human lung library (67), displayed the highest level of expression in the kidney and peripheral blood leukocytes, with high levels of expression in the pancreas, spleen, thymus, and lung and significant expression in a number of other tissues.

Recently a second EP receptor has been described which causes vasodilatation yet is not stimulated by the classical EP_2 agonists (1,38). This novel vasorelaxant receptor, which stimulates adenylyl cyclase, has been termed EP_4. The anomalous ligand binding and tissue distribution of the cloned (so-called) EP_2 receptor raises the possibility that this receptor is the EP_4 receptor rather than the EP_2 receptor. Alternatively, these discrepancies may be due to interspecies variation, as the mouse EP receptors are uncharacterized in vivo.

There is functional evidence that an $EP_{2/4}$ receptor is present in multiple sites along the nephron. Prostaglandin E_2 stimulates cAMP generation when added to preglomerular microvasculature, where this mechanism is thought to be responsible for the glomerular vasodilator effect of PGE_2 (61,68,69). It has been suggested that impaired PGE_2-dependent vasodilatation is a component of the hypertension in spontaneously hypertensive rats (69,70). Alterations of EP receptor expression in this animal model of hypertension remain to be demonstrated.

There are also well-documented stimulatory effects of PGE_2 on cAMP in tubule segments. Prostaglandin E_2 has been shown to stimulate cAMP generation in thin descending limbs in the rat (71). Other studies demonstrate significant stimulation of cAMP generation in both rabbit and rat medullary and cortical TAL (72,73). The functional significance of these cAMP-stimulating EP receptors in these segments of the nephron remains to be characterized. Prostaglandin E_2 also stimulates a receptor coupled to cAMP generation in the cortical and medullary collecting duct (41,44,72,74). Stimulation of this EP receptor increases water reabsorption (44,74) and could conceivably stimulate Na+ absorption by this segment of the nephron (75).

EP Receptors in Renal Disease

The in vivo response to PGE_2 may significantly vary depending on the physiological state of the animal. Dexamethasone has been shown to markedly alter the renal vascular response to PGE_2 from vasodilatation to vasoconstriction (76). The authors suggest that it is consistent with changes in receptor-ligand interactions. A shift in receptor subtype expressed, such as a decrease in EP_2 or an increase in $EP_{1/3}$ receptors induced by dexamethasone, is consistent with this observation. In the Dahl salt-sensitive (DS) rat model of hypertension, salt loading is not accompanied by the increase in EP receptor density observed in salt-resistant rats (DR) (77). As noted above PGE_2 modulates sodium transport along the nephron, and the inability to regulate EP receptor levels in the DS rats could contribute to their salt-induced hypertension. A second rat model of hypertension is the SHR (spontaneously hypertensive rat). These animals have altered reactivity to PGE_2 relative to control animals, though PGE_2 binding is unchanged. Indomethacin treatment abolishes this strain difference (69,70). Inappropriate expression of receptor subtypes in the SHR might account for this pathophysiological condition. In support of this, Good et al. have recently found that PGE_2 fails to inhibit ion transport in medullary TALs dissected from SHRs but potently inhibits ion transport in medullary TALs from control Wistar-Kyoto rats (78). These results suggest that a defect in EP-dependent signaling may exist in the TALs of SHRs and could contribute to the pathogenesis of hypertension in this animal model of hypertension.

FP RECEPTOR

The cloned EP and TP receptors have two regions displaying a high degree of sequence similarity; the second extracellular loop, containing the sequence PG(T/S)WCF, and the seventh transmembrane domain, containing the sequence NQILDPWVY. Abramovitz and coworkers designed a degenerate oligonucleotide probe based upon the conserved sequence in the seventh transmembrane domain sequence and used this to isolate the cDNA encoding the $PGF_{2\alpha}$ receptor from a human kidney cDNA library (79). This cDNA, encoding a protein of 359 aa, conferred $[^3H]PGF_{2\alpha}$ binding on membranes isolated from transfected COS-M6 cells with a K_D of 1 nM. This $[^3H]PGF_{2\alpha}$ binding was displaced by a panel of ligands with a typical agonist order of potency: $PGF_{2\alpha}$ = fluprostenol > PGD_2 > PGE_2 > U46619 > iloprost. When expressed in oocytes, $PGF_{2\alpha}$or fluprostenol induced a Ca^{2+}-dependent Cl^- current, strongly suggesting that this receptor signals in mammalian cells by raising $[Ca^{2+}]i$.

The role of FP receptors in regulating renal function remains unclear. Prostaglandin $F_{2\alpha}$ increases Ca^{2+} in cultured glomerular mesangial cells, and there was no evidence for homologous desensitization by TxA2 or PGE_2. This suggests that an FP receptor may modulate glomerular contraction. While $PGF_{2\alpha}$ also raises intracellular Ca^{2+} in the cortical collecting duct, possibly contributing to its capacity to inhibit water permeability in this nephron segment (28), the FP-selective agonist fluprostenol was without effect on intracellular Ca^{2+}. Furthermore pretreatment with PGE_2 similarly raised intracellular Ca^{2+} and desensitized the CCD to the Ca^{2+} effects of $PGF_{2\alpha}$ (65). Since $PGF_{2\alpha}$ can bind to the EP_1 and EP_3 receptors (46,47,58), the above data suggests that the effects of $PGF_{2\alpha}$ in the CCD are mediated via an EP receptor. Thus a role for the FP receptor in renal tubule cells remains to be established.

PROSTACYCLIN (IP) RECEPTORS

The cDNA sequence of the prostacyclin receptor (IP), has recently been reported (80). Like other receptors, this cDNA encodes a protein with seven transmembrane domains. While expression of the IP receptor in mouse kidney was not observed, there is good functional evidence for the existence of IP receptors in the kidney. Recently, the human IP homologue was cloned from a lung library and demonstrated to have the highest level of expression in the kidney, suggesting that there are significant differences between human and mouse receptor distribution (81).

The IP receptor is selectively activated by the analogue cicaprost (2). Most evidence suggests the PGI_2 receptor signals via stimulation of cAMP generation; however, the cloned mouse PGI_2 receptor also signaled via phosphatidylinositol hydrolysis. Of note, a 10,000-fold higher PGI_2 concentration was required to stimulate phosphatidylinositol hydrolysis (10^{-7} M) in CHO cells transfected with the IP receptor than the concentrations required (10^{-11} M) to stimulate cAMP accumulation in the same cells (80). It remains unclear whether phosphatidylinositol hydrolysis plays any significant role in the physiological actions of PGI_2.

Prostacyclin I_2 has been demonstrated to play an important vasodilator role in the glomerular microvasculature (68,82). The effects of PGI_2 and PGE_2 to stimulate cAMP generation in the glomerular microvasculature were distinct and additive (61), demonstrating that the effects of these two prostanoids are mediated via separate receptors. Renal epithelial effects of PGI_2 have also been reported, but these are less well established. Hébert demonstrated that the PGI_2 analogues iloprost and carbacyclin inhibit water permeability and increase intracellular Ca^{2+} in the isolated perfused cortical collecting duct (83). In contrast to PGE_2, iloprost alone failed to increase basal water permeability, suggesting that, at least in the CCD, the receptor with which it interacts is not coupled to cAMP generation. Because iloprost has also been shown to be an agonist at EP_1 receptors (2), it remains unclear whether these effects prostacyclin analogues are mediated via an IP receptor coupled to IP_3 generation or via an EP_1 receptor. There is also evidence that PGI_2 stimulates cAMP generation in cultured rat inner-medullary collecting ducts; however, these studies have not been confirmed in freshly isolated tissue (84). In summary, while IP receptors appear to play in important vasodilator role in the kidney, their role in regulating renal epithelial function remains to be clearly established.

DP RECEPTORS

Prostaglandin D_2 is a major cyclooxygenase product of pulmonary mast cells (85) and possibly tracheal epithelial cells (86); however, it appears to be a minor product of intrarenal arachidonate metabolism (33). At the time of writing, the cloning of the DP receptor and the tissue distribution of its mRNA has not been reported. Like IP and $EP_{2/4}$ receptors, the DP receptor is thought to couple primarily to increased cAMP generation. Intrarenal infusion of PGD_2 resulted in dose-dependent increase in renal artery flow, urine output, creatinine clearance, and sodium and potassium excretion (87). DP-selective PGD_2 analogues, including the agonist BW 245C and the antagonist BW A868C (2,88), should help clarify whether these renal effects of PGD_2 are mediated by authentic DP receptors.

SUMMARY AND CONCLUSIONS

In summary, the kidney is not only an abundant source for cyclooxygenase products of arachidonate metabolism but also an important biological target for these prostaglandins. There is good functional evidence for the existence of thromboxane A_2, prostacyclin, PGE_2, $PGF_{2\alpha}$, and PGD_2 receptors in the kidney. The corresponding data demonstrating the presence of the receptors at the molecular level are just now evolving. These studies have to date demonstrated that EP_1, EP_2 and EP_3 receptors are present in the kidney, as well as the IP receptor. The intrarenal distribution of the other prostanoid receptors remains to be demonstrated. The availability of molecular probes (both cDNAs and antibodies) will add a new dimension to our understanding of the role of the prostaglandins in the regulation of renal function in salt and water balance in both health and disease.

REFERENCES

1. Lawrence RA, Jones RL. Investigation of the prostaglandin E (EP-) receptor subtype mediating relaxation of the rabbit jugular vein. Br J Pharmacol 1992; 105:817–824.
2. Coleman RA, Kennedy I, Humphrey PPA, et al. Prostanoids and their receptors. In Emmet JC, ed. Comprehensive Medicinal Chemistry. Oxford, Pergamon Press, 1990:643–714.
3. Gardiner PJ. Classification of prostanoid receptors. Adv Prost Thromb Leuk Res 1990; 20:110–118.
4. Haga T, Ross EM, Anderson HJ, Gilman AG. Adenylate cyclase permanently uncoupled from hormone receptors in a novel variant of S49 mouse lymphoma cells. Proc Natl Acad Sci USA 1977; 74:2016–2020.
5. Lefkowitz RJ, Mulliken D, Wood CL, et al. Regulation of prostaglandin receptors by prostaglandins and guanine nucleotides in frog erythrocytes. J Biol Chem 1977; 252:5295–5303.
6. Watanabe T, Umegaki K, Smith WL. Association of a solubilized prostaglandin E_2 receptor from renal medulla with a pertussis toxin-reactive guanine nucleotide regulatory protein. J Biol Chem 1986; 261:13430–13439.
7. Henderson R, Unwin PNT. Three dimensional model of purple membrane obtained by electron microscopy. Nature 1975; 257:28–32.
8. Henderson R, Baldwin JM, Ceska TA, et al. Model for the structure of bacteriorhodopsin based on high-resolution electron cryo-microscopy. J Mol Biol 1990; 213:899–929.
9. Schertler GFX, Villa C, Henderson R. Projection structure of rhodopsin. Nature 1993; 362:770–772.
10. Dixon RAF, Sigal IS, Strader CD. Structure-function analysis of the β-adrenergic receptor. In: Molecular Biology of Signal Transduction, Cold Spring Harbor Symposia on Quantitative Biology. 1988; LIII:487–497.

11. O'Dowd BF, Lefkowitz RJ, Caron MG. Structure of the adrenergic and related receptors. Annu Rev Neurosci 1989; 12:67–83.
12. Hausdorf WP, Caron MG, Lefkowitz RJ. Turning off the signal: Desensitization of β-adrenergic receptor function. FASEB J 1990; 4:2881–2889.
13. Bouvier M, Hausdorf WP, Deblasi A, et al. Removal of phosphorylation sites from the β2-adrenergic receptor delays onset of agonist-promoted desensitization. Nature 1988; 333:370–373.
14. Hausdorf WP, Campbell PT, Ostrowski J, et al. A small region of the β-adrenergic receptor is selectively involved in its rapid regulation. Proc Natl Acad Sci USA 1991; 88:2979–2983.
15. Furci L, Fitzgerald DJ, Fitzgerald GA. Heterogeneity of prostaglandin H_2/thromboxane A_2 receptors: Distinct subtypes mediate vascular smooth muscle contraction and platelet aggregation. J Pharmacol Exp Ther 1991; 258:74–81.
16. Hirata M, Hayashi Y, Ushikubi F, et al. Cloning and expression of cDNA for a human thromboxane A2 receptor. Nature 1991; 349:617–620.
17. Ushikubi F, Nakajima M, Hirata M, et al. Purification of the thromboxane A_2/prostaglandin H_2 receptor from human blood platelets. J Biol Chem 1989; 264:16496–16501.
18. Namba T, Sugimoto Y, Hirata M, et al. Mouse thromboxane A2 receptor: cDNA cloning, expression and Northern blot analysis. Biochem Biophys Res Commun 1992; 184:1197–1203.
19. Taketo M, Rochelle JM, Sugimoto Y, et al. Mapping the genes encoding mouse thromboxane A2 receptor and prostaglandin E receptor subtypes EP2 and EP3. Genomics 1994; 19:585–588.
20. Abe T, Takeuchi K, Abe K. Rat kidney thromaboxane A2 receptor: Molecular cloning and expression. J Am Soc Nephrol 1993; 4:481.
21. Nusing RM, Hirata M, Kakizuka A, et al. Characterization and chromosomal mapping of the human thromboxane A2 receptor gene. J Biol Chem 1994; 268:25253–25259.
22. Dorn GW. Distinct platelet thromboxane A_2/prostaglandin H_2 receptor subtypes. J Clin Invest 1989; 84:1883–1891.
23. Wilkes BM, Solomon J, Maita M, Mento PF. Characterization of glomerular thromboxane receptor sites in the rat. Am J Physiol 1989; 256:F1111–F1116.
24. Spurney RF, Onorato JJ, Albers FJ, Coffman TM. Thromboxane binding and signal transduction in rat glomerular mesangial cells. Am J Physiol 1993; 264:F292–299.
25. Badr KF. Sepsis-associated renal vasoconstriction: Potential targets for future therapy. Am J Kidney Dis 1992; 20:207–213.
26. DeRubertis FR, Craven PA. Activation of protein kinase C in glomerular cells in diabetes: Mechanisms and potential links to the pathogenesis of diabetic glomerulopathy. Diabetes 1994; 43:1–8.
27. Spurney RF, Ruiz P, Pisetsky DS, Coffman TM. Chronic thromboxane receptor blockade reduces renal injury in murine lupus nephritis. Kidney Int 1992; 41:973–982.
28. Stokes JB. Modulation of vasopressin-induced water permeability of the cortical collecting tubule by endogenous and exogenous prostaglandins. Miner Electrolyte Metab 1985; 11:240–248.
29. Toto RD, Anderson SA, Brown-Cartwright D, et al. Effects of acute and chronic dosing of NSAIDs in patients with renal insufficiency. Kidney Int 1986; 30:760–768.
30. Sedor JR, Davidson EW, Dunn MJ. Effects of nonsteroidal anti-inflammatory drugs in healthy subjects. Am J Med 1986; 81:58–70.
31. Schlondorff D. Renal complications of nonsteroidal anti-inflammatory drugs. Kidney Int 1993; 44:643–653.
32. Patrono C, Dunn MJ. The clinical significance of inhibition of renal prostaglandin synthesis. Kidney Int 1987; 32:1.
33. Bonvalet JP, Pradelles P, Farman N. Segmental synthesis and actions of prostaglandins along the nephron. Am J Physiol 1987; 253:F377–F387.
34. Eriksen EF, Richelsen B, Gesser BP, et al. Prostaglandin E2 receptors in the rat kidney: Biochemical characterization and localization. Kidney Int 1987; 32:181–186.
35. Eriksson LO, Larsson B, Hedlund H, Andersson KE. Prostaglandin E2 binding sites in human renal tissue: Characterization and localization by radioligand binding and autoradiography. Acta Physiol Scand 1990; 139:393–404.
36. Eriksson LO, Larsson B, Andersson KE. Biochemical characterization and autoradiographic localization of ^{3}[H]PGE_2 binding sites in rat kidney. Acta Physiol Scand 1990; 139:405–415.
37. Armstrong R, Matthews J, Jones R, Wilson N. Characterization of PGE_2 receptors mediating increased vascular permeability in inflammation. Adv Prost Thromb Leuk Res 1990; 21:375–378.
38. Louttit JB, Head SA, Coleman RA. AH23848B: A selective blocking drug at EP-receptors in pig saphenous vein? The 8th International Conference of Prostaglandins and Related Compounds. 1992:67.
39. Louttit JB, Head SA, Coleman RA. Prostanoid EP receptors in pig saphenous vein. The 8th International Conference on Prostaglandins and Related Compounds. 1992:68.
40. Sonnenburg WK, Zhu J, Smith WL. A prostaglandin E receptor coupled to a pertussis toxin sensitive

guanine nucleotide regulatory protein in rabbit cortical collecting tubule cells. J Biol Chem 1990; 265:8479–8483.
41. Sonnenburg WK, Smith WL. Regulation of cyclic AMP metabolism in rabbit cortical collecting tubule cells by prostaglandins. J Biol Chem 1988; 263:6155–6160.
42. Yamaguchi DT, Hahn TJ, Beeker TG, et al. Relationship of cAMP and calcium messenger systems in prostaglandin-stimulated UMR-106 cells. J Biol Chem 1988; 263:10745–10753.
43. Hebert RL, Jacobson HR, Breyer MD. Prostaglandin E2 inhibits sodium transport in the rabbit CCD by raising intracellular calcium. J Clin Invest 1991; 87:1992–1998.
44. Hebert RL, Jacobson HR, Fredin D, Breyer MD. Evidence that separate PGE2 receptors modulate water and sodium transport in rabbit cortical collecting duct. Am J Physiol 1993; 265:F643–F650.
45. Watson S, Abbot A. Trends in Pharmacological Sciences. Receptor Nomenclature Supplement.
46. Breyer RM, Emeson RB, Tarng J-L, et al. Alternative splicing generates multiple isoforms of a rabbit prostaglandin E2 receptor. J Biol Chem 1994; 269:6163–6169.
47. Sugimoto Y, Namba T, Negishi M, et al. Cloning and expression of a cDNA for mouse prostaglandin E receptor EP3 subtype. J Biol Chem 1992; 267:6463–6466.
48. Sugimoto Y, Negishi M, Hayashi Y, et al. Two isoforms of the EP3 receptor with different carboxyl-terminal domains. J Biol Chem 1993; 268:2712–2718.
49. Negishi M, Sugimoto Y, Irie A, et al. Two isoforms of prostaglandin E receptor EP3 subtype: Different COOH-terminal domains determine sensitivity to agonist-induced desensitization. J Biol Chem 1993; 268:9517–9521.
50. Irie A, Sugimoto Y, Namba T, et al. Third isoform of the prostaglandin-E-receptor EP3 subtype with different C-terminal tail coupling to both stimulation and inhibition of adenylate cyclase. Eur J Biochem 1993; 217:313–318.
51. Namba T, Sugimoto Y, Negishi M, et al. Alternative splicing of C-terminal tail of prostaglandin E receptor subtype EP3 determines G-protein specificity. Nature 1993; 365:166–170.
52. Adam M, Boie Y, Rushmore TH, et al. Cloning and expression of three isoforms of the human EP3 prostanoid receptor. FEBS Lett 1994; 338:170–174.
53. Yang J, Xia M, Goetzl E, Songzhu A. Cloning and expression of the EP3-subtype of human receptors for prostaglandin E2. Biochem Biophys Res Commun 1994; 198:999–1006.
54. Takeuchi K, Takahashi N, Abe T, Abe K. Two isoforms of the rat kidney EP3 receptor derived by alternative splicing: Intrarenal expression and co-localization. Biochem Biophys Res Commun 1994; 199:834–840.
55. Breyer MD, Jacobson HR, Davis LS, Breyer RM. In situ hybridization and localization of mRNA for the rabbit prostaglandin EP3 receptor. Kidney Int 1993; 43:1372–1378.
56. Takeuchi K, Abe T, Takahashi N, Abe K. Molecular cloning and intrarenal localization of rat prostaglandin E2 receptor EP3 subtype. Biochem Biophys Res Commun 1993; 194:885–891.
57. Stokes JB. Effect of prostaglandin E2 on chloride transport across the rabbit thick ascending limb of Henle. J Clin Invest 1979; 64:495–502.
58. Funk C, Furchi L, FitzGerald G, et al. Cloning and expression of a cDNA for the human prostaglandin E receptor EP1 subtype. J Biol Chem 1993; 268:26767–26772.
59. Watabe A, Sugimoto Y, Honda A, et al. Cloning and expression of CDNA for a mouse EP1 subtype of prostaglandin E receptor. J Biol Chem 1993; 268:20175.
60. Chaudhari A, Kirschenbaum MA. Specific prostaglandin E2 binding sites in isolated rat glomeruli: Evidence for glomerular PGE receptors. Prost Leuk Med 1985; 20:55.
61. Chaudhari A, Gupta S, Kirschenbaum M. Biochemical evidence for PGI2 and PGE2 receptors in the rabbit renal preglomerular microvasculature Biochim Biophys Acta 1990; 1053:156–161.
62. Kirschenbaum MA. Prostanoids and Renal Failure: A hypothetical role for prostanoids in progressive renal disease. Contrib Nephrol 1986; 50:36.
63. Plante GE, Breyer MD, Jacobson HR, Heber RL. Distinct effects of PGE2 and the receptor selective PGE2 analog sulprostone (SLP) on renal hemodynamics, urine volume and Na+ excretion in the rabbit (abstr). J Am Soc Nephrol 1991; 2:525.
64. Mene P, Simonson MS, Dunn MJ. Physiology of the mesangial cell. Physiol Rev 1989; 69:1347–1424.
65. Breyer MD, Jacobson HR, Noland TD, et al. Evidence that separate prostaglandin E2 (PGE2) receptors couple to cyclic AMP (cAMP) generation and intracellular calcium ([Ca++]i) in the rabbit cortical collecting duct. J Am Soc Nephrol 1992; 3:452.
66. Honda A, Sugimoto Y, Namba T, et al. Cloning and expression of a cDNA for mouse prostaglandin E receptor EP2 subtype. J Biol Chem 1993; 268:759–762.
67. An S, Yang J, Xia M, Goetzl EJ. Cloning and expression of the EP2 subtype of human receptors for prostaglandin E2. Biochem Biophys Res Commun 1993; 197:263–270.
68. Edwards RM. Effects of prostaglandins on vasoconstrictor action in isolated renal arterioles. Am J Physiol 1985; 248:F779–F784.

69. Chatziantoniou C, Arendshorst WJ. Impaired ability of prostaglandins to buffer renal vasoconstriction in genetically hypertensive rats. Am J Physiol 1992; 32:F573–F580.
70. Chatziantoniou C, Arendshorst WJ. Renal vascular reactivity to vasodilator prostaglandins in genetically hypertensive rats. Am J Physiol 1992; 31:F124–F130.
71. Torikai S, Kurokawa K. Effect of PGE_2 on the cell cyclic AMP content in the thin descending limb of henle of the rat. Miner Electrolyte Metab 1984; 10:21–25.
72. Torikai S, Kurokawa K. Distribution of prostaglandin E2-sensitive adenylate cyclase along the rat nephron. Prostaglandins 1981; 21:427.
73. Nakao A, Allen ML, Sonnenburg WK, Smith WL. Regulation of cAMP metabolism by PGE_2 in cortical and medullary thick ascending limb of Henle's loop. Am J Physiol 1989; 256:C652–C657.
74. Grantham JJ, Burg MB. Effect of prostaglandin E1 on the permeability response of the isolated collecting tubule to vasopressin, adenosine 3′5′-monophosphate, and theophylline. J Clin Invest 1968; 47:1154–1161.
75. Schafer JA, Troutman SL. cAMP mediates the increase in apical membrane $Na+$ conductance produced in rat CCD by vasopressin. Am J Physiol 1990; 259:F823–F831.
76. Sessa WC, Lin L, Nasjletti A. Reciprocal effects of dexamethasone on vasodilatory responses to arachidonic acid and prostanoids in the isolated perfused kidney. Hypertension. 1990; 15(suppl I):I93–I96.
77. Limas C, Limas CJ. Up-regulation of renal prostaglandin receptors in genetic salt-dependent hypertension. Hypertension 1986; 8:566–571.
78. Good DW, George T, Caflisch CR. Prostaglandin E_2 (PGE_2) regulation of ion transport is absent in medullary thick ascending limbs (MTAL) from spontaneously hypertensive rats (SHR) (abstr). J Am Soc Nephrol 1993; 4:512.
79. Abramovitz M, Boie Y, Nguyen T, et al. Cloning and expression of a cDNA for the human prostanoid FP receptor. J Biol Chem 1994; 269:2632–2636.
80. Namba T, Oida H, Sugimoto Y, et al. cDNA cloning of a mouse prostacyclin receptor: Multiple signaling pathways and expression in thymic medulla. J Biol Chem 1994; 269:9986–9992.
81. Bastien L, Sawyer N, Grygorczyk R, et al. Cloning, functional expression, and characterization of the human prostaglandin E2 receptor EP2 subtype. J Biol Chem 1994; 269:11873–11877.
82. Bolger PM, Einser GM, Ramwell PW, et al. Renal action of prostacyclin. Nature 1978; 271:467–469.
83. Hebert RL, Lajeunesse D. Functional and biochemical evidence that prostacyclin (PGI2) inhibits the hydraulic conductivity (Lp) by a different receptor than PGE2 in rabbit cortical collecting duct (CCD) (abstr). J Am Soc Nephrol 1993; 4:454.
84. Veis JH, Dillingham MA, Berl T. Effects of prostacyclin on the cAMP system in cultured rat inner medullary collecting duct cells. Am J Physiol 1990; 258:F1218–1223.
85. Lewis RA, Soter NA, Diamond PT, et al. Prostaglandin D2 generation after activation of rat and human mast cells with anti-IgE. J Immunol 1982; 129:1627–1631.
86. Eling TE, Danilowicz RM, Henke DC. Arachidonic acid metabolism by canine tracheal epithelial cells: Product formation and relationship to chloride secretion. J Biol Chem 1986; 261:12841–12849.
87. Rao PS, Cavanagh D, Dietz JR, et al. Dose-dependent effects of prostaglandin D2 on hemodynamics renal function, and blood gas analyses. Am J Obstet Gynecol 1987; 156:843–851.
88. Leff P, Giles H. Classification of platelet and vascular prostaglandin D2 (DP) receptors: Estimation of affinities and relative efficacies for a series of novel bicyclic ligands. Br J Pharmacol 1992; 106:996–1003.

17

Receptors for Parathyroid Hormone and Parathyroid Hormone–Related Peptide

Gino V. Segre
Massachusetts General Hospital, Harvard Medical School, Boston, Massachusetts

INTRODUCTION

Parathyroid hormone (PTH) is the most critical acute regulator of extracellular calcium and phosphorus through its binding to cell-surface receptors on renal tubule cells and on osteoblasts (1). Chase and Aurbach's observation that PTH increased urinary cAMP immediately before it elicited its classic phosphaturic response was seminal, because it indicated that PTH acts by stimulating adenylyl cyclase (2). Biochemical and pharmacological characterization of PTH's mode of action soon became possible when stimulation of adenylyl cyclase by PTH was shown in both renal and bone cell preparations in vitro (3,4). Understanding of the mechanisms by which the activated PTH receptor signals intracellular effector molecules was complicated subsequently by the discovery of heterotrimeric guanyl nucleotide-binding proteins (G proteins) that transduce signals from cell-surface receptors, such as the PTH receptor, to adenylyl cyclase, and amplify them.

The agonist-occupied receptor must have two general properties: it must modulate events that alter the biological actions of the cell while also initiating processes to terminate these events and to restore the cell's capacity to respond to subsequent stimulation. The following cascade of events is thought to occur when all G protein–coupled receptors, including the PTH receptor, are occupied by agonists: the agonist-occupied receptor activates a G protein, a process during which GDP bound to the G protein's α subunit is exchanged for GTP. This, in turn, results in the dissociation of the α subunit from the β-γ subunits that remain bound to each other; an effector system is then activated or inhibited by the GTP-occupied Gα subunit. Most of PTH's distal actions, if not all, were thought to be the consequence of PTH's capacity to activate the stimulatory G protein (Gs) and the subsequent stimulation of adenylyl cyclase by the dissociated, activate Gα subunit. More recently, however, hormonal stimulation of PTH receptors also has been shown to activate phospholipase C, as evidenced by hormone-stimulated increases of intracellular free calcium ($[Ca^{2+}]i$) and accelerated rates of phosphoinositide hydrolysis (5–11). PTH also promotes Ca^{2+} entry through the cell's plasma membrane (10) and may have direct effects on phospholipase A_2 (12,13). Whether activation of these multiple effector pathways is the direct consequence of productive coupling of receptors through different transducer molecules linked to specific effectors is uncertain. Recent observations in our laboratory conclusively demonstrate, however, that PTH activates both adenylyl cyclase and phospholipase C through interactions with distinct G proteins (unpublished observations, A. Iida-Klein and G. V. Segre). Further work is necessary to determine whether all PTH responses are primary or whether some are secondary, the consequences of postreceptor "cross talk" among different effector-activated pathways. Additionally, the physiological relevancy of the complex cellular responses to PTH that occur pharmacologically is not known.

Direct analysis of PTH/receptor interactions lagged behind those of most other receptors because developing high specific-activity PTH ligands was a formidable problem; several approaches eventually succeeded. The PTH receptor's properties have been characterized primarily using ^{125}I-labeled amino-terminal PTH fragments and its analogues as radioligands, rather than intact hormone. This limitation must be kept in mind, particularly because of data suggesting putative receptors that bind intact hormone but not amino-terminal fragments (see below). Nonetheless, receptors that bind these shortened molecules also bind the full-length, 84–amino acid hormone, and the biological actions of these analogues are largely indistinguishable from those of intact PTH (1). Studies of endogenous receptors by radioreceptor assay and by affinity cross-linking of the ligand to its receptor have defined many of its pharmacological and physicochemical properties. Mostly kidney and bone cells, traditional PTH targets, have been studied, although it is now quite clear that PTH also binds to a variety of other cells or preparations of their plasma membranes. These include fibroblasts (14), circulating lymphocytes (15), chondrocytes (16), vascular smooth muscle (17), fat cells (18), and placental trophoblasts (19). Receptors in these nonclassic locations appear to be authentic, as their activation by PTH is associated with increased cAMP production, and ligand-receptor cross-linking studies do not distinguish these receptors from those present in bone and kidney, when such studies have been performed (14). The issue of whether osteoclasts directly respond to PTH is still controversial, although several lines of evidence suggest that mature osteoclasts do not have PTH receptors and respond to PTH only indirectly (20,21). Additional cell-surface proteins that bind portions of the PTH sequence carboxy terminal to position 53 with high affinity have been reported, however, based on competitive radioreceptor assays that used biologically active PTH (1–84) as the radioligand. Whether these "carboxyl-terminal PTH receptors" are, in fact, authentic receptors is not known, because their occupancy by hormone has not been convincingly linked to activation of any effector system or changes in second-messenger concentrations (22,23).

PARATHYROID HORMONE–RELATED PEPTIDE

As discussed more extensively below, all PTH receptors thus far cloned also bind a second peptide, parathyroid hormone–related peptide (PTHrP), with the same or closely similar affinity. Detailed description of PTHrP's structure and function is beyond the scope of this chapter, although a discussion of the PTH/PTHrP receptor's biological properties requires at least a brief description of PTHrP. PTHrP was originally identified in tumor extracts from cancer patients with elevated blood calcium levels (24–26). It is now recognized to be the factor responsible for most instances of hypercalcemia associated with malignancies, perhaps the most common human paraneoplastic syndrome. In this capacity, PTHrP functions principally as a circulating hormone. It also appears to circulate in the blood of patients without malignancies, although its functions in normal human adult physiology are unknown (27,28). PTH and PTHrP share identical amino acids at 8 of their 13 most amino-terminal positions, although the remainder of their sequences are completely different. Northern blot analyses of PTHrP mRNA, prepared from human cancers, reveal multiple transcripts that are due to alternative mRNA splicing, while others may derive from other mechanisms, such as initiation of transcription from more than one promoter. If all these mRNAs are translated, they would encode peptides that are about 50 to 90 amino acids longer than PTH (29). The capacity of both PTH and PTHrP peptides to bind to the same receptor and for PTHrP to mimic PTH's hypercalcemic actions undoubtedly relate to this limited homology in their amino-terminal sequences. (30). PTHrP is thought to function primarily, however, as a local paracrine or autocrine factor, a hypothesis that stems mainly from its expression and the expression of a PTH/PTHrP receptor, usually in neighboring cells, particularly in many fetal tissues (30).

PTHrP's activation of its receptors plays a critical role in embryogenesis. Homologous recombination has been used to remove the major coding exon from one copy of the mouse PTHrP gene. Homozygous mutants, the products of matings between heterozygotic animals that transmit the mutant allele through their germ lines, die soon after birth and have a multitude of skeletal anomalies (31). More recently, mice with deletion of their PTH/PTHrP receptor have also been developed. Their phenotypes have not yet been fully characterized, however, since the mutation is lethal in utero; the mice die on approximately day 8 of gestation (personal communication, B. Lanske and H. M. Kronenberg). The importance of activated PTH/PTHrP receptors in early fetal development can also be inferred from the wide distribution of PTHrP in all three germ layers and from PTHrP's expression in trophectoderm cells in the morula stage in mice embryos, where it has been proposed to serve a paracrine/autocrine role in the development of parietal endoderm (32). Additionally, mice bearing a transgene consisting of the PTHrP coding sequence driven by a keratin promotor display disturbed hair-follicle development, particularly on the ventral surface of their bodies (112). Perhaps, PTHrP's best-defined and most unique physiological property is to actively transport calcium across the placenta from the ewe to the lamb, against a calcium gradient. This action of PTHrP, however, is hormonal and does not occur through a paracrine or autocrine interaction (33). Most of PTHrP's roles in development and physiology await precise definition (30,33).

Although PTHrP plays a role in controlling fetal blood calcium levels, it is not adequate to regulate blood calcium levels after birth. The profound hypocalcemia that accompanies total parathyroidectomy demonstrates that PTHrP cannot serve as a surrogate for PTH. PTHrP's distribution in many tissues, however, has fueled speculation that receptors in these unorthodox targets might serve to mediate PTHrP's actions, rather than actions of PTH; evidence in supporting these hypotheses is only currently becoming available.

PROPERTIES OF PTH/PTHrP RECEPTORS

The properties of PTH receptors were first characterized using renal cortical plasma membranes and radioligands of the amino-terminal portion of the PTH molecule. For example, all earlier studies and most recent experiments from this laboratory have used [Nle^{8}, Nle^{18}, Tyr^{34}]bovine PTH (1–34) amide, a ^{125}I-labeled sulfur-free PTH analogue, as the radioligand (34,35). PTH receptors were shown to be of high affinity (K_ds between 0.8 to 5 n*M*) and linked to adenylyl cyclase activation, as evidenced by direct measurements of hormonally stimulated enzyme activity or increased intracellular cAMP in plasma cell membrane preparations and in intact cells, respectively (34–36). Further, addition of nonhydrolyzable GTP analogues to membrane preparations accelerated dissociation of the ligand, a characteristic of G protein–coupled receptors (37).

Responses to PTH are determined in large part, of course, by its circulating blood level. The agonist-occupied receptor's second major role, to set in motion mechanisms that regulate cellular responsiveness to further exposure to the ligand, is also thought to be key. The cell regulates its responsiveness by many mechanisms, which include modulating the number of functional receptors, and by influencing postreceptor events important to its mechanism of action. In intact animals with induced primary and secondary hyperparathyroidism, functional PTH receptors are diminished in number when expressed per milligram of renal membrane protein, but have unaltered affinity (38,39). Resistance to PTH action is well recognized, especially in patients with chronic renal failure, who also have elevated PTH levels (40). This decreased responsiveness may be due, at least in part, to agonist-induced downregulation of their PTH receptors, which, in turn, may be due to reduced translation from lower levels of receptor mRNA (see below).

Decreased PTH binding and desensitization of adenylyl cyclase responsiveness to a subsequent PTH challenge occur in vitro in a dose- and time-dependent manner, when cells expressing endogenous PTH receptors are continuously treated with PTH agonists (34,41–45). Interestingly, homologous downregulation of PTH receptors in ROS 17/2.8 cells occurs with hormonal concentrations too low to be measured by competitive radioreceptor assays (34), supporting the notion that certain cellular responses occur with very low levels of receptor occupancy. Our laboratory has recently shown that lower levels of receptor occupancy are necessary to achieve maximal stimulation of adenylyl cyclase than phospholipase C (86). Both differences in receptors occupancy as they relate to effectors and variation in the desensitization of effectors, a consequence of receptor activation, are likely to influence which effector pathways and "downstream" events are modulated.

The mechanisms that underlie these regulatory phenomena are just beginning to be understood. Homologous downregulation in clonal ROS 17/2.8 and OK cells is primarily determined at the posttranscriptional level, because functional PTH receptors are markedly diminished over the first 2 days of hormonal treatment but steady-state levels of receptor mRNA are not altered (46). These data confirm and extend the earlier report by Teitelbaum et al. (47), which showed markedly reduced PTH binding by pretreatment of primary avian bone cells with compounds that interfere with receptor recycling and the lack of effect on PTH binding by inhibitors of protein synthesis. Acutely, homologous PTH receptor downregulation in primary bone cells appeared to be largely dependent on internalization and intracellular processing of ligand-receptor complexes, and subsequent catabolism or reinsertion of PTH receptors into the plasma membrane, rather than to rely on new receptor synthesis. Teitelbaum et al. also showed that internalization of PTH-receptor complexes was agonist-induced and energy-dependent (47). In vivo, Urena et al. have recently shown downregulation of PTH/PTHrP receptor mRNA levels and diminished basal and PTH-sensitive adenylyl cyclase activity in rats with modest levels of experimentally induced renal failure. The high correlation between the levels of blood creatinine and steady-state levels of PTH/PTHrP mRNA, but not between circulating PTH levels and these mRNA levels, suggested that factors other than PTH are responsible (113).

Heterologous regulation of the PTH receptor, that is, regulation by factors other than PTH and PTHrP, also occurs in a dose- and time-dependent manner. Glucocorticoids dramatically increase the number of PTH receptors in osteoblast-like ROS 17/2.8 osteosarcoma cells (48), and they decrease PTH receptor number in OK cells (49). Both retinoic acid (50) and $1,25(OH)_2D$ (51) downregulate PTH receptors in ROS 17/2.8 cells. In the examples thus far studied, heterologous regulation is associated with parallel changes in the steady-state levels of receptor mRNA, in contrast to homologous downregulation of PTH receptors (Ref. 46 and unpublished data, G. V. Segre).

PHYSICOCHEMICAL PROPERTIES

The physicochemical properties of PTH receptors have been partially characterized by affinity cross-linking radioiodinated PTH ligands to them, solubilizing the ligand-receptor complex, and identifying the receptor as a radioactively-labeled band after SDS polyacrylamide gel electrophoresis. These receptors are glycoproteins with a molecular size of about 80,000 Da; the peptide backbone accounts for approximately 59,000 Da and the remainder is due to asparagine-linked oligosaccharides (52–54). Essentially, two principal methods have been used: (a) *N*-hydroxysuccinimidyl-4-azidobenzoate, a heterobifunctional reagent, has been used to cross link ^{125}I-PTH (1–34) bound to its receptor [this method also demonstrated the extraordinary susceptibility of the receptor to proteolysis (55)] and (b) binding of photoreactive derivatives of amino-terminal analogues of both PTH and PTHrP that were first covalently modified by addition of 4-fluoro-3-nitrophenylazide to the α-amino group of the first amino acid or to ϵ-amino functions of lysine residues, then radioiodinated, and finally incubated with intact cells before cross-linking them to receptors with UV light. The biological properties of the family of derivatived PTH and PTHrP analogues have been characterized in detail, after their separation by high-performance liquid chromatography (HPLC). Characterization of the properties of these analogues has identified residues in the ligand that are important for its function, by distinguishing analogs that retained activity from those where modifications of the molecule impaired hormonal activity (56–58).

Amino-terminal analogues of PTHrP, which subsequently became available and could also be made photoreactive, allowed comparisons between the binding properties of PTH (1–34) and PTHrP (1–36) or PTHrP (1–40). Receptors bound the two peptides with the same affinity, the receptors that bound either ligand were of the same apparent molecular size, and both PTH and PTHrP downregulated receptors that bound either ligand (59,60) (Figs. 1 and 2). These studies provided strong evidence that the same receptor binds both ligands, an issue that was definitively resolved when cloned opossum renal and rat bone receptors were shown to bind amino-terminal PTH and PTHrP analogues with equal affinity (5,61). The cloned human receptor also binds both peptides, although it prefers PTH (62). All the actions of PTH and PTHrP, however, may not be mediated through PTH/PTHrP receptors that have been cloned. Receptor mRNAs with differing lengths have been identified in several tissues and organs (63) (Fig. 3), and, as mentioned above, there may be receptors that specifically bind carboxyl-terminal portions of the PTH molecule. Additional PTHrP receptors that do not share binding with PTH or preferentially bind PTHrP seem likely to exist (30,33).

The recent cloning of cDNAs encoding PTH receptors has allowed studies of its ligand-binding and signal-transduction properties in much greater detail through experiments in which receptors are expressed, transiently or stably, in "neutral" cells that do not endogenously express PTH receptors. The availability of cloned receptor cDNAs has also permitted detection of PTH receptor mRNA by both Northern blotting and in situ nucleotide hybridization. These studies have characterized the size and distribution of receptor mRNA. The tissue and cellular locations of receptor transcripts, in

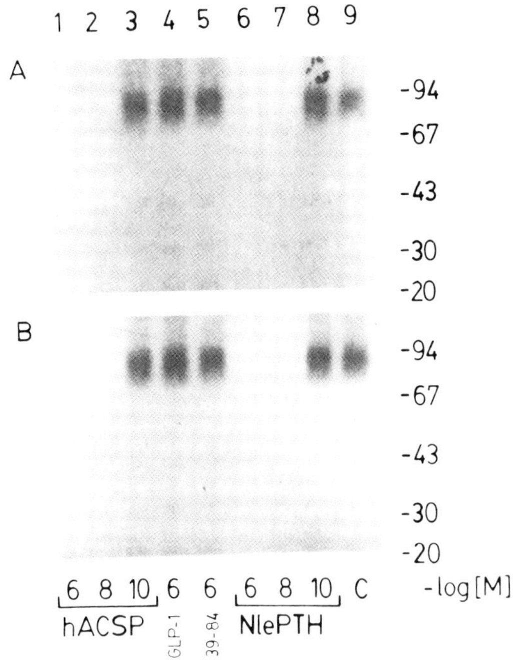

Figure 1 Photoaffinity labeling of ROS 17/2.8 cell PTH receptors. ROS 17/2.8 cells were incubated in the dark (4hr, 15°C) with either (*A*) ^{125}I-photoreactive [Nle^{8,18},Tyr^{34}] bovine PTH (1-34) amide or (*B*) ^{125}I-photoreactive[Tyr^{36}]human PTHrP (1-36) amide (above, labeled "hASCP"). Competing unlabeled ligands are [Tyr^{36}] human PTHrP (1-36) amide range 10^{-6}-10^{-10} M, lanes 1–3), GLP-1 (10^{-6} M, lane 4), human PTH (53-84) (10^{-6} M, lane 5, or [Nle^{8,18},Tyr^{34}]bovine PTH (1-34) amide (range 10^{-6}-10^{-10} M, lanes 6–8). Incubation of the cells in the presence of either photoligand alone is shown in lane 9 (*C*, control). After rinsing, photolysis, and solubilization, the samples were analyzed by SDS-PAGE with subsequent autoradiography. (From Ref. 59.)

particular, have raised many provocative questions concerning potential functions of these receptors in signal transduction, embryogenesis, cell proliferation, and cell differentiation.

The cDNAs encoding opossum renal and rat bone PTH/PTHrP receptors were independently cloned by minor modifications of the mammalian expression methods described by Gearing et al. in their successful cloning of the GM-CSF receptor (64). This technique relies on identifying COS-7 cells that transiently express the receptor of interest by their capacity to bind the relevant radiolabeled ligand, which is then detected by emulsion autoradiography. This approach, which has now been used to clone a large number of cell-surface receptors, has three essential requirements: (a) an appropriate plasmid vector, (b) a high-efficiency expression system, and (c) a highly selective screening system. Additionally, the method's efficiency is enhanced through the use of non-self-annealing adapters and a high-quality, size-selected cDNA library. The plasmid vector CDM-8 (65), which is commercially available as pcDNA 1, was used to clone cDNAs encoding several PTH/PTHrP receptors (5,61). This plasmid features a tyrosine tRNA amber suppressor gene, a polylinker for insertion of the DNAs, a bacterial origin of replication for efficient cloning of the plasmid, a SV40 viral origin of replication that permits rapid multiplication of plasmids in mammalian cells, a strong promoter derived from CMV to drive transcription of DNA inserted in the polylinker, and an M13 origin of replication that permits rapid single-strand DNA sequencing.

To isolate cDNAs that encode PTH receptors, cDNA libraries were prepared from poly-A$^+$ RNAs, which were independently extracted from a clonal opossum kidney (OK) and clonal rat osteosarcoma (ROS 17/2.8) cells. After second-stranding the DNAs, the libraries were independently ligated to Bst-XI non-self-annealing adapters. (Use of these adapters avoids adapter-adapter and

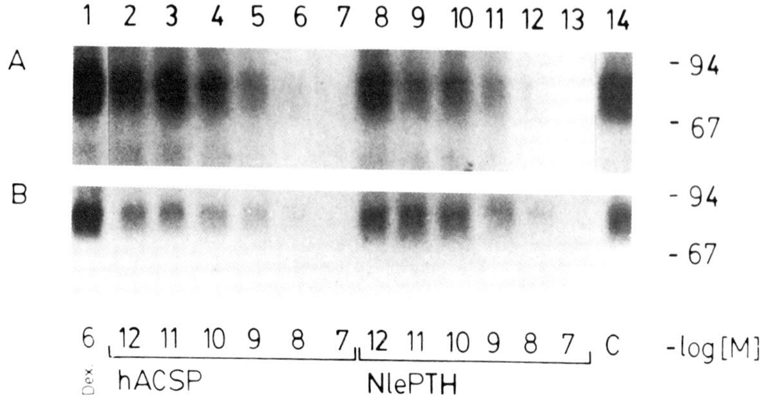

Figure 2 Regulation of ROS 17/2.8 cell receptors by NlePTH, [Tyr^{36}]human PTHrP (1-36) amide, and dexamethasone. ROS 17/2.8 cells were initially treated for 3 days with either [Tyr^{36}] human PTHrP (1-36) amide (above labeled, "hACSP"), 10^{-12}-10^{-7}M, lanes 2–7). NlePTH (10^{-12}-10^{-7} M), lanes 8–13), dexamethasone (10^{-6} M, lane 1), or vehicle alone (lane 14). The cells were then incubated in the dark (4 hr, 15°C), with either (*A*). ^{125}I-photoreactive [Nle^{8,18},Tyr^{34}] bovine PTH (1-34) amide (NlePTH) or (*B*), ^{125}I-photoreactive [Tyr^{36}]human PTHrP (1-36) amide. After rinsing, photolysis, and solubilization, the samples were analyzed by SDS-PAGE with subsequent autoradiography. (From Ref. 59.)

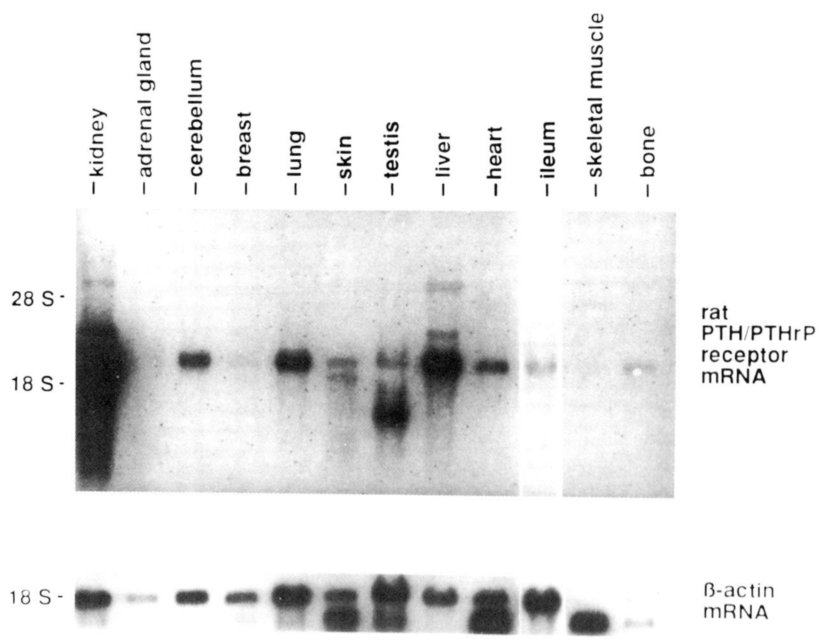

Figure 3 Northern blot analysis of poly (A)+ RNA prepared from different rat tissues. Approximately 5 μg of poly (A)$^{+}$RNA was loaded in each lane, hybridized with the cDNA probe and washed at high stringency conditions; 30 min at 42°C with 300 ml of 1× SSC and 0.1% SDS, and 30 min at 65°C with the same solution. The autoradiograph was developed after 7 days exposure at –80°C. After hybridization with the PTH/PTHrP receptor probe and exposure, the filter was washed and rehybridized with the β-actin probe and then exposed for 20 hr at –80°C. (From Ref. 62.)

DNA-DNA polymers and improves yield because dephosphorylation is not required.) These libraries were then size-selected for DNAs >700 bp in length and used to transform *Escherichia coli*, which contain the amber mutation encoding resistance to ampicillin and tetracycline. Plasmid cDNA pools from approximately 10,000 independent bacterial colonies were transfected into subconfluent COS-7 cells, which were grown in "slideflasks." After a 48-hr incubation to permit maximal expression of the cDNAs, cells were incubated with ^{125}I-[Tyr^{36}] PTHrP (1–36) amide. The slides then were washed with appropriate buffer, the cells fixed with glutaraldehyde, and the slides then were dipped in photoemulsion for autoradiography. Slides were developed after 2 to 4 days and examined by microscopy (dark-field is more efficient than bright-field). The bacterial pools responsible for generating the positive autoradiographic signals were then sequentially subdivided and screened until clones that expressed PTH/PTHrP receptors were isolated (5,61). Complementary DNAs encoding rat renal and human renal and bone PTH/PTHrP receptors were subsequently cloned by standard nucleotide hybridization techniques in which phage cDNA libraries, which had been synthesized from poly-A$^+$ RNA isolated from the respective organs, were screened initially with portions of the rat receptor sequence (62).

The cDNAs encoding these PTH/PTHrP receptors predict them to have general topographic features common to other members of the G protein–linked receptor superfamily; an amino-terminal extracellular region with an amino terminus containing a sequence likely to encode a signal peptide (although not all G protein–linked receptors have a signal sequence), three extracellular loops, three intracellular loops, and a carboxyl-terminal cytoplasmic region. These relatively hydrophilic regions are linked by seven relatively hydrophobic membrane-spanning helices (Figs. 4 and 5).

The PTH/PTHrP receptors's amino acid sequences are highly homologous, and their lengths vary from 585 to 594 amino acids (5,61,62). Rat and mouse PTH/PTHrP receptors are 99% identical

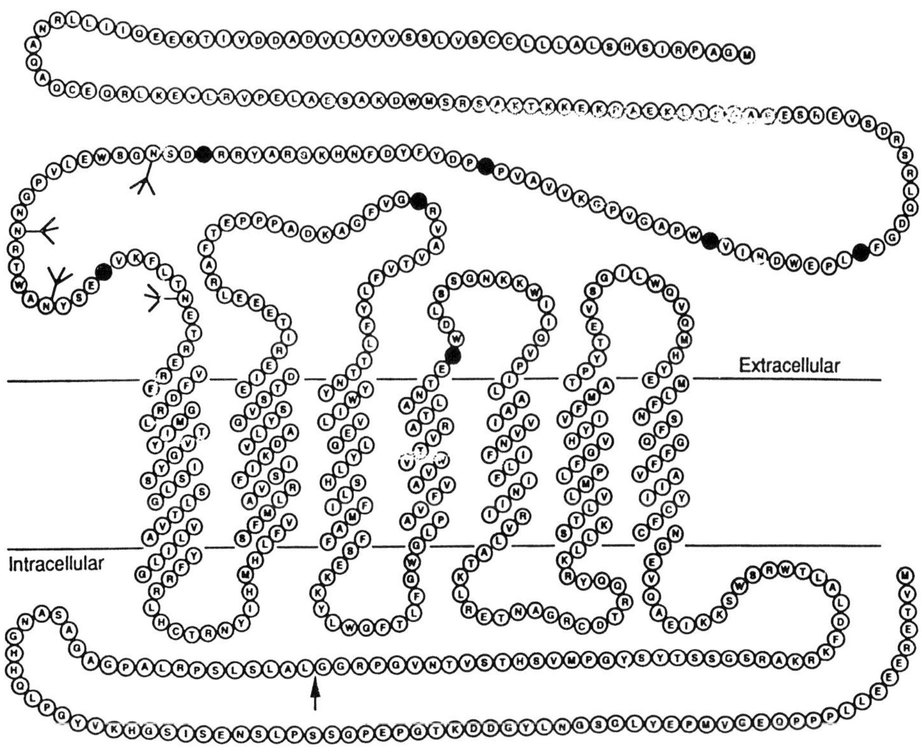

Figure 4 Schematic representation of the opossum PTH/PTHrP receptor. The amino-terminus is extracellular; potential glycosylation sites and conserved cysteines (●) are indicated. In OK-H, a carboxyl-terminally truncated receptor, residues 508-515 (to the left of the arrow) are WPCPSALD. This mutant receptor ends eight residues after the arrow. (From Ref. 60.)

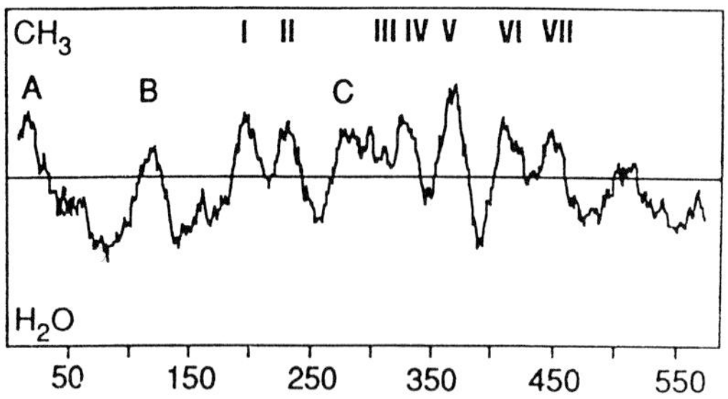

Figure 5 Hydrophobicity plot of the deduced opossum PTH/PTHrP receptor sequence with a 20-residue window. The seven-membrane-spanning helices are indicated as are additional hydrophobic regions A, B, and C. (From Ref. 60.)

at the amino acid level and the human and rat PTH/PTHrP receptors are 91% identical; opossum and rat receptors, whose amino acids are 78% identical, are the most widely divergent of the sequences thus far reported. This phylogenetic conservation across such distantly related mammals is striking. The greatest amino-acid differences among these receptors are in discrete portions of their amino-terminal extracellular regions and their first extracellular loops, and in their carboxyl-terminal intracellular sequences; other portions of their amino-terminal extracellular region and the sequences that putatively span the membrane are especially highly conserved (Fig. 6). All PTH receptors have three additional hydrophobic regions; the location and sequence of the first suggests that it is a signal peptide, although whether it is retained in the mature peptide or cleaved during processing is unknown; the second lies within the amino-terminal extracellular region, and the third within the first putative extracellular loop (Fig. 5). Ten cysteine residues (including two in the putative signal sequence, six in the amino-terminal extension, and one in each of the first two extracellular loops), several charged amino acids and prolines within the receptor's membrane-spanning portions, and four potential glycosylation sites in the amino-terminal extension all are positioned identically (Fig. 6). Although the nucleotide sequences encoding human and rat PTH/PTHrP receptors differ, renal and bone receptors are identical within each species, indicating that the same receptor transcript is present in these two traditional PTH targets. Of course, other receptors that might bind PTH or PTHrP exclusively or preferentially are not excluded, as these may not have been detected by the methods employed (62).

G PROTEIN–LINKED RECEPTORS

PTH/PTHrP receptors are now appreciated to belong to a newly discovered and growing family within the very large superfamily of G protein–linked receptors. Other members of this family, all of which have been cloned in the last 3 years, include receptors for secretin (66), calcitonin (67), vasoactive intestinal peptides 1 (68) and 2 (113), glucagon-like peptide 1 (69), glucagon (70), growth hormone–releasing hormone (71), pituitary adenylyl cyclase–activating peptide (114), gastric inhibitory peptide (115), and corticotrophin releasing hormone (116). Additionally, an insect diuretic hormone (117) and a partial genomic clone from *Caenorhabitidis elegans* (118) are homologous, indicating that this newly discovered family is widely conserved through evolution. Classifying these receptors as members of a distinct G protein–coupled receptor family is warranted because they have no significant sequence identity (<12%) with the other G protein–linked receptors presently in data banks (72,73). Sequence alignment of members of this receptor family shows them to be highly homologous with many identical or highly conserved amino acids (Fig. 7). All members have relatively long amino-terminal, extracellular extensions, a highly conserved pattern of cysteine residues in the amino-terminal extension and in each of the first two putative extracellular loops, and multiple potential asparagine-linked glycosylation sites. Their last membrane-spanning domain and the initial portion of their carboxyl-terminal intracellular region are especially highly conserved;

```
                   **                                                  *
H  MGTARIAPGL ALLLCCPVLS SAYALVDADD VMTKEEQIFL LHRAQAQCEK   50
R  ..A.....S. .......... .......... .F........ ........D.   50
O  ..AP..SHS. ......S... .V........ .I......I. .RN......Q   50

H  RLKEVLQRPA SIMESDKGWT SASTSGKPRK DKASGKLYPE SEEDKEAPTG  100
R  L.....HTA. N......... P......... E.....F... .K.N.DV...  100
O  ......RV.  ELA..A.D.   M.R.A.TK. E.PAE...SQ A..SR.VSDR   97
         *         *                 *                 *
H  SRYRGRPCLP EWDHILCWPL GAPGEVVAVP CPDYIYDFNH KGHAYRRCDR  150
R  ..R....... ...N.V.... .......... .......... ..........  150
O  ..LQDGF... ...N.V...A .V..K..... .......... ..R......S  147
   $          $    $   *     $                   I
H  NGSWELVPGH NRTWANYSEC VKFLTNETRE REVFDRLGMI YTVGYSVSLA  200
R  .....V.... .......... L..M...... .......... ......M...  200
O  .........N .......... .......... .......... ......I..G  197
                                           II
H  SLTVAVLILA YFRRLHCTRN YIHMHLFLSF MLRAVSIFVK DAVLYSGATL  250
R  .......... .......... .....M.... ....A..... .......F..  250
O  .........G .......... .......V.. ........I. .......VST  247
                                    *
H  DEAERLTEEE LRAIAQAPPP PATAAAGYAG CRVAVTFFLY FLATNYYWIL  300
R  .......... .HI...V... ..A..V.... .......... ..........  300
O  ..I..I.... ...FTE  .. .. DK..FV. ......V... ..T.......  294
     III                                 IV
H  VEGLYLHSLI FMAFFSEKKY LWGFTVFGWG LPAVFVAVWV SVRATLANTG  350
R  .......... .......... .....I.... .......... G.........  350
O  .......... .......... .....L.... .......... T........E  344
   *                          V
H  CWDLSSGNKK WIIQVPILAS IVLNFILFIN IVRVLATKLR ETNAGRCDTR  400
R  .......H.. .......... V......... .I........ ..........  400
O  .......... .........A ..V....... .I........ ...... ...  394
                    VI
H  QQYRKLLKST LVLMPLFGVH YIVFMATPYT EVSGTLWQVQ MHYEMLFNSF  450
R  .......R.. ...V...... .T....L... ........I. ..........  450
O  .......... .......... .......... ....I..... ..........  444
    VII
H  QGFFVAIIYC FCNGEVQAEI KKSWSRWTLA LDFKRKARSG SSSYSYGPMV  500
R  .......... .......... R......... .......... ..........  500
O  .......... .......... .......... .......... ..T.......  494

H  SHTSVTNVGP RVGLGLPLSP RLLPTAT  T NGHPQLPGHA KPGTPALETL  548
R  .......... .A..S..... ..P. ..  . ...S...... ...A..T..   546
O  .......... .G..A.S... ..A.G.GASA ...H....YV .H.SISENS.  544

H  ETTPPAMAAP KDDGFLNGSC SGLDEEASGP ERPPALLQEE WETVM        593
R  ..L.VT..V. .......... ......... A...P..... .....        591
O  PSSG.E PGT ....Y....    ..Y.PMV. .Q..P..E.. R....        585
```

Figure 6 Alignment of the human(H), rat(R), and opossum(O) PTH/PTHrP receptors. Identical amino acids between the human and rat, or human and opossum receptors (·); conserved extracellular cysteines (*); conserved extracellular potential glycosylation sites ($); and putative membrane-spanning regions (underlined, I-VII) are indicated. (From Ref. 61.)

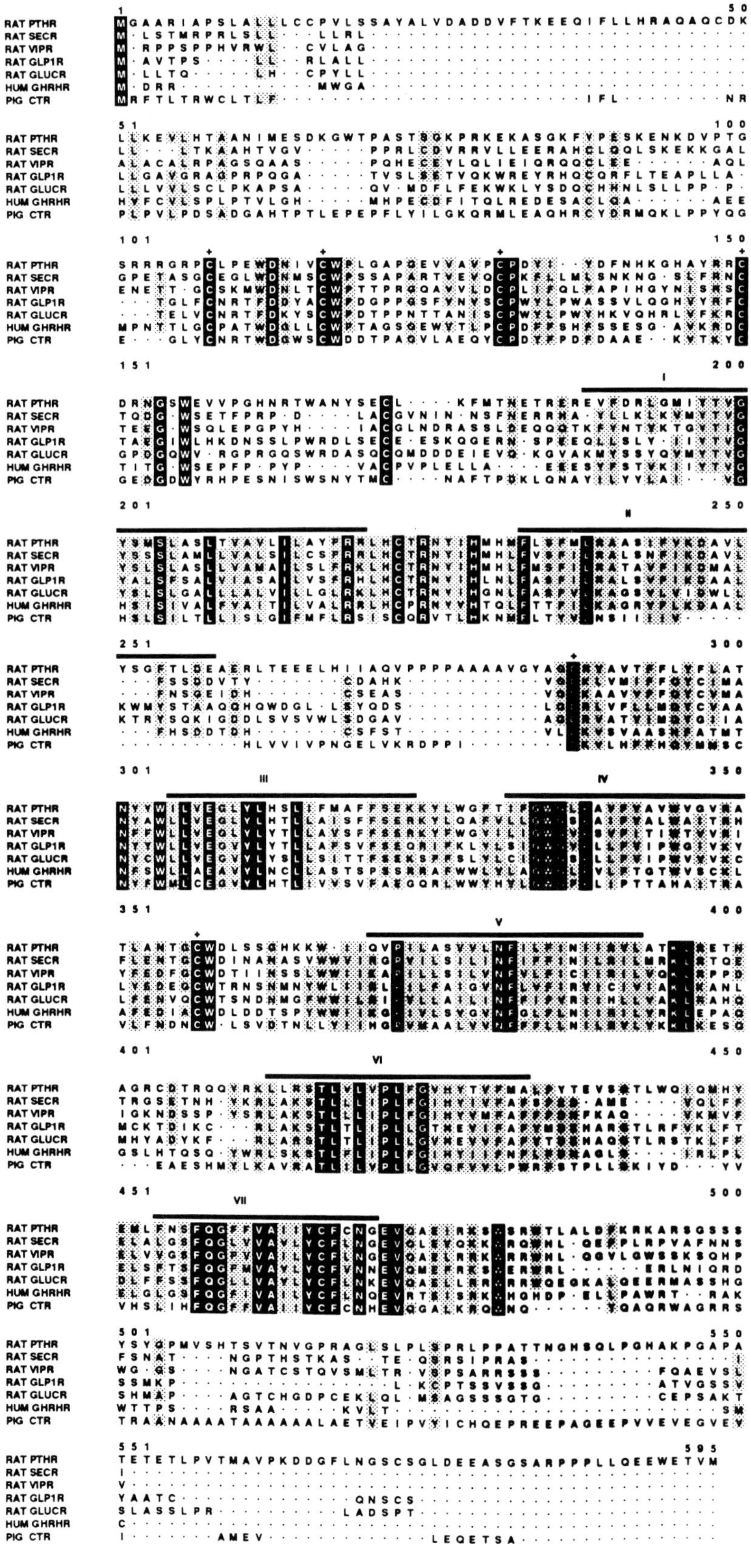
RAT PTHR
RAT SECR
RAT VIPR
RAT GLP1R
RAT GLUCR
HUM GHRHR
PIG CTR

16 of 18 and 17 of 18 amino acids in this region are identical between secretin and PTH/PTHrP receptors and between calcitonin and PTH/PTHrP receptors, respectively.

The unexpectedly close relationships among these receptors and their respective ligands have interesting implications and they lead to some provocative speculations. For example, when animals moved from an oceanic environment, which contains abundant calcium, to terrestrial habitats, where calcium is in short supply, a hormonal system for preventing hypocalcemia would have provided a clear evolutionary advantage. The similarities between the genes encoding PTH and PTHrP suggest that they evolved from a common ancestral molecule by a translocation event and that PTHrP is likely to be the older gene. Chromosomal translocations also are thought to explain the evolutionary relationship among ligands that belong to the secretin/glucagon family of peptides. The existence of a remote common ancestor for the superfamily of G protein–coupled receptors is quite plausible, and the interrelationships among members of this newly discovered family, based on their relative homologies, is consistent with the G protein–coupled seven-membrane–spanning receptor phylogenetic tree presented in Fig. 8. Other receptors belonging to this family certainly will be identified, and their properties will further clarify the evolutionary and functional relationships among its members.

The enormous array of critical roles served by the G protein–linked receptor superfamily is especially noteworthy; receptors that share this common motif of seven membrane-spanning helices are found both in invertebrates and vertebrates, including mammalian as well as submammalian species. Their versatility is exemplified by their capacity to be activated by such diverse stimuli as photons, odors, opioids, catecholamines, prostaglandins, compounds important for cellular metabolism (such as glutamate and adenosine), thrombin, cAMP (in *Dictyostelium discoideum*), mating factor (in yeast), large glycopeptide hormones (such as TSH, LH/hCG, and FSH), and small peptide hormones, including somatostatin, vasopressin, oxytocin, and a rapidly growing number of others (for review, see Refs. 74 to 77).

SPECIFIC MOLECULAR DETERMINANTS

The specific molecular determinants required for PTH/PTHrP-receptor and receptor-G protein interactions are under intense investigation. It will be a difficult task to determine the three-dimensional structures of each of these moieties, and the modifications that occur when they bind each other. Interactions between PTH (and PTHrP) and its receptor(s) are undoubtedly complex, as they occur between ligands that are at least 84 amino acids in length, and highly ordered seven-membrane–spanning receptors consisting of about 590 amino acids. Receptor-transducer interactions are also likely to be very complex because of the myriad of potential interaction sites between these large molecules. Additionally, the cloned, activated PTH/PTHrP receptors all stimulate multiple effectors, including both adenylyl cyclase and phospholipase C, which we have recently shown to be through productive coupling of the receptor to different G proteins (5) (unpublished observation, A. Iida-Klein and G. V. Segre; Fig. 9). This property is shared with at least some other members of this newly discovered receptor family (78–80) and may be common to all of them. It is also a property of activated LH (81) and TSH (82) receptors.

Some of the PTH/PTHrP receptor's ligand-binding domains have been deduced by characterizing the interactions among synthetic PTH and PTHrP fragments and analogues with wild-type and mutant receptors (those with truncations, deletions, and single and clustered substitutions). Additionally, insights have come from studies of these peptides with hybrid receptors. The latter, in which homologous portions of PTH/PTHrP receptors from different species have been exchanged, are particularly powerful because they allow analysis of changes that result in "gain of function" as well as "loss of function." To assess whether a loss-of-function mutation is due to poor or no expression

Figure 7 Analysis of amino acid sequence similarities among the members of this newly discovered G protein–linked receptor family. Sequences were aligned with the GAP program of the Genetics Computer Group (Madison, WI). Solid bars over sequences indicate putative membrane-spanning helices. Among the seven receptors, blackened amino acids are identical and shaded amino acids are similar. (+) indicates conserved cysteine residues; (·) indicate gaps in the sequence. (From Ref. 109.)

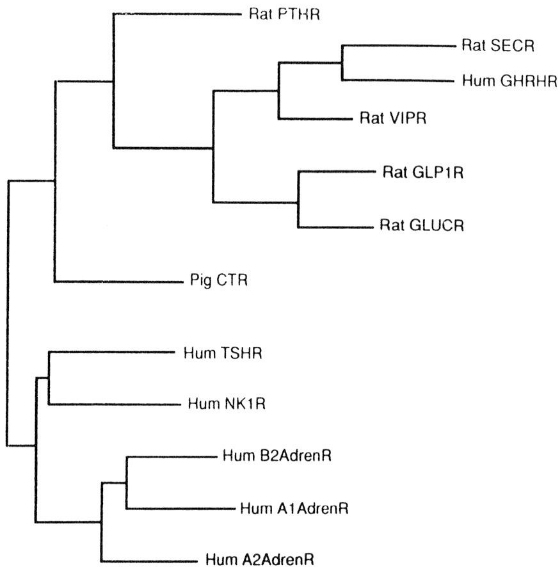

Figure 8 Plausible phylogeny of the G protein–receptor superfamily. The upper portion depicts the seven receptor members of this newly discovered receptor family. Hum TSHR, Hum NK1R, Hum B2AdrenR, Hum A1AdrenR, and Hum A2AdrenR refer to the human homologues of receptors for thyroid stimulating hormone, neurokinen 1, and B2, A1, and A2 adrenergic compounds. (From Ref. 109.)

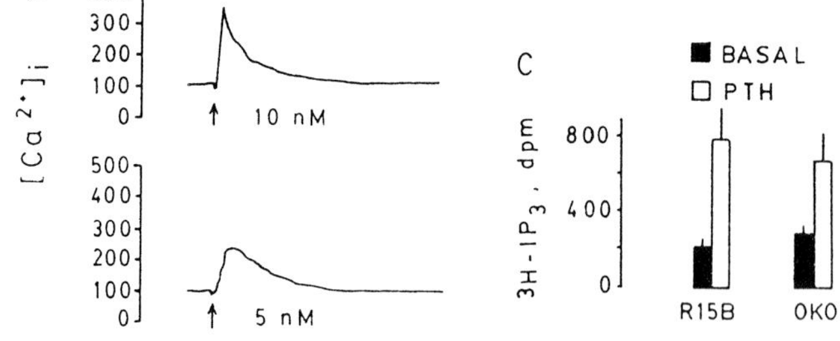

Figure 9 PTH- and PTHrP-stimulated increases of intracellular free $[Ca^{2+}]$ transients and total inositol phosphate production in COS-7 cells transiently expressing either the rat or opossum PTH/PTHrP receptors. Increases in intracellular free $[Ca^{2+}]$ or the rate of inositol phosphate hydrolysis stimulated by either PTH (1-34) amide or PTHrP (1-36) amide were measured in COS-7 cells expressing either the rat or opossum PTH/PTHrP receptor. (*A*) Effects of PTH (1-34) amide (5, 10, 100 n*M*) on intracellular free $[Ca^{2+}]$ in COS-7 cells expressing the rat receptor. (*B*) Effects of PTHrP (1-36) (100 n*M*) on intracellular free $[Ca^{2+}]$ in COS-7 cells expressing either the rat or opossum receptor. (*C*) Stimulation of total inositol phosphate production (60 sec, 37°C, 5 m*M* LiCl) by PTH (1-34) amide in COS-7 cells expressing either rat or opossum receptors. (From Ref. 5.)

or is the result of altered binding or signal transduction from a well-expressed receptor, an epitope such as a short DNA sequence encoding a portion of the MYC protein was incorporated into the receptor's amino-terminal extracellular region.

Some of the extracellular regions are required for ligand binding, but not all of them. Receptors with deletions of many segments of the amino-terminal extracellular extension either fail to be expressed and/or fail to bind. However, receptors in which 45 amino acids of the amino-terminal region (the portion encoded by the E-2 exon, see below) was deleted are fully expressed, bind well, and activate adenylyl cyclase. Through use of discrepancies in binding of amino-terminal fragments to PTH/PTHrP receptors from different species and to chimeric receptors between these different PTH receptors, the receptor's amino-terminal extracellular domain has been shown to largely determine binding specificity and affinity for amino-terminally truncated forms of PTH (1–34), such as PTH (7–34) and PTH (15–34,119). Recent studies have also shown that residues near the amino-terminus of the receptor and within the third extracellular loop are necessary for ligand binding. Receptors in which any one of the five cysteines in the PTH/PTHrP receptor's amino-terminal extension (excluding the two in the signal peptide) are mutated are not expressed. Mutating the first cysteine residue in the amino-terminal portion or either cysteine residue in the putative first or second extracellular loop markedly lowers expression. Proper processing, folding, and membrane insertion of the receptor appear to rely on the integrity of these cysteine residues (83–85). These data complement and extend the previous report that showed complete loss of ligand binding with treatment of renal plasma membranes with reducing agents, suggesting that the PTH receptor's functional integrity requires intact cysteine bonds (37).

The PTH/PTHrP receptor's membrane-spanning helices, which are strongly conserved across species, are clearly essential for signal transduction across the cell's plasma membrane. Analyses of mutant and chimeric PTH/PTHrP receptors have generated a partial map of the receptor's ligand-binding domains and have partially distinguished them from determinants required to induce an "active" receptor conformation, one that allows the receptor to couple productively with G proteins. Extensive studies with chimeric receptors and an analogue of PTH,[Arg^2]PTH (1–34), have pointed to three discrete sites in the fifth and sixth transmembrane segments that are crucial for ligand binding and coupling to Gs (120). As with other hormones and their G protein–linked receptors (74), distinct amino acids and/or portions of the PTH/PTHrP receptor's membrane-spanning helices are critical for PTH binding and receptor activation. From these initial structure/function studies, it is clear that multiple receptor regions are involved both in ligand binding and receptor activation; the former requires at least portions of the amino-terminal extracellular region and the third extracellular loop and/or adjacent membrane-spanning regions, while the latter appears to require regions of the receptor that reside within portions of the fifth and sixth membrane-spanning helices, putatively near its extracellular face (84,85).

Epitope-tagged PTH/PTHrP receptors, also, have been used to define the PTH/PTHrP receptor's general topographical features. Most of the PTH/PTHrP receptor's extracellular and intracellular assignments that had been predicted from computer algorithms of its hydrophobic and hydrophilic amino acids have been determined experimentally, by inserting the epitope into stretches of DNA encoding the many putative extracellular and intracellular regions, expressing these modified sequences, and then reacting the cells with labeled second antiserum with or without permeabilizing the cells with detergent. Definitive data concerning positioning of all the loops is not available, because mutant constructs containing the epitope inserted into all the putative loop regions were not expressed (personal communication, A-B. Abou-Samra).

The activated PTH/PTHrP receptor's capacity to stimulate multiple second-messenger pathways, which was initially reported with COS-7 cells transiently expressing them, has recently been confirmed and extended by studies with stably transfected LLC-PK_1 cells. These porcine cells lack endogenous PTH/PTHrP receptors but express abundant calcitonin receptors and have many biological features indicating that they originated from proximal renal tubular epithelial cells. Subclones of LLC-PK_1 cells expressing either the rat or opossum receptor exhibited high affinity PTH binding and dose-dependent activation by PTH of both cAMP accumulation and increased release of cytosolic [Ca^{2+}] from intracellular stores. The EC_{50} of the cAMP response was 20- to 50-fold lower, however, than the intracellular [Ca^{2+}] response. As with calcitonin treatment of these cells, PTH reduced the rate of cell proliferation and augmented the rate of inorganic phosphate transport. The effect on cell growth was mimicked by cAMP analogues, forskolin, phorbol esters, and calcium ionophores. Regulation of phosphate transport, however, was mimicked only by phorbol esters. Thus, cloned PTH/PTHrP receptors stably expressed at near-physiological levels mediate more than one second-messenger response, as they did when transiently expressed at high receptor copy number in COS cells. Modulation of phosphate transport by agonist occupancy of the same receptor also provides strong evidence that activation of pathways other than those dependent on cAMP is relevant to cellular physiology (86).

Scanning mutagenesis of the receptor's putative intracellular regions, which is in its preliminary stages, has defined a few intracellular regions critical for both receptor expression and G protein coupling. Alanine-scanning in the highly conserved putative first intracellular loop—that is, examining the properties of mutant receptors in which each naturally occurring amino-acid is individually replaced with alanine—reduced receptor binding, presumably because these modifications interfere with receptor processing, folding, or membrane insertion (121). Extensive characterization of mutant rat PTH/PTHrP receptors with carboxyl-terminally truncations of 111 and 78 amino acids of the 591 amino acid glycopeptide, R480 and R513, have revealed the tail portion to have several interesting properties. These truncated receptors have identical potencies, as does the wild-type receptor, but they activate adenylyl cyclase with much higher efficacy, although the EC_{50} of this response was not changed. These and other findings suggest that sequences in the carboxyl-terminal portion of the receptor has several important functions. They lower the affinity of the wild-type receptor for agonist (compared with either R480 or R513), contain domains distal to amino acid 513, contain sequences that interact or allow the receptor to interact with a pertussis toxin–sensitive G protein that inhibits adenylyl cyclase, and increase the efficacy with which the receptor couples to Gs (unpublished data, A. Iida Klein and G. V. Segre). Our earlier preliminary studies, suggesting that OK-H, a mutant receptor with a 70 amino acid deletion of its carboxyl-terminal tail, had unimpaired capacity to stimulate adenylyl cyclase and reduced capacity to stimulate phospholipase C, were misinterpreted because we failed to adequately control for efficiency of receptor expression (83,84). We now appreciate the properties of OK-H to be essentially indistinguishable from those of R513, its rat homologue.

Other data from studies of wild-type and mutant receptors that are equally well expressed do not indicate that the tail region is required for activation of phospholipase C. They do suggest, however, that one or more putative intracellular loops are required to stimulate phospholipase C, that different portions of the receptor intracellular regions are involved in activating adenylyl cyclase and phospholipase C, and that regions critical for PTH/PTHrP receptor coupling to transducer molecules are quite likely to differ from those of the adrenergic and muscarinic receptors, the most thoroughly explored models (unpublished data, A. Iida-Klein and G. V. Segre). Clearly, much more work is needed before structural determinants that are responsible for the PTH/PTHrP receptor's ligand-binding and G protein activation are completely understood. Unraveling the specific intermolecular events that occur between the activated PTH/PTHrP receptors and transducer molecules and between activated G proteins and effectors will be a difficult task. These studies must consider the involvement of the PTH/PTHrP receptors with more than one G protein and must take into consideration the complexities among the G protein subunits and multiple effector molecules. For example, the number of G protein α, β, and γ subunits is growing (74,87), as are the number of different adenylyl cyclases (88–90), and there are at least 12 phospholipase-C enzymes that have been classified into four groups (91). Additionally, G protein $\beta\gamma$ complexes act catalytically under certain circumstances (92,93).

PTH/PTHrP receptors with other sequences also may exist, although the renal and osseous receptors thus far cloned in humans and rats are identical within each species. Northern blot analyses show considerable receptor mRNA heterogeneity that appears to be tissue-specific (Fig. 3). Although a common 2.3-kb transcript is expressed in many tissues, larger-sized transcripts are present in the kidney and liver and smaller-sized transcripts in kidney, skin, and testes (63). These alternatively sized mRNAs may represent transcription from multiple genes and/or alternatively processed mRNAs from one or more genes. Whether any of these alternative transcripts are translated remains to be determined.

Most G protein–coupled receptors, however, exist in several receptor subtypes, either as products of different genes or from alternative splicing of their mRNAs; multiple adrenergic (94), dopaminergic (95–97), muscarinic (98), serotoninergic (99,100), vasopressin (101,102), and angiotensin II (103–106) receptor subtypes are encoded by more than one gene, and alternatively spliced receptors have been reported for LH/hCG (107,108) and dopamine (109) receptors. Receptor subtypes often can provide functional and tissue specificity in complex hormonal systems. Current data are consistent, however, with only a single receptor: cDNAs cloned from both bone and kidney are the same in both rats and humans; homology is close among rat, human, opossum, and mouse receptors; and there is only one copy of the PTH/PTHrP receptor gene, which has been mapped to the short arm of chromosome 3 (personal communication, H. Heath). Nonetheless, the diversity of PTH- and PTHrP-mediated effects mandates a careful search for multiple PTH/PTHrP receptor subtypes that might mediate these many biological actions.

TISSUE LOCALIZATION OF mRNA ENCODING THE PTH/PTHrP RECEPTOR

The results of studies localizing PTH/PTHrP receptor transcripts by in situ hybridization have raised many provocative issues, particularly concerning the functions of the receptor mRNA in kidney and bone, as well as in other organs. In the rat kidney, PTH/PTHrP receptor transcripts localized to convoluted and straight proximal tubules, the cortical portion of thick ascending limbs and distal convoluted tubules, but not to the thin limbs of Henle's loop or the collecting ducts. Interestingly, there were high levels of receptor mRNA in glomeruli, the distribution of which was consistent with expression in podocytes, rather that mesangial cells (Figs. 10 and 11; K. Lee and G. V. Segre, unpublished observations). Studies with primary and immortalized human visceral epithelial cells and mesangial cells confirmed the presence of PTH/PTHrP receptors in podocytes. These receptors, however, bind amino-terminal analogues of PTHrP more effectively that PTH, and, when treated with PTHrP, they increase intracellular [Ca^{2+}] but not cAMP. Additionally, Northern blot analysis reveals that these cells express a 4.0-kb receptor transcript, which is quite distinct from the 2.4-kb transcript, the dominant transcript in whole kidney and in most tissues (P. Ureña, personal communication). The function of these receptors in podocytes is at present unknown.

High levels of PTH/PTHrP receptor mRNA were seen in a highly discrete portion of the rat long-bone growth plate, in the lower proliferative and upper hypertrophic chondrocyte layers, in mononuclear cells that line bony trabeculae, in cortical endosteal and periosteal surfaces, and in some marrow stromal cells (21) (Figs. 12 and 13). Histological examination of "PTHrP-less"

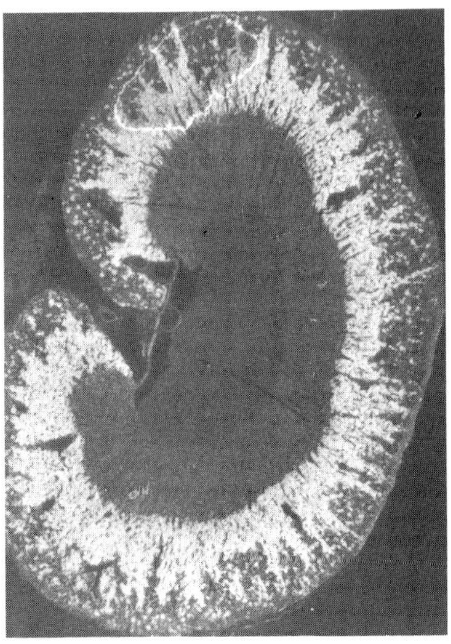

Figure 10 Localization of PTH/PTHrP receptor mRNA in whole rat kidney. Kidney sections from 4-week-old rats were hybridized with ^{35}S-labeled antisense PTH/PTHrP receptor cRNA, and hybridization signals were detected by x-ray autoradiography. A dark-field image is shown.

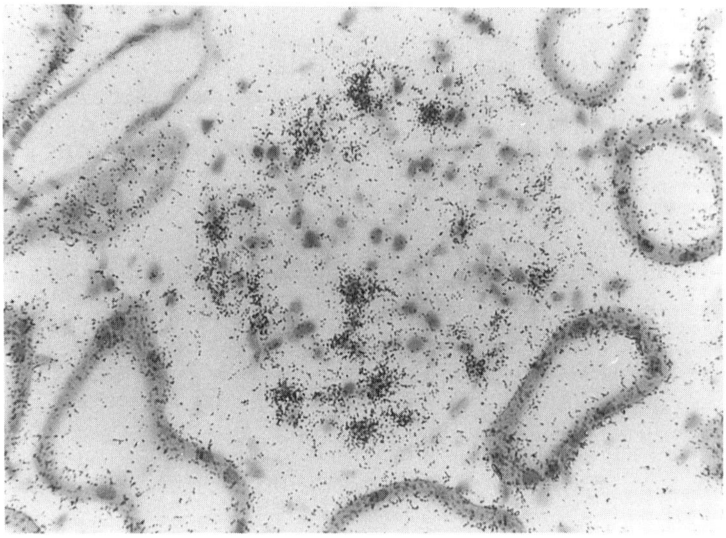

Figure 11 PTH/PTHrP receptor transcripts in the kidney of 4-week-old rats. Paraffin embedded kidney sections from 4-week-old rats were hybridized with ^{35}S-labeled antisense PTH/PTHrP receptor cRNA and hybridization signals were detected by emulsion autoradiography.

mice, who die immediately after birth from yet to be determined causes, show that the PTHrP and its receptor system are critical for normal endochondral bone formation. Homozygous mutants have many skeletal abnormalities, including widespread, premature skeletal mineralization and abnormal chondrocyte development that is most evident in endochondral bone. The mutant animal's deformed long bones are shorter in length and wider than those of normal litter mates and show short, disorganized columns of proliferative growth-plate chondrocytes and distorted remnants of calcified cartilage. In situ hybridization with cRNAs for the PTH/PTHrP receptor, and several chondrocyte and bone cell marker RNAs show that the layer of less differentiated, receptor-negative chondrocytes in the growth plate that express type II collagen to be dramatically reduced, but that the thickness of the hypertrophic chondrocyte layer containing cells that express both type II and X collagen to be normal (Fig. 13). Since cells that do not express PTH/PTHrP receptor mRNA show the most obvious abnormalities, these morphological data suggest that the development of these receptor-negative cells may be regulated directly or indirectly by adjacent chondrocytes that express receptors and thus can respond to PTHrP (110,111). Additionally, the widely distributed PTH/PTHrP receptor mRNA expression in many organs other than bone and cartilage (Fig. 14) suggests that activated PTH/PTHrP receptors have more general and critical roles in embryogenesis.

THE PTH/PTHrP RECEPTOR GENE

The organization of PTH/PTHrP receptor gene is quite distinct from that of the genes of other G protein–linked receptor families. The structure of PTH/PTHrP receptor genes from rat, mouse, and human has been partially determined. The genes in all three are very similar; they extend over 22 kb and contain at least 15 exons and 14 introns. The most 5′ exon thus far detected is upstream from the initiator methionine, the amino-terminal extracellular domain is encoded by four exons, membrane-spanning helices 1 to 4 and portions of their connecting extracellular and intracellular sequences are encoded by 4 exons, while the second extracellular loop and portions of the fourth and fifth membrane-spanning domains are encoded by one exon. The fifth membrane-spanning domain and a portion of third intracellular loop, the sixth and part of the seventh membrane-spanning helices and the intervening third extracellular region, the remaining portion of the seventh

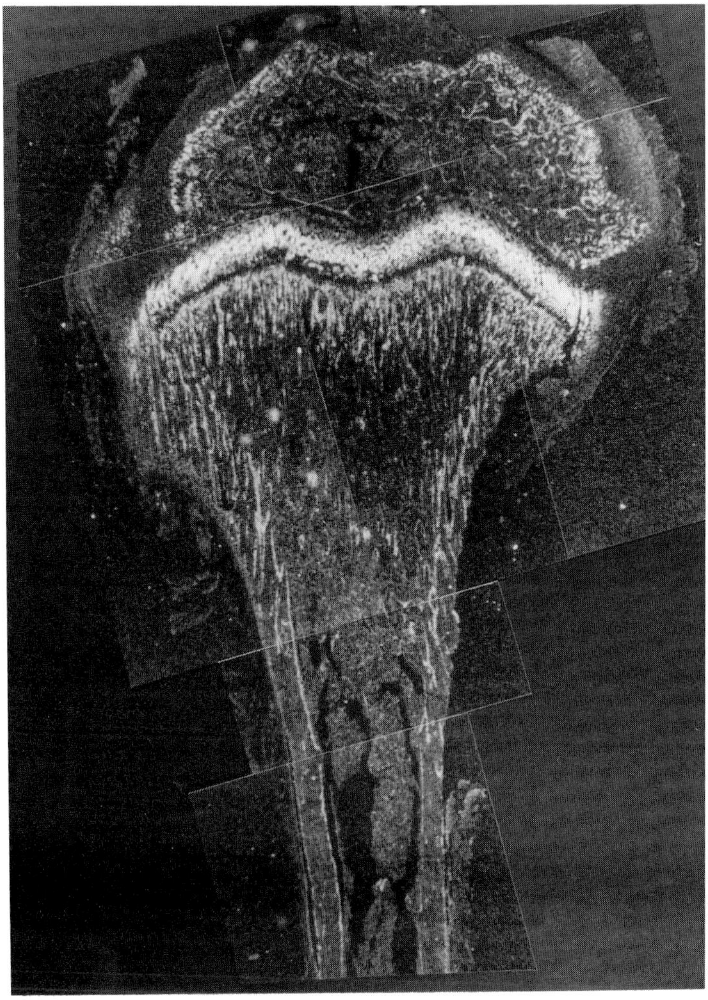

Figure 12 PTH/PTHrP receptor mRNA expression in the tibia of a 4-week-old rat. Paraffin sections of tibias from 4-week-old rats were hybridized with ^{35}S-labeled antisense PTH/PTHrP receptor cRNA, and hybridization signals were detected by emulsion autoradiography. Overlapping dark-field images of the proximal portion of the tibia are shown. The bar represents 1 mm. (From Ref. 106.)

membrane-spanning region, and the carboxy-terminal tail and the 3′-untranslated region, each are encoded by separate exons. Interestingly, the 3′ untranslated region does not contain a classic polyadenylation signal. Many exons are quite short and intronic sequences range considerably in size, with some at short as a 100 base pairs (122) (Fig. 15). This organization differs from those of other members of the G protein–coupled receptor superfamily. Adrenergic receptors and many other related receptors, for example, are intronless. Both PTH/PTHrP and adrenergic receptor genes are organized differently from the receptors for the glycoprotein hormones TSH, FSH, and LH, which have multiple introns in the portions of their genes that encode their amino-terminal extracellular extensions but have only a single exon that encodes their membrane-spanning helices (74). The PTH/PTHrP receptor gene's novel and complex organization will require considerable effort to understand. The presence of relatively short intronic/exonic sequences obviously complicates analysis of the receptor mRNAs because splicing variants may yield multiple transcripts of similar lengths but containing different sequences.

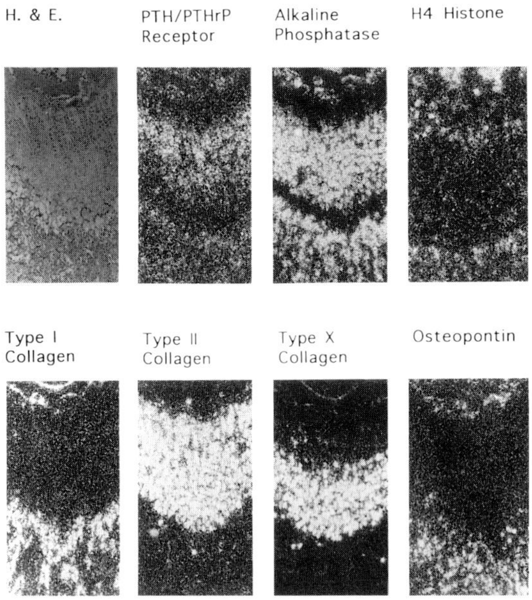

Figure 13 Localization of various osseous cell "marker" mRNAs in the growth plate of the 4-week-old rat tibia. Sequential paraffin-embedded sections of a 4-week-old rat tibia were hybridized with ^{35}S-labeled antisense cRNAs for the various proteins. Dark-field views of hybridized sections are shown with a hematoxylin and eosin staining of the section hybridized with PTH/PTHrP receptor cRNA (H&E). The bar represents 250 μm. (From Ref. 106.)

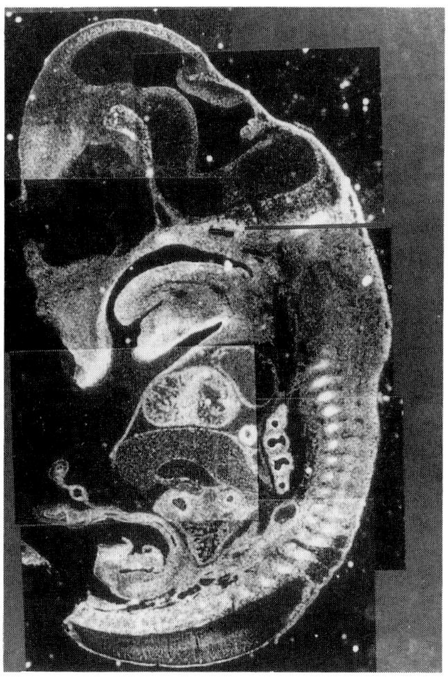

Figure 14 Expression of PTH/PTHrP receptor mRNA in 15-day-old rat fetus. Midline paraffin sections of a 15-day-old rat fetus were hybridized with ^{35}S-labeled antisense PTH/PTHrP receptor cRNA, and hybridization signals were detected by emulsion autoradiography. Note extensive expression in many organs and tissues, which is most intense in vertebrae, skin, bowel walls, heart, and tooth bud. Overlapping dark-field images of the whole fetus are shown.

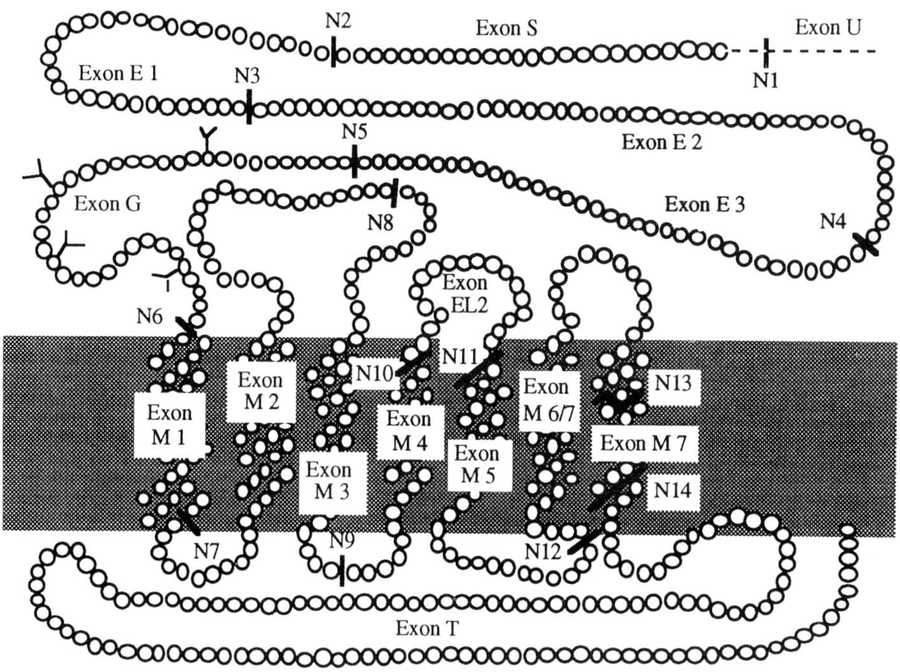

Figure 15 Schematic representation of the rat PTH/PTHrP receptor gene. The rat PTH/PTHrP receptor gene is highly complex with 14 exons encoding the receptor protein and an additional two exons in the 5′ upstream portion of the gene.

CONCLUSION

Future experiments will define the functional characteristics that are determined by the many novel structural features of this PTH/PTHrP receptor, as well as the properties that are associated with its complex gene organization. These studies will broaden our understanding of this particular receptor, its roles in kidney physiology and bone development, in calcium homeostasis and embryogenesis, and in the physiology and development of other tissue and organs in which receptor transcripts are widely distributed after birth. Additionally, defining the properties of PTH/PTHrP receptors will contribute to knowledge concerning this newly discovered G protein–linked receptor family and the evolutionary and functional relationships among its members.

ACKNOWLEDGMENTS

Portions of this chapter previously appeared in Chapter 14, *The Parathyroids: Basic and Clinical Concepts*, JP Bilezikian, R Marcus, and MA Levine, eds. Raven Press, NY 1994. They are reprinted here with permission. I am grateful to A-B. Abou-Samra, T. Gardella, A. Iida-Klein, H. Jüppner, P. Ureña, L. F. Kolakowski, Jr., H. M. Kronenberg, C. W. Lee, and K. Lee for sharing unpublished data and their figures. This work was supported in part by NIH Grants DK-11794, DK-47034, and DK 47237.

REFERENCES

1. Rosenblatt M, Kronenberg HM, Potts JT Jr. Parathyroid hormone physiology, chemistry, biosynthesis, secretion, metabolism and mode of action. In: DeGroot LJ, ed. Endocrinology. Vol. II. Philadelphia: Saunders, 1989:848–891.
2. Chase LR, Aurbach GD. Parathyroid function and the renal secretion of 3′,5′-adenylic acid. Proc Natl Acad Sci USA 1967; 58:518–525.

3. Marcus R, Aurbach GD. Bioassay of parathyroid hormone in vitro in a stable preparation of adenyl cyclase from rat kidney. Endocrinology 1969; 85:801–810.
4. Rodan SB, Rodan GA. The effect of parathyroid hormone and thyrocalcitonin on the accumulation of cyclic 3′-5′-monophospate in freshly isolated bone cells. J Biol Chem 1974; 249:3068–3074.
5. Abou-Samra AB, Jüppner H, Force T, et al. Expression cloning of a common receptor for parathyroid hormone and parathyroid hormone-related peptide from rat osteoblast-like cells: A single receptor stimulates intracellular accumulation of both cAMP and inositol trisphosphates and increases intracellular free calcium. Proc Natl Acad Sci USA 1992; 89:2732–2736.
6. Civitelli R, Fujimori A, Bernier SM, et al. Heterogeneous intracellular free calcium responses to parathyroid hormone correlate with morphology and receptor distribution in osteogenic sarcoma cells. Endocrinology 1992; 130:2392–2400.
7. Dunlay R, Hruska K. PTH receptor coupling to phospholipase C is an alternate pathway of signal transduction in bone and kidney. Am J Physiol 1990; 258:F223–F231.
8. Rappaport MS, Stern PH. Parathyroid hormone and calcitonin modify phospholipid metabolism in fetal rat limb bones. J Bone Min Res 1986; 2:173–179.
9. Cosman F, Morrow B, Kopal M, Bilezikian JP. Stimulation of inositol phosphate formation in ROS 17/2.8 cell membranes by guanine nucleotide, calcium and parathyroid hormone. J Bone Min Res 1989; 4:413–420.
10. Yamaguchi TD, Hahn TJ, Iida-Klein A, et al. Parathyroid hormone–activated calcium channels in an osteoblast-like clonal osteosarcoma cell line—cAMP independent calcium channels. J Biol Chem 1987; 262:7711–7718.
11. Donahue HJ, Fryer MJ, Eriksen EF, Heath H. Differential effects of parathyroid hormone and its analogues on cytosolic calcium ion and cAMP levels in cultured osteoblast-like cells. J Biol Chem 1988; 263:13522–13527.
12. Feyen JHM, van der Wilt G, Moonen P, et al. Stimulation of arachidonic acid metabolism in primary cultures of osteoblast-like cells by hormones and drugs. Prostaglandins 1984; 28:769–781.
13. MacDonald BR, Gallagher JA, Ahnfelt-Ronne I, et al. Effects of bovine parathyroid hormone and 1,25-dihydroxyvitamin D on the production of prostaglandins by cells derived from human bone. FEBS Lett 1984; 169:49–52.
14. Goldring SR, Tyler GA, Krane SM, et al. Photoaffinity labeling of parathyroid hormone receptors: Comparison of receptors across species and target tissues and after desensitization to hormone. Biochemistry 1984; 23:498–502.
15. Yamamoto I, Potts JT Jr, Segre GV. Circulating bovine lymphocytes contain receptors for parathyroid hormone. J Clin Invest 1983; 71:404–407.
16. Enomoto M, Kinashita A, Pan HO, et al. Demonstration of receptors for parathyroid hormone on cultured rabbit costal chondrocytes. Biochem Biophys Res Commun 1989; 162:1222–1229.
17. Mok LL, Nickols GA, Thompson JC, Cooper CW. Parathyroid hormone as a smooth muscle relaxer. Endocr Rev 1989; 10:420–436.
18. Taniguchi A, Kataoka K, Kono T, et al. Parathyroid hormone-induced lipolysis in human adipose tissue. J Lipid Res 1987; 28:490–494.
19. Lafond J, Auger D, Fortier J, Brunetta MG. Parathyroid hormone receptor in human syncytotrophoblast brush border and basal plasma membranes. Endocrinology 1988; 123:2834–2840.
20. McSheehy PMJ, Chambers TJ. Osteoblastic cells mediate osteoclastic responsiveness to parathyroid hormone. Endocrinology 1986; 118:824–828.
21. Lee K, Deeds JD, Chiba S, et al. Parathyroid hormone induces sequential c-fos expression in bone cells in vivo: In situ localization of its receptor and c-fos mRNAs. Endocrinology 1994; 134:441–450.
22. Rao LG, Murray TM. Binding of intact parathyroid hormone to rat osteosarcoma cells: Major contribution of binding sites for the carboxyl-terminal region of the hormone. Endocrinology 1985; 117:1632–1638.
23. McKee MD, Murray TM. Binding of intact parathyroid hormone to chicken renal membranes: Evidence for a second binding site with carboxyl-terminal specificity. Endocrinology 1985; 117:1930–1939.
24. Suva LJ, Winslow GA, Wettenhall RE, et al. A parathyroid hormone–related protein implicated in malignant hypercalcemia: Cloning and expression. Science 1987; 237:893–896.
25. Strewler GJ, Stern PH, Jacobs JW, et al. Parathyroid hormone–like protein from human renal carcinoma cells. Structural and functional homology with parathyroid hormone. J Clin Invest 1987; 80:1803–1807.
26. Mangin M, Webb AC, Dreyer BE, et al. Identification of a cDNA encoding a parathyroid hormone–like peptide from a human tumor associated with humoral hypercalcemia of malignancy. Proc Natl Acad Sci USA 1988; 85:597–601.
27. Burtis WJ, Brady TG, Orloff JJ, et al. Immunochemical characterization of circulating PTHrP in patients with humeral hypercalcemia of malignancy. N Engl J Med 1990; 322:1106–1112.
28. Pandian MR, Morgan CH, Carlton E, Segre GV. Modified immunoradiometric assay of PTHrP: Clinical application in the differential diagnosis of hypercalcemia. Clin Chem 1992; 28:282–288.

29. Mangin M, Ikeda K, Dreyer B, Broadus AE. Isolation and characterization of the human PTH-like peptide gene. Proc Natl Acad Sci USA 1989; 86:2408–2412.
30. Orloff JJ, Wu TL, Stewart AF. Parathyroid hormone-like protein: biochemical responses and receptor interactions. Endocr Rev 1989; 10:476–495.
31. Karaplis AC, Luz A, Glowacki J, Bronson RT, Tybulewicz VLJ, Kronenberg HM, Mulligan RC. Lethal skeletal dysplasia from targeted disruption of the parathyroid hormone-related peptide gene. Genes Dev 1994; 8:277–289.
32. van de Stolpe A, Karperien M, Lowik CWGM, et al. Parathyroid hormone–related peptide as an endogenous inducer of parietal endoderm differentiation. J Cell Biol 1993; 120:235–243.
33. Martin TJ, Moseley JM, Gillespie MT. Parathyroid hormone–related protein, biochemistry and molecular biology. Crit Rev Biochem Mol Biol 1991; 26:377–395.
34. Yamamoto I, Shigeno C, Potts JT Jr, Segre GV. Characterization and agonist-induced down-regulation of parathyroid hormone receptors in clonal rat osteosarcoma cells. Endocrinology 1988; 122:1208–1217.
35. Segre GV, Rosenblatt M, Reiner BL, et al. Characterization of parathyroid hormone receptors in canine renal critical plasma membranes using a radioiodinated sulfin-free hormone analogue: Correlation of binding with adenylate cyclase activity. J Biol Chem 1979; 254:6980–6986.
36. Nissenson RA, Arnaud CD. Properties of the parathyroid hormone receptor-adenylate cyclase system in chicken renal plasma membranes. J Biol Chem 1979; 254:1469–1475.
37. Teitelbaum AP, Nissenson RA, Arnanud CD. Coupling of the canine renal parathyroid hormone receptor to adenylate cyclase: Modulation by guanyl nucleotides and *N*-ethylmaleimide. Endocrinology 1982; 111:1524–1533.
38. Mahoney CA, Nissenson RA. Canine renal receptors for parathyroid hormone: Downregulation in vivo by exogenous parathyroid hormone. J Clin Invest 1983; 72:411–421.
39. Forte LR, Langeluttig SG, Foelling RE, Thomas ML. Renal parathyroid hormone receptors in the chick: Downregulation in secondary hyperparathyroid animal models. Am J Physiol 1982; 243:E154–E163.
40. Quarles LD, Lobaugh B, Murphy G. Intact parathyroid hormone overestimates the presence and severity of parathyroid-mediated osseous abnormalities in uremia. J Clin Endocrinol Metab 1992; 75:145–150.
41. Pun KK, Ho PWM, Nissenson RA, Arnaud CD. Desensitization of parathyroid hormone receptors on cultured bone cells. J Bone Min Res 1990; 5:1193–1200.
42. Mitchell J, Goltzman D. Mechanisms of homologous and heterologous regulation of parathyroid hormone receptors in the rat osteosarcoma cell line UMR-106. Endocrinology 1990; 126:2650–2660.
43. Hanai H, Brennan DP, Cheng L, et al. Downregulation of parathyroid hormone receptors in renal membranes from aged rats. Am J Physiol 1990; 259:F444–F450.
44. Ikeda K, Sugimoto T, Fukase M, Fujita T. Protein kinase C is involved in PTH-induced homologous desensitization by directly affecting PTH receptor in the osteoblastic osteosarcoma cells. Endocrinology 1991; 128:2901–2906.
45. Abou-Samra AB, Zajac JD, Schiffer AD, et al. Cyclic adenosine 3′,5′-monophosphate (cAMP)-dependent and cAMP-independent regulation of parathyroid hormone receptors on UMR 106-01 osteoblastic osteosarcoma cells. Endocrinology 1991; 129:2547–2554.
46. Ureña P, Iida-Klein A, Kong XF, et al. Regulation of parathyroid hormone (PTH)/PTH-related peptide receptor mRNA by glucocorticoids and PTH in ROS 17/2.8 and OK cells. Endocrinology 1994; 134:451–456.
47. Teitelbaum AP, Silve CM, Nyiredy KO, Arnaud CD. Down-regulation of parathyroid hormone (PTH) receptors in cultured bone cells is associated with agonist-specific intracellular processing of PTH-receptor complexes. Endocrinology 1986; 118:595–602.
48. Yamamoto I, Potts JT Jr, Segre GV. Glucocorticoids increase parathyroid hormone receptors in osteoblastic osteosarcoma cells (ROS 17/2). J Bone Min Res 1988; 3:707–712.
49. Teitelbaum AP, Stewler GJ. Parathyroid hormone receptors couple to cyclic adenosine monophosphate in an established renal cell line. Endocrinology 1984; 114:980–985.
50. Schneider HG, Allan EH, Moseley JM, et al. Specific down-regulation of parathyroid hormone (PTH) receptors and responses to PTH by tumour necrosis factor alpha and retinoic acid in UMR 106-06 osteoblast-like osteosarcoma cells. Biochem J 1991; 280:451–457.
51. Titus L, Jackson E, Nanes MS, et al. 1,25-dihydroxyvitamin D reduces parathyroid hormone receptor number in ROS 17/2.8 cells and prevents the glucocorticoid-induced increase in these receptors: Relationship to adenylate cyclase activation. J Bone Min Res 1991; 6:631–637.
52. Karpf DB, Arnaud CD, King K, et al. The canine renal parathyroid hormone receptor is a glycoprotein: Characterization and partial purification. Biochemistry 1987; 26:7825–7833.
53. Shigeno C, Hiraki Y, Westerberg DP, et al. Parathyroid hormone receptors are plasma membrane glycoproteins with asparagine-linked oligosaccharides. J Biol Chem 1988; 263:3872–3878.
54. Shigeno C, Hiraki Y, Westerberg DP, et al. Photoaffinity labeling of parathyroid hormone receptors in clonal rat osteosarcoma cells. J Biol Chem 1988; 263:3864–3871.

55. Karpf DB, Arnaud CD, Bambino T, et al. Structure properties of the renal parathyroid hormone receptor: Hydrodynamic analysis and protease sensitivity. Endocrinology 1988; 123:2611–2619.
56. Shigeno C, Hiraki Y, Stern AM, et al. Preparation of a photoactive analog of parathyroid hormone, [Nl3^{8}, Lys(N-ϵ-4-azido-2-nitrophenyl)^{13}Nle^{18}, Tyr^{34}] bovine parathyroid hormone-(1-34)NH2, a selective, high-affinity ligand for characterization of parathyroid hormone receptors. Anal Biochem 1989; 179:268–273.
57. Jüppner H, Abou-Samra AB, Uneno S, et al. Preparation and characterization of [Nα-(4-azido-2 nitrophenyl)Ala^{1}Tyr^{36}] parathyroid hormone-related peptide (1-36) amide: A high affinity, partial agonis having high cross-linking efficiency with its receptors on ROS 17/2.8 cells. Biochemistry 1990; 29:6941–6946.
58. Jüppner H, Abou-Samra AB, Uneno S, et al. Properties of amino-terminal parathyroid hormone-related peptides modified at positions 11-13. Peptides 1990; 11:1139–1142.
59. Nissenson RA, Diep D, Strewler GJ. Synthetic peptides comprising the amino-terminal sequence of a parathyroid hormone-like protein from human malignancies: Binding to parathyroid hormone receptors and activation cyclase in bone cells and kidney. J Biol Chem 1988; 263:12866–12871.
60. Jüppner H, Abou-Samra AB, Uneno S, et al. The parathyroid hormone-like peptide associated with humoral hypercalcemia of malignancy and parathyroid hormone bind to the same receptor on the plasma membrane of ROS 17/2.8 cells. J Biol Chem 1988; 263:8557–8560.
61. Jüppner H, Abou-Samra AB, Freeman M, et al. A G protein-linked receptor for parathyroid hormone and parathyroid hormone-related peptide. Science 1991; 254:1024–1026.
62. Schipani E, Karga H, Karaplis AC, et al. Identical cDNAs encode a human renal and bone parathyroid hormone/parathyroid hormone-related peptide receptor. Endocrinology 1993; 132:2157–2165.
63. Urena P, Kong XF, Abou-Samra AB, et al. Parathyroid hormone (PTH)/PTH-related peptide (PTHrP) receptor mRNA is widely distributed in rat tissues. Endocrinology 1993; 133:617–623.
64. Gearing DP, King JA, Gough NM, Nicola NA. Expression cloning of a receptor for human granulocyte-macrophage colony-stimulating factor. EMBO J 1989; 8:3667–3676.
65. Seed B, Aruffo A. Molecular cloning of the CD2 antigen, the T-cell erythrocyte receptor by a rapid immunoselection procedure. Proc Natl Acad Sci USA 1987; 84:3365–3369.
66. Ishihara T, Nakamura S, Kaziro Y, et al. Molecular cloning and expression of a cDNA encoding the secretin receptor. EMBO J 1991; 7:1635–1641.
67. Lin HY, Harris TL, Flannery MS, et al. Expression cloning of an adenylate cyclase–coupled calcitonin receptor. Science 1991; 254:1022–1024.
68. Ishihara T, Shigemoto R, Mori K, et al. Functional expression and tissue distribution of a novel receptor for vasoactive intestinal polypeptide. Neuron 1992; 8:811–819.
69. Thorens B. Expression cloning of a pancreatic β cell receptor for the gluco-incretin hormone, glucagon-like peptide 1. Proc Natl Acad Sci USA 1992; 89:8641–8645.
70. Jelinek LJ, Lok S, Rosenberg GB, et al. Expression cloning and signalling properties of the rat glucagon receptor. Science 1993; 259:1614–1616.
71. Mayo KE. Molecular cloning and expression of a pituitary-specific receptor for growth hormone-releasing hormone. Mol Endocrinol 1992; 6:1734–1744.
72. Attwood TK, Eliopoulos EE, Findlay JB. Multiple sequence alignment of protein families showing low sequence homology: A methodological approach using database pattern-matching discriminators for G-protein-linked receptors. Gene 1991; 98:153–159.
73. Probst WC, Snyder LA, Schuster DI, et al. Sequence alignment of the G-protein coupled receptor superfamily. DNA Cell Biol 1992; 11:1–20.
74. Dohlman HG, Thorner J, Caron MG, Lefkowitz RJ. Model systems for the study of seven-transmembrane-segment receptors. Annu Rev Biochem 1991; 60:653–688.
75. Reed RR. Signaling pathways in odorant detection. Neuron 1992; 8:205–209.
76. O'Dowd BF, Lefkowitz RJ, Caron MG. Structure of the adrenergic and related receptors. Annu Rev Neurosci 1989; 12:67–83.
77. Segre GV, Goldring SR. Receptors for secretin, calcitonin, parathyroid hormone (PTH)/PTH-related peptide, vasoactive intestinal peptide, glucagon-like peptide 1, growth hormone-releasing hormone, and glucagon belong to a newly discovered G protein-linked receptor family. Trends Endocrinol Metab 1993; 4:309–314.
78. Chabre O, Conklin BR, Lin HY, et al. A recombinant calcitonin receptor independently stimulates cAMP and calcium/inositol phosphate signalling pathways. Mol Endocrinol 1992; 6:551–556.
79. Force T, Bonventre JV, Flannery MR, et al. A cloned porcine renal calcitonin receptor couples to adenyl cyclase and phospholipase C. Am J Physiol 1992; 262:F1110–F1115.
80. Wheeler MB, Lu M, Dillon JS, et al. Functional expression of the rat glucagon-like peptide-I receptor, evidence for coupling to both adenylyl cyclase and phospholipase-C. Endocrinology 1993; 133:57–62.
81. Gudermann T, Nichols C, Levy FO, et al. Calcium mobilization by the LH receptor expressed in xenopus oocytes independent of cAMP formation: Evidence for parallel activation of two signalling pathways. Mol Endocrinol 1992; 6:272–278.

82. Sande JV, Raspe E, Lejeune PC, et al. Thyrotropin activates both the cyclic AMP and the PIP2 cascades in CHO cells expressing the human cDNA of TSH receptor. Mol Cell Endocrinol 1990; 74:R1–R6.
83. Kronenberg HM, Abou-Samra AB, Jüppner H, et al. Characterization of a receptor that binds both PTH and PTHrP. In: Cohn DV, Gennari C, Tashjian AH Jr, ed. Proceedings of the XIth International Conference on Calcium Regulating Hormones, Florence, Italy. Amsterdam: Elsevier Science Publishers BV, 1992:79–82.
84. Segre GV, Abou-Samra AB, Gardella TJ, et al. Structural analysis of the PTH/PTHrP receptor's functional domains. In: Cohn DV, Gennari C, Tashjian AH Jr., eds. Proceedings of the XIth International Conference on Calcium Regulating Hormones, Florence, Italy, Amsterdam: Elsevier Science Publishers BV, 1992: 92–96.
85. Lee CW, Gardella TJ, Abou-Samra AB, et al. Role of the extracellular regions of the PTH/PTHrP receptor in hormone binding. Endocrinology 1994; 135:1488–1495.
86. Bringhurst FR, Jüppner H, Guo J, et al. Cloned, stably expressed parathyroid hormone (PTH)/PTH-related peptide receptors activate multiple messenger signals and biologic responses in LLC-PK1 kidney cells. Endocrinology 1993; 132:2090–2098.
87. Simon MI, Strathmann MP, Gautam N. Diversity of G proteins in signal transduction. Science 1991; 252:802–808.
88. Tang WJ, Gilman AG. Type-specific regulation of adenylyl cyclase by G protein beta gamma subunits. Science 1991; 254:1500–1503.
89. Tang WJ, Krupinski J, Gilman AG. Expression and characterization of calmodulin-activated (type I) adenylyl cyclase. J Biol Chem 1991; 266:8595–8603.
90. Tang WJ, Gilman AG. Adenylyl cyclases. Cell 1992; 70:869–872.
91. Rhee SG, Ryu SH, Lee KY, Cho KS. Assays of phosphoinositide-specific phospholipase C and different modes of activation. Methods Enzymol 1991; 197:502–511.
92. Birmbaumer L. Receptor-to-effector signalling through G proteins: Roles for beta-gamma dimers as well as alpha subunits. Cell 1992; 71:1069–1072.
93. Federman AD, Conklin BR, Schrader KA, et al. Hormonal stimulation of adenylyl cyclase through Gi-protein beta gamma subunits. Nature 1992; 356:159–161.
94. Bylund DB. Subtypes of alpha 1- and alpha 2-adrenergic receptors. FASEB J 1992; 6:832–839.
95. Monsma FJ Jr, Mahan LC, McVittie LD, et al. Molecular cloning and expression of a D1 dopamine receptor linked to adenylyl cyclase activation. Proc Natl Acad Sci USA 1990; 87:6723–6727.
96. Van THH, Bunzow R, Guan HC, et al. Cloning of the gene for a human dopamine D4 receptor with high affinity for the antipsychotic clozapine. Nature 1991; 350:610–614.
97. Weinshank RL, Adham N, Macchi M, et al. Molecular cloning and characterization of a high affinity dopamine receptor (D1 beta) and its pseudogene. J Biol Chem 1991; 266:22427–22435.
98. Bonner TI, Buckley NJ, Young AC, Brann MR. Identification of a family of muscarinic acetylcholine receptor genes. Science 1987; 237:527–532.
99. Levy FO, Gudermann T, Birnbaumer M, et al. Molecular cloning of a human gene (S31) encoding a novel serotonin receptor mediating inhibition of adenylyl cyclase. FEBS Lett 1992; 296:201–206.
100. Saudou F, Boschert U, Amlaiky N, et al. A family of Drosophila serotonin receptors with distinct intracellular signalling properties and expression patterns. EMBO J 1992; 11:7–17.
101. Lolait SJ, O'Caroll AM, McBride OW, et al. Cloning and characterization of a vasopressin V2 receptor and possible link to nephrogenic diabetes insipidus. Nature 1992; 357:336–339.
102. Birnbaumer M, Seibold A, Gilbert S, et al. Molecular cloning of the receptor for human antidiuretic hormone. Nature 1992; 357:333–335.
103. Takayanagi R, Ohnaka K, Sakai Y, et al. Molecular cloning, sequence analysis and expression of a cDNA encoding human type-1 angiotensin II receptor. Biochem Biophys Res Commun 1992; 183:910–916.
104. Sasaki K, Yamano Y, Bardhan S, et al. Cloning and expression of a complementary DNA encoding a bovine adrenal angiotensin II type-1 receptor. Nature 1991; 351:230–233.
105. Murphy TJ, Alexander RW, Griendling KK, et al. Isolation of a cDNA encoding the vascular type-1 angiotensin II receptor. Nature 1991; 351:233–236.
106. Iwai N, Yamano Y, Chaki S, et al. Rat angiotensin II receptor: cDNA sequence and regulation of the gene expression. Biochem Biophys Res Commun 1991; 177:299–304.
107. Ji I, Ji TH. Exons 1-10 of the rat LH receptor encode a high affinity hormone binding site and exon 11 encodes G-protein modulation and a potential second hormone binding site. Endocrinology 1991; 128:2648–2650.
108. Loosfelt H, Misrahi M, Atger M, et al. Cloning and sequencing of porcine LH-hCG receptor cDNA: Variants lacking transmembrane domain. Science 1989; 245:525–528.
109. Monsma FJ Jr, McVittie LD, Gerfen CR, et al. Multiple D2 dopamine receptors produced by alternative RNA splicing. Nature 1989; 342:926–929.
110. Amizuka N, Warshawsky H, Goltzman D, Karaplis AC. Morphological analysis of endochondral bone formation in normal and PTHrP-deficient fetal mice. J Bone Min Res 1993; 8 (suppl 1):S148.

111. Wysolmerski JJ, Broadus AE, Zhou J, et al. Overexpression of parathyroid hormone-related protein in the skin of transgenic mice interferes with hair follicle development. Proc Natl Acad Sci USA 1994; 91:1133–1137.
112. Ureña P, Kubrusly M, Mannstadt M, et al. The renal PTH/PTHrP receptor is down-regulated in rats with chronic renal failure. Kidney Int 1994; 45:605–611.
113. Lutz EM, Sheward WJ, West KM, et al. The VIP2 receptor: Molecular characterization of a cDNA encoding a novel receptor for vasoactive intestinal peptide. FEBS Lett 1993; 334:3–8.
114. Wank SA, Pisegna JR. Molecular cloning and functional expression of the pituitary adenylate cyclase activating polypeptide (PACAP) type I receptor. Proc Natl Acad Sci USA 1993; 90:6345–6349.
115. Usdin TB, Mesey E, Button DC, et al. Gastric inhibitory polypeptide receptor, a member of the secretin-vasoactive intestinal peptide receptor family, is widely distributed in peripheral organs and the brain. Endocrinology 1993; 133:2861–2870.
116. Chen R, Lewis KA, Perrin MH, Vale WW. Expression cloning of a human corticotropin-releasing factor receptor. Proc Natl Acad Sci USA 1993; 90:8967–8971.
117. Reagan JD. Expression cloning of an insect diuretic hormone receptor: A member of the calcitonin/secretin receptor family. J Biol Chem 1994; 269:9–12.
118. Sulston J, Du Z, Thomas K, et al. The C. elegans genome sequencing project: A beginning. Nature 1992; 356:37–41.
119. Jüppner H, Schipani E, Bringhurst FR, et al. The extracellular amino-terminal region of the parathyroid hormone (PTH)/PTH-related peptide receptor determines the binding affinity for carboxyl-terminal fragments of PTH (1-34). Endocrinology 1994; 134:879–884.
120. Gardella TJ, Jüppner H, Wilson AK, et al. Determinants for[Arg^2]PTH-binding and signaling in the transmembrane region of the parathyroid hormone receptor. Endocrinology 1994; 135:1186–1194.
121. Drake M, Gardella T, Abou-Samra AB, Segre GV. Mutational analysis of the rat PTH/PTHrP receptor: Structural determinants for activation of the stimulatory G protein. J Bone Min Res 1993; 8(suppl 1):S128.
122. Kong XF, Schipani E, Lanske B, et al. The rat, mouse and human genes encoding the receptor for parathyroid hormone and parathyroid hormone-related peptide are highly homologous. Biochem Biophys Res Commun 1994; 200:1290–1299.
123. Iida-Klein A, Guo J, Xie LY, et al. Truncation of the carboxy-terminal region of the rat parathyroid hormone (PTH)/PTH-related peptide receptor enhances PTH stimulation of adenylyl cyclase but not phospholipase C. J Biol Chem 1995 (in press).
124. Gelbert L, Schipani E, Jüppner H. et al. Chromosomal localization of the parathyroid hormone/parathyroid hormone-related peptide receptor gene to human chromosome 3q21.1–21.3. J Clin Endocrinol Metab 1994; 79:1046–1048.
125. Amizuka N, Warshawsky Henderson JE, Goltzman D, Karaplis AC. Parathyroid hormone-related peptide-depleted mice show abnormal endochondral cartilage development and altered endochondral bone. J Cell Biol 1994; 126:1611–1623.

18

Recent Progress in the Cloning and Characterization of Calcitonin Receptor cDNAs

Steven R. Goldring
Harvard Medical School, New England Deaconess Hospital, and Massachusetts General Hospital, Boston, Massachusetts

INTRODUCTION

Calcitonin (CT) was originally identified as a hypocalcemic factor produced by the parafollicular cells of the thyroid gland in response to hypercalcemia (1,2). In mammals, these effects on extracellular calcium levels can be attributed to inhibition of osteoclast-mediated bone resorption and stimulation of renal calcium excretion (3–5). In subsequent studies, CT has been shown to exhibit a broad and diverse spectrum of biological and pharmacological activities, including effects on many different organ systems not directly involved with the regulation of mineral ion homeostasis. These include effects on the gastrointestinal system, central nervous system, and the immune and cardiovascular systems (6). The physiological relevance of many of these activities remains uncertain, but the capacity of CT administration to produce favorable clinical effects on these organs has been exploited in the treatment of disorders such as peptic ulcer disease, pancreatitis, and intractable pain (6).

The introduction of radioligand binding and tissue autoradiographic techniques using iodinated salmon CT permitted the definitive identification and localization of the tissue and cellular distribution of CT receptors and provided the first insights into the mechanisms responsible for the unexpected diversity of CT effects. These studies revealed that CT receptors were widely distributed in diverse tissues in addition to bone and kidney, including the central nervous system (7,8), placenta (9), ovary (6), testis (10), spermatozoa (11), and lymphocytes (12) as well as certain malignant cell lines (13–18). The presence of high-affinity receptors for CT in these tissues and organs provided further evidence that CT might possess relevant physiological extraskeletal and renal effects. In fact, several lines of evidence indicate that certain actions of CT may have predated its function in mineral ion metabolism. The first is provided by the demonstration of the presence of CT in the central nervous system of the chordate *Ciona intestinalis* and in the brain of the cyclostome *Myxine* (6). The second comes from studies that indicate a role for CT in early stages of vertebrate development. In *Xenopus* embryos, addition of CT to the ambient water of the developing eggs produces larvae with narrowed interocular distances (synophthalmia) (19,20). These findings are consistent with faulty neural induction. It is interesting to speculate that these effects may be analogous to the inhibition of formation of polykaryons by CT during the generation of osteoclasts from mononuclear hematopoietic progenitors (21). Calcitonin not only inhibits bone-resorbing activities of mature osteoclasts but may also function as a regulatory hormone during osteoclast differentiation (22).

As further studies were performed using tissue emulsion autoradiography and radioligand binding with iodinated CT from different species, it became increasingly clear that CT receptors were functionally heterogeneous, particularly in the central nervous system, where CT receptors are present in very high numbers in specific regions of the brain (7,8,23). Using membranes prepared from brain tissues, Nakamuta et al. (24) were able to demonstrate two binding-site subtypes with radioiodinated analogues of salmon CT that exhibited differential capacity to form alpha helices. Additional support for the existence of CT receptor subtypes comes from the mapping of CT binding and calcitonin gene-related peptide (CGRP) binding sites in brain tissues. The α-CGRP is a product of the CT gene produced by tissue-specific alternative splicing of the CT gene (25). This 37–amino acid vasoactive peptide is produced in the central nervous system and in peripheral nerves, where it acts as a neurotransmitter. A second form of CGRP, β-CGRP, which is a product of a separate gene and differs from α-CGRP by three amino acids, has also been described (26). In most regions of the brain, the binding patterns of CT and CGRP are distinct; however, in certain restricted areas, there is high-affinity binding of both ligands (23), suggesting the existence of a unique CT-like receptor [termed C3 by Sexton et al. (23)] with the capacity to bind both ligands with comparable affinity. The final evidence supporting the existence of CT receptor subtypes comes from analysis of the functional properties of CT receptors from different tissues. Analysis of the coupling of CT receptors from kidney (27), osteoclasts (28), and cell lines from many different tissues to second-messenger signal transduction systems indicates that the CT receptor is coupled to increases in adenylate cyclase activity. In contrast, binding of CT to receptors in brain tissues inhibits adenylate cyclase activity (29). The recent cloning and characterization of CT receptors has provided direct evidence for the existence of CT receptor isoforms with distinct functional properties. With the reagents derived from these cloned receptors, it will now be possible to determine the molecular basis for the previously reported heterogeneity in CT receptor function.

In addition to widespread tissue distribution and evidence of binding-site heterogeneity, the CT receptor has been shown to exhibit several distinctive functional properties (Table 1). These include the capacity to couple to at least two guanine-nucleotide–binding regulatory G proteins, resulting in activation of different signal transduction pathways, including those involving adenylate cyclase, protein kinase C, and phospholipase C (30,31). In the LLC-PK_1 porcine renal tubular cell line, differential G protein coupling to the receptor appears to be dependent upon the stage of the cell cycle (30). These previous investigations did not establish that a single CT receptor type accounted for stimulation of adenylate cyclase and increases in intracellular free calcium ($[Ca^{2+}]i$). The availability of cloned CT receptor cDNAs has resolved this issue and demonstrated that a single CT receptor can couple to different signaling pathways (32,33).

Examination of the kinetics of hormone binding during continuous exposure to CT has revealed another unusual property of this receptor, especially with respect to binding to salmon and related forms of teleost-derived CTs (28,34,35). These studies demonstrate that the binding of salmon CT to cells or membrane preparations is accompanied by very slow ligand dissociation. This pattern of ligand-receptor interaction appears to be unique to the CT receptor, since with other G protein–coupled receptors, agonist binding leads to a rapid decrease in receptor affinity and either dissociation of the ligand or receptor desensitization (36–40). In our own studies with LLC-PK_1 cells, this persistent receptor occupancy is accompanied by sustained adenylate cyclase activation (34). The structural basis for this unique property of the CT receptor is unclear. One possible explanation is that salmon CT, because of its strong hydrophobic nature, remains bound to the receptor in a membrane-associated "compartment." Unlike the agonist-induced sequestration proposed for the β-adrenergic receptor, in the salmon CT-induced state of receptor occupancy, the ligand-receptor complex remains coupled, presumably through Gsα, to adenylate cyclase. In preliminary studies, we have determined that the cloned CT receptor cDNAs retain this property after transfection into CT receptor-negative cells.

To determine the structural basis for these unique functional properties of the CT receptor,

Table 1 Distinctive Characteristics of the Calcitonin Receptor

Widespread tissue and cellular distribution, including organs not involved directly in regulation of calcium homeostasis
Capacity to couple to multiple signal transduction pathways
Differential G protein–coupling during cell cycle
Slow ligand dissociation with sustained adenylate cyclase activation

Moseley et al. used covalent cross-linking techniques with photoreactive radioiodinated CT analogues and ion exchange chromatography to characterize the CT receptor (41,42). With these techniques, they demonstrated that the CT receptor was a single glycosylated polypeptide of 70,000 to 90,000 Da. These approaches failed, however, to purify sufficient amounts of the CT receptor to obtain amino acid sequences, and it was for this reason that in recent years several laboratories turned to the techniques of molecular biology to clone cDNAs encoding functional CT receptors.

CALCITONIN RECEPTOR CLONING AND CHARACTERIZATION

In order to isolate and characterize the CT receptor, we utilized a mammalian expression system in COS cells (43,44). For these studies, a cDNA library was prepared from the LLC-PK_1 cell line in the mammalian expression vector pcDNA-1 (Invitrogen). We had previously shown that these porcine renal epithelial cells express large numbers of high-affinity CT receptors and that the receptor was functionally coupled to adenylate cyclase (45). The library was size-fractionated and divided into pools of cDNA containing 10,000 recombinants, and these pools were transfected into COS cells and screened for binding of iodinated salmon CT by emulsion autoradiography using dark-field microscopy. Nontransfected COS cells, or COS cells transfected with a plasmid containing the β-galactosidase gene, did not bind CT. A total of 30 pools of cDNA representing 3×10^5 clones were screened, and from these pools two positive clones capable of imparting CT binding to the COS cell transfectants, one of 2.2 kb and the other of 4.0 kb, were isolated. Restriction map and sequence analysis of these clones revealed that they both encoded the same open reading frame and that the smaller clone was a truncated version of the larger clone. In transient tranfection studies in COS cells, both clones exhibited similar functional properties, and subsequent functional analyses were conducted with the smaller clone.

Transfection of the 2.2-kb clone into COS cells resulted in expression of large numbers of high-affinity CT receptors. Scatchard analysis of iodinated salmon CT binding was consistent with the presence of a single class of CT receptors with a K_d for salmon CT of ~6 nM, similar to the properties of the CT receptor in the native LLC-PK_1 cells. We next examined the coupling of the expressed receptor to specific signal transduction pathways. Previous investigations had indicated that the CT receptor could couple to different signaling pathways, although these studies did not establish whether these effects were mediated by a single CT receptor or the presence of individual CT receptor subtypes, each coupled to a different signaling pathway (30,31). Initial studies were conducted with COS cells transiently transfected with the CT receptor cDNA. These results indicated that the expressed receptor was coupled to adenylate cyclase and that exposure to salmon CT produced a concentration-dependent increase in cAMP (43,44).

Because of problems in obtaining consistent results with measurements of intracellular free calcium in the transient transfectants, we created cell lines stably expressing the porcine CT receptor using cotransfection of a murine osteoblast-like cell line, MC-3T3/E1, with the porcine CT receptor and a plasmid that imparted resistance to neomycin. After selection in G418, several different clones expressing CT receptors were isolated and used for further characterization (32). As in the transient transfections, incubation of the cell lines with salmon CT induced a concentration-dependent increase in cAMP levels. In addition, the expressed receptor was coupled to increases in cytosolic free [Ca^{2+}] ([Ca^{2+}]i) and inositol phosphate production. These findings are consistent with association of a single high-affinity CT receptor with G proteins coupled to two independent signaling pathways, one linked to adenylate cyclase and the other to phospholipase C (Fig. 1). It is of interest that the concentration of hormone that elicits a half-maximal response (EC_{50}) for these two pathways differs. The lower EC_{50} for stimulation of adenylate cyclase indicates that the activation of this pathway may occur at a lower receptor occupancy compared to the signal pathway involving phospholipase C. This also could be related to a more efficient interaction with the G protein that couples the occupied receptor to adenylate cyclase (presumably Gsα).

As described in the opening paragraphs of this chapter, in vivo evaluation of the responses to CT have demonstrated effects on diverse organs and tissues in addition to those that are involved in the regulation of mineral ion and bone metabolism. In part, this is related to the widespread distribution of CT receptors, which has been documented by radioligand-binding studies and in situ tissue autoradiography with radioiodinated CT. Also, there is evidence that CT has the capacity to

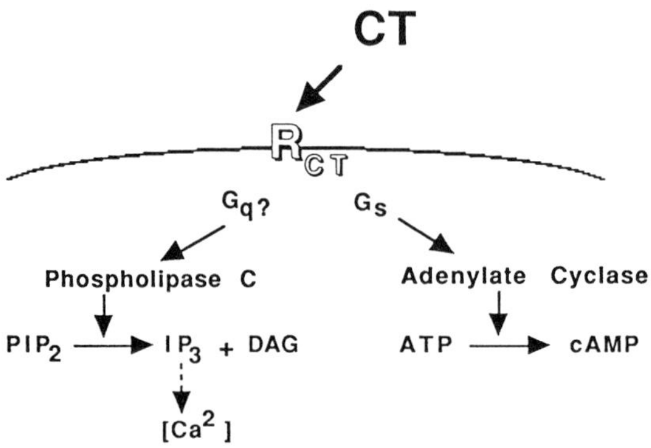

Figure 1 Coupling of the CT receptor to two independent signal transduction pathways. Binding of CT to the cell surface CT receptor results in coupling of the bound receptor to two distinct G proteins [Gs and Gq (or a related G protein)]. The binding of the α-subunit of the heterotrimeric G proteins to distinct effector systems, adenylate cyclase, or phospholipase C, results in activation of these enzymes and production of second-messenger molecules.

interact (with low-affinity binding) to receptors for structurally related ligands (6,46). These ligands, CGRP (which is a potent vasodilator), and amylin (a hormone that elevates blood glucose levels) exhibit similar cross-reactivity with the CT receptor. The availability of the cloned CT receptor has permitted us to examine directly the basis for this unusual overlap in biological activities among these ligands, each of which exhibits its own distinct spectrum of biological and pharmacological effects.

To test directly the capacity of CGRP and amylin to bind to the CT receptor and transduce second-messenger responses, cell lines stably expressing the CT receptor were incubated with these ligands and the binding kinetics and the pattern of coupling to different signaling pathways evaluated. As shown in Fig. 2, incubation of a cell line, PC-1, stably transfected with the porcine CT receptor, with amylin or CGRP results in a concentration-dependent increase in cAMP levels. Although the cAMP response to maximal stimulatory concentrations of these ligands was comparable to the maximal response to CT, the EC_{50}s for CGRP and amylin were almost two orders of magnitude higher. Binding studies with iodinated salmon CT confirm that these ligands bind to the CT receptor with very low affinity compared to CT. Although these ligands can bind to the CT receptor and elicit a response that involves coupling to adenylate cyclase (presumably involving interaction with

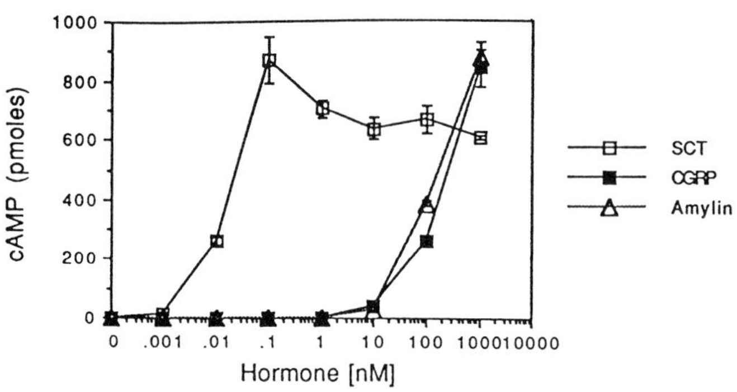

Figure 2 Dose-dependent effects of salmon CT (SCT), calcitonin gene–related peptide (CGRP) or amylin on cAMP levels in a cell line (PC-1) stably transfected with the porcine CT receptor. Cells incubated with increasing concentrations of the three ligands produce a dose-dependent increase in cAMP levels. The EC_{50} for SCT is almost two orders of magnitude lower than that for the two related ligands.

Gsα), neither hormone produces significant effects on $[Ca^{2+}]$i or inositol phosphate levels (32). Furthermore, these ligands fail to affect these other second-messenger molecules, even at concentrations that produce maximal increases in intracellular cAMP content, providing indirect evidence that the effects of CT on phospholipase C and $[Ca^{2+}]$i are not mediated by changes in cAMP levels. More importantly, these results indicate that the interaction of CGRP and amylin (and perhaps other potential cross-reacting ligands) with the CT receptor can result in differential coupling to specific signaling pathways.

STRUCTURAL FEATURES AND DISTRIBUTION OF CT RECEPTORS

Analysis of the predicted amino acid sequence of the cloned CT receptor cDNA revealed that it was structurally related to the recently cloned receptor for parathyroid hormone/parathyroid hormone–related peptide (PTH/PTHrP). Although these receptors exhibit topographical, organization, and functional properties suggesting that they belong to the superfamily of G protein–coupled receptors that have seven transmembrane-spanning domains, the CT and PTH/PTHrP receptors are less than 12% related to the other members of this large family of ligand-binding proteins. Because the CT and PTH/PTHrP receptors differ from these other receptors, the structural features that determine the functional properties of these receptors are not known. To begin to investigate these "structure-function" relationships, in collaboration with Dr. Harald Jüppner (47), we have constructed chimeric CT-PTH/PTHrP receptors to map the ligand-binding domains and to define the regions of the receptors involved in binding to the distinct G proteins. In initial studies, unique restriction sites were introduced into various regions of both receptors to permit ligation of individual portions of either receptor to each other. In addition, new as well as existing restriction sites were also used to create receptors that were truncated at either the amino- or carboxyl-terminal ends. Preliminary results of these studies have been presented (47) and indicate that a chimeric CT-PTH/PTHrP receptor containing the amino-terminal portion of the CT receptor ligated to the PTH/PTHrP receptor at amino acid position 380 in the fifth transmembrane spanning region when expressed in COS cells retains the capacity to bind salmon CT (Fig. 3). This chimera is also able to transduce an increase in cAMP levels in response to treatment with salmon CT. These results, as well as additional results with other chimeric receptors, provisionally localize the minimal ligand-binding domains of the CT receptor to the amino-terminal extension and the first two extracellular loops between the second and third and fourth and fifth transmembrane-spanning domains. Further studies are under way to more rigorously determine the regions of the receptor that define ligand-binding specificity and binding to G proteins.

In recent studies, we have used Northern analysis with ^{32}P-labeled restriction fragments prepared from the porcine CT receptor to determine the distribution and characteristics of the CT receptor in different tissues. Transcripts that hybridize with these CT receptor probes are widely distributed in

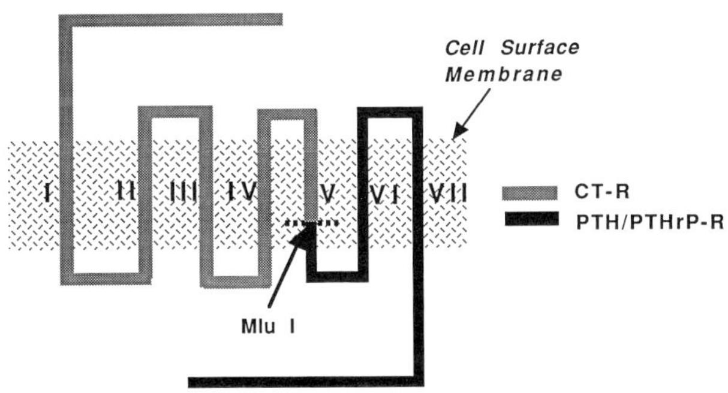

Figure 3 Structural features of a chimeric CT-PTH/PTHrP receptor. A *Mlu* 1 restriction site was created in the fifth transmembrane-spanning domains in the two receptors and used to ligate the amino-terminal portion of the CT receptor to the carboxyl-terminal portion of the PTH/PTHrP receptor. This chimeric cDNA was then transfected into COS cells and binding kinetics and cAMP responses assessed.

many different tissues, including the brain, spinal cord, bone marrow, stomach, ovary, testis, skeletal muscle, and uterus. These results are consistent with radioligand-binding studies that indicate the presence of high-affinity CT receptors in diverse organs, including some in which the functional role for this ligand has not been established, such as the ovary, testis and placenta. With the exception of the stomach, the probe hybridizes to a transcript of comparable mobility (~ 4.2 kb), which is similar to the size of the transcript in the LLC-PK_1 cells. Somewhat surprising is the widespread distribution of the CT receptor message in the brain, even in regions which, based on previous ligand binding studies in other species (7,8), would not be predicted to express high levels of CT receptor mRNA. In part, this could be related to differences in the distribution of CT receptor expression among species. We have used tissue autoradiography with iodinated salmon CT and in situ hybridization with ^{32}P-labeled cRNA probes prepared from the porcine CT receptor to correlate directly ligand binding and CT receptor mRNA expression. These approaches are now being used to map the distribution of CT receptors in the pig and compare the patterns to that observed in other species.

CLONING AND CHARACTERIZATION OF HUMAN AND MURINE CT RECEPTOR cDNAS

We have recently reported the cloning of a human CT receptor from a small-cell carcinoma cell line, BIN-67 (48). These cells, which express large numbers of CT receptors ($>1 \times 10^5$/cell), were used to construct a size-fractionated cDNA library in the expression vector, pcDNA-1 (Invitrogen). The library was screened by low-stringency cross-hybridization with a ^{32}P-labeled restriction fragment prepared from the porcine CT receptor. A single positive clone of 3588 bp was isolated from the initial screening of 55,000 colonies. Analysis of this clone predicted a polypeptide of 490 amino acids which overall exhibited 73% identity and 89% similarity to the porcine CT receptor. The human CT receptor demonstrated many of the structural features characteristic of the porcine CT receptor, including seven hydrophobic domains, an attentuated third intracellular loop, and a long amino-terminal presumed exocytoplasmic stretch with a hydrophobic N-terminal putative signal sequence. The cysteines in the N-terminal region and the first and second extracellular loops, as well as three of the N-linked glycosylation sites, were also conserved. The major area of divergence between the receptors was in the first intracellular loop, where the human CT receptor contained an insert of 16 amino acids not present in the porcine CT receptor (Fig. 4).

Despite the highly conserved sequences of the human and porcine CT receptors, the human ovarian CT receptor after expression in COS cells exhibits higher affinity for human or salmon CT compared to the porcine receptor. That the presence of the 16–amino acid sequence in the first

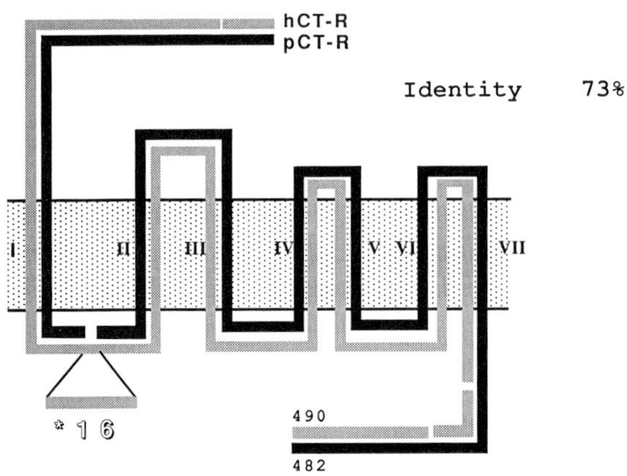

Figure 4 Comparison of the human ovarian (hCT-R) and the porcine renal (pCT-R) CT receptors. Overall the predicted polypeptides were 73% identical at the amino acid level. The major structural difference was the presence in the hCT-R of a 16–amino acid insert (between the first and second transmembrane domains) that was not present in the pCT-R.

intracellular loop can modify ligand binding has been established more definitively by the recent cloning of two CT receptor cDNAs from a library constructed from RNA isolated from a human giant-cell tumor of bone (49). The first form, similar to the human ovarian CT receptor but unlike the porcine CT receptor, contains a 16–amino acid insert in the first intracellular loop. The amino acids are identical to the residues in the ovarian-derived receptor. In the 5′-region, this cDNA differs from the ovarian form of the receptor in that it lacks a 71-bp segment that contains the first (more 5′-) of two in-frame AUG codons. The second human giant-cell tumor CT receptor cDNA also lacks this 71-bp 5′-insert. This clone is similar in structure to the porcine renal CT receptor because it lacks the sequence of 48 nucleotides that encode the 16–amino acid insert in the putative first intracellular domain.

Since the cDNAs cloned from the giant-cell tumor are identical except for the presence or absence of the 16–amino acid insert in the predicted first intracellular loop, they provide an excellent model for defining the functional role of this sequence. Ligand binding and cAMP responses of the expressed giant-cell tumor CT receptor isoforms differ markedly. The cDNA containing the 16–amino acid insert exhibits higher binding affinity for salmon and human CT compared to the form without the 16 amino acids. Because of its predicted intracellular location, it is unlikely that the region of the receptor containing the amino acid insert interacts directly with the ligands. It is more likely that the presence of this additional amino acid sequence somehow alters the conformation of the receptor in such a way as to enhance its ability to bind the ligands.

Analysis of the CT-induced cAMP responses in COS cells transfected with each of the cDNAs yielded quite unexpected results. Despite the lower CT binding affinity of the cDNA lacking the amino acid insert, it exhibits a markedly greater CT-induced cAMP response compared to the cDNA containing the additional 16 amino acids. The amino acids in this insert do not demonstrate the characteristic motif of a G protein binding domain (50–52); therefore, it is unlikely that the reduced magnitude of the hormone-induced cAMP response in this receptor isoform is related to binding of a G protein that inhibits adenylate cyclase (i.e. Giα). It is more probable that the absence of this sequence modifies the receptor conformation in such a way as to improve the efficiency of coupling of other intracellular domains of the receptor to G proteins.

In other studies (Orcel et al., unpublished), we have used the insulin-like growth factor II (IGF II) receptor cDNA to construct a chimeric receptor in which oligonucleotides encoding the putative G protein binding sequences from the porcine CT receptor were substituted for the Giα binding region of the IGF II receptor. These oligonucleotides corresponded to sequences in the intracellular domain between the fifth and sixth transmembrane-spanning helices and the proximal portion of the carboxyl-terminal tail of the CT receptor. Transfection of these chimeric receptors into COS cells resulted in expression of a functional receptor that was coupled to increases in adenylate cyclase, providing direct evidence that these regions of the CT receptor were authentic G protein binding domains.

More recently, we have identified and characterized a mouse brain CT receptor cDNA. This cDNA encodes a receptor protein that, after expression, exhibits high-affinity binding to salmon CT ($K_d \sim 12.5$ n*M*) and is coupled to increases in cAMP levels. The binding affinity of this expressed receptor for salmon CT is lower than that described for the cloned porcine renal and human ovarian CT receptors but is similar to the recently described rat brain CT receptor that has been designated the C1b form (53,54). Structural analysis of the mouse brain CT receptor reveals that it is very highly related to the other CT receptor cDNAs. The major structural feature that distinguishes the mouse cDNA clone from the other CT receptors is the presence of a consecutive 111-bp nucleotide sequence that encodes a 37–amino acid sequence that is predicted to localize to the first extracellular loop between the second and third transmembrane-spanning domains (Fig. 5). The rat C1b receptor contains a similar 37–amino acid cassette. Comparison of the binding kinetics of the mouse brain receptor to the rat C1a receptor, which lacks the 37–amino acid insert, reveals that the presence of these amino acids markedly affects hormone-binding affinity. These conclusions are supported by the results of binding studies with the chimeric CT/PTHrP receptors that also indicate the importance of the extracellular loop between the second and third transmembrane spanning domains for interaction with ligands that bind to the CT receptor.

Further evidence that the first extracellular loop of the CT receptor affects the specificity of ligand binding is provided by results of studies with CT from different species and with peptide hormones that exhibit biological cross-reactivity with CT, namely amylin and CGRP. In contrast to

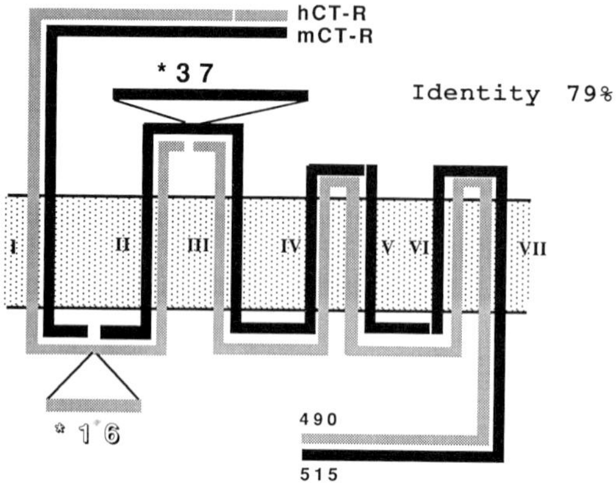

Figure 5 Comparison of the human ovarian (hCT-R) and the mouse brain (mCT-R) CT receptors. Overall the predicted polypeptides were 79% identical at the amino acid level. The major structural differences were the presence in the mCT-R of a 37–amino acid insert (between the second and third transmembrane spanning domains) that was not present in the hCT-R and a 16–amino acid insert (between the first and second transmembrane domains) that was unique to the hCT-R.

results with the expressed human and porcine CT receptor and the rat C1a CT receptor, cells transfected with the mouse CT receptor cDNA do not increase cAMP levels after incubation with rat or human CT, amylin, or CGRP. The absence of the 37–amino acid domain in the first extracellular loop results in restoration of adenylate responses to these ligands (53,54). The failure of rat CT to bind to the mouse CT receptor cDNA is particularly surprising, since this species of CT would be expected to represent the principal endogenous ligand for the receptor. Our results and those reported by Sexton et al. with the C1b rat brain CT receptor suggest that this form of the receptor may function as a binding protein for some as yet unidentified neurotransmitter (53). The existence of a salmon CT-like peptide has been described in the human brain (8), and it is possible that this (or a related peptide) could function as the natural ligand for this isoform of the brain CT receptor. The results of Northern analysis indicate that the CT receptor cDNA that we cloned is not the predominant form of CT receptor in the brain or kidney. Albrandt et al. and Sexton et al. (53,54) reached similar conclusions based on results of RT-PCR using RNA from rat kidney and various regions of rat brain. Although their approaches were not strictly quantitative, they did identify specific areas of the brain, namely the nucleus accumbens, in which the form of the CT receptor containing the 37–amino acid insert appeared to be more highly expressed.

We have used the mouse CT receptor cDNA to undertake preliminary characterization of the CT receptor gene. Southern analysis of the restriction fragments and partial sequencing of subclones from a genomic library identified four putative exons based on the presence of appropriate exon/intron junctional motifs and sequence identities to the mouse CT receptor cDNA (55). The four exons were located in the 5′-end of the open reading frame and were separated by lengthy introns of >2 kb. Thus far, we have not yet identified the sequences that encode the equivalent 16–amino acid cassette that characterizes the human ovarian CT receptor or the 111-bp cassette that is present in the mouse brain receptor. Additional analyses, therefore, will be necessary to prove that these "cassettes" represent the products of separate exons. Southern analysis of genomic DNA by Sexton et al. supports our initial findings regarding the CT receptor gene structure (53). Based on Southern hybridization of the CT receptor cDNA to genomic DNA, they estimated that the rat CT receptor gene is very lengthy, spanning at least 50 kb.

We have used the technique of interspecific back-cross analysis (56) to localize the CT receptor to the proximal region of mouse chromosome 6, where it is linked to three previously characterized genes, *Met*, *Ptn*, and *Terb* (57,58). Comparison of our interspecific map of chromosome 6 with a composite mouse linkage map that reports the location of many uncloned mouse mutations (compiled by M. T. Davisson, T. H. Roderick, A. L. Hillyard, and D. P. Doolittle and provided from GBASE, a computerized database maintained at The Jackson Laboratory, Bar Harbor, Maine) revealed that the CT receptor mapped in a region of the composite map that contains one mutation, sightless (*Sig*). Heterozygotes for this mutation have open eyes at birth and display slight hydrocephaly. Homozygotes die at birth with more pronounced hydrocephaly and sometimes with hind-foot anomalies, especially syndactyly (59). The region to which the CT receptor gene localizes on mouse chromosome 6 shares homology with human chromosome 7q. Recently, we have used PCR and in situ hybridization techniques to confirm the location of the human CT receptor gene on 7q. These results indicate that the gene resides on chromosome 7q at band q22. Additional studies will be required to determine a possible association with other genes that function as specific disease markers.

THE CT RECEPTOR AND RELATED RECEPTOR FAMILY

As described in the preceding section, analysis of the predicted structural organization of the cloned CT receptor cDNAs indicates that they belong to the so-called *superfamily* of G protein–coupled receptors (60–63). Two characteristics distinguish the G protein–coupled receptor superfamily from other protein superfamilies. The first is the presence in these receptors of seven hydrophobic segments that are predicted to form transmembrane spanning α-helices. The second feature is their capacity, after agonist binding, to accelerate the exchange of bound GDP for GTP on specific G protein α subunits that are associated with the individual receptor proteins. Formal proof of the organization of these receptor proteins into membrane-spanning domains has been hampered by the inability to crystallize these proteins. A low-resolution model for bovine rhodopsin has been developed and it is consistent with a seven-transmembrane-spanning topography, but high-resolution modeling will be required to formally test these structural predictions (64,65). The assignment of the CT receptor to this superfamily is based on the presence in the predicted structures of the cloned CT receptor cDNAs of seven hydrophobic segments as well as the functional capacity of the expressed receptors to couple to intracellular signaling systems through interactions with G proteins.

As stated above, the grouping of the G protein–coupled receptors into a superfamily is based on the presence in their predicted protein structures of common structural or functional features. This association does not require an obvious similarity in amino acid sequence, although sequence similarities and identities have been useful in assigning the individual receptors to separate *families*. Within a family, in addition to a conservation of amino acid similarity ($\geq$20%) there are structural and functional themes that distinguish the individual families. These similarities (e.g., a commonality in gene structure and organization) have been useful in determining the evolutionary origins as well as the relationships among the individual receptor proteins and their families.

A general functional property shared by the G protein–coupled receptors is their role in the transduction of extracellular signals across the lipid bilayer of the cell surface and transfer of these signals to intracellular effector systems that result in modulation of cell function. The actual coupling of the activated receptor to the intracellular signal transduction pathways is accomplished by interaction and activation of heterotrimeric G proteins that associate with distinct topographical domains within the intracellular regions of the receptors (66–68). These G proteins consist of α, β, and γ subunits, each of which is structurally distinct. As a family, these G proteins and their subunits are now known to be quite diverse, and this heterogeneity is clearly important in permitting these molecules to interact with the many different types of receptors and distinct effector systems. In the absence of an extracellular signal, the receptor-associated G proteins are in an inactive state in which their α subunits are occupied by GDP. After activation by the appropriate extracellular signal, the GDP is dissociated from the α subunit and replaced by GTP. This results in dissociation of the complex into α and β-γ subunits after which the α subunit interacts with specific effectors such as adenylate cyclase or phospholipase C or may directly associate with and modulate the activity of membrane-bound ion channels (66–68).

A remarkable feature of the G protein–coupled receptors is the extreme diversity of exogenous signals that they are capable of transducing. These stimuli include, for example, photons, organic molecules that are responsible for odor detection and discrimination, opioids, catecholamines and indoleamines, eicosanoid hormones, purines such as adenosine, cAMP, calcium, and a wide spectrum of peptides and glycoprotein hormones (60–63). Within the individual families of the G protein–coupled receptors, it is possible to identify certain common themes in terms of the properties of the ligands or extracellular signals and the G protein selectivities. This is probably accounted for by the similarities in the primary amino acid sequence and structural organization that define the separate families.

As described in the preceding section, based on similarities in amino acid sequences in recently cloned receptor cDNAs, the CT receptor can be grouped into a new family that is distinct from other members of the superfamily of G protein–coupled receptors. This family contains, in addition to the CT and PTH/PTHrP receptors, the receptors for the glucagon family of peptides, glucagon (69), secretin (70), vasoactive intestinal peptide (71), glucagon-like peptide 1 (72), growth hormone–releasing hormone (73) and pituitary adenylate cyclase activating peptide (74). The most recent addition to this family is the so-called insect diuretic hormone receptor from adult *Manduca sexta*, which stimulates fluid secretion and cAMP synthesis in the Malphighian tubules (75). The peptide that activates this receptor belongs to the corticotropin-releasing factor peptide family.

The ligands for the individual members of the CT receptor family are all relatively small peptide hormones. Many of the ligands, namely the members of the glucagon family, are structurally related and exhibit overlap in physiological properties. The receptors themselves, although exhibiting considerable differences in their amino acid sequences, share certain common structural and functional motifs. For example, they all contain an extended N-terminal domain containing conserved cysteines and several potential N-linked glycosylation sites. The receptors for the glycoprotein hormones exhibit a similar organization, although the N-terminal extracellular extension is even more lengthy, exceeding almost 400 amino acids in the thyroid hormone–stimulating receptor (76). Construction of chimeric receptors with other glycoprotein hormone receptors and receptor mutants with amino acid substitutions or deletions has helped to localize the ligand-binding domain to this extracellular region of the glycoprotein hormone receptors. The ligand-binding domain in the receptors in the CT family has not been firmly established, but amino acid truncations in the PTH/PTHrP receptors and the construction of chimeric CT-PTH/PTHrP receptors indicate the importance of this region in ligand binding (47). It is likely, however, that the other extracellular loops are also involved in this interaction.

All members of the CT receptor family interact with the Gsα transducer molecule through which they are coupled to adenylate cyclase. Binding of their respective ligands results in activation of this enzyme and increases in intracellular levels of cAMP. The distinct structural organization of these receptors probably underlies their capacity to couple, in addition to adenylate cyclase, to signal pathways that increase intracellular free calcium and inositol phosphate hydrolysis (32,33,77). As discussed in the preceding section, we have used a chimeric CT-IGF II receptor to identify at least two distinct segments of the CT receptor that have the capacity to interact with G proteins and transduce distinct second-messenger responses (Orcel et al., unpublished). The capacity of G protein–coupled receptors to activate both adenylate cyclase and phospholipase C is not unique to the CT receptor family. For example, the TSH receptor has been shown to increase adenylate cyclase activity and activate phospholipase C (76), and the m^2-muscarinic (78) and α-2 adrenergic receptors (79) mediate both adenylate cyclase inhibition and stimulation of phospholipase C.

The origins and evolution of the CT receptor and the receptors for the other members of this peptide hormone receptor family is not known. There is, however, evidence concerning the evolution of the ligands. For example, it has been suggested that PTH evolved from an ancestral PTHrP gene by a translocation event. Similar translocations are also implicated in the diversification of the ligands that belong to the glucagon family of peptides. In contrast, CT and calcitonin gene-related peptide are products of the same gene produced by alternative RNA processing. The mechanisms underlying the evolution and diversification of the receptors for the members of the CT receptor family are not known. The selection pressures for these events may have been provided when life forms moved from the oceans to the land environment in which calcium was not immediately available from the acqueous surroundings. In the terrestrial habitats, new hormonal systems were necessary for rigorously regulating extracellular calcium levels, and these hormones and their receptors may have evolved to accomodate these unique demands.

REFERENCES

1. Copp DH, Cameron EC, Cheney BA, et al. Evidence for calcitonin—A new hormone from the parathyroid that lowers blood calcium. Endocrinology 1962; 70:638–649.
2. Hirsch PF, Voelkel EF, Munson PL. Thyrocalcitonin: Hypocalcemic, hypophosphatemic principle of the thyroid gland. Science 1964; 146:412–413.

3. Friedman J, Raisz LG. Thyrocalcitonin: Inhibitor of bone resorption in tissue culture. Science 1965; 150:1465–1467.
4. Raisz LG, Niemann I. Early effects of parathyroid hormone and thyrocalcitonin on bone in organ culture. Nature 1967; 214:486–487.
5. Warshawsky H, Goltzman D, Rouleau MF, Bergeron JJM. Direct in vivo demonstration by radioautography of specific binding sites for calcitonin in skeletal and renal tissues of the rat. J Cell Biol 1980; 85:682–694.
6. Azria M. The Calcitonins: Physiology and Pharmacology. Basel: Karger, 1989.
7. Goltzman D. Interaction of calcitonin and calcitonin gene-related peptide at receptor sites in target tissues. Science 1985; 227:1343–1345.
8. Fischer JA, Tobler PH, Kaufmann et al. Calcitonin: Regional distribution of the hormone and its binding sites in the human brain and pituitary. Proc Natl Acad Sci USA 1981; 78:7801–7805.
9. Nicholson GC, D'Santos CS, Evans T, et al. Human placental calcitonin receptors. Biochem J 1988; 250:877–882.
10. Chausmer A, Stuart C, Stevens M. Identification of testicular cell plasma membrane receptors for calcitonin. J Lab Clin Med 1980; 96:933–938.
11. Silvestroni L, Menditto A, Frajese G, Gnessi L. Identification of calcitonin receptors in human spermatozoa. J Clin Endocrinol Metab 1987; 65:742–746.
12. Marx SJ, Aurbach GD, Gavin JR, Buell DW. Calcitonin receptors on cultured human lymphocytes. J Biol Chem 1974; 249:6812–6816.
13. Upchurch KS, Parker LM, Scully RE, Krane SM. Differential cyclic AMP responses to calcitonin among human ovarian carcinoma cell lines: A calcitonin-responsive line derived from a rare tumor type. J Bone Min Res 1986; 1:299–304.
14. Findlay DM, DeLuise M, Michelangeli VP, et al. Properties of a calcitonin receptor and adenylate cyclase in BEN cells, a human cancer cell line. Cancer Res 1980; 40:1311–1317.
15. Findlay DM, Michelangeli VP, Moseley JM, Martin TJ. Calcitonin binding and deregulation by two cultured human breast cancer cell lines (MCF7 and T47D). J Biochem 1981; 196:513–520.
16. Gattei V, Bernabei PA, Pinto A, et al. Phorbol ester induced osteoclast-like differentiation of a novel human leukemic cell line (FLG 29.1). J Cell Biol 1991; 116:437–447.
17. Binet E, Laurent P, Evain-Brion D. F-9 embryonal carcinoma cells autocrine system: Correlation between immunoreactive calcitonin secretion and calcitonin receptor number. J Cell Physiol 1985; 124:288–292.
18. Evain D, Binet E, Anderson WB. Alterations in calcitonin and parathyroid hormone responsiveness to adenylate cyclase in F-9 cells treated with retinoic acid and dibutryl cyclic AMP. J Cell Physiol 1981; 109:453–459.
19. Burgess AMC. The effect of calcitonin on the prechordal mesoderm, neural plate and neural crest of Xenopus embryos. J Anat 1985; 140:49–55.
20. Burgess AMC. The developmental effect of calcitonin on the interocular distance in early Xenopus embryos. J Anat 1982; 135:745–751.
21. Vaes G. Cellular biology and biochemical mechanisms of bone resorption: A review of recent developments on the formation, activation and mode of action of osteoclasts. Clin Orthop Rel Res 1988; 231:239–271.
22. Suda T, Takahashi N, Martin TJ. Modulation of osteoclast differentiation. Endocr Rev 1992; 13:66–80.
23. Sexton PM. Central nervous system binding sites for calcitonin and calcitonin gene-related peptide. Mol Neurobiol 1991; 5:251–273.
24. Nakamuta H, Orlowski RC, Epand RM. Evidence for calcitonin receptor heterogeneity: Binding studies with nonhelical analogs. Endocrinol 1990; 127:163–169.
25. Rosenfeld MG, Mermod JJ, Amara SG, et al. Production of a novel neuropeptide encoded by the calcitonin gene via tissue-specific processing. Nature 1983; 304:129–135.
26. Brain S, MacIntyre I, Williams TJ. A second form of human calcitonin gene-related peptide which is a potent vasodilator. Eur J Pharm 1986; 124:349–352.
27. Goldring SR, Dayer J-M, Russell RGG, et al. Response to hormones of cells cultured from human giant cell tumors of bone. J Clin Endocrinol Metab 1978; 46:425–433.
28. Nicholson GC, Moseley JM, Yates JP, Martin TJ. Control of cyclic adenosine 3′,5′-monophosphate production in osteoclasts: Calcitonin-induced persistent activation and homologous desensitization of adenylate cyclase. Endocrinology 1987; 120:1902–1908.
29. Rizzo AJ, Goltzman D. Calcitonin receptors in the central nervous system of the rat. Endocrinology 1981; 108:1672–1677.
30. Chakraborty M, Chatterjee D, Kellokumpu S, et al. Cell cycle-dependent coupling of the calcitonin receptor to different G proteins. Science 1991; 251:1078–1082.
31. Zaidi M, Datta HK, Moonga BS, MacIntyre I. Evidence that the action of calcitonin on rat osteoclasts is mediated by two G proteins acting via separate post-receptor pathways. J Endocrinol 1990; 126:473–481.
32. Force T, Bonventre JV, Flannery MR, et al. A cloned porcine renal calcitonin receptor couples to adenylyl cyclase and phospholipase C. Am J Physiol 1992; 262:F1110–F1115.

33. Chabre O, Conklin BR, Lin HY, et al. A recombinant calcitonin receptor independently stimulates cAMP and Ca^{2+}/inositol phosphate signaling pathways. Mol Endocrinol 1992; 6:551–556.
34. Heron J-F, Dayer J-M, Goldring SR, Krane SM. Factors modulating the response of a porcine renal tubular cell line to calcitonin and antidiuretic hormone. Calcif Tiss 1981; 33:41–50.
35. Lamp SJ, Findlay DM, Moseley JM, Martin TJ. Calcitonin induction of a persistent activated state of adenylate cyclase in human breast cancer cells (T 47D). J Biol Chem 1981; 256:12269–12274.
36. Lohse MJ, Benovic JL, Caron MG, Lefkowitz RJ. Multiple pathways of rapid β_2-adrenergic receptor desensitization. J Biol Chem 1990; 265:3202–3209.
37. Lohse MJ, Andexinger S, Pitcher J, et al. Receptor-specific desensitization with purified proteins. J Biol Chem 1992; 267:8558–8564.
38. Lohse MJ, Benovic JL, Codina J, et al. β-Arrestin: A protein that regulates β-adrenergic receptor function. Science 1990; 248:1547–1550.
39. Hausdorff WP, Caron MG, Lefkowitz RJ. Turning off the signal: Desensitization of β-adrenergic receptor function. FASEB J 1990; 4:2881–2889.
40. Pitcher J, Lohse MJ, Codina J, et al. Desensitization of the isolated β_2-adrenergic receptor by β-adrenergic receptor kinase, cAMP-dependent protein kinase, and protein kinase C occurs via distinct molecular mechanisms. Biochemistry 1992; 31:3193–3197.
41. Moseley JM, Smith P, Martin TJ. Identification of the calcitonin receptor by chemical cross-linking and photoaffinity labeling in human cancer cell lines. J Bone Min Res 1986; 1:293–297.
42. Moseley JM, Findlay DM, Martin TJ, Gorman JJ. Covalent cross-linking of a photoactive derivative of calcitonin to human breast cancer cell receptors. J Biol Chem 1982; 257:5846–5851.
43. Lin HY, Harris TL, Flannery MS, et al. Expression cloning of an adenylate cyclase-coupled calcitonin receptor. Science 1991; 254:1022–1024.
44. Lin HY, Harris TL, Flannery MS, et al. Expression cloning and characterization of a porcine renal calcitonin receptor. Trans Assoc Am Phys 1991; 104:265–272.
45. Goldring SR, Dayer J-M, Ausiello DA, Krane SM. A cell strain cultured from porcine kidney increase cyclic AMP content upon exposure to calcitonin or vasopressin. Biochem Biophys Res Commun 1978; 83:434–440.
46. Wimalawansa SJ. Calcitonin: Molecular biology, physiology, pathophysiology and its therpeutic uses. In: Pecile A, Barnard B, eds. Advances in Bone Regulatory Factors: Morphology, Biochemistry, Physiology and Pharmacology. England: Plenum Press, 1990;121–160.
47. Jüppner H, Flannery MS, McClure I, et al. Chimeras between the receptors for calcitonin (CTR) and parathyroid hormone (PTH)/PTH related peptide (PTHrP) define functionally important domains. J Bone Min Res 1993; 8:S183.
48. Gorn AH, Lin HY, Yamin M, et al. The cloning, characterization and expression of a human calcitonin receptor from an ovarian carcinoma cell line. J Clin Invest 1992; 90:1726–1735.
49. Gorn AH, Rudolf SM, Yamin M, et al. The cloning of a human osteoclast calcitonin receptor from a giant cell tumor of bone (osteoclastoma). J Bone Min Res 1993; 8:S384.
50. Okamoto T, Katada T, Murayama Y, et al. A simple structure encodes G protein–activating function of the IGF II/mannose 6-phosphate receptor. Cell 1990; 62:709–717.
51. Okamoto T, Nishimoto I. Analysis of stimulation—G protein subunit coupling by using active insulin-like growth factor II receptor peptide. Proc Natl Acad Sci USA 1991; 88:8020–8023.
52. Okamoto T, Nishimoto I. Detection of G protein–activator regions in M4 subtype muscarinic, cholinergic and α-adrenergic receptors based upon characteristics in primary structure. J Biol Chem 1992; 267:8342–8346.
53. Sexton PM, Houssami S, Hilton JM, et al. Identification of brain isoforms of the rat calcitonin receptor. Mol Endocrinol 1993; 7:815–821.
54. Albrandt K, Mull E, Brady EMG, et al. Molecular cloning of two receptors from rat brain with high affinity for salmon calcitonin. FEBS Lett 1993; 325:225–232.
55. Yamin M, Flannery MR, Tapp DR, et al. Analysis of a unique murine brain calcitonin receptor (CTR) cDNA and preliminary characterization of the murine CTR gene: Evidence for the existence of functionally distinct isoforms of the CTR. J Bone Min Res 1993; 8:S129.
56. Copeland NG, Jenkins NA. Development and applications of a molecular genetic linkage map of the mouse genome. Trends Genet 1991; 7:113–118.
57. Li Y-S, Hoffman RM, Le Beau MM, et al. Characterization of the human pleiotrophin gene. J Biol Chem 1992; 267:26011–26016.
58. Li E, Beston TH, Jaenisch R. Targeted mutation of the DNA methyltransferase gene results in embryonic lethality. Cell 1992; 69:915–926.
59. Searle AG. Mouse News Lett 1965; 33:29.
60. Strosberg AD. The molecular biology of receptors: Techniques and applications of receptor research. New York: Ellis Harwood, 1987.

61. Strosberg AD. Structure/function relationship of proteins belonging to the family of receptors coupled to GTP-binding proteins. Eur J Biochem 1991; 196:1–10.
62. Dohlman HG, Thorner J, Caron MG, Lefkowitz RJ. Model systems for the study of seven-transmembrane-segment receptors. Annu Rev Biochem 1991; 60:653–688.
63. Dohlman HG, Bouvier M, Benovic JL, et al. The multiple membrane spanning topography of the β-2 adrenergic receptor. J Biol Chem 1987; 262:14282–14288.
64. Baldwin JM. The probable arrangement of the helices in G protein–coupled receptors. EMBO J 1993; 12:1693–1703.
65. Shertler GF, Villa C, Henderson R. Projection structure of rhodopsin. Nature 1993; 362:770–772.
66. Simon MI, Strathmann MP, Gautam N. Diversity of G proteins in signal transduction. Science 1991; 252:802–808.
67. Gilman AG. G proteins: transducers of receptor-generated signals. Annu Rev Biochem 1987; 56:615–649.
68. Birnbaumer L. Receptor-to-effector signaling through G proteins: Roles for $\beta\gamma$ dimers as well as α subunits. Cell 1992; 71:1069–1072.
69. Jelinek LJ, Lok S, Rosenberg GB, et al. Expression cloning and signalling properties of the rat glucagon receptor. Science 1993; 259:1614–1616.
70. Ishihara T, Nakamura S, Kaziro Y, et al. Molecular cloning and expression of a cDNA encoding the secretin receptor. EMBO J 1991; 10:1635–1641.
71. Ishihara T, Shigemoto R, Mori K, et al. Functional expression and tissue distribution of a novel receptor for vasoactive intestinal polypeptide. Neuron 1992; 8:811–819.
72. Thorens B. Expression cloning of the pancreatic β-cell receptor for the gluco-incretin hormone glucagon-like peptide 1. Proc Natl Acad Sci USA 1992; 85:8641–8645.
73. Mayo KE. Molecular cloning and expression of a pituitary-specific receptor for growth hormone-releasing hormone. Mol Endocrinol 1992; 6:1734–1744.
74. Pisegna JR, Wank SA. Molecular cloning and functional expression of the pituitary adenylate cyclase-activating peptide type I receptor. Proc Natl Acad Sci USA 1993; 90:6345–6349.
75. Reagan JD. Expression cloning of an insect diuretic hormone receptor. J Biol Chem 1994; 269:1–4.
76. Nagayama Y, Rapoport B. The thyrotropic receptor 25 years after its discovery: New insights after its molecular cloning. Mol Endocrinol 1992; 6:145–156.
77. Abou-Samra AB, Jüppner H, Force T, et al. Expression cloning of a PTH/PTHrp receptor from rat osteoblast-like cells: A single receptor stimulates intracellular accumulation of both cAMP and inositol triphosphates and increases intracellular free calcium. Proc Natl Acad Sci USA 1992; 89:2732–2736.
78. Hosey MM. Diversity of structure, signaling and regulation within the family of muscarinic cholinergic receptors. FASEB J 1992; 6:845–852.
79. Lomasney JW, Cotecchia S, Lefkowitz RJ, Caron MG. Molecular biology of α-adrenergic receptors: Implications for receptor classification and for structure-function relationships. Biochem Biophysica Acta 1991; 1095:127–139.

19

Vitamin D and the Plasma Membrane Calcium Pump

Rajiv Kumar, Emanuel E. Strehler, and Qiang Cai
Mayo Clinic and Foundation
Rochester, Minnesota

INTRODUCTION

In this chapter, we will discuss recent insights concerning the structure and function of the plasma membrane calcium pump and its regulation by vitamin D. The actions of vitamin D include an increase in the expression of several genes involved in calcium transport, including the gene for one of the plasma membrane calcium pump isoforms. The net effect of the increase in the synthesis of various proteins involved in calcium translocation is an increase in the absorption of calcium in the intestine and the reabsorption of calcium from the tubule in the kidney.

VITAMIN D PHYSIOLOGY AND THE SYNTHESIS OF 1,25-DIHYDROXYVITAMIN D_3

It is now well established that the increase in efficiency of intestinal calcium absorption during states of dietary calcium deprivation is mediated by the active metabolite of vitamin D, 1,25-dihydroxy-vitamin D (Refs. 1 to 6 and references therein). It is also clear that the reabsorption of calcium in the renal tubule is influenced in part by 1,25-dihydroxyvitamin D. The metabolites of vitamin D in conjunction with parathyroid hormone (PTH) and calcitonin comprise the "vitamin D-endocrine system," and the regulation of the synthesis of 1,25-dihydroxyvitamin D synthesis by PTH and other factors results in a net increase in the retention of calcium by the organism.

Vitamin D_3 is formed in the skin as a result of the conversion of 7-dehydrocholesterol to previtamin D_3 by ultraviolet light present in sunlight (7–11). A wide range of wavelengths will efficiently transform 7-dehydrocholesterol to previtamin D_3. Factors influencing the extent of formation of previtamin D_3 include the duration of exposure to sunlight, the spectral properties of the incident light, pigmentation in skin, and other factors that might influence the penetration of ultraviolet light into the lower portions of the skin that contain 7-dehydrocholesterol (9,10). Previtamin D_3 is subsequently transformed at body temperature to vitamin D_3. Vitamin D_3 binds more tightly to a sterol-binding globulin, vitamin D-binding protein, than does previtamin D_3, and this property allows the preferential movement of vitamin D_3 out of the skin into the circulation (7–12). Vitamin D_2 is also present in the diet, is absorbed in the intestine, and is metabolized in a manner similar to that of cutaneously derived vitamin D_3. Vitamin D_2 is obtained from a plant sterol, ergosterol, and is available only in dietary products. It is not formed endogenously in the skin. Therefore, plasma concentrations of vitamin D_2 are an index of orally absorbed vitamin D, whereas concentrations of vitamin D_3 reflect endogenous synthesis as well as dietary intake.

Vitamin D_3 is transported to the liver, where it is converted by a microsomal cytochrome

P-450–containing vitamin D_3 25-hydroxylase into 25-hydroxyvitamin D_3 (13–17). The activity of the microsomal vitamin D_3 25-hydroxylase enzyme is regulated by preexisting concentrations of 25-hydroxyvitamin D_3 and D_3. The K_m of this enzyme is relatively low compared to that of another enzyme capable of transforming vitamin D_3 to 25-hydroxyvitamin D_3, the mitochondrial vitamin D_3 25-hydroxylase (15,16). The latter enzyme has a higher K_m for vitamin D_3 than does the microsomal enzyme and is not inhibited by vitamin D stores. Therefore, the administration of large amounts of exogenous vitamin D_3 or vitamin D_2 is associated with large increases in plasma 25-hydroxyvitamin D concentrations. Plasma 25-hydroxyvitamin D concentrations are an accurate measure of vitamin D stores.

25-Hydroxyvitamin D_3 is the major circulating form of vitamin D in the blood in states in calcium and phosphorus demands. It is metabolized to 1,25-dihydroxyvitamin D_3 by a multicomponent enzyme containing a cytochrome P-450, in mitochondria of the proximal tubule of the kidney (1–6,18–33). In situations where calcium and phosphorus are not needed, 25-hydroxyvitamin D_3 is metabolized to 24R,25-dihydroxyvitamin D_3 and several other metabolites (1–6,18–33). Other factors are known to control the biological activity of the 25-hydroxyvitamin D_3 1α-hydroxylase enzyme. These have been reviewed extensively elsewhere and will not be discussed further.

THE MECHANISM OF ACTION OF VITAMIN D INVOLVES NONGENOMIC AND GENOMIC EVENTS

Vitamin D_3 via its active metabolite, $1,25(OH)_2D_3$, plays a vital role in the regulation of calcium absorption in the intestine and the kidney, the mineralization of bone in vivo, and the maintenance of normal growth (Refs. 1 to 6. Please see references in these reviews for original articles). In addition, it alters the growth rate of various cells in vitro and in many instances causes cells to differentiate (34,35). The actions of $1,25(OH)_2D_3$ at the cellular level are mediated by both genomic and nongenomic mechanisms (1–6). Nongenomic actions include an increase in the uptake of calcium at the apical surface of the intestinal cell and the rapid movement of calcium into cells and across intestinal preparations maintained ex vivo (36–40). The genomic effects that are dependent upon receptors for $1,25(OH)_2D_3$ include increases in the synthesis of various proteins, such as the vitamin D-dependent calcium binding proteins, the 25-hydroxyvitamin D 24-hydroxylase, the $1,25(OH)_2D_3$ receptor, the plasma membrane calcium pump, osteocalcin, osteopontin, and ornithine decarboxylase, among others (1–6,41–75). In addition, $1,25(OH)_2D_3$ decreases the synthesis of proteins such as collagen and parathyroid hormone (76–79). Of the various proteins whose synthesis is controlled by $1,25(OH)_2D_3$, the plasma membrane calcium pump (PMCA) is of great importance, as it controls the rate of exit of calcium from the basolateral membrane into the extracellular fluid space, and thus increases the rate of accretion of the calcium by the organism (64–66).

THE MOVEMENT OF CALCIUM ACROSS CELL MEMBRANES AND EPITHELIA DEPENDS UPON THE ACTIVITY OF CALCIUM CHANNELS, PUMPS, AND EXCHANGERS

As shown in Fig. 1, calcium moves in and out of the cell and intracellular compartments through the action of various channels, pumps, and exchangers (80–83). Calcium channels allow the ingress of calcium into the cell, whereas calcium is extruded from the cell by the plasma membrane calcium pump and/or by the action of the sodium-calcium exchanger.

In considering the manner in which calcium moves across epithelia, it is important to remember that the movement of calcium into the cell is down an electrical and concentration gradient. The extrusion of calcium from the interior of the cell into the extracellular fluid space is against a concentration and electrical gradient and requires the expenditure of energy. The thermodynamic considerations in the movement of calcium across the intestinal epithelial cell layer are shown schematically in Fig. 2 (84). On reviewing these aspects of cellular calcium extrusion, it is clear that the PMCA plays an extremely important role in the absorption of calcium.

The PMCA has an Mr of 135 to 140,000 and exists as an integral plasma membrane protein that is located in most transporting epithelia along the basolateral aspect of the cell (85–95). In

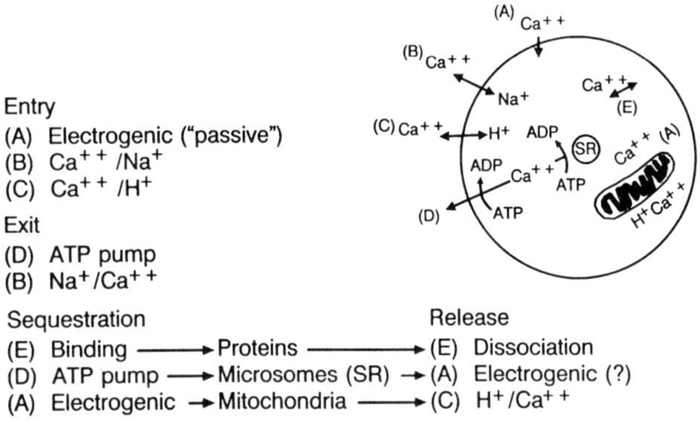

Figure 1 Options in the cellular movement of calcium. (From Ref. 80)

certain instances, as in the mammalian choroid plexus or in the avian shell gland, it is located on the apical membrane of the cell (87,94). In these tissues, however, the PMCA is appropriately located for the extrusion of calcium into the cerebrospinal fluid and the eggshell, respectively. The PMCA forms a calcium-sensitive, lanthanum-stabilized, acid-stable acyl phosphate intermediate that can be visualized on gels following the rapid labeling of membranes with γ ^{32}P ATP (81–83,96,97). This intermediate forms as a result of the transfer of the γ phosphate group from ATP to the carboxyl side chain of an aspartyl residue in the enzyme. ATP utilization and Ca^{2+} transport are tightly coupled in the pump; one ATP is split for each Ca^{2+} ion transported (83). Upon movement of calcium across the membrane, the acyl-phosphate obligatory bond is broken down to release inorganic phosphate. The acyl-phosphate obligatory intermediate of the PMCA reaction cycle is to be distinguished from the more stable phosphate intermediates formed by the phosphorylation of serine and threonine residues. The PMCA binds calmodulin in a calcium-dependent way, and this property has been used to purify the pump from various tissues (81,97–99). The PMCA is stimulated by calcium, calmodulin, proteolysis, and phosphatidyl inositol diphosphate (81–83,96,97,100,101). In

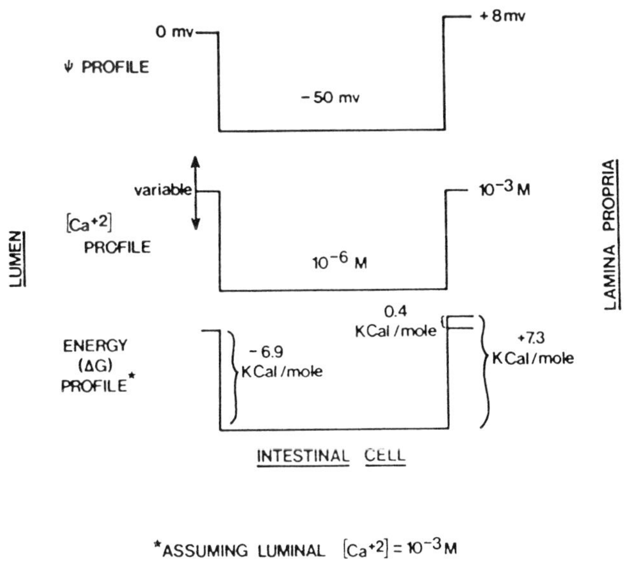

Figure 2 Thermodynamic considerations in the movement of calcium across an epithelial cell. (From Ref. 84.)

cardiac muscle, the pump is stimulated by the catalytic unit of cyclic AMP protein kinase, whereas cyclic GMP protein kinase may play a similar role in smooth muscle (101–106). Stimulation of the pump has also been observed as a consequence of phosphorylation by protein kinase C (107–109). The PMCA is inhibited by vanadate and oxalate. A calcium adenosine triphosphatase is also present in microsomes; however, it has a lower molecular weight than the PMCA, belongs to the subclass of ER/SR-calcium pumps, and is not inhibited by oxalate. We have recently cloned several isoforms of the PMCA from diverse human tissues and from normal human osteoblasts (110–113). The main structural features of the pump are shown in Fig. 3.

The Plasma Membrane Calcium Pump Is Present in Calcium Transporting Epithelia

Using immunohistochemical techniques, we have demonstrated that the PMCA is present in all calcium-transporting tissues analyzed so far (85–95). The pump is oriented in such a fashion as to allow the movement of calcium from within the cell into either the extracellular fluid space or the cerebrospinal fluid or the chick eggshell. These data supplement other, more extensive data demonstrating pump activity by biochemical means. The calcium-transporting tissues in which the PMCA has been detected by immunohistochemistry are shown in Table 1.

Analysis of the Structure of the Plasma Membrane Calcium Pump Reveals Specific Domains and Isoforms

Our laboratories have been responsible for isolating and sequencing cDNAs for several isoforms of the PMCA (96,110–113). Direct protein sequencing and exhaustive cDNA library screening data have shown that the human plasma membrane calcium pump is encoded by a multigene family consisting of at least four separate members. Additional isoform complexity is generated through alternative RNA splicing occurring at several "hot spots" in the primary gene transcripts (96,114–117). Table 2 summarizes the current state of knowledge regarding the various PMCA isoforms in different tissues.

Analysis of the Structure of the Human Plasma Membrane Calcium Pump Isoform 1 Gene

Analysis of the hPMCA-1 gene demonstrates that it occupies well over 100 kb of genomic DNA on chromosome 12q21-q23 (118) and contains 22 exons interrupted by introns varying in length from

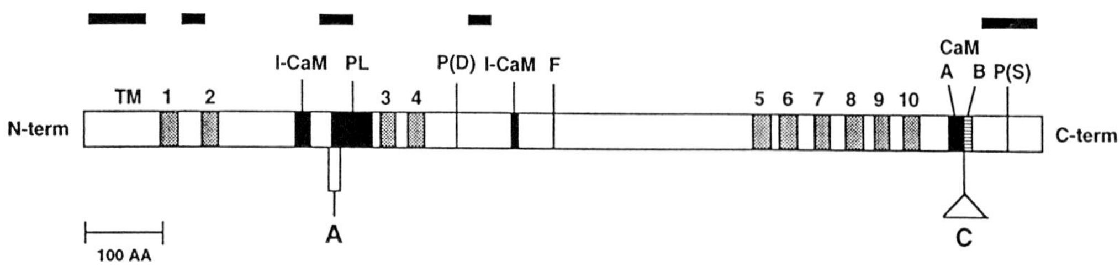

Figure 3 Domain assignment in the plasma membrane calcium pump and location of isoform variable regions. Top: Scheme of a PMCA (isoform type hPMCA1b), showing the location of known important domains, the areas of particularly high sequence divergence (black bars) among isoforms encoded by different genes and the sites (A and C) of possible alterations generated by translation of alternatively spliced mRNAs. Abbreviations: TM, putative transmembrane domain; PL, putative acidic phospholipid-sensitive region; P(D), site (aspartate residue) of acylphosphate formation; I-CaM, "inhibitory" regions that interact with the calmodulin binding region in the absence of Ca^{2+}/calmodulin; F, fluorescein isothiocyanate (FITC) binding site (= part of the ATP binding region); CaM, calmodulin binding region, separated into subdomains A and B; P(S), site (serine residue) of phosphorylation by the cAMP-dependent protein kinase. (From Ref. 96.)

Table 1 Distribution of PMCA in Transporting Epithelia as Assessed by Immunohistochemistry

Tissue	Source	Cell type	Location in cell	Reference
Kidney	Rat, human	Distal convoluted tubule, principal cell	Basolateral	85,90
Liver	Rat	Hepatocyte	Basolateral	95
Intestine	Rat, chick	Absorptive cell	Basolateral	92
Trophoblast	Rat, human	Syncytiotrophoblast	Basal	86,88
Choroid plexus	Cat Human	Choroid plexus secretory cell	Apical	87
Shell gland	Chick	Principal cell	Apical	94
Osteoblasts	Human	Osteoblasts	Not vectorially oriented	89
Osteoclast	Chick	Osteoclasts	Not vectorially oriented	Preliminary data

less than 100 bp to well over 30 kb (119). Large segments of the gene have been sequenced; in particular, more than 1 kb of the 5′ flanking (putative promoter) region has been analyzed in detail. Of substantial interest has been the finding that two purely 5′ untranslated exons appear to be alternatively used, indicating alternative promoter usage for the transcription of this gene. At least one sequence with resemblance to a vitamin D–regulatory element has been described in the 5′ region of this gene.

The Plasma Membrane Calcium Pump Protein Is Regulated in Vivo by Vitamin D and Dietary Calcium and Phosphorus

We have shown that the PMCA is regulated by $1,25(OH)_2D_3$ (65). When vitamin D–deficient chicks are given vitamin D_3, there is an increase, shortly after the administration of the vitamin, in the amount of PMCA pump present in the intestinal cells of these animals, as demonstrated by Western blot analysis. This is shown in Fig. 4.

In addition, the administration of a low-calcium or low-phosphorus diet to animals fed adequate amounts of vitamin D also results in an increase in the amount of PMCA protein (65) in the duodena of chicks maintained on such a diet. Figure 5 demonstrates the regulation of the plasma membrane calcium pump protein by calcium and phosphorus deficiencies.

VITAMIN D AND ADAPTATION TO DIETARY CALCIUM AND PHOSPHATE DEFICIENCIES INCREASE INTESTINAL PLASMA MEMBRANE CALCIUM PUMP ISOFORM 1 GENE EXPRESSION

We examined the effect of vitamin D and other variables on the synthesis of the chick intestinal PMCA mRNA (Fig. 6) (64). The DNA probe for Northern analysis was obtained by reverse transcription and PCR with intestinal poly A^+ RNA using two 20 mer oligonucleotides homologous to the 3′ coding region of the human PMCA isoform 1. We demonstrated by Northern analysis that the repletion of vitamin D-deficient chicks with vitamin D increases PMCA isoform 1 mRNA in the duodenum, jejunum, ileum, and colon. After the injection of $1,25(OH)_2D_3$ into vitamin D–deficient chicks, duodenal PMCA isoform 1 mRNA increased by 2 hr, reached a maximum at about 16 hr, and returned to baseline at 48 hr.

Adaptation of chicks to either a calcium- or a phosphorus deficient diet resulted in a two- to threefold increase in duodenal PMCA mRNA. These results indicate that vitamin D and specific

Table 2 cDNA Deduced Data on Mammalian Plasma Membrane Ca^{2+}-Pump Isoforms[a]

Isoform designation	Source	Splicing variants[b]	Length in amino acid residues	Calculated M_r
PMCA 1	Rat, human rabbit, pig	1a	1176	129,500
		1b	1220	134,700
		1c	1249	137,800
		1d	1258	138,800
		1e	1171	129,200
PMCA 2	Rat, human	2a/2z	1154	127,400
		2b/2z	1198	132,600
		2a/2x	1168	128,800
		2b/2x	1212	134,000
		2a/2w	1199	131,600
		2b/2w	1243	136,800
PMCA 3	Rat, human	3a/3z	1145	125,800
		3b/3z	1192	131,400
		3e/3z	1140	125,300
		3g/3z	1115	122,900
		3a/3x	1159	127,300
		3b/3x	1206	132,900
		3e/3x	1154	126,800
		3g/3x	1129	124,400
PMCA 4	Human, bovine, rat	4a/4z	1158	128,100
		4b/4z	1193	132,600
		4a/4x	1170	129,400
		4b/4x	1205	133,900

[a]Not all splice combinations have actually been detected as contiguous cDNAs. See Keeton et al. (116) and Stauffer et al. (117) for more details.
[b]The nomenclature for alternatively spliced isoform variants uses lowercase letters added to the corresponding isoform gene number (1, 2, 3, etc.). The lettering follows a somewhat arbitrary "historical" pattern of the detection of alternative splicing variants.

variables that affect calcium absorption through the vitamin D endocrine system increase intestinal PMCA gene expression.

In summary, we have shown that the PMCA, isoform 1, is regulated by vitamin D, and that the movement of calcium from the intestinal lumen across epithelial cells and the basolateral membrane into the extracellular fluid space is greatly enhanced by vitamin D, due to its effect on the synthesis of calcium binding proteins and the synthesis and the activity of the PMCA (4,5,64–66). A scheme depicting the events in calcium transport in the vitamin D–deplete and replete states are shown in Fig. 7.

VITAMIN D REGULATORY ELEMENTS ARE PRESENT IN THE GENES OF VITAMIN D–REGULATED PROTEINS

Several proteins are regulated by $1,25(OH)_2D_3$ in vivo and in cell culture systems. As noted earlier, $1,25(OH)_2D_3$ not only induces but, in some instances, decreases the synthesis of various proteins.

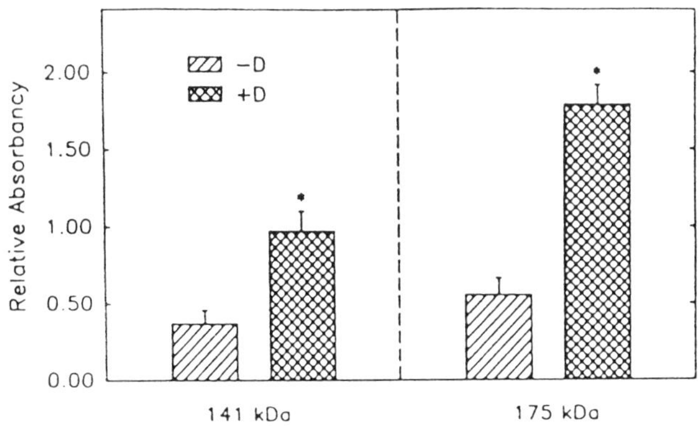

Figure 4 Effect of vitamin D_3 on the duodenal Ca^{2+}-pump epitope. Densitometric assessment of the 141- and 175-kDa bands on Western blots probed with antibody 5F10 against the plasma membrane calcium pump. For the 141-kDa band, the mean ±SE of the –D and +D bands are 0.37 ± 0.09 and 0.97 ± 0.13, respectively, with a p value of 0.03. For the 175-kDa band, the mean ±SE of the –D and +D bands are 0.56 ± 0.11 and 1.79 ± 0.13, respectively, with a p value of 0.01. (From Ref. 65).

The 5′ regulatory regions of the rat and human osteocalcin gene, the mouse and the pig osteopontin gene, and the rat 9K calbindin gene (120–132) have been studied for the presence of vitamin D–regulatory elements. A summary of the minimal sequence structures of the vitamin D regulatory elements (VDREs) of the osteocalcin, osteopontin and 9K calbindin VDREs is shown in Table 3. Although the vitamin D–regulated promoters initially identified are longer than the regions listed in Table 3, the structures shown are effective in generating hormone-stimulated increases in the activity of reporter genes placed 3′ of the promoter elements. In addition, the VDREs bind to the hormone-occupied VDR in the presence of a cell nuclear extract. As noted by Umesono and others (123), the AGGTCA half site, when present as a direct repeat, can function as a response element for triiodothyronine, vitamin D, or retinoic acid. The critical difference is the presence of a spacer element between the direct repeat hormone response elements. Thus, a three nucleotide spacer is effective as a VDRE; a four-nucleotide spacer converts the direct repeat to a thyroid response element; and a five-nucleotide spacer will convert the direct repeat to a retinoic acid response element (the "3-4-5 rule"). The promoters of the osteocalcin and osteopontin genes are direct repeats (imperfect repeats for osteocalcin) in which the half sites are separated by three bases.

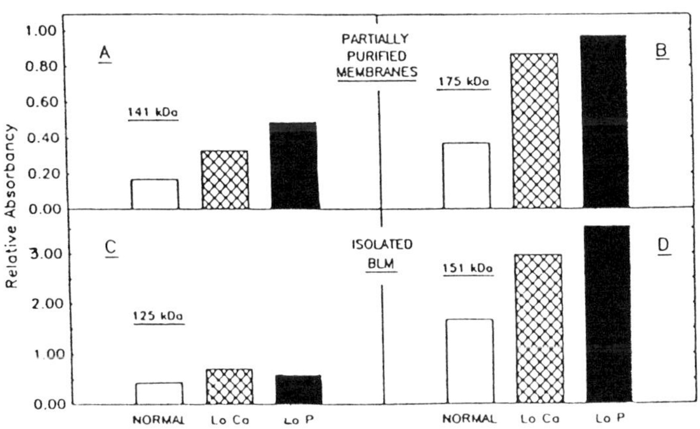

Figure 5 Effect of Ca and P deficiencies on the duodenal Ca^{2+}-pump epitope. Densitometric assessment of the 141- and 175-kDa bands. (From Ref. 65.)

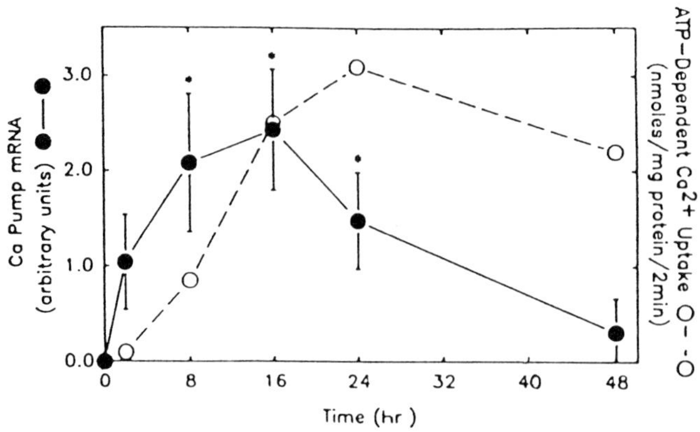

Figure 6 Temporal pattern of response of the duodenal PMCA-1 mRNA to $1,25(OH)_2D_3$. $1,25(OH)_2D_3$ (0.5 μg) was intravenously injected into vitamin D–deficient chickens at zero time. The number of replicate experiments for the time periods 0, 2, 8, 16, and 24 hr was 8 and that for 48 hr was 6. Each time point in each experiment represents the Northern blot analysis of total duodenal RNA (10 μg) from a pool of three animals. The probe was the cloned PMCA-1 cDNA. Values at 8, 16, and 24 hr by densitometric analysis were greater than the zero-time control value at $p < 0.05$. The p value for the 2-hr time point was 0.076; at 48 hr, $p > 0.5$. For comparison, previously published data on the ATP-dependent uptake of ^{45}Ca by isolated basolateral membrane vesicles (BLMVs) from a similar protocol are shown. The values, for comparative purposes, are given as [(density at time t)/(density at zero time)] −1 ●, Ca^{2+} pump mRNA: ○, BLMV Ca^{2+} uptake. (From Ref. 64.)

Although the so-called "3-4-5 rule" is operative in the instances noted above, it is clear that other VDREs are present in the human osteocalcin promoter that do not follow the 3-4-5 rule. Carlberg and colleagues (132) have recently demonstrated that a second class of VDREs is present in the osteocalcin gene and that these operate in a manner different than that noted for the VDREs described in Table 3. The sequence PuGGTCA arranged as a direct repeat with spacing of six nucleotides or as a palindrome without spacing also functions as a VDRE. The difference between the classes of VDREs lies in the nature of the factors needed to bind to and activate the VDRE (see below). While the direct repeat sequences separated by three nucleotides can be activated only by the vitamin D receptor *and* retinoic acid–X receptor together, the second class of VDREs can be activated by VDR alone. This would suggest that multiple types of VDREs exist in various vitamin D–regulated genes.

Promoter elements have been sought in the 5′ region of the 28K CaBP gene. Using computer algorithms, Minghetti et al. located a potential VDRE between −350 and −299 bp upstream of the transcription start site of the chick calbindin gene (133). Experiments using a reporter construct containing approximately 2,100 bp 5′ of the transcription start site showed high levels of basal chloramphenicol acetyl-transferase (CAT) activity and a twofold induction in CAT activity following the addition of $1,25(OH)_2D_3$. A shorter construct containing 924 bp 5′ to the transcription start site showed a smaller induction of reporter gene activity following the addition of $1,2\ (OH)_2D_3$. A construct containing 679 bp of DNA 5′ to the transcription start site, however, demonstrated significant reduction in reporter gene activity (134). DNase 1 footprinting experiments showed two prominent areas of protection against DNase 1 digestion upon the addition of intestinal nuclear extracts (135). These areas are located at −592 to −572 bp and −372 to −337 bp 5′ to the transcription start site. Ferrari and others were unable to demonstrate a VDRE in the region of the chick calbindin 28K gene between nucleotides −451 and +46. Using a construct that extended from bp −2200 to +46 (136), these authors were unable to demonstrate an increase in reporter gene activity in several cell lines following the addition of $1,25(OH)_2D_3$. This data is in contrast to that reported by Minghetti et al. (133). Therefore, at the present time, it is unclear where vitamin D regulatory elements reside in the 28K CaBP gene. Certainly, the degrees of induction noted in some of the reports are much less than the degrees of induction noted in vivo. Recently, Gill and Christakos reported on the presence of a VDRE in the 5′ region of the mouse $calbindin_{28K}$ gene (137). The effect of the VDRE

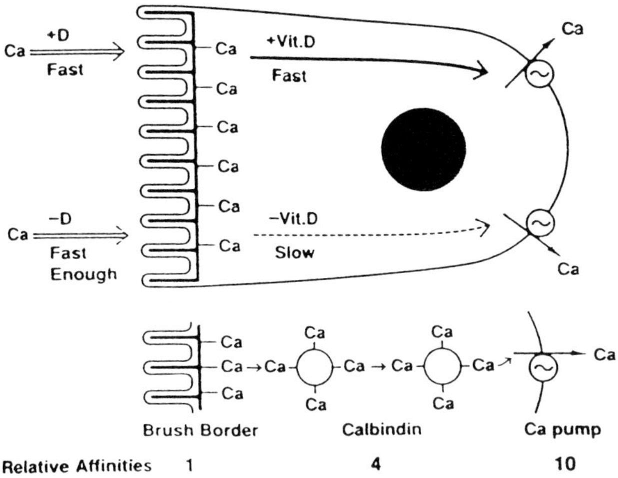

Figure 7 The transcellular diffusional-active transport model of Ca^{2+} absorption. (From Ref. 66.)

(i.e., an increase in the activity of the reporter gene in the presence of $1,25(OH)_2D_3$) was seen in the presence of butyrate. This VDRE, however, does not follow the 3-4-5 rule, as noted above for some of the other VDREs, as the spacer element is made up of four bases. The sequence of this element is:

−200 −160
ct GGGGGA tgtg AGGAGA aa TGAGT ctg AGCAAGCTCCAA
VDRE BUTYRATE RESPONSE ELEMENT

$1,25(OH)_2D_3$ not only induces the synthesis of various proteins but also suppresses the synthesis of other proteins in other cell types. Lichtler and others isolated the rat $\alpha 1$ (I) collagen promoter and cloned a 3.6 kb upstream DNA fragment 5′ to the chloramphenicol acetyl transferase reporter gene in a CAT expression vector (138). The chimeric plasmid was used to transfect ROS 17/2.8 cells. The expression of the reporter gene was diminished upon the addition of $1,25(OH)_2D_3$ to these cells. A 5′-flanking portion of the human PTH gene also contains a vitamin D response element that results in a decrease in the level of RNA initiated from the human PTH gene promoter following treatment with $1,25(OH)_2D_3$ (139,140). Recent experiments have localized this VDRE to a fragment of DNA

Table 3 Minimal Vitamin D Regulatory Elements Present in Vitamin D–Regulated Genes

Minimal vitamin D regulatory element	aggtca	agg	aggtca
Rat osteocalcin gene VDRE	gggtga	atg	aggaca
Human osteocalcin gene VDRE	gggtga	acg	ggggca
Mouse osteopontin gene VDRE	ggttca	cga	ggttca
9K calcium binding protein	gggtgt	cgg	aagccc

Source: Ref. 123.

between −125 to −101 bp 5′ of the transcription start site. The sequence of the VDRE is TATGTGTCTGC **TTTGAACCTA** TAGTT and contains a sequence (bold print, opposite strand) that is similar to that found in the VDRE of the osteopontin gene.

The VDREs bind specifically to the 1,25$(OH)_2D_3$ receptor, a ~ Mr 48,000 protein that has homology with thyroid hormone and retinoic acid receptors (68–75,141). Other proteins also bind to sequences within or close to the VDRE for the osteocalcin gene. An AP-1 binding site is present in the VDRE of the osteocalcin gene and binds c-*fos* and c-*jun* (129,142,143). In addition, cotransfection experiments with plasmids expressing c-*fos* and c-*jun* and an osteocalcin VDRE reporter construct reduces the basal and 1,25$(OH)_2D_3$–stimulated expression of the CAT gene, suggesting that c-*fos* and c-*jun* bind to the AP-1 binding site and reduce the ability of the VDRE to either bind to or stimulate the osteocalcin VDRE. The requirement of additional factors to ensure optimal binding of the VDR to VDREs suggested that an accessory nuclear factor was necessary for the optimal binding of protein to DNA (144–147). This factor has been recently identified as RXR (148). RXR enhances the binding of VDR to the osteocalcin VDRE as noted above.

The regulation of the PMCA isoform 1 gene is very likely to also involve the interaction of the vitamin D receptor with vitamin D regulatory elements present in the 5′ region of this gene. Further analysis of binding of regulatory factors to control elements in this gene should provide interesting information concerning the regulation of calcium flux across the basolateral membrane of calcium transporting epithelia.

CONCLUSIONS

1,25-Dihydroxyvitamin D_3 increases the activity of genes involved in calcium transport. At the apical surface of a transporting cell, the sterol increases permeability of the membrane to calcium. An increase in the synthesis of calcium-binding protein within the cell probably promotes calcium movement toward the basolateral membrane of the cell. At the same time as the increases in calcium movement are noted in the apical and main portion of the cell, there is a 1,25-dihydroxyvitamin D_3–mediated increase in calcium pump synthesis and activity at the basolateral portion of the cell. The changes in synthesis of proteins involved in calcium transport are mediated by the interaction of 1,25-dihydroxyvitamin D_3 and its receptor with response elements in the appropriate genes.

REFERENCES

1. DeLuca HF. The vitamin D story: A collaborative effort of basic science and clinical medicine. FASEB J 1988; 2:224–236.
2. Minghetti PP, Norman AW. 1,25$(OH)_2$-vitamin D_3 receptors: Gene regulation and genetic circuitry. FASEB J 1988; 2:3043–3053.
3. Kumar R. The metabolism of 1,25-dihydroxyvitamin D_3. Physiol Rev 1984; 64:478–504.
4. Gross MD, Kumar R. The physiology and biochemistry of vitamin D-dependent calcium binding proteins. Am J Physiol 1990; 259:F195–209.
5. Kumar R. Vitamin D and calcium transport. Kidney Int 1991; 40:1177–1189.
6. Lowe KE, Maiyar AC, Norman AW. Vitamin D-mediated gene expression. Crit Rev Eukaryotic Gene Exp 1992; 2:65–109.
7. Windaus A, Schenck F, von Weder F. Uber das antirachitisch wirksame bestrahlungs-produkt aus 7-dehydro-cholesterin. Hoppe-Seylers Z Physiol Chem 1936; 241:100–103.
8. Esvelt RP, Schnoes HK, DeLuca HF. Vitamin D_3 from rat skins irradiated in vitro with ultraviolet light. Arch Biochem Biophys 1978; 188:282–286.
9. Holick MF, McLaughlin JA, Clark MB, et al. Photosynthesis of previtamin D_3 in human skin and the physiologic consequences. Science 1980; 210:203–205.
10. Clemens TL, Henderson SL, Adams JS, Holick MF. Increased skin pigmentation reduces the capacity of skin to synthesize vitamin D_3. Lancet 1982; 1:74–76.
11. McLaughlin JA, Anderson RR, Holick MF. Spectral character of sunlight modulates photosynthesis of previtamin D_3 and its photoisomers in human skin. Science 1982; 216:1001–1003.
12. Haddad JG. Nature and functions of the plasma binding protein for vitamin D and its metabolites. In: Kumar R, ed. Vitamin D: Basic and Clinical Aspects. Boston: Martinus Nijhoff, 1984:383–396.
13. Ponchon G, DeLuca HF. The role of the liver in the metabolism of vitamin D. J Clin Invest 1969; 48:1273–1279.

14. Bhattacharyya MH, DeLuca HF. Subcellular location of rat liver calciferol-25-hydroxylase. Arch Biochem Biophys 1974; 160:58–62.
15. Bjorkhem I, Holmberg I. On the 25-hydroxylation of vitamin D_3 in vitro studied with a mass fragmentographic technique. J Biol Chem 1979; 254:9518–9524.
16. Yoon PS, DeLuca HF. Resolution and reconstitution of soluble components of rat liver microsomal vitamin D_3-25-hydroxylase. Arch Biochem Biophys 1980; 203:529–541.
17. Masumoto O, Ohyama Y, Okuda K. Purification and characterization of vitamin D 25-hydroxylase from rat liver mitochondria. J Biol Chem 1988; 263:14256–14260.
18. Holick MF, Schnoes HK, DeLuca HF, et al. Isolation and identification of 1,25-dihydroxycholecalciferol: A metabolite of vitamin D active in intestine. Biochemistry 1971; 10:2799–2804.
19. Haussler MR, Boyce DW, Littledike ET, Rasmussen H. A rapidly acting metabolite of vitamin D_3. Proc Natl Acad Sci USA 1971; 68:177–181
20. Norman AW, Myrtle JF, Midgett RJ, et al. 1,25-Dihydroxycholecalciferol: Identification of the proposed active form of vitamin D_3 in the intestine. Science 1971; 173:51–54.
21. Lawson DEM, Fraser DR, Kodicek E, et al. Identification of 1,25-dihydroxycholecalciferol, a new kidney hormone controlling calcium metabolism. Nature 1971; 230:228–230.
22. Fraser DR, Kodicek E. Unique biosynthesis by kidney of a biologically active vitamin D metabolite. Nature 1970; 228:764–766.
23. Gray RW, Omdahl JL, Ghazarian JG, DeLuca HF. 25-Hydroxycholecalciferol-1-hydroxylase: Subcellular location and properties. J Biol Chem 1972; 247:7528–7532.
24. Akiba T, Endou H, Koseki C, et al. Localization of 25-hydroxyvitamin D_3-1α-hydroxylase activity in the mammalian kidney. Biochem Biophys Res Commun 1980; 94:313–318.
25. Brunette MG, Chan M, Ferriere C, Roberts KD. Site of 1,25$(OH)_2$ vitamin D_3 synthesis in the kidney. Nature 1978; 276:287–289.
26. Kawashima H, Torikai S, Kurokawa K. Localization of 25-hydroxyvitamin D_3 1α-hydroxylase and 24-hydroxylase along the rat nephron. Proc Natl Acad Sci USA 1981; 78:1199–1203.
27. Ghazarian JG, Jefcoate CR, Knutson JC, et al. Mitochondrial cytochrome P450: A component of chick kidney 25-hydroxycholecalciferol-1α-hydroxylase. J Biol Chem 1974; 249:3026–3033.
28. Ghazarian JG, DeLuca HF. 25-Hydroxycholecalciferol-1-hydroxylase: A specific requirement of NADPH and a hemoprotein component in chick kidney mitochondria. Arch Biochem Biophys 1974; 160:63–72.
29. Pedersen JI, Ghazarian JG, Orme-Johnson NR, DeLuca HF. Isolation of chick renal mitochondrial ferredoxin active in the 25-hydroxyvitamin D_3-1α-hydroxylase system. J Biol Chem 1976; 251:3933–3941.
30. Yoon PS, DeLuca HF. Purification and properties of chick renal mitochondrial ferredoxin. Biochemistry 1980; 19:2165–2171.
31. Yoon PS, Rawlings J, Orme-Johnson WH, DeLuca HF. Renal mitochondrial ferredoxin active in 25-hydroxyvitamin D_3-1α-hydroxylase: Characterization of the iron-sulfur cluster using interprotein cluster transfer and electron paramagnetic resonance spectroscopy. Biochemistry 1980; 19:2172–2176.
32. Paulson SK, DeLuca HF. Subcellular location and properties of rat renal 25-hydroxyvitamin D_3-1α-hydroxylase. J Biol Chem 1985; 260:11488–11492.
33. Fraser DR: Regulation of the metabolism of vitamin D. Physiol Rev 1980; 60:551–613.
34. Gross M, Bollman-Kost S, Ennis B, et al. Effect of 1,25-dihydroxyvitamin D_3 on mouse mammary tumor (GR) cells: Evidence for receptors, cellular uptake, inhibition of growth and lateration in morphology at physiologic concentrations of hormone. J Bone Min Res 1986; 1:457–467.
35. Bar-Shavit Z, Teitelbaum SL, Reitsma P, et al. Induction of monocyte differentiation and bone resorption by 1,25-dihydroxyvitamin D_3. Proc Natl Acad Sci USA 1983; 80:5907–5911.
36. Rasmussen H, Matsumoto T, Fontaine O, Goodman DBP. Role of changes in membrane lipid structure in the action of 1,25-dihydroxyvitamin D_3. Fed Proc 1982; 41:72–77.
37. Fontaine O, Matsumoto T, Goodman DBP, Rasmussen H. Liponomic control of Ca^{2+} transport: Relationship to mechanism of action of 1,25-dihydroxyvitamin D_3. Proc Natl Acad Sci USA 1981; 78:1751–1754.
38. Baran DT, Kelly AM. Lysophosphatidylinositol: A potential mediator of 1,25-dihydroxyvitamin D-induced increments in hepatocyte cytosolic calcium. Endocrinology 1988; 122:930–934.
39. Norman AW, Nemere I, Muralidharan KR, Okamura WH. 1β,25(OH)2-vitamin D_3 is an antagonist of 1α,25(OH)2-vitamin D_3 stimulated transcaltachia (the rapidd hormonal stimulation of intestinal calcium transport). Biochem Biophys Res Commun 1992; 189:1450–1456.
40. Farach-Carson MC, Sergeev I, Norman AW. Nongenomic actions of 1,25-dihydroxyvitamin D_3 in rat osteosarcoma cells. Structure-function studies using ligand analogs. Endocrinology 1991; 129:1876–1884.
41. Wasserman RH, Corradino RA, Taylor AN. Vitamin D-dependent calcium-binding protein: Purification and some properties. J Biol Chem 1968; 243:3978–3986.
42. Wasserman RH, Taylor AN. Vitamin D-dependent calcium-binding protein: Response to some physiological and nutritional variables. J Biol Chem 1968; 243:3987–3993.

43. Thomasset M, Parkes CO, Cuisinier-Gleizes P. Rat calcium-binding proteins: Distribution, development, and vitamin D dependence. Am J Physiol 1982; 243:E483–E488.
44. Christakos S, Friedlander EJ, Frandsen BR, Norman AW. Studies on the mode of action of calciferol: XIII. Development of a radioimmunoassay for vitamin D-dependent chick intestinal calcium binding protein and tissue distribution. Endocrinology 1979; 104:1495–1503.
45. Shinki T, Takahashi N, Miyaura C, et al. Ornithine decarboxylase activity in chick duodenum induced by 1,25-dihydroxycholecalciferol. Biochem J 1981; 195:685–690.
46. Steeves RM, Lawson DEM. Effect of 1,25-dihydroxyvitamin D on S-adenosyl-methionine decarboxylase in chick intestine. Biochim Biophys Acta 1985; 841:292–298.
47. DeJonge HR, Ghijsen WEJ, Van Os CH. Phosphorylated intermediates of Ca^{2+}-ATPase and alkaline phosphatase in plasma membranes from rat duodenal epithelium. Biochim Biophys Acta 1981; 647:140–149.
48. Price PA, Baukol SA. 1,25-dihydroxyvitamin D_3 increases synthesis of the vitamin K-dependent bone protein by osteosarcoma cells. J Biol Chem 1980; 255:11660–11663.
49. Effect of vitamin D status on vitamin K-dependent osteocalcin formation. Nutr Rev 1982; 40:249–250.
50. Chang PL, Prince CW. 1α,25-dihydroxyvitamin D_3 stimulates synthesis and secretion of nonphosphorylated osteopontin (secreted phosphoprotein 1) in mouse JB6 epidermal cells. Cancer Res 1991; 51:2144–2150.
51. Prince CW, Butler WT. 1,25-dihydroxyvitamin D_3 regulates the biosynthesis of osteopontin, a bone-derived cell attachment protein, in clonal osteoblast-like osteosarcoma cells. Coll Relat Res 1987; 7:305–313.
52. Wilson PW, Lawson DEM. Incorporation of ^{3}H-leucine into an actin-like protein in response to $1,25(OH)_2D_3$ in chick intestinal brush borders. Biochem J 1978; 173:627–631.
53. Lane SM, Lawson DEM. Differentiation of the changes in alkaline phosphatase from calcium ion-activated adenosine triphosphatase activities associated with increased calcium absorption in chick intestine. Biochem J 1978; 174:1067–1070.
54. Ghijsen WEJM, Van Os CH. 1,25-Dihydroxyvitamin D_3 regulates ATP-dependent calcium transport in basolateral plasma membranes of rat enterocytes. Biochim Biophys Acta 1982; 689:170–172.
55. Meyer SA, Wasserman RH. Vitamin D_3 increases ATP-dependent calcium transport of chick duodenal basolateral membranes. Fed Proc 1983; 42:1367.
56. Ghijsen WEJM, Van Os CH, Heizmann CW, Murer H. Regulation of duodenal Ca^{2+} pump by calmodulin and vitamin D-dependent Ca^{2+}-binding protein. Am J Physiol 1986; 251:G223–G229.
57. Morgan DW, Welton AF, Heick AE, Christakos S. Specific in vitro activation of Ca,Mg-ATPase by vitamin D-dependent rat renal calcium binding protein (calbindin D_{28K}). Biochem Biophys Res Commun 1986; 138:547–553.
58. Walters JR. Calbindin-D9K stimulates the calcium pump in rat enterocyte basolateral membranes. Am J Physiol 1989; 256:G124–G128.
59. Varghese S, Deaven LL, Huang YC, et al. Transcriptional regulation and chromosomal assignment of the mammalian calbindin-D28K gene. Mol Endocrinol 1989, 3:495–502.
60. Clemens TL, McGlade SA, Garrett KP, et al. Extracellular calcium modulates vitamin D-dependent calbindin-D28K gene expression in chick kidney cells. Endocrinology 1989; 124:1582–1584.
61. Varghese S, Lee S, Huang YC, Christakos S. Analysis of rat vitamin D-dependent calbindin-D28K gene expression. J Biol Chem 1988; 263:9776–9784.
62. Dupret JM, Brun P, Perret C, et al. Transcriptional and post-transcriptional regulation of vitamin D-dependent calcium-binding protein gene expression in the rat duodenum by 1,25-dihydroxycholecalciferol. J Biol Chem 1987; 262:16553–16557.
63. Theofan G, Nguyen AP, Norman AW. Regulation of calbindin-D28K gene expression by 1,25-dihydroxyvitamin D_3 is correlated to receptor occupancy. J Biol Chem 1986; 261:16943–16947.
64. Cai Q, Chandler JS, Wasserman RH, et al. Vitamin D and adaptation to dietary calcium and phosphate deficiencies increase intestinal plasma membrane calcium pump gene expression. Proc Natl Acad Sci USA, 1993; 90:1345–1349.
65. Wasserman RH, Smith CA, Brindak ME, et al. Vitamin D and mineral deficiencies increase the plasma membrane calcium pump of chicken intestine. Gastroenterology 1992; 102:886–894.
66. Wasserman RH, Chandler JS, Meyer SA, et al. Intestinal calcium transport and calcium extrusion processes at the basolateral membrane. J Nutr 1992; 122:662–671.
67. Kumar R, Schnoes HK, DeLuca HF. Rat intestinal 25-hydroxyvitamin D_3 and 1α,25-dihydroxyvitamin D_3-24-hydroxylase. J Biol Chem 1978; 253:3804–3809.
68. Pike JW: Vitamin D_3 receptors: structure and function in transcription. Annu Rev Nutr 1991; 11:189–216.
69. Baker AR, McDonnell DP, Hughes MR, et al. Cloning and expression of full-length cDNA encoding human vitamin D receptor. Proc Natl Acad Sci USA 1988; 85:3294–3298.
70. Berger U, Wilson P, McClelland RA, et al. Immunocytochemical detection of 1,25-dihydroxyvitamin D receptors in normal human tissues. J Clin Endocrinol Metab 1988; 67:607–613.

71. Brumbaugh PF, Haussler MR. 1,25-Dihydroxycholecalciferol receptors in intestine. Temperature-dependent transfer of the hormone to chromatin via a specific cytosol receptor. J Biol Chem 1974; 249:1258–1262.
72. Brumbaugh PF, Haussler MR: 1,25-Dihydroxycholecalciferol receptors in intestine: Association of 1,25-dihydroxycholecalciferol with intestinal mucosa chromatin. J Biol Chem 1974; 249:1251–1257.
73. Brumbaugh PF, Haussler MR. Specific binding of 1,25-dihydroxycholecalciferol to nuclear components of chick intestine. J Biol Chem 1975; 250:1588–1594.
74. Burmester JK, Maeda N, DeLuca HF. Isolation and expression of rat 1,25-dihydroxyvitamin D_3 receptor cDNA. Proc Natl Acad Sci USA 1988; 85:1005–1009.
75. Burmester JK, Wiese RJ, Maeda N, DeLuca HF. Structure and regulation of the rat 1,25-dihydroxyvitamin D_3 receptor. Proc Natl Acad Sci USA 1988; 85:9499–9502.
76. Silver J, Naveh-Many T. Mayer H, et al. Regulation by vitamin D metabolites of parathyroid hormone gene transcription in vivo in the rat. J Clin Invest 1986; 78:1296–1301.
77. Russell J, Lettieri D, Sherwood L. Suppression by $1,25(OH)_2D_3$ of transcription of the pre-proparathyroid hormone gene. Endocrinology 1986; 119:2864–2866.
78. Genovese C, Rowe D, Kream BE. Construction of DNA sequences complementary to rat $\alpha 1$ and $\alpha 2$ collagen mRNA and their use in studying the regulation of type I collagen synthesis by 1,25-dihydroxyvitamin D. Biochemistry 1984; 23:6210–6215.
79. Kream BE, Rowe DW, Gworek SC, Raisz LG. Parathyroid hormone alters collagen synthesis and procollagen mRNA levels in fetal rat calvaria. Proc Natl Acad Sci USA 1980; 77:5654–5648.
80. Racker E. Fluxes of Ca^{2+} and concepts. Fed Proc 1980; 39:2422–2426.
81. Carafoli E. Intracellular calcium homeostasis. Annu Rev Biochem 1987; 56:395–433.
82. Penniston JT. Plasma membrane Ca^{2+}-ATPases as active Ca^{2+} pumps. In: Cheung WY, ed. Calcium and Cell Function. New York: Academic Press, 1983; 4:99–149.
83. Carafoli E. Calcium pump of the plasma membrane. Physiol Rev 1991; 71:129–153.
84. Wasserman R, Fullmer CS, Shimura F. Calcium absorption and the molecular effects of vitamin D_3. In: Kumar R, ed. Vitamin D: Basic and Clinical Aspects. Boston: Martinus Nijhoff, 1984:233–257.
85. Borke JL, Caride A, Verma AK, et al. Plasma membrane calcium pump and 28 kDa calcium binding protein in cells of rat kidney distal tubules. Am J Physiol 1989; 257:F842–849.
86. Borke JL, Caride A, Verma AK, et al. Calcium pump epitopes in placental trophoblast membranes. Am J Physiol 1989; 257:C341–C346.
87. Borke JL, Caride AJ, Yaksh TL, et al. Cerebrospinal fluid calcium homeostasis: Evidence for a plasma membrane Ca^{++}-pump in mammalian choroid plexus. Brain Res 1989; 489:355–360.
88. Kelley LK, Borke JL, Verma AK, et al. The calcium transporting ATPase and the calcium or magnesium dependent nucleotide phosphatase activities of human placental trophoblast basal plasma membrane are separate enzyme activities. J Biol Chem 1990; 265:5453–5459.
89. Borke JL, Eriksen EF, Minami J, et al. Epitopes to the human erythrocyte Ca^{++}-Mg^{++} ATPase pump in human osteoblast-like cell plasma membranes. J Clin Endocrinol Metab 1988; 67:1299–1304.
90. Borke JL, Minami J, Verma A, et al. Monoclonal antibodies to human erythrocyte membrane Ca^{++}-Mg^{++} adenosine triphosphatase pump recognize an epitope in the basolateral membrane of human kidney distal tubule cells. J Clin Invest 1987; 80:1225–1231.
91. Borke JL, Minami J, Verma AK, Penniston JT, Kumar R. Co-Localization of erythrocyte Ca^{++}-Mg^{++} ATPase and vitamin D-dependent 28-kilodalton-calcium binding protein in the cells of human kidney distal tubules. Kidney Int 1988; 34:262–267.
92. Borke JL, Caride A, Verma AK, et al. Cellular and segmental distribution of Ca^{++}-pump epitopes in rat intestine. Pflugers Arch 1990; 417:120–122.
93. Borke JL, Penniston JT, Kumar R. Recent advances in calcium transport by the kidney. Semin Nephrol 1990; 10:15–23.
94. Wasserman RH, Smith CA, Smith CM, et al. Immunohistochemical localization of a calcium pump and calbindin-D_{28K} in the oviduct of the laying hen. Histochemistry 1991; 96:413–418.
95. Kessler F, Bennardini F, Bachs O, et al. Partial purification and characterization of the Ca^{2+}-pumping ATPase of the liver membrane. J Biol Chem 1990; 265:16012–16019.
96. Strehler EE. Recent advances in the molecular characterization of plasma membrane Ca^{2+} pumps. J Membrane Biol 1991; 120:1–15.
97. Carafoli E, Zurini M. The Ca^{2+}-pumping ATPase of plasma membranes: Purification, reconstitution and properties. Biochim Biophys Acta 1982; 683:279–301.
98. Niggli V, Penniston JT, Carafoli E. Purification of the (Ca^{2+}-Mg^{2+})-ATPase from human erythrocyte membranes using a calmodulin affinity column. J Biol Chem 1979; 254:9955–9958.
99. Hakim G, Itano T, Verma AK, Penniston JT. Purification of the Ca^{2+}- and Mg^{+} requiring ATPase from rat brain synaptic plasma membrane. Biochem J 1982; 207:225–231.
100. Michalak M, Famulski K, Carafoli E. The Ca^{2+}-pumping ATPase in skeletal muscle sarcolemma:

Calmodulin dependence, regulation by cAMP-dependent phosphorylation, and purification. J Biol Chem 1984; 259:15540–15547.
101. Choquette D, Hakim G, Filoteo AG, et al. Regulation of plasma membrane Ca^{2+} ATPases by lipids of the phosphatidylinositol cycle. Biochem Biophys Res Comm 1984; 125:908–915.
102. Caroni P, Zurini M, Clark A, Carafoli E. Further characterization and reconstitution of the purified Ca^{2+}-pumping ATPase of heart sarcolemma. J BioL Chem 1983; 258:7305–7310.
103. DeSchutter G, Wuytack F, Verbist J, Cateels R. Tissue levels and purification by affinity chromatography of the calmodulin-stimulated Ca^{2+}-transport ATPase in pig arterial smooth muscle. Biochim Biophys Acta 1984; 773:1–10.
104. Furukawa N, Nakamura H. Characterization of the (Ca^{2+}-Mg^{2+}) ATPase purified by calmodulin-affinity chromatography from bovine aortic smooth muscle. J Biochem (Tokyo) 1984; 96:1343–1350.
105. Sarkadi B, Enyedi A, Foldes-Papp Z, Gardos G. Demonstration of two distinct calcium pumps in platelet membrane vesicles. J Biol Chem 1986; 261:9552–9557.
106. Caroni P, Carafoli E. Regulation of Ca^{2+}-pumping ATPase of heart sarcolemma by a phosphorylation-dephosphorylation process. J Biol Chem 1981; 256:9371–9373.
107. Wang KK, Wright LC, Machan CL, et al. Protein kinase C phosphorylates the carboxyl terminus of the plasma membrane Ca^{2+}-ATPase from human erythrocytes. J Biol Chem 1991; 266:9078–9085.
108. Furukawa K, Tawada Y, Shigekawa M. Protein kinase C activation stimulates plasma membrane Ca^{2+} pump in cultured vascular smooth muscle cells. J Biol Chem 1989; 264:4844–4849.
109. Smallwood JI, Gugi B, Rasmussen H. Regulation of erythrocyte Ca^{2+} pump activity by protein kinase C. J Biol Chem 1988; 263:2195–2101.
110. Verma AK, Filoteo AG, Stanford DR, et al. Complete primary structure of a human plasma membrane Ca^{2+} pump. J Biol Chem 1988; 263:14152–14159.
111. Strehler EE, James P, Fischer R, et al. Peptide sequence analysis and molecular cloning reveal two calcium pump isoforms in the human erythrocyte membrane. J Biol Chem 1990; 265:2835–2842.
112. Heim R, Hug M, Iwata T, et al. Microdiversity of human-plasma-membrane calcium-pump isoform 2 generated by alternative RNA splicing in the N-terminal coding region. Eur J Biochem 1992; 205:333–340.
113. Kumar R, Haugen JD, Penniston JT. The molecular cloning of a plasma membrane calcium pump from human osteoblasts. J Bone Min Res 1993; 8:505–413.
114. Strehler EE, Strehler-Page M-A, et al. mRNAs for plasma membrane calcium pump isoforms differing in their regulatory domain are generated by alternative splicing that involves two internal donor sites in a single exon. Proc Natl Acad Sci USA 1989; 86:6908–6912.
115. Kessler F, Falchetto R, Heim R, et al. Study of calmodulin binding to the alternatively spliced C-terminal domain of the plasma membrane Ca^{2+} pump. Biochemistry 1992; 31:11785–11792.
116. Keeton TP, Burk SE, Shull GE. Alternative splicing of exons encoding the calmodulin-binding domains and C-termini of plasma membrane Ca^{2+}-ATPase isoforms 1, 2, 3, and 4. J Biol Chem 1993; 268:2740–2748.
117. Stauffer TP, Hilfiker H. Carafoli E, Strehler EE. Quantitative analysis of alternative splicing options of human plasma membrane calcium pump genes. J Biol Chem 1993; 268:25993–26003 (correction J Biol Chem 1994; 269:32022).
118. Olson S, Wang MG, Carafoli E, et al. Localization of two genes encoding plasma membrane Ca^{2+}-transporting ATPase to human chromosomes 1q25-32 and 12q21-23. Genomics 1991; 9:629–641.
119. Hilfiker H, Strehler-Page M-A, Stauffer TP, et al. Structure of the gene encoding the human plasma membrane calcium pump isoform 1. J Biol Chem 1993; 268:19717–19725.
120. Kerner SA, Scott RA, and Pike JW. Sequence elements in the human osteocalcin gene confer basal activation and inducible response to hormonal vitamin D_3. Proc Natl Acad Sci USA 1989; 86:4455–4459.
121. McDonnell DP, Scott RA, Kerner SA, et al. Functional domains of the human vitamin D_3 receptor regulate osteocalcin gene expression. Mol Endocrinol 1989; 3:635–644.
122. Terpening CM, Haussler CA, Jurutka PW, et al. The vitamin D-responsive element in the rat bone gla protein gene is an imperfect direct repeat that cooperates with other Cis-elements in 1,25-dihydroxyvitamin D_3-mediated transcriptional activation. Mol Endocrinol 1991; 5:375–385.
123. Umesono K, Murakami KK, Thompson CC, Evans RM. Direct repeats as selective response elements for the thyroid hormone, retinoic acid and vitamin D_3 receptors. Cell 1991; 65:1255–1266.
124. Demay MB, Gerardi JM, DeLuca HF, Kronenberg HM. DNA sequences in the rat osteocalcin gene that bind the 1,25-dihydroxyvitamin D_3 receptor and confer responsiveness to 1,25-dihydroxyvitamin D_3. Proc Natl Acad Sci USA 1990; 87:369–373.
125. Darwish HM, DeLuca HF. Identification of a 1,25-dihydroxyvitamin D_3-response element in the 5′-flanking region of the rat calbindin D-9k gene. Proc Natl Acad Sci USA 1992; 89:603–607.
126. Noda M, Vogel RL, Craig AM, et al. Identification of a DNA sequence responsible for binding of the 1,25-dihydroxyvitamin D_3 receptor and 1,25-dihydroxyvitamin D_3 enhancement of mouse secreted phosphoprotein 1 (Spp-1 or osteopontin) gene expression. Proc Natl Acad Sci USA 1990; 87:9995–9999.

127. Zhang Q, Wrana JL, Sodek J. Characterization of the promoter region of the porcine opn (osteopontin, secreted phosphoprotein 1) gene. Eur J Biochem 1992; 207:649–659.
128. Ozono K, Liao J, Kerner SA, et al. The vitamin D-responsive element in the human osteocalcin gene. J Biol Chem 1990; 265:21881–21888.
129. Own TA, Bortell R, Yocum SA, et al. Coordinate occupancy of AP-1 sites in the vitamin D-responsive and CCAAT box elements by Fos-Jun in the osteocalcin gene: Model for phenotype suppression of transcription. Proc Natl Acad Sci USA 1990; 87:9990–9994.
130. Markose ER, Stein JL, Stein GS, Lian JB. Vitamin D-mediated modifications in protein-DNA interactions at two promoter elements of the osteocalcin gene. Proc Natl Acad Sci USA 1990; 87:1701–1705.
131. Bortell R, Owen TA, Bidwell JP, et al. Vitamin D-responsive protein-DNA interactions at multiple promoter regulatory elements that contribute to the level of rat osteocalcin gene expression. Proc Natl Acad Sci USA 1992; 89:6119–6123.
132. Carlberg C, Bendik I, Wyss A, et al. Two nuclear signalling pathways for Vitamin D. Nature 1993; 361:657–660.
133. Minghetti PP, Gibbs PEM, Norman AW. Computer analysis of 1,25-dihydroxyvitamin D_3-receptor regulated promoters: Identification of a candidate D_3-response element. Biochem Biophys Res Comm 1989; 162:869–875.
134. Maiyar AC, Minghetti PP, Norman AW. Transfection of avian vitamin D-dependent calbindin-D_{28K} 5′ flanking promoter sequence in primary chick kidney cells. Mol Cell Endocrinol 1991; 78:127–135.
135. Boland R, Minghetti PP, Lowe KE, Norman AW. Sequences near the CCAAT region and putative 1,25-dihydroxyvitamin D_3-response element and further upstream novel regulatory sequences of calbindin-D_{28K} promoter show DNase I footprinting protection. Mol Cell Endocrinol 1991; 75:57–63.
136. Ferrari S, Battini R, Pike WJ. Functional analysis of the promoter region of the gene encoding chicken calbindin D28K. Adv Exp Med Biol 1990; 269:21–25.
137. Gill RK, Christakos S. Identification of sequence elements in mouse calbindin-D_{28K} gene that confer 1,25-dihydroxyvitamin D_3- and butyrate-inducible responses. Proc Natl Acad Sci USA 1993; 90:2984–2988.
138. Lichtler A, Stover ML, Angilly J, et al. Isolation and characterization of the rat α1(I) collagen promoter. J Biol Chem 1989; 264:3072–3077.
139. Okazaki T, Igarashi T, Kronenberg HM. 5′-Flanking region of the parathyroid hormone gene mediates negative regulation by $1,25(OH)_2D_3$ vitamin D_3. J Biol Chem 1988; 263:2203–2208.
140. Demay MB, Kiernan MS, DeLuca HF, Kronenberg HM. Sequences in the human parathyroid hormone gene that bind the 1,25-dihydroxyvitamin D_3 receptor and mediate transcriptional repression in response to 1,25-dihydroxyvitamin D_3. Proc Natl Acad Sci USA 1992; 89:8097–8101.
141. McDonnel DP, Mangelsdorf DJ, Pike JW, et al. Molecular cloning of complementary DNA encoding the avian receptor for vitamin D. Science 1987; 235:1214–1217.
142. Schule R, Umesono K, Mangelsdorf DJ, et al. Jun-Fos and receptors for vitamins A and D recognize a common response element in the human osteocalcin gene. Cell 1990; 61:497–504.
143. The osteocalcin gene promoter: Stimulated by vitamins A and D, inhibited by cell-growth factors Jun-Fos. Nutr Rev 1991; 49:308–309.
144. Ross TK, Moss VE, Prahl JM, DeLuca HF. A nuclear protein essential for binding of rat 1,25-dihydroxyvitamin D_3 receptor to its response elements. Proc Natl Acad Sci USA 1992; 89:256–260.
145. Liao J, Ozono K, Sone T, et al. Vitamin D receptor interaction with specific DNA requires a nuclear protein and 1,25-dihydroxyvitamin D_3. Proc Natl Acad Sci USA 1990; 87:9751–9755.
146. Sone T, Ozono K, Pike JW. A 55-kilodalton accessory factor facilitates vitamin D receptor DNA binding. Mol Endocrinol 1991; 5:1578–1586.
147. Sone T, Kerner S, Pike JW. Vitamin D receptor interaction with specific DNA. J Biol Chem 1991; 266:23296–23305.
148. Yu VC, Delsert C, Andersen B, et al. RXRβ: a coregulator that enhances binding of retinoic acid, thyroid hormone, and vitamin D receptors to their cognate response elements. Cell 1991; 67:1251–1266.

20
Molecules Involved in Proximal Tubular Apical Na/Pi Cotransport

J. Biber and H. Murer
Institute of Physiology, University of Zurich, Zurich, Switzerland

INTRODUCTION

Renal handling of phosphate represents an important determinant in maintaining the concentration of inorganic phosphate (P_i) in the plasma within a fairly narrow range (phosphate homeostasis). Under normal conditions, the freely filtered inorganic P_i is reabsorbed to a large extent (up to 80%) in the proximal tubules. The highest rates of P_i reabsorption are observed within the pars convoluta of the proximal tubules (for review, see Ref. 1). Proximal tubular reabsorption of P_i is transcellular and is accomplished by phosphate transport systems located in the brush border and basolateral membrane of the polarized proximal tubular cell. At the apical cell surface, P_i is taken up via an obligatory sodium-dependent P_i-transport system (Na/P_i-cotransport). Exit of P_i at the basolateral cell surface most likely occurs via an anion exchange mechanism (for review, see Ref. 2).

In the last few years, it has become clear that proximal tubular apical Na/P_i cotransport represents a major target for the physiological/pathophysiological regulation of renal P_i reabsorption. Using intact tubular systems, isolated brush border membranes, and cultured renal epithelial cells, it has been demonstrated that hormonal (e.g., parathyroid hormone) and nonhormonal factors (e.g., phosphate diet) that control proximal tubular P_i reabsorption also influence the rate of apical Na/P_i cotransport (1–3). These factors often provoke a change in the maximal transport capacity (V_{max}) of the apical Na-dependent P_i-transport step. It has therefore been suggested that they alter the number of Na/P_i cotransporters residing within the apical membrane.

Regulation of apical Na/P_i cotransport was studied mainly by functional parameters and in part also by the use of competitive inhibitors such as phosphonoformic acid (4). Recently, we have succeeded in cloning several cDNAs encoding renal Na/P_i-cotransport systems. In this article, we will discuss some aspects of the newly cloned Na/P_i cotransporters, their localization within the nephron, and their possible role in the physiological and pathophysiological regulation of renal P_i reabsorption.

IDENTIFICATION AND CHARACTERIZATION OF CLONED Na/P_i-COTRANSPORT SYSTEMS

Identification

Biochemical approaches to identify Na/P_i-cotransport systems have failed mainly because of the lack of suitable high-affinity probes. Phoshonoformic acid and its derivatives have been used as inhibitors of apical Na/P_i cotransport. However, the specificity of phosphonoformic acid binding to brush border membranes is still controversial (3). A more direct approach to identify membrane transport systems became possible using *Xenopus laevis* oocytes as an expression system (5). Based on the observations that injection of poly(A)$^+$RNA isolated from the kidney cortex of the rabbit into oocytes results in expression of Na/P_i-cotransport activity (6), we have recently cloned several Na/P_i-cotransport systems from kidney cortex cDNA libraries of various species (Na$P_{i\text{-}x}$; see Table 1).

Originally, a system named NaP_{i-1} was isolated from a rabbit kidney cortex cDNA library (7). Based on nucleotide-sequence homologies, similar Na/P_i cotransporters have also been identified in the mouse and human genomes (M. Hughes; personal communication). In addition, the expression cloning strategy has identified two other systems in rat (NaP_{i-2}) and human (NaP_{i-3}) kidney cortex cDNA libraries (8). Using a hybridization approach, a Na/P_i cotransporter homologous to the $NaP_{i-2/3}$ systems was also identified in a cDNA library from OK cells (NaP_{i-4}; Ref. 9). Sequence comparison of the deduced amino acid sequences revealed that the renal Na/P_i cotransporters cloned so far belong to two different types (families) of transporters, a type I (NaP_{i-1}) and a type II (NaP_{i-2}) family (see Table 1). There is only 20% identity between the type I and type II transporters. To date, these two types of renal Na/P_i cotransporters do not seem to belong to a described family of mammalian or nonmammalian membrane transport systems (10).

The proteins encoded by the cloned cDNAs were identified by Western blots using polyclonal antibodies raised against synthetic peptides based on the deduced N- and C-terminal amino acid sequences. In brush border membranes isolated from rabbit kidney cortex, the NaP_{i-1} system appeared as a protein of 60 to 64 kDa (11), and in brush border membranes isolated from rat kidney cortex, the NaP_{i-2} system appeared as a 80- to 90-kDa protein (12). These values seem to be in agreement with predicted molecular weights and with the fact that renal Na/P_i cotransporters of both types are N-glycosylated (7,8).

Structural Aspects

Based on hydropathy analysis of the deduced amino acid sequences, it is evident that both types of Na/P_i cotransporters exhibit several (at least eight) transmembrane-spanning domains; proposed secondary structures are illustrated in Fig. 1. According to these models, the N terminus of both types of Na/P_i cotransporters would be positioned at the cytoplasmic surface, whereas the C termini would be of opposite orientation. In in vitro translation experiments performed in the presence of pancreatic microsomes, core glycosylation of both transporters was observed (7,8). The N-glycosylation sites likely to be used are indicated (Fig. 1). Furthermore, the deduced amino acid sequences contain several potential phosphorylation sites for protein kinase C. Phosphorylation of renal apical Na/P_i cotransporters has been discussed with respect to the regulation of proximal apical Na/P_i cotransport, as by parathyroid hormone (for review, see Ref. 3). However it remains to be shown

Table 1 Comparison of Cloned Renal Na/P_i Cotransporters[a]

Transporter	Source	Identity (%)	Similarity (%)	Amino acids encoded
Type I				
NaP_{i-1}	Rabbit kidney	100	100	465
NaP_{i-1M}	Mouse kidney	64.3	81	465
NaP_{i-1H}	Human kidney	69.7	84	465
NaP_{i-2}	Rat kidney	100	100	637
Type II				
NaP_{i-3}	Human kidney	91.2	94.8	639
NaP_{i-4}	OK cells	81.3	88.5	653

[a]The BESTFIT algorithm of the GCG-program package was used to align the sequences. Sequence comparisons are relative to the NaP_{i-1} system in type I transporters and relative to the NaP_{i-2} system in type II transporters. GenBank accession numbers are M76466 for NaP_{i-1}, L13257 for NaP_{i-2}, L13258 for NaP_{i-3}, and L26308 for NaP_{i-4}.

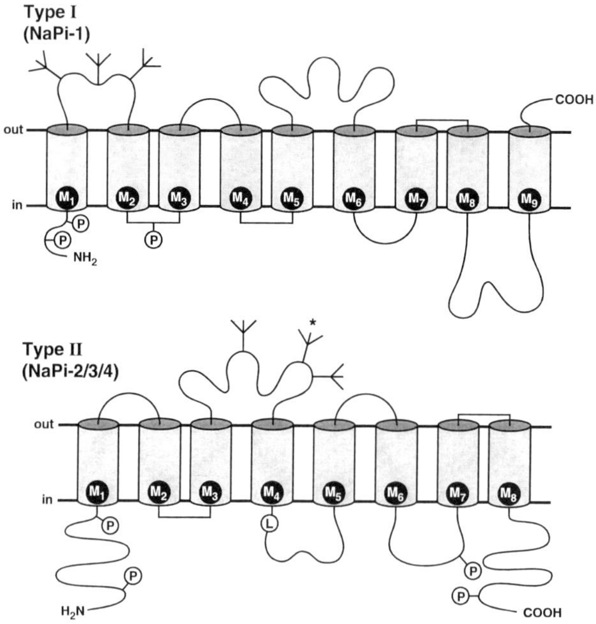

Figure 1 Proposed secondary structures of type I and type II renal apical Na/P_i cotransporters. The most likely used N-glycosylation sites used are indicated; (*) indicates an additional N-glycosylation site in $NaP_{i\text{-}3}$ and $NaP_{i\text{-}4}$ compared to $NaP_{i\text{-}2}$. Potential protein kinase C phosphorylation sites are indicated by P.

that phosphorylation of Na/P_i cotransporters by, for example, parathyroid hormone indeed occurs and that such phosphorylation reactions alter the function of the protein.

Functional Characterization

Cloned Na/P_i cotransporters were functionally characterized after injection of the corresponding cRNAs into oocytes. These studies demonstrated that expressed activities exhibit kinetic characteristics similar to those described for Na/P_i cotransport in isolated proximal tubular brush border membrane vesicles (1–3). For example, $NaP_{i\text{-}2}$ cRNA–induced expression of Na/P_i cotransport exhibited an apparent K_m for P_i of 0.13 m*M* and a constant for Na-interaction of 43 m*M*. The Hill coefficient of the latter interaction was around 2, suggesting that at neutral pH, Na/P_i cotransport is electroneutral (2 $Na^+/HPO_4^=$). However, recent electrophysiological measurements performed with oocytes injected with the $NaP_{i\text{-}2}$ cRNA revealed that Na/P_i transport is electrogenic (18). These functional characteristics are typical for the $NaP_{i\text{-}2}$, $NaP_{i\text{-}3}$, and $NaP_{i\text{-}4}$ systems. Injection of $NaP_{i\text{-}1}$ cRNA into oocytes resulted in expression of Na/P_i-cotransport activity that lacked a dependence on sodium or pH, as observed with the $NaP_{i\text{-}1/2}$ system, yet it exhibited a K_m value for P_i of 0.1 m*M*. Currently the exact role of the type I Na/P_i-cotransport system (e.g., $NaP_{i\text{-}1}$ of rabbit) in renal P_i-reabsorption is not known.

NEPHRON LOCALIZATION

By Northern blot analysis with mRNA isolated from different tissues of various species, the cloned renal Na/P_i-cotransport systems are predominantly expressed in renal cortical tissue. There are two exceptions: $NaP_{i\text{-}1}$–related mRNA was also detected in liver tissue (7) and $NaP_{i\text{-}3}$– related mRNA was also detected in mRNA derived from human lung tissue (8). The functional significance of these findings has not been investigated. To further localize the cloned Na/P_i-cotransport system in kidney tissue, reverse-transcribed mRNA from single microdissected nephron segments was used as the template for the PCR reaction (RT-PCR). Immunohistochemical methods were also employed. In rabbit kidney, the $NaP_{i\text{-}1}$ system was found to be expressed in proximal tubules by both methods

(11,13). By immunohistochemistry, the NaP_{i-1} protein was found in the brush border membrane. Notably, the NaP_{i-1} protein was uniformly distributed in convoluted and straight proximal tubules of both superficial and deep nephrons. In contrast, in normal rat kidney, immunolocalization of the NaP_{i-2} protein suggests that expression of the NaP_{i-2} protein in proximal tubules is heterogeneous (Fig. 2). The highest expression was observed in convoluted straight proximal tubules (12). In all proximal tubular segments, NaP_{i-2}–related immunofluorescence was localized exclusively to the brush border membrane of proximal tubular cells and often in subapical vesicles belonging to the endocytic apparatus.

All together, the data available so far indicate that the sites of the expression of the cloned Na/P_i cotransporters (specifically of the type II system) coincide with the previously described nephron sites for P_i reabsorption (1).

ROLE OF CLONED Na/P_i COTRANSPORTERS IN PHYSIOLOGICAL AND PATHOPHYSIOLOGICAL REGULATION OF RENAL P_i REABSORPTION

Adaption

Reabsorption of phosphate is decreased in animals fed a high-phosphate diet, whereas animals with a low intake of phosphate reabsorb almost 100% of the filtered load of phosphate (1). The proximal tubule seems to be the major site for this adaption phenomenon. As demonstrated in microperfusion studies and experiments with isolated brush border membrane vesicles, the rate of apical Na/P_i cotransport is markedly increased in phosphate-deprived animals (for review, see Refs. 1 to 3). This proximal tubular response to a low-P_i diet is independent of other factors such as parathyroid hormone or vitamin D (1) and therefore appears intrinsic to the proximal tubular cell.

Analysis of mRNA isolated from the kidney cortex of rats chronically (several days) fed a low-P_i diet showed a higher content of Na/P_i cotransporter-(NaP_{i-2}) related mRNA compared to mRNA isolated from control animals. Parallel analysis of brush border membranes isolated from the kidney cortex of adapted and control animals by Western blots using anti-(NaP_{i-2}) antibodies revealed that

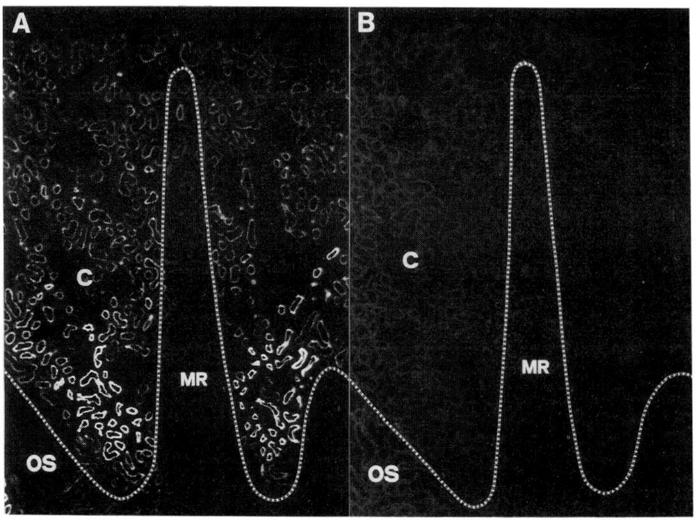

Figure 2 Intrarenal distribution of the NaP_{i-2} protein as revealed by immunofluorescence using anti-(NaP_{i-2}) antibodies. (A) Strong immunostaining was observed in the pars convoluta of proximal tubules (particularly of deep nephrons). C, cortex; MR, medullary rays; OS, outer stripe. (B) Immunostaining after pretreatment of the antiserum with the antigenic peptide (peptide protection).

the abundance of NaP_{i-2} protein is increased by a factor of 3 to 4. Both observations are consistent with the working hypothesis that the observed increase of the V_{max} of apical Na/P_i cotransport is due to an increased number of Na/P_i-cotransport systems (NaP_{i-2}).

Similar adaptation experiments have been performed with rabbits, in which kidney cortex mRNA and brush border membranes were analyzed for NaP_{i-1} by Northern and Western blot analysis. In contrast to the NaP_{i-2} system of rat kidney cortex, low-P_i diet did not alter either the content of NaP_{i-1} mRNA or the amount of NaP_{i-1} protein (14).

These observations (although made in different species) suggest that the two types of Na/P_i-cotransport systems (NaP_{i-1}/rabbit and NaP_{i-2}/rat) might play different roles in the intrinsic adaptive response of proximal tubular cells to a low P_i-diet. The mechanism(s) by which a low P_i-diet induces a change of Na/P_i-cotransporter mRNA content remain to be elucidated.

X-Linked Hypophosphatemia

The X-linked Hyp mouse represents a well-studied model for the X-linked human disorder of phosphate homeostasis (i.e., X-linked hypophosphatemia or (XLH). Hyp mice are characterized by increased fractional excretion of phosphate and by an impaired metabolism of vitamin D (15). With respect to the renal handling of phosphate, the defect seems to manifest itself at the level of the brush border Na/P_i cotransport. Kinetic studies indicate that the maximal rate (V_{max}) of Na/P_i cotransport in brush border membranes of Hyp mice is half of that observed in brush border membranes of normal mice, while the apparent K_m for P_i is indistinguishable. The decrease of V_{max} in Hyp mice could not be attributed to an impaired response of the transporter to the Na-gradient driving force, membrane potential, or pH (15). Therefore it has been suggested that the loss of Na/P_i cotransport in Hyp mice may be attributed to a decreased number of transporters in the brush border membrane.

Recently, NaP_{i-2}–derived probes (cDNA and antibodies) have been used to investigate the basis for the specific reduction in Na/P_i cotransport in renal brush border membranes of Hyp mice. These studies provided evidence that the abundance of NaP_{i-2}–related mRNA and protein is proportionally reduced (approximately by a factor of 2) in the mutant strain (16). These results imply that the genetic defect underlying X-linked hypophosphatemia may not be at the level of the structure of the Na/P_i-cotransport system (NaP_{i-2}–like) but rather would be related to a factor controlling the stability or rate of transcription of the Na/P_i-cotransporter mRNA Interestingly, the $NaP_{i-2/3}$ gene has recently been localized on chromosome 5q35 (17), suggesting that, in X-linked hypophosphatemia, an X-linked factor might be involved in the control of transcription/stability of mRNA coding for apical Na/P_i-cotransport systems (NaP_{i-2}–like).

SUMMARY

Two types of renal Na/P_i-cotransport systems (type I and type II) have recently been identified by expression cloning. Both types of Na/P_i cotransporters appear to be involved in the proximal tubular apical Na-dependent transport of phosphate, as suggested by studies on the localization of the corresponding mRNAs (by RT-PCR) and proteins (by immunohistochemistry).

Initial experiments concerning possible roles of clones Na/P_i cotransporters in the physiological and pathophysiological regulation of proximal tubular absorption of phosphate indicate that the type II (e.g., NaP_{i-2}/rat) system is involved in the control of renal P_i absorption by low-P_i diet as well as in X-linked hypophosphatemia. It remains to be shown how the newly identified Na/P_i cotransport systems might eventually be involved in the control of renal P_i-reabsorption by the various other factors such a parathyroid hormone. Also, the genomic organization of cloned Na/P_i cotransporters remains to be elucidated.

ACKNOWLEDGMENTS

We thank Drs. A. Werner, S. Magagnin, D. Markovich, and V. Sorribas for the cloning experiments and Drs. B. Kaissling, M. Custer, and M. Lötscher for the RT-PCR and immunohistochemical studies. Also, we thank Drs. M. Levi (Dallas) and S. A. Kempson (Indianapolis) for the low P_i-diet studies and Dr. S. Tenenhouse for the studies on the Hyp mouse model. The continuous financial support from the Swiss National Funds is gratefully acknowledged.

REFERENCES

1. Berndt TJ, Knox FG. Renal regulation of phosphate excretion. In: Seldin GW, Giebisch G, eds. The Kidney, Physiology and Pathophysiology. New York: Raven Press, 1992:2511–2532.
2. Murer H, Biber J. Renal tubular phopshate transport. In: Seldin DW, Giebisch G, eds. The Kidney, Physiology and Pathophysiology. New York: Raven Press, 1992:2481–2509.
3. Murer H, Werner A, Reshkin S, et al. Cellular mechanisms in proximal tubular reabsorption of inorganic phosphate. Am J Physiol 1991; 260:C885–C899.
4. Kempson SA. Novel specific inhibitors of epithelial phosphate transport. News Physiol Sci 1988; 3:154–157.
5. Hediger MA, Coaday MJ, Ikeda TS, Wright EM. Expression cloning and cDNA sequencing of the Na/glucose cotransporter. Nature 1987; 330:379–381.
6. Werner A, Biber J, Forgo J, et al. Expression of renal transport systems for inorganic phosphate and sulfate in Xenopus laevis oocytes. J Biol Chem 1990; 265:12331–12336.
7. Werner A, Moore ML, Mantei N, et al. Cloning and expression of cDNA for a Na/P_i cotransport system of kidney cortex. Proc Natl Acad Sci USA 1991; 88:9608–9612.
8. Magagnin S, Werner A, Markovich D, et al. Expression cloning of human and rat renal cortex Na/P_i cotransport. Proc Natl Acad Sci USA 1993; 90:5979–5983.
9. Sorribas V, Markovich D, Hayes G, et al. Cloning of a Na/P_i-cotransporter from opossum kidney cells. J Biol Chem 1994; 269:6615–6621.
10. Murer H, Biber J. Renal sodium-phosphate cotransport. Curr Opin Nephrol 1994; 3:504–510.
11. Biber J, Custer M, Werner A, et al. Localization of NaP_{i-1}, a Na/P_i-cotransporter, in rabbit kidney proximal tubules. Part II: Localization by immunohistochemistry. Pflugers Arch 1993; 424:210–215.
12. Custer M, Lötscher M, Biber J, et al. Expression of Na/P_i-cotransport (NaP_{i-2}) in rat kidney: Localization by RT-PCR and immunohistochemistry. Am J Physiol 1994; 266:F767–F774.
13. Custer M, Meier F, Schlatter E, et al. Localization of NaP_{i-1}, a Na/P_i-cotransporter, in rabbit kidney proximal tubules. Part I: mRNA-localization by RT-PCR. Pflugers Arch 1993; 424:203–209.
14. Werner A, Kempson SA, Biber J, Murer H. Alteration of Na/P_i-cotransport to low P_i-diet. J Biol Chem 1994; 269:6637–6639.
15. Tenenhouse HS, Martel J. Renal adaption to phosphate deprivation: Lessons from the X-linked Hyp mouse. Pediatr Nephrol 1993; 7:312–318.
16. Tenenhouse HS, Werner A, Biber J, et al. Renal Na-phosphate cotransporter immunoreactive protein and mRNA is reduced in X-linked Hyp mice. J Clin Invest 1994; 93:671–676.
17. Kos CH, Tihy F, Lemieux C, et al. Localization of the sodium phosphate cotransporter gene to human chromosome 5q35. Genomics 1994; 19:176–177.
18. Busch A, Waldegger S, Herzer T, et al. Electrophysiological analysis of Na/P_i-cotransport mediated by a transporter cloned from rat kidney and expressed in *Xenopus* oocytes. Proc Natl Acad Sci USA 1994; 81:8205–8208.

21
Molecular Biology of Chloride Channels

Klaus Steinmeyer and Thomas J. Jentsch
Center for Molecular Neurobiology, Hamburg University, Hamburg, Germany

INTRODUCTION

Chloride channels represent an important class of membrane proteins and are present in the membranes of virtually every cell. They are involved in a myriad of physiological functions, ranging from participation in intracellular pH regulation to cell volume regulation (1–3). More specialized functions include transepithelial transport and regulation of excitability in nerve and muscle.

Chloride is often distributed close to its electrochemical equilibrium (4), which, in turn, lies close to the membrane potential. In excitable cells, chloride channels contribute to the stabilization of the resting membrane potential; in skeletal muscle, chloride conductance helps to repolarize the membrane after an action potential. In inhibitory synapses, activation of chloride channels associated with GABA and glycine receptors suppresses the generation of action potentials. In epithelial cells, the intracellular Cl^- concentration is often kept above its electrochemical equilibrium. This is achieved by coupling the influx of chloride to the transport of other ions (e.g., by $Na^+/K^+/2Cl^-$ cotransport, or Cl^-/HCO_3^- exchange). Opening of Cl^-channels then results in a net chloride efflux, and transport direction will depend on the polarized expression (apical or basolateral) of the channel. To maintain electroneutrality, cations are transported in parallel. The resultant osmotic gradient drives transepithelial water movement.

Chloride secretion may be found in airway epithelia as well as the colon. A decrease in airway chloride transport is the basis of cystic fibrosis, whereas secretory diarrhea is due to an excessive secretion. Accordingly, in these tissues the main secretory chloride channel, CFTR, is expressed in the apical membrane. The situation is reversed in the kidney. Here, basolaterally localized chloride channels, coupled to the activity of transporters such as $Na^+/K^+/2Cl^-$, Na^+/Cl^- and K^+/Cl^- cotransport mechanisms as well as Cl^-/HCO_3^- exchangers (3,5), contribute to the reabsorption of 99% of Cl^- present in the primary filtrate. In addition to these transcellular pathways are paracellular shunts, the mechanisms of which are understood poorly. Although chloride transport in kidney is mainly reabsorptive, there are also apically localized Cl^- channels, suggesting a physiological role for Cl^- secretion in kidney (6).

Mirroring their functional diversity, Cl^- channels with various electrophysiological, pharmacological, and regulatory properties have been characterized in renal epithelia (7) and also in many other tissues and organs (8–12). This variability suggests that they are derived from different genes. Due to the impact of molecular cloning techniques, the work during the past few years has resulted in the molecular identification of several distinct putative chloride channel gene families. So far these structural classes include (a) the ligand-gated channel superfamily (GABA and glycine receptors) (13,14); (b) the ClC family of voltage-gated chloride channels (15–18); (c) the I_{Cln} chloride channel (19); (d) phospholemman (20,21); (c) ABC transporters (CFTR, 22 and MDR1) (23); and (f) p64 (24). However, it is not yet clear for some of these genes (or gene families) whether they actually encode channels or are activators of channels endogenous to the cells used for expression.

The field of renal chloride channels is still in its infancy. Although molecular information on chloride channels expressed in the kidney is available, some of these are expressed more or less ubiquitously (and thus also in the kidney). Most likely we still miss genes for most chloride channels expressed in the kidney.

While this review stresses the relevance of chloride channels for renal physiology, it also covers the molecular biology of chloride channels in general.

THE ClC FAMILY OF VOLTAGE-GATED CHLORIDE CHANNELS

ClC-0: The *Torpedo* Chloride Channel

The first member of this gene family to be cloned (15) was ClC-0, the voltage-gated chloride channel from *Torpedo* electric organ. It is a protein of 805 amino acids with a predicted molecular weight of ~89 kDa. Twelve hydrophobic domains are hypothesized (25) to span the lipid bilayer. Patch-clamp analysis of ClC-0 expressed in *Xenopus* oocytes revealed (26) a "double-barreled" structure, which is typical for this channel. In the model proposed by Miller (27), the channel is a functional dimer of two protochannels (of about 10 pS unitary conductance) which can open and close independently of each other but can also be closed simultaneously by a common gate. The protein encoded by the single cloned cDNA is sufficient to generate a channel with such complex properties. It is likely that this can be achieved only in a (homo)multimeric complex, the stoichiometry of which remains to be determined. ClC-0 is localized in the noninnervated membrane (28,29) of the electrocyte opposite the nicotinic acetylcholine receptor. It functions in stabilization of the membrane potential of the noninnervated cell surface during the discharge of the electric organ, a role necessary for efficient current generation. Immunofluorescence studies (29) as well as Northern analysis (K. Steinmeyer and T. J. Jentsch; unpublished) indicated that expression of ClC-0 is not restricted to the electric organ. It also is present in skeletal muscle and brain, although to a much lesser degree.

Interestingly, a "double-barreled" chloride channel with similar kinetics and voltage dependencies (30) was identified by patch-clamp studies in basolateral membranes of the rabbit cortical collecting duct principal cells. This channel has a larger unitary conductance (23 vs. 10 pS). Pharmacological properties and ion selectivity have not yet been reported for this channel, making further comparison impossible. Since double-barreled structure and channel behavior are quite unusual, this may indicate that it is a member of the ClC chloride channel family. However, at this point it is not yet clear whether all ClC members have this property, as single-channel data so far are available only for ClC-0.

ClC-1: The Major Skeletal Muscle Chloride Channel

The major mammalian skeletal muscle chloride channel, ClC-1 was cloned by homology screening using ClC-0 cDNA (16). The complete cDNA sequences of rat and human ClC-1, as well as their genomic structure, are now known (31,32). These channel proteins are larger than their *Torpedo* counterparts, having about 890 amino acids (M_r of ~110 kDa). Although ClC-1 is expressed predominantly in skeletal muscle, weak expression is detected also in smooth muscle, heart, liver, and kidney. In skeletal muscle, ClC-1 is developmentally regulated. After birth, ClC-1 mRNA levels increase steeply (16). Electrophysiology and pharmacology of ClC-1 are fully consistent with the known properties of macroscopic muscle chloride conductance. In skeletal muscle membrane, chloride conductance is unusually high and accounts for about 80% of resting muscle membrane conductance (8). This suggests that ClC-1 must be highly expressed in the muscle membrane. However, there are no reports of ClC-1 single-channel currents in intact skeletal muscle. This could be explained either by its expression predominantly in T tubules (which are not accessible for the patch pipette) (33–35) and/or by a very small single-channel conductance. Noise-analysis measurements (36) of ClC-1–transfected mammalian cells indeed revealed a very small single-channel conductance of only 1 pS, which is below the limit of resolution of current patch-clamp technology.

The cause of myotonia, a hereditary disease in both humans and animals, is a defect in ClC-1. It is characterized by overexcitability of the muscle membrane (37). A role for ClC-1 was first demonstrated in the myotonic mouse strain ADR (38); its gene was destroyed structurally by the insertion of a transposon (39). Disease-causing mutations have now been identified in other myotonic mouse strains (40). While myotonia is a recessive disease in mice, in humans both recessive (Becker, 41) and dominant (Thomsen, 42) forms of myotonia exist. The human ClC-1 gene is located on chromosome 7q35 (43). The CLC-1 locus was linked tightly to both recessive and dominant forms of human myotonia (43–45). Several different point mutations were identified in families with recessive and dominant forms of the disease: a Phe to Cys exchange (F413C) in putative transmembrane domain D8 causes myotonia (43) in some Becker myotonia families. An exchange of Gly to Glu (G230E) between D3 and D4 was detected in Canadian Thomsen families (46), whereas a Pro to Leu exchange (P480L) in a putative loop connecting D9 and D10 is the cause of myotonia in Thomsen's own family (31). When these mutations were introduced in the human ClC-1 cDNA and the mRNA was then expressed in *Xenopus* oocytes, chloride currents were abolished. In addition, when coexpressed with the wild-type protein, the mutants found in dominant myotonia suppressed the currents of the normal channel. This fully reproduces the disease phenotype in vitro (31). The fact that different mutations in a single gene can lead to recessive and dominant patterns of inheritance has interesting implications for channel structure. The existence of recessive mutations indicates that a 50% loss of channel function is not sufficient to cause myotonia. Accordingly, in vitro studies have also shown that muscle Cl^- conductance must be reduced to at least 30% to induce sufficient electrical instability (47). This excludes a gene dosage effect of the mutated allele. A dominant phenotype can be explained by a model proposing a homomultimeric structure for the channel. In this model, a dominant mutation leads to a defective subunit which associates with the normal one (encoded by the other allele of a heterozygous patient) and functionally inactivates it. As an independent confirmation of this model, coexpression of G230E mutant ClC-1 with the normal channel generated currents with altered kinetics and ion selectivity. By titrating the wild-type with the mutant channel, a predicted ClC-1 subunit stoichiometry was derived, strongly suggesting that the channel consists of more than two (possibly four) subunits. Such a structure is likely to apply for the other members of this protein family.

ClC-2: A Volume-Regulated Chloride Channel

Using a ClC-1 cDNA probe under low stringency, ClC-2 was cloned from rat brain (17). It is about 50% identical to either ClC-1 or ClC-0. Northern analysis and cDNA cloning revealed an ubiquitous distribution. Expression was found in every tissue (e.g., in rat skeletal muscle, heart, brain, lung, pancreas, stomach, intestine, and liver) and cell line examined. ClC-2 is expressed in the kidney as well as in the renal cell lines MDCK, LLC-PK1, COS, and BSC1 (17). This channel is closed in oocytes under resting conditions but can be activated by unphysiologically strong hyperpolarization (in excess of –100 mV). Once activated, it has a slightly inwardly rectifying current-voltage relationship and a chloride-over-iodide ion selectivity. Its ubiquitous expression suggests an important housekeeping role and hence a mechanism of activation other than hyperpolarization. Gründer et al. (25) found that ClC-2 could be activated by hypotonicity when expressed in *Xenopus* oocytes, implicating a role in regulatory volume decrease (RVD). Previously, physiological studies revealed a parallel opening of potassium and chloride channels in various cell types (1–3), though the characteristics of these chloride channels (outward rectification, iodide-over-chloride selectivity) often differed from those of ClC-2. The slow activation kinetics upon exposure to hypotonicity is consistent with activation by a slow volume increase in these large cells. Extensive mutagenesis and electrophysiological analysis (25) identified structures important for the activation by voltage and cell volume. Two functionally distinct but adjacent regions (an "essential" and a "modulating" one) were found at the N terminus. Deletions in the essential region produced constitutively open channels that were unresponsive to both voltage and medium tonicity; those in the modulating region produced channels that look like partially volume-activated channels (intermediate phenotype). These latter mutant channels can be further activated by hypotonicity. In contrast to wild-type ClC-2, intermediate phenotype channels could also be closed by hypertonicity. The structural requirements on these domains are relaxed, since several point mutations in the essential region had no effect. Remarkably, these domains are position-independent, as they can be transplanted to different parts of the channel protein without loss of function. A model similar to but distinct from the "ball and chain" model for cation channels was envisaged: an N-terminal–inactivating particle binds to a putative receptor on the channel molecule at rest and closes it (48). The affinity of this putative "receptor" domain is decreased by hyperpolarization or by cell swelling, releasing the inactivating particle and opening the channel. Identification of this binding site and an understanding of the mechanism by which cell swelling leads to a change in the affinity of this receptor will no doubt be of great interest and importance.

The ClC-K Subfamily of Kidney Chloride Channels

Using RT-PCR and degenerate primers based on conserved regions of ClC-0, ClC-1, and ClC-2, Uchida et al. (18) cloned another member of the ClC-family from rat kidney mRNA. This channel, termed ClC-K1, is about 40% identical to the other ClC channels. It is a protein of 686 amino acids and expression of its cRNA in *Xenopus* oocytes was reported to lead to slightly outwardly rectifying chloride currents. In contrast to ClC-0, ClC-1, and ClC-2, which show a $Cl^- > Br^- > I^-$ selectivity, ClC-K1 is more permeable for Br^- than for Cl^-. Considering the high homology to ClC-0, ClC-1, and ClC-2, the lack of any voltage-dependence of ClC-K1 is surprising.

ClC-K1 is predominantly expressed in the kidney, especially in the inner medulla. Analysis by RT-PCR of microdissected nephron segments identified the thin ascending limb (TAL) of Henle's loop as site of highest expression. Moderate expression of ClC-K1 was found in the inner medullary collecting duct, the thin descending limb of Henle's loop, and the cortical collecting duct. It is only weakly expressed in the proximal convoluted tubule. The TAL has the highest Cl^- permeability among the nephron segments (49) and, together with the inner medullary collecting duct, is part of the countercurrent system for urine concentration. Interestingly, ClC-K1 mRNA levels increase after dehydration of rats (18). Taken together with the RT-PCR data, these observations suggest the involvement of ClC-K1 in the high chloride permeability of the TAL.

Kieferle et al. (50) combined RT-PCR and hybridization approaches to clone two closely related (~80% identity) ClC channels from the rat kidney. One of these (rClC-K1) is very similar to ClC-K1 [if a sequence mistake in the published sequence (18) is taken into account] and might be identical to it. The other channel was named rClC-K2. Both channels are expressed nearly exclusively in the kidney, and expression of their mRNA was found in cortex as well as in medulla. Both channels are expressed differently along the nephron, as demonstrated by RT-PCR of microdissected nephron segments. While rClC-K1 is expressed strongly in the cortical thick ascending limb and the distal convoluted tubule and less strongly in the S3 segment of the proximal tubule and the cortical collecting tubule, rClC-K2 is expressed additionally in glomerula and the S2 segment of the proximal tubule. Using rClC-K2 as a probe, two additional, closely related ClC channels were isolated from a human kidney cDNA library (hClC-Ka and hClC-Kb). The human channels are about 80% identical to the rat ClC-K channels but more than 90% identical to each other. The high intraspecies homology does not allow us to classify one particular human channel as the species homologue of the corresponding rat channel. Though highly related to each other, they originate from different genes. Unfortunately, both rClC-K1, -K2, and hClC-Ka, -Kb, could not be functionally expressed in *Xenopus* oocytes or other expression systems. This is in contrast to the expression of ClC-K1 published by Uchida et al. (18). The reason for this discrepancy is unclear. In vitro translation data indicated that the proteins were inserted into membranes and glycosylated. Their glycosylation is not consistent with the current topological model for ClC channels, since all putative N-linked glycosylation sites are predicted to be intracellular. Mutation of a highly conserved N-linked glycosylation site (located between domains D8 and D9) abolished core glycosylation of ClC-K channels in vitro, suggesting that this segment must be extracellular.

I_{Cln}

Paulmichl et al. (19) implemented expression cloning to isolate a novel putative chloride channel (I_{Cln}) from messenger RNA of the Madin Darby canine kidney epithelial cell line (MDCK). Expression of I_{Cln} in *Xenopus* oocytes results in a strongly outwardly rectifying chloride conductance. I_{Cln} currents rise instantaneously after voltage steps and deactivate slowly at voltages higher than +40 mV. However, at physiological voltages, currents are generally quite small. The currents are independent of internal calcium and can be blocked by known inhibitors or chloride channels (NPPB, 5-nitro-2-(3-phenylpropylamino)benzoic acid; DIDS, 4,4′-diisothiocyanatostilbene-2,2′-disulfonic acid). Interestingly, I_{Cln} can be inhibited by extracellular nucleotides—including ATP, ADP, GTP, cAMP, and cGMP—in rather high concentrations (19). The rather small protein encoded by the cDNA (235 amino acids, predicted M_r ~26 kDa) does not possess any hydrophobic domains predicted to span the lipid bilayer as a α-helix. Paulmichl et al. (19) proposed a model in which functional I_{Cln} channels consist of two subunits, each having four amphipathic β-strands that cross the membrane. A common pore is assumed to be formed by an eight-stranded β-barrel. A similar model has been proposed for the voltage-dependent anion channel (VDAC) from yeast mitochondria. However, there is no sequence homology to VDAC, nor to any other known protein.

The sequence predicts a nucleotide-binding domain (GXGXG), modeled to be on the external side of the membrane. Mutations in that domain indeed altered the sensitivity of I_{Cln} to extracellular nucleotides. Additionally, they also altered gating kinetics of the expressed currents and conferred external calcium sensitivity. The simplest explanation for these observations is that the I_{Cln} protein resides in the plasma membrane and functions by itself as a chloride channel.

The I_{Cln} mRNA is expressed in various cell types of different species (19,51,52), and homologous proteins have now been cloned from rat kidney cells (51) and rat heart cells (53). Such proteins have also been cloned from *Xenopus* oocytes (53). The ubiquitous expression pattern of I_{Cln} indicates that it may have a housekeeping function, such as volume regulation. This would also be consistent with its distribution in the kidney, where it is expressed in the cortex as well as in the medulla (51). In contrast to ClC-K1, its expression is not altered when rats are dehydrated (51). Indeed, currents resembling I_{Cln} have been induced by cell swelling in different epithelial cells (54,55), in fibroblasts (56), and in *Xenopus* oocytes (57). In NIH 3T3 cells, I_{Cln}-like Cl^- currents are also inhibited by extracellular nucleotides, although the sensitivity to individual nucleotides is completely reversed. An involvement of I_{Cln} in cell volume regulation during RVD is strongly suggested by two experiments: (a) introduction of antisense oligonucleotides derived from the MDCK I_{Cln} channel into 3T3 fibroblasts suppressed the swelling-induced Cl^- currents together with a reduction of the endogenous I_{Cln} protein (56) and (b) injection of oocytes with antibodies against the *Xenopus* protein also blocked the native hypotonicity-induced chloride current (53).

Immunofluorescence and cell fractionation studies of oocytes and cardiac myocytes demonstrated that the majority of endogenous I_{Cln} is localized within the cytoplasm, where it interacts with cytoskeletal proteins (53). This is an unexpected and puzzling result, since such a localization is inconsistent with the proposed function of I_{Cln} as a chloride channel. It suggests that I_{Cln} is a protein that may rather activate an endogenous Cl^- channel during cell swelling via cytoskeletal interactions. However, this interpretation is difficult to reconcile with the mutagenesis studies. In *Xenopus* oocytes, swelling-induced Cl^- current is only detectable in freshly defolliculated oocytes and decays over time until it is undectable 6 days later (57), implying that the capability of the channel to respond to cell swelling depends somehow on the presence of the follicular cell layer. It will be interesting to see whether injection of I_{Cln} cRNA is able to restore the lost endogenous hypotonicity-activated Cl^- conductance. A positive result would argue for a direct role of I_{Cln} as a Cl^- channel. Certainly further experiments, such as reconstitution of the purified protein in artificial lipid bilayer, are needed to clarify this point.

PHOSPHOLEMMAN

Phospholemman (PLM) was originally identified as a major target for phosphorylation in the sarcolemma of the myocardium (hence its name) (20). It is a small polypeptide of 72 amino acids with a single predicted transmembrane span and is expressed in heart and skeletal muscle as well as in stomach, esophagus, aorta, and liver. No expression was found in kidney (20). Phospholemman displays sequence homology to the γ-subunit of the Na^+, K^+-ATPase, the function of which is unclear. It came as a surprise that phospholemman induces chloride currents when expressed in *Xenopus* oocytes (21). Currents activate very slowly with strong hyperpolarization, superficially resembling ClC-2 currents. However, in contrast to ClC-2, PLM-induced chloride currents display a $I^- > NO_3^- > Br^- > Cl^-$ ion selectivity (58). It does not depend on intracellular calcium, arguing against activation of the endogenous oocyte Ca-dependent chloride channel. It seems unlikely that PLM mediates cAMP-stimulated cardiac chloride currents, which closely resemble CFTR currents (59). Indeed CFTR is also expressed in the heart (59). Mutating two amino acids in the predicted transmembrane span slightly altered channel kinetics (21), suggesting that PLM is a Cl^- channel and not a channel-modulating molecule.

Several more recent observations cast some doubts on a direct role if PLM as a chloride channel. Oocytes have an endogenous hyperpolarization-activated Cl^- conductance, which has the same ion selectivity ($I^- > Cl^-$) as PLM-induced Cl^- currents (58). Moreover, PLM-induced Cl^- currents are detected only when high concentrations of its cRNA are expressed in oocytes.

I_{sk} (60) is thought to be a potassium channel which is slowly activated after depolarization. A Cl^- current with nearly identical properties can be induced when the I_{sk} protein is overexpressed in oocytes (61). While both proteins have a single transmembrane span, they do not show any sequence identity. In addition, slowly activating Cl^- currents have been recorded at very negative voltages in oocytes after expression of high amounts of a nonfunctional ClC-1 mutant. In contrast to wild-type ClC-1, these currents are more selective for I^- than for Cl^- (31). These results raise the possibility that PLM is a regulator of an endogenous Cl^- channel that is activated in an unphysiological manner as a consequence of overexpression of exogenous membrane proteins. Unfortunately, although quite abundantly expressed in heart, PLM channel activity has not yet been recorded from this organ, making it difficult to correlate these data. More work is needed to explain all these interesting although contradictory observations.

CHLORIDE CHANNELS OF THE ABC TRANSPORTER FAMILY

The Cystic Fibrosis Transmembrane Conductance Regulator (CFTR)

The protein associated with cystic fibrosis (CF) is CFTR (22). The most common inherited lethal disease, CF is caused by defective Cl^- transport in secretory epithelia. The CFTR protein shows structural similarity to the ABC (ATP-binding cassette) family of transporters that function as ATP-dependent solute pumps (62). This initially raised doubts that CFTR itself mediates the epithelial cAMP-regulated Cl^- transport. This question is now settled, and there is no reasonable argument against this point of view. It is beyond the scope of this article to mention all the work that has contributed to this knowledge; interested readers are referred to corresponding reviews (63–65).

Briefly, mutations in CFTR alter ion selectivity (66) and single-channel conductance (67,68), which are both intrinsic properties of a channel pore. Moreover, highly purified CFTR protein has been successfully reconstituted into lipid bilayers (69), and biophysical analysis demonstrated typical chloride currents sensitive to protein kinases. This leaves virtually no doubt that CFTR is a chloride channel.

Two mouse models of CF have been generated by knockout of CFTR (70–72). In one transgenic line, symptoms are more variable and more benign, which may be due to a remaining very low level of functional CFTR expression (71). With both lines, chloride transport was impaired (71,73).

Previous results suggested that several mutant forms of CFTR do not reach the plasma membrane (74). However, functional expression of the most frequent CFTR mutant (ΔF508) was recently observed in oocytes (75) and in Vero cells (76). This can now be explained in part by the temperature-sensitivity of CFTR mutants. In cell lines transfected with the ΔF508 mutant, CFTR is correctly processed at 30°C but not at 37°C (77).

Previous work on excised patches indicated that after phosphorylation of CFTR, additional ATP hydrolysis was required to open the channel (66). A study on permeabilized sweat duct cells (78) now suggests that nonhydrolytic binding of ATP (in the millimolar range) is sufficient and necessary for opening. This may couple chloride channel function to the energy state of the cell (78). More work is needed to explain this apparent discrepancy which may be due in part to the use of different experimental systems.

In addition to functioning as a chloride channel, CFTR has also been suggested to play a role in plasma membrane recycling (79) as well as to be a regulator of an outwardly rectifying chloride channel (80,81), which was believed to be defective in cystic fibrosis several years ago. This theory has been put aside after expression of CFTR yielded very different, linear channels. It has also been suggested that CFTR is a cAMP-dependent water channel (82). All these intriguing and somewhat confusing results will require independent confirmation. It remains to be seen whether CFTR has some function in addition to being a chloride channel. Perhaps, like other members of the ABC transporter superfamily, CFTR may actively transport as yet unknown substances.

As shown by Northern analysis (22), in situ hybridization (83), and immunocytochemistry (84), CFTR is present in epithelial cells of many different organs. Further, a recent patch-clamp study (85) reports frequent observation of "CFTR-like" chloride channels in several nonepithelial cell lines, suggesting that CFTR is also expressed (although at a very low level) in these cells.

In lung, expression of CFTR protein is relatively low, which is unexpected, since this organ together with airway epithelia is severely affected in cystic fibrosis. In contrast, CFTR protein is abundantly expressed in proximal and distal tubules of the kidney (84), which is not a site of prominent clinical symptoms. However, it has been reported that some CF patients show increased Na^+ reabsorption in the proximal tubule, leading to impairment of renal diluting capacity (86,87). This might suggest that Cl^- secretion by CFTR normally plays a role in the kidney. Consistent with this, in the renal epithelium, CFTR is localized in apical membranes. In addition, CFTR is also found in membranes of intracellular vesicles below this face of the plasma membrane (84). A cAMP-regulated Cl^- conductance has indeed been demonstrated in endocytic vesicles from the proximal tubule of the kidney (88). There is some evidence that CF is associated with a defective acidification of endosomes and other intracellular organelles (89). However, a recent study failed to show a role of CFTR in acidification of lysosomes (90). Future studies will be needed to reveal the precise function of CFTR in the kidney. Since the CFTR-associated Cl^- channel is activated by cAMP, it might be the target of hormones that are known to regulate renal transport via this intracellular second messenger (6).

The P-Glycoprotein (Multidrug-Resistance Protein)

P-glycoprotein is another member of the ABC transporter superfamily, and its overexpression is responsible for the multidrug resistance of cancer cells (91). The human 170-kDa P-glycoprotein, also termed MDR1, has a similar overall structure as CFTR, with 12 transmembrane domains and two ATP-binding domains that couple ATP hydrolysis to drug transport.

P-glycoprotein is expressed in the epithelia of several tissues, including pancreas, colon, kidney, adrenal gland, intestine, liver, and reproductive organs (uterus and testis) (92–95). In these tissues, MDR1 is localized in apical membranes, suggesting a role in the secretion of metabolites and drugs into bile, urine, and gastrointestinal tract. Both MDR and CFTR seem to have complementary patterns of epithelial expression (95). In some tissues (intestine and gravid uterus), a switch in expression from one gene to another was even observed (95), suggesting that they serve distinct physiological roles. However, in certain cultured cells, such as T84 colon cells, both genes are simultaneously expressed (22,96). The complementary expression may also not apply to the kidney, where both MDR1 and CFTR are expressed in epithelial cells of the proximal tubules (84,92,95). It has been shown that secretion of digoxin in the proximal tubule is mediated by P-glycoprotein (97–99).

Triggered by the finding that CFTR is a chloride channel, MDR1 was tested for channel function. Its overexpression in two different cell lines led indeed to hypotonicity-activated, ATP-dependent chloride currents (23), with voltage- and time-dependencies similar to those of currents previously observed in different cell types (54,100). These currents could be inhibited by several known inhibitors of P-glycoprotein transport (forskolin, 1,9-dideoxyforskolin, and verapamil) and by chloride channel blockers (NPPB, DIDS). Whereas active transport required hydrolyzable intracellular ATP, ATP binding was sufficient to activate chloride currents (23). Active transport and channel function could be affected differentially by transportable substances and mutations in the nucleotide binding fold (101). MDR1 cannot perform simultaneously active transport and serve as a chloride channel (101), suggesting that it can exist in two mutually exclusive and interconvertible configurations. However, the physiological role of MDR1 in volume regulation is unclear. In human T84 colon cells that express MDR1, 1,9-dideoxyforskolin effectively inhibited transport of vinblastine but did not affect volume-stimulated Cl^- secretion (102). This is in contrast to the data obtained for the volume-activated Cl^- conductance in MDR1-transfected cell lines (23). In addition, some cells that displayed secretion of the drug failed to express a volume-stimulated Cl^- secretion, suggesting that there is no correlation of volume-activated chloride current and MDR-mediated vinblastine secretion in this cell line (102). Finally, while volume-regulated chloride currents originally were seen only in MDR1-transfected NIH 3T3 cells and not in nontransfected cells, recent work has shown that the same cells actually do exhibit a very similar endogenous volume-sensitive chloride current

Table 1 Cloned Chloride Channels (or Chloride Channel Activators)

Protein	Amino acids	Tissue distribution	Structure	Function	References
ClC-0	805	Torpedo electric organ, skeletal muscle, brain	12 TMDs, N and C termini intracellular	Stabilization of V_m	15, 25, 29 (unpublished results)
ClC-1	994	Skeletal muscle, smooth muscle, heart	"	Stabilization of V_m Defect: myotonia	16, 31, 36, 39, 40, 43, 45, 46
ClC-2	907	ubiquitous	"	Volume regulation?	17
ClC-K1	686	Kidney	"	Cl^- reabsorption?	18, 50
ClC-K2	686	Kidney	"	Cl^- reabsorption?	50
I_{Cln}	235	Ubiquitous	β-barrel, N- and C-terminus intracellular	Volume-regulation?	19, 51, 52, 56
Phospholemman	72	Heart, muscle, stomach, aorta, liver, esophagus	1 single TMD, N terminus extracellular, C terminus intracellular	?	20, 21
CFTR	1480	Pancreas, sweat gland, kidney, colon, lung, liver, intestine, salivary gland, and others	12 TMDs, 2 NBFs, 1 R-domain, N and C termini intracellular	Cl^- secretion	22, 83, 84, 94, 95
MDR1	1280	Adrenal gland, kidney, lung, liver, colon, and others	12 TMDs, 2 NBFs, N and C termini intracellular	Drug extrusion, volume regulation?	23, 92, 93, 94, 95, 106, 107, 108
p64	437	Ubiquitous	1-4 TMDs	?	24

TDM, transmembrane domain; NBF, nucleotide (ATP)-binding fold; R-domain, regulatory domain.

(56). Thus, very similar chloride currents that are provoked by overexpression of MDR1 in 3T3 cells and by I_{Cln} in oocytes seem to be intrinsic to these cells.

Since mutagenesis studies of CFTR indicate that some of the hydrophobic putative transmembrane domains participate in forming the pore, it is puzzling that expression of MDR1, which has no sequence homology to CFTR in these domains, also results in chloride currents. Clearly, definitive proof that P-glycoprotein is a Cl^- channel by itself awaits further work, such as identification of mutants with altered ion selectivity or functional reconstitution in lipid bilayers. It will be interesting to see whether overexpression of other members of this gene family also leads to ion currents.

p64

The indanyloxyacetic acid derivative IAA-94 is a potent inhibitor of Cl^- uptake in bovine renal microsomes (inhibition constant, K_i of $1 \mu M$) (103). Using it as a ligand, four major proteins were affinity-purified from solubilized bovine kidney cortex microsomes and from tracheal apical membranes. Reconstitution of the purified proteins into liposomes and planar lipid bilayer gave rise to Cl^- channel activity (104). At the single-channel level, at least three different chloride channels could be detected. Sequencing of the eluted proteins excluded two, namely the α-subunit of the Na, K-ATPase and glutathione-S-transferase, as possible candidates for chloride channel proteins (105). Since it seems unlikely that the different chloride conductances seen after reconstitution are mediated by the remaining two, contamination with minor proteins of the eluate may be in part responsible for the observed chloride channel activity. This is also consistent with the observation that the reconstituted chloride channel activity is not sensitive to IAA (104). However, antibodies raised against one, a 64-kDa protein (p64), were able to deplete this Cl^- channel activity from solubilized kidney membranes (105). When solubilized kidney vesicles were immunoprecipitated with anti-p64 antibodies, no chloride channels could be measured after reconstitution of the immunodepleted protein in liposomes. The antibodies detected proteins in several cell types from different species and later were used to clone the corresponding protein from a kidney cDNA library (24). The cloned sequence predicts a protein of 437 amino acids with a calculated M_r of 49 kDa, but its translation product migrates as a 64-kDa protein when analyzed on SDS-PAGE. The sequence predicts two (or possibly four) putative transmembrane domains and contains consensus sites for phosphorylation by different protein kinases. Northern analysis again showed a ubiquitous expression of p64, with highest expression in kidney cortex, skeletal muscle, and heart, and at lower levels in kidney medulla, adrenal, and brain. Immunofluorescence revealed that p64 is mainly present in perinuclear vesicles (105), suggesting that it might be the Cl^- channel of intracellular organelles. This would explain the failure of p64 to induce Cl^- channel activity in *Xenopus* oocytes. However, the only evidence for p64 being a Cl^- channel itself is the capability of anti-p64 antibodies to deplete Cl^- channel activity from solubilized kidney vesicles. Attempts to reconstitute functional Cl^- channels from affinity-purified p64 were unsuccessful. This may be explained by the stringent conditions necessary to elute the protein from the columns. Cloning of the p64 cDNA should allow purification of the protein from more suitable protein overexpression systems.

CONCLUSIONS

Within the past few years, members of six different gene families have been cloned that generate chloride currents when expressed in appropriate cells. Except for the family of neuronal ligand-gated chloride channels, members of the other families are in addition to other tissues also expressed in the kidney. Kidney-specific expression has so far only be observed for ClC-K channels of the voltage-gated ClC chloride channel family. Certainly, more gene families with chloride channel function will emerge, and undoubtedly (as for the ClC family) more members of such families will be identified. In the cases of CFTR and ClC-1, disease models have provided important insights into the physiological functions of the affected Cl^- channels. However, while plentiful information has accumulated from electrophysiological studies of many different chloride channels, our knowledge of the molecular structure of these proteins is still poor. We do not know the physiological function of most of them, and in some cases a definitive proof that these molecules are real channel proteins is still missing. Answers to these questions will require a thorough characterization of these proteins by combined molecular biological, biochemical, and electrophysiological techniques.

REFERENCES

1. Hoffmann EK, Simonsen LO. Membrane mechanisms in volume and pH regulation in vertebrate cells. Physiol Rev 1989; 69:315–382.
2. Hoffmann EK, Ussing HH. Membrane mechanisms in volume regulation in vertebrate cells and epithelia. In: Schafer JA, Ussing HH, Kristensen P, Giebisch GH, eds. Membrane Transport in Biology. Vol. 5. Berlin: Springer-Verlag, 1992.
3. Cala PM. Principles of cell volume regulation: Ion flux pathways and the roles of anions. In: Alvarez-Leefmans FJ, Russell JM, eds. Chloride Channels and Carriers in Nerve, Muscle, and Glial Cells. New York: Plenum Press, 1990: 67–83.
4. Hille B. Ionic Channels of Excitable Membranes. Sunderland, MA: Sinauer, 1992.
5. Russell JM, Boron WF. Chloride transport in the squid giant axon. In: Alvarez-Leefmans FJ, Russell JM, eds. Chloride Channels and Carriers in Nerve, Muscle, and Glial Cells. New York: Plenum Press, 1990: 85–107.
6. Simmons NL: Renal epithelial Cl^- secretion. Exp Physiol 1993; 78:117–137.
7. Reeves WB, Andreoli TE. Renal epithelial chloride channels. Annu Rev Physiol 1992; 54:29–50.
8. Bretag AH. Muscle chloride channels. Physiol Rev 1987; 67:618–724.
9. Blatz AL. Chloride channels in skeletal muscle. In: Alvarez-Leefmans FJ, Russell JM, eds. Chloride Channels and Carriers in Nerve, Muscle, and Glial Cells. New York: Plenum Press, 1990:407–420.
10. Gögelein H. Chloride channels in epithelia. Biochim Biophys Acta 1988; 947:521–547.
11. Liedtke CM. Regulation of chloride transport in epithelia. Annu Rev Physiol 1989; 51:43–60.
12. Dawson DC. Ion channels and colonic salt transport. Annu Rev Physiol 1991; 53:321–339.
13. Schofield PR, Darlison MG, Fujita N, et al. Sequence and functional expression of the $GABA_A$ receptor shows a ligand-gated receptor superfamily. Nature 1987; 328:221–227.
14. Grenningloh G, Rienitz A, Schmitt B, et al. The strychnine-binding subunit of the glycine receptor shows homology with nicotinic acetylcholine receptor. Nature 1987; 328:215–220.
15. Jentsch TJ, Steinmeyer K, Schwarz G. Primary structure of Torpedo marmorata chloride channel isolated by expression cloning in Xenopus oocytes. Nature 1990; 348:510–514.
16. Steinmeyer K, Ortland C, Jentsch TJ. Primary structure and functional expression of a developmentally regulated skeletal muscle chloride channel. Nature 1991; 354:301–304.
17. Thiemann A, Gründer S, Pusch M, Jentsch TJ. A chloride channel widely expressed in epithelial and non-epithelial cells. Nature 1992; 356:57–60.
18. Uchida S, Sasaki S, Furukawa T, et al. Molecular cloning of a chloride channel that is regulated by dehydration and expressed predominantly in kidney medulla. J Biol Chem 1993; 268:3821–3824.
19. Paulmichl M, Li Y, Wickman K, et al. New mammalian chloride channel identified by expression cloning. Nature 1992; 356:238–241.
20. Palmer CJ, Scott BT, Jones LR. Purification and complete sequence determination of the major plasma membrane substrate for cAMP-dependent protein kinase and protein kinase C in myocardium. J Biol Chem 1991; 266:11126–11130.
21. Moorman JR, Palmer CJ, John JE, et al. Phospholemman expression induces a hyperpolarization-activated chloride current in Xenopus oocytes. J Biol Chem 1992; 267:14551–14554.
22. Riordan JR, Rommens JM, Kerem BS, et al. Identification of the cystic fibrosis gene: cloning and characterization of complementary DNA. Science 1989; 245:1066–1073.
23. Valverde MA, Díaz M, Sepúlveda FV, et al. Volume-regulated chloride channels associated with the human multidrug-resistance P-glycoprotein. Nature 1992; 355:830–833.
24. Landry S, Sullivan S, Nicolaides M, et al. Molecular cloning and characterization of p64, a chloride channel protein from kidney microsomes. J Biol Chem 1993; 268:14948–14955.
25. Gründer S, Thiemann A, Pusch M, Jentsch TJ. Regions involved in the opening of ClC-2 chloride channel by voltage and cell volume. Nature 1992; 360:759–762.
26. Bauer CK, Steinmeyer K, Schwarz JR, Jentsch TJ. Completely functional double-barreled chloride channel expressed from a single Torpedo cDNA. Proc Natl Acad Sci USA 1991; 88:11052–11056.
27. Miller C, White MM. Dimeric structure of single chloride channels from Torpedo electroplax. Proc Natl Acad Sci USA 1984; 81:2772–2775.
28. Jentsch TJ, Pusch M, Rehfeldt A, Steinmeyer K. The ClC family of voltage-gated chloride channels: structure and function. In: Higashida H, Yoshioka T, Mikoshibak, eds. Molecular Basis of Ion Channels and Receptors Involved in Nerve Excitation, Synaptic Transmission and Muscle Contraction. Ann NY Acad Sci Vol. 707. New York, 1993:285–293.
29. Ortland C. Klonierung und Charakterisierung eines Chloridkanals der Skelettmuskelfaser der Ratte. Ph.D. dissertation, Bochum University, Bochum, FRG, 1993.
30. Sansom SC, La B-Q, Carosi SL. Double-barreled chloride channels of collecting duct basolateral membrane. Am J Physiol 1990; 259:F46–F52.

31. Steinmeyer K, Lorenz C, Pusch M, et al. Multimeric structure of ClC-1 chloride channels as revealed by mutations in dominant myotonia congenita (Thomsen). EMBO J 1994; 13:737–743.
32. Lorenz C, Meyer-Kleine C, Steinmeyer K, et al. Genomic organization of the human muscle chloride channel ClC-1 and analysis of novel mutations leading to Becker type myotonia. Hum Mol Genet 1994; 3:941–946.
33. Palade PT, Barchi RL. Characteristics of the chloride conductance in muscle fibers of the rat diaphragm. J Gen Physiol 1977; 69:325–342.
34. Dulhunty AF. Effect of chloride withdrawal on the geometry of the t-tubules in amphibian and mammalian muscle. J Membr Biol 1982; 67:81–90.
35. Heiny JA, Valle JR, Bryant SH. Optical evidence for a chloride conductance in the T-system of frog skeletal muscle. Pflugers Arch. 1990; 416:288–295.
36. Pusch M, Steinmeyer K, Jentsch TJ. Low single channel conductance of the major skeletal muscle chloride channel, ClC-1. Biophys J 1994; 66:149–152.
37. Rüdel R, Lehmann-Horn F. Membrane changes in cells from myotonia patients. Physiol Rev 1985; 65:310–356.
38. Mehrke G, Brinkmeier H, Jockusch H. The myotonic mouse mutant ADR: Electrophysiology of the muscle fiber. Muscle Nerve 1988; 11:440–446.
39. Steinmeyer K, Klocke R, Ortland C, et al. Inactivation of muscle chloride channel by transposon insertion in myotonic mice. Nature 1991; 354:304–308.
40. Gronemeier M, Condie A, Prosser J, et al. Nonsense and missense mutations in the muscular chloride channel gene Clc-1 in mytotonic mice. J Biol Chem 1994; 269:5963–5967.
41. Becker PE. Myotonia Congenita and Syndromes Associated with Myotonia: Clinical-Genetic Studies of the Non-dystrophic Myotonias. Stuttgart: Georg Thieme, 1977.
42. Thomsen J. Tonische Krämpfe in willkürlich beweglichen Muskeln in Folge von ererbter psychischer Disposition. Arch Psychiatr Nervenkrankh 1876; 6:702–718.
43. Koch MC, Steinmeyer K, Lorenz C, et al. The skeletal muscle chloride channel in dominant and recessive human myotonia. Science 1992; 257:797–800.
44. Abdalla JA, Casley WL, Cousin HK, et al. Linkage of Thomsen disease to the T-cell receptor beta (TCRB) locus on chromosome 7q35. Am J Hum Genet 1992; 51:579–584.
45. Koch MC, Ricker K, Otto M, et al. Evidence for genetic homogeneity in autosomal recessive generalized myotonia (Becker). J Med Genet 1993; 30:914–917.
46. George AL Jr, Crackower MA, Abdalla JA, et al. Molecular basis of Thomsen's disease (autosomal dominant myotonia congenita). Nature Genet 1993; 3:305–310.
47. Kwiecinski H, Lehmann-Horn F, Rüdel R. Drug-induced myotonia in human intercostal muscle. Muscle Nerve 1988; 11:576–581.
48. Hoshi T, Zagotta WN, Aldrich RW. Biophysical and molecular mechanisms of shaker potassium channel inactivation. Science 1990; 250:533–538.
49. Imai M, Kokko JP. Sodium chloride, urea, and water transport in the thin ascending limb of Henle. J Clin Invest 1974; 53:393–402.
50. Kieferle S, Fong P. Bens M, et al. Two highly homologous members of the ClC chloride channel family in both rat and human kidney. Proc Natl Acad Sci USA 1994; 91:6943–6947.
51. Ishibashi K, Sasaki S, Uchida S, et al. Tissue expression of mRNA of chloride channel from MDCK cells and its regulation by protein kinases. Biochem Biophys Res Commun 1993; 192:561–567.
52. Abe T, Takeuchi K, Ishii K, Abe K. Molecular cloning and expression of a rat cDNA encoding MDCK-type chloride channel. Biochim Biophys Acta 1993; 1173:353–356.
53. Krapivinsky GP, Ackerman MJ, Gordon EA, et al. Molecular characterization of a swelling-induced chloride conductance regulatory protein, pI_{Cln}. Cell 1994; 76:439–448.
54. Worrell RT, Butt AG, Cliff WH, Frizzell RA. A volume-sensitive chloride conductance in human colonic cell line T84. Am J Physiol 1989; 256:C1111–C1119.
55. Solc CK, Wine JJ. Swelling-induced and depolarization induced Cl^-channels in normal and cystic fibrosis epithelial cells. Am J Physiol 1991; 261:C658–C674.
56. Gschwentner M, Nagl UO, Wöll E, et al. Antisense oligonucleotides suppress cell volume-induced activation of chloride channels. Pflúgers Arch. In press.
57. Ackerman MJ, Wickman KD, Clapham DE. Hypotonicity activates a chloride current in Xenopus oocytes. J Gen Physiol 1994; 103:153–179.
58. Kowdley GC, Ackerman SJ, John JE, et al. Hyperpolarization activated chloride currents in Xenopus oocytes. J Gen Physiol 1994; 103:217–230.
59. Nagel G, Hwang TC, Nastiuk KL, et al. The protein kinase A-regulated cardiac Cl^- channel resembles the cystic fibrosis transmembrane conductance regulator. Nature 1992; 360:81–84.
60. Takumi T, Ohkubo H, Nakanishi S. Cloning of a membrane protein that induces a slow voltage-gated potassium channel. Science 1988; 242:1042–1045.

61. Attali B, Guillemare E, Lesage F, et al. The protein IsK is a dual activator of K^+ and Cl^-channels. Nature 1993; 365:850–852.
62. Higgins CF. ABC transporters: From microorganisms to man. Annu Rev Cell Biol 1992; 8:67–113.
63. Welsh MJ, Anderson MP, Rich DP, et al. Cystic fibrosis transmembrane conductance regulator: A chloride channel with novel regulation. Neuron 1992; 8:821–829.
64. Fuller CM, Benos DJ. CFTR! Am J Physiol 1992; 263:C267–C286.
65. Riordan JR. The cystic fibrosis transmembrane conductance regulator. Annu Rev Physiol 1993; 55:609–630.
66. Anderson MP, Gregory RJ, Thompson S, et al. Demonstration that CFTR is a chloride channel by alteration of its anion selectivity. Science 1991; 253:202–205.
67. Sheppard DN, Rich DP, Ostedgaard LS, et al. Mutations in CFTR associated with mild-disease-form Cl^-channels with altered pore properties. Nature 1993; 362:160–164.
68. Tabcharani JA, Rommens JM, Hou Y-X, et al. Multi-ion pore behaviour in the CFTR chloride channel. Nature 1993; 366:79–82.
69. Bear CE, Li C, Kartner N, et al. Purification and functional reconstitution of the cystic fibrosis transmembrane conductance regulator (CFTR). Cell 1992; 68:809–818.
70. Snouwaert JN, Brigman KK, Latour AM, et al. An animal model for cystic fibrosis made by gene targeting. Science 1992; 257:1083–1088.
71. Dorin JR, Dickinson P, Alton EWFW, et al. Cystic fibrosis in the mouse by targeted insertional mutagenesis. Nature 1992; 359:211–215.
72. Colledge WH, Ratcliff R, Foster D, et al. Cystic fibrosis mouse with intestinal obstruction. Lancet 1992; 340:680.
73. Clarke LL, Grubb BR, Gabriel SE, et al. Defective epithelial chloride transport in a gene-targeted mouse model of cystic fibrosis. Science 1992; 257:1125–1128.
74. Cheng SH, Gregory RJ, Marshall J, et al. Defective intracellular transport and processing of CFTR is the molecular basis of most cystic fibrosis. Cell 1990; 63:827–834.
75. Drumm ML, Wilkinson DJ, Smit LS, et al. Chloride conductance expressed by ΔF508 and other mutant CFTRs in Xenopus oocytes. Science 1991; 254:1797–1799.
76. Dalemans W, Barbry P, Champigny G, et al. Altered chloride ion channel kinetics associated with the ΔF508 cystic fibrosis mutation. Nature 1991; 354:526–528.
77. Denning GM, Anderson MP, Amara JF, et al. Processing of mutant cystic fibrosis transmembrane conductance regulator is temperature sensitive. Nature 1992; 358:761–764.
78. Quinton PM, Reddy MM. Control of CFTR chloride conductance by ATP levels through non-hydrolytic binding. Nature 1992; 360:79–81.
79. Bradbury NA, Jilling T, Berta G, et al. Regulation of plasma membrane recycling by CFTR. Science 1992; 256:530–532.
80. Egan M, Flotte T, Aflone S, et al. Defective regulation of outwardly rectifying Cl^- channels by protein kinase A corrected by insertion of CFTR. Nature 1992; 358:581–584.
81. Guggino WB. Outwardly rectifying chloride channels and CF: A divorce and remarriage. J Bioenerg Biomembr 1993; 25:27–35.
82. Hasegawa H, Skach W, Baker O, et al. A multifunctional aqueous channel formed by CFTR. Science 1992; 258:1477–1479.
83. Trezise AEO, Buchwald M. In vivo cell-specific expression of the cystic fibrosis transmembrane conductance regulator. Nature 1991; 353:434–437.
84. Crawford I, Maloney PC, Zeitlin PL, et al. Immunocytochemical localization of the cystic fibrosis gene product CFTR. Proc Natl Acad Sci USA 1991; 88:9262–9266.
85. Gabriel SE, Price EM. Boucher RC, Stutts MJ. Small linear chloride channels are endogenous to non-epithelial cells. Am J Physiol 1992; 263:C708–C713.
86. Robson AM, Tateishi S, Ingelfinger JR, et al. Renal function in patients with cystic fibrosis. J Pediatr 1971; 79:42–50.
87. Stenvinkel P, Hjelte L, Alván G, et al. Decreased renal clearance of sodium in cystic fibrosis. Acta Paediatr Scand 1991; 80:194–198.
88. Bae H-R, Verkman AS. Protein kinase A regulates chloride conductance in endocytic vesicles from proximal tubule. Nature 1990; 348:637–639.
89. Barasch J, Kiss B, Prince A, et al. Defective acidification of intracellular organelles in cystic fibrosis. Nature 1991; 352:70–73.
90. Van Dyke RW, Root KV, Schreiber JH, Wilson JM. Role of CFTR in lysosome acidification. Biochem Biophys Res Commun 1992; 184:300–305.
91. Higgins CF. The multidrug resistance P-glycoprotein. Curr Opin Cell Biol 1993; 5:684–687.
92. Thiebaut F, Tsuruo T, Hamada H, et al. Cellular localization of the multidrug-resistance gene product P-glycoprotein in normal human tissues. Proc Natl Acad Sci USA 1987; 84:7735–7738.

93. Arceci RJ, Croop JM, Horwitz SB, Housman D. The gene encoding multidrug resistance is induced and expressed at high levels during pregnancy in the secretory epithelium of the uterus. Proc Natl Acad Sci USA 1988; 85:4350–4354.
94. Bremer S, Hoof T, Wilke M, et al. Quantitative expression patterns of multidrug-resistance P-glycoprotein (MDR1) and differentially spliced cystic-fibrosis transmembrane-conductance regulator mRNA transcripts in human epithelia. Eur J Biochem 1992; 206:137–149.
95. Trezise AEO, Romano PR, Gill DR, et al. The multidrug resistance and cystic fibrosis genes have complementary patterns of epithelial expression. EMBO J 1992; 11:4291–4303.
96. Hunter J, Hirst BH, Simmons NL. Epithelial secretion of vinblastine by human intestinal adenocarcinoma cell (HCT-8 and T84) layers expressing P-glycoprotein. Br J Cancer 1991; 64:437–444.
97. Tanigawara Y, Okamura N, Hirai M, et al. Transport of digoxin by human P-glycoprotein expressed in a porcine kidney epithelial cell line (LLC-PK1). J Pharmacol Exp Ther 1992; 263:840–845.
98. Hori R, Okamura N, Aiba T, Tanigawara Y. Role of P-glycoprotein in renal tubular secretion of digoxin in the isolated perfused rat kidney. J Pharmacol Exp Ther 1993; 263:840–845.
99. Okamura N, Hirai M, Tanigawara Y, Tanaka K, et al. Digoxin-cyclosporin A interaction: Modulation of the multidrug transporter P-glycoprotein in the kidney. J Pharmacol Exp Ther 1993; 266:1614–1619.
100. Rasola A, Galietta LJV, Gruenert DC, Romeo G. Ionic selectivity of volume-sensitive currents in human epithelial cells. Biochim Biophys Acta 1992; 1139:319–323.
101. Gill DR, Hyde SC, Higgins CF, et al. Separation of drug transport and chloride channel functions of the human multidrug resistance P-glycoprotein. Cell 1992; 71:23–32.
102. McEwan GTA, Hunter J, Hirst BH, Simmons NL. Volume-activated Cl^- secretion and transepithelial vinblastine secretion are not correlated in cultured human T84 intestinal epithelial layers. FEBS Lett 1992; 304:233–236.
103. Landry DW, Reitman M, Cragoe EJ Jr, Al-Awqati Q. Epithelial chloride channel: Development of inhibitory ligands. J Gen Physiol 1987; 90:779–798.
104. Landry DW, Akabas MH, Redhead C, et al. Purification and reconstitution of chloride channels from kidney and trachea. Science 1989; 244:1469–1472.
105. Redhead CR, Edelman AE, Brown D, et al. A ubiquitous 64-kDa protein in a component of a chloride channel of plasma and intracellular membranes. Proc Natl Acad Sci USA 1992; 89:3716–3720.
106. Gros P, Croop J, Housman DE. Mammalian multidrug resistance gene: Complete cDNA sequence indicating strong homology to bacterial transport proteins. Cell 1986; 47:371–380.
107. Chen C-J, Chin JE, Ueda K, et al. Internal duplication and homology with bacterial transport proteins in the mdrl (P-glycoprotein) gene from multidrug-resistant human cells. Cell 1986; 47:381–389.
108. Fojo AT, Ueda K, Slamon DJ, et al. Expression of a multidrug-resistance gene in human tumors and tissues. Proc Natl Acad Sci USA 1987; 84:265–269.

22

Anion Exchangers

Mary Jo Godinich and Michael L. Jennings
The University of Texas Medical Branch, Galveston, Texas

INTRODUCTION

The amino acid sequences and tissue distributions have been determined for many different transport proteins by the use of recombinant DNA technology. Within this group are the coupled anion exchangers, of which the Na^+-independent Cl^--HCO_3^- exchanger is the most thoroughly characterized. It is the focus of this chapter. The following terminology has evolved for the anion exchanger (AE) family, which consists of genes denoted *AE1*, *AE2*, and *AE*3 (1,2). The respective products of these genes are the *AE1*, *AE2*, and *AE3* proteins. The erythrocyte *AE1* gene product is also called "band 3" for its position on SDS-polyacrylamide gels (3). Because the erythrocyte and kidney *AE1* polypeptides are similar, the term "band 3" is sometimes used in reference to kidney *AE1*. Throughout this chapter, however, "band 3" will be used only in reference to erythrocyte *AE1*.

Historically, much of the information prior to the cloning of the mouse erythroid Cl^--HCO_3^- exchanger (4) was derived from biochemical studies of the human band-3 protein (5). Recombinant DNA techniques, however, have made it possible to define, manipulate, and express anion exchange proteins from tissues and species in which biochemical information would be difficult or impossible to obtain. Table 1 lists the mammalian Cl^--HCO_3^- exchange proteins for which the cDNA sequence is known.

This chapter summarizes what is known about electroneutral Na^+-independent Cl^--HCO_3^- exchangers and describes how molecular characteristics have added to the understanding of cellular function. It is not intended to be a comprehensive review of the literature on anion exchange proteins; readers are referred to recent review articles for more detailed information (1,2,6–13).

SEQUENCE AND HOMOLOGIES

The erythroid *AE1* proteins of various species range in size from 848 to 929 amino acid residues with molecular mass of 93 to 102 kDa. The *AE2* and *AE3* proteins are slightly larger and range from 1227 to 1237 residues in length, with a molecular mass of 135 kDa. On the basis of hydropathy plots (2,4,14,15), each protein can be divided into two major domains of roughly equal mass: a hydrophilic N-terminal cytoplasmic domain and a hydrophobic membrane-spanning domain. A small third domain is defined by the 25 hydrophilic residues at the C terminus of the protein. Both the C terminus and the N terminus are on the cytoplasmic side of the membrane (16). Sequence homology among AE proteins within a given species and among different species is much greater in the membrane-spanning domain (64–97%) than in the N-terminal cytoplasmic domain (36–91%) (Table 2). The membrane domains of *AE1*, *AE2*, and *AE3* have very similar hydropathy plots (Fig. 1), indicating multiple membrane-spanning segments. It is worth mentioning that, even though there are pharmacological similarities (block by stilbenedisulfonates) between anion exchangers and some anion channels, there is no significant sequence homology between Cl^--HCO_3^- exchangers and Cl^- channels (17–20).

Table 1 Known Anion Exchanger Sequences

Date	Exchanger	Species	Tissue	Cloning strategy	Ref.
1985	*AE1*	Mouse	Erythrocyte	Polyclonal antibody screening of splenic cDNA library	4
1986	*AE2*	Human	Cell line	Mouse band-3 probe used to screen cDNA library from K562 cell line	115
1988	*AE1*	Human	Erythrocyte	Human K562 probe used to screen human fetal liver cDNA library	104
1988	*AE2*	Mouse	Kidney	Murine band-3 probe used to screen murine kidney cDNA library	32
1988	*AE1*	Chicken	Erythrocyte	Band-3 cDNA clone used to screen chick erythroid cDNA library	157
1988	*AE1*	Chicken	Erythrocyte	Mouse band-3 probe used to screen chick erythrocyte cDNA library	26
1989	*AE1*	Human	Erythrocyte	Mouse band 3 used to probe fetal liver cDNA library	158
1989	*AE1*	Mouse, rat	Kidney	Murine band-3 probes used to screen mouse kidney library, demonstrating truncation of renal form	31
1989	*AE1*	Rat	Kidney	Mouse band-3 probe used to screen rat kidney cDNA library	27
1989	*AE3*	Mouse	Brain	Murine probes derived from genomic library used to screen mouse brain cDNA library	14
1990	*AE2*	Rat	Choroid plexus	Mouse AE1 probe used to screen rat choroid plexus cDNA library	35
1990	*AE2* *AE3*	Rat	Stomach, brain	Rat kidney AE1 probe used to screen brain, kidney, stomach cDNA libraries	15
1992	*AE2*	Rabbit	Ileum	Degenerative primers derived from mammalian clones used to PCR overlapping segments of mRNA	34
1992	*AE2*	Human	Kidney	PCR amplification of human kidney mRNA	33
1992	*AE1*	Trout	Erythrocyte	Murine band-3 probe used to screen trout splenic cDNA library	117

THE *AE1* GENE AND TRANSCRIPTS

The *AE1* gene has been localized in humans to chromosome 17q21 → qter by in situ hybridization (21); the *AE2* gene is in region 7q35 → 7q36 (22). The chromosomal location of human *AE3* has not been determined. Of the three, the *AE1* gene has been the most extensively studied.

There appears to be a single copy of the *AE1* gene in the mouse (23), human (21,24), chicken (25,26), and rat (27). The 17-kb murine gene has been extensively characterized and found to be composed of 20 exons, the first 19 ranging in size from 73 to 253 bp, and 19 introns ranging in size from 79 bp to 3.9 kb (Fig. 2).

Exon 1 from the mouse gene codes for most of the 5′ untranslated band 3 transcript, while exon 2 contains a portion of the untranslated 5′ region and the first five codons of band 3 (23). Extensive mapping of a 5′ partial sequence from a rat genomic library demonstrates the same organization of

Table 2 Sequence Comparison Between Anion Exchangers[a]

	AE1				AE2			
	Human		Rodent		Human		Rodent	
	NH_2	COOH	NH_2	COOH	NH_2	COOH	NH_2	COOH
AE1								
Human	—	—	—	—	—	—	—	—
Rodent	73	92	92	97	—	—	—	—
AE2								
Human	38	71	36	68	—	—	—	—
Rodent	37	71	36	68	92	94	91	97
AE3								
Rodent	41	67	37	64	49	70	50	69

[a]The sequence comparison of carboxyl- and amino-terminal portions of anion exchanger isoforms is expressed as percent amino acid identity. Because rat and mouse sequences are very similar, a comparison of mouse with rat for a given protein is not included. Instead, the entries in rows and columns denoted "rodent" are averages of the values obtained for mouse and rat. The boundary between the amino- and carboxyl-terminal domains is (somewhat arbitrarily) defined as the position corresponding to human Arg 387. The program *PC/Gene* (Intelligenetics) was used to make the comparisons.

the first 5 exons as in the mouse (28). Murine exons 3 to 20 code for the remainder of the translated band-3 protein; exon 20 includes the 3′ untranslated region.

Of the 19 murine introns, 17 have been sequenced and their donor splice sites determined (23). Comparison to a hydropathy map of the band-3 protein (Fig. 1) suggests that the intron/exon boundaries exist in areas that encode the hydrophilic segments of the protein; that is, the introns are between rather than within membrane-spanning domains. A similar relationship holds true for the introns mapped thus far in the human *AE1* gene (21,29).

The 5′ end of the murine gene does not contain common promoter signals in the form of TATA or CCAAT sequences proximal to the sites of erythroid or kidney transcription initiation. There are, however, several G-rich regions and multiple repeats that may play a role in the regulation of transcription (30). Similarly, there are no recognized promoter sequences proxiaml to the erythroid initiation sites in rat (28). However, unlike the murine counterpart, there is a potential TATA signal 25 nucleotides upstream to the proposed kidney initiation site in the rat, as well as recognized hormone-receptor binding sites further upstream (28).

At the 3′ end of the murine gene, a single polyadenylation site, AATAAA, exists 12 bp upstream from the poly(A+) tail. When the cDNA of this segment is aligned with the *AE1* gene, there are no additional polyadenylation sites 110 nucleotides 3′ to the AATAAA polyadenylation signal, indicating that this region codes for the termination of the *AE1* transcript (14).

The only difference between the erythroid and renal *AE1* gene products is that the renal polypeptide lacks the first 79 amino acids of band 3 (31). The mRNA for this "truncated" form is observed as a 4.2-kb product on Northern plots of murine poly(A^+) RNA (27,31), as compared to the larger 4.5-kb erythroid product. Murine kidney mRNA lacks the sequences from exons 1 to 3 and introns 1 to 3 of the *AE1* gene. Likewise, rat kidney poly (A^+) RNA lacks nucleotides from exons 1 to 3 but does contain sequences from the third intron of the *AE1* gene (27,31). These renal and erythroid transcriptional differences are thought to be tissue-specific.

Transcriptional initiation sites have been mapped for mouse and rat erythrocyte and kidney mRNAs (27,28,30). For the erythrocyte, there are several "clusters" of initiation sites within exon 1 that span 43 nucleotides in the mouse and 120 nucleotides in the rat. In both species, erythrocyte

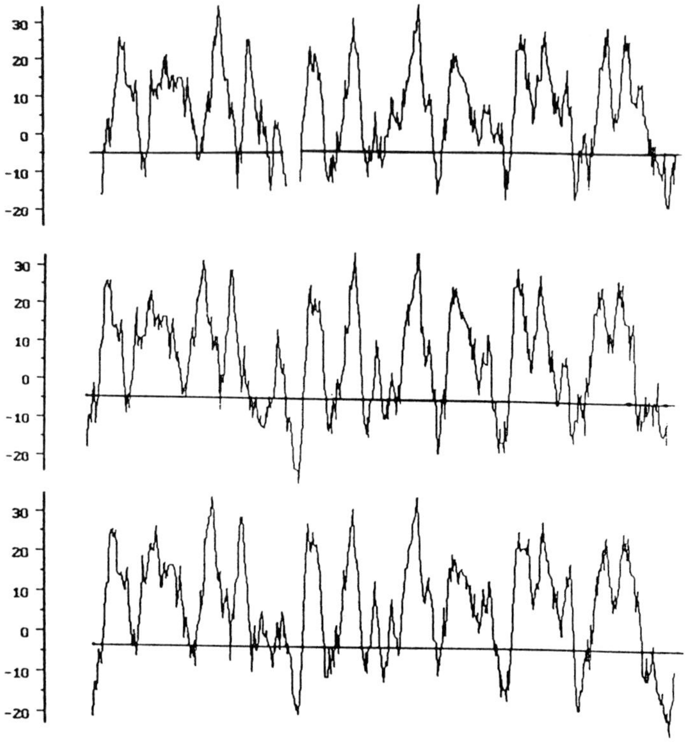

Figure 1 The hydropathy (159) profiles of the membrane domains of *AE1*, *AE2*, and *AE3*, with a window of nine residues. Similar comparison of hydropathy profiles has been presented by Kopito (14). From top to bottom, plots represent *AE1*, *AE2*, and *AE3*, beginning at the position of human Arg 387. The break in the *AE1* plot represents the position of the Z-loop insertion found in *AE2* and *AE3*.

initiation is within 200 bases of the translation initiator codon. In kidney mRNA, however, only one transcription initiation site has been determined in both mouse and rat. In the mouse, the site lies 5′ to erythroid initiation sites within exon 1, while in the rat, it lies 3′ in relation to erythroid initiation sites within the third intron (Fig. 2).

A number of minor *AE1* transcripts have been identified in kidney. In the rat, their sizes are 3.6 kb (15), 4.1 kb (27), 4.5 kb, and 4.7 kb (31), and in the mouse, 4.5 kb (31). Whether these transcripts are a result of the alternate promoters or of alternate splicing of the *AE1* gene has yet to be determined.

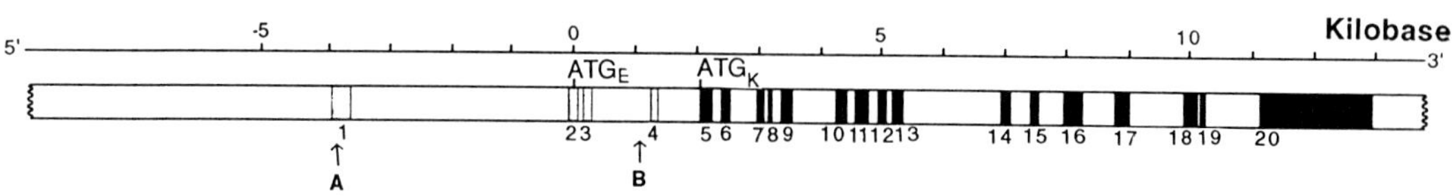

Figure 2 The *AE1* gene: Black boxes represent exons that encode amino acid sequences common to both erythroid and renal *AE1* proteins. Gray boxes represent exons that encode sequences found only in erythrocyte *AE1*. ATG_E represents the location of the initiator codon of erythrocyte *AE1*, while ATG_K represents the location for coding of Met 1 of renal *AE1* (Met 80 of erythroid *AE1*). (A) Site for murine and rat erythrocyte and murine kidney transcription initiation. (B) Site of rat kidney transcription initiation.

THE *AE2* GENE AND TRANSCRIPTS

The product of *AE2* gene transcription has been identified in the kidney of mouse, rat, and human (15,32,33), with recent identification in rabbit ileum (34) as well as a number of other tissues (see below). Rat *AE2* is quite abundant in choroid plexus and is 98.6% identical to murine kidney *AE2* (35). The differences between the two species occurs in the nucleotide sequence of the Z loop (see below).

The *AE2* transcripts of various species studied to date have similar characteristics, including an untranslated 5′ sequence between 64 and 200 bases in size, an open reading frame of approximately 3700 nucleotides, and a 3′ untranslated sequence of 134 to 192 bases.

The 5′-untranslated region of rat and mouse *AE2* cDNAs are 99% identical. The GCC sequence immediately before the presumed initiator ATG is consistent with the eukaryotic consensus sequence for translation initiation (36). It is identical in rabbit ileum (34), rat stomach (15), and murine kidney (32). The 5′-untranslated portion of cDNA also contains in-frame stop codons for each species.

The 3′-untranslated sequence has a high degree of similarity between mouse and rat and is very short compared to that of *AE1*. In mouse, rat, rabbit, and human, the 3′ untranslated region lacks the typical polyadenylation signal but possesses the sequence AATAATTTAAA upstream from the poly(A^+) tract (15,32–34) and may therefore be the signal for termination of transcription.

THE *AE3* GENE AND TRANSCRIPTS

The *AE3* gene is 12 kb in size and includes 24 exons (37). The mapped junctions between introns and exons conform to established consensus sequences. The major products of the *AE3* gene are found in the heart and brain and are of different sizes (discussed below). The first six exons of the gene code for the 5′ untranslated sequence and the first 270 codons of brain mRNA while exons 7 to 23 contain the coding and 3′-untranslated sequences common to brain and cardiac mRNAs (Fig. 3). The intron between exons 6 and 7 contains the coding sequence of the 5′-untranslated and N-terminal coding sequences of cardiac mRNA and is where transcription is initiated in this product (37).

No TATA element is located upstream from the cardiac transcription initiation site, but there are sequences that conform to cap site consensus sequences, promoter sequences, and a transcription factor. For example, there is a single copy of CATTCCT, a sequence found in promoters of muscle-specific genes referred to as the M-CAT sequence (38). There is also a potential binding site for the transcription factor Sp1 upstream from the cardiac initiation sites (37). At the 3′-terminal portion of the transcript, the cardiac *AE3* lacks a consensus AATAAA polyadenylation signal, but three poly(A^+) addition sites are observed (37).

Two major *AE3* gene transcripts have been described in the rat (15,37) and mouse (14). The larger transcript is 4.0 kb in the mouse (14) and 4.4 kb in the rat (15). This transcript is found predominantly in brain, though it is a minor component of cardiac mRNA (15) and even less a component of kidney mRNA (14,15). The size of the smaller transcript is 3.4 kb in mouse (14) and 3.8 kb in rat (37) and is detected only in cardiac tissue. The difference in the 5′ region between cardiac and brain transcripts is not explained by truncation, as in the erythrocyte and kidney *AE1* products. Rather, the 844 nucleotides of the 5′ terminus of the brain transcript are replaced in the

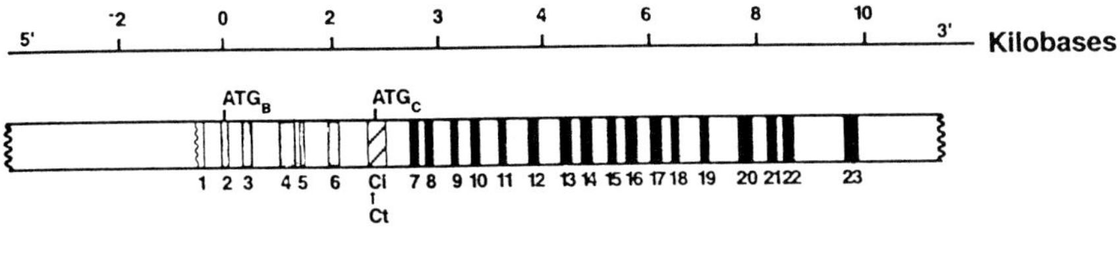

Figure 3 The *AE3* gene: Black boxes represent exons that encode amino acid sequences common to both brain and cardiac proteins. Gray boxes represent exons that encode only for sequences found in brain *AE3* protein. Open box represents the incompletely mapped first exon. ATG_B is the location of the initiator codon of brain *AE3*. ATG_C is the codon for Met 1 of cardiac *AE3*. Striped box represents brain intron 6 (C_i) in which cardiac transcription initiation (C_t) takes place.

cardiac transcript by 376 nucleotides of little similarity. The open reading frames of the two products are in phase.

In rat, the cardiac transcriptional initiation site has been localized to a position 196 bases 5′ to the first base of the probable translation initiation codon (37). Another signal occurs at position −163 and may represent the initiation site of a minor transcript. The transcriptional initiation site has not been identified in the larger *AE3* gene transcript.

TISSUE DISTRIBUTION

As outlined in Table 1, mRNAs for anion exchangers have been detected in various tissues in different species. In a comprehensive survey, Kudrycki et al. (15) determined the tissue distribution of *AE1*, *AE2*, and *AE3* in rat. Using a probe from the 3′-untranslated region of rat *AE1* cDNA, *AE1* mRNA was found at high levels in rat spleen and kidney, with much lower levels in uterus, skeletal muscle, heart, brain, lung, liver, stomach, and large intestine. Probes from both 3′-coding and 3′-untranslated sequences detected *AE2* mRNA, with greatest abundance in rat stomach; intermediate levels in large intestine, lung, and uterus; and smaller levels in kidney and liver. In addition to the above tissues, *AE2* has been detected in murine choroid plexus (35) and a human lymphoid cell line (32). At minimal autoradiographic exposure, *AE3* was seen in heart, brain, and uterus and at longer exposure, in skeletal muscle, lung, stomach, small intestine, large intestine, and kidney (15).

RENAL LOCALIZATION

The collecting duct plays a major role in acid/base homeostasis and is the primary renal location of Na^+-independent Cl^--HCO_3^- exchange, as indicated by functional studies and immunohistochemical staining with anti–band-3 antibodies (39–42). In addition, there is functional evidence for Cl^--HCO_3^- exchange in the thick ascending loop of Henle (TALH) (43,44) and mesangial cells (45). Morphological differences exist in cellular composition of tubules between rat and rabbit, the two species in which the majority of functional studies have been performed. These differences have caused difficulty in establishing general functional characteristics of the anion exchanger as well as the molecular identities of exchanger subtypes. These species differences in morphology have been described in detail in recent reviews (39–42).

The collecting duct can be divided both functionally and histologically into three segments: the cortical collecting tubule (CCT); the outer medullary collecting duct (OMCD), which in turn is subdivided into outer and inner stripes; and the inner medullary collecting duct (IMCD). Each segment displays cellular heterogeneity. The CCT is composed of principal cells (65%), and alpha (α) and beta (β) intercalated cells (ICs) (35%). The OMCD is composed of principal cells (60–65%), and α-ICs (35–40%). In the rat, the IMCD consists of principal cells and α-IC cells in the initial segment and IMCD cells in the terminal portion. The rabbit IMCD is composed only of IMCD cells. Other differences between cellular composition of the collecting duct of rat and rabbit include predominance of β-ICs in the rabbit initial CCT, which decrease in number axially, so that α-ICs predominate at the corticomedullary junction (46–48).

In the CCT (49–52) and both stripes of the OMCD (50,53,54) of rat and rabbit, functional evidence supports the presence of Cl^--HCO_3^- exchange on the basolateral side of the α-IC. Basolateral Cl^- is necessary both for HCO_3^- transport (54–59) and recovery of the α-IC from an acid load (57,60–62). Anion exchange also is sensitive to DIDS (4,4′-diisothiocyanatostilbene-2,2′-disulfonate), with an IC_{50} similar to band 3 (56,63). Antibodies derived from various epitopes of band 3 have been used to further localize *AE1* in rat (64–68), rabbit (69,70), and human collecting duct (71). These studies demonstrate *AE1* antibody binding to the basolateral side of α-ICs of the CCT and OMCD in each species.

Apical Cl^--HCO_3^- exchange of the β-IC differs from basolateral Cl^--HCO_3^- exchange of the α-IC not only in its membrane localization (61,69) but also in its reduced DIDS sensitivity (55,72) and its ability to catalyze Cl^- self-exchange at a faster rate than Cl^--HCO_3^- exchange (73–75). In addition, no antibodies prepared to date against *AE1* or *AE2* bind to the apical side of the β-IC of the CCT despite functional evidence of Cl^--HCO_3^- exchange in this membrane (66,67,69). Therefore, the molecular identity of this exchanger remains in question. However, a recent study using recombinant

DNA technology and band-3 antibody staining of β-IC membrane vesicles suggests that this exchanger is *AE1* (76). The authors suggest that the inability of available *AE1* antibodies to bind apically to β-ICs is due to conformational masking of epitopes, which may also affect DIDS binding. Additional studies will be necessary to clarify the molecular identity of the apical anion exchanger in the β-IC.

The remaining cells in the collecting duct also fail to bind available band-3 antibodies, but functional studies support the presence of basolateral Cl^--HCO_3^- exchange in the principal cells of the CCT and OMCD in both rat and rabbit (77–79). Both α-ICs and IMCD cells in the initial IMCD demonstrate Cl^--HCO_3^- exchange as well (80). Molecular identity of the proteins responsible for Cl^--HCO_3^- exchange in these cells would be of interest because (a) neither *AE2* nor *AE3* has been localized to any nephron segments and (b) mRNA for *AE2* and *AE3* has been detected in the kidney (15).

The presence of Cl^--HCO_3^- exchange in the TALH remains uncertain. Functional studies of murine cortical TALH suggest parallel apical membrane Cl^--HCO_3^- and Na^+-H^+ exchange (43). This model has been challenged by recent studies, which show Na^+ and Cl^- fluxes to be independent of CO_2 and HCO_3^- (81). In the medullary TALH, functional studies support a role for basolateral Cl^--HCO_3^- as well as Na^+-H^+ exchange in cell-volume regulation (44). While no immunohistochemical studies have identified an AE isoform in this nephron segment, preliminary studies using in situ hybridization with probes to segments of band 3 demonstrate the presence of band-3 mRNA in medullary TALH (82). It is also interesting to note that the *AE2* cDNA was prepared from a mouse kidney cell line derived from immortalized medullary TALH cells (32). Further studies are necessary to demonstrate conclusively functional Cl^--HCO_3^- exchange in the TALH and identify the AE isoform(s) responsible for anion exchange in these segments.

STRUCTURAL DOMAINS

Cytoplasmic Domain

The cytoplasmic domains of *AE2* and *AE3* are approximately 240 residues longer than that of erythroid *AE1* and are more similar to each other than to the *AE1* protein. Because of the amino acid variability among the cytoplasmic domains and the ability of truncated AEs to transport Cl^- and HCO_3^- (14,35,83), the cytoplasmic domain is believed not be necessary for anion transport. The most thoroughly characterized function of the cytoplasmic domain of band 3 is to provide an attachment site for the erythrocyte membrane skeleton (84,85). The cytoplasmic domain of human band 3 also serves as a binding site for glycolytic enzymes and hemoglobin (84,86).

The isolated cytoplasmic domain of human and band 3 is a highly elongated dimer (87). The cytoplasmic domain binds the skeletal protein ankyrin with high affinity (85). The structural basis of this binding has been characterized by Low and coworkers (86); a "hinge" region between residues 175 and 200 represents one of several points of interaction with ankyrin. The cytoplasmic domain undergoes a set of pH-dependent conformational changes that involve deformation of this hinge region. These conformational changes are associated with the interconversion of the cytoplasmic domain among high-affinity, low-affinity, and nonbinding states for ankyrin binding (86).

Band-3 binding also occurs to the red cell membrane skeletal proteins 4.1 (88) and 4.2 (89). Two sites have been identified in the cytoplasmic domain that might cooperate to form a binding site for band 4.1 (90). In the rat kidney there is basolateral colocalization of band 3 with ankyrin and spectrin in intercalated cells (64), but detailed evaluation of the assembly of this complex has not been performed. It would be very interesting to compare the structures of the erythrocyte band 3 membrane skeleton/band 3 complex with that formed with collecting duct *AE1*, which has a truncated cytoplasmic domain.

The cytoplasmic domain of human red cell band 3 also binds the glycolytic enzyme glyceraldehyde-3-phosphate dehydrogenase (GAPDH) (91). The binding is associated with the highly acidic amino terminus and is believed to have a role in the regulation of glycolysis in human red cells, mediated by the phosphorylation of a tyrosine located 8 residues from the N terminus (86). It is as yet unclear whether this regulatory role applies to other species, because the tyrosine within a highly acidic N-terminal sequence is not conserved in band 3 of other mammalian species (e.g., mouse) (4). Recent work has demonstrated that GAPDH colocalizes with band 3 in erythrocytes and with *AE1* in the renal medulla of the rat (68). These findings suggest that a GAPDH binding site exists that is different from the acidic amino terminus or that the GAPDH antibody binds to a protein structure complex to which *AE1* antibody also binds. The possible interaction of glycolytic enzymes with *AE2* or *AE3* has not been explored.

Membrane Domain

Sequence and Structure

The membrane-spanning domains of the AE proteins are all approximately the same length and contain many highly conserved sequences (1,11). The membrane domain is very hydrophobic and has a net positive charge. The structure of the membrane domain is usually modeled as a bundle of α helices, based on the sequence and on circular dichroism measurements showing that the erythrocyte band-3 membrane domain is highly α helical (92). The exact number of transmembrane helices is unknown but is at least 10 and possibly as many as 14 (Fig. 4) (9,13,93). The sequences of most of the transmembrane helices are conserved throughout the AE family members; there is less conservation of the sequences of the surface connecting loops. About half the charged residues in the membrane domain are conserved and are found mainly in hydrophilic surface connector loops. However, some charged residues are very likely within the membrane, as would be expected for an ion transport protein.

New techniques have allowed the reconstitution of purified band 3 into two-dimensional crystals (94,95). Native and deglycosylated membrane domains were reconstituted with phospholipid and cholesterol, and negatively stained specimens were examined by electron microscopy (95). Projection maps at 20 Å based on image analyses of these negatively stained crystals reveal the dimeric nature of the protein, which had been strongly suggested by numerous biochemical studies (96–99). The dimer consists of two (apparently) identical subunits related by twofold rotational symmetry. There are three subdomains within each subunit. A pore at the dimer interface probably represents an access

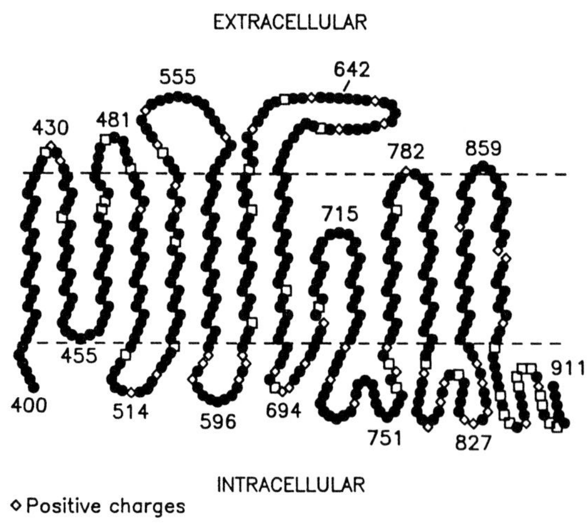

Figure 4 Two-dimensional folding model of *AE1*. The model is based on sequence, chemical modification, in situ proteolysis, and antibody binding (5,9,13,29,93). The positions of positive (Arg, Lys, His) and negative (Asp, Glu) residues are indicated. The topology of the first eight membrane spans is reasonably well established. Lys 430 can be labeled from the extracellular medium (93), indicating that the first transmembrane helix is very likely the first hydropathy peak in Fig. 1. The loop centered at about Tyr 555 is definitely extracellular and contains several cleavage sites for extracellular proteases. The consensus N-glycosylation site at Asn 642 is indeed glycosylated (160) and extracellular. The arrangement of the remainder of the protein is much less certain.

channel for anion transport. The shape, size, and position of two subdomains and a central depression are very similar when the two-dimensional sheet and tubular crystals are superimposed. The third subdomain may change position conformationally from an extended to a more compact form; the role of this subdomain in transport is not known.

The C-terminal truncated polypeptides consisting of only the membrane domains of *AE1* (83), *AE2* (35) and *AE3* (14) have been expressed and shown to be able to transport $^{36}Cl^-$ or to mediate intracellular pH changes that reflect Cl^--HCO_3^- exchange. These studies demonstrate that the cytoplasmic domain is not necessary for anion exchange, in agreement with earlier biochemical studies on erythrocyte band 3 (100,101).

Inhibitor Binding

Many different substances are known to inhibit anion exchange in red blood cells and other tissues. Cabantchik and Gregor (102) have recently reviewed the properties of these inhibitors. The present discussion is confined to the stilbenedisulfonate derivatives, which include SITS (4-acetamido-4′-isothiocyanato-stilbene-2,2′-disulfonate), DIDS, H_2DIDS(4,4′-diisothiocyanatostilbene-2,2′-disulfonate), and DNDS (4,4′-dinitrostilbene-2,2′-disulfonate). In discussing the inhibition of transport by stilbenedisulfonate derivatives, it is important to make a distinction between covalent and noncovalent binding (5). Stilbenedisulfonates bind reversibly to a pocket in the protein that is accessible from the extracellular but not the intracellular medium. The affinity of reversible binding is determined by both electrostatic and hydrophobic interactions (102). Reversible binding, at least for some stilbenedisulfonates, appears to take place in two stages: a rapid initial attachment and a slower process (still noncovalent) that locks the inhibitor in a high-affinity site (103). In this context, the "site" for reversible binding consists of all the amino acid residues that surround the bound stilbenedisulfonate.

Some stilbenedisulfonate derivatives (including DIDS and H_2DIDS) have an isothiocyanate group that can react covalently with lysine side chains. Both DIDS and H_2DIDS react covalently with lysine residues in red cell band 3. Early biochemical studies indicated that the site of most rapid covalent reaction corresponds to Lys 539 or 542 of the human AE1 sequence (5,104). Site-directed mutagenesis of Lys 539 does not inhibit anion transport (105–107); however, it does prevent covalent binding of H_2DIDS at neutral pH (105,106), suggesting that Lys 539 is the primary site of covalent H_2DIDS binding. A somewhat different result was obtained by Garcia and Lodish, who found that mutation of Lys 539 to any of several residues does not prevent covalent DIDS binding (107). This difference possibly can be explained by the higher reactivity of DIDS than H_2DIDS for covalent binding in native band 3 (108) and the possibility that DIDS reacts covalently with an alternative lysine when Lys 539 is not available. Lys 539 is conserved in all known anion exchanger sequences.

A bifunctional reagent, H_2DIDS is capable of forming two covalent bonds in a single band-3 polypeptide, and the binding of H_2DIDS to both Lys 539 and a second Lys results in the cross-linking of the two major chymotryptic fragments of band 3 (109). Direct sequencing of fragments cross-linked with H_2DIDS indicates that Lys 851 is the second Lys (110). Lys 851 had previously been shown to react with pyridoxal phosphate, another inhibitor of anion exchange (111).

All members of the anion-exchanger family are sensitive to the inhibitory effects of DIDS and H_2DIDS. However, *AE1* demonstrates 100-fold greater sensitivity to DIDS than *AE2* (31,35). The sensitivity of *AE3* to DIDS is closer to that of *AE1*, although covalent reaction with either *AE2* or *AE3* takes place at similar rates (112). Substitution of methionine for Lys 869 in murine band 3 (human Lys 851), results in a significantly reduced affinity for DIDS (113) or DNDS (114). It is of interest that, like *AE1*, *AE3* has a lysine in this position, but *AE2*, which is less sensitive to DIDS, has a methionine in this position. Therefore, the amino acid in the position of human Lys 851 appears to be a determinant of affinity for reversible stilbenedisulfonate binding.

Z Loop

One of the significant differences between *AE1* and the other members of the anion-exchanger family is an insertion in the latter of approximately 30 amino acid residues between membrane-spanning helices 5 and 6. The 30 residues are hydrophilic and lie close to the extracellular chymotrypsin cleavage site at position 555 of human *AE1* (Figs. 1 and 4). The sequence of this insertion, known as the "Z loop" (115), is not conserved between mouse and rat (15,32) and is unlikely to be necessary for transport. When amino acids from mouse *AE2* are placed in a similar position in mouse *AE1*, neither transport nor stilbenedisulfonate inhibition is affected (116). Interestingly, while the Z loop is unique to the mammalian *AE2* and *AE3* transporters, it has also been identified in trout *AE1* (117).

TRANSPORT KINETICS

The kinetics of band-3–mediated anion exchange have been extensively characterized in red blood cells. Work in several laboratories has established that the Cl^- conductance of the membrane is a very small fraction (less than 0.1%) of what would be predicted on the basis of the tracer flux of Cl^- (118–120). That is, the tracer flux consists almost entirely of an obligatory 1:1 exchange. The conventional method for measuring anion exchange is a so-called self-exchange experiment under conditions of no net anion movement. It is also possible to measure net anion exchange. In either case, for every Cl^- ion that moves in one direction, some other anion must move in the opposite direction. This requirement for exchange is not a consequence of a transmembrane electrical constraint, because the same requirement exists if the membrane permeability for cations (Na^+ and/or K^+) is drastically increased with ionophores. Thus, a very important functional characteristic of red cell band 3 is that it is an exchanger rather than a Cl^- channel. It may turn out that band 3 has some structural features in common with channels, but functionally it behaves very differently from a channel.

Although band-3–mediated anion exchange is a tightly coupled process, it is also rapid, at least for the physiological substrates Cl^- and HCO_3^-. The maximum flux for each of these anions (measured as Cl^--Cl^-, HCO_3^--HCO_3^-, or Cl^--HCO_3^- exchange) is about 50,000 ions per band-3 polypeptide per second (121). This turnover number is quite fast compared with other non-channel-transport proteins, such as the sodium pump (100/s) (122), Na-K-2Cl cotransporter (4000/s) (123), or Na^+-Ca^{2+} exchanger (5000/s) (124). The turnover numbers of *AE2* and *AE3* are not known, but if they are similar to that of *AE1*, the Cl^--HCO_3^- exchange requirements of most cells can be met with a relatively small number of copies of the protein.

As pointed out by Rothstein et al. (125), several years ago, there are two general mechanisms by which a protein could catalyze a 1:1 exchange. The first is denoted "ping-pong," using the terminology of Cleland (126) for two-substrate enzymes. In the ping-pong mechanism, the anions take turns crossing the membrane. The catalytic cycle is the following: an intracellular anion binds to an inward-facing transport site, is transported outward by way of a conformational change in the protein, and is released into the extracellular medium. Following release of the anion, the protein cannot transport another intracellular anion outward until it is reset by the extracellular binding, inward translocation, and intracellular release of an initially extracellular anion. In the ping-pong mechanism, the coupling between anion efflux and influx requires that there be two structurally distinct state of the transporter: inward-facing and outward facing. The rapid conformational transition between these states requires the presence of a transportable anion.

The other possible general mechanism for coupled anion exchange involves a ternary complex among the protein and the two exchanging anions, one of which originates on each side of the membrane. In this mechanism, the catalytic cycle consists of the binding of each of the exchange partners, either randomly or in some order (e.g., intracellular first), followed by a conformational change that allows the two anions to exchange places. Models of this sort are denoted "simultaneous," because both substrates must bind before either is transported.

There is considerable evidence that red cell band 3 catalyzes anion transport by way of a ping-pong mechanism, summarized by Jennings (9). It should be emphasized, however, that the kinetics of anion exchange are complex, and it is possible that the actual mechanism is not ping-pong in its simplest form. For example, the catalytic cycle may consist of internal binding and outward translocation, as in the ping-pong model, but external release may require binding of an external anion (127). This model represents a hybrid between ping-pong and simultaneous because it involves distinct inward-facing and outward-facing states (as in ping-pong), but it also includes a ternary complex with the inward-going and outward-going anions (as in simultaneous). Many other hybrid models are possible, none of which has been rigorously tested experimentally.

In summary, it is reasonably well established that band 3 can exist in at least two transport-related conformations and that the proportions of the conformations are influenced by anion gradients, as would be expected from a ping-pong model. However, that actual transport mechanism may be more complicated. An additional complexity is that high concentrations of anions actually inhibit anion exchange (5). The site responsible for this self-inhibition has been called the "modifier site" and, for Cl^-, is located on the cytoplasmic side of the membrane (128). The relation between the modifier site and the transport site(s) is not known.

The kinetics of anion exchange in nonerythroid cells have not been examined in as much detail, but there is evidence that, in HL60 cells, Cl^--Cl^- exchange obeys simultaneous rather than ping-pong kinetics (129,130). These cells are known to express *AE2* rather than *AE1* (115). The implication of these findings is that the catalytic cycle for *AE2* is simultaneous, where as that for *AE1* is ping-pong. It seems unlikely that two proteins of such similar structure (judged by hydropathy profile) would have fundamentally different catalytic mechanisms. However, the disagreement between results in red cells and in cells expressing *AE2* may only be apparent. It may be that the catalytic mechanisms of *AE1* and *AE2* are actually similar and that each includes features of both ping-pong and simultaneous models.

INTRACELLULAR pH DEPENDENCE

Red Cells

Because a major physiological function of Cl^--HCO_3^- exchange is the regulation of pH, it is of interest to determine the effect of pH on anion exchange mediated by *AE1*, *AE2*, and *AE3*. In red cells, the anion permeability is much higher than the Na^+ and K^+ permeabilities (131), and the membrane potential is equal to the equilibrium potential for Cl^-,HCO_3^-, and H^+. The intracellular pH of red cells can therefore be manipulated easily by changing the extracellular pH and then allowing the intracellular pH to equilibrate by way of downhill Cl^--HCO_3^- exchange. Alternatively, in the presence of low HCO_3^- concentrations of low temperatures, the extracellular pH can be changed to some desired value and Cl^--Cl^- exchange measured before appreciable pH equilibration. In this manner the effects of intracellular and extracellular pH on red cell anion exchange may be studied independently.

There is a sizable literature on the pH dependence of anion exchange in red cells, especially the differences in pH dependences of monovalent and divalent anions (5). For the present purposes, the discussion is confined to the effects of pH on Cl^- transport. Bilateral acidification (pH < 7) causes inhibition of Cl^--Cl^- exchange (132). In resealed red cell ghosts, in which the intracellular Cl^- concentration is not dependent on pH, the Cl^--Cl^- exchange flux at 150 m*M* Cl^- is essentially constant between pH 7 and 9 (133). In intact cells, intracellular alkalinization actually inhibits the Cl^--Cl^- exchange flux (132), although the inhibition can be explained on the basis of the lower intracellular Cl^- concentration at alkaline intracellular pH. Thus, unlike anion exchange in some nonerythroid cells (see below), intracellular alkalinization does not activate red cell Cl^--Cl^- exchange.

Nonerythroid Cells

In vitro microperfusion studies of the rabbit CCT have examined the effects of intracellular pH (pH_i) changes on Cl^--HCO_3^- exchange in both principal cells and beta intercalated cells (β-IC) (77). In principal cells, reduction of CO_2 in the peritubular solution from 5% (25 m*M* HCO_3^-) to 2% (25 m*M* HCO_3^-) resulted in an immediate intracellular alkalinization followed by slow pH_i recovery. Subsequent removal of external Cl^- again resulted in intracellular alkalinization, which was reversed upon readdition of peritubular Cl^-. Thus, the Cl^- dependence of pH_i recovery under these conditions was consistent with Cl^--HCO_3^- exchange. The authors explained the slow pH_i recovery as an activation of Cl^--HCO_3^- exchange in response to acute alkalinization.

The pH_i dependence of Cl^--HCO_3^- exchange in the β-IC was studied in a similar manner. The Cl^- dependence of the apical Cl^--HCO_3^- exchanger was characterized following a reduction of peritubular CO_2 from 5% to 2% (at constant 25 m*M* HCO_3^-), which resulted in a rapid intracellular alkalinization of the β-IC. Unlike the principal cell, however, there was no pH_i recovery from the alkaline load induced by these conditions. From the results of the latter experiment, it was concluded that the β-IC apical anion exchanger is not activated under conditions of acute intracellular alkalinization, suggesting that this exchanger is not affected by increases in pH_i.

The pH_i-dependence of Na^+-independent anion exchange in mesangial cells has also been examined (45). Cultured rat mesangial cells were perfused with solutions containing 5% CO_2 (25 m*M* HCO_3^-). The effects of Cl^- removal and addition on pH_i were evaluated in Na^+-free solutions. Removal of Cl^- from the perfusing solution resulted in a rapid and sustained intracellular alkalinization, which reversed when Cl^- was reintroduced. These findings are consistent with Na^+-independent anion exchange. A plot of the initial base efflux following readdition of Cl^- versus pH_i at the time of the maneuver suggests that the activity of Na^+-independent anion exchange is dependent on pH_i. That is, the exchanger is relatively inactive at pH_i less than 7.2 and increases in activity with pH_i values greater than 7.2.

Similar approaches have been used to evaluate the effect of pH_i on anion-exchanger isoforms in expression systems (113). Human 293 cells transfected with cDNAs of *AE2* or *AE3* demonstrated intracellular alkalinization after removal of external Cl^- and intracellular acidification upon reintroduction of Cl^-. Plots of initial H^+ flux observed when Cl^- was reintroduced vs. pH_i are consistent with an activation of *AE2* and *AE3* by high intracellular pH (113).

It is often difficult to determine whether increased Cl^--HCO_3^- exchange fluxes at alkaline pH_i are due to actual activation of transport activity or to the elevated HCO_3^- concentration gradient brought about by the experimental maneuver. Since the Cl^--HCO_3^- exchanger is capable of performing Cl^--Cl^- exchange, it is possible to study the effects of pH_i on anion exchange by measuring Cl^- influx or Cl^- efflux. Experiments by Olsnes and coworkers characterized the effect of pH_i on Cl^- self-exchange in African green monkey kidney cells (Vero cells) (134–137). Confluent cell cultures were incubated in HCO_3^--free (Hepes-buffered) solutions with a pH range of 6.7 to 7.8. Intracellular pH values measured in cells incubated in these solutions were similar to external pH values. In the absence or presence of external unlabeled Cl^-, DIDS-sensitive $^{36}Cl^-$ uptake was greater in cells incubated in solutions of pH above 7.0 than in solutions with a lower pH. Chloride efflux was evaluated in a similar manner. The results demonstrate that efflux of $^{36}Cl^-$ from cells bathed in solutions with a pH above 7.0 was greater than from cells bathed in more acidic solutions.

The studies by Olsnes et al. suggest that DIDS-sensitive Cl^- flux is stimulated by an increase in pH_i above 7.2 and are consistent with reported pH_i-dependence for anion transporters in principal cells (77), mesangial cells (45), and for *AEs* expressed in cultured cells (113). However, the molecular identity of the anion exchanger in Vero cells is not known. It is interesting to note that the apical exchanger of the renal CCTβ-IC appears not to be stimulated by alkaline PH_i, unlike the rest of the Na^+-independent AEs thus far studied. The reason for this difference in pH_i activation remains unclear.

CLINICAL SIGNIFICANCE

The response of renal Cl^--HCO_3^- exchange to systemic acidosis or alkalosis has been studied using functional, immunohistochemical, and—to a limited extent—recombinant DNA techniques. These acid/base effects have been the subject of recent reviews (39–42).

Initial microperfusion studies of the rabbit CCT demonstrated that this segment can either reabsorb or excrete bicarbonate (138–140). Increased HCO_3^- reabsorption was observed in tubules dissected from acid-loaded rabbits. Conversely, increased HCO_3^- excretion occurred in tubules dissected from alkali-loaded rabbits. These initial studies were later confirmed in rabbit and rat under a variety of conditions (50,52,53,55,141,142).

At the cellular level, the rate of Cl^- self-exchange mediated by the apical anion exchanger of β-ICs decreased with acid loading and increased with alkali loading in rabbit (73). The decreased activity observed with in vivo acid-loading was later confirmed with in vitro microperfusion studies (143). Under conditions of in vivo chloride-depletion metabolic alkalosis, morphological changes suggest increased transport activity of the apical exchanger in rat (41). In α-ICs, basolateral staining with *AE1* antibody increased with metabolic acidosis in rat (144), which agrees with studies that show increased cortical mRNA for *AE1* induced by chronic respiratory acidosis (145). The above studies demonstrate the ability of the CCT to compensate for disturbances in normal acid/base homeostasis.

The response of the anion exchanger to changes in external pH varies among nephron segments, consistent with the heterogenous cellular composition along the nephron. In the OMCD (outer and inner stripe), functional, immunocytochemical, and Northern hybridization data differ in the response of this segment to changes in external pH. For example, chronic respiratory acidosis results in a twofold increase in steady-state *AE1* mRNA in rat medulla (145). Since *AE1* has been localized only to the basolateral α-IC in medulla (66,67), the increase in message indicates an increase in synthesis of basolateral anion exchanger (145). Oral acid loading has also resulted in increased intensity of basolateral *AE1* antibody staining in rat OMCD a-ICs (146). The above studies, however, do not agree with functional studies that fail to show increased HCO_3^- reabsorption with acidosis induced by oral ammonium chloride loading in rabbits (50). Conversely, decreased HCO_3^--reabsorption does not occur with oral alkali loading in either rabbit or rat (50,53,54). This discrepancy between HCO_3^- reabsorption and changes in anion-exchanger mRNA levels remains to be resolved; for further discussion, see Schuster (40).

There are other clinical situations in which renal anion exchange can be important. For example, oxalate flux in human red cell membranes is significantly higher in patients with idiopathic nephrolithiasis when compared with controls (147). The oxalate flux is inhibited by DIDS and is thought to occur via anion exchange (148,149). In a subset of these patients, there is familial clustering of calcium oxalate stone formation expressed as an autosomal dominant trait with variable penetrance. The authors suggest that nephrolithiasis may occur by increased oxalate transport through abnormal function of the anion exchanger in the kidney.

As described earlier, mutations in band 3 have been used to determine the DIDS binding site. The effect of naturally occurring gene mutations of the AEs would therefore be of clinical interest. Several variants of band 3 have been described with varying effects on transport function, including band 3 Memphis (150) and Southeast Asian ovalocytosis (SAO) (151–153). In band 3 Memphis, there is a point mutation (Lys-56 → Glu), which does not confer abnormal properties to red cells but does demonstrate altered (slower) mobility of the protein on an SDS-polyacrylamide gel (154). In SAO, however, not only is there the same Lys-56 → Glu point mutation, but there is also the deletion of 27 bp that results in a deletion of amino acids 400 to 408 (155). This deletion occurs at the boundary between the cytosol and first transmembrane segment and is felt responsible for the characteristics of SAO, including resistance to malaria, a rigid, oval-shaped erythrocyte, altered glycosylation, and reduced inhibitor binding (151–153,156). The only known humans with the SAO mutation are heterozygous for the variant. The kidneys of these individuals would be expected to express some normally functioning *AE1* as well as nonfunctional *AE1* with the SAO deletion. The presence of nonfunctioning *AE1* in the kidney could result in diminished transport and metabolic acidosis. It is possible, however, that normal renal Cl^--HCO_3^- transport can be achieved with altered *AE1* present or by compensatory changes elsewhere in the nephron. Functional studies in individuals with band-3 variants will help resolve these questions.

REFERENCES

1. Kopito RR. Molecular biology of the anion exchanger gene family. Int Rev Cytol 1990; 123:177–199.
2. Alper SL. The band 3-related anion exchanger (AE) gene family. Annu Rev Physiol 1991; 53:549–564.
3. Fairbanks G, Steck TL, Wallach DFH. Electrophoretic analysis of the major polypeptides of the human erythrocyte membrane. Biochemistry 1971; 10:2606–2616.
4. Kopito RR, Lodish HF. Primary structure and transmembrane orientation of the murine anion exchange protein. Nature 1985; 316:234–238.
5. Passow H. Molecular aspects of band 3 protein-mediated anion transport across the red blood cell membrane. Rev Physiol Biochem Pharmacol 1986; 103:62–203.
6. Jennings ML. Structure and function of the red blood cell anion transport protein. Annu Rev Biophys Chem 1989; 18:397–430.
7. Salhany JM. Erythrocyte Band 3 Protein. Boca Raton, FL: CRC Press, 1990.
8. Jennings ML. Cellular Anion Transport. In: Seldin DW, Giebisch G, eds. The Kidney: Physiology and Pathophysiology. New York: Raven Press, 1992:113–145.
9. Jennings ML. Anion Transport Proteins. In: Seldin DW, Giebisch G, eds. The Kidney: Physiology and Pathophysiology. New York: Raven Press, 1992:503–535.
10. Passow H. The band 3 proteins: An introduction. In: Bamberg E, Passow H, eds. The Band 3 Proteins: Anion Transporters, Binding Proteins, and Senescent Antigens. Amsterdam: Elsevier, 1992:1–6.
11. Wood PG. The anion exchange proteins: homology and secondary structure. In: Bamberg E, Passow H,

eds. The Band 3 Proteins: Anion Transporters, Binding Proteins, and Senescent Antigens. Amsterdam: Elsevier, 1992:325–352.
12. Alper SL. Molecular and cell biological aspects of the AE anion exchanger gene family. In: Bamberg E, Passow H, eds. The Band 3 Proteins: Anion Transporters, Binding Proteins, and Senescent Antigens. Amsterdam: Elsevier, 1992:9–15.
13. Reithmeier RAF. The erythrocyte anion transporter (band 3). Curr Opin Struct Biol 1993; 3:515–523.
14. Kopito RR, Lee BS, Simmons DM, et al. Regulation of intracellular pH by a neuronal homolog of the erythrocyte anion exchanger. Cell 1989; 59:927–937.
15. Kudrycki KE, Newman PR, Shull GE. cDNA cloning and tissue distribution of mRNAs for two proteins that are related to the band 3 chloride/bicarbonate exchanger. J Biol Chem 1990; 265:462–471.
16. Lieberman DM, Reithmeier RAF. Localization of the carboxyl terminus of band 3 to the cytoplasmic side of the erythrocyte membrane using antibodies raised against a synthetic peptide. J Biol Chem 1988; 263:10022–10028.
17. Bauer CK, Steinmeyer K, Schwarz JR, Jentsch TJ. Completely functional double-barreled chloride channel expressed from a single *Torpedo* cDNA. Proc Natl Acad Sci USA 1991; 88:11052–11056.
18. Jentsch T, Steinmeyer K, Schwarz G. Primary structure of *Torpedo marmorata* chloride channel isolated by expression cloning in *Xenopus oocytes*. Nature 1990; 348:510–514.
19. Abe T, Takeuchi K, Ishii K, Abe K. Molecular cloning and expression of a rat cDNA encoding MDCK-type chloride channel. Biochim Biophys Acta 1993; 1173:353–356.
20. Thiemann A, Gründer S, Pusch M, Jentsch T. A chloride channel widely expressed in epithelial and non-epithelial cells. Nature 1992; 356:57–60.
21. Showe LM, Ballantine M, Huebner K. Localization of the gene for the erythroid anion exchange protein, band 3, to human chromosome 17. Genomics 1987; 1:71–76.
22. Palumbo AP, Isobe M, Huebner K, et al. Chromosomal localization of a human band 3-like gene to region 7q35-7q36. Am J Hum Genet 1986; 39:307–316.
23. Kopito RR, Andersson M, Lodish HF. Structure and organization of the murine band 3 gene. J Biol Chem 1987; 262:8035–8040.
24. Stewart EA, Kopito R, Bowcock AM. A PstI polymorphism for the human erythrocyte surface protein band 3 (EPB3) demonstrates close linkage of EPB3 to the nerve growth factor receptor. Genomics 1989; 5:633–635.
25. Cox JV, Moon RT, Lazarides E. Anion transporter: highly cell-type-specific expression of distinct polypeptides and transcripts in erythroid and nonerythroid cells. J Cell Biol 1985; 100:1548–1557.
26. Kim H-RC, Yew NS, Ansorge W, et al. Two different mRNAs are transcribed from a single genomic locus encoding the chicken erythrocyte anion transport proteins (band 3). Mol Cell Biol 1988; 8:4416–4424.
27. Kudrycki KE, Shull GE. Primary structure of the rat kidney band 3 anion exchange protein deduced from a cDNA. J Biol Chem 1989; 264:8185–8192.
28. Kudrycki KE, Shull GE. Rat kidney band 3 Cl^-/HCO_3^- exchanger mRNA is transcribed from an alternative promoter. Am J Physiol 1993; 264:F540–F547.
29. Tanner MJA, Wainwright SD, Martin P. Structure, molecular genetics and topology of the human red cell anion transporter (AE1). In: Bamberg E, Passow H, eds. The Band 3 Proteins: Anion Transporters, Binding Proteins, and Senescent Antigens. Progress in Cell Research Vol. 2. Amsterdam: Elsevier, 1992:17–22.
30. Kopito RR, Andersson MA, Lodish HF. Multiple tissue-specific sites of transcriptional initiation of the mouse anion antiport gene in erythroid and renal cells. Proc Natl Acad Sci USA 1987; 84:7149–7153.
31. Brosius FC, III, Alper SL, Garcia AM, Lodish HF. The major kidney band 3 gene transcript predicts an amino-terminal truncated band 3 polypeptide. J Biol Chem 1989; 264:7784–7787.
32. Alper SL, Kopito RR, Libresco SM, Lodish HF. Cloning and characterization of a murine band 3–related cDNA from kidney and from a lymphoid cell line. J Biol Chem 1988; 263:17092–17099.
33. Gehrig H, Müller W, Appelhans H. Complete nucleotide sequences of band 3 related transport protein AE2 from human kidney. Biochim Biophys Acta 1992; 1130:326–328.
34. Chow A, Dobbins JW, Aronson PS, Igarashi P. cDNA cloning and localization of a band 3–related protein from ileum. Am J Physiol 1992; 263:G345–G352.
35. Lindsey AE, Schneider K, Simmons DM, et al. Functional expression and subcellular localization of anion exchanger cloned from choroid plexus. Proc Natl Acad Sci USA 1990; 87:5278–5282.
36. Kozak M. An analysis of 5′-noncoding sequences from 699 vertebrate messenger RNAs. Nucl Acids Res 1987; 15:8125–8148.
37. Linn SC, Kudrycki KE, Shull GE. The predicted translation product of a cardiac AE3 mRNA contains an N terminus distinct from that of the brain AE3 Cl^-/HCO_3^- exchanger. J Biol Chem 1992; 267:7927–7935.
38. Mar JH, Ordahl CP. A conserved CATTCCT motif is required for skeletal muscle-specific activity of the cardiac troponin T gene promoter. Proc Natl Acad Sci USA 1988; 85:6404–6408.
39. Schuster VL. Organization of collecting duct intercalated cells. Kidney Int 1990; 38:668–672.

40. Schuster VL. Function and regulation of collecting duct intercalated cells. Annu Rev Physiol 1993; 55:267–288.
41. Verlander JW, Madsen KM, Tisher CC. Structural and functional features of proton and bicarbonate transport in the rat collecting duct. Semin Nephrol 1991; 11:465–477.
42. Hamm LL, Weiner ID, Vehaskari VM. Structural-functional characteristics of acid-base transport in the rabbit collecting duct. Semin Nephrol 1991; 11:453–464.
43. Friedman PA, Andreoli TE. Co_2-stimulated NaCl absorption in the mouse renal cotical thick ascending limb of Henle. J Gen Physiol 1982; 80:683–711.
44. Hebert SC. Hypertonic cell volume regulation in mouse thick limbs II. Na^+-H^+ and Cl^--HCO_3^- exchange in basolateral membranes. Am J Physiol 1986; 250:C920–C931.
45. Boyarsky G, Ganz MB, Sterzel RB, Boron WF. pH regulation in single glomerular mesangial cells: II. Na^+-dependent and -independent Cl^--HCO_3^- exchangers. Am J Physiol 1988; 255:C844–C856.
46. Ridderstrale Y, Kashgarian M, Koeppen B, et al. Morphological heterogeneity of the rabbit collecting duct. Kidney Int 1988; 34:655–670.
47. Emmons C, Matsuzaki K, Stokes JB. Axial heterogeneity of cortical collecting duct cell types (abstr). Kidney Int 1989; 35:453.
48. Tisher CC, Madsen KM. Anatomy of the kidney. In: Brenner BM, Rector FC, eds. The Kidney. Philadelphia, PA: Saunders, 1991:3–75.
49. Laski ME, Kurtzman NA. Characterization of acidification in the cortical and medullary collecting tubule of the rabbit. J Clin Invest 1983; 72:2050–2059.
50. Lombard WE, Kokko JP, Jacobson HR. Bicarbonate transport in cortical and outer medullary collecting tubules. Am J Physiol 1983; 244:F289–F296.
51. Breyer MD, Kokko JP, Jacobson HR. Regulation of net biacarbonate transport in rabbit cortical collecting tubule by peritubular pH, carbon dioxide tension, and bicarbonate concentration. J Clin Invest 1986; 77:1650–1660.
52. Hamm LL, Hering-Smith KS, Vehaskari VM. Control of bicarbonate transport in collecting tubules from normal and remnant kidneys. Am J Physiol 1989; 256:F680–F687.
53. Atkins JL, Burg MB. Bicarbonate transport by isolated perfused rat collecting ducts. Am J Physiol 1985; 249:F485–F489.
54. McKinney TK, Davidson KK. Bicarbonate transport in collecting tubules from outer stripe of outer medulla in rabbit kidneys. Am J Physiol 1987; 253:F816–F822.
55. Star RA, Burg MB, Knepper MA. Bicarbonate secretion and chloride absorption by rabbit cortical collecting ducts: Role of chloride/bicarbonate exchange. J Clin Invest 1985; 76:1123–1130.
56. Stone DK, Kokko JP, Jacobson HR. Anion dependence of rabbit medullary collecting duct acidification. J Clin Invest 1983; 71:1505–1508.
57. Breyer MD, Jacobson HR. Regulation of rabbit medullary collecting duct cell pH by basolateral Na^+/H^+ and Cl^-/base exchange. J Clin Invest 1989; 84:996–1004.
58. Weiner ID, Hamm LL. Use of fluorescent dye BCECF to measure intracellular pH in cortical collecting tubule. Am J Physiol 1989; 256:F957–F964.
59. Hays SR, Alpern RJ. Basolateral membrane sodium-independent, chloride/bicarbonate exchange in the inner stripe of the rabbit outer medullary collecting tubule. J Gen Physiol 1990; 95:347–367.
60. Zeidel ML, Silva P, Seifter JL. Intracellular pH regulation in rabbit renal medullary collecting duct cells: Role of chloride-bicarbonate exchange. J Clin Invest 1986; 77:1682–1688.
61. Schwartz GJ, Satlin LM, Bergman JE. Fluorescent characterization of collecting duct cells: A second H^+-secreting type. Am J Physiol 1988; 255:F1003–F1014.
62. Hays SR, Alpern RJ. Na-independent Cl-HCO_3 exchange is the major basolateral membrane HCO_3 transport mechanism in the outer medullary collecting tubule. Kidney Int 1989; 35:455.
63. Janoshazi A, Ojcius DM, Kone B. Relation between the anion exchange protein in kidney medullary collecting duct cells and red cell band 3. J Membr Biol 1988; 103:181–189.
64. Drenckhahn D, Schluter K, Allen DP, Bennett V. Colocalization of band 3 with ankyrin and spectrin at the basal membrane of intercalated cells in the rat kidney. Science 1985; 230:1287–1289.
65. Verlander JW, Madsen KM, Tisher CC. Effect of acute respiratory acidosis on two populations of intercalated cells in rat cortical collecting duct. Am J Physiol 1987; 253:F1142–F1156.
66. Verlander JW, Madsen KM, Low PS, et al. Immunocytochemical localization of band 3 protein in the rat collecting duct. Am J Physiol 1988; 255:F115–F125.
67. Alper SL, Natale J, Gluck S, et al. Subtypes of intercalated cells in rat kidney collecting ducts defined by antibodies against erythroid band 3 and renal vacuolar H^+-ATPase. Proc Natl Acad Sci USA 1989; 86:5429–5433.
68. Ercolani L, Brown D, Stuart-Tilley A, Alper SL. Colocalization of GAPDH and band 3 (AE1) proteins in the rat erythrocytes and kidney intercalated cell membranes. Am J Physiol 1992; 262:F892–F896.

69. Schuster VL, Bonsib SM, Jennings ML. Two types of collecting duct mitochondria-rich (intercalated) cells: Lectin and band 3 cytochemistry. Am J Physiol 1986; 251:C347–C355.
70. Schuster VL, Fejes-Toth G, Naray-Fejes-Toth A, Gluck S. Colocalization of H^+-ATPase and band 3 anion exchanger in rabbit collecting duct intercalated cells. Am J Physiol 1991; 260:F506–F517.
71. Drenckhahn D, Merte C. Restriction of the human kidney band 3–like anion exchanger to specialized subdomains of the basolateral plasma membrane of intercalated cells. Eur J Cell Biol 1987; 45:107–115.
72. van Adelsberg J, Edwards JC, Herzlinger D, et al. Isolation and culture of HCO_3^--secreting intercalated cells. Am J Physiol 1989; 256:C1004–C1011.
73. Tago K, Schuster VL, Stokes JB. Regulation of CL^- self-exchange by cAMP in cortical collecting tubule. Am J Physiol 1986; 251:F40–F48.
74. Tago K, Warden DJ, Schuster VL, Stokes JB. Effects of inhibitors of Cl^- conductance on Cl^- self-exchange in rabbit cortical collecting tubule. Am J Physiol 1986; 251:F1009–F1017.
75. Schuster VL, Stokes JB. Chloride transport by the cortical and outer medullary collecting duct. Am J Physiol 1987; 253:F203–F212.
76. van Adelsberg JS, Edwards JC, Al-Awqati Q. The apical Cl/HCO_3 exchanger of beta intercalated cells. J Biol Chem 1993; 268:11283–11289.
77. Weiner ID, Hamm LL. Regulation of intracellular pH in the rabbit cortical collecting tubule. J Clin Invest 1990; 85:274–281.
78. Wang X, Kurtz I. H^+/base transport in principal cells characterized by confocal fluorescence imaging. Am J Physiol 1990; 259:C365–C373.
79. Kuwahara M, Sasaki S, Marumo F. Cl/HCO3 exchange and Na-HCO3 symport in rabbit outer medullary collecting duct cells. Am J Physiol 1991; 260:F635–F642.
80. Star RA. Basolateral membrane sodium-independent Cl^-/HCO_3^- exchange in rat inner medullary collecting duct cell. J Clin Invest 1990; 85:1959–1966.
81. DiStefano A, Greger R, de Fouffignac D, Wittner M. Active NaCl transport in the cortical thick ascending limb of Henle's loop of the mouse does not require the presence of bicarbonate. Pflugers Arch 1992; 420:290–296.
82. Fryer JN, Weld MM, Okawara Y, Levine DZ. In situ hybridization studies of band 3 anion exchanger mRNA in rat kidney tubules (abstr). J Am Soc Nephrol 1993; 4:838.
83. Lepke S, Becker A, Passow H. Mediation of inorganic anion transport by the hydrophobic domain of mouse erythroid band 3 protein expressed in oocytes of *Xenopus laevis*. Biochim Biophys Acta 1992; 1106:13–16.
84. Low PS. Structure and function of the cytoplasmic domain of band 3: Center of erythrocyte membrane-peripheral protein interactions. Biochim Biophys Acta 1986; 864:145–167.
85. Bennett V. The membrane skeleton of human erythrocytes and its implications for more complex cells. Ann Rev Biochem 1985; 54:273–304.
86. Low PS. Band 3: Calorimetry, cytoskeletal associations, role in metabolic regulation, and role in aging. In: Bamberg E, Passow H, eds. The Band 3 Proteins: Anion Transporters, Binding Proteins, and Senescent Antigens. Amsterdam: Elsevier, 1992:219–225.
87. Appell KC, Low PS. Partial structural characterization of the cytoplasmic domain of the erythrocyte membrane protein, band 3. J Biol Chem 1981; 256:11104–11111.
88. Pasternack GR, Anderson RA, Leto TL, Marchesi VT. Interactions between protein 4.1 and band 3: An alternative binding site for an element of the membrane skeleton. J Biol Chem 1985; 260:3676–3683.
89. Korsgren C, Cohen CM. Associations of human erythrocyte band 4.2: Binding to ankyrin and to the cytoplasmic domain of band 3. J Biol Chem 1988; 263:10212–10218.
90. Jons T, Drenckhahn D. Identification of the binding interface involved in linkage of cytoskeleton protein 4.1 to the erythrocyte anion exchanger. EMBO J 1992; 11:2863–2867.
91. Tsai I, Murthy P, Steck TL. Effect of red cell membrane binding on the catalytic activity of glyceraldehyde-3-phosphate dehydrogenase. J Biol Chem 1982; 257:1438–1442.
92. Oikawa K, Lieberman DM, Reithmeier RAF. Conformation and stability of the anion transport protein of human erythrocyte membranes. Biochemistry 1985; 24:2843–2848.
93. Jennings ML, Anderson MP, Monaghan R. Monoclonal antibodies against human erythrocyte band 3 protein: Localization of proteolytic cleavage sites and stilbenedisulfonate-binding lysine residues. J Biol Chem 1986; 261:9002–9010.
94. Dolder M, Walz T, Hefti A, Engel A. Human erythrocyte band 3 solubilization and reconstitution into two-dimensional crystals. J Mol Biol 1993; 231:119–132.
95. Wang DN, Kuhlbrandt W, Sarabia VE, Reithmeier RAF. Two dimensional structure of the membrane domain of human band 3, the anion transport protein of the erythrocyte membrane. EMBO J 1993; 12:2233–2239.
96. Steck TL. Cross-linking the major proteins of the isolated erythrocyte membrane. J Mol Biol 1972; 66:295–305.

97. Staros JV, Kakkad BP. Cross-linking and chymotryptic digestion of the extracytoplasmic domain of the anion exchange channel in intact human erythrocytes. J Membr Biol 1983; 74:247–254.
98. Schubert D. The relationships between oligomeric structure and function of band 3 protein from human erythrocyte membranes: Present knowledge and suggestions for further experiments. Molec Aspects Med 1988; 10:233–237.
99. Casey JR, Reithmeier RAF. Analysis of the oligomeric state of band 3, the anion transport protein of the human erythrocyte membrane, by size exclusion high performance liquid chromatography. J Biol Chem 1991; 266:15726–15737.
100. Lepke S, Passow H. Effects of incorporated trypsin on anion exchange and membrane proteins in human red cell ghosts. Biochim Biophys Acta 1976; 455:353–370.
101. Grinstein S, Ship S, Rothstein A. Anion transport in relation to proteolytic dissection of band 3. Biochim Biophys Acta 1978; 507:294–304.
102. Cabantchik ZI, Greger R. Chemical probes for anion transporters of mammalian cell membranes. Am J Physiol 1992; 262:C803–C827.
103. Verkman AS, Dix JA, Solomon AK. Anion transport inhibitor binding to band 3 in red blood cell membranes. J Gen Physiol 1983; 81:421–449.
104. Tanner MJA, Martin PG, High S. The complete amino acid sequence of the human erythrocyte membrane anion-transport protein deduced from the cDNA sequence. Biochem J 1988; 256:703–712.
105. Bartel D, Lepke S, Layh-Schmitt G, et al. Anion transport in oocytes of *Xenopus laevis* induced by expression of mouse erythroid band 3 protein—Encoding cRNA and of a cRNA derivative obtained by side-directed mutagenesis at the stilbene disulfonate binding site. EMBO J 1989; 8:3601–3609.
106. Bartel D, Hans H, Passow H. Identification by site-directed mutagenesis of Lys-558 as the covalent attachment site of dihydro DIDS in the mouse erythroid band 3 protein. Biochim Biophys Acta 1989; 985:355–358.
107. Garcia AM, Lodish HF. Lysine 539 of human band 3 is not essential for ion transport or inhibition by stilbene disulfonates. J Biol Chem 1989; 264:19607–19613.
108. Lepke S, Fasold H, Pring M, Passow H. A study of the relationship between inhibition of anion exchange and binding to the red blood cell membrane of 4,4′-diisothiocyanodihydrostilbene-2,2′-disulfonic acid (DIDS) and its dihydro derivative (H_2DIDS). J Membr Biol 1976; 29:147–177.
109. Jennings ML, Passow H. Anion transport across the erythrocyte membrane, in situ proteolysis of band 3 protein, and cross-linking of proteolytic fragments by 4,4′-diisothiocyano-dihydrostilbene-2,2′-disulfonate. Biochim Biophys Acta 1979; 554:498–519.
110. Okubo K, Kang D, Hamasaki N, Jennings ML. Red blood cell band 3: Lysine-539 and lysine 851 react with the same 4,4′-diisothiocyanodihydrostilbene-2,2′-disulfonate molecule. J Biol Chem 1994; 269:1918–1926.
111. Kawano Y, Okubo K, Tokunaga F, et al. Localization of the pyridoxal phosphate binding site at the COOH-terminal region of erythrocyte band 3 protein. J Biol Chem 1988; 263:8232–8238.
112. Alpern RJ. Apical membrane chloride/base exchange in the rat proximal convoluted tubule. J Clin Invest 1987; 79:1026–1030.
113. Lee BS, Gunn RB, Kopito RR. Functional differences among nonerythroid anion exchangers expressed in a transfected human cell line. J Biol Chem 1991; 266:11448–11454.
114. Wood PG, Müller H, Sovak M, Passow H. Role of Lys 558 and Lys 869 in substrate and inhibitor binding to the murine band 3 protein: A study of the effects of site-directed mutagenesis of the band 3 protein expressed in the oocytes of *Xenopus laevis*. J Membr Biol 1992; 127:139–148.
115. Demuth DR, Showe LC, Ballantine M, et al. Cloning and structural characterization of a human non-erythroid band 3–like protein. EMBO J 1986; 5:1205–1214.
116. Karbach D, Hanke-Baier P, Wendel J, et al. Anion transport in the red blood cell of the mouse and in erythroleukemic K562 cells. In: Bamberg E, Passow H, eds. The Band 3 Proteins: Anion Transporters, Binding Proteins, and Senescent Antigens. Progress in Cell Research Vol. 2. Amsterdam: Elsevier, 1992:295–305.
117. Hübner S, Michel F, Rudloff V, Appelhans H. Amino acid sequence of band-3 protein from rainbow trout erythrocytes derived from cDNA. Biochemistry 1992; 285:17–23.
118. Knauf PA, Fuhrmann GF, Rothstein S, Rothstein A. The relationship between exchange and red anion flow across the human red blood cell membrane. J Gen Physiol 1977; 69:363–386.
119. Knauf PA, Law F-Y, Marchant P. Relationship of net chloride flow across the human erythrocyte membrane to the anion exchange mechanism. J Gen Physiol 1983; 81:95–126.
120. Fröhlich O. Relative contributions of the slippage and tunneling mechanisms to anion net efflux from human erythrocytes. J Gen Physiol 1984; 84:877–893.
121. Brahm J. Temperature-dependent changes of chloride transport kinetics in human red cells. J Gen Physiol 1977; 70:283–306.
122. DeWeer P. Cellular sodium-potassium transport. In: Seldin DW, Giebisch G, eds. The Kidney, Physiology and Pathophysiology. New York: Raven Press, 1992:93–112.

123. Haas M, Forbush B III. [3H] bumetanide binding to duck red cells: Correlation with inhibition of (Na + K + 2 Cl) co-transport. J Biol Chem 1986; 261:8434–8441.
124. Reeves JP. Molecular aspects of sodium-calcium exchange. Arch Biochem Biophys 1992; 292:329–334.
125. Rothstein A, Cabantchik ZI, Knauf P. Mechanism of anion transport in red blood cells: Role of membrane proteins. Fed Proc 1976; 35:3–10.
126. Cleland WW. The kinetics of enzyme-catalyzed reactions with two or more substrates or products: I. Nomenclature and rate equations. Biochim Biophys Acta 1963; 67:104–137.
127. Salhany JM, Rauenbuehler PB. Kinetics and mechanism of erythrocyte anion exchange. J Biol Chem 1983; 258:245–249.
128. Knauf PA, Mann NA. Location of the chloride self-inhibitory site of the human erythrocyte anion exchange system. Am J Physiol 1986; 251:C1–C9.
129. Restrepo D, Kozody DJ, Spinelli LJ, Knauf PA. Cl-Cl exchange in promyelocytic HL-60 cells follows simultaneous rather than ping-pong kinetics. Am J Physiol 1989; 257:C520–C527.
130. Restrepo D, Cronise BL, Snyder RB, et al. Kinetics of DIDS inhibition of HL-60 cell anion exchange rules out ping-pong model with slippage. Am J Physiol 1991; 260:C535–C544.
131. Sachs JR, Knauf PA, Dunham PB. Transport through red cell membranes. In: Surgenor DMacN, ed. The Red Blood Cell. New York: Academic Press, 1975:613–702.
132. Gunn RB, Dalmark M, Tosteson DC, Wieth JO. Characteristics of chloride transport in human red blood cells. J Gen Physiol 1973; 61:185–206.
133. Funder J, Wieth JO. Chloride transport in human erythrocyte and ghosts: A quantitative comparison. J Physiol (Lond) 1976; 262:679–698.
134. Olsnes S, Tønnessen TI, Sandvig K. pH-regulated anion antiport in nucleated mammalian cells. J Cell Biol 1986; 102:967–971.
135. Olsnes S, Tønnessen TI, Ludt J, Sandvig K. Effect of intracellular pH on the rate of chloride uptake and efflux in different mammalian cell lines. Biochemistry 1987; 26:2778–2785.
136. Tønnessen TI, Ludt J, Sandvig K, Olsnes S. Bicarbonate/chloride antiport in Vero cells: I. Evidence for both sodium-linked and sodium-independent exchange. J Cell Physiol 1987; 132:183–191.
137. Tønnessen TI, Aas AT, Ludt J, et al. Regulation of Na^+/H^+ and Cl^-/HCO_3^- antiports in Vero cells. J Cell Physiol 1990; 143:178–187.
138. McKinney TD, Burg MB. Bicarbonate transport by rabbit cortical collecting tubules: Effect of acid and alkali loads in vivo on transport in vitro. J Clin Invest 1977; 60:766–768.
139. McKinney TD, Burg MB. Bicarbonate absorption by rabbit cortical collecting tubules in vitro. Am J Physiol 1978; 234:F141–F145.
140. McKinney TD, Burg MB. Bicarbonate secretion by rabbit cortical collecting tubules in vitro. J Clin Invest 1978; 61:1421–1427.
141. Levine DZ, Iacovitti M, Nash L, Vandorpe D. Secretion of bicarbonate by rat distal tubules in vivo: Modulation by overnight fasting. J Clin Invest 1988; 81:1873–1878.
142. Garcia-Austt J, Good DW, Burg MB, Knepper MA. Deoxycorticosterone-stimulated bicarbonate secretion in rabbit cortical collecting ducts: Effects of luminal chloride removal and in vivo acid loading. Am J Physiol 1985; 249:F205–F212.
143. Satlin LM, Schwartz GJ. Cellular remodeling of HCO_3^- secreting cells in rabbit renal collecting duct in response to an acidic environment. J Cell Biol 1989; 109:1279–1288.
144. Kim J, Shami H, Tixher CC, Madsen KM. Immunocytochemical response of intercalated cells in rat collecting duct to metabolic acidosis and hypokalemia (abstr). J Am Soc Nephrol 1991; 2:270.
145. Teixeira da Silva JC, Perrone RD, et al. Rat kidney band 3 mRNA modulation in chronic respiratory acidosis. Am J Physiol 1991; 260:F204–F209.
146. Alper SL, Sabolic I, Tyszkowski R, Brown D. Metabolic acidosis and alkalosis modulate anion exchange (AE1) expression in kidney collecting ducts (abstr). J Am Soc Nephrol 1991; 2:263.
147. Baggio B, Giovanni G, Marchini F, et al. An inheritable anomaly of red-cell oxalate transport in "primary" calcium nephrolithiasis correctable with diuretics. N Engl J Med 1986; 314:599–604.
148. Bambaro G, Baggio B. Idiopathic calcium oxalate nephrolithiasis: A cellular disease. Scan Micro 1992; 6:247–254.
149. Baggio B, Gambaro G, Marchini F, et al. Raised transmembrane oxalate flux in red blood cells in idiopathic calcium oxalate nephrolithiasis. Lancet 1984; 2:12–13.
150. Mueller TJ, Morrison M. Detection of a variant of protein 3, the major transmembrane protein of the human erythrocyte. J Biol Chem 1977; 252:6573–6576.
151. Sarabia VE, Casey JR, Reithmeier RAF. Molecular characterization of the band 3 protein from Southeast Asian ovalocytes. J Biol Chem 1993; 268:10676–10680.
152. Schofield AE, Reardon DM, Tanner MJA. Defective anion transport activity of the abnormal band 3 in hereditary ovalocytic red blood cells. Nature 1992; 355:836–838.

153. Moriyama R, Ideguchi H, Lombardo CR, et al. Structural and functional characterization of band 3 from Southeast Asian ovalocytes. J Biol Chem 1992; 267:25792–25797.
154. Yannoukakos D, Vasseur C, Draincourt C, et al. Human erythrocyte band 3 polymorphism (Band 3 Memphis): characterization of the structural modification (Lys 56 → Glu) by protein chemistry methods. Blood 1991; 78:1117–1120.
155. Tanner MJA, Bruce L, Martin PG, et al. Melanesian hereditary ovalocytes have a deletion in red cell band 3. Blood 1991; 78:2785–2787.
156. Mohandas N, Lie-Injo LE, Friedman M, Mak JW. Rigid membranes of Malayan ovalocytes: A likely genetic barrier against malaria. Blood 1984; 63:1385–1392.
157. Cox JV, Lazarides E. Alternative primary structures in the transmembrane domain of the chicken erythroid anion transporter. Mol Cell Biol 1988; 8:1327–1335.
158. Lux SE, John KM, Kopito RR, Lodish HF. Cloning and characterization of band 3, the human erythrocyte anion-exchange protein (AE1). Proc Natl Acad Sci USA 1989; 86:9089–9093.
159. Kyte J, Doolittle RF. A simple method for displaying the hydropathic character of a protein. J Mol Biol 1982; 157:105–132.
160. Jay DG. Glycosylation site of band 3, the human erythrocyte anion-exchange protein. Biochemistry 1986; 25:554–556.

23
Organic Anion Transporters

Victor L. Schuster
Albert Einstein College of Medicine, Bronx, New York

INTRODUCTION: RENAL TRANSPORT OF INORGANIC VS. ORGANIC ANIONS

The last decade has witnessed the start of an explosion in our understanding of the molecular mechanisms of renal inorganic anion transport. The cloning of the erythrocyte Cl-HCO_3 exchanger (band 3, now called *AE1*) (1) led to the rapid localization and identification of truncated forms of the same gene expressed in the kidney (2–5). Other anion exchangers have also been identified molecularly in the kidney (*AE2*) (6). Following the cloning of a family of chloride channels by Jentsch et al., an increasing number of renal Cl channels have been identified by homology cloning (for example, Ref. 7). Finally, renal transporters for inorganic sulfate (8) and phosphate (9,10) were recently expression- and homology-cloned.

In the face of this excellent progress on inorganic anion transporters, there has been relative neglect of the molecular study of renal transport of organic anions. There are probably several reasons for this. First, expression cloning is more difficult with organic anions because there is usually a large degree of nonionic diffusion of the protonated species. This means that a strong and specific inhibitor must be found if one is to separate carrier-mediated transport from the background "leak." Second, since it is only very recently that any such transporters have been cloned, homology cloning is only now possible.

THE RENAL ORGANIC ANION SECRETORY SYSTEM: HISTORY AND UBIQUITY

It has been recognized since 1874 that the kidney secretes organic anions (11). In fact, Marshall's famous experiments in 1928 (i.e., to show that the proximal tubules of aglomerular goosefish secrete phenol red), were the first to clearly establish the physiological principle of tubular secretion (12). Since then, a large experimental literature has described the tubular secretion of a myriad of organic acids that are anionic at physiological pH (for a list that exceeds 200 compounds, see Ref. 13). The phenomenon has been described in almost all nonmammalian vertebrates and in crustaceans (14). The site of highest secretion is variable along the proximal tubule, including the late portion (snakes, most mammals), the early and midportion (frogs, pigs), and any portion (flounder) (15). In the rabbit, secretion rates are ranked: S2 > S3 > S1 (16). In the rat, transport across the basolateral membrane (slice uptakes) suggests that the S3 (outer medulla) has the highest transport (17,18). Table 1 lists a few representative substrates (adapted from Ref. 19).

THE MOLECULARLY NEGLECTED RENAL ORGANIC ANION SECRETORY SYSTEM

There are at least five reasons why renal organic anion secretory transporters should be understood at a molecular level. (a) Hundreds of xenobiotics (i.e., environmental chemicals derived from plants,

Table 1 Substrates Transported by the Renal Organic Anion Secretory Pathway

Endogenous compounds	Drugs
Amino acids	Acetazolamide
Benzoate	Cephalothin
Bile salts	Chlorothiazide
Cyclic AMP	Cimetidine (cation)
Long-chain fatty acids	Ethacrynic acid
Hippurate	Fluoresceinate
Hydroxybenzoates	Furosemide
Hydroxyindoleacetic acid	Indomethacin
Oxalate	Penicillin G
Prostaglandins	Probenecid
Steroid hormones	Saccharin
Urate	Salicylate

animals, and industrial chemistry) are secreted by this system (20). Although some of these compounds existed in prehistory, scores of new xenobiotic organic anions are created yearly. (b) Many clinically important drugs are secreted by this system. For example, diuretics in general are secreted into the lumen of the proximal tubule and subseqently act on more distal nephron segments (acetazolamide, chlorothiazide, ethacrynic acid, furosemide). (c) Some endogenous hormones (steroids, prostaglandins), metabolic intermediates (oxalate), and end products (hippurate) are secreted by this system, but the details are poorly understood. (d) Recent evidence suggests that organic anion secretion may play a role in fluid accumulation within the cysts in renal cystic disease (21) (e) Because the system accepts structurally diverse substrates, it presents an intriguing transport problem. Is the organic anion transport "system" made up of multiple proteins with overlapping specificities? If so, can a given transporter be induced by exposure to a given substrate, as with clonal expansion in the immunoglobulin system? Or is the number of transporters much more limited? If so, how can so many diverse substrates be transported by so few proteins?

Despite the broad significance of understanding the organic anion secretory system, there is surprisingly little successful work on the molecular cloning or expression of these renal transporters.

PAH: THE PROTOTYPICALLY SECRETED SUBSTRATE

If hundreds of diverse substrate are secreted by this "system," how is one to approach it experimentally or conceptually? Fortunately, some order out of confusion has come from the many careful micropuncture studies of Ullrich et al (22–27). Their strategy has been to first measure uptake of isotopic organic anions from the peritubular capillary into the proximal tubule, and then determine whether other compounds compete for *p*-aminohippurate (PAH) uptake. They have proposed that the transporters can be functionally grouped into three classes: (a) an exchange system for sulfate and oxalate; (b) a cotransport system for Na^+ and dicarboxylates; and (c) an exchange system for hydrophobic anions and long-chain fatty acids.

In their hands, the last of these has been evaluated experimentally by assaying a test compound for its ability to compete with PAH uptake. Upon evaluating a broad range of aromatic and aliphatic compounds as potential inhibitors of PAH uptake, they concluded that a typical inhibitor (substrate candidate) for this system has (a) a negative or partial negative charge that is optimally 6 to 7 angstroms from a second negative charge and (b) a hydrophobic region, optimally 8 to 10 angstroms long (23,26).

From subsequent vesicle studies, it is now clear that PAH is taken up across the basolateral membrane of the proximal tubule in exchange for α-ketoglutarate (αKG), the outward gradient of which derives from Na-coupled uptake and the Krebs cycle (28–30). The apical exit step in PAH secretion is phenomenologically less well understood, but vesicle studies suggest that it probably involves PAH/OH exchange (31,32). Figure 1 summarizes these aspects of the PAH system.

These experiments give direction to investigators who plan to clone and express "the PAH system" at a molecular level. Indeed, although the transporter(s) has (have) not yet been cloned, PAH transport from kidney mRNA has been expressed in *Xenopus* oocytes by two groups (33,34). In each case, *Xenopus* oocytes were injected with size-fractionated mRNA, either from the renal cortex of rabbits (33) or from whole rat kidney (34). In expression using rabbit mRNA by Kwon et al., PAH uptake was 8–45-fold that of water-injected controls. The apparent K_m was ~300 μM, similar to that in intact kidneys. In this study, PAH transport was probenecid-insensitive. The sucrose fraction of greatest activity corresponded to mRNA of 0.7 to 1.3 kb (33). In *Xenopus* expression using mRNA derived from whole rat kidney by Wolff et al., PAH transport was found to be probenecid-sensitive (1 m*M*), as it is in the intact tubule. The mRNA fraction yielding the greatest degree of PAH uptake in this study corresponded to a size of 1.8 to 3.2 kb (34). The reason(s) for the discrepancies in size and inhibitor sensitivity between the two studies are not known.

Despite Ullrich's emphasis on PAH as a prototypical anion, it is almost certainly an over-simplification to equate an understanding of PAH uptake across the basolateral membrane with an understanding of the whole of renal organic anion secretion. Some compounds fail to interact with any of Ullrich's three basolateral "systems" yet are clearly secreted across the tubule (e.g., 4-aminobenzoate) (13,26). This indicates that other transporters must exist outside of this framework. A recent review on renal organic anion transport states that "both the number of systems and their relative contributions to the handling of a given organic anion remain areas of uncertainty" (29).

GLYCOLYSIS AND RENAL TUBULE LACTATE TRANSPORT

In several renal epithelia, Na,K-ATPase is tightly coupled to glycolysis (35–40). There is also evidence suggesting coupling of H^+ATPases to glycolysis in the S3 proximal tubule (41) and in the collecting duct of the outer medulla (outer stripe) (42). In fact, the freshly isolated collecting duct is one of the few mammalian cell types to produce lactate at high rates under aerobic conditions (40,43,44). Single dissected rat and mouse cortical collecting ducts (CCDs) and outer medullary collecting ducts (OMCDs) have very high glycolytic capacities (44,45). In contrast, in the proximal tubule, glycolysis is low and gluconeogenesis high (46). Indeed, histochemical and immunocytochemical data indicate that enzymes of glycolysis (e.g., hexokinase, phosphofructokinase, and pyruvate kinase) are distributed preferentially in the collecting duct (46–50). In the rabbit, these enzymes increase in parallel along the whole distal nephron (51).

Intercalated cells of the α subtype (52) appear to be particularly glycolytic. Functional studies reveal that glycolysis maintains normal cellular ATP levels at least as well as oxidative phosphory-

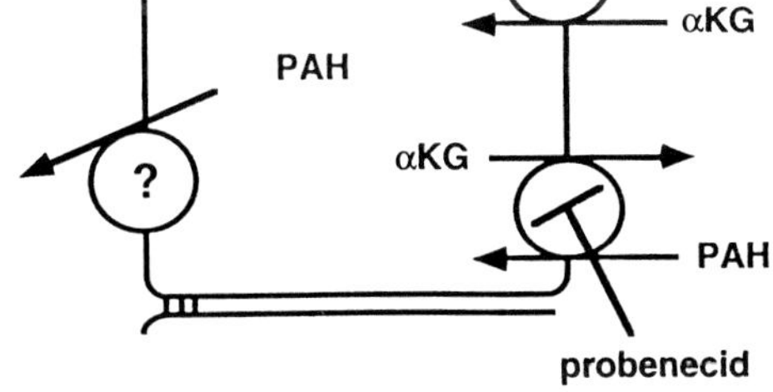

Figure 1 Cellular mechanism of tubular secretion of PAH by the proximal tubule anion secretory pathway. Na-dependent cotransport of α-ketoglutarate raises its concentration above equilibrium within the cell. The resulting outwardly directed gradient drives PAH entry across the basolateral membrane via probenecid-inhibitable exchange. The mechanism of apical exit of PAH is unclear but probably occurs by facilitated diffusion.

lation in rabbit and mouse OMCDi tubules (42,45), and immunocytochemical staining for the glycolytic enzyme hexokinase I in the rat outer medullary collecting duct is strongest in mitochondria-rich (α) intercalated cells (48). Glyceraldehyde phosphate dehydrogenase (GAPDH) also colocalizes with *AE1* in the basolateral membrane of medullary α intercalated cells (53).

Glycolysis of one glucose molecule generates two lactate anions and two ATPs (54). Given that the cell ATP/ADP ratio usually remains constant, the ATPs will be hydrolyzed to ADP and P_i, accompanied by the release of two H^+ (55). The net effect of glycolysis is thus the generation of two lactic acids per glucose molecule metabolized. There is thus a need for facilitating lactate efflux from renal epithelial cells, presumably in proportion to the rate of lactate generation by each segment.

Three observations suggest that lactate generated in collecting duct cells effluxes down a concentration gradient across the basolateral membrane into the plasma: (a) Urine lactate concentrations are low (56,57); (b) measurements of renal tissue (lactate) suggest that cell-to-plasma concentration gradients are ~3:1 in the cortex and ~8:1 in the inner medulla (56–58); (c) lactate effluxes preferentially across the basal membrane of the toad (59,60) and turtle bladder (61,62); of mouse (63), rabbit (64), and canine (MDCK) collecting duct cell lines (39,65); and of freshly isolated rabbit cortical collecting duct cells grown in primary culture (66).

Lactate/H^+ cotransporters have been functionally described at the basolateral membrane of the proximal tubule (67,68) and the medullary thick ascending limb (69). When the whole kidney is isolated and perfused, metabolic labeling studies reveal that lactate production and consumption (gluconeogenesis) are occurring simultaneously. This means that lactate produced by "distal nephron" segments is being taken up by the proximal tubule for gluconeogenesis, and the resulting glucose is being utilized by "distal" segments for glycolysis (an "intrarenal Cori cycle") (70).

Taken together, all of these functional studies indicate that a basolateral lactate/H^+ cotransporter is probably expressed in many different tubule cell types. The relationship of lactate generation to efflux in a generic renal tubule cell is shown in Fig. 2. As discussed below, one version of a lactate/H^+ cotransporter (probably the first member of a family) now appears to have been cloned.

"MONOCARBOXYLATE TRANSPORTER-1"

The first monocarboxylate transporter (*MCT1*) has just been recognized as such by Garcia et al. in the laboratory of Brown and Goldstein (71). The story of the cloning of the lactate/pyruvate transporter illustrates both the serendipity and persistence necessary to clone organic anion transporters. Studies were under way to understand the molecular mechanisms of mevalonate transport. A mevalonate transporter (*MEV*) was expression-cloned from a mutant Chinese hamster ovary (CHO) cell line. The *MEV* differed from the wild-type transporter (*Mev*-wt) by a single base-pair substitution (71). This produced a single amino acid change that resulted in a large gain of function, i.e. mevalonate

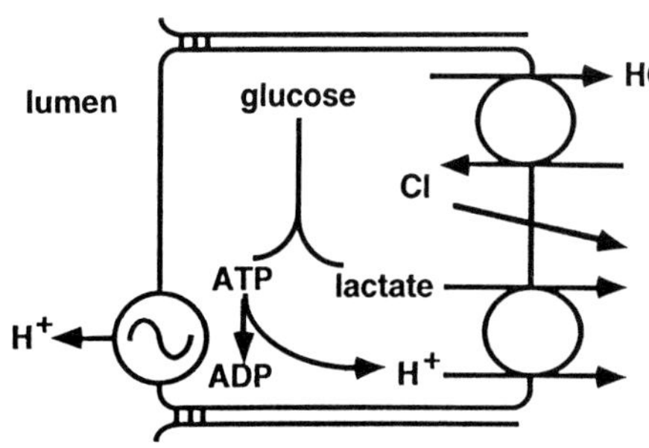

Figure 2 Glycolysis in a collecting duct cell of the alpha subtype. The ATP generated by glycolysis is utilized for H^+ secretion by an apical H^+ ATPase. The resulting bicarbonate anion crosses the basolateral membrane via the *AE1* anion exchanger, with recycling of chloride across the basolateral membrane. The H^+ released by ATP hydrolysis, and the lactate anion generated from glycolysis, exit across the basolateral membrane via a lactate/H^+ cotransporter.

transport. Since the *MEV*-wt transporter did not transport mevalonate at significant rates yet was a classic 12-membrane-domain-spanning protein (i.e., a transporter), function of *Mev*-wt was pursued.

The *Mev*-wt transporter was found to catalyze ^{14}C-pyruvate transport when stably expressed (71). As is true for monocarboxylate transporters in general (72), ^{14}C-pyruvate transport was inhibited by α-cyanocinnamates and by phloretin, and to a lesser extent by the disulfonic stilbene DIDS. The calculated K_m for pyruvate was 0.9 m*M*. Imposition of pH gradients caused changes in pyruvate transport by *MCT1* consistent with either pyruvate/H^+ cotransport or pyruvate/OH exchange. As predicted by these results, collapse of the pH gradient across the cell membrane inhibited pyruvate transport. Preloading of transfected cells with either pyruvate or lactate resulted in transstimulation of transport, i.e., increased uptake of labeled pyruvate. An anti-*MCT1* antibody labeled basolateral membranes of a number of epithelial cells, including a "subset of proximal and distal convoluted tubule cells" as well as a number of other tissues (71).

It will be of interest to see whether the renal expression of *MCT1* can account for all known lactate/H^+ cotransport along the nephron, since the latter has been phenomenologically described in several renal tubule epithelia, including the apical membrane of the proximal tubule (28).

Studies from the author's laboratory have also been directed at lactate/H^+ transport. Starting with antibodies directed against the gel-purified fraction of rabbit erythrocyte membranes containing the rabbit *MCT* homologue, we cloned and expressed an immunoglobulin-like integral membrane protein ("*L6*") that appears to be closely associated with *MCT1*. Under a variety of conditions, *L6* copurifies with rabbit *MCT1* and is immunologically localized in areas that also appear to be sites of *MCT1* expression (73,74). Substantial further work will be required to determine whether *L6* and *MCT1* are truly colocalized, whether they are specifically associated with each other, and whether such an association has any functional consequences.

THE HEPATIC APPROACH TO RENAL ORGANIC ANION TRANSPORT: ORGANIC ANION TRANSPORTING POLYPEPTIDE ("OATP")

The liver and kidney share common probenecid-sensitive organic anion transport of sulfonamides (75), beta-lactam antibiotics (e.g. penicillin) (76), phenol red derivatives (77), steroidal hormones (78), and sulfonic acid dyes (79). Both organs also share transport of bromosulfophthalein (BSP), a typical organic anion dye that circulates tightly bound to albumin and thus is secreted mostly by the liver (in contrast, PAH, which is not tightly bound, is secreted predominantly by the kidney). Hepatic BSP uptake is the basis of the time-honored BSP test of liver function in humans. In liver disease, plasma BSP levels are elevated after injection. During these high plasma levels, urinary BSP excretion increases dramatically and is probenecid-inhibitable (80), indicating that BSP undergoes renal tubular secretion by an organic anion secretory pathway. In the rabbit, BSP is comparable to probenecid as an inhibitor of PAH transport (81).

To understand hepatic BSP transport further, Wolkoff et al. first functionally characterized BSP uptake in rat hepatocytes (82). Subsequently, Jacquemin et al. used this information in the *Xenopus* oocyte expression system to clone the transporter (83). The transporter is termed "organic anion transport polypeptide" or OATP. Oocyte studies show that OATP mediates Na-independent uptake of BSP, taurocholate, and cholate (83).

The author's laboratory has further studied OATP expression in the kidney. In unpublished studies, we find that OATP mRNA is strongly expressed in rat kidney outer medulla and, to a lesser degree, in the cortex. Moreover, several renal mRNA bands hybridize to the OATP probe, depending on the Northern blot stringency, indicating that there are several forms of OATP-related messages expressed in rat kidney. Further Northern blots have indicated that OATP is under tight control by testosterone but not estrogen or glucocorticoids. Immunocytochemical studies using an antibody directed at the C terminus of OATP show that this protein is localized to the apical membrane of the S3 proximal tubule. Several organic anions appear to be good substrates for OATP when it is expressed in heterologous systems. Taken together, these studies suggest that OATP represents at least one of several possible apical exit steps for organic anions after they are brought into the proximal tubule cell across the basolateral membrane by the "PAH system."

THE MUTANT SOUTHDOWN SHEEP

Defects in the hepatic and renal transport of organic anions have been described in a naturally occurring autosomal recessive mutation. Southdown lambs develop photosensitivity upon eating grass at weaning, due to the inability of the liver to take up and clear an alkaloid anion (phylloerythrin) derived from chlorophyll. Renal clearances of PAH, bilirubin, BSP, rose bengal, and indocyanine green are substantially reduced, and plasma levels of coproporphyrin and cholic acid are elevated (84–87).

Kidney failure in Southdown sheep occurs at 2 to 5 years of age (88). In younger animals, the major histological finding is proximal tubule accumulation of bilirubin globules and loss of proximal tubule brush borders. In later stages, multifocal fibrosis develops around various nephron segments in the medullary rays (89–92). An attractive hypothesis is that the Southdown mutation results in defective transport from the proximal tubule cell of toxic bile salts or conjugated organic anions. As organic anion transporters are cloned, the Southdown sheep should be explored as a model system.

URATE TRANSPORTER(S)

Urate is an organic anion that has a complex pattern of reabsorption and secretion along the length of the proximal tubule (19). Recently, Knorr et al. have generated antibodies against pig uricase and have shown strong labeling at the brush border of the rat proximal tubule brush border (93). The same antibodies were able to immunodeplete electrogenic urate transport from isolated rat renal brush border membrane vesicles. Therefore, it appears that the electrogenic urate transporter shares homology, or is identical with, uricase. These antibody reagents should now allow the successful cloning of cDNA(s) for at least one of the components of renal urate transport.

PROXIMAL TUBULE FORMATE AND OXALATE TRANSPORTERS

Karniski and Aronson first reported the provocative finding of a formate-Cl exchange process in rabbit proximal tubule brush border membrane vesicles (94). These investigators offered a hypothesis whereby formate anion and protonated formic acid undergo cycling. In this scheme, formate anion would be secreted into the urine via a formate-Cl exchanger, the formate would be protonated in the more acid lumen, and the formic acid (protonated) would reenter the cell via nonionic diffusion (94). Subsequent experiments were performed in which the rate of cell swelling was determined after adding formate to the perfusate of isolated perfused rabbit proximal tubules. The results were consistent with the existence of an apical formate-Cl exchanger (95).

In the rat, in situ micropuncture and microperfusion experiments in the accessible proximal tubule confirmed that addition of physiological formate concentrations to the luminal perfusate resulted in a substantial increase in the reabsorptive rate of fluid from a Cl-rich, HCO_3-poor perfusate (96). Similar results were later reported for the early distal tubule, i.e., that luminal formate lead to an increase in Cl reabsorption via a thiazide-insensitive mechanism, presumably formate-Cl exchange (97).

Although the formate-Cl exchanger has not yet been cloned, substantial progress has been made toward this goal. Soleimani and coworkers have recently used stilbene affinity chromatography to partially purify a 162-kDa protein from rabbit kidney cortex. Reconstitution of the proteins eluted from the affinity column and incorporation into liposomes showed that this protein catalyzes Cl-Cl anion exchange (and presumably Cl-formate exchange) (98). Further experiments by the same laboratory provided stronger evidence, in that the agent phenylglyoxal blocked proximal tubule brush border Cl-Cl exchange, and labeled phenylglyoxal also bound in a specific fashion to the same 160-kDa protein as above (99). Further purification of this 160-kDa protein and library or PCR screening using degenerate oligonucleotide probes should permit cloning of the cDNA for this important transporter as well.

RENAL BILE SALT TRANSPORTERS

Bile salts are organic anions at physiological pH. The major bile acids, cholic acid and chenodeoxycholic acid, are conjugated in the liver with either glycine or taurine to produce the respective bile salts (100). Bile acid levels in the peripheral circulation are usually $\leq 10\ \mu M$. Nonetheless, the daily filtered load of 0.5 g dictates that sulfated and nonsulfated bile salts must be reabsorbed to avoid depletion of the bile salt pool. Proximal reabsorption of bile acids is Na-coupled and >95% efficient (101–103). Molecularly, the mechanism of the apical entry step for bile acids into the proximal tubule cell is not yet completely clear. Meier et al. recently expression-cloned the rat liver Na-dependent bile acid transporter (104). Northern blot analysis revealed expression of a Na-dependent bile acid transporter transcript in the rat kidney. It remains to be determined whether this represents the same transporter as expressed in the liver and whether the transporter is localized at the apical membrane of the proximal tubule.

As with most Na-coupled proximal tubule reabsorptive processes, Na-coupled apical entry probably raises intracellular bile salt concentrations inside the proximal tubule cell. Bile salts do not readily cross cell membranes. As detergents, bile acids at high concentrations are clearly toxic to renal tubules (105). Therefore, the cell presumably has mechanisms for basolateral bile salt efflux, although these have not been identified at a molecular level.

SUMMARY AND CONCLUSIONS

It is clear that some progress has been made toward a molecular understanding of renal organic anion transporters. As exemplified by Na/H exchangers, Cl-HCO_3 exchangers, facilitated glucose transporters, and chloride channels, cloning the first member of a gene family is the initial (and most arduous) step in finding related transporters. Since the number of different kinds of organic anions transported by kidney tubules is far greater than that of inorganic anions and since some progress has now been made in cloning, we can expect that the next few years will witness a similar explosion in the molecular identification and study of renal organic anion transporters.

REFERENCES

1. Kopito RR, Lodish HF. Primary structure and transmembrane orientation of the murine anion exchange protein. Nature (London) 1985; 316:234–238.
2. Schuster VL, Bonsib SM, Jennings ML. Two types of collecting duct mitochondria-rich (intercalated cells): Lectin and band 3 cytochemistry. Am J Physiol (Cell Physiol) 1986; 251:C347–C355.
3. Kudrycki KE, Shull GE. Primary structure of the rat kidney band 3 anion exchange protein deduced from a cDNA. J Biol Chem 1989; 264:8185–8192.
4. Brosius FC III, Alper SL, Garcia AM, Lodish HF. The major kidney band 3 gene transcript predicts an amino-truncated band 3 polypeptide. J Biol Chem 1989; 264:7784–7787.
5. Kudrycki KE, Shull GE. Rat kidney band 3 Cl^-/HCO_3^- exchanger mRNA is transcribed from an alternative promoter. Am J Physiol (Renal Fluid Electrolyte Physiol) 1993; 264:F540–F547.
6. Alper SL, Kopito R, Lodish HF. A molecular biological approach to the study of anion transport. Kidney Int 1987; 32(suppl 23):S117–S128.
7. Uchida S, Sasaki S, Furukawa T, et al. Molecular cloning of a chloride channel that is regulated by dehydration and expressed predominantly in kidney medulla. J Biol Chem 1993; 268:3821–3824.
8. Markovich D, Forgo J, Stange G, et al. Expression cloning of rat renal Na^+/SO_4^{2-} cotransport. Proc Natl Acad Sci USA 1993; 90:8073–8077.
9. Magagnin S, Werner A, Markovich D, et al. Expression cloning of human and rat renal cortex Na/Pi cotransport. Proc Natl Acad Sci (USA) 1993; 90:5979–5983.
10. Werner A, Moore ML, Mantei N, et al. Cloning and expression of cDNA for a Na/Pi cotransport system of kidney cortex. Proc Natl Acad Sci USA 1991; 88:9608–9612.
11. Heidenhain R. Versuche über den Vorgang der Harnabsonderung. Pflugers Arch 1874; 9:1–27.
12. Marshall EK Jr, Grafflin AL. The structure and function of the kidney of *Lophius piscatorius*. Bull Johns Hopkins Hosp 1928; 43:205–235.
13. Møller JV, Sheikh I. Renal organic anion transport system: Pharmacological, physiological, and biochemical aspects. Pharmacol Rev 1983; 34:315–358.
14. Pritchard JB, Miller DS. Comparative insights into the mechanisms of renal organic anion and cation secretion. Am J Physiol (Reg Physiol) 1991; 261:R1329–R1340.
15. Dantzler WH. Comparative aspects of renal function. In: Seldin DW, Giebisch G, eds. The Kidney: Physiology and Pathophysiology. New York: Raven Press, 1992:885–942.
16. Shimomura A, Chonko AM, Grantham JJ. Basis for heterogeneity of para-aminohippurate secretion in rabbit proximal tubules. Am J Physiol (Renal Fluid Electrolyte Physiol) 1981; 240:F430–F436.

17. Sheikh MI, Møller JW. Renal handling of phenol red. IV. Tubular localization in rabbit and rat kidney in vivo. Am J Physiol (Renal Fluid Electrolyte Physiol) 1980; 238:F159–F165.
18. Sottiurai V, Longley JB. Quantitation of functional differences between the two segments of the rat proximal tubule in the handling of chlorphenol red and hippuran ^{131}I. Q J Exp Physiol 1970; 55:193–201.
19. Grantham JJ, Chonko AM. Renal handling of organic anions and cations: Excretion of uric acid. In: Brenner BM, Rector FC, eds. The Kidney. Philadelphia, PA: Saunders, 1991:483–509.
20. Kluwe WM, Hook JB. Effects of environmental chemicals on kidney metabolism and function. Kidney Int 1980; 18:648–655.
21. Sliman GA, Sweeney WE, Avner ED. Organic anion uptake and chloride secretion mediate tubular cyst formation in murine metanephric organ culture. J Am Soc Nephrol 1993; 4:824.
22. Ullrich KJ, Rumrich G, Fritzsch G, Klöss S. Contralateral para-aminohippurate (PAH) transport in the proximal tubule of the rat kidney: II. Specificity: aliphatic dicarboxylic acids. Pflugers Arch 1987; 408:38–45.
23. Fritzsch G, Rumrich G, Ullrich KJ. Anion transport through the contralateral cell membrane of renal proximal tubule. The influence of hydrophobicity and molecular charge distribution on the inhibitory activity of organic anions. Biochim Biophys Acta 1989; 978:249–256.
24. Ullrich KJ, Rummel W, Papavassiliou F, Hierholzer K. Contralateral *p*-aminohippurate transport in the proximal tubule of the rat kidney: VIII. Transport of corticosteroids. Pflugers Arch 1991; 418:371–382.
25. Ammer U, Natochin Y, Ullrich KJ. Tissue concentration and urinary excretion pattern of sulfofluorescein by the rat kidney. J Am Soc Nephrol 1992; 3:1474–1487.
26. Ullrich KJ, Rumrich G. Contraluminal transport systems in the proximal renal tubule involved in secretion of organic anions. Am J Physiol (Renal Fluid Electrolyte Physiol) 1988; 254:F453–F462.
27. Ullrich KJ, Rumrich G. Renal contraluminal transport systems for organic anions (paraaminohippurate, PAH) and organic cations (N1-methyl-nicotinamide, NMeN) do not see the degree of substrate ionization. Pflugers Arch 1992; 421:286–288.
28. Aronson PS. The renal proximal tubule: A model for diversity of anion exchangers and stilbene-sensitive anion transporters. Annu Rev Physiol 1989; 51:419–441.
29. Pritchard JB, Miller DS. Proximal tubular transport of organic anions and cations. In: Seldin DW, Giebisch G, eds. The Kidney: Physiology and Pathophysiology. New York: Raven Press, 1992:2921–2945.
30. Sullivan LP, Grantham JJ. Specificity of basolateral organic anion exchanger in proximal tubule for cellular and extracellular solutes. J Am Soc Nephrol 1992; 2:1192–1200.
31. Steffens TG, Holohan PD, Ross CR. Operational modes of the organic anion exchanger in canine renal brush-border membrane vesicles. Am J Physiol (Renal Fluid Electrolyte Physiol) 1989; 256:F596–F609.
32. Blomstedt JW, Aronson PS. pH gradient-stimulated transport of urate and *p*-aminohippurate in dog renal microvillus membrane vesicles. J Clin Invest 1993; 65:931–934.
33. Kwon O, Kwon HM, Hong SK, Goldinger JM. Size-selected mRNA induces expression of *p*-aminohippurate transport in Xenopus oocytes. Proc Soc Exp Biol Med 1989; 192:205–208.
34. Wolff NA, Philpot RM, Miller DS, Pritchard JB. Functional expression of renal organic anion transport in *Xenopus laevis* oocytes. Mol Cell Biochem 1992; 114:35–41.
35. Balaban R, Bader JP. Studies on the relationship between glycolysis and ($Na^+ + K^+$)-ATPase in cultured cells. Biochim Biophys Acta 1984; 804:419–426.
36. Lynch RM, Balaban RS. Coupling of aerobic glycolysis and Na^+-K^+-ATPase in renal cell line MDCK. Am J Physiol (Cell Physiol) 1987; 253:C269–C276.
37. Kone BC, Kikeri D, Zeidel ML, Gullans SR. Cellular pathways of potassium transport in renal inner medullary collecting duct. Am J Physiol (Cell Physiol) 1989; 256:C823–C830.
38. Lynch RM, Balaban RS. Energy metabolism of renal cell lines, A6 and MDCK: Regulation by Na-K-ATPase. Am J Physiol (Cell Physiol) 1987; 252:C225–C231.
39. Kurtz A, Pfeilschifter J, Malmstrom K, Wodson RD, et al. Mechanism of NaCl transport-stimulated prostaglandin formulation in MDCK cells. Am J Physiol (Cell Physiol) 1987; 252:C307–C314.
40. Grupp C, Pavenstadt-Grupp I, Grunewald RW, et al. A Na-K-Cl cotransporter in isolated rat papillary collecting duct cells. Kidney Int 1989; 36:201–209.
41. Kurtz I. Apical Na^+/H^+ antiporter and glycolysis-dependent H^+-ATPase regulate intracellular pH in the rabbit S_3 proximal tubule. J Clin Invest 1987; 80:928–935.
42. Zeidel ML, Silva P, Seifter JL. Intracellular pH regulation and proton transport by rabbit renal medullary collecting duct cells: Role of plasma membrane proton adenosine triphosphatase. J Clin Invest 1986; 77:113–120.
43. Krebs HA. The Pasteur effect and the relations between respiration and fermentation. Essays Biochem 1972; 8:1–34.
44. Bagnascao S, Good D, Balaban R, Burg M. Lactate production in isolated segments of the rat nephron. Am J Physiol (Renal Fluid Electrolyte Physiol) 1985; 248:F522–F526.
45. Uchida S, Endou H. Substrate specificity to maintain cellular ATP along the mouse nephron. Am J Physiol (Renal Fluid Electrolyte Physiol) 1988; 255:F977–F983.

46. Wirthensohn G, Guder WG. Renal substrate metabolism. Physiol Rev 1986; 66:469–497.
47. Gstraunthaler G, Pfaller W, Kotano P. Biochemical characterization of renal epithelial cell cultures (LLC-PK$_1$ and MDCK). Am J Physiol (Cell Physiol) 1985; 248:F536–F544.
48. Lawrence GM, Trayer IP. Histochemical and immunohistochemical localization of hexokinase isoenzymes in rat kidney. Histochem J 1984; 16:697–708.
49. Lawrence GM, Jepson MA, Trayer IP, Walker DG. The compartmentation of glycolytic and gluconeogenic enzymes in rat kidney and liver and its significance to renal and hepatic metabolism. Histochem J 1986; 18:43–53.
50. Schmid H, Mall A, Scholz M, Schmidt U. Unchanged glycolytic capacity in rat kidney under conditions of stimulated gluconeogenesis: Determination of phosphofructokinase and pyruvate kinase in microdissected nephron segments of fasted and acidotic animals. Hoppe-Seylers Z Physiol Chem 1980; 361:819–827.
51. Guder WG, Ross BD. Enzyme distribution along the nephron. Kidney Int 1984; 26:101–111.
52. Schuster VL. Function and regulation of collecting duct intercalated cells. Annu Rev Physiol 1993; 55:267–288.
53. Ercolani L, Brown D, Stuart-Tilley A, Alper SL. Colocalization of GAPDH and band 3 (AE1) proteins in rat erythrocytes and kidney intercalated cell membranes. Am J Physiol (Renal Fluid Electrolyte Physiol) 1992; 262:F892–F896.
54. Stryer L. Biochemistry. San Francisco, CA: Freeman, 1981:1–949.
55. Madias NE. Lactic acidosis. Kidney Int 1986; 29:752–774.
56. Dell RB, Winters RW. Lactate gradients in the kidney of the dog. Am J Physiol 1967; 213:301–307.
57. Scaglione PR, Dell RB, Winters RW. Lactate concentration in the medulla of rat kidney. Am J Physiol 1965; 209:1193–1198.
58. Capraro V, Valzelli G, DeAgostini C. Lactic acid concentration in the kidney of the golden hamster, *Mesocricetus auratus,* in different conditions of diuresis. Nature (London) 1961; 190:178–179.
59. Leaf A, Page LB, Anderson J. Respiration and active sodium transport of isolated toad bladder. J Biol Chem 1959; 234:1625–1629.
60. Leaf A. The mechanism of the asymmetrical distribution of endogenous lactate about the isolated toad bladder. J Cell Comp Physiol 1959; 54:103–108.
61. Steinmetz PR, Husted RF, Mueller A, Beauwens R. Coupling between H^+ transport and anaerobic glycolysis in turtle bladder: Effects of inhibitors of H^+ ATPase. J Membr Biol 1981; 59:27–34.
62. Arruda JAL, Sabatini S, Westenfelder C. Serosal Na/Ca exchange and H^+ and Na^+ transport by the turtle and toad bladders. J Membr Biol 1982; 70:135–146.
63. Stoos BA, Náray-Fejes-Tóth A, Carretero OA, et al. Characterization of a mouse cortical collecting duct cell line. Kidney Int 1991; 39:1168–1175.
64. Bello-Reuss E, Cabell-Kluch L. Membrane voltages and polarity of acid and lactate secretion by a peanut-lectin positive cell line (RCCT-28A). Kidney Int 1990; 37:533.
65. Rosenberg SO, Fadil T, Schuster VL. A basolateral lactate/H^+ co-transporter in Madin-Darby canine kidney (MDCK) cells. Biochem J 1993; 289:263–268.
66. Fejes-Tóth G, Náray-Fejes-Tóth A. Differentiated transport functions in primary cultures of rabbit collecting ducts. Am J Physiol (Renal Fluid Electrolyte Physiol) 1987; 253:F1302–F1307.
67. Siebens AW, Boron WF. Effect of electroneutral luminal and basolateral lactate transport on intracellular pH in salamander proximal tubules. J Gen Physiol 1987; 90:799–831.
68. Murer H, Barac-Nieto M, Ullrich KJ, Kinne R. Renal transport of lactate. In: Greger R, Lang F, Silbernagl S, eds. Renal Transport of Organic Substances. New York: Springer-Verlag, 1981:211–223.
69. Vinay P, Sénécal J, Noël J, et al. Basolateral transport of lactate in dog thick ascending limbs. Am J Physiol (Renal Fluid Electrolyte Physiol) 1990; 258:F1042–F1053.
70. Bartlett S, Espinal J, Janssens P, Ross BD. The influence of renal function on lactate and glucose metabolism. Biochem J 1984; 219:73–78.
71. Garcia CK, Goldstein JL, Pathak RK, et al. Molecular characterization of a membrane transporter for lactate, pyruvate, and other monocarboxylates: Implications for the Cori cycle. Cell 1994; 76:865–873.
72. Poole RC, Halestrap AP. Transport of lactate and other monocarboxylates across mammalian plasma membranes. Am J Physiol (Cell Physiol) 1993; 264:C761–C782.
73. Schuster VL, Bao Y, Fritz PH, Jennings ML. Immunological identification of a basolateral lactate-H^+ co-transporter in rabbit kidney. J Am Soc Nephrol 1991; 2:711.
74. Lu R, Kanai N, Bao Y, et al. cDNA cloning, expression, and regulation of an immunoglobulin-like basolateral membrane protein expressed in rabbit kidney tubules. J Am Soc Nephrol 1993; 4:617.
75. Despopoulos A, Sonnenberg H. Congruence of excretory functions of liver and kidney: Sulfonamides. Am J Physiol 1967; 212:1117–1122.
76. Tsuji A, Terasaki T, Tamai I, Takeda K. In vivo evidence for carrier-mediated uptake of beta-lactam antibiotics through organic anion transport systems in rat kidney and liver. J Pharmacol Exp Ther 1990; 253:315–320.

77. Kim JH, Hong SK. Urinary and biliary excretions of various phenol red derivatives in the anesthetized dog. Am J Physiol 1962; 202:174–178.
78. Despopoulos A. Excretory physiology of steroidal hormones in liver. J Pharmacol Exp Ther 1970; 173:43–47.
79. Despopoulos A. Congruence of renal and hepatic excretory functions: Sulfonic acid dyes. Am J Physiol 1971; 220:1755–1758.
80. Blondheim SH. Effect of probenecid on excretion of bromosulfophthalein. J Appl Physiol 1955; 7:529–532.
81. Park YS, Yoo HS, Hong SK. Kinetic studies on transport of organic acids in rabbit kidney slices. Am J Physiol 1971; 220:95–99.
82. Min AD, Johansen KL, Campbell CG, Wolkoff AW. Role of chloride and intracellular pH on the activity of the rat hepatocyte organic anion transporter. J Clin Invst 1991; 87:1496–1502.
83. Jacquemin E, Hagenbuch B, Stieger B, et al. Expression cloning of a rat liver Na^+-independent organic anion transporter. Proc Natl Acad Sci USA 1994; 91:133–137.
84. Engelking LR, Gronwall R. Bile acid clearance in sheep with hereditary hyperbilirubinemia. Am J Vet Res 1979; 40:1277–1280.
85. Dhumeaux D, Berthelot P. Chronic hyperbilirubinemia associated with hepatic uptake and storage impairment: A new syndrome resembling that of the mutant Southdown sheep. Gastroenterology 1975; 69:988–993.
86. Gronwall R, Sulfobromophthalein sodium excretion and hepatic storage in Corriedale and Southdown sheep with inherited hepatic dysfunction. Am J Vet Res 1970; 31:2131–2133.
87. Cornelius CE, Gronwall RR. Congenital photosensitivity and hyperbilirubinemia in Southdown sheep in the United States. Am J Vet Res 1968; 29:291–295.
88. Jamieson ND, Swan JB. Photosensitive diseases in New Zealand: VI. Some liver function tests on congenitally photosensitive Southdown, normal Southdown, and normal Romney sheep. NZ J Sci Technol 1952; 34:354–359.
89. McGavin MD, Gronwall RR, Cornelius CE, Mia AS. Renal radial fibrosis in mutant Southdown sheep with congenital hyperbilirubinemia. Am J Pathol 1972; 67:601–607.
90. McGavin MD, Cornelius CE, Gronwall RR. Lesions in Southdown sheep with hereditary hyperbilirubinemia. Vet Pathol 1972; 9:142–151.
91. Cuppage FE, Shimamura T, McGavin MD. Nephron obstruction in mutant Southdown sheep. Vet Pathol 179; 16:483–485.
92. Filippich LJ, English PB, Seawright AA. Comparison of renal function in a congenital hyperbilirubinaemic Southdown sheep and normal sheep. Res Vet Sci 1977; 23:204–212.
93. Knorr BA, Lipkowitz MS, Potter BJ, et al. Isolation and immunolocalization of a rat renal cortical membrane urate transporter. J Biol Chem 1994; 269:6759–6764.
94. Karniski LP, Aronson PS. Anion exchange pathways for Cl transport in rabbit renal microvillus membranes. Am J Physiol (Renal Fluid Electrolyte Physiol) 1987; 253:F513–F521.
95. Schild L, Aronson PS, Giebisch G. Effects of apical membrane Cl(-)-formate exchange on cell volume in rabbit proximal tubule. Am J Physiol 1990; 258:F530–F536.
96. Wang T, Giebisch G, Aronson PS. Effects of formate and oxalate on volume absorption in rat proximal tubule. Am J Physiol 1992; 263:F37–F42.
97. Wang T, Agulian SK, Giebisch G, Aronson PS. Effects of formate and oxalate on chloride absorption in rat distal tubule. Am J Physiol 1993; 264:F730–F736.
98. Soleimani M, Bizal GL, Anderson CC. A protein with anion exchange properties found in the kidney proximal tubule. Kidney Int 1993; 44:565–573.
99. Soleimani M, Hattabaugh YJ, Bizal GL. Identification and covalent modification of a renal brush-border anion exchanger. Biochim Biophys Acta 1993; 1149:127–134.
100. Goad LF. Cholesterol synthesis and metabolism. In: Makin HLJ, ed. Biochemistry of Steroid Hormones. St. Louis, MO: Blackwell Scientific Publications, 1984:20–70.
101. Barnes S, Gollan JL, Billings BH. The role of tubular reabsorption in the renal excretion of bile acids. Biochem J 1977; 166:65–73.
102. Wilson FA, Burckhardt G, Murer H, et al. Sodium-coupled taurocholate transport in the proximal convolution of the rat kidney in vivo and in vitro. J Clin Invest 1981; 67:1141–1150.
103. Weiner IM, Glasser JE, Lack L. Renal excretion of bile acids: Taurocholic, glycocholic, and cholic acids. Am J Physiol 1993; 207:964–970.
104. Hagenbuch B, Stieger B, Foguet M, et al. Functional expression cloning and characterization of the hepatocyte Na^+/bile acid cotransport system. Proc Natl Acad Sci USA 1991; 88:10629–10633.
105. Aoyagi T, Lowenstein L. The effect of bile acids and renal ischemia on renal function. J Lab Clin Med 1968; 71:686–694.

24
Molecular Biology of Renal Sodium-Conducting Ion Channels

David E. McCoy and Bruce A. Stanton
Dartmouth Medical School, Hanover, New Hampshire

INTRODUCTION

Two major classes of sodium (Na^+)-conducting ion channels have been identified in renal epithelial cell plasma membranes by the patch-clamp technique. Those classes are distinguished primarily by their unitary conductance, ionic selectivity, and sensitivity to amiloride. One class, composed of amiloride-sensitive, Na^+-selective channels, mediates transepithelial sodium absorption across the collecting duct (Table 1) through low-conductance (~4 pS) highly sodium-selective channels and higher conductance (~8 pS) relatively poorly Na^+-selective channels. The other class, composed of nonselective cation channels, can be subdivided into two groups (Table 2): (a) amiloride-insensitive, nonselective cation channels, which are expressed in a variety of nephron segments and may subserve a number of cellular functions, including cell volume regulation, initiation of cell proliferation, and receptor-mediated calcium entry, and (b) amiloride-sensitive, nonselective cation channels, which are inhibited by cGMP and mediate transepithelial sodium reabsorption across the inner medullary collecting duct (IMCD). The diversity of Na^+-conducting ion channels in the kidney may result from multiple genes, alternative splicing of one or more genes, diverse posttranslational events modifying channel properties, and/or by different combinations of heterogeneous channel-forming proteins or the differential expression of regulatory protein subunits (see below).

Recently, several excellent and comprehensive reviews have described the biophysical and biochemical properties of renal Na^+-conducting ion channels (1–7). Accordingly, those properties are reviewed here only briefly. The aim of this chapter is to review the literature on the molecular biology of *renal Na^+-conducting ion channels*. The reader is also referred to several recent articles that review the molecular biology of epithelial sodium channels and cGMP-gated, nonselective cation channels (4,5,8,9).

BIOPHYSICAL AND BIOCHEMICAL PROPERTIES OF NA^+-CONDUCTING ION CHANNELS IN THE KIDNEY

Amiloride-Sensitive, Na^+-Selective Channels

Amiloride-sensitive, Na^+-selective channels are expressed predominantly in the collecting duct and A6 cells (Table 1), where they mediate sodium uptake across the apical cell membrane. Highly Na^+-selective ($P_{Na+}:P_{K+} > 20:1$), low-conductance (~4–5 pS) channels are thought to be responsible for most, if not all, sodium absorption across the cortical collecting duct (CCD) and A6 cells, especially when sodium absorption is stimulated by aldosterone (2,3,10). This channel has very long opening and closing kinetics, and the channel-open probability (Po) is reduced by protein kinase C (11) and a fall in cytoplasmic pH. The channel Po is not regulated directly by voltage or calcium

Table 1 Characteristics and Distribution of Sodium-Selective Ion Channels Along the Nephron[a]

	PT, rat[b]	PST, rabbit	CCD, rat, mouse	CCD, rabbit	CCD, rabbit	IMCD, cow	A6, frog	A6, frog	A6, frog
Technique	Patch	Patch	Patch	Patch	Patch	Bilayer	Bilayer	Patch	Patch
γ (pS)	15	12	5	4	9	8, 45	~4–80	~4	8
I-V plot	Linear	Linear	Linear	Nonlinear	Linear	Linear	Linear	Nonlinear	Linear
P_{Na^+}/P_{K^+}	10	19	>10	>19	<4	~8	2	20	3
P_{cat}/P_{an}	10	—	+>>>–	+>>>–	—	+>>>–	+>>>–	+>>>–	—
Amiloride sensitive	—	Yes	Yes	Yes	Yes	Yes	Yes	Yes	Yes
K_i, amiloride	—	—	<1 μM	<1 μM	<1 μM	<1 μM	<1 μM	<1 μM	<1 μM
Inhibitors	—	—	↓pH	—	—	—	—	PKC	—
Voltage-activated	No	No	No	No	Yes, hyper.	No	No	Yes, hyper.	Yes, hyper.
Calcium-activated	No	—	Yes[c]	No	No	—	—	—	—
Mean open time	17 ms 74 ms	—	1.0 sec	2.1 sec	50 ms	—	5 sec	20 ms	43 ms
Mean closed time	13 ms 112 ms	—	1.2 sec	0.3 sec 5.2 sec	0.1 sec 3.4 sec	—	<200 ms	86 ms	97 ms
Reference	53	54	44,55–57	58,59	59	60	61	11,62	62

[a] γ(pS) is the single-channel conductance; P_{Na^+}/P_{K^+} is the permeability ratio of Na^+ to K^+; P_{cat}/P_{an} is the permeability ratio of cations to anions; +>>>– indicates that the channel is more permeable to cations than anions; the voltage dependence was modest, hyperpolarizing voltages increased the Po; — indicates not reported.

[b] Channels were studied in brush border membrane vesicles.

[c] The channel was inhibited by increased calcium, but only in cell-attached patches and not in inside-out patches, indicating that calcium inhibits the channel indirectly, most likely by activating protein kinase C[11]. The A6 cell line is thought to be derived from the distal nephron of frog kidney. The variability in the biophysical characteristics of Na^+ channels suggests that several genes may encode for amiloride-sensitive Na^+-selective channels or that Na^+ channels are composed of several protein subunits and that the characteristics of a particular channel depends on the combinatorial assembly of the subunits. It also must be considered that some of the differences may be related to methodological approaches.

Table 2 Characteristics and Distribution of Cation-Selective Ion Channels Along the Nephron[a]

	PT,[b] rat	PT,[c] Necturus	PCT rabbit	PST[d] rabbit	cTAL[d] mouse	bDCT, rabbit	CCD, rabbit	CCD, mouse	CCD, mouse	IMCD, rat, mouse	A6, frog	A6, frog
Technique	Patch, bilayer	Patch	Patch	Patch	Patch	Patch	Patch	Patch	Patch	Patch	Patch	Patch
γ (pS)	~50	18	25	28	27	21	~30	34	26	28	21	1
I-V	Linear	Linear	Linear	Linear	Linear	Linear	Linear	Linear	Linear	Linear	Linear	Linear
P_{Na^+}/P_{K^+}	~1	~1	1	1	1	1	~1	1	1	1	1.5	1
P_{cat}/P_{an}	10	9	+>>>–	2	+>>>–	—	10	11–48	18	10–13	>45	+>>>–
Amiloride-sensitive	—	—	—	No	—	—	No	—	No	Yes	No	—
K_i, amil.	—	—	—	—	—	—	—	—	—	<1 μM	—	—
Inhibitors	—	Gadol[e]	—	DPC[f] NPPB[g] SITS[h]	ATP[i]	DPC[f]		cGMP	Flufen[j] ATP	cGMP[k] ATPγS[l] PMA[l]	—	cGMP[m]
Voltage-activated	No	No	No	Yes depol.	No	Yes, depol.	No	Yes, depol.	Yes, depol.	No	Yes, depol	—
Calcium-activated	No	No	Yes	—	Yes	—	No	Yes	Yes	Yes		No
Mean open time	4 ms 156 ms	3.6 ms	—	2 ms 6.7 ms	—	—	1.6 sec	—	—	38 ms	6 ms	
Mean closed times	4 ms 74 ms	2 ms 786 ms	—	2.0 ms 9.6 ms	—	—	3.4 sec 5.8 sec	—	—	50 ms	3 ms 19 ms	
Reference	53	63,64	65	66	67,68	69	58,59	36,44	37	39–42,70	71	72

[a] γ(pS) is the single-channel conductance; P_{Na^+}/P_{K^+} is the permeability ratio of Na^+ to K^+; P_{Cat}/P_{An} is the permeability ratio of cations to anions; +>>>– indicates that the channel was more permeable to cations than anions; the voltage dependence of some channels was modest; — indicates not reported.

[b] Channels were studied in brush border membranes.

[c] Channel is stretch-activated and equally permeable to Ca^{2+} and Na^+.

[d] Channel is located in the basolateral membrane.

[e] Gadol. is gadolinium, an inhibitor of mechanosensitive channels.

[f] DPC is diphenylamine carboxylic acid, a nonspecific inhibitor of some chloride and cation channels

[g] NPPB is 5-Nitro-2-(3phenylpropylamino)-benzoic acid.

[h] SITS is 4-acetamido-4'-isothiocyanatostilbene-2,2'-disulfonic acid.

[i] ATP, ADP, AMP, and ATPγS inhibit the channel.

[j] Flufen is Flufenamic acid.

[k] cGMP and cGMP-dependent protein kinase inhibit the channel (39,40,42).

[l] ATPγS (100 μ*M*; *n* = 7) and PMA (phorbol 12-myristate 13-acetate 10 n*M*; *n* = 4) inhibited the channel (D. Light and B. Stanton, unpublished observations).

[m] cGMP activates the channel.

(Table 1). Aldosterone stimulates sodium absorption across CCD and A6 cells by increasing the Po of channels already present in the membrane (5,12). This early (~45 min) increase in sodium transport may result from the methylation of the ~90-kDa channel subunit (Table 3) and by the new synthesis of the 70-kDa aldosterone-induced protein (Table 3). In the late stage of aldosterone stimulation of sodium absorption, the hormone may also increase the synthesis and expression of new sodium channels (5). In contrast, ADH increases transepithelial sodium absorption by causing the fusion of channels from an intracellular pool into the apical membrane (5,13) and by increasing the Po of individual channels by protein kinase A–mediated phosphorylation (14–16).

The ~4 pS Na^+-selective channel has been purified from bovine renal papilla (i.e., most likely IMCD) and from A6 cells by Benos and Kleyman and their colleagues (see Table 3). The channel is ~730 kDa in size and is composed of six heterogeneous subunits. Table 3 summarizes our current understanding of the functions of each channel subunit. Most notably, the ~150-kDa subunit is thought to have an amiloride binding site on the extracellular domain and an ankyrin binding site on the cytoplasmic domain. Recent evidence suggests that the ~150-kDa subunit may form the channel pore (17) and that other subunits may play important roles in regulating the ability of the ~150-kDa subunit to conduct sodium (see Table 3).

A second type of Na^+-selective channel has been identified in CCD, IMCD, and A6 cells (Table 1). This channel exhibits a single-channel conductance of ~8 pS, is poorly selective to sodium over potassium (P_{Na+}:P_{K+} ~2:1), and has faster kinetics than the 4-pS channel. Because macroscopic sodium currents across A6 cells are most similar to currents carried by the 4-pS channel and because aldosterone increases transepithelial sodium absorption across A6 cells by increasing the number of active 4-pS channels in the membrane without changing the number of active 8-pS channels, it is assumed that the 8-pS channel does not contribute significantly to transepithelial sodium reabsorption (2). Although the

Table 3 Subunits of the ~730-kDa Renal Amiloride-Sensitive Sodium Channel and Their Possible Function

Subunit M_r (kDa)	Function	Ref.
~315 (260–230)[a]	Effector protein of ADH: cAMP-mediated phosphorylation (stimulates channel activity).	14,73,74
~150 (140–110)[a]	Subunit may form channel pore: Amiloride and ankyrin binding subunit. Protein kinase C–mediated phosphorylation (inhibits channel activity).	14,17,73,75–77
~95–90	Methylated following increased aldosterone. Methylation stimulates channel activity. ADP-ribosylated (may stimulate channel activity).	78–80
~70	Aldosterone-induced protein (increases channel activity).	81,82
~55	Amiloride-binding protein. Protein kinase C–mediated phosphorylation (inhibits channel activity).	14,73,77
~41–40	α_{1-3} subunit of Gi protein: inhibits 4 pS and stimulates 8 pS Na^+ channel activity.	79,83

[a]Kleyman et al. (73) used a monoclonal anti-idiotypic antibody (RA 6.3) to immunoprecipitate the Na^+ channel. The antibody precipitated a 725-kDa protein, which under reducing conditions dissociated into four polypeptides of 260–230, 180, 140–110, and 70 kDa. The 140–110 kDa subunit binds amiloride. The discrepancy in the molecular masses in channel subunits between the reports of Benos et al. (84) and those reported by Kleyman et al. may be related to differences in the composition of the reducing sample buffers.

Source: From Ref. 84.

physiological role of the 8-pS channel is not clear at this time, it has been suggested that the 4-pS and 8-pS channels represent two states of the same protein that interconvert following protein degradation (2,18,19). Alternatively, the 4-pS and 8-pS channels may be encoded by different genes or may result from differences in subunit composition of a multimeric channel complex. At the present time these hypotheses cannot be evaluated experimentally without the cloning of the relevant protein subunits.

Finally, Na^+-conductive ion channels have been identified in the apical membrane of the proximal tubule (Table 1). Those channels are characterized by (a) a single channel conductance of 10 to 12 pS; (b) high selectivity for Na^+ over K^+ ($P_{Na+}:P_{K+} > 10:1$); and (c) amiloride sensitivity. In light of the observation that μM concentrations of amiloride do not inhibit sodium reabsorption across the proximal tubule, the physiological role of these channels is presently unknown.

Nonselective Cation Channels

Nonselective cation channels are a large and heterogeneous group of channels that are found in a wide variety of cell types. In the broadest sense, the group includes but is not limited to nicotinic acetylcholine receptors, gap junctions, glutamate receptors, mechanosensitive (i.e., stretch-activated) channels, cyclic nucleotide (e.g., cAMP and cGMP)-gated cation channels, cation channels found in peptidergic nerve terminals and subcellular organelles, major intrinsic polypeptides (MIP) in lens fiber cell membranes, cation channels involved in taste reception, and cation channels involved in receptor-mediated calcium entry (7). Nonselective cation channels are involved in a variety of cellular functions, including volume regulation, transepithelial sodium absorption, initiation of cell proliferation, receptor-mediated calcium entry, excitation-contraction coupling, generation and maintenance of action potentials in Purkinje fibers, and secretion in exocrine cells (7). A well-defined subgroup of nonselective cation channels, referred to as NSC channels, includes channels that do not discriminate between sodium and potassium, are activated by intracellular calcium, and are rather impermeable to divalent cations (7). Some nonselective cation channels—especially those in olfactory, lingual, auditory, and visual epithelia, which play important roles in sensory perception—are regulated by amiloride and analogues of amiloride (4).

Renal Nonselective Cation Channels

Nonselective cation channels are expressed in every nephron segment and in A6 cells (Table 2). In general, they are characterized by a single channel conductance of ~28 pS and an inability to discriminate between sodium and potassium. They are also highly selective for cations vs. anions and, with one notable exception, are not permeable to divalent cations. Most of the channels are insensitive to amiloride and, again with one exception (see below) have relatively fast kinetics. Some but not all of these channels are activated by increased cellular calcium levels. The function of cation channels in the kidney is largely unknown except for the stretch-activated 25-pS channel, which appears to be involved in cell volume regulation in *Necturus* proximal tubule and the cGMP-gated, nonselective cation channel that mediates transepithelial sodium absorption in the IMCD (Table 2). To date, cDNA clones have been isolated for only the cGMP-gated, nonselective cation channel (see below).

Renal cGMP-Gated, Nonselective Cation Channels

The only renal nonselective cation channel that is inhibited by amiloride is the cGMP-gated nonselective cation channel located in the IMCD and CCD (Table 2). This channel is active in cell-attached patches of isolated rat IMCDs and in rat and mouse IMCD cells in culture (20). The channel has a single-channel conductance of 28 pS, is activated by increased cell calcium levels, and is inhibited by micromolar concentrations of amiloride ($K_i < 0.1$ μM), cGMP, cGMP-dependent protein kinase, protein kinase C, and ATP (Table 2). In contrast to other nonselective cation channels, the channel in IMCD cells is not inhibited by DPC (Table 2). Atrial natriuretic peptide (ANP), via its second-messenger cGMP, completely inhibits amiloride-sensitive sodium absorption across the IMCD (20,21). Because neither ANP nor cGMP inhibit the 4-pS sodium-selective channel (N. Kizer and B. Stanton; unpublished observations) it is reasonable to conclude that the cGMP-gated, nonselective cation channel is responsible for all electrogenic sodium absorption across the IMCD.

Although amiloride-sensitive, Na^+-selective channels have been isolated from the IMCD (22), these channels have not been observed by the patch-clamp technique in this segment.

cGMP-gated cation channels are also expressed in several nonrenal cell types including photoreceptor epithelia (23). Striking similarities exist between photoreceptor and renal cGMP-gated cation channels, including similar single-channel conductances (28 pS in the absence of calcium), similar ion selectivity for monovalent cations, linear single-channel I-V relationships, increased Po at depolarizing voltages, and inhibition by amiloride and derivatives of amiloride (23). Notable differences between photoreceptor and renal cGMP-gated cation channels include the following: (a) cGMP increases the Po of channels in photoreceptor cells whereas cGMP decreases the Po of channels in CCD and IMCD cells (Table 2) and (b) increased calcium decreases the single-channel conductance of channels in photoreceptor cells whereas calcium increases the Po of the channel in CCD and IMCD cells (Table 2). Full-length cDNA clones encoding the photoreceptor and renal cGMP-gated nonselective cation channels have been isolated (see below).

MOLECULAR BIOLOGY OF AMILORIDE-SENSITIVE, SODIUM-SELECTIVE CHANNELS

Recently, Lingueglia et al. (24) and Canessa et al. (25) isolated cDNAs from rat colon libraries that encode an amiloride-sensitive sodium channel. Both groups isolated cDNA clones that are almost identical in that they differ by only one amino acid located at the N terminus. However, the two groups have proposed very different two-dimensional structures (see below). Lingueglia et al. (24) report that the cDNA contains an open reading frame of 2097 nucleotides (nt) encoding a polypeptide of 699 amino acids with a predicted molecular weight of 79 kDa. In vitro translation experiments performed in the absence of microsomes resulted in the translation of a polypeptide of 75 kDa. However, when translation was performed in the presence of microsomal membranes, the apparent molecular mass of the polypeptide increased to 92 kDa. The authors report that hydropathy analysis suggests the presence of six, 20 amino acid transmembrane spanning domains (Fig. 1A). In addition, sequence analysis suggested the presence of two putative extracellular N-glycosylation sites and several putative intracellular phosporylation sites for protein kinase A, protein kinase C, and casein kinase II. Electrophysiological and $^{22}Na^+$ flux studies demonstrated that the cDNA encodes a protein that manifests biophysical and pharmacological properties similar to native, highly Na^+-selective channels. For example, the ED_{50}s for amiloride and amiloride derivatives is similar to that described for sodium channels in rat colon. The cDNA encoding the rat colon sodium channel shares no sequence homology with previously cloned channels. Interestingly, however, sequence homology was found between the cloned sodium channel and the mec4 and deg1 gene products, which encode transmembrane proteins, degenerins, which are involved in sensory touch transduction in *Caenorhabditis elegans* (26). A mutation in degenerin causes neural degeneration (26). It has been suggested that degenerin may be an ion channel that, when mutated, induces deleterious increases in intracellular ionic content.

Canessa et al. (25,27,28) have isolated a sodium channel cDNA, termed αrENaC, from a rat colon library that contains a 2094-nt open reading frame encoding a 698 amino acid protein with a predicted molecular weight of 79 kDa. Northern blot analysis revealed that the clone hybridized to a 3.5-kb mRNA transcript isolated from rat kidney cortex and medulla, distal colon, and stomach. Moreover, in situ hybridization results indicate that αrENaC mRNA is expressed in the rat CCD (27). Oocytes injected with cRNA transcribed from αrENaC express amiloride-sensitive sodium currents that are similar to native sodium channels. However, sodium currents in injected oocytes are smaller than those observed in oocytes injected with size-fractionated mRNA, thereby leading to the speculation that the 79 kDa protein is only one of several subunits that may be involved in sodium channel function.

In recent communications, Canessa et al. (27,28) report that αrENaC is a 5 pS sodium channel and that two additional cDNAs, βrENaC and γrENaC, have been isolated that are homologous (~40% amino acid identity) to αrENaC. βrENaC and γrENaC are expressed in renal cortex and medulla but they do not code for sodium channels. Interestingly, however, when the cRNAs from βrENaC and γrENaC are coinjected into oocytes with the cRNA from αrENaC, the amiloride-sensitive sodium current is increased severalfold above the level seen in oocytes injected with αrENaC alone. These results suggests that the sodium channel is a heteromultimeric protein consisting of at least three protein subunits and that αrENaC encodes the pore-forming unit. However, the molecular mass of αrENaC is predicted to be 79 kDa when unglycosylated and 92 kDA when glycosylated, whereas biochemical and patch-clamp studies suggest that the ion-conducting protein subunit is ~150 kDa (see Table 3). Although an explanation for this apparent discrepancy is not currently available, it is tempting to speculate that more complete glycosylation of the 79-kDa subunit may increase the molecular mass to ~150 kDa or, alternatively, that αrENaC may be a dimer.

In contrast to the conclusion by Lingueglia et al. (24) that αrENaC encodes for a protein with six, 20 amino acid transmembrane spanning domains (Fig. 1A), Canessa et al. (25,27) propose that the channel has two hydrophobic regions that form transmembrane domains or two transmembrane hairpin loops (Fig. 1B). Canessa et al. have proposed that most of αrENaC is extracellular and located between the hydrophobic membrane spanning domains. The amino terminal 110 amino acids lack a signal sequence and have been assigned to the cytoplasm. This amino terminal region has a consensus sequence (Gly-X-Gly-X-Gly) that may be involved in nucleotide binding. The extracellular domain contains six putative glycosylation sites. According to this model, however, all potential cyclic nucleotide–dependent protein kinase phosphorylation sites are located on the extracellular side

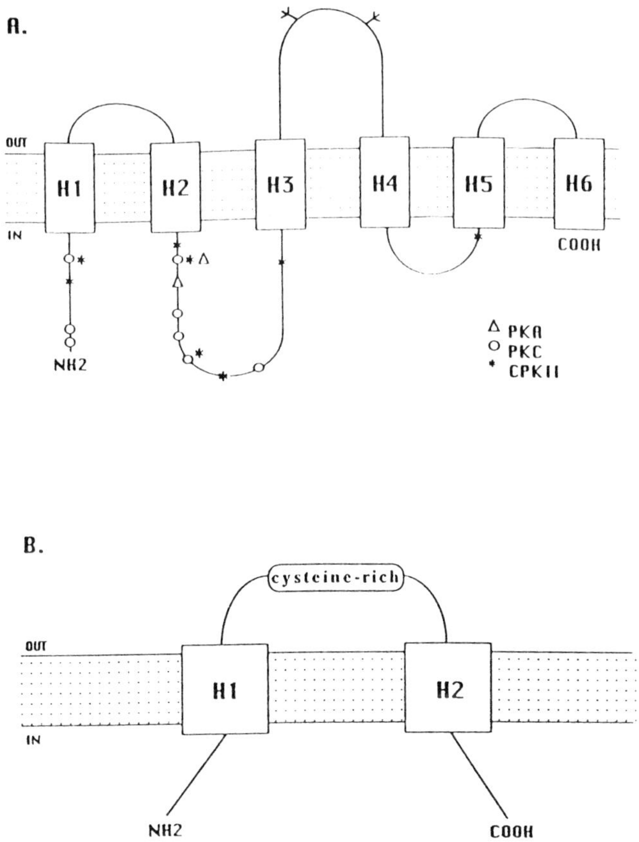

Figure 1 (A) Putative structural model of the amiloride-sensitive sodium channel as proposed by Lingueglia et al. (24). There are two putative extracellular N-linked glycosylation sites, two potential consensus phosphorylation sites for PKA, eight potential consensus phosphorylation sites for PKC, and eight potential consensus phosphorylation sites for casein kinase II. (B) Putative structural model of the amiloride-sensitive sodium channel as proposed by Canessa et al. (25,27). Membrane-spanning or membrane-hairpin loops are labeled H1 and H2. A cysteine-rich box is shown located extracellularly. These models are based on amino acid sequence.

of the plasma membrane. Verification of the models proposed by Lingueglia et al. and Canessa et al. must await experimental support.

Several other cDNAs have been isolated that may encode proteins playing a role in sodium channel function. A cDNA isolated from a human kidney library has been shown to code for an amiloride-binding protein (ABP) (29). The 2396-nt open reading frame of ABP encodes a 694 amino acid protein with a predicted molecular mass of 79 kDa; ~100 kDa when the cDNA is expressed in mammalian cells. ABP shares no similarity to αrENaC. Northern blot analysis demonstrates that the ABP mRNA is 2.4 kb in length in human kidney, whereas mouse and pig kidney ABP mRNA are significantly larger (4.4 kb and 3.3 kb, respectively). In expression studies, the pharmacological profiles of amiloride and amiloride analogue binding in cells transfected with human kidney ABP cDNA are similar to that found in pig kidney cell membranes. However, the protein has equal affinities for amiloride and EIPA, an analogue of amiloride that has a low affinity for Na^+-selective channels. Moreover, in cells expressing ABP, amiloride-sensitive sodium channel activity could not be demonstrated during patch-clamp analysis. The authors concluded that the cDNA may not code for the pore-forming structure of the channel. ABP may be a regulatory subunit that requires other subunits for functional expression of the channel.

Additional ABPs have been cloned from rat colon and lung tissues (30). Proximal and distal colon, duodenum, liver, placenta, and thymus cDNAs have a 2668-nt open reading frame that encodes a protein of 746 amino acids with a calculated molecular mass of 85 kDa. These cDNAs share 81% amino acid identity with the human kidney ABP homologue described above. Although a rat ABP probe was shown to hybridize to a 2.7-kb transcript in rat distal colon, duodenum, liver, placenta, and thymus, an ABP could not be detected by Northern blot analysis of rat kidney poly(A^+) RNA. However, ABP was detected in rat kidney by polymerase chain reaction (PCR). Moreover, the rat probe hybridized with a 2.4-kb transcript of poly (A^+) RNA isolated from human kidney. The amiloride binding profile for the 85 kDa ABP encoded by the 2.7-kb cDNA is similar to that observed in pig and human kidney and is characteristic of an epithelial sodium channel. In lung, placenta, colon, and spleen, a 1.2-kb transcript corresponding to the 3′ terminus of the 2.7-kb transcript has been detected by Northern blot analysis. The predicted molecular mass for this short ABP is 25 kDa. The amiloride binding profile for the protein encoded by the 1.2-kb cDNA is similar to that observed for an amiloride binding protein in pneumocytes.

While it is not yet known what if any role ABPs play in sodium channel function, it is possible that they represent one of the necessary protein subunits required for channel function. Because amiloride binds to a wide variety of proteins in addition to sodium channels, such as the Na^+-K^+-ATPase, the Na^+/H^+ exchanger, the Ca^{2+}/Na^+ exchanger, and other proteins unrelated to sodium transport (31), it is possible that the cDNA encoding for ABPs may be unrelated to sodium channels.

Another protein that participates in amiloride-sensitive sodium channel activity is apical protein *Xenopus* (APX), a protein located in the apical membrane of A6 cells (32). The cDNA encoding APX was isolated by screening an expression library with antisera against the α subunit of the Na^+-K^+-ATPase (32). In addition to recognizing Na^+-K^+-ATPase in the basolateral membrane, the antisera labeled an apical membrane protein in A6 cells (32). The cDNA encoding APX has a 4260-nt open reading frame coding for a 1420 amino acid, ~160-kDa protein that shares no similarity with other sequenced proteins. The APX cDNA was shown to hybridize to a 5.2-kb transcript on Northern blots of poly(A^+) RNA isolated from A6 cells and *Xenopus* kidney. Although injection of APX cRNA alone into *Xenopus* oocytes did not induce an amiloride-sensitive current, antisense APX RNA or antisense oligonucleotides specific for the APX cDNA sequence inhibited amiloride-sensitive sodium current induced by injection of A6 poly(A^+) RNA into *Xenopus* oocytes (32). Furthermore, an antibody raised against an APX-fusion protein reacted with the sodium channel complex (130-kDa subunit) isolated from A6 cells. Thus, APX appears to play an important role in the functional expression of the multimeric, amiloride-sensitive sodium channel complex.

Finally, in a preliminary communication, Cunningham et al. (33) report the isolation of a 6.5-kb cDNA clone that encodes the 55 kDa subunit of the sodium channel. That cDNA clone was isolated by screening a bovine papillary expression library with a polyclonal antibody that recognizes the 315-, 150-, and 55-kDa subunits of the epithelial amiloride-sensitive sodium channel. The cDNA was shown to react with two mRNA species of 7 and >9.5 kb on Northern blots. Sense cRNA transcribed from the clone and injected into *Xenopus* oocytes induced the expression of sodium currents that were *insensitive* to amiloride. Western blot analysis of oocytes injected with cRNA demonstrated specific antibody reactivity to a 55-kDa protein. Those observations suggest that the 55-kDa protein may play an important role in the formation of the sodium-conducting pore of the sodium channel.

FUTURE DIRECTIONS

The efforts of investigators to describe the mechanisms of renal sodium transport across the collecting duct have shed considerable light on the structure and function of renal Na^+-selective and nonselective ion channels. However, many questions remain unanswered: (a) What role do ABPs and APX play in channel function? (b) What is the functional significance of ABP and APX expression in cells that do not express amiloride-sensitive sodium channels? (c) What roles do the six channel subunits play in channel structure and function? (d) Why does the cloned αrENaC sodium channel cDNA encode a protein of 79 to 92 kDa whereas the amiloride binding protein that forms channels in bilayer membranes in 110 to 180 kDa in size? To answer these questions, it is necessary to clarify the functions of the different channel subunits and to provide experimental verification of the two-dimensional models of channel structure.

MOLECULAR BIOLOGY OF AMILORIDE-SENSITIVE, NONSELECTIVE CATION CHANNELS

Nonselective cation channels are present in a variety of excitable and nonexcitable tissues, including many epithelia (7). The molecular cloning of the cGMP-gated cation channel expressed in the bovine rod outer segment (34) led to the subsequent discovery of related gene products in olfactory epithelia, olfactory neurons, pineal gland, heart, aorta, brain, and kidney (6,9,23). In the kidney, the presence of mRNA that hybridizes to a retinal cGMP-gated nonselective cation channel probe (35) is of particular interest in light of the observations that (a) nonselective cation channels are expressed in the proximal tubule, cortical thick ascending limb, distal convoluted tubule, CCD, IMCD, and A6 cells (Table 2) and (2) cGMP-gated, nonselective cation channels are expressed in the CCD, IMCD, and A6 cells (Table 2). The physiological role of nonselective cation channels in the proximal tubule, cortical thick ascending limb, and distal convoluted tubule is not yet understood and the effects of cGMP on those channels has not been reported. These channels may be involved in cell volume regulation, cell proliferation, sodium reabsorption, and/or calcium entry. As noted above, the cGMP-gated, nonselective cation channels in the IMCD mediate virtually all transepithelial sodium reabsorption across the IMCD.

The first molecular evidence that the kidney expresses a gene related to the photoreceptor cGMP-gated nonselective cation channel came from a study by Ahmad et al. in 1990 (35). By Northern blot analysis, those investigators reported that a rat photoreceptor cGMP-gated cation channel probe hybridized to poly(A^+) RNA (3.2 kb) isolated from M1 CCD cells. Subsequently, the same group isolated partial cDNAs encoding for putative cGMP-gated cation channels in M1 CCD cells (36). Two partial cDNA clones were isolated: one that differs from the cGMP-gated cation channel in rat photoreceptor by 1 nt out of 426 nt and one that differs from the rat photoreceptor sequence by 20 nt out of 426 nt. A third partial cDNA clone was obtained from a rat kidney cDNA library using PCR. That cDNA clone differed by only 1 nt out of 426 nt from the rat photoreceptor sequence. All base pair differences were in redundant positions; thus, the deduced amino acid sequences for all the clones were identical to the rat photoreceptor channel. Because the two different sequences were identified in M1 CCD cells, a cell line that expresses cGMP-gated nonselective cation channels (36), it was suggested that M1 CCD cells and perhaps CCD cells in vivo express more than one gene coding for cGMP-gated, nonselective cation channels. That hypothesis is consistent with patch-clamp studies in M1 CCD cells reporting the presence of cGMP-gated nonselective cation channels as well as nonselective cation channels that are inhibited by ATP but are not regulated by cGMP (36,37) (Table 2).

Our laboratory has a long-standing interest in the biophysics and molecular biology of the renal cGMP-gated, nonselective cation channel (21,38–49). As a first step toward isolating a full-length cDNA clone coding for this channel, we used RT-PCR of poly(A^+) RNA to isolate partial cDNAs encoding this channel in rat and mouse IMCD cells. Oligonucleotide primers were designed from conserved regions flanking the cGMP binding domain, which is highly conserved among the cGMP-gated cation channels that have been cloned (23). PCR products of 790 bp and 524 bp were identified and found to hybridize to rat retinal cation channel probes by Southern blot analysis (45,47,48). Northern blot analysis of poly(A^+) RNA isolated from IMCD cells using the 790-bp PCR product as a probe revealed several bands, including one at 3.2 kb (45), the same size as the retinal and olfactory cGMP-gated cation channel transcript. Northern blot analysis of mouse kidney poly(A^+) RNA using the 524 bp PCR product as a probe identified a similar 3.2-kb band (47,48). The 524-bp cDNA isolated from mouse IMCD has significant sequence identity with the mouse photoreceptor cGMP-gated cation channel; i.e., only three base-pair differences resulting in two amino acid changes, one conserved (47). In contrast, the 790-bp cDNA is significantly different from the mouse photoreceptor, thereby suggesting that the IMCD may express several genes encoding nonselective cation channels.

Recently, we have obtained the full-length sequence of a cDNA clone encoding a cGMP-gated, nonselective cation channel in IMCD (49). The open reading frame is 2055 nt long and encodes a protein with a calculated molecular mass of 79 kDa. The deduced amino acid sequence is ~95% identical to the mouse photoreceptor cGMP-gated cation channel (50). The cDNA encoding the channel shares no sequence homology with the sodium-selective channels cloned by Lingueglia et al. (24) and Canessa et al. (27). The putative two-dimensional structure of the renal cGMP-gated cation channel, which is in general agreement with the structure of the photoreceptor channel (23), is depicted in Fig. 2. The N terminus of the protein is located on the cytoplasmic side of the membrane. There are six hydrophobic transmembrane domains, H1 through H5, followed by a long cytoplasmic domain containing an 80 amino acid region near the C terminus that shares sequence identity with the cyclic nucleotide binding domain of the photoreceptor channel.

Within the two-dimensional structure of the renal cGMP-gated cation channel are two sequence motifs reminiscent of voltage-gated potassium channels. One, S4, has arginine residues at every third position and has been proposed to serve as the voltage sensor in voltage-gated channels. However, cGMP-gated channels, including the renal channel, are only weakly voltage-dependent (23). Because the S4 motif in cGMP-gated channels has only four positively charged residues compared with a maximum of seven in voltage-gated channels, the functional significance of the S4 motif in cGMP-gated channels is unclear. A second sequence motif sharing significant homology with the putative pore region of voltage-gated potassium channels is located between H4 and H5. This segment of 20 amino acids spans the membrane twice in a hairpin-like β sheet and is thought to form the ion-conducting pore.

Additional full-length cDNA clones have been isolated in our laboratory and sequence analysis indicates that two notable differences exist between mouse IMCD cDNA clones and the cDNA encoding the mouse photoreceptor channel. First, one cDNA clone has a 28 amino acid insertion in

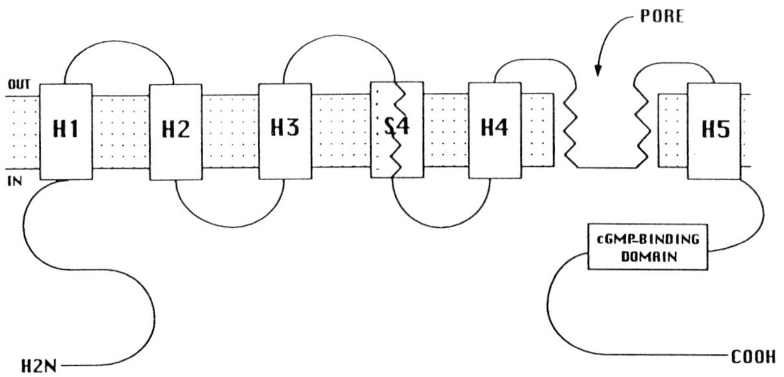

Figure 2 Putative structural model of the renal cGMP-gated, nonselective cation channel. Shown are the five transmembrane-spanning domains, H1–H3, S4, H4, and H5 and the membrane-spanning pore region. The cGMP-binding domain is located intracellularly near the carboxyl terminus. (From Ref. 23.)

the 5′ cytoplasmic domain that is absent in photoreceptor channels. Second, we have identified a second isoform that has a deletion in the H2 domain. This 107 bp deletion is encoded by exon 9 of the gene. The functional significance of the 28 amino acid insertion in the N-terminal cytoplasmic domain as well as the H2 deletion is unknown. It is tempting to speculate, however, that they may account for some of the observed differences between cGMP-gated channels in photoreceptor and IMCD cells (See above). Moreover, the presence of two or more alternatively spliced gene products in the IMCD suggests that the cGMP-gated cation channel may be a heteromultimeric structure. Experiments currently in progress are evaluating the biophysical characteristics of channels encoded by the renal IMCD channel cDNA clones and are testing the hypothesis that the cGMP-gated cation channel in the IMCD is a heteromultimeric structure.

Recent evidence suggests that the cGMP-gated cation channel in photoreceptor is alternatively spliced and that the channel may be heteromultimeric (51). Chen et al. isolated two cDNA clones (hRCNC2a and hRCNC2b) differing only at their 5′ ends from the human retinal cDNA (hRCNC1) that codes for a functional cGMP-gated cation channel. Genomic cloning and sequence analysis demonstrated that the two clones are alternatively spliced products of the same gene and differ only at their N termini. The proteins encoded by these cDNAs contain 623 amino acids (hRCNC2a) and 909 amino acids (hRCNC2b). Immunocytochemistry localized hRCNC2a to the rod outer segment, whereas hRCNC2b was localized to the outer plexiform layer. The authors concluded that hRCNC2a is the alternatively spliced variant in rod cells. Interestingly, whereas patch-clamp recordings of hRCNC2a-transfected embryonic kidney cells revealed that hRCNC2a fails to encode functional channels, cells cotransfected with hRCNC1 (the human rod cGMP-gated channel: 686 amino acids) and hRCNC2a, show channel activity with kinetic and pharmacological properties similar to cGMP-gated cation channels. Moreover, an in-frame deletion of exon 8, which encodes H1 in the human cGMP-gated cation channel, does not encode a functional channel (52). Thus, it is possible that variant forms of the cGMP-gated channel protein complexes with the full-length protein. Taken together, these observations suggest that hRCNC1 encodes the pore-forming subunit of the channel, whereas hRCNC2a and possibly hRCNC2b encode regulatory subunits that may be involved in regulating channel opening and closing and sensitivity to diltiazem, an inhibitor of channel activity.

Our laboratory has also examined the distribution of the renal cGMP-gated cation channel along the nephron by RT-PCR of proximal straight tubule (PST), medullary thick ascending limb (mTAL), CCD, and distal collecting tubule (DCT) cell poly(A^+) RNA (48). Oligonucleotide primers used to amplify a 524-bp cDNA in IMCD cells amplified 524-bp cDNAs in all nephron segments examined. Southern blot analysis, restriction digest analyses, and sequence analysis confirmed the identity of the 524-bp cDNAs as the cGMP-gated cation channel. Additional support for the expression of a cGMP-gated cation channel or a related gene product in these nephron segments was provided by Western blot analysis using an antipeptide monoclonal antibody directed against a highly conserved region of the cGMP-binding domain of the channel. The antibody specifically reacted with a single 50-kDa protein in all nephron segments studied and with a 63-kDa protein in bovine rod outer segment (49). The expression of the 63-kDa protein in photoreceptors cells is due to a 98 amino acid deletion from the N-terminal end of the 79-kDa protein. Accordingly, the differences in molecular mass between the IMCD and photoreceptor cGMP-gated cation channel may result from tissue-specific differences in posttranslational events. Taken together, these observations suggest that a cGMP-gated cation channel or a related gene product may be expressed in all nephron segments. Although the role of cGMP-gated cation channels in nephron segments proximal to the IMCD is unknown, it is tempting to speculate that hormones that increase cGMP, such as ANP and nitric oxide (NO), may regulate sodium and perhaps calcium uptake in these nephron segments. The physiological implications of such an action remains to be evaluated.

FUTURE DIRECTIONS

Although it is known that nonselective cation channels in IMCD mediate sodium absorption, the physiological role of nonselective cation channels in more proximal nephron segments remains poorly understood. To define the structural and functional roles of these channels in renal ion transport, the following experimental considerations must be addressed: (a) expression of full-length renal cDNA sequences of cGMP-gated cation channels and functional studies that evaluate the biophysical properties of the translated protein; (b) the identification of genes encoding regulatory subunits of these channels; (c) determine whether alternative splicing, posttranslational modifications, gene mutations, and/or tissue-dependent expression is responsible for the functional differences between photoreceptor and kidney cGMP-gated nonselective cation channels; (d) determine whether nonselective cation channels interact with any of the sodium channel subunits and whether sodium-selective and cation-selective channels are coexpressed in the same cell; (e) determine what factor(s) may regulate tissue-specific expression of cation channel genes: and (f) determine the function and physiological role of cation channels in proximal tubule, medullary thick ascending limb, distal tubule, and cortical collecting duct. The answers to these questions together with the information described in this chapter will provide valuable insights into the physiological role of sodium-conducting ion channels and renal function.

NOTE ADDED IN PROOF

Since this review was written (January 1994), significant advances have been made with regard to the molecular biology of sodium-conducting ion channels. References 85–88, although not a comprehensive list, describe recent work in this area. The reader is encouraged to review recent publications for the most current information on renal sodium-conducting ion channels.

ACKNOWLEDGMENTS

We thank those investigators who provided reprints and preprints of their work in press. Unfortunately, due to page limitations, we could not cite all of the manuscripts submitted. We also thank our colleagues, Katherine Karlson, Flora Ciampolillo-Bates, Neil Kizer, and Robery Molday for their insight and dedication to the project of isolating the cDNAs encoding the renal cGMP-gated cation channel. Work in the author's laboratory cited in this review was supported by NIH grants DK-34533 (B.S.) and DK-08689 (D.M.) and a grant from the American Heart Association Grant-In-Aid (B.S.).

REFERENCES

1. Smith PR, Benos DJ. Epithelial Na^+ channels. Annu Rev Physiol 1991; 53:509–530.
2. Palmer LG. Epithelial Na channels: Function and diversity. Annu Rev Physiol 1992; 54:51–66.
3. Duchatelle P, Ohara A, Ling BN, et al. Regulation of renal epithelial sodium channels. Mol Cell Biochem 1992; 114:27–34.
4. Benos DJ. Cunningham S, Baker RR, et al. Molecular characteristics of amiloride-sensitive sodium channels. Rev Physiol Biochem Pharmacol 1992; 120:32–113.
5. Horisberger J-D, Canessa C, Rossier BC. The epithelial sodium channel: Recent developments. Cell Physiol Biochem 1993; 3:283–294.
6. Korbmacher C, Barnstable CJ. Renal epithelial cells show nonselective cation channel activity and express a gene related to the cGMP-gate photoreceptor channel. In: Sieman D, Hescheler J, eds. Nonselective Cation Channels. Basel: Birkhäuser Verlag, 1993:147–164.
7. Siemen D. Nonselective cation channels. In: Sieman D, Heschler J, eds. Nonselective Cation Channels: Pharmacology, Physiology and Biophysics. Basel: Birkhäuser Verlag, 1993:3–25.
8. Garty H. Molecular properties of epithelial, amiloride-blockade Na^+ channels. FASEB J 1994; 8:522–528.
9. Barnstable CJ. Cyclic nucleotide-gated nonselective cation channels: A multifunctional gene family. In: Sieman D, Heschler J, eds. Nonselective Cation Channels. Basel: Birkhäuser Verlag, 1993:121–134.
10. Kramer RH, Siegelbaum SA. Intracellular Ca^{2+} regulates the sensitivity of cyclic nucleotide-gated channels in olfactory receptor neurons. Neuron 1992; 9:897–906.
11. Ling BN, Eaton DC. Effects of luminal Na^+ on single Na^+ channels in A6 cells, a regulatory role for protein kinase C. Am J Physiol (Renal Fluid Electrolyte Physiol) 1989; 256:F1094–F1103.
12. Kemendy AE, Kleyman TR, Eaton DC. Aldosterone alters the open probability of amiloride-blockade sodium channels in A6 epithelia. Am J Physiol (Cell Physiol) 1992; 263:C825–C837.
13. Marunaka Y, Eaton DC. Effects of vasopressin and cAMP on single amiloride-blockade Na channels. Am J Physiol (Cell Physiol) 1991; 260:C1071–C1084.
14. Oh Y, Smith PR, Bradford AL, et al. Regulation by phosphorylation of purified epithelial Na^+ channels in purified lipid bilayers. Am J Physiol (Cell Physiol) 1993; 265:C85–C91.
15. Prat AG, Ausiello DA, Cantiello HF. Vasopressin and protein kinase A activate G protein-sensitive epithelial Na^+ channels. Am J Physiol (Cell Physiol) 1993; 265:C218–C223.

16. Prat AG, Bertorello AM, Ausiello DA, Cantiello HF. Activation of epithelial Na^+ channels by protein kinase A requires actin filaments. Am J Physiol (Cell Physiol) 1993; 265:C224–C233.
17. Sariban-Sohraby S, Abramow M, Fisher RS. Single-channel behavior of a purified epithelial Na^+ channel subunit that binds amiloride. Am J Physiol (Cell Physiol) 1992; 263:C1111–C1117.
18. Lewis SA, Alles WP. Urinary kallikrein: A physiological regulator of epithelial Na absorption. Proc Natl Acad Sci USA 1986; 83:5345–5348.
19. Zweifach A, Lewis SA. Characterization of a partially degraded Na^+ channel from urinary tract epithelium. J Membr Biol 1988; 101:49–56.
20. Stanton BA. Molecular mechanisms of ANP inhibition of renal sodium transport. Can J Physiol Pharmacol 1991; 69:1546–1552.
21. Kizer N, Ciampolillo F, Stanton BA. Characterization of an inner medullary collecting duct cell line isolated from a transgenic mouse (abstr). FASEB J 1992; 6:A1194.
22. Sariban-Sohraby S, Benos DJ. Detergent solubilization, functional reconstitution, and partial purification of epithelial amiloride-binding protein. Biochemistry 1986; 25:4639–4646.
23. Eismann E, Bönigk W, Kaupp UB. Structural features of cyclic nucleotide-gated channels. Cell Physiol Biochem 1993; 3:332–351.
24. Lingueglia E, Voilley N, Waldmann R, et al. Expression cloning of an epithelial amiloride-sensitive Na^+ channel: A new channel type with homologies to *Caenorhabditis elegans* degenerins. FEBS Lett 1993; 318:95–99.
25. Canessa CM, Horisberger J, Rossier BD. Epithelial sodium channel related to proteins involved in neurodegeneration. Nature 1993; 361:467–470.
26. Driscoll M, Chalfie M. The mec-4 gene is a member of a family of Caenorhabditis elegans genes that can mutate to induce neuronal degeneration. Nature 1991; 349:588–593.
27. Canessa CM, Merillat A-M, Horisberger J-D, Rossier BC. Identification of N-glycosylation sites of α-rENaC, a subunit of the epithelial Na^+ channel (abstr). J Am Soc Nephrol 1994; 4:864.
28. Canessa CM, Schild L, Buell G, et al. The amiloride-sensitive epithelial sodium channel is made of three homologous subunits. Nature 1994; 367:463–467.
29. Barbry P, Champe M, Chassande O, et al. Human kidney amiloride-binding protein: cDNA structure and functional expression. Proc Natl Acad Sci USA 1990; 87:7347–7351.
30. Lingueglia E, Renard S, Voilley N, et al. Molecular cloning and functional expression of different molecular forms of rat amiloride-binding proteins. Eur J Biochem 1993; 216:679–687.
31. Goldstein O, Asher C, Barbry P, et al. An epithelial high-affinity amiloride-binding site, different from the Na^+ channel. J Biol Chem 1993; 268:7856–7862.
32. Staub O, Verrey F, Kleyman TR, et al. Primary structure of an apical protein from *Xenopus laevis* that participates in amiloride-sensitive sodium channel activity. J Cell Biol 1993; 119:1497–1506.
33. Cunningham SA, Clements ML, Arrate MP, et al. Cloning and expression of the 55 kDa subunit of the epithelial amiloride-sensitive sodium channel (abstr). J Cell Biol 1990; 111:63a.
34. Kaupp UB, Niidome T, Tanabe T, et al. Primary structure and functional expression from complementary DNA of the rod photoreceptor cyclic GMP-gated channel. Nature 1989; 342:762–766.
35. Ahmad I, Redmond LJ, Barnstable CJ. Developmental and tissue-specific expression of the rod photoreceptor cGMP-gated ion channel gene. Biochem Biophys Res Commun 1990; 173:463–470.
36. Ahmad I, Korbmacher C, Segal AS, et al. Mouse cortical collecting duct cells show nonselective cation channel activity and express a gene related to the cGMP-gated rod photoreceptor channel. Proc Natl Acad Sci USA 1992; 89:10262–10266.
37. Korbmacher C, Volk T, Segal AS, et al. ATP and calcium modulate a non-selective cation channel in M-1 mouse CCD cells (abstr). J Am Soc Nephrol 1993; 4:870.
38. Stanton BA. Characterization of apical and basolateral membrane conductances of rat inner medullary collecting duct. Am J Physiol (Renal Fluid Electrolyte Physiol) 1989; 256:F862–F868.
39. Light DB, Ausiello DA, Stanton BA. Guanine nucleotide-binding protein, α*i-3, directly activates a cation channel in rat renal inner medullary collecting duct cells. J Clin Invest 1989; 84:352–356.
40. Light DB, Corbin JD, Stanton BA. Dual ion-channel regulation by cyclic GMP and cyclic GMP-dependent protein kinase. Nature 1990; 344:336–339.
41. Light DB, McCann FV, Keller TM, Stanton BA. Amiloride-sensitive cation channel in rat inner medullary collecting duct cells. Am J Physiol (Renal Fluid Electrolyte Physiol) 1988; 255:F278–F286.
42. Light DB, Schwiebert EM, Karlson KH, Stanton BA. Atrial natriuretic peptide inhibits a cation channel in rat inner medullary collecting duct. Science 1989; 243:383–385.
43. DePalo D, Karlson K, Stanton B. Expression of amiloride-sensitive sodium conductance in Xenopus oocytes injected with mRNA from rat kidney (abstr). FASEB J 1990; 4:A267.
44. Kizer N, Hu J-M, Fejes-Toth G, Stanton BA. Whole cell conductances and single channel analysis of a cortical collecting duct cell line isolated from a transgenic mouse (abstr). FASEB J 1991; 5:A869.
45. Stanton BA, Karlson K. Molecular cloning of a cGMP-gated renal cation channel cDNA (abstr). FASEB J 1992; 6:A1808.

46. Kizer N, Lewis B, Ciampolillo F, Stanton B. Aldosterone and AVP stimulate electrogenic sodium reabsorption in an inner medullary collecting duct (IMCD) cell line isolated from a transgenic mouse (abstr). J Am Soc Nephrol 1992: 3:811.
47. Stanton BA, Kizer N, McCoy D, et al. Molecular cloning of a cGMP-gated cation channel cDNA in IMCD (abstr). J Am Soc Nephrol 1993; 4:880.
48. McCoy DE, Karlson K, Molday RS, Stanton BA. Polymerase chain reaction (PCR) localization of an amiloride-sensitive, non-selective cGMP-gated cation channel in mouse kidney (abstr). J Am Soc Nephrol 1993; 4:874.
49. Stanton B, McCoy D, Kizer N, et al. Molecular cloning of cGMP-gated cation channel cDNAs in kidney. FASEB J. In press.
50. Pittler SJ, Lee AK, Altherr MR, et al. Primary structure and chromosomal localization of human and mouse rod photoreceptor cGMP-gated cation channel. J Biol Chem 1992; 267:6257–6262.
51. Chen T-Y, Peng Y-W, Dhallan RS, et al. A new subunit of the cyclic nucleotide-gated cation channel in retinal rods. Nature 1993; 362:764–767.
52. Dhallan RS, Macke JP, Eddy RL, et al. Human rod photoreceptor cGMP-gated channel: Amino acid sequence, gene structure, and functional expression. J Neurosci 1992; 12:3248–3256.
53. Marom S, Dagan D, Winaver J, Palti Y. Brush-border membrane cation conducting channels from rat kidney proximal tubules. Am J Physiol 1989; 257:F328–F335.
54. Gogelein H, Greger R. Na^+ selective channels in the apical membrane of rabbit late proximal tubules (pars recta). Pflugers Arch 1986; 406:198–203.
55. Palmer LG, Frindt G. Amiloride-sensitive Na channels from the apical membrane of the rat cortical collecting tubule. Proc Natl Acad Sci USA 1986; 83:2767–2770.
56. Palmer LG, Frindt G. Effects of cell Ca and pH on Na channels from rat cortical collecting tubule. Am J Physiol 1987; 253:F333–F339.
57. Palmer LG, Frindt G. Conductance and gating of epithelial Na channels from rat cortical collecting tubule: Effects of luminal Na and Li. J Gen Physiol 1988; 92:121–138.
58. Laskowski FH, Christine CW, Gitter AH, et al. Cation channels in he apical membrane of collecting duct principal cell epithelium in culture. Renal Physiol Biochem 1990; 13:70–81.
59. Ling BN, Hinton CF, Eaton DC. Amiloride-sensitive sodium channels in rabbit cortical collecting tubule primary cultures. Am J Physiol (Renal Fluid Electrolyte Physiol) 1991; 261:F933–F944.
60. Oh Y, Benos DJ. Single-channel characteristics of a purified bovine renal amiloride-sensitive Na channel in planar lipid bilayers. Am J Physiol (Cell Physiol) 1993; 264:C1489–C1499.
61. Sariban-Sohraby S, Latorre R, Burg M, et al. Amiloride-sensitive epithelial Na^+ channels reconstituted into planar lipid bilayer membranes. Nature 1984; 308:80–82.
62. Hamilton KL, Eaton DC. Single-channel recording from two types of amiloride-sensitive epithelial Na^+ channels. Membr Biochem 1986; 6(2):149–171.
63. Filipovic D, Sackin H. A calcium-permeable stretch-activated cation channel in renal proximal tubule. Am J Physiol (Renal Fluid Electrolyte Physiol) 1991; 260:F119–F129.
64. Filipovic D, Sackin H. Stretch- and volume-activated channels in isolated proximal tubule cells. Am J Physiol (Renal Fluid Electrolyte Physiol) 1992; 262:F857–F870.
65. Merot J, Bidet M, Gachot B, et al. Patch clamp study on primary culture of isolated proximal convoluted tubules. Pflugers Arch 1988; 413:51–61.
66. Gogelein H, Greger R. A voltage-dependent ionic channel in the basolateral membrane of late proximal tubules of the rabbit kidney. Pflugers Arch 1986; 407(suppl 2):S142–S148.
67. Paulais M, Teulon J. A cation channel in the thick ascending limb of Henle's loop of the mouse kidney: Inhibition by adenine nucleotides. J Physiol (London) 1989; 413:315–327.
68. Teulon J, Paulais M, Bouthier M. A Ca^2-activated cation-selective channel in the basolateral membrane of the cortical thick ascending limb of Henle's loop of the mouse. Biochim Biophys Acta 1987; 905:125–132.
69. Poncet V, Merot J, Poujeol P. A calcium-permeable channel in the apical membrane of primary cultures of the rabbit distal bright convoluted tubule. Pflugers Arch 1992; 422:112–119.
70. Ono S, Mougouris T, Dubois TD Jr., Sansom SC. ATP and calcium modulation of mechanosensitive nonselective cation channels of IMCD cells. Am J Physiol (Renal Fluid Electrolyte Physiol) 1994; 267:F558–F565.
71. Hamilton KL, Benos DJ. A non-selective cation channel in the apical membrane of cultured A6 kidney cells. Biochim Biophys Acta 1990; 1030:16–23.
72. Marunaka Y, Ohara A, Matsumoto P, Eaton DC. Cyclic GMP-activated channel activity in renal epithelial cells (A6). Biochim Biophys Acta Bio-Membr 1991; 1070:152–156.
73. Kleyman TR, Kraehenbuhl J-P, Ernst SA. Characterization and cellular localization of the epithelial Na^+ channel: Studies using an anti-Na^+ channel antibody raised by an antiidiotypic route. J Biol Chem 1991; 266:3907–3915.

74. Sariban-Sohraby S, Sorscher EJ, Brenner BN, Benos DJ. Phosphorylation of a single subunit of the epithelial Na^+ channel protein following vasopressin treatment of A6 cells. J Biol Chem 1988; 263:13875–13879.
75. Kleyman TR, Cragoe EJ Jr, Kraehenbuhl JP. The cellular pool of Na^+ channels in the amphibian cell line A6 is not altered by mineralocorticoids: Analysis using a new photoactive amiloride analog in combination with anti-amiloride antibodies. J Biol Chem 1989; 264:11995–12000.
76. Smith PR, Saccomani G, Joe E-H, et al. Amiloride-sensitive sodium channel is linked to the cytoskeleton in renal epithelial cells. Proc Natl Acad Sci USA 1991; 88:6971–6975.
77. Benos DJ, Saccomani G, Sariban-Sohraby S. The epithelial sodium channel: Subunit number and location of amiloride binding site. J Biol Chem 1987; 262:10613–10618.
78. Sariban-Sohraby S, Burg M, et al. Methylation increases sodium transport into A6 apical membranes vesicles: Possible mode of aldosterone action. Science 1984; 225:745–746.
79. Ausiello DA, Stow JL, Cantiello HF, et al. Purified epithelial Na^+ channel complex contains the pertussis toxin-sensitive $G\alpha_{i\text{-}3}$ protein. J Biol Chem 1992; 267:4759–4765.
80. Sariban-Sohraby S, Fisher RS, Abramow M. Aldosterone-induced and GTP-stimulated methylation of a 90 kDa polypeptide in the apical membrane of A6 epithelia. J Biol Chem 1994; 268:26613–26617.
81. Szerlip HM, Weisberg L, Clayman M, et al. Aldosterone-induced proteins: Purification and localization of GP65,70. Am J Physiol 1989; 256:C865–C872.
82. Blazer-Yost BL, Fesseha Y, Cox M. Aldosterone-mediated Na^+ transport in renal epithelia: Time-course of induction of a potential regulatory component of the conductive Na^+ channel. Biochem Int 1992; 26:887–897.
83. Mohrmann M, Cantiello HF, Ausiello DA. Inhibition of epithelial Na^+ transport by atriopeptin, protein kinase *c*, and pertussis toxin. Am J Physiol (Renal Fluid Electrolyte Physiol) 1987; 253:F372–F376.
84. Smith JJ, Welsh MJ. Fluid and electrolyte transport by cultured human airway epithelia. J Clin Invest 1993; 91:1590–1597.
85. Karlson KH, Ciampollilo-Bates F, McCoy DE, Kizer NL, Stanton BA. Cloning of a cGMP-gated cation channel from mouse kidney inner medullary collecting duct. Biochem Biophys Acta. In press.
86. Rotin D, Bar-Sagi D, O'Brodovich H, Merilainen J, Lehto VP, Canessa CM, Rossier BC, Downey GP. An SH3 binding region in the epithelia Na^+ channel (αrENaC) mediates its localization at the apical membrane. EMBO J 1994; 13:4440–4450.
87. Duc C, Farman N, Canessa CM, Bonvalet J-P, Rossier BC. Cell-specific expression of epithelial sodium channel α, β, and γ subunits in aldosterone-responsive epithelia from the rat: Localization by in situ hybridization and immunocytochemistry. J Cell Biol 1994; 127:1907–1921.
88. Lingueglia E, Renard S, Waldmann R, Voilley N, Champigny G, Plass H, Lazdunski M, Barbry P. Different homologous subunits of the amiloride-sensitive Na^+ channel are differently regulated by aldosterone. J Biol Chem 1994; 269:13736–13739.

25

Renal Potassium Channels

Mirian A. Boim
Paulista School of Medicine, São Paulo, Brazil

Steven C. Hebert
Brigham and Women's Hospital and Harvard Medical School, Boston, Massachusetts

INTRODUCTION: GENERAL CHARACTERISTICS OF POTASSIUM CHANNELS

Potassium channels in the kidney play diverse physiological roles, including the regulation of cell volume, the maintenance of cell potential, and the transepithelial transport of potassium. Over the past few years, the cDNAs encoding many K^+ channels have been isolated, but only a few of these appear to be significantly expressed in the kidney. Structural models of these channels have been proposed (Fig. 1) (1–3) and several experimental strategies have been employed to define certain functional domains (e.g., components of the ion pore and voltage sensor) within these channels. Despite this important progress, we know very little about the biochemical regulation of these K^+ channels and even less regarding transcriptional regulation. But given recent progress in the molecular identification of new K^+ channels that exhibit significant expression in the kidney (e.g., Refs. 2–5), such information should be forthcoming. In this chapter we provide an overview of some of the types of K^+ channels that have been identified in the mammalian kidney, discuss their role in mediating renal potassium excretion, and describe recent and exciting information on the molecular characterization of these channels.

Potassium handling by the kidney depends the coordinated functioning of different cell types in several distinct segments of the nephron (6). The interaction of potassium transporters, pumps, and channels working in a complex interaction in apical and basolateral membranes determines the direction and the magnitude of potassium transport in such nephron segments. Potassium recycling occurs across the basolateral membrane of proximal tubules and the apical membrane of thick ascending limbs. In mammalian proximal tubules, potassium is accumulated into cells via Na^+,K^+-ATPase located in the basolateral membrane (6). This action is opposed by two pathways that mediate K^+ efflux (recycling) from the cell to extracellular fluid: K^+-Cl^- cotransporters and K^+ channels (7–9). Two different types of K^+ channels appear to be involved in basolateral K^+ recycling. The activity of low-conductance (20 pS) voltage-gated K^+ channels apparently parallels Na^+,K^+-ATPase activity (10,11) (probably coupled to the changes in membrane potential), since basolateral membrane conductance decreases when the pump is inhibited by ouabain (12). In addition, it has been suggested that K^+ recycling across the basolateral membrane of the proximal tubule can be accomplished by ATP-sensitive K^+ channels (K_{ATP}), which are modulated by Na^+,K^+-ATPase-mediated changes in intracellular levels (13). Microelectrode analysis in the isolated perfused rabbit proximal tubule have provided evidence that K_{ATP} channels are a major determinant of the macroscopic K^+ conductance of basolateral membranes (13).

Potassium recycling also occurs in the thick ascending limb, where Na^+, K^+, and Cl^- are absorbed via Na-K-2Cl cotransport. However, the net reabsorption of K^+ is much less than Na^+

and Cl^- because K^+ is recycled across the luminal membrane. Patch-clamp studies using cultured cells have identified different types of K^+ channels in this segment, either in the apical and basolateral membranes (14–18). Ca^{2+}-activated and voltage-dependent K^+ channels have been described; however, only K_{ATP}-type K^+ channels are found in apical membranes of native TAL cells. This latter K^+ channel has a high open probability, is voltage- and calcium-independent, and inhibited by millimolar concentrations of ATP (13,14,16).

Potassium is secreted mainly by the distal tubule and collecting duct (6,19,20). Two classes of K^+ channel have been described in this region. One class is characterized by a high single-channel conductance (42 to 180 pS), exhibits sensitivity to calcium, and is voltage-gated such that the open probability increases with membrane depolarization (21–23). The other class of K^+ channel has a lower single-channel conductance (4 to 9 pS), is calcium- and voltage-insensitive, has a high open probability (24,25), and is sensitive to pH and ATP (26,27).

CLASSIFICATION AND STRUCTURAL CHARACTERISTICS OF RENAL POTASSIUM CHANNELS

Ion channels are transmembrane proteins that form narrow, hydrophilic pores through which ions can diffuse passively. Normally channels can transport ions at a higher rate than exchangers, cotransporters, or pumps. Fluxes as high as 1 million ions/sec can be achieved by channels (28). Thus ion channels can catalize ion fluxes into and out of the cell and, to operate sensibly, they must open or close rapidly in response to biological signals. This occurs because channel proteins can switch rapidly between conducting and nonconducting conformations. This mechanism of control of the channel by biological stimuli is referred as "gating." Another important characteristic of ion channels is their selectivity. This property permits channels to distinguish or discriminate among ions. There are some cases where potassium, for instance, permeates the pore at a rate 10^4-fold higher than the rate for Na^+, which is smaller than K^+ ion. Thus, one of the most important goals of ion channel research is to understand the two crucial functions of gating and ionic selectivity.

Based on these properties, K^+ channels can be classified into five broad categories: (a) voltage-gated K^+ (K_V) channels can open or close in response to changes in membrane potential; (b) calcium-activated K^+ (K_{Ca}) channels are modulated by changes in the intracellular calcium concentration; (c) ligand-gated K^+ channels are controlled by neurotransmitters (serotonin), hormones (norepinhephrine and acetylcholine), or cyclic nucleotides (cyclicGMP); (d) ATP-sensitive K^+ (K_{ATP}) channels are regulated by the intracellular concentration of ATP; and (e) stretch-controlled (K_{str}) channels are modulated by mechanical forces.

Ion channels vary considerably in their electrophysiological and pharmacological properties, even within a single class of channels. Thus, K^+ channels can also be categorized, based on the characteristics of their ionic current profile, as delayed or outward rectifiers and inward rectifiers.

Delayed Rectifiers

Delayed-rectifier K^+ channels exhibit slowly activating outward currents with time constants on the order of hundreds of milliseconds. Several members of voltage-gated K^+ channels present delayed rectification, including the slow-activating voltage-dependent K^+ channel (I_{sK}) and those from the *Shaker* superfamily (29). Although both types of K^+ channel are delayed rectifiers, the molecular models proposed for these channels are remarkably different, as shown in Fig. 1.

The voltage-gated *Shaker*-type K^+ channels show a highly conserved core region, which contains six hydrophobic α helical segments (S1–S6) proposed to span the membrane, flanked by variable amino and carboxyl termini. The putative pore-forming region (H5) is located between the S5 and S6 segments (30–32). *Xenopus laevis* oocyte expression studies have provided evidence that these channels are formed by homomultimeric assembly (33,34) with four identical subunits joining together to create a single active channel (1) (see Fig. 1). Moreover, the existence of heteromultimeric channels has been suggested (35,36), which could create K^+ channels with different properties compared with homultimeric channels. This type of assembly would increase the possibilities for expression of channels with more diverse properties than predicted based just on the number of channel proteins encoded in the genome (37).

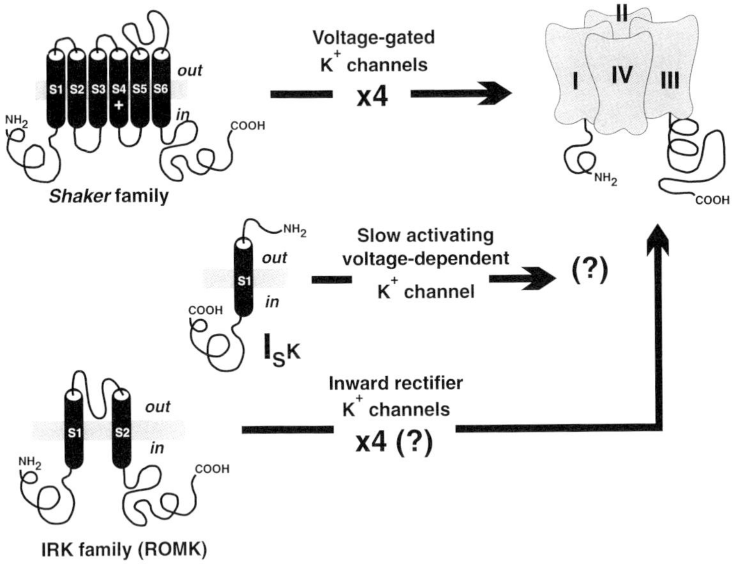

Figure 1 The proposed topology of renal potassium channels. The cylinders represent putative membrane-spanning α helices and are numbers S1 to S6 from the amino-(NH_2) terminus to the carboxyl-(COOH) terminus. See text for discussion.

The second class of delayed rectifiers includes the slow voltage-gated K^+ channels. A channel protein showing a slow voltage-gated K^+ current was recently cloned from rat kidney (2). The cloned cDNA encodes a membrane protein (I_{sK}) of 130 amino acids, which forms a channel that differs structurally from *Shaker* channels as well as from other cloned K^+ channels (ATP-sensitive and IRK1) (Fig. 1). The predicted structural model of the I_{sK} channel presents only a single membrane-spanning domain, with the NH_2-terminus located in the extracellular site and the carboxyl end inside the cell. Of interest, the I_{sK} channel has no recognizable H5-like region. This has called into question whether the I_{sK} protein is in fact capable of forming the ion-conducting portion of an ion channel. In this regard, a recent study has suggested that I_{sK} may encode a regulatory protein rather than a specific ion channel (38). In this study, K^+-channel activity was observed in *Xenopus laevis* oocytes injected with a low amount of synthetic messenger RNA (complementary RNA, cRNA) transcribed from the I_{sK} cDNA, while Cl^- channels were expressed in oocytes injected with larger amounts of I_{sK} cRNA. A single polypeptide that forms the ionic pore of a channel could not account for such a dramatic change in ionic selectivity.

Inward Rectifiers

Channels showing inward current rectification permit a greater influx of an ion at hyperpolarized membrane potential than efflux during depolarization. They are characterized by a lack of significant voltage gating and by their ability to transport potassium more readily in the inward than outward direction (39,40). Inward rectifiers include the classic (strong) inwardly rectifying (IRK) K^+ channels, which exhibit little or no conductance above a certain threshold potential, and the "weakly" inwardly rectifying ATP-sensitive K^+ (K_{ATP}) channels which show a reduced but significant conductance at depolarizing potentials. The structural model suggested for the inward rectifiers differs from that for voltage-gated K^+ channels (see Fig. 1); the inward rectifiers have only two membrane-spanning domains (M1 and M2). However, these channels (IRK and K_{ATP}), in sharp contrast to the I_{sK} channel (see discussion above), conserve the amino acid segment that is homologous to the pore-forming H5 region of the voltage-gated K^+ channel. The conservation of an H5-like region would be consistent with the IRK and K_{ATP} proteins forming the ion-conducting pore of the K^+ channel. However, it is not known if the IRK channel is assembled in the same fashion as *Shaker*-type channels, that is, if it is composed of several identical subunits (homomultimeric). In addition, the possibility of heteromultimeric complexes should not be excluded, since variable electrophysiological profiles have been found for K_{ATP} channels in the mammalian nephron (reviewed in Ref. 41), which could be explained by different isoforms of the channel assembling into functional units.

ELECTROPHYSIOLOGICAL CHARACTERISTICS AND LOCALIZATION OF RENAL POTASSIUM CHANNELS

As discussed above, ion channels exhibit a high degree of diversity, varying in their electrophysiological and pharmacological properties. However, channels belonging to a specific class present certain general characteristics that make it possible to categorize them. Table 1 summarizes these general characteristics and localizations along the mammalian nephron. The slow-activating voltage-dependent K^+ channels (I_{sK}) show slow activation of K^+ currents after membrane polarization, lasting for at least 20 min (2), suggesting that the channel responsible for the outward current does not undergo inactivation. In addition, the outward K^+ current induced by I_{sK} is reduced in the presence of the K^+ channel blockers, tetraethylammonium (TEA) and Ba^{2+}. Immunohistochemical analysis has shown that the I_{sK} protein (channel or channel regulator, see above) is present in apical membranes of proximal tubule cells (5).

The voltage-gated K^+ channels (K_V channels; also referred as *Shaker*-type in Table 1) can close or open in response to changes in the membrane potential. They are characterized by single ion transport rates in the range of 10^7 per sec, high ion selectivity, and a steep voltage sensitivity of their ion conductance (23). The ion conductance of K_V channels is basically controlled by two processes: (a) voltage-dependent activation, which controls the time- and voltage-dependence of the ion channel opening in response to changes in membrane potential, and (b) an inactivation process, which controls the rate and extent of ion-channel closure during a maintained depolarization. In addition, the ion conductance activity of these channels is modulated by protein dephosphorylation and interaction with guanyl nucleotide binding (G) proteins (42). Voltage-sensitive K^+ channels can be inhibited by several agents. Charybdotoxin and its many isoforms are known to block several types of K^+ channels, including the K_V-type channels. This toxin is thought to act by physically plugging the channel's pore. On the other hand, agents like tetraethylammonium (TEA^+) have a different mechanism of inhibition since, unlike peptide toxins, which are too large to permeate the

Table 1 Renal Localization of K^+ Channel Types

Type	Localization	General characteristics
I_{SK}	Proximal tubule	Voltage-gated Delayed rectifier Slow activation of K^+ current Inhibited by TEA^+ and Ba^{2+}
Shaker-type	Cortical collecting duct Distal tubule	Voltage-gated Delayed rectifier High conductance K^+ selectivity Inhibited by TEA^+, charybdotoxin
IRKs (K_{ATP})	Proximal tubule Thick ascending limb Cortical collecting duct	High K^+ selectivity Inward rectification Sensitive to sulfonylurea Inhibited by Ba^{2+} but not TEA^+ Rundown reversed by Mg-ATP

narrower parts of the pore, TEA^+ is believed to partially enter the ion pore when it blocks the channel (43).

Shaker-like cDNA clones have recently been identified in rabbit kidney and renal epithelial cell lines (LLC-PK1, pig proximal tubule), and M1-CCD, cortical collecting duct) by using the polymerase chain reaction (PCR) with *Shaker*-specific oligonucleotide primers (44). One of these clones (KC22) is highly expressed in the rabbit kidney and cell cultures from rabbit distal tubule (4). Recently, a K^+ channel with features of both *Shaker* and cyclic nucleotide-gated (K_{cn}) K^+ channels has been identified (45). The deduced K_{cn} protein shows 45% amino acid homology with the *Shaker* superfamily; however, unlike *Shaker* channels, the K_{cn} channel contains a putative cyclic nucleotide-binding domain. Northern analysis showed that the K_{cn} channel is importantly expressed in the mammalian kidney.

As shown in Table 1, the inward-rectifying channels (IRK and K_{ATP}) are characterized by high open probability, low-to-moderate conductance at a physiological K^+ concentration of 5 m*M*, and inward rectification (28). The inward rectification is independent on blockade of outward current by internal cations. Magnesium is the cytoplasmic cation that gives rise to the inward rectification. Mg^{2+} can apparently enter ion inner vestibule of the channel but cannot diffuse through the channel (28,40). Patch-clamp experiments, have shown that the outward current becomes noisy in the presence of 100 μM Mg^{2+} (28), consistent with a flickery-type block. The Mg^{2+} block is dependent on both concentration (activity) and voltage (46). Thus, internal Mg^{2+} can modulate channel conductance, inducing rectification, which is abolished in the absence of Mg^{2+}. In addition, there is an interaction of inward rectifier channels with permeant ions through multiple binding sites present in the pore (28). These permeant ions—such as Ba^{2+}, Na^+, and Cs^+—can either slowly permeate or block the pore and are believed to be responsible for the K^+ conductance not increasing linearly with K^+ concentration (47).

The activity of the K_{ATP}-type inward rectifying K^+ channel is inhibited by increasing intracellular ATP concentrations, which can vary from μM to m*M*, depending on the subtype of channel (41,48). Actually, the ADP/ATP ratio appears to be even more important in regulating the channel activity than ATP per se (49). K_{ATP} channels are calcium- and voltage-insensitive, being highly sensitive to changes in pH in the rat but not in the rabbit thick ascending limb (16,50). In addition to ATP, the channel activity is also blocked by hypoglycemic agents (sulfonylureas) glibenclamide, tolbutamide, and glyburide (48). K_{ATP} channels also display rundown (loss of channel activity) after membrane patch excision, which can be reversed by Mg-ATP (Table 1). Although IRK and K_{ATP} channels show inward rectification, the IRK channels are stronger rectifiers compared with the weakly rectifying ATP-sensitive K^+ channel. Moreover, IRK channels, unlike K_{ATP} channels, are insensitive to sulfonylureas and the channel rundown is not prevented by internal Mg-ATP (51).

K_{ATP} channels are found in several sites along the nephron (Fig. 2). K_{ATP} channels displaying a 50-pS conductance have been found in the basolateral membrane of the proximal tubule, where they appear to play an important role in the obligate K^+ recycling associated with Na^+,K^+-ATPase activity (52). In the apical membrane of the thick ascending limb of Henle, at least two types of K_{ATP} channels have been described: channels with either 20-pS and 60-pS conductances. Both K_{ATP} channels appear to be involved in the Na^+-K^+-$2Cl^-$ cotransporter function, promoting K^+ recycling from cell to lumen (16,53). K_{ATP} channels have also been found in both apical and basolateral membranes of principal cells of the cortical collecting duct, playing a key role in K^+ secretion (6,50).

MOLECULAR CHARACTERIZATION OF POTASSIUM CHANNELS

Although the patch-clamp technique has proved to be an invaluable tool for evaluation of the kinetic and the pharmacological properties of single ion channels, it was quite limited in providing a detailed biochemical or molecular characterization of channels. However, with the advent of molecular biology approaches, like expression cloning and cloning by homology, our understanding of K^+ channels has been greatly advanced. Some general aspects of our current understanding of the molecular features of K^+ channels are presented below.

Voltage-Gated K Channels

A major advance in understanding the functioning, biochemistry, and molecular structure of the voltage-gated K (K_V) channels was achieved in 1987, when the *Shaker* gene which encodes K_V

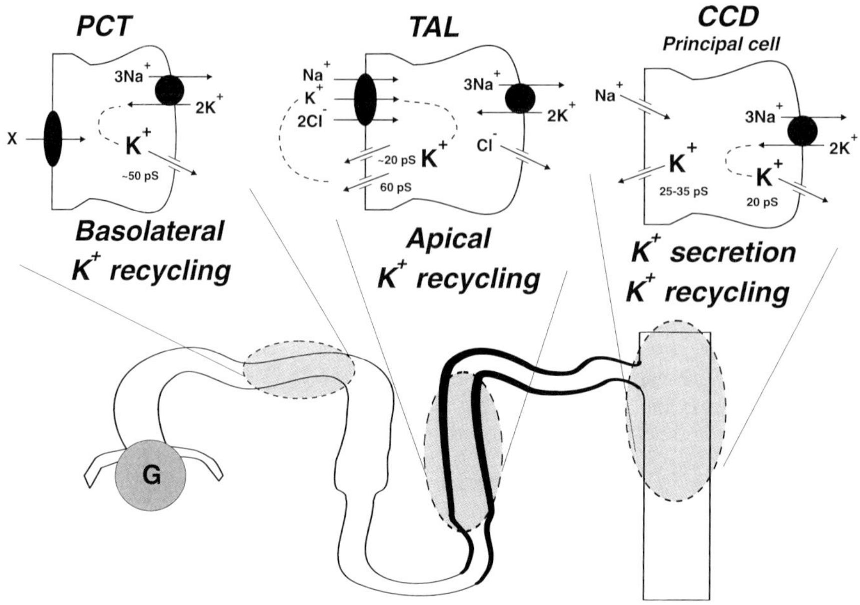

Figure 2 Distribution of ATP-sensitive (K_{ATP}) potassium channels in the mammalian nephron. Abbreviations: PCT, proximal convoluted tubule; TAL, thick ascending limb of Henle; CCD, cortical collecting duct. (From Ref. 41.)

channels was cloned from *Drosophila melanogaster* (54). Four distinct *Shaker* genes have been identified: *Shaker*, *Shab*, *Shaw*, and *Sha I*. Molecular analysis of the *Shaker* locus indicates that some of these genes produce alternatively spliced transcripts, giving rise to a greater molecular diversity of related channels (55,56). Mammalian homologues for all of the *Drosophila* K^+ channel genes have been isolated from rat, mouse, and humans (57–60). Injection of cRNAs transcribed from the cloned cDNAs into *Xenopus laevis* oocytes have led to the successful expression of the K_V channels.

The *Shaker* channel proteins and the homologous vertebrate voltage-gated channels have a number of common molecular features (see Fig. 1). The conserved S4 membrane-spanning segment is arginine-rich and represents a major part of the apparatus that senses changes in membrane voltage (61). Of particular interest are the NH_2- and COOH-termini, which have been implicated in the inactivation of the channel. Two mechanisms have been proposed for *Shaker* channel inactivation, a fast N-type inactivation, probably involving the NH_2 terminus, and a slow C-type inactivations involving the COOH terminus (62,63). It has been shown that the N-type of inactivation acts like a "ball and chain" mechanism, where the NH_2 terminal ball swings into the internal mouth of the channel and blocks the channel from the inside (64,65). This type of inactivation is sensitive to tetraethylammonium (TEA^+) applied internally. The C-type inactivation is suggested to be due to closure of the external mouth of the channel. This latter mechanism is unaffected by internal TEA^+ but it is sensitive to the presence of external TEA^+ (62).

As discussed above, voltage-gated K^+ channels can be inhibited by several agents. Experiments involving mutating the channel protein have provided some insights into the molecular mechanism by which these molecules interact with and block the channel. For example, TEA^+ blocks the channel by interacting with the pore (43). The threonine at position 32 alters K^+ channel blockade by external TEA^+, and changing this residue to lysine, arginine, glutamine, or valine makes the channel essentially insensitive to TEA^+. Moreover, substituting tyrosine, a different aromatic amino acid, at this same position enhanced the blocking affinity 50-fold, suggesting that the amino acid at position 32 is specifically involved in binding of external TEA (32,43). Of interest in this regard, the pore forming H5 region of *Shaker* channels is rich in aromatic residues. Recently, a computational model based on the interaction between monovalent cations and the π electrons of the benzene ring present in the aromatic amino acids has been used to explain the selectivity of *Shaker* channels to K^+ over Na^+, Rb^+, and Li^{2+}. The model predicts that in an aqueous environment, the interaction between these residues and the cation is influenced by solvation. In the complex benzene-litium for instance, the cation is small enough that no water molecules can solvate the Li^+. On the other hand, for the complex benzene-K^+, solvation occurs and the energy necessary to remove the cation is smaller; thus K^+ would be preferred (66) over Li^+ or Na^+.

ATP-Sensitive K^+ Channels

ATP-sensitive K^+ (K_{ATP}) channels have been identified in several excitable cells such as pancreatic β cells, central neurons, cardiac, skeletal, and smooth muscle, as well as nonexicatable systems such as respiratory and tubular epithelia (48). Thus these channels are involved in several different functions, as diverse as glucose-stimulated insulin release, muscle relaxation, and regulation of urinary K^+ secretion. Although K_{ATP} channels present in different cells share several properties, some differences have been observed among channels from different tissues or even from different portions of the same tissue (41,48). These divergent characteristics (e.g., differences in single-channel conductances) suggest that different isoforms of K_{ATP} channels may exist.

Table 2 shows some functional features of renal K_{ATP} channels, including ROMK1, a recently cloned ATP-regulated K^+ channel from rat kidney thought to represent a renal K_{ATP} channel (see below). While renal K_{ATP} channels share many properties and characteristics of K_{ATP} found in other tissues, such as pancreatic β cells and cardiac muscle cells (48), they lack sensitivity to external TEA^+, exhibit a lower sensitivity to sulfonylurea-type inhibitors, and require higher ATP concentrations (millimolar vs. micromolar in β cells) to inhibit channel activity (41,53). Variable conductances, sensitivities to ATP, pH and sulfonylureas have been observed. Moreover, the K_{ATP} channel type found in excitable cells (e.g., pancreatic β cells and myocytes) is highly sensitive to metabolic alterations, responding to substrates such as glucose, while the channel type found in renal epithelia appears to be modulated mainly by hormones via second messengers (53).

While sensitivity to ATP is a basic characteristic of all K_{ATP} channels, some controversy has centered around the physiological relevance of ATP in modulating channel activity. This is especially true for K_{ATP} channels found in excitable cells where the ATP concentration necessary to close the channel (micromolar) is much lower than measured cytosolic ATP concentration (millimolar). It is quite clear, however, that the concentration of ATP required to effect channel closure in mammalian renal K_{ATP} channels is within the range of ATP concentrations observed in renal epithelial cells [K_i

Table 2 Characteristics of K_{ATP} Channels in Kidney

	ROMK1	Rat TALH	Rabbit TALH	Rat CCD
Single-channel conductance, γ (pS)	≈40	≈60	10–27	25–35
Inward rectifier	Yes	Yes	Yes	Yes
Open probability, P_0	High	High	High	High
ATP inhibits		Yes	Yes	Yes
↓ Po by ↑ ATP or ↑ (ADP/ATP)	±	At [m*M*]	At [m*M*]	$K_i \approx 0.5–1$ m*M*
Inhibited by glyburide	No	No	Yes High μM	Yes High μM
Ion selectivity	$K^+ >> Na^+$	$K^+ = Rb^+ = NH_4^+ = Cs^+ >> Na^+$	$K^+ >> Na^+$ (20:1)	$K^+ >> Na^+$ (20:1)
pH_i-dependence (↓ pH_i reduces P_0)	?	Yes	No	Yes
↑ $[Ca^{2+}]_i$ inhibits	?	Yes	No	No

for channel closure ≈ 0.6 to 1.0 m*M* (67); cell (ATP) 1 to 3 m*M* (68,69)]. Moreover, the gating kinetics for ATP can be modulated by ADP such that ADP increases the K_i for ATP possibly by competition for an ATP binding site on the channel or an associated subunit. Thus, increasing the activity of membrane ATPases would reduce ATP and increase ADP (or increase the ADP/ATP ratio) and thereby enhance K_{ATP} channel activity. Such a mechanism could account for the functional coordination of basolateral Na^+,K^+-ATPase activity and K_{ATP} channels in proximal tubules (13,41,53).

The mechanism(s) for ATP-ADP modulation of K_{ATP} channel activity is also not clear. In pancreatic β cells and myocytes, nonhydrolyzable ATP analogues are as effective as ATP in effecting channel closure and ATP can close the channel in the absence of Mg^{+2}, indicating that phosphorylation of the channel or an associated subunit is not required for the ATP sensitivity of this type of K_{ATP} channel (48,49,70). Phosphorylation-dephosphorylation processes have, however, been implicated in regulating K_{ATP} channel activity. Trube and coworkers have shown that exposure of K_{ATP} channels from pancreatic β cells to micromolar concentrations of Mg-ATP induces reactivation of channel activity after rundown, whereas the removal of Mg^{2+} or replacement of ATP with nonhydrolyzable analogue results in rapid channel rundown (71,72). Moreover, in addition of the protein kinase A inhibitor (PKI) to the cytosolic face of a membrane patch from β cells reduces whereas exposure to the catalytic subunit of cAMP-dependent protein kinase stimulates channel activity (72). Based on these data Ribalet and coworkers have suggested a different mechanism for K_{ATP} channel regulation by ATP (73): the cAMP-dependent protein kinase activity is increased at low concentrations of ATP and reduced at higher concentrations due to the binding of ATP to PKI, whose activity is thereby enhanced. In other words, low levels of ATP provides substrate for protein kinase A, which hydrolyzes ATP, producing phosphorylation and channel opening. Higher concentrations of ATP activate PKI, preventing channel phosphorylation and resulting in channel closure. Wang and Giebisch have proposed a similar mechanism for channel gating by ATP of the apical K_{ATP} channel from principal cells of cortical collecting ducts (67).

Cloning of the Putative Renal K_{ATP} Channel

A channel with high K^+ selectivity was recently cloned from the outer medulla of rat kidney (3). The cDNA, ROMK1, predicts a 45-kDa channel protein with a novel topology (Figs. 3 and 4). Unlike voltage-gated K^+ channels, the ROMK1 protein exhibits only two membrane-spanning domains (M1 and M2). This channel exhibits inward rectification, high K^+ selectivity when expressed in *Xenopus laevis* oocytes, and belongs to the newly described family of inward rectifiers (IRK family) (51,74).

The expression of the ROMK1 protein in *Xenopus* oocytes gives rise to channels with the following properties: (a) a conductance of 30 to 40 pS with high K^+:Na^+ selectivity; (b) weak inward rectification in the presence of cytosolic-side Mg^{2+}; (c) sensitivity to external Ba^{2+} but not TEA^+; (d) "rundown" or loss of channel activity in the absence of MgATP; and (e) reactivation of channels after rundown by reexposure to MgATP. Based on these general properties, this channel has been proposed to form, or provide the pore-forming component of, the renal ATP-sensitive potassium channels. Recent studies examining the nephron distribution of mRNAs encoding this channel would be consistent with this possibility.

The ROMK1 channel conserves an amino acid segment between the two putative membrane spanning helices that is homologous to the pore-forming H5 region of the voltage-gated K^+ channel (59% similarity; see Fig. 4). This is of considerable importance, not only because it suggests that ROMK1 and the 6-membrane spanning segments-type voltage-gated channels evolved from a common ancestral gene but also because it supports an important role for the H5 region in forming the channel pore. In addition, this region contains the Gly-Try-Gly triplet, which is conserved in all channels with high K^+ selectivity (75) (interestingly, the triplet is absent from the I_{sK}-type channel).

One of the cardinal features of the K_{ATP} channel, found in apical membranes of principal cells in the cortical collecting duct, is a lack of sensitivity to external TEA^+ (24,26,41,50), which is also a feature of the K^+ secretory channel in this nephron segment (18,26,41). ROMK1 also exhibits not significant TEA^+ sensitivity (up to 15 m*M*) when expressed in *Xenopus laevis* oocytes (3). On the other hand, the presence of an aromatic amino acid, Phe, at position 148 within the H5 region would be expected to impart significant sensitivity to external TEA^+ in ROMK1. Site-directed mutagenesis

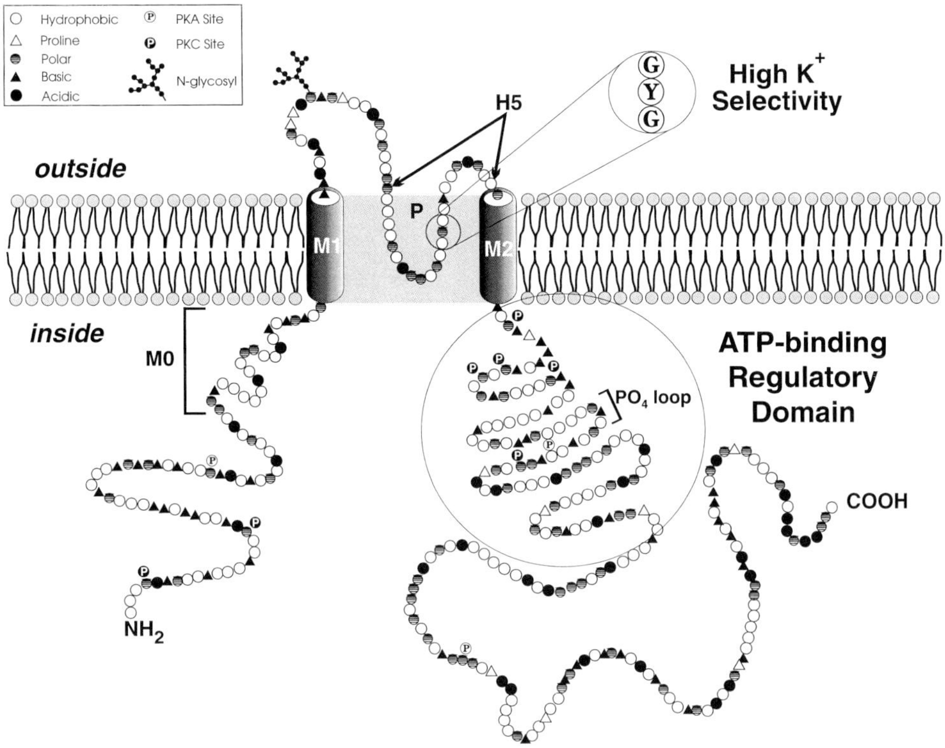

Figure 3 Structural model of the ROMK1-channel protein. Each symbol represents a single amino acid. The H5 region contains the putative channel pore labeled "P". M1 and M2 are putative membrane-spanning a helices. The M0 region is an amphipathic region. The potential kinase A (PKA; open circles with "P") and kinase C (PKC; solid circles with "P") phosphorylation sites are indicated. The single possible N-linked glycosylation (N-glycosyl) site is shown.

studies in *Shaker* channels have shown that substitution of an aromatic amino acid at a similar position confers a high sensitivity to external TEA^+. We have argued that the positively charged amino acid arginine (R) at position 147 (see Fig. 4) would be expected to interfere with TEA^+ binding and thus could explain the lack of high TEA^+ sensitivity in the ROMK1 channel (3). In addition, we have suggested that two other differences in the H5 region between the *Shaker*-type channels and ROMK1 may affect ROMK1 channel function: positions occupied by Val 140 and Ile 142 in ROMK1 (see Fig. 4) have been shown in *Shaker*-type channels to alter NH_4^+ and K^+/Rb^+ conductances. Specific mutagenesis studies of the ROMK1 pore will be required to substantiate these possibilities.

The ROMK1 channel protein appears to be glycosylated at Asn 117, which would be consistent with an extracellular location for the segment linking the first membrane-spanning helix, M1, and the channel pore, P. An amphipathic region, MO, which is adjacent to M1 on the NH_2-terminal side of the ROMK1 channel protein (Figs. 3 and 4) has 36% similarity to the S4 region of voltage-gated ion channels. This region in ROMK1, however, lacks the typical S4 arginine-rich segment and the basic amino acid at every third position thought to provide the voltage sensor for *Shaker* channels. The net charge of +1 on ROMK1 versus +8 for the *Shaker* A-type channel would be consistent with the virtual voltage insensitivity of the ROMK1 channel (3).

In view of the effects of ATP on renal K_{ATP} channel function, the finding of a potential nucleotide-binding site on ROMK1 has provided further support for the possibility that the ROMK channel can function as an ATP-sensitive K^+ channel. As shown in Figs. 3 and 4, a region following the M1 region contains a Walker type A site motif within a so-called PO_4 or P loop (Fig. 3) that has been linked to ATP binding in many other proteins. Further support for the possibility that this

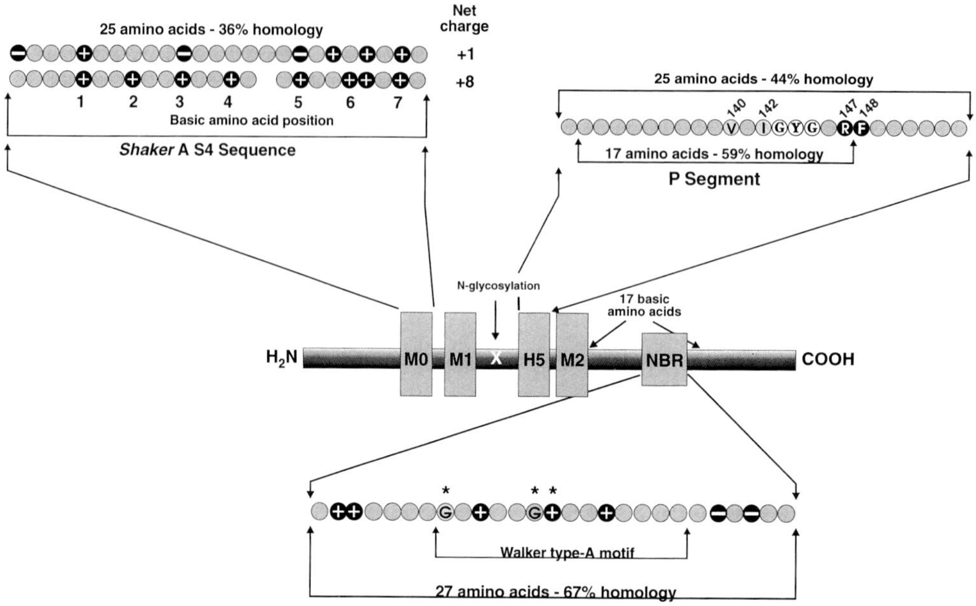

Figure 4 Similarity of defined regions on the ROMK1 channel protein to other proteins. The boxed regions, M0, M1, H5, M2, and NBR (potential nucleotide-binding region) are shown. Each circle represents a single amino acid. Abbreviations: G, glycine, Y, tyrosine; R, arginine; F, phenylalanine; positive sign, arginine or lysine; negative sign, acidic residue. See Ref. 3.

region might be involved in nucleotide binding was provided by the finding that a larger, 27–amino acid region containing the Walker type A site, exhibits high homology to the catalytic subdomain I of ERBB3, a member of the epidermal growth factor (EGF) receptor tyrosine kinase family. In addition, several potential protein kinase A and protein kinase C phosphorylation sites are present on the ROMK1 channel protein. Interestingly, some of these potential phosphorylation sites are within a region that has been postulated to form an ATP-binding regulatory region containing a high density of basic (positively charged) amino acids (see Fig. 3). Based on these structural considerations, two possible mechanisms have been proposed for ATP-dependent regulation of ROMK1 channel activity (3). First, the potential PKA sites in the ROMK1 channel protein may be involved in the Mg-ATP-dependent reactivation after the channel rundown. Second, the channel activity may involve regulation by highly positively charged ATP-binding regulatory domain in a manner similar to that proposed for the "ball and chain" mechanism (28,76) or suggested for the "R" domain of the cystic fibrosis transmembrane conductance regulator, CFTR, Cl^- channel (77–79). Further studies will be required to explore these possibilities.

ACKNOWLEDGMENTS

This work was supported in part by a grant to S.C.H. from the National Institutes of Health (DK37605). M.B. was supported by a grant from CAPES—Brazil (1393/92-3).

REFERENCES

1. MacKinnon R. Determination of the subunit stoichiometry of a voltage-activated potassium channel. Nature 1991; 350:232–235.
2. Takumi T, Ohkubo H, Nakanishi S. Cloning of a membrane protein that induces a slow voltage-gated potassium current. Science 1988; 242:1042–1045.

3. Ho K, Nichols G, Lederer WJ, et al. Cloning and expression of an inwardly rectifying ATP-regulated potassium channel. Nature 1993; 362:31–38.
4. Desir GV, Velázquez H. Identification of a novel K-channel gene (KC22) that is highly expressed in distal tubule of rabbit kidney. Am J Physiol 1993; 264:F128–F133.
5. Sugimoto T, Tanabe Y, Shigemoto R, et al. Immunohistochemical study of a rat membrane protein which induces a selective potassium permeation: Its localization in the apical membrane portion of epithelial cells. J Membr Biol 1990; 113:39–47.
6. Stanton BA, Giebisch GH. Renal potassium transport. In: Windhager EE, ed. Handbook of Physiology, Renal Physiology. New York: Oxford University Press, 1992:813–874.
7. Sackin H, Palmer LG. Basolateral potassium channels in renal proximal tubule. Am J Physiol 1987; 253:F476–F487.
8. Parent L, Cardinal J, Sauve R. Single-channel analysis of a K channel at basolateral membrane of rabbit proximal convoluted tubule. Am J Physiol 1988; 254:F105–F113.
9. Palmer LG, Sackin H. Regulation of renal ion channels. FASEB J 1988; 2:3061–3065.
10. Gogelein H, Greger R. Potassium selective channels in the basolateral and luminal membranes of the late proximal tubule of the rabbit kidney. Pflugers Arch 1987; 410:288–295.
11. Gogelein H, Greger R. Single channels recordings from basolateral and apical membranes of the renal proximal tubules. Pflugers Arch 1984; 401:424–426.
12. Messner G, Wang W, Paulmichl M, et al. Ouabain decreases apparent potassium conductance in proximal tubule of the amphibian kidney. Pflugers Arch 1985; 404:131–137.
13. Tsuchiya K, Wang W, Giebisch GH, Welling PA. ATP is a coupling modulator of parallel Na,K-ATPase-K-channel activity in the renal proximal tubule. Proc Natl Acad Sci USA 1992; 89:6418–6422.
14. Merot J, Pocet V, Bidet M, Tauc M, Poujeol P. Apical membrane ionic channels in the rabbit cortical thick ascending limb in primary culture. Biochem Biophys Acta 1991; 1070:387–400.
15. Bleich M, Schlatter E, Greger R. The luminal K^+ channel of the thick ascending limb of Henle's loop. Pflugers Arch 1990; 415:449–460.
16. Wang WH, White S, Geibel J, Giebisch GH. A potassium channel in the apical membrane of rabbit thick ascending limb of Henle's loop. Am J Physiol 1990; 258:F244–F253.
17. Taniguchi J, Guggino WB. Membrane stretch: a physiological stimulator of Ca^{2+}-activated K^+ channels in thick ascending limb. Am J Physiol 1989; 257:F347–F352.
18. Gogelein H, Greger R. Role of K conductive pathways in the nephron. Kidney Int 1987; 31:1055–1064.
19. Shimizu T, Yoshitomi K, Tanigushi J, et al. Effect of high NaCl intake on Na and K transport in the rabbit distal convoluted tubule. Pflugers Arch 1989; 414:500–508.
20. Malnic G, Berlirner RW, Giebisch G. Flow dependence of K secretion in cortical distal tubules of the rat. Am J Physiol 1989; 256:F932–F941.
21. Frind G, Palmer LG. Ca-activated K channels in apical membrane of mammalian CCT and their role in K secretion. Am J Physiol 1987; F458–F467.
22. Gitter AH, Beyenbach KW, Christine CW, et al. High-conductance K channels in apical membranes of principal cells cultured from rabbit cortical collecting duct anlagen. Pflugers Arch 1987; 408:282–290.
23. Hunter M, Lopes A, Boulpaep E, Giebisch G. Regulation of single K-channels from apical membrane of rabbit collecting tubule. Am J Physiol 1986; 251:F725–F733.
24. Frindt G, Palmer L. Low-conductance K channels in apical membrane of rat cortical collecting tubule. Am J Physiol 1989; 256:F143–F151.
25. Wang WH, Henderson RM, Giebel J, et al. Mechanism of aldosterone-induced increase of K conductance in early renal tubule cells of the frog. J Membr Biol 1989; 11:277–289.
26. Wang W, Giebel J, Giebisch G. Regulation of small conductance K channel in the apical membrane of rat cortical collecting tubule. Am J Physiol 1990; 259:F494–F502.
27. Wang W, Giebel J, Giebisch G. The role of intracellular pH in aldosterone induced increase in K conductance in early distal tubule cells of frogs. Kidney Int 1989; 36:491.
28. Hille B. Ionic Channels of Exitable Membranes. Sunderland, MA: Sinauer, 1992.
29. Wei A, Covarrubias M, Butler A, et al. K^+ current diversity is produced by an extended gene family conserved in *Drosophila* and mouse. Science 1990; 248:599–603.
30. Miller C. 1990. Annus mirabilis of potassium channels. Science 1991; 252:1092–1096.
31. Hartmann HA, Kirch GE, Drewe JA, et al. Exchange conduction pathways between two related K channels. Science 1991; 251:942–944.
32. Yellen G, Jurman ME, Abramson T, MacKinnon R. Mutations affecting internal TEA blockade identify the probable pore forming region of a K^+ channel. Science 1991; 251:939–941.
33. Timpe LC, Schwartz TL, Tempel BL, et al. Expression of functional potassium channels from *Shaker* cDNS in *Xenopus* oocytes. Nature 1988; 331:143–145.
34. Iverson LE, Tanouye MA, Lester HA, et al. A-type potassium channel expressed from *Shaker* locus cDNA. Proc Natl Acad Sci USA 1988; 85:5723–5727.

35. Sheng M, Liao YJ, Jan YN, Jan LY. Presynaptic A-current based on heteromultimeric K^+ channels detected in vivo. Nature 1993; 365:75–75.
36. Wang HW, Kunkel DD, Martin TM, et al. Heteromultimeric K^+ channels in terminal and juxtaparanodal regions of neurons. Nature 1993; 365:75–79.
37. Pongs O. Molecular biology of voltage-dependent potassium channels. Physiol Rev 1992; 72:S69–S78.
38. Attal B, Guillemare E, Lesage F, et al. The protein I_{sK} is a dual activator of K^+ and Cl^- channels. Nature 1993; 365:850–852.
39. Kurachi Y. Voltage-dependent activation of the inward-rectifier potassium channel in the ventricular cell membrane of the guinea-pig heart. J Physiol 1985; 366:365–385.
40. Matsuda H. Magnesium gating of the inwardly rectifying K^+ channel. Annu Rev Physiol 1991; 53:289–298.
41. Wang W, Sackin H, Giebisch G. Renal potassium channels and their regulation. Annu Rev Physiol 1992; 54:81–96.
42. Catterall WA. Structure and function of voltage-sensitive ion channels. Science 1988; 242:50–61.
43. MacKinnon R, Yellen G. Mutations affecting TEA blockade and ion permeation in voltage-activated K^+ channels. Science 1990; 250:276–279.
44. Desir GV, Hamlin E, Puente AH, et al. Isolation of putative voltage-gated epithelial potassium channel isoforms from rabbit kidney and LLC-PK1 cells. Am J Physiol 1992; 262:F151–F157.
45. Desir GV, Welling P, Engel D, Zhang J. Molecular cloning and expression of a cyclic nucleotide-gated K^+ channel. 26th Annual Meeting of the American Society of Nephrology, Boston, MA, Nov 14–17, 1993.
46. Matsuda H. Voltage-dependent block of cardiac inwardly rectifying K^+ channels by internal Mg^{+2}. In: Strata P, ed. Mg^{+2} and Excitable Membranes. Heidelberg: Springer-Verlag, 1990.
47. Sakamnn B, Trube G. Conductance properties of single inwardly rectifying potassium channels in ventricular cells from guinea-pig heart. J Physiol 1984; 347:641–657.
48. Ashcroft SJH, Ashcroft FM. Properties and functions of ATP-sensitive K-channels. Cell Signal 1990; 2:197–214.
49. Misler S, Falke LC, Gillis K, McDaniels MA. Metabolic regulated potassium channel in dispersed rat pancreatic β cells. Proc Natl Acad Sci USA 1986; 83:19–23.
50. Wang W, Shwab A, Giebisch G. Regulation of small-conductance K^+ channel in apical membrane of rat cortical collecting tubule. Am J Physiol 1990; 259:F494–F502.
51. Kubo Y, Baldwin TJ, Jan JN, Jan L. Primary structure and functional expression of a mouse inward rectifier potassium channel. Nature 1993; 362:127–132.
52. Tsuchiya K, Wang W, Giebisch G, Welling PA. ATP is a coupling modulator of parallel Na,K-ATPase-K-channel activity in the renal proximal tubule. Proc Natl Acad Sci USA 1992; 89:6418–6422.
53. Misler S, Giebisch G. ATP-sensitive potassium channels in physiology, pathophysiology, and pharmacology. Curr Opin Nephrol Hypertens 1992; 1:21–33.
54. Papazian DM, Schwarz TL, Tempel BL, et al. Cloning of genomic and complementary DNA from Shaker, a putative potassium channel gene from *Drosophila*. Science 1987; 237:749–753.
55. Kamb A, Tseng-Grank J, Tanouye MA. Multiple products of the *Drosophila* Shaker gene may contribute to potassium channel diversity. Neuron 1988; 1:421–430.
56. Schwarz TL, Tempel BL, Papazian DM, et al. Multiple potassium-channel components are produced by alternative splicing at the Shaker locus in *Drosophila*. Nature 1988; 331:137–142.
57. Tempel BL, Jan YN, Jan LY. Cloning of a probable K^+ channel gene from mouse brain. Nature 1988; 331:143–145.
58. Baumann A, Grupe A, Ackermann A, Pongs O. Structure of the voltage-dependent K^+ channel is conserved from *Drosophila* to vertebrate central nervous system. EMBO J 1988; 7:24570–2463.
59. Christie MJ, Adelman JP, Douglas J, North RA. Expression of a cloned rat brain potassium channel in *Xenopus* oocytes. Science 1988; 244:221–224.
60. McKinnon D. Isolation of a cDNA clone coding for a putative second potassium channel indicates the existence of a gene family. J Biol Chem 1989; 264:8230–8236.
61. Liman ER, Hess P, Weaver F, Koren G. Voltage-sensing residues in the S4 region of a mammalian K^+ channel. Nature 1991; 253:752–756.
62. Choi KL, Aldrich RW, Yellen G. Tetraethylammonium blockade distinguishes two inactivation mechanisms in voltage-activated K^+ channels. Proc Natl Acad Sci USA 1992; 88:5092–5095.
63. Hoshi T, Zagotta WN, Aldrich RW. Two types of inactivation in *Shaker* K^+ channels: effects of alterations in the carboxy-terminal region. Neuron 1991; 7:547–556.
64. Hoshi T, Zagotta WN, Aldrich RW. Biophysical and molecular mechanism of *Shaker* potassium channel inactivation. Science 1990; 250:533–538.
65. Zagotta WN, Hoshi T, Aldrich RW. Restoration of inactivation in mutants of *Shaker* potassium channels by a peptide derived from *Sh*B. Science 1990; 250:568–570.
66. Kumpf R, Dougherty DA. A mechanism of ion selectivity in potassium channels: Computational studies of cation-π interactions. Science 1993; 261:1708–1710.

67. Wang W, Giebisch G. Dual effect of adenosine triphosphate on the apical small conductance K^+ channel of the rat cortical collecting duct. J Gen Physiol 1991; 98:35–61.
68. Uchida S, Endou H. Substrate specificity to maintain cellular ATP along the mouse nephron. Am J Physiol 1988; 255:F977–F983.
69. Torikai S. Dependency of microdissected nephron segments upon oxidative phosphorylation and exogenous substrates: A relationship between tubular anatomical location in the kidney and metabolite activity. Clin Sci 1989; 77:287–295.
70. Ashcroft FM. Adenosine 5′-triphosphate-sensitive potassium channels. Annu Rev Neurosci 1988; 11:97–118
71. Rorsmann P, Trube G. Glucose dependent K^+-channels in pancreatic β cells are regulated by intracellular ATP. Pflugers Arch 1985; 37:495–498.
72. Ohno-Shosaku T, Zunkler BJ, Trube G. Dual effects of ATP on K^+ currents of mouse pancreatic β cells. Pflugers Arch 1987; 408:133–138.
73. Ribalet B, Ciani S, Eddlestone GT. ATP mediates both activation and inhibition of K^+ (ATP) channel activity via cAMP-dependent protein kinase in insulin-secreting cell lines. J Gen Physiol 1989; 94:693–717.
74. Kubo Y, Reuveny E, Slesinger PA, et al. Primary structure and functional expression of a rat G-protein-coupled muscarinic potassium channel. Nature 1993; 364:802–806.
75. Heginbotham L, Abramson T, MacKinnon R. A functional connection between the pores of distantly related ion channels as revealed by mutant K^+ channels. Science 1992; 258:1152–1155.
76. Armstrong CM, Bezanilla F. Inactivation of the sodium channel: II. Gating current experiments. J Gen Physiol 1977; 70:567–590.
77. Anderson MP, Welsh MJ. Regulation by ATP and ADP of CFTR chloride channels that contain mutant nucleotide-binding domains. Science 1992; 257:1701–1704.
78. Rich DP, Gregory RJ, Anderson MP, et al. Effect of deleting the R domain on CFTR-generated chloride channels. Science 1991; 253:205–207.
79. Anderson MP, Berger HA, Rich DP, et al. Nucleoside triphosphates are required to open the CFTR chloride channel. Cell 1991; 67:775–784.

26

Structure and Regulation of Na,K-ATPase in the Kidney

Peter L. Jørgensen, Li Mei Meng, and Per Amstrup Pedersen
August Krogh Institute, Copenhagen University, Copenhagen, Denmark

INTRODUCTION

Na,K-ATPase in the nephron couples the chemical energy in ATP to transport of Na^+ and other solutes across the tubular epithelium. As the Na,K pump in kidney, it is responsible for the primary active transport of half of net Na^+ reabsorption and the secondary active transport of a number of solutes in the proximal tubules. Practically all Na^+ reabsorption in the thick ascending limbs of Henle (TAL), distal convoluted tubules (DCT), and collecting tubules (CT) is driven by the Na,K pump. In proximal tubules (PCT), the Na, K pump transports about one-third of the filtered Na^+ that enters the cytoplasmic region of low electrochemical potential for Na^+ via Na^+-coupled cotransporters for glucose, amino acids, phosphate etc., or countertransport systems for Ca^{2+} or H^+ (1,2) (see Fig. 1). The Na,K pump thus supplies the energy for active transport processes of widely different characteristics in the discrete nephron segments, but this diversity does not reside within the Na,K pump per se. The main function of the Na,K pump appears to be the same in all nephron fragments; to maintain electrochemical gradients for Na^+ across the cell membrane (1–4).

Regulation of the Na,K pump in kidney and other epithelia bordering the extracellular fluid space is decisive for establishing and maintaining constant osmolality of the body fluids and for adaptation to changes in salt and water intake. Mechanisms have evolved allowing for rapid, acute adaptation of the activity of existing pumps or for slow, chronic adaptation of the number of pump sites in a given nephron segment (1,2,5–10). Provided that the supply of metabolic energy is sufficient, the capacity for active transtubular solute reabsorption is determined by the concentration of Na,K pump sites (5–7). The nature and direction of the transtubular transport processes depend on the Na^+-coupled transport elements in the cell membranes in conjunction with the conductances of the cell membranes and their junctions and basement membrane.

Purification and crystallization of Na,K-ATPase from kidney (11) and cloning of the $\alpha 1$ subunit and $\beta 1$-subunit genes (12–14) have formed the basis for a more detailed analysis of the mechanisms for control of the activity and concentration of Na,K pumps in the kidney tubules. Cloning of the genes has permitted new molecular biological approaches to the study of the regulation of the Na,K pump: the analysis of gene transcription and translation of mRNA, the hybridization techniques for identification of the α- and β-subunit isoforms in kidney, and very sensitive PCR techniques for analysis of mRNA in single microdissected nephron segments.

It is a major purpose of this review to examine how the avalanche of information about the molecular biology of the Na,K pump in kidney can be put together into a coherent picture to provide answers to some of the important questions concerning the regulation of the Na,K pump in kidney tubules. Another important contribution of the molecular biological approach is the possibility of establishing structure-function relationships through the work on mutant pumps and constructs of

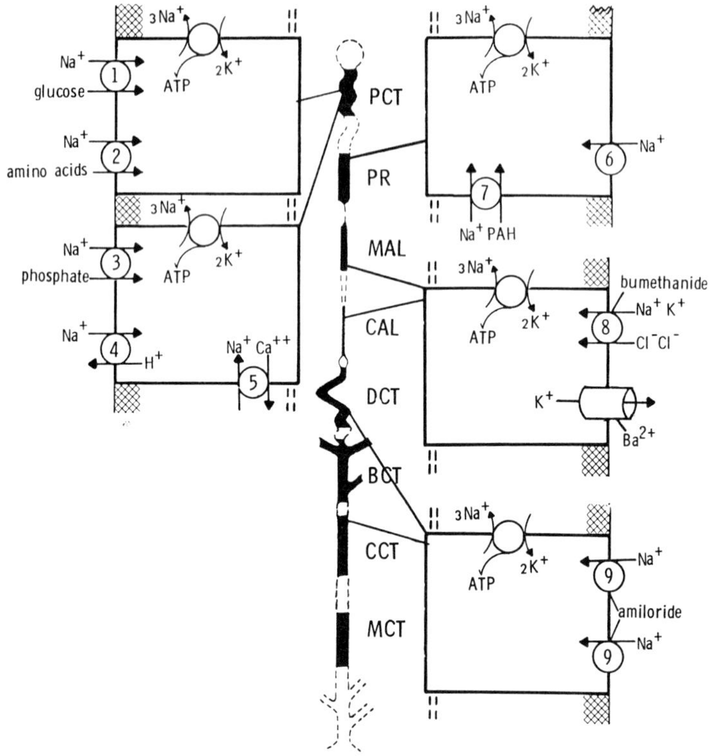

Figure 1 Model for the function of Na,K-ATPase along the nephron. In PCT and PR, the Na,K-pump maintains electrochemical gradients for Na^+ ($\Delta\mu Na^+$) for utilization in secondary active solute transport by Na-coupled carriers that are numbered 1 through 7 (see Refs. 1 and 2 and references therein). In MAL and CAL, transcellular NaCl transport consist of primary active Na^+ transport and secondary active transport of Cl^- through the Na,K, Cl cotransport system in the luminal membrane. Recycling of K^+ through the K channel maintains the membrane potential and the driving force for the flux of Cl^- from cytoplasm to blood. In the CCT, the primary active Na^+ transport is coupled to passive conductance flux of Na^+ ions into the cytoplasm through the amiloride-sensitive Na^+ channel in the luminal membrane.

chimeras with other cation pump proteins. To examine this, we will first consider the distribution of the Na,K pump along the nephron, its localization in the cell, and its association with the cytoskeleton. Next, we will review the structure of the purified Na,K-ATPase and the organization of the $\alpha 1$ and $\beta 1$ subunit genes and their regulation in the kidneys, by ions, and by the hormones that are active in regulation of sodium reabsorption.

Recent Review Articles on the Structure and Function of the Na,K Pump

The expansion of our knowledge of the structure and function of Na,K-ATPase is reflected in a rapid succession of recent reviews on Na,K-ATPase genes and regulation of expression (13), subunit assembly and functional maturation (15), the isozymes of Na,K-ATPase (16), structure and transport mechanism (17), physiological aspects and regulation of Na,K-ATPase (18), reconstitution and cation exchange (19), chemical modification (20), occlusion of cations (21), and structure-function relationships of cation binding (22). Other valuable sources are the review articles and recent developments reported at the international Na,K pump conferences in 1990 (23,24) and 1993 (25).

Na,K-ATPASE IN THE NEPHRON

Distribution of Na,K-ATPase Along the Nephron

Enzyme assays in microdissected segments and histochemical or immunocytochemical analysis show that the highest concentration of Na,K-pump sites per cell or per unit tubule length is found in nephron segments with a high capacity for Na^+ reabsorption. In the TAL and the distal convoluted tubule, the concentration of Na,K-pump sites amounts to 40 to 50 million per cell, while the concentrations are much lower in the thin limbs of Henle (near the detection limit) and in the collecting ducts (3 to 8 million per cell) (see Fig. 1). There are a considerable number of Na,K-pump sites in the proximal convoluted tubule (25 million per cell), but the number drops on advancing to the proximal straight tubule (10 million per cell) (3). These estimates of the apparent number of Na,K-pump sites on the cell surface are obtained by [^{3}H]-ouabain binding in medium containing Mg^{2+} and vanadate or phosphate (3,11). Permeabilization by osmotic or thermic shock does not seem to affect the determination of the number of [^{3}H]-ouabain binding sites (3), while the permeabilization increases Na,K-ATPase activity greatly. In A6 epithelial cells, a considerable pool of latent, presumably intracellular sites can be demasked with optimum concentrations of detergent ($NaDodSO_4$) (26), as in *Xenopus laevis* oocytes (27).

Histochemical analysis shows that the reaction deposit for the ouabain-sensitive K^+ *p*-nitrophenyl phosphatase (K^+-*p*NPPase) is demonstrated only at the inside of the infoldings of the basal lateral membrane, while the deposit is absent from the luminal membrane and the part of the surface membrane facing the contraluminal basement membrane (28). The immunogold- or peroxidase-labeled antibody demonstrated labeling confined to the protoplasmic aspect of the basal lateral membrane (29). In the PCT, no evidence of specific binding to the luminal brush border membrane was found. The binding of the lateral membrane ended sharply at the intracellular junctional complex and distinctly separated the two major cellular membrane domains (29). The intensity of labeling of the basal lateral membrane is uneven, with the most intense labeling in complex invaginated regions. Reaction product was most intense in the basal lateral infoldings of the membranes of the TAL, and also in this segment the luminal membrane was devoid of labeling.

Expression of α-Subunit Isoforms of Na,K-ATPase Along the Nephron

The identification of several isoforms of the α subunit ($\alpha1$, $\alpha2$, $\alpha3$) (12) and β subunit ($\beta1$, $\beta2$) (14,30) has been a major contribution of the molecular biological approach. The $\alpha1\beta1$-isozyme of Na,K-ATPase is ubiquitous and constitutively expressed in most cells. It is predominant in mammalian and amphibian kidney (*Xenopus laevis* and *Bufo marinus*). N-terminal sequencing identified the $\alpha1\beta1$-unit as the isozyme of Na,K-ATPase that has been purified from the outer renal medulla (31). This is confirmed by Northern blot analysis of mRNA (32). Extensive in situ hybridization using isoform-specific cDNA probes reveals the presence of $\alpha1$-subunit mRNA in all nephron segments of the rat, including the CCD, while the $\alpha2$- and $\alpha3$-subunit mRNA cannot be detected (33). Adrenalectomy reduces the $\alpha1$ isoform of Na,K-ATPase in distal rat nephron (34), and aldosterone exclusively alters the pool of the $\alpha1$ isoform in CCD (35).

However, titration of microdissected segments with ouabain (36) and immunological studies have suggested that other isoforms of Na,K-ATPase could be present in the rabbit collecting duct, where Na,K-ATPase is more sensitive to ouabain and to Na^+ than in more proximal tubule segments (36). Heterogeneity with detection of small amounts of the $\alpha2$- or $\alpha3$-subunit isoforms has been demonstrated in rabbit and rat kidney using antibodies with α-subunit isoform specificity (37,38). Two monoclonal antibodies with specificity to the $\alpha1$ or $\alpha3$ isoforms were shown to distinguish Na,K-ATPase in the CCD. The antibody with specificity to the $\alpha1$ isoform inhibited Na,K-ATPase in all segments of the nephron except the CCD, while the antibody with specificity to the $\alpha3$ isoform inhibited Na,K-ATPase only in the CCD. Another attraction is that the presence of an isoform with high sensitivity to ouabain in the CCD would make the CCD a preferential site of action of the endogenous ouabain (39). Unexpectedly, however, the $\alpha3$ isoform mRNA could not be detected in the CCD by PCR on whole kidney RNA or in RNA from microdissected segments (40). To explain the previous detection of a high sensitivity to ouabain for Na,K-ATPase in microdissected CCD, it has been proposed that an $\alpha3$-like isoform is present in the CCD, and several laboratories are engaged in a search for such a new pump isoform. At this point, the conclusion is therefore that the $\alpha 1$ isoform is found in all segments of the kidney including the CCD and that the other known α-subunit isoforms, $\alpha 2$ and $\alpha 3$, are not demonstrable in significant amounts in rat kidney.

Cytoskeletal Associations and Polarity of the Na,K Pump in Kidney Tubules

In the polarized tubule cells of mammalian kidney, the specific associations of Na,K-ATPase with cytoskeletal components and the cell-cell contacts appear to be important for the induction of polarity of the $\alpha\beta$ unit between luminal and basal lateral membranes. The epithelial cell adhesion molecule (CAM) uvomorulin (cadherin) functions as an inducer of cell polarity for the constitutively expressed $\alpha 1\beta 1$ units through cytoplasmic linkage to the membrane cytoskeleton. One link to the cytoskeleton is a high-affinity binding site for ankyrin ($K_d = 10^{-8}$ *M*) that has been demonstrated in the purified renal Na,K-ATPase (41). A fraction of the $\alpha 1\beta 1$-units seems to be associated in Na,K-ATPase-ankyrin-fodrin complexes, with similarity to the capnophorin-ankyrin-spectrin complexes in the cytoskeleton of the human erythrocyte. Induction of cell-cell contact alters the properties and distribution of these proteins. Before contact between the epithelial cells, the ankyrin-fodrin tetramers form complexes with the membrane proteins, either Na,K-ATPase or uvomorulin. On cell-cell contact, uvomorulin seems to mediate redistribution, so that the Na,K-ATPase-ankyrin-fodrin complexes accumulate at the sites of cell-cell contact (42). It is proposed that the cell-cell contacts via uvomorulin induce the specific distribution at the cell surface of Na,K-ATPase during development of the polarized epithelial cells. Once polarity has been established, the proteins are replaced by targeting to the appropriate membrane from the Golgi complex.

Loss of polarity with incorrect localization of Na,K-ATPase to apical membranes has been associated with a number of diseases including polycystic kidney disease (43). Maldistribution of the Na,K-ATPase also accompanies the syndrome of acute renal failure (44), which is seen as a consequence of renal ischemia with low cytoplasmic ATP concentration. After ischemia, the decrease in oxygen uptake in kidney tubules is related to a decline in functional Na,K pumps, while Na,K-ATPase activity measured under V_{max} conditions shows no significant change. After recovery from ischemia, marked changes in ultrastructure of PCT with loss of brush border and loss of the polar distribution of α and β subunits of Na,K-ATPase are revealed by immunocytochemical techniques. The subunits are also present in lumenal membranes and subapical membrane vesicles, and the redistributed Na,K-ATPase remains functional (45,46). There is a similar loss of the polar distribution of ankyrin and fodrin. In the postischemic tubule cells, these cytoskeletal proteins are no longer associated with Na,K-ATPase along the basal lateral infoldings but distributed diffusely throughout the cytosol.

PURIFIED RENAL Na,K-ATPase

Purification and Structure of Renal $\alpha 1\beta 1$ Isozyme of Na,K-ATPase

The procedure for purification of Na,K-ATPase in membrane-bound form from the outer renal medulla of mammalian kidney provides an opportunity for exploring the structure of the Na,K-pump proteins in their native membrane environment. The Na,K-pump protein remains embedded in the membrane bilayer throughout the purification procedure, thus maintaining the asymmetric orientation of the protein in the basolateral membrane of the kidney cell in the purified preparation (11). The selective detergent treatment in the presence of ATP and EDTA removes cytoskeletal and extraneous proteins, while Na,K-ATPase is protected and remains in the membrane. This preparation has been particularly useful in studies of ultrastructure and protein conformation and for the identification of sites for binding of ATP and cations (17,47). A further advantage is that the preparation from outer medulla contains essentially only the ($\alpha 1\beta 1$)-isozyme of Na,K-ATPase, while preparations from most other tissues consist of two or three α- and β-subunit isoforms.

In the pure preparation of Na,K-ATPase from outer renal medulla, the $\alpha 1$-subunit forms 65–70% of the total protein and the molar ratio of α to β is 1:1, corresponding to a mass ratio of about 3:1 (1,5). Functionally the preparation is fully active, in the sense that each $\alpha\beta$-unit binds ATP, P_i, cations, and the inhibitors vanadate and ouabain. The molecular activity is close to a maximum value of 7000–8000 P_i/min. The highest reported binding capacities for ATP and phosphate are in the range of 5 to 6 nmol/mg protein and close to one ligand per $\alpha\beta$ unit (11,48) when fractions with maximum specific activities of Na,K-ATPase (40 to 50 μmol P_i/min/mg protein) are selected for assay. In these preparations the ion-binding capacity was 10 nmol/mg protein for ^{86}Rb and 15 to 17 nmol/mg protein for ^{22}Na.

The membrane-bound preparation from kidney is easily solubilized in nonionic detergent, and analytical ultracentrifugation shows that the preparation consists predominantly (80–85%) of soluble $\alpha\beta$ units with M_r 143,000. The soluble $\alpha\beta$ unit maintains full Na,K-ATPase activity and undergoes the cation- or nucleotide-induced conformational transitions that are observed in the membrane-bound preparation. A cavity for occlusion of 2 K^+ or 3 Na^+ ions can be demonstrated within the structure of the soluble $\alpha\beta$ unit as an indication that the cation pathway is organized in a pore through the $\alpha\beta$ unit rather than in the interphase between subunits in an oligomer (17,48).

Crystal formation is induced by incubation of membrane-bound Na,K-ATPase from kidney with vanadate or other ligands that stabilize the protein in the E_2 conformation. In Na,K-ATPase, the predominant crystal form has the two-sided plane group symmetry, p1, and the unit cell contains one protomeric $\alpha\beta$ unit with a height of 120 μm (Fig. 2). It is asymmetrically inserted into the membrane, protruding about 60 Å on the cytoplasmic surface and only 20 Å at the extracytoplasmic face. This can be inferred from the uneven mass distributions of the α and β-subunits. The α subunit protrudes with a major portion of its mass to form a cytoplasmic protrusion with approximate dimensions 45 × 65 Å in the plane of the membrane (49). The bulk of the hydrophobic residues of the β subunit are exposed to the extracellular surface.

Organization of the α Subunit and Structure of Cation Sites in the Membrane

Selective cleavage and labeling studies established preliminary structure-function correlates for some of the domains formed by the α subunit at the cytoplasmic surface (48) (Fig. 3). Within the large central protrusion comprising 434 residues, cleavage of T1 (at 438, Fig. 3) separates the phosphorylation site (D-369) from other segments that may be involved in ATP binding: a segment contributing a hydrophobic pocket formed by Ile, Val, His and Leu residues for accommodation of adenine and ribose moieties of ATP and the segments around residues that are covalently labeled by ATP analogues (For reference, see Ref. 48). The cytoplasmic loop between transmembrane segment M2 and M3 has been shown to be important for transmission of a conformational change from the ATP site to the cation sites in the membrane interior through selective cleavage of bond C3 or T3. Cleavage of bond T2 near the N terminus releases a segment of 30 residues, and the

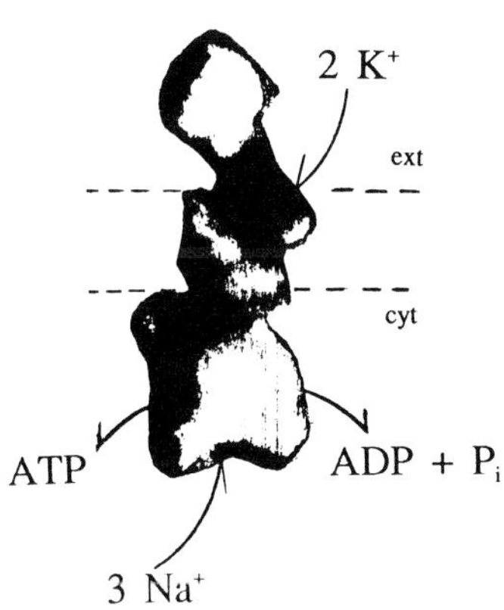

Figure 2 Coupled Na,K transport in a model redrawn from a three-dimensional model of the $\alpha\beta$ unit reconstructed from an electron microscope tilt series of a protomer p1 crystal of Na,K-ATPase induced with Mg^{2+}-vanadate (see Refs. 11 and 28). The position of the lipid bilayer is suggested by the dotted lines.

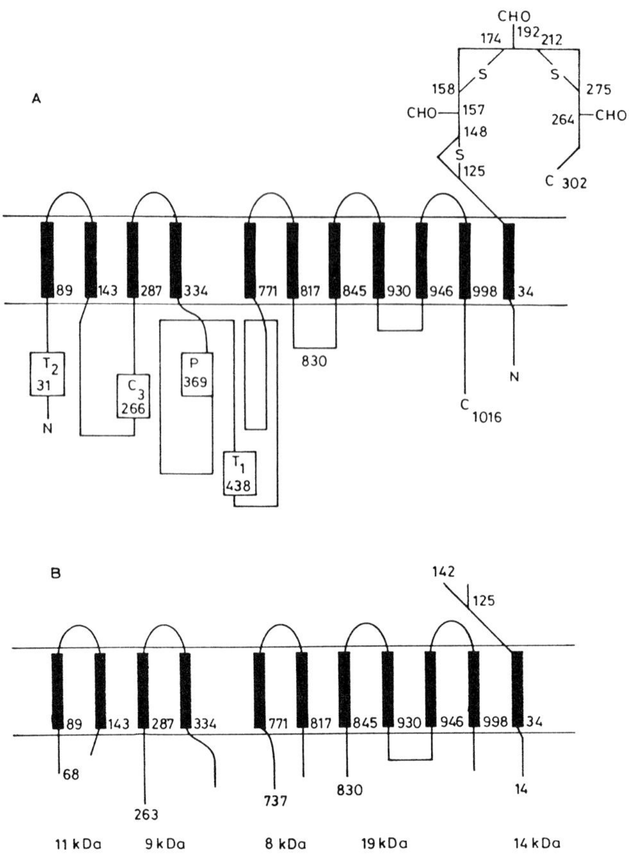

Figure 3 (A) Disposition of the $\alpha\beta$ unit in the membrane, based on sequence information, selective proteolytic digestion of the α subunit, and hydrophobic labeling (48). The model for the β subunit is based on sequencing of surface peptides and identification of S-S bridges (55,56). T1, T2, and C3 show the location of proteolytic splits. The CHO are glycosylated asparagines in the β-subunit. (B) Peptide fragments remaining in the membrane after extensive tryptic digestion of the membrane-bound Na,K-ATPase from outer medulla of pig kidney as described by Karlish et al. (50).

truncated enzyme has an altered conformational equilibrium with altered function of cation and nucleotide sites as an indication that the N terminus is involved in regulation of the conformational equilibrium but that it is not directly involved in formation of sites for ligand binding (48). Little is known about the catalytic functions of the cytoplasmic domains of the C-terminal half of the α subunit, but a segment near the C terminus participates in associations with the β subunit (see below).

The cation sites appear to be located to the intramembraneous part of the α subunit, since it is possible to shave off all of the cytoplasmic protrusion of the α subunit by extensive proteolysis without affecting occlusion of Rb^+ or Na^+ (50). In the membrane model of Fig. 3, there are seven negatively charged residues localized in transmembrane segments of the α subunit. The amino acids with negatively charged or oxygen-containing side chains can be important for binding or translocating the positively charged Na^+ and K^+ ions. Proteolytic digestion and chemical modification suggested that E953 and possibly E954 could be involved in cation binding (50).

Heterologous expression and site-directed mutagenesis has led to identification of a number of potentially important residues, but the development of suitable expression systems has been complicated mainly because most eukaryote cells express high levels of endogenous Na,K-ATPase. Expression in COS-1 (51) and HeLa cells (52,53) has taken advantage of the fact that the Na,K-ATPase activity of the rodent $\alpha1\beta1$ isoform is much more resistant to ouabain than the endogenous enzyme activity. The ouabain sensitive α subunit was modified (L111R and N122D) to encode an ouabain resistant isoform and thus allowing the cells to grow in 1 μM ouabain. The abundance of expressed Na,K-ATPase is relatively low and the system does not allow a thorough characterization of the mutant proteins, since only cells transfected with a functional ouabain-resistant α-subunit allele can be selected and characterized. This approach identifies several carboxyl-containing amino acid residues in the transmembrane region as being critical for overall enzyme function. The carboxyl-containing residues of E327 and D925 are not absolutely essential, but modification of E778, D803, and D807 completely abolishes the activity (52). Further studies are required to see whether this is due to interference with insertion of the protein into the membranes or if the substituted residues are in fact essential for cation binding. Modification of D953 and D954 reduces the specific activity of Na,K-ATPase and alters the apparent affinities for cation activation, but these residues are not essential for the overall Na,K-ATPase activity (52,53).

Structure of the β Subunit of Na,K-ATPase

The Na,K-ATPase and H,K-ATPase are unique in the family of cation pumps in requiring a β subunit for catalytic activity. The β subunit contributes to protein stability and folding and it plays an important role in the functional maturation of the $\alpha\beta$ unit in the endoplasmic reticulum and for intracellular transport to the plasma membrane (15).

The bulk of hydrophilic residues of the β subunit are exposed on the extracellular surface (54), with three sites of complex glycosylation at Asn-157, 192, and 264. The β-subunit sequence has one hydrophobic segment (Ile^{34}-Leu^{58}), which is labeled from the bilayer by light-activated hydrophobic labeling (For references, see Ref. 48). In the β1-subunit isoform, three disulfide bonds are formed by residues Cys^{125}-Cys^{148}, Cys^{158}-Cys^{174}, and Cys^{212}-Cys^{275} (55,56) (Fig. 3), and their reduction is accompanied by loss of Na,K-ATPase activity (55,57). The β subunit is not as well conserved as the α subunit, with 91% overall homology between β subunit of sheep, pig, and human and 61% between β subunit of human and *Torpedo*. The consensus sequences in beta signatures 1 and 2 (58) are preserved in the β-subunit isoforms and β subunit of H,K-ATPase as an indication that the positions of tryptophans and cysteins are well-conserved elements. The β2-subunit isoform has a function as a recognition element for cell adhesion in the brain (30), but this isoform is not expressed in kidney, where interactions with the cytoskeletal elements are mediated through the binding of ankyrin to the α subunit.

ACUTE REGULATION OF THE Na,K-PUMP IN KIDNEY TUBULES

Regulation by Ions and ATP

Acute adaptation within minutes of the turnover rate of existing Na,K pumps is possible because they are working way below their maximum capacity (V_{max}) in the conditions of the kidney tubules. The activities of cytoplasmic ATP and extracellular K^+ are saturating, and pump activity depends on the intracellular $[Na^+]_{cyt}$ activity. This can be explained from the reaction scheme in Fig. 3 (48), showing the relationships between ion movements, phosphoryl transfer, and E_1-E_2 transition. In the normal clockwise operation, the major structural transitions between E_1 and E_2 forms of the $\alpha\beta$ unit constitute the cation translocation steps, Na extrusion involving the E_1P-E_2P transitions and K uptake the E_1K-E_1ATP transition. Na^+ and K^+ are transported in sequence, Na^+ first and then K^+ in a "ping-pong," sequential reaction.

In the reaction cycle in Fig. 4, the rate-limiting step is the conformational transition, E_1-E_2, and these steps are also the control points of the reaction cycle in the tubule cells. At low concentrations of ATP, the rate limiting steps are the transition from E_2K to E_1KATP and the release of K^+ from the occluded state. In conditions where cytoplasmic K^+ increases or the substrate ATP is in short supply, this mechanism will slow the rate of ion movements (47,48). This is illustrated by the decrease in rate at a given Na/K ratio when ATP drops from 1 to 0.2 m*M* (Fig. 5), while a variation of ATP concentration in the range 1 to 3 m*M* has little influence on the rate of ATP splitting. The concentration of ATP in the cytoplasm (2 to 3 mmol/L) is therefore close to saturating the pump. Studies of cation stimulation show that the extracellular K^+ concentration of 4 to 5 mmol/L is sufficient for saturation of K^+-ion sites and the pump rate is determined by the cytoplasmic Na/K

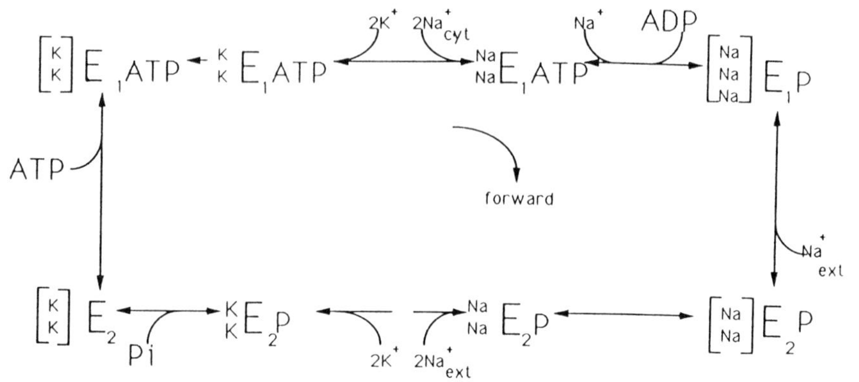

Figure 4 Reaction cycle of the Na,K pump with four major occluded conformations and "ping-pong" sequential cation translocation. The phosphoforms can occlude Na^+ and dephosphoforms can occlude K^+ or Rb^+. Na^+ and K^+ without brackets are cations bound to an open form, and they can exchange with medium cations. $[Na^+]$ or $[K^+]$ within brackets are occluded and prevented from exchanging with medium cations. Note that the charge-translocating step with release of Na^+_{ext} is coupled to transition from $E_1P[3Na]$ to $E_2P[2Na]$ (see Ref. 48 and references therein).

ratio. At the relatively low ratios of 10Na/140K or 20Na/130K in the tubule cells, the data in Fig. 5 predict that the molecular activity of the pump should be only 5–20% of V_{max}. The dependence of pump rate on $[Na^+]_{cyt}$ is steep, and even modest changes in ion activity from 15 to 24 m*M* Na^+ are sufficient for doubling the Na,K-pump's activity (1,5). These predictions from the behavior of isolated Na,K-ATPase have been confirmed in experiments on isolated proximal tubules with measurements of the cation dependence of oxygen uptake (59). There is also a quantitative correlation between the amounts of Na,K-ATPase that can be isolated from the kidney tissue and the transport capacities in the nephron (1).

In the PCT, Na^+ only enters the cytoplasmic space of low electrochemical potential for Na^+ via the Na-coupled cotransport systems for secondary active transport of glucose, phosphate, amino acids, Ca^{2+}, or protons (see Fig. 1). The rate of net solute reabsorption therefore depends on the load of these solutes, and the maximum capacity of the transport systems will be limited by the number of Na,K pumps in the given transport segment (1).

In the medullary TAL, the important function is to dilute the tubule fluid by reabsorbing NaCl in excess of water and thus providing osmotic gradients for concentrating or diluting the urine. The transcellular transport of NaCl consists of secondary active transport of Cl^- in coupling with the entry of Na^+ and K^+ across the lumenal membrane through the Na,K,Cl-cotransport system and primary active Na^+-transport driven by the Na,K pump (1). The Na,K,Cl-cotransport system is inhibited by cytoplasmic Na^+, and the recent cloning and sequencing of its protein confirms that it is a substrate for protein kinases and sensitive to cAMP (60). Regulation of K conductance is important for maintaining the membrane potential close to the magnitude of the equilibrium potential for K^+, providing a driving force for conductance flux of Cl^- from cytoplasm to blood. A Ca^{2+}-activated K channel in the lumenal membrane may also form an important link between second-messenger systems (Ca^{2+}, cAMP dependent protein kinases, and protein phosphatases) and membrane conductance (61).

The rate-limiting steps for transcellular Na^+ transport across the CCD are the passive conductance flux of Na^+ ions into the cytoplasm through amiloride-sensitive Na^+ channels in the lumenal membrane and the active Na^+ transport from cytoplasm to blood which is driven by the Na,K pump. Provided that the supply of ATP is sufficient, the Na,K pump is capable of matching the active flux of Na^+ across the basolateral membrane to the apical sodium conductance. In the early or acute aldosterone-induced response, the turnover rate of existing Na,K pumps in the basolateral membrane is increased in response to upregulation of the lumenal membrane sodium conductance through activation of preexisting latent Na^+-channels (5,6).

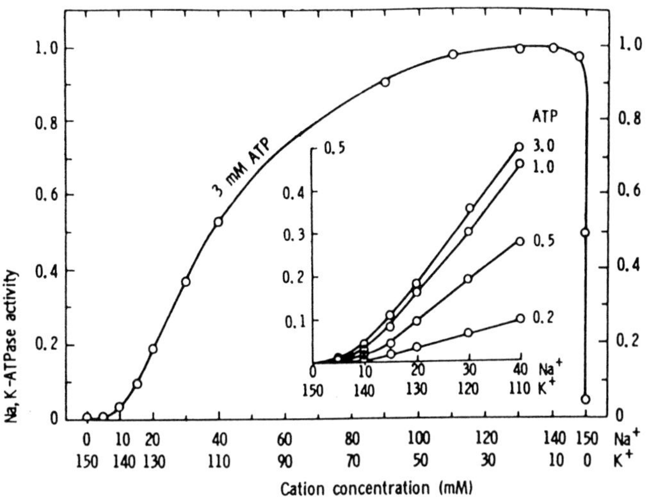

Figure 5 Activity of purified renal Na,K-ATPase as a function of Na^+, K^+, and ATP. In the principal curve, ATPase activity was measured in the presence of 3 m*M* of ATP and variable concentrations of Na^+ and K^+, with the sum of their concentrations being 150 m*M*. In the inset curve, stimulation of Na,K-ATPase at low Na/K ratios was determined at low ATP concentrations (1,2).

Regulation by Protein Kinases, Epinephrine, and Dopamine

A variety of other mechanisms for fast kinetic control of the activity of Na,K pumps in kidney tubules have been proposed mainly as a result of studies on microdissected tubule segments—e.g., direct effects of dopamine and phosphorylation by cAMP-dependent protein kinase A (PKA) or protein kinase C (PKC) (4,8–10). These factors are also known modifiers of channel and carrier proteins and may thus alter the cation conductances of the cell membranes. It is a problem to distinguish direct effects on the Na,K pump from changes in activity that are secondary to altered ion activities in the cytoplasm. Fast changes in the number of Na,K-pump sites may also result from translocation of pumps from intracellular pools at the surface membrane (3,14).

In kidney cell lines in culture, inhibition of ouabain-sensitive Rb^+ uptake is seen after incubation with phorbol ester, and the effect seems to correlate with phosphorylation of the α subunit of Na,K-ATPase (9). Consensus sequences (933-KTRRNS-938) for PKC and PKA phosphorylation are found in the last cytoplasmic loop before the C terminus of the $\alpha 1$ isoform of Na,K-ATPase. Demonstration of phosphorylation of the α subunit by PKA and PKC in isolated Na,K-ATPase has raised hopes that these kinases serve as receptors for a variety of first messengers (prostaglandin E_2, endothelin, adenosine, insulin, norepinephrine, and dopamine) that would inhibit Na,K-ATPase in proximal tubules. The functional significance of these phosphorylation experiments is questionable, because phosphorylation of the α subunit in isolated Na,K-ATPase requires Triton-X-100 (0.1–0.2%) in concentrations in excess of the critical micelle concentration of the detergent, sufficient to completely denature and inactivate Na,K-ATPase (22).

Even more complex interactions involving bidirectional regulation by dopamine and α-adrenergic agonists have been observed in isolated proximal convoluted tubules. Dopamine (10 μM) inhibited Na,K-ATPase in the presence but not in the absence of the α-adrenergic agonist oxymetazoline (1 μM). Na,K-ATPase was stimulated (+20%) by oxymetazoline at Na^+ 10–30 m*M* but not at 50 to 70 m*M* Na^+. Dopamine inhibited (–45%) at 50 to 70 m*M* Na, while at 10 to 30 m*M* Na^+ dopamine inhibited (–35%) only in the presence of oxymetazoline (8,10). Needless to say, these observations involve very complex patterns for activation of the Na,K-ATPase by Na^+. The authors propose that the explanation could be that Na^+ acts not only as an activator and substrate but also as a regulator of the phosphorylation state of the enzyme.

Modulation of Na,K-pump or Na,K-ATPase activity by different intracellular messenger systems can be demonstrated in intact or partially disrupted renal tubules but not in the isolated preparations of Na,K-ATPase from renal tissues (10). The regulators of GTP-binding proteins, the cAMP-PKA or PKC systems, and metabolites of the arachidonic cascade are all known to affect the opening probability of various membrane ion channels and cotransport or countertransport systems. Operationally, it is therefore difficult to discern direct effects on the Na,K pump from indirect effects via altered transepithelial or transmembrane potentials or altered ion activities in the cell cytoplasm.

The question can be raised whether the observed modulation of Na,K-ATPase by the different messengers and protein kinases or phosphatase systems in experiments on microdissected single tubule segments reflect problems in assaying Na,K-ATPase in the complex structure of a partially intact tubule after permeabilization procedures that may leave the enzyme with different concentrations of Mg^{2+}, ATP, Na^+, K^+ or ouabain, depending on ligand activities and the nature of the membrane in the particular tubule segment. Kidney membranes are tight and they show a remarkable tendency for vesiculation (11,56) in the medullary TAL, with formation of right-side-out vesicles with latent Na,K-ATPase activity. In other tubule segments, the tendencies for vesicle formation could be different, leading to formation of mixtures of inside-out and right-side-out vesicles. A variety of artifacts may arise if the access of ligands to the cytoplasmic or extracellular aspects of Na,K-ATPase are limited by vesiculation. The conditions for assay of ion transport, the number of Na,K-pump sites, or of demasked Na,K-ATPase activity therefore have to be strictly defined, to exclude the possibility that some of the unexpected observations based on assays of Na,K-ATPase in intact tubules may be due to unspecific phenomena.

CHRONIC REGULATION OF THE NUMBER OF Na,K-PUMP SITES IN KIDNEY TUBULES

Genes of the Na,K-Pump Proteins

The molecular signals responsible for mediating the specific and highly variable expression of the $\alpha1\beta1$ unit along the nephron of the kidney are not known. Explanations of the nephron-specific expression of the α- and β-subunit genes and the details of the developmental and hormonal regulatory influences have to await detailed analysis of gene expression. Examination of the 5′ end of the $\alpha1$- and $\beta1$-subunit genes may reveal sites for binding of factors and hormone receptor elements that are potentially available in kidney tubules.

Structure and Regulation of the α1-Subunit Gene

On the basis of primer extension and S1 nuclease protection analysis, the transcription initiation site of the $\alpha1$-subunit gene appears to be located between nucleotides-273 and –270 relative to the translation start site (ATG) (62). Exon 1 encodes the first four amino acids (MGKG) of the primary translation product. The first intron is approximately 11 kb in length, and it should be remembered that regulatory sequences can also be found in this region of a gene. A potential TATA box—ATATTTT—is located 27 bp upstream of the transcription initiation site.

In addition to being predominant in the kidney, the $\alpha1$ gene is expressed ubiquitously and thus has the features of a housekeeping gene. As in other constitutively expressed genes, the 5′ portion of the $\alpha1$ gene is rich in G+C exhibiting 67% G+C. The 5′ untranslated region has 75% G+C and the first 900 bp of intron A has 69% G+C. Numerous potential Sp1 transcription factor recognition sequences (GGGCGG) are present in the 5′ flanking region (five sites) and in the 5′ untranslated region (three sites). A potential Sp1 binding site (GGGCGG) is located 18 bp upstream of the apparent TATA box in the position where CCAAT sequences are frequently found. Binding of the selective protein as an oligomer to the Sp1 site in the promoter region can increase transcription many times, and this complex can in part substitute for the function of the TATA box (14,62).

The 5′ flanking regions were examined for potential hormone response elements because the Na,K-ATPase activity in kidney is modulated by hormones, including adrenocortical steroids and thyroid hormone. The glucocorticoid response element consists of a hexanucleotide core TGTTCT, forming a 15-bp dyad symmetry element (62). Regions in the $\alpha1$ gene exhibit a match to the core element, but for each homology to the entire 15 bp, palindrome sequence is low. The $\alpha1$ 5′ flanking region contain sequences matching the core pentanucleotide CACCC, part of an upstream element acting synergistically with the glucocorticoid receptor binding site, but it is not located near a potential glucocorticoid response element.

In the $\alpha 1$ gene, there are only sequences with limited similarity to the consensus sequences of thyroid hormone response elements, while these are observed frequently in the $\beta 1$ gene. Sequence elements that may mediate responses to cAMP and Ca^{2+} are observed in the $\alpha 1$ gene. The promoter region contains a TGACGTTT sequence of –657 that exhibits perfect identity to the sequence that mediates transcriptional activation by Ca^{2+}. The $\alpha 1$ gene also has a sequence resembling binding sites for AP1, AP-2, and AP-3, cellular factors mediating transcriptional activation in response to the phorbol ester stimulated protein kinase C (63). The presence of an AP-1 site raises the possibility that the Na,K-pump gene may be regulated by the *jun* and *fos* oncogenes. Expression of *fos* and *jun* genes is known to be increased by extracellular stimuli such as phorbol esters, tissue growth factors, and ion activities.

Structure of the β1-Subunit Gene

Several β-subunit genes have been characterized (14,64), but only the β1 gene seems to be expressed in kidney tubules. The β1-subunit gene has 6 exons and a 5′ flanking region containing a potential TATA box and several putative CAAT and GC boxes (65). Potential binding sites for thyroid and glucocorticoid receptors were identified together with multiple sequence motifs that exhibit homology to calcium- and serum-responsive elements. Activation of the β1-subunit gene was shown to be mediated by a transcriptional process. Examination of the 5′ flanking region of the β1-subunit gene reveals three potential thyroid hormone response elements (TRE) at positions –455, –226, and –99. T3 regulation of the β1-subunit Na,K-ATPase gene has been studied in an intestinal epithelial cell line where T3 (50 n*M*) stimulates mRNA levels threefold after 24 hr. Transient infection with plasmids containing the β1 promoter and varying length of 5′ flanking region fused to a luciferase reporter gene showed that the TRE at –455 is functional in the β1 gene (66). Using 5′ deletions and site-directed mutagenesis, the sequence spanning 22 bp from –459 to –438 is identified as that required for transactivation by T3. The antisense strand of the sequence contains two hexamers (5′GA*AGGTCA*CTCC*GGGACG*CCGGA 3′). That agrees with the consensus half-binding site (AGGT(C/A)A) of the T3 receptor; one of the half sites in the β1-subunit gene is an exact match, while the other only is a three-sixths match. They are separated by a 4-bp nucleotide spacing, which is required for the specific binding of the thyroid hormone receptor.

Translational Regulation of α- and β-Gene Expression

In several tissues, the abundance of α-subunit mRNA exceeds that of β-subunit mRNA, raising the possibility that β-subunit mRNA plays a limiting role in the rate of Na,K-pump biosynthesis. Regulation of gene expression at the level of translation is becoming widely appreciated as an important modulator of protein synthesis. For Na,K-ATPase, it is important to be aware of the role of translational regulation of subunit synthesis, since association of the α and β subunits in the endoplasmic reticulum is required for transport via the Golgi apparatus to the plasma membrane (67). Studies of α- and β-subunit synthesis in a cell-free system showed that α1 mRNA was translated less efficiently than β1 mRNA. The subunit mRNAs were equally stable in the system, but α1 mRNA was consistently translated less efficiently than β1 mRNA. The prediction of a complex mRNA secondary structure in the 5′UT region of the α1 mRNA (Fig. 6) provides a potential explanation for translational inhibition. This mechanism could account for equal accumulation of the two subunit proteins in tissues where α1 mRNA is more abundant than β1 mRNA. Translational control could also explain why some systems display only modest changes in amount of functional αβ unit in spite of significant induction of α1 mRNA levels.

Biosynthesis and Assembly of Na,K-ATPase α and β Subunits

The αβ heterodimer is the minimal functional unit of the Na,K pump (48). Correct assembly of an α and a β subunit and transport of the αβ heterodimer from the endoplasmic reticulum (ER) via the Golgi to the plasma membrane is a prerequisite for obtaining a functional enzyme unit. The α and β subunits are synthesized without cleavable N-terminal signal peptides and are cotranslationally inserted into the ER in a signal-recognition-particle–dependent manner (15,68–72).

Proteolytic removal of the five N-terminal residues during or shortly after biosynthesis is the only observed modification of the α subunit (15). The role of the five N-terminal amino acids remains

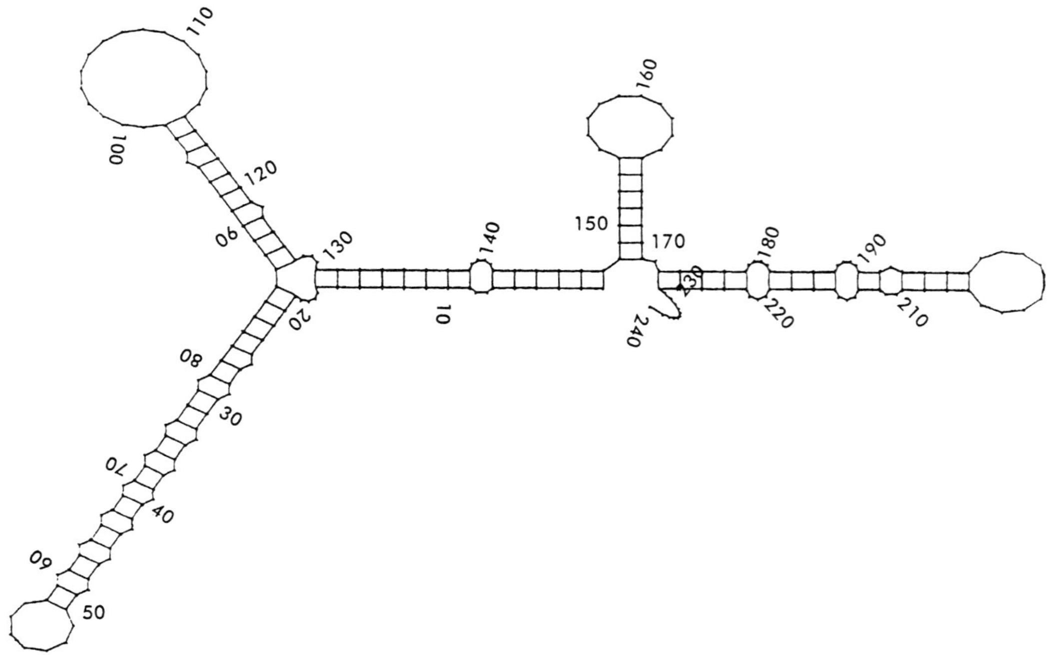

Figure 6 Predicted secondary structure of the 5′ UT region of $\alpha1$ mRNA from the nucleotide sequence analyzed by the FOLD program. This prediction of a complex secondary structure with four stem loops provides a potential explanation for inhibition of translation (67).

unknown with respect to membrane insertion and subunit assembly. The signal for membrane insertion of the α subunit has been mapped to the first four transmembrane segments (73).

The mature β subunit is N-glycosylated at three positions and contains three disulfide bonds. The β subunit is therefore subject to extensive processing during its synthesis and intracellular transport to the plasma membrane (15). A 16-residue-long stretch of amino acids in the transmembrane segment has been shown to be necessary and sufficient for membrane insertion of the β subunit (71). The formation of $\alpha\beta$ heterodimers has primarily been studied in *Xenopus* oocytes and mouse L cells. Both systems express endogenous Na,K-ATPase activity but possess the capacity to express additional pumps. In mouse L cells, advantage is taken of the fact that the endogenous activity is ouabain-resistant (71). Transfection of mouse L cells with α-cDNA derived from an ouabain-sensitive isoform results in the appearance of ouabain-sensitive Na,K-ATPase activity in the plasma membrane. The difference in ouabain sensitivity permits discrimination of the endogenous activity from the transfected activity. In transfected mouse L cells, the ouabain-sensitive enzyme is a hybrid between the endogenous β subunit and the transfected α subunit. These experiments demonstrate that the α and β subunits from different species are able to assemble, strongly indicating that regions in the α and β subunits required for heterodimer formation have been well conserved during evolution.

In contrast to the situation in mouse L cells, functional expression of exogenous pumps at the plasma membrane could only be observed in *Xenopus* oocytes after injection of both α and β mRNA (74). In *Xenopus* oocytes, the endogenous α subunit is synthesized in excess of the endogenous β subunit (75). The overexpressed α subunit exists in an immature trypsin-sensitive form that is confined to the ER and slowly degraded (76). When $\beta 1$ or $\beta 3$ subunits are overexpressed relative to the α subunit, they remain in a coreglycosylated form and are slowly degraded in what seems to be the ER (77). Simultaneous biosynthesis of endogenous α subunits and exogenous $\beta 1$ or $\beta 3$ subunits renders the oocyte α subunit trypsin-resistant, extends the biological half-lives of the α and β subunits, and increases the number of functional Na,K-pumps at the plasma membrane.

Studies in *Xenopus* oocytes using antisense oligonucleotides complementary to either the endogenous α or β subunit have shown that α and β subunits are inserted independently into the ER and retain their ability to assemble into functional Na,K pumps for an extended period of time (78). These experiments demonstrate that the $\alpha\beta$ heterodimer is the only transport competent form of the α and β subunits. The specific amino acid interactions between the α and β subunits required for subunit assembly have not yet been defined.

Experiments using transfected mouse L cells have shown that β subunits lacking the cytoplasmic domain are able to assemble with the endogenous α subunit, and the assembled hybrid pumps are transported to the plasma membrane. The β subunits with transmembrane deletions that do not prevent insertion into the ER also assemble with the endogenous α subunits.

Transfection of HeLa cells with cDNA-encoding chimeras between the intact or C-terminal-deleted extracellular domain of the β subunit and the cytoplasmic and membrane domains of the dipeptidyl peptidase IV has identified the 96 residues of the extracellular domain as the region required for assembly with the α subunit (79). However, the assembled α and β subunits are confined to the ER and consequently do not exist in a transport-competent form.

Chimeric Na,K-ATPase/Ca-ATPase α subunits have revealed that the 161 carboxyl-terminal amino acids of the chicken $\alpha 1$ subunit are required and sufficient for assembly with the chicken β subunit (80). Immunoprecipitation of β subunits with anti-α antibodies was the criterion used for assembly in these studies.

Ion Regulation of Gene Expression and Biosynthesis

The amount of Na,K-ATPase in cell membranes is modulated according to the demand for transport capacity through effects of Na^+ concentrations in cytoplasm on transcription or biosynthesis rates. This feedback regulation of the amount of Na,K-ATPase protein in the cells was proposed as a hypothesis for explaining adaptive changes in amount of Na,K-ATPase following changes in supply of Na^+ to adrenalectomized rats (5). In this model, a sustained change in Na/K ratio in cytoplasm following an increased influx of Na^+ results in adaptive increases in the amount of Na,K-ATPase that appear slowly after 16 to 24 hr in vivo. As illustrated in Fig. 7, the feedback cycle is completed when the capacity for active Na,K transport has been increased to a level (from $V_m = 1$ to $V_m = 2$) allowing the increased flux rates to be maintained at the original levels of cytoplasmic Na/K

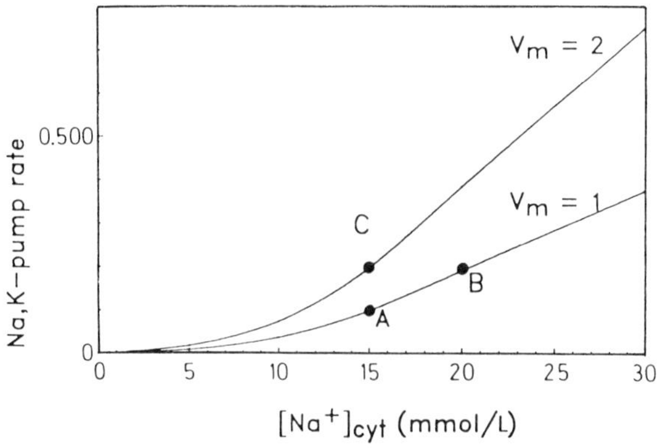

Figure 7 Na,K-pump rate as a function of $[Na^+]$ activity in the cell cytoplasm before (V_m = 1) and after (V_m = 2) adaptation of the amount of Na,K-ATPase to a twofold higher level. The actute adaptation following an increased rate of Na^+ influx and a rise of $[Na^+]_{cyt}$ from 15 mmol/l (A) to 20 mmol/l (B) causes an increase in the turnover rate of existing pumps from 0.1 to 0.2. After chronic adaptation involving a doubling of the amount of Na,K-ATPase (corresponding to an increase from V_m = 1 to V_m = 2), the increased turnover rate (0.2) of Na,K pumping can be sustained at the original level of $[Na^+]_{cyt}$.

activities. Induction of Na,K-ATPase is also elicited after incubation of cultured cells in ouabain or low-K media (81,82). In suspensions of kidney tubule cells (83), an increase in Na/K ratio after 2 to 4 hr triggers a marked increase in rate of synthesis of Na,K-ATPase protein. Quantification of mRNA by hybridization with $[^{32}P]$-cDNA shows an early rise in amount of specific mRNA followed by a late increase in rate of synthesis of the α and β subunits and in abundance of $\alpha\beta$ units in the cells (84–86). Data on kidney cells (87) and cultured muscle (88) show that changes of $[Na^+]_{cyt}$ predominantly affect the level of $\beta1$ mRNA. The time required for effecting a change in amount of Na,K-ATPase (16 to 24 hr) agrees with the rate of change in response to in vivo changes in Na^+ load. Rates of degradation of $\alpha\beta$ units are slow, with T1/2 = 20 to 40 hr. It has been proposed that Ca^+ is involved in mediating the effect of $[Na^+]_{cyt}$ (89), but ion response elements have not been identified and little is known about the molecular mechanism of these ion effects on biosynthesis. On the basis of minor changes in activity during in vitro incubation, a defective homeostatic response of Na,K-ATPase to salt induction has been related to the pathogenesis of hypertension (90).

Thyroidal Regulation of Na,K-ATPase Gene Expression in Kidney

Thyroid hormone stimulation of respiration and the rate of thermogenesis is associated with enhanced rates of active Na,K transport in kidney cortex. The degree of saturation of T3 receptors in kidney cortex correlates well with enhancement of Na,K-ATPase activity and energy consumption coupled to Na,K transport (91). Increments of α- and β-subunit synthesis can largely account for the increased abundance of the enzyme, mediated by transcriptional mechanisms leading to an enhanced number of Na,K-pump sites. Administration of T3 to hypothyroid rat induced renal Na,K-ATPase activity that is associated with increased $\alpha1$ and $\beta1$ mRNA levels and elevated transcription rates (66,91). These findings indicate that T3 might regulate $\alpha1$ and $\beta1$ gene expression at the transcriptional level through direct interaction of T3 and the T3 receptor with a *cis*-acting T3 response element (TRE) on the $\alpha1$ and $\beta1$ genes, although posttranscriptional processes may also contribute to the overall regulation.

Interestingly, three TRE-like sequences have been found in the promoter region of human Na,K-ATPase $\beta1$ gene (66). However, only one of these sequence elements is well conserved in the promoter region of rat $\beta1$ gene. Deletion and mutation analysis confirmed that this element is a functioning thyroid hormone receptor element (see above). It has not been established whether the primary effect of T3 induction of transcription of the $\alpha1$ gene in kidney involves direct interaction of a nuclear T3-receptor complex with *cis*-acting regulatory elements of $\alpha1$ gene or whether the induction is secondary to T3 induction of other regulatory proteins that mediates enhanced transcription of the Na,K-ATPase genes. Functional TRE sequences for the $\alpha 1$ gene of Na,K-ATPase have not been identified.

Differential Regulation by Aldosterone and Thyroid Hormone

Chronic adaptation of the amount of Na,K-pump protein (2,5) and the area of basolateral membrane per cell (92) is a slow process developing over several days in response to a sustained increase in aldosterone secretion and in transepithelial Na^+ flux across the epithelium (93). The question is whether the effect of aldosterone on the biosynthesis of Na,K-ATPase is direct or indirect. A direct effect implies interaction of aldosterone with hormone-receptor elements interacting with promoter elements in the genes of Na,K-ATPase to accelerate transcription. Alternatively, aldosterone could have a direct effect on the splicing or the stability of mRNA or on the process of translation of mRNA to protein. An effect of aldosterone on the membrane conductance could be transmitted to an effect on the biosynthesis of Na,K-ATPase through the known effects of Na^+ and K^+ ion activities on the rate of biosynthesis of the pump proteins (discussed above). Aldosterone's effects on the rate of mRNA synthesis have been analyzed in relation to stimulation of Na,K-ATPase synthesis (35). In cortical collecting ducts, aldosterone in the presence of triiodothyronine increases the amount of Na,K-ATPase by de novo synthesis of pump units independent of changes in cytoplasmic Na^+ (94), while changes in Na^+ concentration may stimulate recruitment of a latent pool of Na,K-ATPase independent of protein synthesis.

In the surface cells of the distal colon, Na^+ reabsorption is regulated by aldosterone in the same manner as in the CCD of the kidney. Endogenous aldosterone and thyroid hormone in a physiological range of concentrations modulates the abundance of $\alpha 1$ and $\beta 1$ mRNA and the number of functional Na,K-pump units in these epithelial cells (32). In the range of serum aldosterone concentrations seen during dietary sodium deprivation (0.6 n*M* to 1.4–1.9 n*M*) the hormone effects are mediated through type I mineralocorticoid receptors ($K_{0.5}$ 0.3–3 n*M*), since much higher concentrations are required for binding to type II glucocorticoid receptors ($K_{0.5}$ 25–50 n*M*) (95). The rise in aldosterone leads to marked accumulation of $\alpha 1$ mRNA, a rise of $\beta 1$ mRNA, and to almost a doubling of the abundance of Na,K-pump molecules. In the collecting duct of rabbit kidney, the transcellular Na flux also varies as a function of aldosterone concentration (96) in the same range as that observed here for the colon epithelium, and the time course of the increment of Na,K-ATPase is correlated to the changes in basolateral membrane area (92). Upon exposure to aldosterone, no change is observed after 3 to 4 hr, but the amplification of basolateral membrane area begins within 24 hr and continues at a rapid rate for the first 3 days. A similar time course is seen for the effect of deoxycorticosterone treatment on the Na,K-ATPase activity of the cortical collecting duct (93). The increase in membrane area thus appears to be parallel to the change in number of Na,K-pump sites, with a constant density of pump sites in the newly synthesized membrane.

At low concentrations of thyroid hormone (T3), the response to aldosterone is impaired and a single dose of T3 may restore the aldosterone response to that found in the euthyroid state (32), while T3 given without aldosterone is ineffective (97). Thyroid hormone (T3) also plays a permissive role in the effect of aldosterone on Na,K-ATPase activity in the collecting duct of the rabbit (94). In the amphibian bladder, T3 antagonizes the late response of Na,K-pump synthesis (98). These synergisms or antagonisms can be understood as overlaps between the domains of the two hormones, but the explanation may rather be a differential effect of aldosterone and T3 on the transcription of the $\alpha 1$- and $\beta 1$- subunit genes of Na,K-ATPase. The α and β subunits depend mutually on each other for obtaining the correct configuration required for the $\alpha\beta$ unit to leave the endoplasmic reticulum to reach the Golgi and the plasma membrane (15). A reduction in rate of β-subunit insertion into the endoplasmic reticulum membrane following a reduction in T3 concentration and β mRNA will therefore reduce the half-life of the $\alpha 1$ subunit in the endoplasmic reticulum and lead to reduced overall rates of transfer of $\alpha\beta$ units to the plasma membrane. In addition to the kidney (91,98), differential regulation of Na,K-ATPase subunits by thyroid hormone has been observed in liver, heart, and muscle (98–100).

Mechanism of Escape from the Effect of Hyperaldosteronemia on Na,K-ATPase in Kidney

In spite of a continued elevation of the serum concentrations of aldosterone, escape can be observed with decline of the number of Na,K-pump sites to control levels or less if the synthesis of the $\alpha 1$-

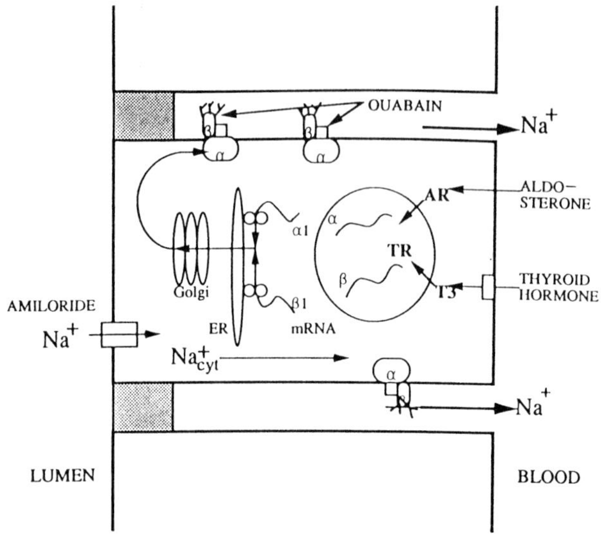

Figure 8 Model of Na,K pump biosynthesis illustrating the possible molecular mechanisms for escape from the effect of aldosterone on the rate of Na,K pump biosynthesis. The α and β subunits emerging from the ribosomes associate in the endoplasmic reticulum (ER) before migration to the Golgi and the basal lateral membrane. Aldosterone increases the rate of $\alpha1\beta1$ unit synthesis, presumably through an effect on the rate of $\alpha1$- and $\beta1$-gene transcription. At high aldosterone, escape is seen when reduced levels of $[Na^+]_{cyt}$ and/or thyroid hormone (T3) limit the rate of β-subunit synthesis (32).

and $\beta1$-subunits is not coordinated. The interactions of aldosterone, thyroid hormone, and $[Na^+]_{cyt}$ in regulation of the α- and β-subunit genes are summarized in Fig. 8, illustrating the possible molecular mechanisms for escape from the effect of aldosterone on the number of Na,K-pump sites. Low $[Na^+]_{cyt}$ levels can interrupt the aldosterone-induced rise in ouabain binding sites with return to control levels of the number of Na,K-pump sites (93). The morphological response to aldosterone treatment was also prevented by a low-Na diet (92). The effect of $[Na^+]_{cyt}$ on the amount of Na,K-ATPase seems predominantly to be due to reduction of the level of $\beta1$ mRNA. In other systems, $[Na^+]_{cyt}$ remains within the normal range on a low-sodium diet (101,102), and low levels of T3 can suppress mRNA levels, in particular for the β subunit, leading to return of Na,K-pump concentrations in the cell to control levels in spite of continued maintenance of aldosterone levels three- to fourfold higher than control. Reduction of T3 and/or $[Na^+]_{cyt}$ serve to limit biosynthesis of Na,K-ATPase in situations of limited energy supply or limited supply of Na^+, a substrate for the pump. They both seem to work at the level of the β-subunit gene, affecting synthesis of the β subunit as a limiting factor for assembly of the $\alpha\beta$ unit and functional maturation of the Na,K pump.

REFERENCES

1. Jørgensen PL. Na,K-ion pump in kidney tubules. Physiol Rev 1980; 60:864–917.
2. Jorgensen PL. Structure, function and regulation of Na,K-ATPase in the kidney. Kidney Int 1986; 29:10–20.
3. Doucet A. Function and control of Na,K-ATPase in single nephron segments of the mammalian kidney. Kidney Int 1988; 34:749–760.
4. Doucet A. Na,K-ATPase in the kidney tubule in relation to natriuresis. Kidney Int 1992; 41:S118–S124.
5. Jørgensen PL. The role of aldosterone in the regulation of Na,K-ATPase in rat kidney. J Steroid Biochem 1972; 3:181–191.
6. Rossier BC, Palmer LG. Mechanism of aldosterone action on sodium and potassium transport. In: Seldin, D.W., Giebish, G. eds. The Kidney, 2d ed. New York: Raven Press, 1992:1373–1409.
7. Rossier BC, Geering K, Kraehenbuhl JP. Regulation of the sodium pump: How and why? Trends Biochem Sci 1987; 12:483–487.

8. Bertorello AM, Aperia A, Walaas SI, Nairn AC, Greengard P. Phosphorylation of the catalytic subunit of Na,K-ATPase inhibits the activity of the enzyme. Proc Natl Acad Sci USA 1991; 88:11359–11362.
9. Middleton JP, Wasiuddin AK, Collinsworth G, et al. Heterogeneity of protein kinase C-mediated rapid regulation of Na,K-ATPase in kidney epithelial cells. J Biol Chem 1993; 268:15958–15964.
10. Bertorello AM, Katz AI. Short-term regulation of renal Na,K-ATPase activity: Physiological relevance and cellular mechanisms. Am J Physiol 1993; 265:F743–F755.
11. Jørgensen PL. Isolation of Na,K-dependent ATPase. Methods Enzymol 1974; 32:277–294 and 1988; 156:29–143.
12. Shull GE, Greeb J, Lingrel JB. Molecular cloning of three distinct forms of Na,K-ATPase α-subunit from rat brain. Biochemistry 1986; 25:8125–8132.
13. Lingrel JB, Orlowski J, Shull MM, Price EM. Molecular Genetics of Na,K-ATPase. Progress in Nucleic Acid Research and Molecular Biology. 1990; 38:37–89.
14. Young RM, Shull GE, Lingrel JB. Multiple mRNAs from rat kidney and brain encode a single Na,K-ATPase beta subunit protein. J Biol Chem 1987; 262:4905–4910.
15. Geering K. Subunit assembly and functional maturation of Na,K-ATPase. J Membr Biol 1990; 115:109–121.
16. Sweadner K. Isozymes of the Na,K-ATPase. Biochim Biophys Acta 1989; 988:185–220.
17. Jorgensen PL. Na,K-ATPase Structure and transport mechanism. In: Schafer JA, ed. Membrane Transport in Biology. Vol. 5. New York: Springer-Verlag, 1992.
18. Horisberger JD, Lemas V, Kraehenbühl JP, Rossier BC. Structure function relationship of Na,K-ATPase. Annu Rev Physiol 1991; 53:565–584.
19. Cornelius F. Functional reconstitution of the sodium pump: Kinetics of exchange reactions performed by reconstituted Na,K-ATPase. Biochim. Biophys. Acta 1991; 1071:19–66.
20. Pedemonte CH, Kaplan JH. Chemical modification as an approach to elucidation of sodium pump structure-function relations. Am J Physiol 1990; 258:C1–C23.
21. Glynn IM, Karlish SJD. Occluded cations in active transport. Annu Rev Biochem 1990; 59:171–205.
22. Vasilets LA, Schwarz W. Structure-function relationships of cation binding in the Na,K-ATPase. Biochim Biophys Acta 1993; 1154:201–222.
23. Kaplan JH, DeWeer P, eds. The Sodium Pump: Structure, Mechanism, and Regulation. New York: Rockefeller University Press, 1991.
24. Kaplan JH, DeWeer P, eds. The Sodium Pump: Recent Developments. New York: Rockefeller University Press, 1991.
25. VIIth Int. Conf. on The Sodium Pump, Todtmoos, Germany, September 1993. Hoppe Seylers Biol Chem 1993; 374:545–624.
26. Nielsen JM, Jorgensen PL. Differential aldosterone effects on epithelial cell pools of $\alpha\beta$-unit binding sites. Hoppe Seylers Biol Chem 1993: 374:576.
27. Schmaltzning G, Kröner S, Passow H. Evidence for intracellular sodium pumps in permeabilized Xenopus laevis oocytes. Biochem J 1989; 260:395–399.
28. Maunsbach AB, Skriver E, Hebert H, Jorgensen PL. The renal Na,K-ion pump: Identification, ultrastructure and cytochemical localization. Verh Anat Ges 1984; 78:S55–S75.
29. Kashgarian M, Biemesderfer D, Caplan M, Forbush B. Monoclonal antibody to Na,K-ATPase: Immunocytochemical localization along nephron segments. Kidney Int 1985; 28:899–913.
30. Gloor SH, Antonicek H, Sweadner KJ, et al. The adhesion molecule on glia [AMOG] is a homologue of the β-subunit of Na,K-ATPase. J Cell Biol 1990; 110:165–174.
31. Jørgensen PL, Collins JH. Tryptic and chymotryptic cleavage sites in the sequence of α-subunit of Na,K-ATPase from outer medulla of mammalian kidney. Biochim Biophys Acta 1986; 860:570–576.
32. Wiener H, Nielsen JM, Klærke DA, Jorgensen PL. Aldosterone and thyroid hormone modulation of α1-, β1-mRNA and Na,K-pump sites in the rabbit distal colon epithelium: Evidence for a novel mechanism of escape from the effect of hyper-aldosteronemia. J Membr Biol 1993; 133:203–211.
33. Farman N, Corthesy-Theulaz I, Bonvalet JP, Rossier BC, Localization of α-isoforms of Na,K-ATPase in rat kidney by in-situ hybridization. Am J Physiol 1991; 260:C468–C474.
34. Farman N, Coutry N, Logvinenko N, et al. Adrenalectomy reduces α1 and not β1 Na,K-ATPase mRNA expression in rat distal nephron. Am J Physiol 1992; 263:C810–C817.
35. Welling PA, Caplan M, Sutters M, Giebisch G. Aldosterone-mediated Na,K-ATPase expression is α1 isoform specific in the renal cortical collecting duct. J Biol Chem 1993; 268:23469–23476.
36. Doucet A, Barlet C. Evidence for differences in the sensitivity to ouabain of Na,K-ATPase along the nephron of rabbit kidney. J Biol Chem 1986; 261:993–995.
37. Arystenhova EA, Lakhtinaa OE, Mydyanov NN. Immunodetection of Na,K-ATPase α-isoform in renal and nerve tissues. FEBS Lett 1989; 250:545–548.
38. Hansen O. Heterogeneity of Na,K-ATPase from kidney Acta Physiol Scand 1991; 146:229–234.
39. Hamlyn JM, Blaustein MP, Bova S, et al. Identification and characterization of a ouabain-like compound from human plasma. Proc Natl Acad Sci USA 1991; 88:6259–6263.

40. Cheval L, Barlet-Bas C, Doucet A. Characterization of molecular isoforms of Na,K-ATPase subunits along the rat nephron by polymerase chain reaction. Hoppe Seylers Biol Chem 1993; 374:604.
41. Nelson WJ, Westnock PJ. Ankyrin binding to Na,K-ATPase and implications for the organization of membrane domains in polarized epithelial cells. Nature 1987; 328:533–535.
42. Nelson WJ, Shore EM, Wang AZ, Hammerton RW. Identification of a membrane-cytoskeletal complex containing the cell adhesion molecule uvomorulin (E-cadherin), ankyrin, and fodrin in Marvin Darby canine kidney cells. J Cell Biol 1990; 110:349–357.
43. Molitoris BA, Chan LK, Shapiro JI, et al. Loss of epithelial polarity: A novel hypothesis for reduced proximal tubule Na transport following ischemic injury. J Membr Biol 1989; 107:119–127.
44. Moliteris BA, Falk SA, Dahl RH. Ischemic induced loss of epithelial polarity. J Clin Invest. 1989; 84:1334–1339.
45. Canfield PE, Gerdes AE, Moliteris BA. Effect of reversible ATP depletion on tight epithelium integrity. Am J Physiol 1991; 262:F1038–F1045.
46. Molitoris BA. Na,K-ATPase that redistributes to apical membrane during ATP depletion remains functional. Am J Physiol 1993; 265:F693–F697.
47. Jorgensen PL. Mechanism of the Na,K-ion pump: Protein structure and conformations of the pure Na,K-ATPase. Biochim Biophys Acta 1982; 694:27–68.
48. Jorgensen PL, Andersen JP. Structural basis for E_1-E_2 conformational transition in Na,K-ATPase and Ca-ATPase. J Membr Biol 1988; 103:95–120.
49. Maunsbach AB, Skriver E, Hebert H. Two-dimensional crystals and three-dimensional structure of Na,K-ATPase analyzed by electron microscopy. Soc Gen Physiol Ser 1991; 46:159–172.
50. Carpasso JM, Hoving S, Tal DM, Goldshleger R, et al. Extensive digestion of Na,K-ATPase by specific and nonspecific proteases with preservation of cation occlusion sites. J Biol Chem 1992; 267:1150–1158.
51. Vilsen B. Glutamate 329 located in the fourth transmembrane segment of the α-subunit of the rat kidney Na,K-ATPase is not an essential residue for active transport of sodium and potassium ions. Biochemistry 1993; 32:13340–13349.
52. Jewell EA, Lingrel JB. Site-directed mutagenesis of the Na,K-ATPase: Consequences of substitutions of negatively charged amino acids localized in the transmembrane domains. Biochemistry 1993; 32:13523–13530.
53. Van Huysse JW, Jewell EA, Lingrel JB. Site-directed mutagenesis of a predicted cation binding site of Na,K-ATPase. Biochemistry 1993; 32:819–826.
54. Dzandzhugazyan KN, Jorgensen PL. Asymmetric orientation of amino groups in α-subunit and β-subunit of Na,K-ATPase in tight right-side-out vesicles of basolateral membranes from outer medulla. Biochim Biophys Acta 1985; 817:165–173.
55. Kirley TL. Determination of three disulfide bonds and one free sulfhydryl in the beta subunit of (Na,K)-ATPase. J Biol Chem 1989; 264:7185–7192.
56. Ohta T, Yoshida M, Nagano K, et al. Structure of the extra-membranous domain of the beta-subunit of (Na,K)-ATPase revealed by the sequences of its tryptic peptides. FEBS Lett 1986; 204:297–301.
57. Esmann M. Disulfide bonds in the β-subunit of Na,K-ATPase. Biochim Biophys Acta 1982; 688:251–259.
58. Bairock A. The ENZYME data bank. Nucleic Acids Res 1993; 21:3155–3156.
59. Mandel LJ. Primary active sodium transport, oxygen consumption, and ATP: Coupling and regulation. Kidney Int 1986; 29:3–9.
60. Xu JC, Lytle C, Zhu TT, et al. Molecular cloning and functional expression of the bumetanide sensitive Na-K-Cl cotransporter. Proc Natl Acad Sci USA 1994; 91:2201–2205.
61. Klærke DA, Wiener H, Zeuthen T, Jorgensen PL. Ca activation and pH dependence of a maxi K channel from rabbit distal colon epithelium. J Membr Biol 1993; 136:9–21.
62. Shull MM, Pugh DG, Lingrel JB. The human Na,K-ATPase $\alpha 1$ gene: Characterization of the 5′flanking region and identification of a restriction fragment length polymorphism. Genomics 1990; 6:451–460.
63. Yagawa Y, Kawakami I, Nagano K. Cloning and analysis of the 5′-flanking region of rat Na,K-ATPase alpha 1 subunit gene. Biochim Biophys Acta 1990; 1049:286–292.
64. Lane LK, Shull MM, Whitmer KR, Lingrel JB. Characterization of two genes for the human Na,K-ATPase beta subunit. Genomics 1990; 5:445–453.
65. Liu B, Gick G. Characterization of the 5′ flanking region of the rat Na+/K(+)-ATPase beta 1 subunit gene. Biochim Biophys Acta 1992; 1130:336–338.
66. Feng J, Orlowski J, Lingrel JB. Identification of a functional thyroid hormone response element in the upstream flanking region of the human Na,K-ATPase $\beta 1$ gene. Nucleic Acids Res 1993; 21:2619–2626.
67. Devarajan P, Gilmore-Hebert M, Benz EJ. Differential translation of the Na,K-ATPase subunit mRNAs. J Biol Chem 1992; 267:22435–22439.
68. Caplan, MJ, Palade, G, Jamieson JD, Biosynthesis of the Na,K-ATPase in Madin Darby canine kidney cells: Activation and cell surface delivery. J Biol Chem 1986; 261:2860–2865.
69. Fisher JA, Baxter-Lowe LA, Hokin LE. Regulation of Na,K-ATPase biosynthesis in developing artemia salina. J Biol Chem 1986; 261:515–519.

70. Geering K, Meyer DI, Paccolat MP, et al. Membrane insertion of α and β-subunits of Na,K-ATPase. J Biol Chem 1985; 260:5254–5160.
71. Kawakami K, Nagano K. The transmembrane segment of the human Na,K-ATPase β-subunit acts as the membrane incorporation signal. J Biochem 1988; 103:54–60.
72. Cyanis E, Bayley H, Edelman IS. Cell-free transcription and translation of Na,K-ATPase α- and β-subunit cDNAs. J Biol Chem 1990; 265:10829–10835.
73. Homareda H, Kawakami K, Nagano K, Matsui H. Membrane insertion of α- and β-subunit of human Na,K-ATPase. Progr Clin Biol Res 1988; 268B:77–84.
74. Noguchi S, Mishine M, Kawamura M, Numa S. Functional expression of Na,K-ATPase from cloned cDNA. FEBS Lett 1987; 225:27–52.
75. Geering K, Theulaz I, Verrey F, et al. A role for the β-subunit in the expression of functional Na,K-ATPase in Xenopus oocytes. Am J Physiol 1989; 257:C851–C858.
76. Jaunin P, Horisberger JD, Richter K, et al. Processing, intracellular transport, and functional expression of endogenous and exogenous alpha-beta 3 Na,K-ATPase complexes in Xenopus oocytes. J. Biol Chem 1992; 267:577–585.
77. Ackermann U, Geering K. Mutual dependence of Na,K-ATPase α- and β-subunit for correct posttranslational processing and intracellular transport. FEBS Lett 1990; 269:105–108.
78. Ackermann U, Geering K. β1-subunits and β3-subunits can associate with prehsynthesized α-subunits of Xenopus oocyte Na,K-ATPase J Biol Chem 1992; 267:12911–12915.
79. Horisberger JD, Jaunin P, Good PJ, et al. Coexpression of α1 with putative β3 subunits results in functional Na,K-pumps in Xenopus occytes. Proc Natl Acad Sci USA 1991; 88:8397–8400.
80. Lemas MV, Hamrick M, Emerick M, et al. Structural requirements for the interaction between α- and β-subunits. Hoppe-Seylers Biol Chem 1993; 374:548.
81. Boardman LJ, Huett M, Lamb JF, et al. Evidence for the genetic control of the sodium pump density in HeLa cells. J Physiol 1974; 241:771–794.
82. Wolitzky BA, Fambrough DM. Regulation of the Na,K-ATPase in cultured chick skeletal muscle. J Biol Chem 1986; 261:9990–9999.
83. Rayson BM. Na,K-ATPase regulation in Dahl sensitive and Dahl resistant rats. J Biol Chem 1985; 260:12740–12743.
84. Bowen WJ, McDonough A. Pretranslational regulation of Na,K-ATPase in cultured canine kidney cells by low K. Am J Physiol 1987; 52:C179–C189.
85. Ismail-Beigi F, Pressley TA, Haber RS, et al. Kinetic analysis of Na,K-ATPase induced by low external K^+ in a rat liver cell line. J Biol Chem 1988; 263:8162–8167.
86. Pressley TA, Edelman IS. Reduced ouabain inhibition of Na,K-ATPase in cultured cell recipients of the ouabain resistance gene. J Biol Chem 1986; 261:9779–9786.
87. Lescale-Matys L, Hensley CB, Crnkovic-Markovic R, et al. Low K^+ increases Na,K-ATPase abundance in LLC-PK1/C14 cells by differentially increasing beta and not alpha, subunit mRNA. J Biol Chem 1990; 265:17935–17940.
88. Taormino JP, Fambrough DM. Pre-translational regulation of the Na,K-ATPase in response to demand for ion transport in cultured chicken skeletal muscle. J Biol Chem 1990; 265:4116–4123.
89. Rayson BM. Calcium: A mediator of the cellular response to chronic Na+/K(+)-ATPase inhibition. J Biol Chem 1993; 268:8851–8854.
90. Rayson BM. Na,K-ATPase regulation in Dahl sensitive and Dahl resistant rats. J Biol Chem 1985; 260:12740–12743.
91. Horowitz B, Hensley CB, Quintero M, et al. Differential regulation of Na,K-ATPase α1, α2, and β-subunit mRNA and protein levels by thyroid hormone. J Biol Chem 1990; 265:14308–13314.
92. Wade JB, Kashgarian M, Giebisch G. Morphological and physiological responses to aldosterone: Time course and sodium dependence. Am J Physiol 1990; 259:F88–F94.
93. O'Neil RG, Hayhurst RA. Sodium dependent modulation of the renal Na,K-ATPase: Influence of mineralocorticoids on the collecting duct. J Membr Biol 1985; 85:169–179.
94. Barlet C, Doucet A. Triiodothyronine enhances renal response to aldosterone in the rabbit collecting tubule. J Clin Invest 1987; 79:629–631.
95. Marver D. Assessment of mineralocorticoid activity in the rabbit colon. Am J Physiol 1984; 246:F437–F446.
96. Schwartz GJ, Burg MB. Mineralocorticoid effects on cation transport by cortical collecting tubules in vitro. Am J Physiol 1978; 235:F576–F585.
97. Edmonds CJ, Thompson BD, Marriot J. Interrelationship of the effects of aldosterone and thyroid hormones on sodium transport and electrical properties of rat colon. J Endocrinol 1970; 8:189–197.
98. Geering K, Girardet M, Bron JP, et al. Hormonal regulation of Na,K-ATPase biosynthesis in the toad bladder: Effect of aldosterone and 3,5,3'triodo-L-thyronin. J Biol Chem 1982; 257:10338–10343.
99. Hensley CB, Azuma KM, Ming-jer T, McDonough AA. Thyroid hormone induction of rat myocardial

Na,K-ATPase: $\alpha1$, $\alpha2$, and $\beta1$-mRNA and -protein levels at steady state. Am J Physiol 1992; 262: C484–C492.

100. Melikian J, Ismail-Beigi F. Thyroid hormone regulation of Na,K-ATPase subunit-mRNA expression in neonatal rat myocardium. J Membr Biol 1991; 119:171–177.
101. Schultz SG. Intracellular sodium activities and basolateral membrane potassium conductances of sodium-absorbing epithelial cells. In: Schultz SG, ed. Current Topics in Membranes and Transport. Vol. 34. San Diego: Academic Press, 1989:21–44.
102. Turnheim K, Plass H, Grasl M, et al. Sodium absorption and potassium secretion in rabbit colon during sodium deficiency. Am J Physiol 1986; 250:F235–F245.

27

Renal Plasma Membrane Vacuolar H^+ ATPases

Properties and Function in Acid-Base Homeostasis

Stephen L. Gluck, L. Shannon Holliday, Masahiro Iyori, Tatiana Kostrominova, and Beth S. M. Lee

Washington University School of Medicine, St. Louis, Missouri

SITES OF BICARBONATE REABSORPTION AND GENERATION IN THE NEPHRON AND ROLE OF THE RENAL VACUOLAR H^+ ATPase

In maintaining acid-base balance, the kidney daily reabsorbs the 4500 millimoles of filtered bicarbonate and regenerates the approximately 70 millimoles of bicarbonate consumed by metabolic proton generation (1–11). The renal tubule effects both bicarbonate reabsorption and regeneration by hydrogen ion secretion (1,7). Although the majority of bicarbonate reabsorption is accomplished by Na^+-H^+ exchange in the proximal tubule (12), thick ascending limb (13–16), and distal convoluted tubule (17), vacuolar H^+ ATPases residing on the plasma membrane have an important or essential role in H^+ secretion in both proximal and distal nephron segments (10,12,18–22).

The proximal tubule reabsorbs 80% of the filtered bicarbonate (23). Some 60–70% of the proton secretion in this segment arises from Na^+-H^+ exchange (23); the remaining 30–40% of H^+ secretion is attributable to a brush-border membrane vacuolar H^+ ATPase (19,24). The thick ascending limb reabsorbs 10–15% of the filtered bicarbonate (13). At least 80% of the proton secretion in this segment comes from a Na/H antiporter in the luminal membrane, and up to 20% originates from a luminal membrane vacuolar H^+ ATPase (11,15,16,25). The distal convoluted tubule normally reabsorbs only 1–2% of the filtered bicarbonate. Some 65–80% of the bicarbonate reabsorption is from Na/H antiport (17). The remainder occurs by an amiloride-insensitive mechanism that may represent a vacuolar H^+ ATPase (17,26).

The collecting duct is responsible for reabsorption of the remaining bicarbonate in the tubular fluid and for the secretion of additional hydrogen ion, resulting in the generation of bicarbonate, which is added to the blood. The cortical portion of the collecting duct contains several segments that are morphologically and functionally distinct: the connecting tubule, the initial collecting tubule, and the cortical collecting tubule (27). These segments are a mosaic of two major cell types: the principal cells, comprising about 60% of the cells, and the intercalated cells. The intercalated cells are responsible for most or all of the hydrogen ion transport in these segments* (reviewed in References 29 and 30). In these two segments, there are both acid-secreting (α or type A) and bicarbonate-secreting (β or type B) intercalated cells,† which differ in the type and arrangement of

*With the exception of the inner stripe of the outer medulla in the rabbit kidney, in which the principal cells also have a luminal membrane vacuolar H^+ ATPase and therefore may contribute to H^+ secretion (28).
†Studies indicate that there are more than two different phenotypic forms of intercalated cells (31–33). A newly described functional type of intercalated cell that has Cl^-/HCO_3^- exchange in both the apical and basolateral membranes has been called the γ intercalated cell. (33)

ion transporters they possess. These properties are discussed in greater detail below. The majority of hydrogen ion transport in intercalated cells arises from a vacuolar H^+ATPase, which is abundant in the intercalated cells (26,34,35). The vacuolar H^+ATPase is probably the enzyme responsible for regulation of net acid secretion in the distal nephron (36,37). Intercalated cells also appear to have a H^+,K^+-ATPase, that secretes H^+ in exchange for potassium reabsorption (38). This enzyme probably has an important function in active reabsorption of potassium from the urine during potassium depletion; its role in urinary acidification and acid-base homeostasis is still uncertain.

The outer medullary collecting tubule has two functionally distinct segments, the outer and inner stripes. Like the cortical collecting tubule, the outer medullary collecting tubule epithelium is composed of principal and intercalated cells; however, these segments have only α (acid-secreting) intercalated cells and few or no bicarbonate-secreting cells (reviewed in Reference 30). The inner stripe has the highest rate of H^+ secretion of the collecting duct segments (39).

The inner medullary collecting duct in the rat has a few α intercalated cells in the first third of its length (40) but is otherwise composed of a single cell type—the inner medullary collecting duct cell. These cells secrete hydrogen ion by an unknown mechanism, possibly an H^+,K^+-ATPase (41,42). The inner medullary collecting duct probably contributes significantly to overall net acid secretion, particularly during metabolic acidosis (43–45).

In summary, vacuolar H^+ATPases have an important role in bicarbonate transport in the proximal tubule, distal convoluted tubule, and cortical and outer medullary collecting ducts, and they may contribute to bicarbonate transport in the thick ascending limb.

PROPERTIES OF THE KIDNEY VACUOLAR H^+ATPase AND COMPARISON WITH OTHER VACUOLAR H^+ATPases

Vacuolar H^+ATPases are found in all eukaryotic cells, including fungal, plant, and animal cells, where they function universally in the acidification of intracellular membrane compartments (46,47). In some cell types, such as the macrophage and neutrophil (48), vacuolar H^+ATPases reside on the plasma membrane at relatively low densities and serve in the maintenance and regulation of intracellular pH (pHi). In a small set of specialized cells, including several types of renal tubular epithelial cells and osteoclasts, vacuolar H^+ATPases reside in the plasma membrane in a polarized distribution and at great densities and function in the transport of hydrogen ion across a cell or cell layer.

In this chapter, we will review the general properties of vacuolar H^+ATPases and then review the specialized aspects of their structure and function that pertain to their function in renal acid-base homeostasis.

General Properties of Vacuolar H^+ATPases

Electrogenic proton pumps of the vacuolar system were first found in lysosomes and chromaffin granules (49,50), but these early studies did not examine whether these pumps differed from the mitochondrial H^+ATPase. The first evidence that the vacuolar H^+ATPases were a new class of proton pump came from a characterization of the H^+ATPase responsible for electrogenic hydrogen ion secretion by the turtle urinary bladder (51). The turtle bladder proton pump manifested the distinctive properties of resistance to inhibition by vanadate (an inhibitor of the E_1E_2 or "P-type" ATPases, exemplified by the H^+,K^+-ATPase and Na^+,K^+-ATPase) and resistance to azide and oligomycin (inhibitors of the mitochondrial F_0F_1 or "F-type" H^+ATPase) but exquisite sensitivity to sulfhydryl reagents. The turtle bladder H^+ATPase was also inhibited by the hydrophobic carboxyl-reactive agent dicyclohexylcarbodiimide (DCCD), a high-affinity inhibitor of the F_0F_1 H^+ATPases. All vacuolar H^+ATPases discovered since share these properties* (46,47).

---

*With the possible exception of the vacuolar H^+ATPase from avian osteoclasts (52), in which one study has described vanadate-sensitive proton transport in membrane vesicles from these cells. Other studies have found that the osteoclast H^+ATPase is not inhibited by vanadate (53).

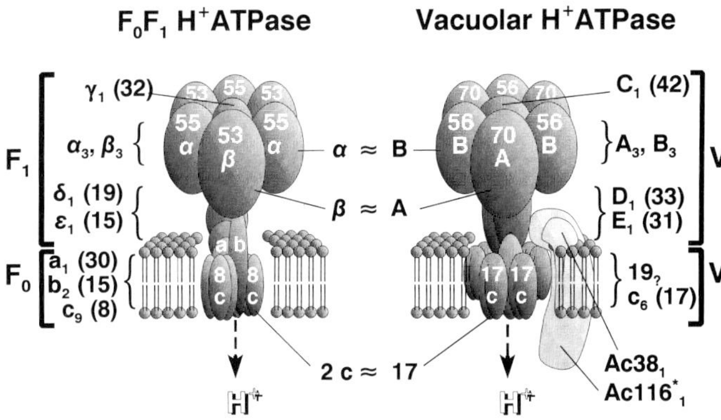

Figure 1 Structure of the vacuolar H$^+$ATPases and comparison with the F_0F_1 H$^+$ATPases.

Enzymatic Properties of the Vacuolar H$^+$ATPases

Vacuolar H$^+$ATPases transport only protons; there is no evidence for cotransport or antiport of any cations or anions (46,47,54). In assays of ATP-driven acidification of membrane vesicles or vacuoles in intact cells, however, the vacuolar H$^+$ATPases require charge movement to shunt the inward-positive potential difference generated from electrogenic proton transport (46,47). This charge movement is provided by entry of a permeant anion, such as chloride, or conductive exit of a cation, such as efflux of potassium, by the exogenously added ionophore valinomycin. The vacuolar H$^+$ATPases also require divalent cations for enzymatic activity; Mg^{2+} normally provides this requirement, although other divalent cations, such as Mn^{2+}, Ca^{2+}, and Fe^{2+}, can support ATPase activity in vitro. Vacuolar H$^+$ATPase activity may be affected by some anions. Several of the vacuolar H$^+$ATPases isolated from plants are activated by chloride ion (55), but, as discussed below, neither the isolated bovine kidney H$^+$ATPase nor the coated vesicle H$^+$ATPase isolated from bovine brain are stimulated by chloride (34,56). Most vacuolar H$^+$-ATPases are inhibited by nitrate anion, (57–62), but their IC_{50} values vary considerably. Nitrate is a chaotropic anion; in the plant vacuolar H$^+$ATPase, nitrate may function by dissociating the cytoplasmic (V_1) domain of the H$^+$-ATPase from the membrane (60). As discussed below, nitrate also inhibits the kidney brush-border vacuolar H$^+$ATPase (62) but not by dissociation of the V_1 domain.

Vacuolar H$^+$ATPases are inhibited by sulfhydryl reagents such as *N*-ethylmaleimide (NEM) and 7-chloro-4-nitrobenz-2-oxa-1,3-diazole (NBD-Cl), with IC_{50} values in the low micromolar range (34,46,62–64). Vacuolar H$^+$ATPases are also uniformly sensitive to submicromolar concentrations of the macrolide antibiotic bafilomycin A1 (65). Vacuolar H$^+$ATPases from mammalian lysosomes, secretory vesicles, endosomes, and other compartments are also inhibited with high affinity by the concanamycins (66–68), which inhibit with IC_{50} values about one-tenth those of bafilomycin A_1.

*Structural Properties of the Vacuolar H$^+$ATPase**

The vacuolar H$^+$ATPases are large, multisubunit enzymes consisting of a cytoplasmic (V_1) domain, or "catalytic sector," composed of peripheral membrane proteins, and a transmembrane (V_0) domain, or "membrane sector," composed of intrinsic membrane proteins (Figure 1). They evolved from an ancient ancestral multisubunit proton pump that engendered several broad classes of H$^+$ATPases (Figure 2).

*The polypeptide composition of vacuolar H$^+$ATPases isolated from different sources shows considerable variability. The structure that is described here derives from the best available information on H$^+$ATPases from mammalian tissues.

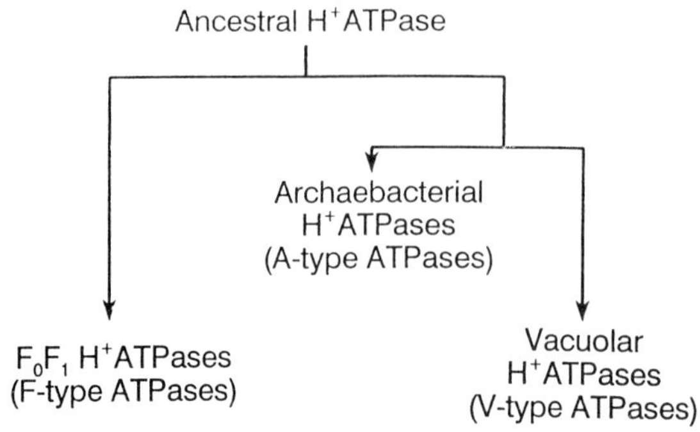

Figure 2 Evolutionary origins of the V-type and F-type ATPases.

Much of our understanding of the vacuolar H^+-ATPase comes from comparisons of the enzyme with the F_0F_1 H^+ATPases, the proton pumps of mitochondria, eubacteria, and chloroplasts. As shown in Figure 1, F_0F_1 H^+ATPases are also large multisubunit enzymes that have two major domains, a catalytic domain (F_1), composed of globular peripheral membrane proteins, and a transmembrane (F_0) domain, composed of intrinsic membrane proteins. The structure of F_1 has been studied extensively by biochemical methods (69,70) and more recently by x-ray crystallography (71). The β and α subunits of the F_1 domain of the F_0F_1 H^+ATPases are present in three copies each, as a hexagon of alternating subunits forming the catalytic "head" of the enzyme, attaching to a central γ subunit (Figure 1). The β subunit is the site of enzymatic ATP hydrolysis, although the actual catalytic site occurs at the interface of the β and α subunits (71). The α subunit, which may have a regulatory function, has a high-affinity nonhydrolytic nucleotide binding site. The β and α subunits are homologues of the A and B subunits of the vacuolar H^+ATPases, with about 25% identity, respectively. The F_0F_1 H^+ATPases have two "stalk" subunits, δ, and ϵ that attach the catalytic head to the membrane (F_0) domain; these stalk subunits are not homologous to any of the vacuolar H^+ATPase subunits.

In the *Escherichia coli* F_0F_1 H^+ATPase, the F_0 domain is composed of three structural polypeptides, a, b, and c, in a stoichiometry of 1:2:9–12 (72). The c subunit, the major structural component, is a M_r 8000 highly hydrophobic protein, or proteolipid, and has homology with a $M_r \sim$ 17,000* proteolipid subunit of the vacuolar H^+ATPase. The M_r 8000 F_0 proteolipid subunit has two membrane-spanning helices and contains a single aspartic acid residue in one of the helices which binds protons during H^+ transport activity and is the residue with which DCCD reacts to inhibit the enzyme. Although the isolated c subunit functions as a proton channel when reconstituted into lipid bilayers (73), the intact F_0 complex has a far lower proton conductance until F_1 is attached (72). In the intact F_0F_1 H^+ATPase, the proteolipid may transmit protons through the membrane by proton binding and release induced by conformational changes in the internal hydrophilic extramembranous loop rather than by acting as a conducting pore (74). The a and b subunits may form a central core, essential for F_1 attachment, around which the c subunits are arrayed (72). The structure of the mitochondrial F_0 domain is far more complex and is composed of as many as nine different polypeptides (75).

How the proton electrochemical gradient induces the F_0F_1 H^+ATPase to synthesize ATP (and the mechanism of ATP-driven H^+ transport) has been studied extensively. The favored mechanism is the rotating three-site model (76), in which ADP and P_i condense spontaneously to form ATP at the active site of a β/α subunit pair. During the catalytic cycle, either the head, the stalk, or the stalk and c subunit rotate, producing conformational changes sequentially at each of the three β/α pairs, which results in the release of ATP. The recent crystallographic structure of mitochondrial F_1 supports this mechanism (75). Although the crystallized F_1 contained the characteristic $\alpha_3\beta_3\gamma\delta\epsilon$ stoichiometry, the diffraction map showed only the hexagonal ring of β/α pairs with only a part of a central γ

*The M_r, originally reported for the kidney H^+ATPase was 15,000 (34), and studies of H^+ATPase from various mammalian preparations have reported values varying from 14,000 to 17,000. Most of the current literature uses a value of 17,000.

subunit (75). This result indicates that δ and ϵ subunits and part of the γ subunit are disordered, consistent with their ability to move in the complex. The visible portion of the γ subunit was asymmetrical in its association with the hexagon of β/α pairs. The results suggest that the "stalk" domain and γ subunit rotate during the course of ATP synthesis (or H$^+$ pumping), causing the asymmetrical γ subunit to induce successive conformational changes in the β/α pairs.

The mechanism by which the proton electrochemical gradient produces this reaction cycle is still unclear. In the bacterial F_0F_1 H$^+$ATPase, it has been proposed that clusters of three proteolipid c subunits use conformational energy, induced by proton binding and unbinding and transmitted through the c subunit hydrophilic loop to drive rotation of the "stalk" (74). If this were the case, the stoichiometry of H$^+$ transported/ATP hydrolyzed (synthesized) could vary depending on the number of H$^+$ binding sites in the c subunit. Alternatively, protons might drive "stalk" rotation more directly in a manner similar to the bacterial flagellar motor (77).

The structure and function of the vacuolar H$^+$ATPases are far less well understood, but they share several features in common with the F_0F_1 H$^+$ATPases. The V_1 cytoplasmic domain is composed of peripheral membrane proteins. It can be stripped from the membrane by alkali or chaotropic ions and is then found as soluble protein complex (62). The number and functions of subunits in this domain are summarized in Table 1. Evidence suggests that the V_1 domain contains A, B, C, D, and E subunits (78,79) with respective sizes of 70, 56, 42, 33, and 31 kDa in a stoichiometry of 3:3:1:1:1 (80). The A and B subunits, which are homologous to the F_0F_1 β and α subunits, are thought to form a hexagon of alternating subunits constituting the catalytic "head" of enzyme, attaching to a central C subunit (80,81), resembling the "head" of the F_0F_1 H$^+$ATPases.

The A and B subunits of the vacuolar H$^+$ATPases are structurally more closely related to the archaebacterial H$^+$ATPases (A-ATPases) than they are to the F_0F_1 H$^+$ATPases (82). The A and B subunits share regions of amino acid sequence identity with each other, with the A and B subunits of the H$^+$ATPase of archaebacteria, and with all β and α subunits of the F_0F_1 ATPases (82). These two subunits probably evolved from a common ancestral gene.

The A subunit is probably the site of ATP hydrolytic activity (83,84). The deduced amino acid sequence of the A subunit (85) contains a "P-loop" nucleotide binding motif (86) that is probably part of the active site; cysteine 254 in this motif is the residue with which NEM reacts to inhibit enzymatic activity (87). The vacuolar H$^+$ATPase B subunit does not have a P-loop motif (88) but may have a noncatalytic nucleotide binding site (89). The function of the B subunit of the vacuolar H$^+$ATPase is uncertain, but it may act as a regulatory subunit that affects the overall enzymatic properties of the H$^+$ATPase (34,88).

There are two isoforms of both the A subunit [the A1 and A2 isoforms; (85,90–92)], and the B subunit [the B1 and B2 isoforms; (88,93–95)] of the mammalian vacuolar H$^+$ATPase, which are all encoded by different genes. The A2 isoform was isolated from a human osteoclastoma cDNA library (92), but there is uncertainty about its role in normal cells. Expression of the A2 subunit transcript has not been detected in normal tissues, and hybridization analysis of genomic DNA with the A1 subunit cDNA probe detects only a single gene (91). cDNA clones for the B1 ("kidney") and B2 ("brain") subunit isoforms were isolated, respectively, from human and bovine kidney and brain cDNA libraries. The deduced amino acid sequence of the two isoforms is more than 90% identical in the mid-coding region (approximately 480 residues); the few amino acid differences are mostly conserved across species. The amino terminal 24-30 residues, and carboxyl terminal 10-18 residues, in contrast, have no identity, but are highly conserved between species (88).

cDNA clones have been reported for the C (96) and E subunits (97,98) of mammalian vacuolar H$^+$ATPase.* Although neither of these exhibits any sequence similarity to subunits of the F_0F_1 H$^+$ATPases, the C subunit is thought to have a role similar to the γ subunit, residing in the "head" of the enzyme. As indicated above, the D and E subunits may reside in a "stalk" domain. By functional analogy with the F_0F_1 H$^+$ATPase, the vacuolar H$^+$ATPase "stalk" likely functions in transmitting energy from conformational changes in the catalytic site to proton binding sites on the proteolipid. It may also have a role in controlling the assembly of the H$^+$ATPase on the membrane (D. M. Underhill and S. L. Gluck, manuscript in preparation).

---

*A cDNA clone has been reported for a "D" subunit (99), but this sequence encodes the human homologue of the bovine Ac38 polypeptide (100).

Table 1 Subunits of the Mammalian Kidney Vacuolar H^+ATPase

Domain	Subunit M_r	Letter/ name(s)	Copies per H^+ATPase	Function	Structural features
		A subunit	3	Site of ATP hydrolysis during catalysis	"P-loop" nucleotide-binding motif (86); ATP-synthase motif (82); homologous to $F_0F_1\beta$ subunit
	70,000	A2 isoform			
		B subunit	3	? Regulatory subunit Influence on enzymatic properties	ATP-synthase motif; homologous to $F_0F_1\alpha$ subunit
	58,000[a]	B1 "kidney" isoform			
	56,000	B2 "brain" isoform			
V_1	42,000	C subunit	1	Unknown function; probably resides in "stalk"	Not homologous to any F_0F_1 subunit
	33,000		1	Unknown function; probably resides in "stalk"	Structure unknown
	31,000	E subunit	1	Unknown function; probably resides in "stalk"	Not homologous to any F_0F_1 subunit
	17,000[b]	Proteolipid c subunit	6	Probably major structural component of "proton channel"	DCCD-reactive glutamate residue; homologous to F_0F_1 proteolipid
V_0	14,000[c]	Name not designated	Unknown	Unknown	Unknown
	12000[c]	Name not designated	Unknown	Unknown	Unknown

[a]Evidence suggests that only three copies of a B1 isoform or three copies of a B2 isoform are present in a single H^+ATPase complex (D.M. Underhill and S.L.G.; unpublished observations).
[b]M_r = 15,000 in the original description of H^+ATPase isolated from bovine kidney (34).
[c]The precise composition of the vacuolar H^+ATPase remains unresolved, and differences in subunit composition have been reported among enzyme purified from mammalian sources. The M_r = 14,000 subunit may be part of the V_1 domain, as reported for the H^+ATPase isolated from insect intestine (369).

The V_0 domain of the vacuolar H^+ATPase, like the F_0 domain, is thought to bind and transmit protons through the lipid bilayer. The precise composition of the membranous V_0 domain of the vacuolar H^+ATPase is uncertain. Experimental evidence indicates that there are 6 copies of the $M_r \sim 17{,}000$ proteolipid subunit in the vacuolar enzyme (80), which are thought to form the major structural component of the V_0 domain. With a stoichiometry of six proteolipid polypeptides, the vacuolar H^+ATPases have two-thirds* the number of proteolipid subunits as in F_0. The vacuolar H^+ATPase proteolipid appears to have evolved from a gene duplication, as both the amino and carboxyl terminal halves of the subunit share homology with the smaller F_0 proteolipid. Like the F_0 proteolipid, the vacuolar H^+ATPase proteolipid reacts covalently with DCCD (101). DCCD may react with a glutamic acid residue in one of the predicted membrane-spanning hydrophobic helices of the vacuolar H^+ATPase M_r 17,000 proteolipid (102). The F_0 domain also has a M_r 19,000 polypeptide subunit, whose stoichiometry and function are presently unknown (103).

In the bacterial F_0F_1 H^+ATPase, which probably has nine proteolipid subunits, the stoichiometry of H^+ transport/ATP hydrolysis of 3:1 is thought to result from coupling of three c subunits (each with a single proton binding site) for each β/α subunit pair (74). It has been proposed that alterations in the number of proteolipid subunits coupled with each pair of catalytic subunits (β/α, or A/B in the vacuolar H^+ATPases) could result in a change in the stoichiometry of proton transport/ATP hydrolysis (104). Thus the vacuolar H^+ATPases, which have six proteolipid subunits each with a single putative H^+-binding residue (102,105), would have two proteolipid subunits for each A/B subunit pair, giving a predicted stoichiometry of 2 H^+ for each ATP hydrolyzed. As discussed below, some experimental evidence in the intact turtle urinary bladder supports a 2:1 stoichiometry (106).

In some mammalian vacuolar H^+ATPase preparations, additional polypeptides are found associated with the H^+ATPases that, in some papers, are considered to be part of the V_0 sector (103,107,108), and in other papers have been termed accessory proteins (109). In mammalian preparations, the H^+ATPase from chromaffin granules has a 38-kDa (Ac38) and 116-kDa polypeptide (Ac116) associated with it, both of which are intrinsic membrane proteins, as in experiments that strip the peripheral membrane proteins off the purified vacuolar H^+ATPase, these polypeptides remain associated with the membrane (103,107,109). The H^+ATPase from coated vesicles has Ac38 and either a 100-kDa (84) or 116-kDa polypeptide (110), which are intrinsic membrane proteins. The cDNA for Ac38 has been isolated (100), but its function remains unknown. The cDNA for Ac116 has been isolated (111) and belongs to a family of conserved proteins that have been identified in the genome of *Caenorhabtidis elegans* (112). A brain-specific isoform of the mammalian Ac116 has been identified that contains an 18–amino acid insert, generated by alternative splicing (113).

The V_0 domain of the H^+ATPase appears to be the site of the inhibition by bafilomycin, which inhibits proton conduction through liposomes containing V_0 subunits (103,108). Some evidence suggests that bafilomycin may bind to Ac100, even though the 17-kDa proteolipid is the principal proton-conductive element (103).

Function of Vacuolar H^+ATPase in Intracellular Organelles

Vacuolar H^+ATPases acidify a variety of intracellular compartments in the endocytic and secretory pathways (46,114,115). In the endocytic pathway, vacuolar acidification is essential for the dissociation of ligands from their receptors in the early endosome, for proteolytic cleavage occurring in the endosome, for the passage of some viruses and toxins from the vacuolar lumen into the cytosol, for activation of a multitude of lysosomal hydrolases, and for export of small solutes generated by degradation from the lysosome (114,115). In the secretory pathway, vacuolar acidification is required for proteolytic cleavage during posttranslational processing, for the accumulation of small solutes in specialized secretory granules such as synaptic vesicles, for the concentration and packing of proteins and solutes in secretory granules, and for targeting secretory products to the proper plasmalemmal domain in polarized cells (116).

The cell maintains a pH gradient in the endosomal and secretory pathways (116). The pH of the early endosome is about 6.1, that of the late endosome is about 5.5, and the pH of the lysosome is 4.7 to 5.2. The trans-Golgi network is the first acidic compartment of the secretory pathway with

*Or one-half, if the stoichiometry of the F_0 proteolipid is c_{12}.

a pH of about 6.3. The pH of secretory vacuoles, such as insulin-containing vesicles or chromaffin granules, is about 5.5. The basis for maintenance of different steady-state pH values of these different compartments is uncertain, although it has been proposed that coexistent Na^+,K^+-ATPase in the compartments limits the pH by generating an adverse electrochemical gradient for electrogenic proton secretion (117,118). The normal function of the pH "gradients" in the endocytic and secretory pathways is uncertain.

Properties of Plasma Membrane Vacuolar H^+ATPases

The plasma membrane vacuolar H^+ATPases differ from vacuolar H^+ATPases of intracellular organelles in several ways. The plasma membrane vacuolar H^+ATPase in hydrogen ion-transporting renal epithelial cells reside at high densities (119), and they have a polarized distribution (26,35) that allows for vectorial secretion of hydrogen ion. The plasma membrane vacuolar H^+ATPases of the nephron are also subject to physiologic regulation (10,22,29), which allows the kidney to preserve acid-base balance.

PROPERTIES OF THE VACUOLAR H^+ATPase IN KIDNEY

Transport Properties of Vacuolar H^+ATPase in Turtle Urinary Bladder

Many of the physiologic properties of H^+ secretion by vacuolar H^+ATPases in urinary epithelia were first elucidated in the turtle urinary bladder, a model epithelium that acidifies its lumen and which has transport properties similar to those of the cortical collecting tubule (29,120). Under short-circuit conditions, after sodium transport is inhibited by ouabain or amiloride, the bladder exhibits lumen-positive current that is identical (in meq/min) to the rate of luminal acidification measured with a pH stat (121), a strong indication that the pump is electrogenic. As noted above, membrane vesicle fractions from the turtle bladder were found to acidify their lumen upon the addition of ATP, indicating that they contained an ATP-driven proton pump (51,122). The rate of acidification was increased by conditions that collapse a potential difference across the vesicle membrane, indicating that the pump was electrogenic. Proton transport was inhibited by DCCD and sulfhydryl reagents but not by the F_0F_1 inhibitors oligomycin and azide or the E_1E_2 inhibitor vanadate (51), demonstrating that the pump had a unique inhibitor sensitivity profile, subsequently shown to be a general characteristic of the vacuolar H^+ATPases. These experiments provided the first direct evidence that the urinary bladder proton pump was an ATPase with properties distinct from the yeast plasma membrane H^+ATPase or the gastric H^+-K^+-ATPase.

Although most of the properties of the vacuolar H^+ATPase of urinary epithelia have been determined from studies of the purified enzyme, the apparent H^+/ATP stoichiometry of the turtle bladder proton pump has been examined in the intact tissue using two different approaches. Dixon and Al-Awqati (123) used measurements of the $\Delta G'_{ATP}$ and the apparent PMF of the pump, extrapolated from a plot of transport rate as a function of the luminal pH gradient, to arrive at a stoichiometry of 3 H^+/ATP. Andersen and Steinmetz (120,124) have pointed out, however, that the apparent PMF obtained in this manner can be misleading if the shape of the pump I-V curve has an inflection near zero. Steinmetz et al. (106) measured the production of lactate as a function of H^+ transport rates in bladders maintained under anaerobic conditions using glucose as a substrate. The measured lactate formation/H^+ transport ratios were constant at 0.55 to 0.58 under a variety of conditions, yielding a calculated stoichiometry at 2 H^+/ATP.

Transport Properties of Vacuolar H^+ATPase in Mammalian Kidney Membranes

Properties of Renal Vacuolar H^+ATPase Revealed from Membrane Vesicle Studies

An ATP-driven proton pump with transport properties identical to those of the proton pump in the turtle urinary bladder was found in membrane vesicles from bovine kidney medulla (125). ATP-induced acidification was not inhibited by several mitochondrial H^+ATPase inhibitors (oligomycin, efrapeptin, and rutamycin) or by 500 μM vanadate, but was eliminated by NEM [K_i = 28 μM (125)], and by Zn^{2+} (K_i = 170 μM (34)]. Proton transport activity in the kidney membranes required ATP and was not supported by any other nucleotide (125). Proton transport activity with nearly identical properties was subsequently described in membranes from rat (126) and human renal medulla (127).

As indicated above, vacuolar H^+ATPases acidify many intracellular compartments in the vacuolar membrane system. Not surprisingly, vacuolar H^+ATPase proton transporting activity was found in a membrane preparation from rat kidney cortex that was enriched for endosomes (128). The ATP-induced proton transport in these membranes had properties typical of other vacuolar H^+ATPases, including sensitivity to NEM, DCCD, and Zn^{2+} and resistance to oligomycin (128). H^+ transport was highly selective for ATP, with a K_m = 77 μM. Acidification required a permeant anion (128, 129), with a rank order of efficacy of $SCN^- > Cl^- > Br^- > I^- >> HPO_4^{2-} > HCO_3^- > F^-$ (129). These membranes had ionophore-stimulated ATPase activity whose spectrum of sensitivity to inhibitors was similar to that for ATP-driven acidification, consistent with the presence of an H^+ATPase whose activity is affected by the proton electrochemical gradient across the vesicle membrane (130). Endosome-enriched membranes from rabbit kidney cortex had ATP-driven proton transport with properties similar to those from rat kidney cortex (131).

In early studies, brush-border membranes were found to have intravesicular ATPase activity in the sealed membranes. The activity was stimulated protonophores and inhibited by DCCD, which was interpreted as representing an H^+ATPase in the membrane (132). Subsequent experiments, however, showed that the protonophore-stimulated ATPase activity was insensitive to high concentrations of NEM (133) and was therefore unlikely to have arisen from vacuolar H^+ATPase activity.

The first evidence for a vacuolar H^+ATPase in renal brush border came from immunocytochemical staining of rat kidney with anti-H^+ATPase antibodies, which demonstrated extensive staining of the brush border (26). Burckhardt and colleagues demonstrated that isolated rat kidney brush border membranes into which ATP and an ATP-regenerating system were introduced by freeze-thawing (134) alkalinized their interior by a DCCD and NEM-inhibitable mechanism and had internal NEM-sensitivie ATPase activity. They later showed that treatment of brush-border membranes with cholate resulted in a reorientation of the membrane, such that addition of ATP to the vesicles resulted in intravesicular acidification (135). Acidification in these reoriented brush-border membranes had an inhibitor sensitivities profile typical of the vacuolar H^+ATPases. It was resistant to azide, oligomycin, and vanadate, but was inhibited by DCCD and Zn^{2+} and had K_i's for NEM and NBD-Cl of 0.77 μM and 0.39 μM. The K_m for ATP was 93 μM, with a substrate preference of ATP>GTP≈ITP>UTP; ADP was a competitive inhibitor of acidification with a K_i = 24 μM. The same laboratory later showed that acidification by the reoriented brush border membranes was highly sensitive to bafilomycin A_1, with a $K_i < 10$ μM (63). These properties are in good agreement with those of the purified bovine brush-border vacuolar H^+ATPase (62) (see below).

Properties of Renal Vacuolar H^+ATPase Isolated from Mammalian Kidney Membranes

The bovine kidney medullary membranes discussed above were found to contain NEM-sensitive ATPase activity that was resistant to oligomycin, azide, and vanadate; this activity was used as an assay for isolation of the bovine kidney vacuolar H^+ATPase (34,54). Kidney vacuolar H^+ATPase was initially isolated from solubilized bovine kidney medullary membranes by precipitation and ion exchange chromatography (54). The isolated bovine H^+ATPase was used to generate a monoclonal antibody to the enzyme (136), which enabled the development of an immunoaffinity method for purifying the active enzyme from solubilized kidney membranes in a single step (34).

Vacuolar H^+ATPase has been isolated by this immunoaffinity technique from bovine kidney microsomal membranes* (from outer medulla and cortex) (34,54), bovine kidney brush-border membranes (62), and bovine kidney cortex lysosomes (137) (Table 2). Like other mammalian vacuolar H^+ATPases (46,47,138), the enzymes isolated from these kidney membranes shared several properties. All of the H^+ATPases were electrogenic; inhibitable by NEM but not by oligomycin, azide, or vanadate, and did not require the presence of specific monovalent ions or cations for activity (34,54,125).

H^+ATPase isolated from microsomes, brush border, and lysosomes differed in several enzymatic

---

*Microsomes are a mixture of different membrane fractions, but the preparation used [the G2 membrane fraction in (125)] is enriched for the B2 or "kidney" isoform of the B subunit, indicating that much of the membrane originates from intercalated cells (see Reference 88).

Table 2 Properties of H^+ATPase in Different Kidney Membrane Fractions

	Membrane fraction		
	Microsome (34,54)	Brush border (62)	Lysosome (137)
pH optimum	6.3	7.4	6.9
Substrate specificity	ATPase:GTPase = 4:1	ATPase:GTPase = 2:1	ATPase:GTPase = 3:1
Lipid effects	Activated by PG > PI >> PC > PS	No lipid activation	No lipid activation
Multivalent cation effects	Zn^{+2}: 100% inhib CU^{+2}: 100% inhib Al^{+3}: 0% inhib	Zn^{+2}: 100% inhib Cu^{+2}: 50% inhib Al^{+3}: 0% inhib	Zn^{+2}: 100% inhib Cu^{+2}: 20% inhib Al^{+3}: 80% inhib
Anion effects	No Cl^- requirement Inhibition by NO_3^-	No Cl^- requirement Inhibition by NO_3^-	No Cl^- requirement Inhibition by NO_3^-
Structure	A subunit: single 70 kDa B subunit: 58 kDa (B1) > 56 kDa (B2) E subunit: single 31 kDa	A subunit: single 70 kDa B subunit: 56 kDa (B2) only E subunit: multiple ~31 kDa	A subunit: single 70 kDa B subunit: 56 kDa (B1) only E subunit: single 31 kDa

properties. The pH optimum of the brush border H^+ATPase was 7.2, close to the steady-state intracellular pH of the proximal tubule cell (23), while that from the microsomes was 6.3, well below the steady-state intracellular pH of about 7.2 in intercalated cells (28,31,139–146). The pH optimum of the brush-border H^+ATPase is therefore poised constitutively for optimal transport in the proximal tubule cell. In contrast, the pH optimum of the microsomal H^+ATPase, which probably comes mostly from intercalated cells, is positioned such that the activity of the H^+ATPase would increase were cytosolic pH to fall, increasing intercalated cell H^+ secretion. The magnitude of such changes would be small, however: only 20–25% over a physiologic pH range of 6.2 to 7.5 (34). The pH optimum of the lysosomal H^+ATPase was 6.9, close to physiologic cell pH.

Vacuolar H^+ATPases isolated from the different kidney membrane fractions differed in other properties (Table 2). The medullary microsomal enzyme activity was activated by phosphatidyl glycerol, phosphatidyl inositol, and phosphatidyl serine (34); in contrast, the activities of the brush-border and lysosomal enzymes were not affected by added lipids (62,137). Several studies have shown that the apical membrane of epithelia maintains a different lipid composition from that of the basolateral membrane and intracellular membrane compartments (147–149). It is possible that changes in the lipid environment of the plasma membrane could be a means for physiologic regulation, although this has not been demonstrated directly.

The H^+ATPases from different membrane compartments varied in their substrate specificity (Table 2), suggesting that they differ in the structure of the catalytic site. As discussed below, the catalytic site probably occurs at the interface of the A and B subunits of the H^+ATPase, implying that variations in structure of either of the subunits could contribute to functional differences. Striking differences among the H^+ATPases from different compartments were also found in the ability of divalent and trivalent cations to support or inhibit ATPase activity (34,62,137). For the microsomal H^+ATPase, the divalent cation preference for activity was Mn,Mg>>Ca>Co>>Ba,Sr, and aluminum did not support activity; for the brush border H^+ATPase, the preference was Mn>>Mg>>Co>Al>Ca>>Ba,Sr. 1 mM Zn^{2+} inhibited both the microsomal and brush border enzymes completely; 1 m*M* Cu^{2+} inhibited 100% of the microsomal H^+ATPase activity, but only 49% of the brush border H^+ATPase activity. Al^{3+} was able to support brush border, but not microsomal, H^+ATPase activity, and inhibited lysosomal H^+ATPase activity (137). The differences in the ability of these ions to support activity suggests that at least some of the effects of the multivalent cations occurs at the active site of the H^+ATPases.

Both ATP-induced acidification and potential generation by the purified, reconstituted H^+ATPase occurred in the absence of chloride (34). Chloride neither stimulated nor was required for either the ATPase or proton transporting activity of the purified H^+ATPase (34). The requirement of chloride, or other permeant anions, for ATP-induced acidification of kidney membrane vesicles (125,126,128,130) discussed above most likely arises from the need for anion entry to collapse an inside-positive potential difference produced by electrogenic H^+ secretion.

H^+ATPase isolated from bovine kidney brush-border membranes was inhibited by nitrate with an IC_{50} of 21 m*M* (62), a concentration much lower than that needed to dissociate the kidney H^+ATPase cytosolic domain subunits (62). Sulfite anion stimulated the H^+ATPase at concentrations in the 1–30 m*M* range and inhibited the enzyme at higher concentrations, with an IC_{50} of 93 m*M*. Both nitrate and sulfite (at concentrations >5 m*M*) both inhibited the H^+ATPase with uncompetitive kinetics (62,137), suggesting that they do not inhibit at the catalytic site. Thus, the kidney H^+ATPase may have a regulatory oxyanion binding site. Bicarbonate, the principal cellular oxyanion, stimulated H^+ATPase activity 33% at 150 m*M* (62).

The vacuolar H^+ATPase inhibitor bafilomycin A_1 inhibited the kidney H^+ATPase with an IC_{50} of 1–2 n*M* and 90% inhibition at 30 n*M* (63,64). Omeprazole, an acid-activated sulfhydryl-reactive inhibitor of the gastric H^+,K^+-ATPase (150), also inhibited the mammalian vacuolar H^+ATPase by reacting with the same sulfhydryl residue as NEM (151). Sch28080, an H^+-K^+-ATPase inhibitor that acts by binding to the external K^+ binding site of the enzyme (152), had no effect on the isolated kidney vacuolar H^+ATPase (S.L.G.; unpublished data). It inhibited vacuolar H^+ATPase-driven acidification of rat renal endosome-enriched membranes by 25%, and the effect was not affected by the presence or absence of potassium (153). Electrogenic H^+ secretion in the intact turtle urinary bladder, a process that is probably derived entirely from a vacuolar H^+ATPase, was also inhibited in a concentration-dependent manner by Sch28080 (154,155), and the effect was the same in the presence and absence of luminal potassium (154). Thus, Sch28080 appears to have indirect effects on intact tissues that may preclude its use to distinguish vacuolar H^+ and H^+,K^+-ATPases.

Structural Properties of H^+ATPase in Kidney

The vacuolar H^+ATPase isolated from bovine kidney membranes by ion-exchange chromatography or immunoaffinity chromatography contained polypeptides at M_r = 70,000, ~56,000 (as a cluster of three to four discrete polypeptides), 45,000, 42,000, 38,000, 33,000, 31,000, 15,000, 14,000, and 12,000 (34,54,62). This composition was similar to that reported for other mammalian vacuolar H^+ATPases (reviewed in Reference 46) but notably lacked the M_r = 110,000 or 116,000 intrinsic membrane polypeptide observed in other H^+ATPase preparations. A summary of the subunits of the mammalian kidney vacuolar H^+ATPase is given in Table 1. The kidney H^+ATPase isolated by ion exchange chromatography exhibited two peaks of ATPase activity (34). These fractions were subjected to polyacrylamide gel electrophoresis under nondenaturing conditions, and two complexes with approximate M_r values of 551,000 and 523,000 were found (54). The polypeptide composition in the two peaks of activity showed some differences. Most notably, two B subunit polypeptides at M_r = 58,000 and 56,000 were found to segregate on the column, each following one of the peaks of ATPase activity eluting from the column (34). These findings were an initial indication that different structural forms of the H^+ATPase might exist containing isoforms of a B subunit.

H^+ATPase was isolated by immunoaffinity chromatography from kidney microsomes and from brush border to examine the possibility that H^+ATPases with different structures were located in different membrane compartments in the kidney. On two-dimensional polyacrylamide gels, both of the enzyme preparations showed a single A subunit polypeptide. In contrast, the enzymes differed substantially in the composition of the B and E subunits. In H^+ATPase from both microsomes and from brush border, the B subunit showed several polypeptides at M_r = 56,000, but the pattern from the two preparations was reproducibly different. Only the microsome-derived H^+ATPase had a prominent polypeptide at M_r = 58,000, which had a pI slightly more acidic than that of the M_r = 56,000 polypeptides (62). In the brush border H^+ATPase, multiple E subunit polypeptides were observed, with M_rs in the 31,000–35,000 range; all of these exhibited immunoreactivity with a monoclonal antibody to the COOH-terminus of the E subunit (98). In contrast, in the microsomal H^+ATPase, only a single E subunit polypeptide was observed. These results suggested that structural variations in the B and/or E subunits might be a basis for differences in enzymatic properties or distribution among vacuolar H^+ATPases.

As discussed above, cDNA clones for the A, B1, B2, and E subunits have been isolated from kidney cDNA libraries (85,88,93,97,98,156). The B1 and B2 subunits represent two isoforms of the B subunit that are encoded by different genes. The predicted protein products of the two cDNAs are 98% identical over most of the protein. They differ markedly, however, in the sequences of the amino-terminal 28 amino acids and the carboxyl-terminal 12 amino acids (88).

The cDNAs for the A and E subunit are expressed in all mammalian tissues (85,91,97) and appear identical to those in the constitutively expressed vacuolar H^+ATPase common to all cells. The B2 isoform is also expressed in all mammalian tissues (88,95) and encodes a subunit probably residing in constitutive forms of the vacuolar H^+ATPase, such as lysosomes and endosomes (137). The B1 isoform, however, is expressed at detectable levels only in the kidney (88) and placenta (R. D. Nelson, S. Bae, and S. L. G.; unpublished observations) and may encode a subunit with cell-specific functions.

Distribution of Vacuolar H^+ATPase in Kidney

Distribution of Vacuolar H^+ATPase by Physiologic Criteria.

Proximal Tubule. Approximately one-third of proximal tubule bicarbonate reabsorption (H^+ secretion) was found to be independent of Na^+-H^+ exchange (12,157,158), indicating that another transporter, such as an H^+ATPase, had a significant role in proximal H^+ secretion. The sodium-independent amiloride-insensitive bicarbonate reabsorption in the rat proximal tubule was inhibited by luminal NEM and DCCD, suggesting that it arose from a vacuolar H^+ATPase (24). In the rabbit (157) and rat (20) proximal tubule, a sodium-independent mechanism for pH_i recovery following acidification with NH_4Cl was found that was inhibited by luminal NEM and DCCD (157) and by inhibitors of ATP production and bafilomycin A_1 (20), properties consistent with a vacuolar H^+ATPase. Several other studies in intact tubules have provided additional physiologic evidence for vacuolar H^+ATPase-driven H^+ secretion in the proximal tubule luminal membrane (159,160).

Distal Tubule. Studies in the rat early distal tubule demonstrated that 20% of the bicarbonate reabsorption was resistant to the Na^+-H^+ antiport inhibitors amiloride and ethylisopropylamiloride (EIPA), and that bafilomycin A_1, inhibited about 36% of bicarbonate reabsorption, consistent with a small contribution of a vacuolar H^+ATPase to overall H^+ secretion (17). In the late distal tubule (corresponding the initial collecting tubule), amiloride and EIPA had no effect on bicarbonate reabsorption, whereas bafilomycin inhibited 47%, indicating that a vacuolar H^+ATPase may be the major transporter responsible for H^+ in this segment (17).

Cortical and Outer Medullary Collecting Duct. The physiologic evidence for a vacuolar H^+ATPase in the cortical and outer medullary collecting tubule is vast. The intact cortical collecting tubule, under suitable conditions, reabsorbs bicarbonate and generates a lumen-positive potential difference in the absence of sodium or presence of luminal amiloride, consistent with a model of luminal H^+ secretion by an electrogenic H^+ATPase (161–166). More direct evidence for a vacuolar H^+ATPase in the plasma membrane of collecting tubule cells has come from studies on regulation of their intracellular pH. After pH_i of individual collecting tubule cells is acidified by the NH_4Cl prepulse technique (167), pH_i recovery proceeds partially by Na^+-H^+ exchange (141–143) and partly by a sodium-independent amiloride-insensitive mechanism that is resistant to the H^+,K^+-ATPase inhibitor Sch28080 (142,144,168) but inhibitable by luminal NEM (144,145,168) thought to represent the luminal vacuolar H^+ATPase.* Until recently, intracellular pH measurements were performed on entire tubules, which presented a major problem of distinguishing H^+ transport in intercalated cells from that in principal cells. This problem has largely been solved by an ingenious method of loading the pH probe BCECF selectively into intercalated cells, developed by Weiner and Hamm (169). Using this method, several investigators have found evidence for vacuolar H^+ATPase-driven pH_i recovery in intercalated cells of the cortical collecting tubule (10,30,170).

*Breyer and Jacobson (141) investigated the recovery of pH_i of outer medullary collecting tubules in CO_2-free buffers following acidification by exposure to NH_4Cl, and found that recovery was blocked by basolateral amiloride and was absolutely dependent on basolateral sodium, indicating sole control by Na^+-H^+ exchange. Several subsequent studies (21,28,142) showed that, in CO_2-free buffers, the rate or time course for activation of sodium-independent recovery is slow, requiring as long as 25 min or more to reach baseline pH; Breyer and Jacobson may have failed to detect this H^+-extrusion mechanism because their experiments were of short duration.

Limited electrophysiologic data on bicarbonate-secreting (β) intercalated cell is consistent with an electrogenic H^+ATPase in the basolateral membrane (170,171).

The outer stripe of the outer medullary collecting tubule has functionally distinct H^+-secreting intercalated cells and Na^+-transporting principal cells (172,173); it reabsorbs bicarbonate by an amiloride-resistant sodium-independent mechanism (172), consistent with H^+ secretion by a vacuolar H^+ATPase. Studies of intracellular pH regulation in individual cells from outer stripe indicate that the intercalated cells, but not the principal cells, have a luminal plasma membrane vacuolar H^+ATPase (144,145).

The inner stripe of the outer medullary collecting tubule (in the rabbit) is significantly different from the outer stripe. The inner stripe does not transport sodium and normally has a lumen-positive potential difference thought to arise from electrogenic proton secretion (36,39,165,166). This segment was once thought to exist of a single cell type (142,174,175), but morphologic (26,176–178) and physiologic evidence (28,168) has shown that there are two functionally distinct cell types. In recent studies, vacuolar H^+ATPase-driven proton extrusion was measured in individual inner stripe intercalated cells from rates of sodium-independent recovery of pH_i following in vitro acid loading (28,168). A minority cell population in the inner stripe, which probably represent intercalated cells, had higher rates of vacuolar H^+ATPase-driven H^+ extrusion than the neighboring majority (principal) cells (28,168), although the latter also appeared to have apical membrane H^+ATPases (28).

Distribution of Vacuolar H^+ATPase by Immunocytochemistry. The immunocytochemical distribution of vacuolar H^+ATPase in the rat nephron (see Table 3), performed using antibodies monospecific to the M_r 70,000, 56,000, and 31,000 subunits (26,35,179), showed a distribution in agreement with (or predictive of) the distribution of the H^+ATPase assessed by physiologic methods (11,15,16,19,24,25,28,142,144,168,180).

In the S1 and S2 segments of the proximal tubule, vacuolar H^+ATPase was found in the

Table 3 Distribution of Vacuolar H^+ATPase in Rat Kidney[a]

Segment	Distribution	Intensity
Proximal tubule: S1	Brush-border microvilli	3+
	Subvillar invaginations and endosomes	2+
Proximal tubule: S2	Brush-border microvilli	2+
	Subvillar invaginations and endosomes	2+
Proximal tubule: S3	Brush-border microvilli	0
	Subvillar invaginations and endosomes	2+
Loop: cortical thin descending limb	Apical membrane	1+
	Basolateral membrane	1+
Loop: medullary thin limb	Apical membrane	0
	Basolateral membrane	0
Loop: thick ascending limb	Apical membrane and apical vesicles	1+
Distal convoluted tubule	Apical membrane	1+
Connecting tubule	Principal cells: Apical membrane	1+
	Intercalated cells (plasma membrane and vesicles)	4+
Cortical collecting tubule	Principal cells:	0
	Intercalated cells (plasma membrane and vesicles)	4+
Outer medullary collecting tubule: outer stripe	Principal cells:	0
	Intercalated cells (plasma membrane and vesicles)	4+
Outer medullary collecting tubule: inner stripe	Principal cells: Apical membrane	0
	Intercalated cells (plasma membrane and vesicles)	4+
Inner medullary collecting tubule	Principal cells: Apical membrane (B1 subunit only)	1+
	Intercalated cells (first third only)	4+

[a]The distribution is derived from immunocytochemical studies in rat kidney (26). The distribution of H^+ATPase in rabbit kidney is largely similar, although differences are present (178).

brush-border microvilli and in the invaginations and vesicles at the base of the microvilli (26). H^+ATPase staining was absent from clathrin-coated pits in this latter region. In the S3 segment, H^+ATPase labeling was again found in the subvillar invaginations of the apical membrane but was absent from the microvilli (26).

In the initial part of the thin descending limb, moderate H^+ATPase labeling was found in both the apical and basolateral membranes; staining was absent from the inner part of the thin limb. Moderate H^+ATPase labeling was observed in the apical membrane and apical vesicles in the medullary and cortical thick ascending limb, and weak to moderate staining was present in the apical membrane of the distal convoluted tubule (26).

In both the connecting tubule and cortical collecting tubule, intense H^+ATPase staining was observed in all of the intercalated cells, with variable distributions in apical membrane, basolateral membrane, or cytosolic vesicles among the cells (26). Six different patterns of H^+ATPase staining were discernible in rat kidney (179): well-polarized apical (WPA; 38%), poorly polarized apical (PPA; 25%), diffuse (D; 9%), bipolar (B-A; 6%), poorly-polarized basolateral (PPB; 21%), and well-polarized basolateral (WPB; 2%). As discussed below, the distribution of H^+ATPase in these cells is dynamic, responding to the acid-base status of the animal.

The principal cells in the connecting tubule had weak to moderate apical membrane H^+ATPase staining, resembling that in the distal convoluted tubule (26). The principal cells in the cortical collecting tubule, however, were devoid of detectable H^+ATPase labeling (26).

In the outer medullary collecting tubule, in both the outer and inner stripe, principal cells had no detectable H^+ATPase staining, and intercalated cells labeled intensively with H^+ATPase antibodies (26). In contrast to the cortex, intercalated cells in the outer medullary segments showed only WPA or PPA H^+ATPase distributions (179), consistent with physiologic evidence that no bicarbonate secretion occurs in these segments (reviewed in Reference 30).

In the inner medullary collecting duct, the intercalated cells (present only in the first third of the segment) had intense H^+ATPase labeling (26) with a WPA distribution (179). The principal cells of the inner medulla showed weak apical staining with antibody of the B1 subunit isoform (181) but no staining with antibodies to the A, E, or proteolipid subunits of the H^+ATPase (181), indicating that functional vacuolar H^+ATPases probably do not reside in the plasma membrane.

Although vacuolar H^+ATPases are on endosomes, lysosomes, trans-Golgi network, and other acidic organelles, where they can be detected immunocytochemically on fixed intact cells (136,182), H^+ATPase staining generally is not demonstrable on these intracellular organelles in sections of kidney tissue (26,35,119). The reason for this apparent discrepancy is probably the relatively low density of H^+ATPases in intracellular organelles. It has been estimated that there are 22 H^+ATPases on a single chromaffin granule (183). Using a value of 0.5 μm for the diameter of a chromaffin granule yields a density of 7 pumps/μm^2 in these organelles. In contrast, proton–secreting urinary epithelial cells have a density of over 14,000 pumps/μm^2 (119). At these enormous densities, H^+ATPases are readily demonstrable on the plasma membrane in several cell types in the kidney.

Cell-Specific Expression of H^+ATPase Subunits

As discussed above, there are two isoforms of the B subunit that are encoded by different genes. Nelson et al. (88) examined the distribution of the B1 and B2 subunit isoform in rat tissues. High levels of B1 subunit mRNA and protein expression were found only in kidney cortex and medulla and not in any other tissues tested. The distribution of the B1 ("kidney") isoform protein was determined by immunocytochemistry in rat kidney and compared with the distribution of the E (Mr 31,000) subunit. The B1 isoform was expressed at high levels in both α and β intercalated cells. In these cells, the distribution of B1 subunit staining was identical to that of E subunit staining, indicating no preferential targeting of the isoform to apical or basolateral poles. As indicated above, the B1 subunit antibody also labeled the apical membrane of inner medullary principal cells, but no other subunits of the vacuolar H^+ATPase were detectable in these cells. Physiologic studies also indicated that H^+ secretion by the inner medullary principal cells was not from a vacuolar-type proton pump (reviewed in Reference 184) but may be from an H-K ATPase (42). No staining with B1 subunit isoform antibody was observed in the proximal tubule, loop of Henle, or distal convoluted tubules.

The B2 subunit isoform mRNA was expressed in all rat tissues tested, with highest levels in brain and adrenal medulla (88). In recent studies, polyclonal antibodies specific for the mammalian

B2 subunit isoform were generated, and the distribution in mammalian kidney was examined (185). Antibodies to the B2 subunit isoform labeled the proximal tubule brush border and subvillar invaginations intensely in a distribution identical in the S1, S2, and S3 segments to that obtained earlier with antibodies to the E subunit (26,179). In the loop of Henle, moderate labeling was found in the apical membrane in thick ascending limb, and slight labeling of the apical membrane in distal convoluted tubule was observed. These staining patterns were also identical to those observed earlier with E subunit antibodies (26,179). In marked contrast, no labeling of cells in the cortical or medullary collecting duct segments was found with the B2 isoform-specific antibody. In experiments with double-label immunocytochemistry with the two isoform-specific antibodies, no segments were detected that showed staining for both the B1 and B2 subunits (185).

Factors That Modulate Vacuolar H^+ATPase Activity

The kidney plasma membrane vacuolar H^+ATPase is subject to physiologic regulation that enables renal epithelial cells to control rates of transepithelial H^+ transport. Although the basis for this control remains largely unknown, two classes of candidates have emerged.

Kidney Cytosolic Proteins That Modulate Vacuolar H^+ATPase Activity. Inhibitors and activators of the purified kidney microsome H^+ATPase were found in cytosol from bovine kidney (186,187). The properties of the inhibitor and activator are summarized in Table 4. The inhibitor was purified to a high degree using several precipitation, ion exchange, and size separation steps (187) and eluted from a gel filtration column with an apparent M_r = 14–20,000. Inhibitor activity was sensitive to treatment with trypsin but was not affected by lipase, carbohydrate hydrolases, or nucleases, indicating that it is a protein. Inhibition was concentration-dependent and required 20 min incubation time or longer to exhibit maximal inhibitory activity. Inhibition was not reversible by washing. Neither various protease inhibitors nor addition of BSA had any effect on inhibitor activity, indicating that the inhibitor is unlikely to be a protease. The inhibitor reduced ATP-driven acidification in bovine kidney membranes by 90%, demonstrating that it is active against the H^+ATPase in its native membraqne state and implying that it interacts with the H^+ATPase on its cytoplasmic domain. The inhibitory effect on the purified H^+ATPase was pH-dependent, showing an increase in the maximum inhibition of the enzyme above pH 7.5. The pH-dependence was poised such that the inhibitor would reduce H^+ATPase activity with an increase in cytosolic pH above the normal physiologic range. The inhibitor was equally effective (at maximal concentrations) on H^+ATPase purified from kidney microsomes, brush-order membranes, and lysosomes (187).

Table 4 Properties of Inhibitor and Activator of Kidney Vacuolar H^+ATPase

	Inhibitor	Activator
Actions	Inhibits solubilized immunoaffinity-purified H^+ATPase Inhibits ATP-dependent proton transport	Activates solubilized immunoaffinity purified H^+ATPase
Mode of action	Saturable effect on H^+ATPase Inhibition requires preincubation with the H^+ATPase. Inhibition is irreversible; activity cannot be restored by washing enzyme at any pH	Saturable effect on H^+ATPase Nonenzymatic effect. Probably works by binding Activator readily washed off, but binds more tightly at pH < 7.5
pH effects	Percent inhibition increases for pH > 7.5	Binding optimum at pH 6.5; percent activation increases for pH < 6.5
Composition	Heat-labile protein. Active M_r of 14–20,000 by gel filtration	Heat-stable protein. Active M_r of ~35,000 by gel filtration
Specificity	Highly specific for vacuolar H^+ATPases. Slight effect on F_0F_1 H^+-ATPase Not selective for subclass of vacuolar H^+ATPase	Highly specific for vacuolar H^+ATPases. Slight effect on F_0F_1 H^+-ATPasc Selective for brush border > microsomal >> lysosomal V-ATPase

The cytosolic H^+ATPase activator was also partially purified by precipitation, ion exchange, and gel filtration chromatography (186) and eluted from a gel filtration column with an apparent M_r = 35,000. Activator activity was concentration-dependent and saturable and was sensitive to treatment with trypsin, indicating that it is a protein. The stimulation of H^+ATPase by the activator was nearly immediate, occurring with 1 min or less of preincubation time. Activation was reversible by washing, but the pH of the buffer greatly affected the ease of removal of the activator. At pH values of 6.5 and below, the activator required 10 min to dissociate from the H^+ATPase; whereas at higher pH values, the dissociation was immediate. Activation of the purified H^+ATPase was also highly pH-dependent. In the pH range ≤6.6, the activator stimulated H^+ATPase activity up to 1200-fold; at pH values ≥6.6, there was only a 1- to 2-fold stimulation of activity. The pH dependence was therefore positioned such that the activator would increase H^+ATPase activity with a decrease in cytosolic pH below the normal physiologic range. The activator showed a more than twofold greater stimulation of microsomal and brush-border H^+ATPase activity than it did on lysosomal H^+ATPase activity, demonstrating a significant selectivity in its effect on different kidney vacuolar H^+ATPases. This implies that the activator could exhibit selective regulatory effects on H^+ATPases residing on the plasma membrane (186).

Other Factors That Modulate ATP-Driven Proton Transport or Vacuolar H^+ATPase Activity. Gurich and Dubose (188) found that in vitro addition of 8-Br-cAMP to endosome-enriched membranes from rabbit kidney cortex affected ATP-driven proton transport. In buffer containing 100 m*M* Cl^-, high concentrations of 8-Br-cAMP (250 μ*M*) inhibited acidification partially in all endosome-enriched membrane fractions from a sucrose density gradient but showed a greater inhibition (up to 60%) in the higher-density fractions. In contrast, low concentrations of 8-Br-cAMP (5 μ*M*) slightly stimulated acidification in the light membrane fractions but still partially inhibited in the higher-density fractions. The results suggest that the vacuolar H^+ATPase in these preparations resides in a heterogenous population of vesicles that may be subject to different regulatory mechanisms, including protein kinases.

In buffers containing only 6 m*M* Cl^-, the baseline rate of ATP-induced acidification was reduced, and 250 μ*M* cAMP inhibited H^+ transport by about 90% in all gradient fractions. The authors interpreted this result to indicate that cAMP exerted a direct suppression of the H^+ATPase-independent of effects on anion permeability and suggested that this might occur through phosphorylation. Their results differ from those of Mulberg et al. (189), who demonstrated that cAMP-dependent protein kinase (PKA) increased ATP-dependent acidification in bovine brain–coated vesicles by increasing the chloride permeability. Gurich and Dubose (188) used only 1 m*M* ATP and no regenerating system in their experiments; it is therefore possible that the observed effects were due to competitive nucleotide substrate interactions.

Gurich et al. (190) found, in a subsequent study, that both GTP and GTP-γ-S stimulated the initial rate of acidification in endosome-enriched membranes from rabbit renal cortex. They demonstrated that the effect was blocked by pretreatment of the membranes with pertussis toxin and suggested that G proteins may be capable of stimulating the vacuolar H^+ATPase in renal cortex endosomes.

PHYSIOLOGIC REGULATION OF THE VACUOLAR H^+ATPase IN URINARY EPITHELIA*

The mammalian kidney has the ability to adjust net acid excretion in response to changes in the physiologic environment of the animal. The physiologic factors that influence or control the rate of H^+ transport may be divided into those that produce rapid or *acute* responses, occurring in minutes to hours and usually readily reversible, and those that produce *chronic* responses, occurring in hours to days and often requiring major changes in cell architecture. Factors that affect H^+ transport may function, in principle, by one (or more) of three possible mechanisms shown in Figure 3: (a) a change in the

*This review does not discuss those aspects of the regulation of bicarbonate secretion directed at control of luminal Cl^-/HCO_3^- exchange. Renal bicarbonate secretion has been the subject of recent excellent reviews (6,30,191–193).

Table 5 ATPase Activity in Individual Microdissected Nephron Segments (pmol/hr/mm)

Segment[a]	Control kidneys[b]			Acid administration[c]			Alkali administration[c]			Mineralocorticoid administration[c]				Adrenalectomy[c]
	Refs. 290,295	Ref. 297	Ref. 306	Ref. 290	Ref. 297	Ref. 301	Ref. 295	Ref. 297	Ref. 301	Ref. 364	Ref. 304	Ref. 294	Ref. 293	Ref. 291
PT-early (PCT)	—	440	550	—	62	90	—	96	88	—	—	—	—	94
PT-late (PST)	—	—	350	—	—	96	—	—	96	—	—	—	—	113
mTAL	720	220	360	—	192	222	108	96	34	—	—	—	—	95
cTAL	1080	340	420	147	94	—	—	71	94	—	—	—	125	107
DCT	2160	—	—	97	—	—	97	—	—	—	—	—	127	ND
CCT	924	280	350	173	186	114	41	107	92	100	161	200	188	38
OMCT	714	220	250	183	140	169	43	115	53	208	191	300	213	41
IMCD	804	320	—	169	100	—	53	76	—	—	—	—	371	—

[a]PT, proximal tubule; PCT, proximal convoluted tubule; PST, proximal straight tubule; mTAL, medullary thick ascending limb; cTAL, cortical thick ascending limb; DCT, distal convoluted tubule; CCT, cortical collecting tubule; OMCT, outer medullary collecting tubule; IMCD, inner medullary collecting duct

[b]Values expressed as pmol/hr/mm.

[c]Values expressed as percent of control activity.

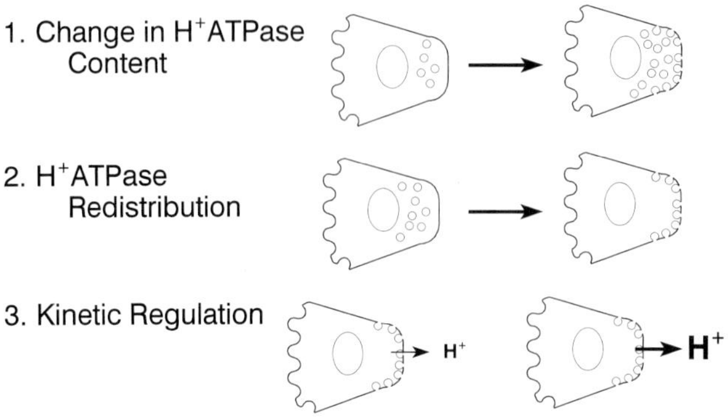

Figure 3 General classes of mechanisms for regulation of epithelial H^+ transport.

kinetics of the H^+ATPase; (b) a change in the number of active H^+ATPases residing on the plasma membrane by redistribution to or from intracellular compartments; and (c) a change in the quantity of the H^+ATPase in the cell without any modification of the relative distribution in the cell.

H^+ secretion by the vacuolar H^+ATPase in several nephron segments is subject to acute regulation by several factors. The most important of these acute factors are the luminal proton electrochemical gradient, the partial pressure of CO_2 (P_{CO_2}), the capacity for basolateral bicarbonate exit, and aldosterone. Many of the details by which acute factors influence the rate of H^+ secretion by vacuolar H^+ATPases in urinary epithelia were first elucidated in the turtle and toad urinary bladder, model epithelia with transport properties similar to those of the cortical collecting tubule (29,120).

Acute Regulation of the Vacuolar H^+ATPase in Toad and Turtle Urinary Bladder

Proton transport in the bladder is performed by a subset of cells containing carbonic anhydrase, which are called CA cells in the turtle bladder (or mitochondria-rich cells in the toad bladder). The bladder CA cells are analogous to the cortical collecting tubule intercalated cells and share many of their characteristics. There are two functional types of CA cells: α cells, which secrete H^+, and β cells, which secrete bicarbonate (194). The α cell has an apical membrane proton pump, belonging to the vacuolar class of H^+ATPases (29,51,195), which acidifies its lumen (121), and a band 3–like Cl^-/HCO_3^- exchanger on the basolateral membrane (196–199). The β cell probably has a basolateral vacuolar H^+ATPase (29,200,201) and a luminal Cl^-/HCO_3^- exchanger (202,203) that differs from the basolateral α cell exchanger (203) (Figure 4).

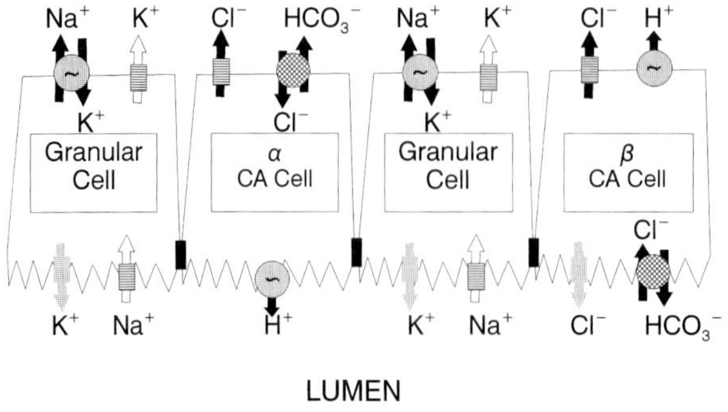

Figure 4 Model for H^+ secretion in the turtle urinary bladder.

Recent experiments suggest that an H^+-K^+-ATPase may account for a significant proportion of net H^+ secretion in the kidney collecting duct (38). Much of the evidence for this rests on the findings that H^+-K^+-ATPase inhibitors, such as Sch28080, substantially reduce collecting duct H^+ secretion (38). These observations prompted a reevaluation of H^+ transport in the bladder for evidence of an H^+-K^+-ATPase (154,155). Although ouabain-sensitive active reabsorption of luminal potassium was found in turtle bladder and had about 14% of the flux of active H^+ secretion (204), there was no evidence for coupling of H^+ secretion to K^+ reabsorption (205). Two groups of investigators (154,155) found that Sch28080 inhibited H^+ secretion in the intact bladder, prompting a reexamination of the possibility of a luminal H^+-K^+-ATPase in the turtle bladder. Careful studies done by Kohn, Steinmetz, and colleagues demonstrated, however, that the inhibitory effect of Sch28080 is not dependent on the presence of luminal potassium and is not blocked by barium, weakening the evidence for a luminal H^+-K^+-ATPase (154). At the present time, it appears that Sch28080 inhibits electrogenic H^+ secretion in the intact turtle bladder by an indirect mechanism.

Acute Regulation by the Luminal Proton Electrochemical Gradient

The most carefully studied factor producing acute changes in H^+ transport is the proton electrochemical gradient across the membrane in which the H^+ATPase resides (120). Proton secretion by the bladder was found to be electrogenic (51,120,205,206) and did not require sodium transport or luminal sodium (205,207,208). Lowering the luminal pH of the bladder slowed the rate of luminal H^+ secretion by imposing an adverse proton electrochemical gradient across the membrane (124, 206,209). Application of a lumen-negative potential difference across the bladder epithelium also stimulated H^+ secretion, and imposition of a lumen-positive potential difference across the epithelium inhibited it (124,206,210). The effect of the proton electrochemical gradient across the luminal membrane on the rate of H^+ secretion was equivalent whether the proton-motive force was generated by pH gradients or electrical gradients (124,206). The relationship between the active proton transport rate and the luminal proton electrochemical gradient was nonlinear, saturating at a proton electrochemical gradient of near zero (124). All of these observations are most readily explained by a model with an electrogenic pump as the predominant proton secretory mechanism.

The observed current-voltage relationship of the bladder fits a mathematical model for the H^+ATPase which assumes that it has a stoichiometry of 2 H^+/ATP and a two-domain structure, with a catalytic "head" and a membrane-spanning proton channel resembling that of the vacuolar and F-ATPases (124), although, as discussed above, the V_0 domain of the vacuolar H^+ATPase may not function as a channel. Studies on the bladder are generally consistent with a model in which the electrochemical gradient affects only the kinetics of the plasma membrane H^+ATPase, without producing changes in the number of H^+ATPases residing on the plasma membrane (124).

Acute Regulation of H^+ Secretion by Intrinsic Regulatory Mechanisms: CO_2, Basolateral Bicarbonate Exit, and the Possible Role of Cell pH

Like most epithelia, the turtle bladder has intrinsic or "homocellular" regulatory mechanisms that couple solute transport by the luminal and basolateral membrane (210a). In the bladder CA cell, luminal H^+ secretion is dependent on basolateral bicarbonate exit. Studies in the turtle bladder over several decades have led to the following overall paradigm for the effects of CO_2, basolateral HCO_3^-, and basolateral Cl^- on H^+ secretion (Figure 4):

Luminal H^+ secretion by an electrogenic pump (vacuolar H^+ATPase) generates intracellular OH^-, which cannot exit the cell. In the absence of CO_2, the OH^- produced by the pump causes intracellular pH to rise, which in turn suppresses luminal H^+ secretion. In the presence of CO_2, carbonic anhydrase catalyzes the combination of OH^- with CO_2 to form bicarbonate, which can then exit the basolateral membrane through a Cl^-/HCO_3^- exchanger. The chloride taken up by this exchange exists through a basolateral membrane chloride channel.

Numerous studies in the turtle bladder support individual aspects of this overall model. The rate of H^+ secretion in the bladder was found to be critically dependent on the availability of CO_2 (211), and the rate of H^+ secretion was greatly stimulated, within seconds, by raising the ambient P_{CO_2} (206,211–214). These findings were interpreted to indicate that CO_2 is required to buffer the OH^- generated by active H^+ secretion, and that in the absence of CO_2, cell pH alkalinizes, suppressing luminal H^+ transport.

Cohen et al. demonstrated, for several values of P_{CO_2}, that raising the basolateral bicarbonate concentration at constant P_{CO_2} inhibits luminal H^+ secretion, and that the inhibition can be prevented by elevating the ambient P_{CO_2} (215). They proposed that H^+ secretion was responding to changes in intracellular pH. When the exit of basolateral bicarbonate through the Cl^-/HCO_3^- exchanger was inhibited with disulfonic stilbenes (196), luminal H^+ secretion was inhibited. Exposure of SITS-treated bladders to 5% CO_2 transiently stimulated H^+ secretion, an effect attributed to an initial reduction in pH_i by CO_2, with a subsequent accumulation of bicarbonate and rise in pH_i (196). Removal of basolateral chloride also inhibited H^+ secretion (198), probably by inhibiting (rather than reversing) basolateral Cl^-/HCO_3^- exchange, since submillimolar chloride concentrations partially restored H^+ secretion. The inhibition of H^+ secretion was attributed to an effect on pH_i, rather than direct inhibition of the H^+ATPase, as increasing the P_{CO_2} in low-chloride buffers transiently stimulated H^+ secretion (198).

Many aspects of this model have withstood experimental scrutiny, but the details of the intracellular mechanisms that control the luminal H^+ATPase remain largely unresolved. The central hypothesis of the model, that pH_i is the primary signal controlling the rate of luminal H^+ secretion (120,215), remains controversial.

CO_2 and some maneuvers predicted to change the pH_i of CA cells exert at least part of their effect by changing the number of luminal H^+ATPases through membrane fusion or endocytic removal (213,214,216,217). Clausen and Dixon (218,219), using impedance analysis, found that the turtle bladder apical membrane capacitance (a direct function of the membrane surface area) changed in response to manipulations that produce acute changes in bladder H^+ secretion, such as treatment with acetazolamide or CO_2. Part of this effect was attributable to alterations in endocytic internalization rates, presumably representing removal of H^+ATPases from the luminal membrane. Dixon et al. (220) later found that azide prevented the reduction in H^+ secretion and luminal membrane capacitance induced by acetazolamide, although it did not affect constitutive dextran internalization rates. This interesting result suggests that the vesicles involved in regulating H^+ transport by internalization and fusion differ from those involved in constitutive membrane turnover and underscores the problems in relating rates of exocytosis and endocytosis to net changes in the number of apical H^+ATPases. No experiments have excluded the possibility that part of the effect of CO_2 is exerted through changes in the kinetics of the H^+ATPase (214).

Role of Intracellular pH in Regulating Luminal H^+ Secretion It has been postulated that CO_2, which stimulates H^+ secretion, and acetazolamide, which inhibits, exert their effects by changing the pH_i of the CA cells, and experimental evidence supports this view (196,211,215). The DMO method (221) used to measure pH_i in these studies, however, yields values indicative of the entire epithelial tissue rather than values specifically from the CA cells. Several ensuing studies examined the hypothesis that cell pH is the immediate signal affecting the CA cell CA, using newer methods for measuring intracellular pH (222–225). Cannon et al. (222) measured the pH_i of individual CA cells in intact bladders with the pH-sensitive probe 6-carboxyfluorescein (222). They found that both CO_2 and the weak acid butyrate lowered pH_i in the CA cells and transiently stimulated both H^+ secretion and lumenal exocytosis by release of previously internalized FITC-dextran into the lumen (213). The authors interpreted these results to indicate that intracellular acidification, rather than CO_2 specifically, was the signal for membrane fusion, but problems undermine this conclusion. The authors found that the CA cells had a resting pH_i 0.5 pH units above the surrounding principal cells, indicating that principal cells have a resting pH_i of as low as 6.0, well out of the normal range, raising doubts about the validity of the measurements. The investigators did not exclude the possibility that butyrate enhanced endogenous CO_2 production—for example, as a substrate—or by uncoupling mitochondrial oxidative phosphorylation. They also did not determine whether raising the serosal bicarbonate concentration to levels that inhibit the H^+ secretory response to CO_2 prevented the fall in pH_i or the release of FITC-dextran. Andersen and Steinmetz (124) showed earlier that lowering luminal pH sufficiently to inhibit H^+ completely produced a transient "overshoot" in H^+ secretion when the luminal pH was raised under CO_2-free conditions but not in the presence of CO_2, presumably because basolateral entry of bicarbonate prevented intracellular acidification.

Graber et al. used 4-methylumbelliferone as a probe for measuring pH_i in individual CA cells in the intact bladder. In contrast to the studies above (222), they found that CA cells had a resting

pH_i of 0.1 pH units above that of principal cells. In a following study, Graber et al. (225) demonstrated that propionate, under appropriate conditions, acidified pH_i in CA cells without producing any increase in H^+ secretion.

Steinmetz proposed in 1969 that acetazolamide inhibits H^+ secretion by preventing the buffering of OH^- and raising pH_i (211), but early evidence from his own laboratory suggested that this might not be the case. Acetazolamide, at concentrations that inhibited 73% of luminal H^+ secretion, was found to produce no detectable change in cell pH by the DMO method (211). Van Adelsberg et al. (223) found that acetazolamide raised pH_i in CA cells by 0.12 pH units and proposed that this was the basis for its inhibition of H^+ secretion. Dixon and colleagues (220) found evidence that acetazolamide inhibits H^+ secretion by inducing luminal membrane internalization, and they found that azide prevented this inhibition. Graber et al. (225) found that acetazolamide inhibition raised pH_i by 0.25 pH units in only a small subpopulation of CA cells yet inhibited 80% of H^+ secretion. In bladders in which pH_i was "clamped" at 7.0 with serosal DMO, acetazolamide still inhibited H^+ transport 74%. They also found that in propionate-treated bladders, in which the pH_i of individual CA cells was acidified by 0.15 pH units, acetazolamide inhibited H^+ transport 100%. These findings indicate that the inhibition of H^+ secretion by acetazolamide probably occurs by stimulating luminal membrane internalization through an effect that is independent of cell pH.

In summary, there is experimental evidence both to support and to dispute intracellular pH as the signal sensed by the CA cell during acute regulatory responses.

If pH_i is an immediate signal controlling luminal H^+ secretion by the vacuolar H^+ATPase, how does it act? It is unlikely that a fall in intracellular pH stimulates the H^+ATPase directly. The curve relating H^+ secretion to apparent pH_i described by Cohen (215) is not at all similar to the pH dependence of ATPase activity of the purified renal enzyme (34). Acidification of intracellular pH in CA cells has been reported to raise intracellular calcium activity; an elevation in intracellular calcium may be required to promote membrane fusion events, as calcium chelators inhibited CO_2 or butyrate-induced H^+ secretion (222,223,226,227). On the other hand, increasing the calcium permeability of the bladder with calcium ionophore inhibited H^+ secretion (228,229). In the mammalian intercalated cell (see below), some maneuvers that raise intracellular calcium, such as removal of basolateral sodium, have no effect on H^+ secretion (21), and the mild elevation of intracellular calcium produced by intracellular acidification appears to inhibit vacuolar H^+ATPase-driven H^+ extrusion (21).

Acute Regulation of H^+ Secretion by Intrinsic Regulatory Mechanisms: Coupling of H^+ Secretion to Metabolism

Luminal H^+ secretion by the bladder is affected by the availability and type of metabolic substrate. Prolonged incubation of bladders in the absence of substrates depleted their endogenous substrate, and reduced H^+ secretion (230–232). In the substrate-depleted bladders, addition of glucose restored H^+ transport to control rates, but addition of pyruvate had no effect (230). Treatment of bladders with the glycolytic inhibitor 2-deoxyglucose had an effect similar to substrate depletion: H^+ secretion was inhibited, and was restored by addition of glucose but not pyruvate (231). These results suggest that the rate of glycolysis, rather than the rate of mitochondrial ATP production, has a strong influence on the rate of H^+ secretion. The mechanism of this effect in the bladder is unknown, but it may indicate that glycolytic enzymes are bound in a close functional association with the luminal H^+ATPase, as has been demonstrated for the anion transporter band 3 and other transport enzymes (233–236). It should be noted, however, that substrate-depleted bladders may be able to use substrates other than glucose (232).

Under anaerobic conditions, the maximal rate of H^+ secretion is achieved with 1% ambient P_{CO_2}; under aerobic conditions, the maximal rate increases nearly fourfold and is reached at 5% ambient P_{CO_2} (212, 231). The basis for the change in the response of the bladder to CO_2 with metabolic state is undetermined; it may reflect a requirement of aerobic metabolism for membrane insertion with CO_2, as discussed above.

Acute Regulation of H^+ Secretion by Hormones

Aldosterone. Studies in the bladder demonstrated that aldosterone stimulates H^+ secretion independent of effects on sodium transport (237–239). The effect occurred within 1 hr and was due to a direct stimulation of the pump and not a secondary to stimulation of the overall metabolic rate (230). Whether the effect is the result of an increase in the number or kinetics of luminal H^+ATPases is unknown. In one study, the RNA transcription inhibitor actinomycin D prevented the response to aldosterone (239), suggesting that new protein synthesis is required for the response, but does not exclude any of the mechanisms shown in Figure 3.

β-Adrenergic Agonists and Cyclic AMP. In the turtle bladder, addition of serosal cAMP, treatment with β-adrenergic agonists and other agents that elevate cAMP (240,241) or treatment with carbachol (242,243) all stimulate bicarbonate secretion. The available evidence indicates that most of this effect is the result of an increase in the number of functional Cl^-/HCO_3^- exchangers and chloride channels in the luminal membrane (presumably of the β CA cells) (194,244) that may occur through membrane fusion events (245,246). At present it is unknown whether any of these agents has a direct effect on the basolateral membrane vacuolar H^+ATPase.

Acute Regulation of the Vacuolar H^+ATPase in Kidney

Acute Regulation by the Luminal Proton Electrochemical Gradient

Initial experiments in the cortical and medullary collecting duct suggested that the α cell closely resembled the CA cell, with an electrogenic H^+ATPase in the luminal membrane, and a Cl^-/HCO_3^- exchanger and chloride channel on the basolateral membrane. Since tubules cannot be studied under voltage-clamped conditions, the evidence for electrogenic H^+ secretion is not as strong as in the turtle bladder. As discussed above, the cortical collecting tubule also secretes bicarbonate, and in early studies of H^+ secretion in this segment, the contribution of bicarbonate secretion to overall rates of bicarbonate reabsorption was not determined. Nevertheless, in intact cortical collecting tubules and outer stripe of the outer medullary, several physiologic studies supported the presence of an electrogenic luminal H^+ATPase that did not require luminal sodium, and in which the transepithelial potential difference, which was determined partly by sodium reabsorption in the cortical collecting tubule and outer stripe, influenced the rate of H^+ secretion (161–166). Sparse electrophysiologic data on bicarbonate-secreting (β) intercalated cells supported a model with an electrogenic H^+ATPase in the basolateral membrane responsible for bicarbonate secretion (170,171). As discussed above, the isolated renal vacuolar H^+ATPase is electrogenic (34,54,125), and several studies have demonstrated by immunocytochemistry that the enzyme resides in the plasma membrane of both α and β intercalated cells (26,35,119,247–249).

The inner stripe of the outer medullary collecting tubule does not transport sodium, and normally has a lumen-positive potential difference thought to arise from electrogenic proton secretion (36,39,165,166). Reducing the luminal pH to <5 in this segment lowered the pH_i of intercalated cells from 7.27 to 7.03, consistent with inhibition of luminal H^+ secretion (31). Depolarizing the tubule cells with K^+ and valinomycin produced a rise in pH_i, consistent with a stimulation of the H^+ATPase (143). Removing basolateral chloride inhibited H^+ secretion, partly by reducing basolateral bicarbonate exit through Cl^-/HCO_3^- exchange, and partly by preventing the normal charge counterbalance to electrogenic H^+ secretion provided by chloride secretion (36). Under chloride-free conditions, the tubule maintained the lumen-positive potential despite reduced H^+ secretion (36,164). In chloride replete conditions, 90–95% or more of outer medullary H^+ secretion was accompanied by chloride secretion rather than K^+ reabsorption (36,37) without any detectable potassium reabsorption (37). These observations produced a model for the inner stripe intercalated cell similar to the turtle bladder CA cell, with an electrogenic H^+ATPase in the luminal membrane, in which H^+ secretion is accompanied by Cl^- secretion (Figure 5).

More recently, the model for the proton-secreting α intercalated cell has become more complex. Wingo and colleagues have proposed that a substantial fraction of tubular H^+ secretion originates from an H^+-K^+-ATPase, and that the lumen-positive potential difference arises from a potassium diffusion potential through luminal membrane potassium channels (38,250). According to this model (Figure 5), net potassium reabsorption is not observed in tubules from normal animals because of potassium recycling through barium-sensitive apical potassium channels. Consistent with this revised model are findings that both luminal Ba^{2+} and the H^+-K^+-ATPase inhibitor Sch28080 eliminated CO_2-stimulated bicarbonate reabsorption in the rabbit cortical collecting duct (251), and that in the rabbit outer medullary collecting tubule inner stripe ($OMCD_i$), luminal perfusion with Ba^{2+}, a potassium channel blocker, and the H^+-K^+-ATPase inhibitors Sch28080, H224/25, and A80915A reduced bicarbonate reabsorption (H^+ secretion) (252). 5 or 10 nM bafilomycin A_1 partially inhibited

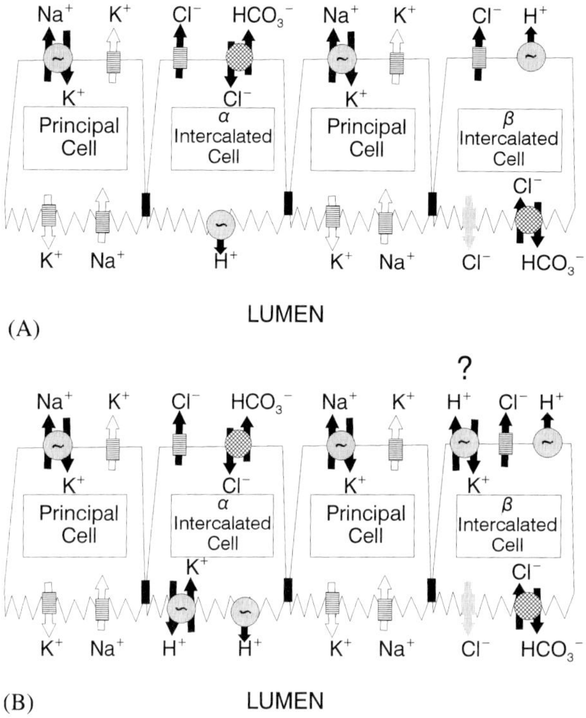

Figure 5 Model for H$^+$ secretion in the mammalian cortical collecting tubule. (A) "Classical" model. (B) "Revised" model with a luminal H$^+$-K$^+$-ATPase.

OMCD$_i$ H$^+$ secretion, and A80915A produced additional inhibition. The interpretation of these findings is complicated by several factors. First, as discussed above, Sch28080 appears to inhibit vacuolar H$^+$ATPase H$^+$ secretion in the intact turtle bladder, and it is not yet certain how specifically it and other agents inhibit the H$^+$,K$^+$-ATPase in renal tubules. Second, it is possible that barium produces an increase in the potential difference across the apical membrane of the cell, which would be expected to reduce the rate of H$^+$ secretion by an electrogenic H$^+$ATPase. Third, the concentrations of bafilomycin used in the studies are well below the concentrations needed to achieve complete H$^+$ATPase inhibition in other systems. Lastly, it is possible that the preparation method required to mount the tubule in a perfusion apparatus has greater adverse effects on the H$^+$ATPase than it does on the H$^+$,K$^+$-ATPase. Studies of H$^+$ transport by individual intercalated cells (employing measurements of intracellular pH recovery) have not found evidence for an H$^+$,K$^+$-ATPase (142,145). Consequently, the importance of the H$^+$,K$^+$-ATPase in H$^+$ secretion in the normal collecting duct remains an unresolved issue.

Both luminal amiloride and removal of luminal sodium inhibit H$^+$ secretion in the cortical collecting duct, probably by reducing the lumen-negative potential difference (161–166). In contrast, amiloride increased bath-to-lumen Rb flux in the rabbit cortical collecting tubule, an effect that was inhibited both by luminal Ba^{2+} and by Sch28080 (253); Wingo and colleagues have proposed that, in the presence of amiloride, K$^+$ secretion through apical potassium channels and reabsorption through the apical H$^+$,K$^+$-ATPase are both increased. However, this model would predict an increase in H$^+$ secretion rather than the observed decrease with amiloride. Thus, for the present time, a model with the luminal electrogenic H$^+$ATPase as the principle proton secretory transporter, whose rate of transport is increased by a more lumen negative potential difference, fits the observed data most closely.

In the proximal tubule, it has been demonstrated that luminal pH has a significant effect on net rates of H$^+$ secretion (23,254,255), but the component of total H$^+$ secretion attributable to the vacuolar H^+ATPase in response to changes in the proton electrochemical gradient under these conditions has not been determined.

Acute Regulation of H^+ Secretion by Intrinsic Regulatory Mechanisms: CO_2, Basolateral Bicarbonate Exit, and the Possible Role of Cell pH

Outer Medullary Collecting Tubule. The outer medullary collecting tubule secrets H^+ without coexisting bicarbonate secretion (36,39). Investigations on the acute regulation of H^+ secretion in this segment are consequently simpler to interpret than those from the cortical collecting tubule (see below).

In the outer stripe of the outer medullary collecting tubule, H^+ secretion resembles electrogenic H^+ secretion in the turtle bladder, with functionally distinct H^+-secreting intercalated cells, and Na^+-transporting principal cells (172,173). The inner stripe of the outer medullary collecting tubule (in the rabbit) is different. It was once thought that the inner stripe existed of a single cell type (142,174,175), but both morphologic and physiologic studies have shown that there are two functionally distinct cell types. (26,28,168,176–178). Studies from Weiner and Hamm have shown that a minority cell population in the inner stripe, probably representing intercalated cells, has higher rates of vacuolar H^+ATPase-driven H^+ extrusion than the neighboring majority cells, although the latter also appear functionally to have apical membrane H^+ATPases (28). These investigators have largely solved the problem of distinguishing H^+ transport in intercalated cells from that in principal cells by a method in which the pH probe BCECF is incorporated selectively into intercalated cells (169).

Many of the characteristics of H^+ secretion by α intercalated cells in the outer medullary collecting tubule resemble H^+ secretion in the turtle bladder. Lowering or raising basolateral bicarbonate at constant P_{CO_2} stimulates or inhibits H^+ secretion, respectively (37), and lowering (37) or raising (256) the P_{CO_2} at a constant basolateral bicarbonate concentration respectively inhibits or stimulates H^+ secretion. Like the turtle bladder α CA cell, the α intercalated cell has a basolateral Cl^-/HCO_3^- exchanger (28,31,32,141,176,257–259) and a basolateral chloride conductance (260). As in the turtle bladder, acetazolamide (39,172), basolateral disulfonic stilbenes (31,36,172), and removal of basolateral chloride (36) all inhibit H^+ secretion.

In several respects, however, the intercalated cells in the outer medullary collecting tubule differ from those reported for the CA cells of the turtle bladder. The intercalated cells have basolateral Na^+-H^+ exchange and Na^+-HCO_3^- cotransport (21,28,141,142,145,168,259), which have not been found in turtle bladder cells (223). As discussed above, there is also evidence for a luminal H^+,K^+-ATPase in intercalated cells (38,250).

Mechanisms for Altering Rates of Luminal H^+ Secretion

A number of studies have provided information on the intrinsic regulatory mechanisms that control vacuolar H^+ATPase-driven H^+ secretion by α intercalated cells. Some of the available evidence suggests that changes in the number of luminal H^+ATPases by membrane fusion or internalization is an important mechanism controlling rates of H^+ secretion in the α intercalated cell. Madsen and Tisher (261) found that acute respiratory acidosis of 5- to 6-hr duration in rats produced an increase in apical surface density and loss of tubulovesicular structures in intercalated cells of the outer medullary collecting tubule, consistent with recruitment of luminal membrane by fusion events. This length of exposure to an elevated P_{CO_2} is probably too short for chronic changes in H^+ transport to have occurred (262) (see below). Schwartz and Al-Awqati (263) found that intercalated cells in rabbit medullary collecting tubules internalized FITC-dextran into acidic compartments, and that a change from CO_2-free to HCO_3^-/CO_2 buffers produced a 24–27% reduction of the fluorescent intensity in the cells in each segment. This was interpreted to represent CO_2-induced release of the dextran by exocytosis because it was inhibited by colchicine, although release of dextran into the lumen was not demonstrated, and other possible causes for loss of fluorescent intensity—such as increased scatter, cell volume changes, or a change in the focal plane of the vesicles—were not excluded. In contrast, McKinney and Davidson (256) showed that elevating the P_{CO_2} stimulated H^+ secretion 46–52%, an effect that was inhibited by colchicine but which did not produce any significant change in intercalated cell apical membrane surface density assessed by electron microscopy. Thus, it is still unclear how much of the intrinsic regulation of vacuolar H^+ATPase in intercalated cells is attributable to changes in numbers of pumps residing on the luminal membrane.

Control of H^+ATPase enzyme kinetics (i.e., the intrinsic rate of ATP hydrolysis in the absence of imposed electrochemical gradients) is another possible mechanism for intrinsic regulation of the luminal vacuolar H^+ATPase. Some evidence suggests that accessory proteins may regulate H^+ATPase kinetics. Fanestil and colleagues found indirect evidence for H^+ATPase inhibitory proteins in the toad bladder when they showed that inhibitors of protein and RNA synthesis stimulated H^+ secretion (238). More recently, bovine kidney cytosol was found to have protein factors (discussed above) that activated (186) or inhibited (87) the purified bovine kidney vacuolar H^+ATPase. The effect of these putative regulatory proteins was found to be highly pH dependent, indicating that they might participate in the intrinsic regulation of the H^+ATPase. The inhibitor reduced ATPase activity of the purified H^+ATPase by 45% over the pH range of 6.0 to 7.5; at pH values above pH 7.5, inhibition increased to 70%. The activator increased activity about 100% over a pH range of 8.0 to 6.6, and below pH 6.6, it increased activity up to 1200%. The pH dependence of the inhibitor and activator activities occur in a physiologic range for cell pH, and, in principle, could serve to stimulate the H^+ATPase during cytosolic acidification, and stimulate the H^+ATPase during cytosolic alkalinization. Gurich and DuBose, as noted above, have found that GTP-binding proteins may be involved in regulating renal endosomal acidification (188,190). At present, it is unknown whether G proteins participate in regulating transepithelial H^+ secretion.

Intracellular Signals Controlling Rates of Luminal H^+ Secretion

Some experimental evidence supports intracellular pH as a primary intracellular signal controlling luminal H^+ secretion. In isolated outer medullary collecting tubules, changing from HCO_3^-/CO_2 buffers to CO_2-free conditions, which inhibits H^+ secretion, raised intracellular pH (28), and lowering basolateral bicarbonate, which stimulates H^+ secretion, decreased cell pH (143,264). Both addition of basolateral DIDS (31,141,264) or removal of basolateral Cl^- (31), which inhibit basolateral Cl^-/HCO_3^- exchange, alkalinized the cytosol and suppressed H^+ secretion, presumably by elevating pH_i.

Other results, however, indicate that factors other than intracellular pH are responsible for the intrinsic regulation of the luminal H^+ATPase. In two studies, no significant differences were observed in the intracellular pH of α intercalated cells in CO_2-free, normal bicarbonate, or high-bicarbonate buffers (144,168). Removal of basolateral sodium did not change the rate of outer medullary collecting tubule H^+ secretion (bicarbonate reabsorption) (164,265) even though, in several studies, removal of basolateral sodium or addition of basolateral amiloride caused an intracellular acidification (21,141,143).

In studies of intracellular pH regulation in intercalated cells, α intercalated cells in rabbit outer medullary collecting tubule, inner stripe, were found to have a sodium-independent amiloride-insensitive mechanism for intracellular pH recovery thought to represent the luminal vacuolar H^+ATPase (28,142,144,145,168). Kuwahara, et al. (144) found that the rate of sodium-independent pH_i recovery in α intercalated cells was no different in the presence or absence of bicarbonate buffers, but the rate of vacuolar H^+-driven proton extrusion again was higher for any value of pH_i in bicarbonate buffer, since the buffering capacity of the cells was higher in bicarbonate buffers. Both Hays and Alpern (21) and Weiner et al. (28) found the rate of recovery of pH_i following intracellular acidification to be greater in the presence of HCO_3^-/CO_2 than in its absence. Weiner et al. found that the rate of sodium-independent pH_i recovery after acidification to pH 6.25 in intercalated cells from the inner stripe of outer medulla was 0.034 pH units/min in CO_2/HCO_3^--free buffers (28). In CO_2/HCO_3^- buffers, Kuwahara et al. (144) found that the rate of sodium-independent pH_i recovery after acidification to pH 6.40 was 0.234 pH units/min, nearly 10-fold higher for the same value of intracellular pH. Weiner and Hamm (266) had shown previously in β intercalated cells that NH_4Cl-induced acidification does not provoke entry of HCO_3^- by reversal of Cl^-/HCO_3^- exchange. Thus, in all of these studies, a faster rate of H^+ secretion was found in the presence of bicarbonate buffers at equal pH_i values, strongly suggesting that CO_2 directly increases vacuolar H^+ATPase-driven H^+ extrusion independent of its effects on pH_i.

In further support of this, Hayashi et al. (168) showed that elevation of basolateral HCO_3^- in vitro for 3 hr, which lowers tubular H^+ secretion, reduced the rate of pH_i recovery from an NH_4Cl

prepulse. The effect was not attributable to a change in buffer capacity or to the degree of initial acidification. This finding indicates that bicarbonate suppresses the intrinsic rate of luminal H^+ secretion independent of its effect on intracellular pH.

These results suggest a model in which H^+ secretion by the luminal vacuolar H^+ATPase responds to relative changes in intracellular pH, but in which the "set point" (or magnitude of proton flux at a given pH) is controlled by other factors, such as the P_{CO_2}. It is unlikely that the luminal H^+ATPase In the intercalated cell has a primary function in regulating or restoring intracellular pH, as the rate of pH_i recovery from basolateral Na^+-H^+ exchange exceeds that from the H^+ATPase (28,141–146). It is still uncertain, however, how accurately the rate of pH_i recovery reflects tubular secretion rates, as the rates of H^+ secretion calculated from these studies are four to five times the measured rate of bicarbonate reabsorption in the outer medullary collecting tubule, assuming that the inner stripe consists of a single cell type (21,259).

Two studies have examined whether intracellular calcium (Ca_i) has a role in regulating the luminal H^+ATPase. Hays and Alpern (21) found that removal of basolateral sodium produced a transient "spike" increase in Ca_i, arising by release from intracellular stores. Following this transient, there was a sustained increase in Ca_i. Their evidence suggested that the sustained elevation in Ca_i inhibited the initial rate of sodium-independent pH_i recovery from intracellular acidification.* Furuya et al. (146), however, demonstrated that the outer medullary collecting tubule has basolateral Ca^{+2}-H^+ exchange (likely arising from a Ca^{+2}-ATPase), which may have been activated by the elevated Ca_i, producing an increase in cellular H^+ entry which would appear as an inhibition of H^+ efflux. The results of Hays and Alpern (21) suggest that changes in Ca_i are not required for activation of the H^+ATPase following a fall in intracellular pH or in response to CO_2.

Cortical Collecting Tubule

Information on the intrinsic regulation of the vacuolar H^+ATPase in the cortical collecting tubule is more difficult to interpret, because of the coexisting processes of H^+ secretion (bicarbonate reabsorption) and bicarbonate secretion, and the failure, in most studies, to distinguish between the two mechanisms. Some evidence is consistent with coupling of the basolateral vacuolar H^+ATPase to luminal bicarbonate entry through the Cl^-/HCO_3^- exchanger. Raising or lowering basolateral bicarbonate was found to suppress or stimulate, respectively, net bicarbonate reabsorption in cortical collecting tubule (267). Removal of basolateral chloride, which stimulates bicarbonate secretion (268), acidified the intracellular pH of the β intercalated cell (139,170,180).

In contrast, lowering the ambient P_{CO_2} in vitro had no effect on net bicarbonate transport in the cortical collecting tubule (267) even though it elevated the intracellular pH of β intercalated cells (266), suggesting that the H^+ATPase was not suppressed by intracellular alkalinization. Acute elevation of the P_{CO_2} in vitro lowered intracellular pH (266) but had no effect on net bicarbonate transport (267), and in vivo elevation of P_{CO_2} for 5–6 hr produced no discernible morphologic changes in β intercalated cells (268a). From the information presently available, it appears likely that the intrinsic regulation of the basolateral membrane H^+ATPase may differ substantially from that controlling the apical H^+ATPase. In the β intercalated cell, basolateral Na^+-H^+ exchange has an even greater role in maintaining pH_i than it does in the α intercalated cell (170,180,269).

Proximal Tubule

Many factors actuely affect rates of H^+ secretion by the proximal tubule (23). In most of the available studies, it has not been determined to what extent these factors affect Na^+-H^+ antiport or the luminal vacuolar H^+ATPase. A few studies do provide evidence for participation of the vacuolar H^+ATPase in acute regulation of proximal H^+ secretion.

Kurtz (157) demonstrated that the S3 portion of the proximal tubule had a sodium-independent mechanism for pH_i recovery (following acidification with NH_4Cl) that was inhibited by luminal

*In this study, the authors proposed that calcium was required for the late recovery of pH_i following intracellular acidification, since the intracellular calcium chelator BAPTA "inhibited" the late recovery of pH_i. However, the resting pH_i level in the presence of BAPTA was 7.6, far above normal, and recovered to the more normal level of pH 7.1 following acidification. Intracellular calcium levels also dropped nearly to zero in the experiments, and this may have produced some nonspecific inhibitory effects.

NEM and DCCD, consistent with the presence of a functional vacuolar H^+ATPase on the plasma membrane. Nakhoul et al. (160) found in the S3 part of proximal tubule that basolateral CO_2/HCO_3^-, but not luminal, induced an intracellular alkalinization that was not attributable to bicarbonate entry, and which appeared to arise from a luminal proton pump. The alkalinization did not occur in response to a fall in intracellular pH induced by luminal CO_2/HCO_3^-, nor was the alkalinization inhibited by acetazolamide, which prevented the fall in pH_i induced by basolateral CO_2/HCO_3^-. These observations indicate that CO_2/HCO_3^- stimulated the presumed H^+ATPase activity directly and independently of effects on intracellular pH.

Schwartz and Al-Awqati (263) demonstrated that the S2 portion of the proximal tubule internalized FITC-dextran into acidic vacuoles. They found that CO_2 produced a colchicine-inhibitable decrease in the fluorescent signal (as described above), which was interpreted to represent release of dextran by exocytosis and presumptive insertion of H^+ATPases into the luminal membrane. Kurtz (157) observed sodium-independent pH_i recovery in the rabbit S2 proximal tubule, interpreted to represent an H^+ATPase. The activity was inhibited by pretreatment of the tubule with colchicine, a result interpreted to indicate that the response might be dependent on membrane fusion. In later studies, colchicine injection was found to induce a loss of H^+ATPase from the brush border membrane in rat proximal tubule by interfering with vesicular traffic (270).

In summary, the proximal tubule S3 segment luminal H^+ATPase is activated by basolateral CO_2/HCO_3^-, and it appears unlikely that this effect is exerted through changes in intracellular pH. Some evidence in the S2 segment suggests that regulation may occur by addition of H^+ATPase through membrane fusion events. As discussed below, however, removal of bicarbonate from the proximal tubule reduces intracellular ATP levels and has other metabolic effects that might affect the vacuolar H^+ATPase. Consequently, the mechanism of activation of the proximal tubule H^+ATPase by CO_2/HCO_3^- remains unclear.

Acute Regulation of H^+ Secretion by Intrinsic Regulatory Mechanisms: Coupling of H^+ Secretion to Metabolism. Information on the influence of cellular metabolism on the plasma membrane vacuolar H^+ATPase in the kidney is scant. The sodium-independent mechanism for pH_i recovery in the S3 portion of the proximal tubule studied by Kurtz (157), thought to represent a vacuolar H^+ATPase, was not affected by the mitochondrial cytochrome inhibitor cyanide, but was reduced markedly by the glycolysis inhibitor iodoacetamide. This suggests that the kidney proximal tubule vacuolar H^+ATPase, like that in the turtle bladder, is coupled preferentially to glycolysis. Vinay and colleagues (271) examined the metabolic cost of the vacuolar H^+ATPase in suspensions of rabbit proximal tubule, and found that only 4.5% of the total phosphorylative respiration was attributed to the vacuolar H^+ATPase (as compared to the 58.8% attributed to the Na^+-K^+-ATPase). Dickman and Mandel (272), investigating metabolic respiration in suspensions of rabbit proximal tubule, got a similar result, finding that bafilomycin A_1 reduced the ouabain-insensitive O_2 consumption by 20%. They observed that removal of CO_2/HCO_3^- also lowered oxygen consumption by 20%, and that the effect originated from a limitation in mitochrondrial substrate uptake. Removal of CO_2/HCO_3^- also reduced cellular ATP content by 50%, and increased cellular lactate production about 10-fold. These impressive metabolic effects of CO_2/HCO_3^- are candidate mechanisms which might influence vacuolar H^+ATPase activity independent of effects on cell pH.

Acute Regulation of H^+ Secretion by Hormones.

Aldosterone. Aldosterone stimulates distal nephron H^+ secretion (2,273). This effect occurs in part because aldosterone increases the lumen-negative potential difference in the distal tubule and collecting duct by increasing lumenal sodium permeability (2,273,274). Aldosterone was found to stimulate H^+ secretion in vitro in the isolated renal outer medullary collecting tubule, inner stripe, a segment that does not transport sodium (259,265). These observations demonstrate that at least part of the acute action of mineralocorticoids is a direct stimulation of H^+ secretion not attributable changes in the collecting tubule potential difference, and independent of effects on sodium transport (265).

The mechanism of the direct stimulation of H^+ secretion remains unknown. A rise in H^+ secretion could occur by increases in the quantity of H^+ATPase protein, by recruitment of preexisting enzyme from an intracellular or inactive pool, or by kinetic activation of the H^+ATPase. Preliminary studies suggest that mineralocorticoids induce a modest overall increase in H^+ATPase protein in both cortex and medulla and a modest increase in H^+ATPase in the luminal membrane of outer medullary α intercalated cells by redistribution (275). A possible effect on the kinetics of the H^+ATPase has not been excluded.

β-Adrenergic Agonists and Cyclic AMP. β-adrenergic agonists, such as isoproterenol, and other agents that elevate cAMP, stimulate H^+ and bicarbonate secretion; isoproterenol was found to elevate cAMP levels in isolated intercalated cells from both cortical (276) and outer medullary collecting tubule (177,277). In the cortical collecting tubule, both isoproterenol and cAMP enhanced bicarbonate secretion (278–280) by increasing luminal Cl^-/HCO_3^- exchange (281) and possibly by opening a luminal anion channel (279). Since these agents decrease the lumen-negative potential in this segment, it has been suggested that they may stimulate the luminal H^+ATPase directly in α intercalated cells (30,280). In the rabbit outer medullary collecting tubule (inner stripe), cAMP and forskolin increased H^+ secretion 34.5% and 39%, respectively (282). The mechanism of these effects is unknown.

Other Hormones. Several peptide hormones exhibit moderate effects on H^+ transport. Vasopressin (283,284) and glucagon (285,286) inhibited bicarbonate secretion (or enhanced H^+ secretion) in the rat cortical collecting tubule and distal convoluted tubule (284). Calcitonin produced an apparent stimulation of H^+ secretion in rat cortical collecting tubule (287). Prostaglandin PGE_2 produced a 12% inhibition of H^+ secretion in the outer stripe of rabbit outer medullary collecting tubule (282). Protein kinase C activators have no effect on net bicarbonate reabsorption in the cortical collecting tubule (288). The effects of all of these agents are of uncertain physiologic significance.

Chronic Regulation of H^+ Secretion by the Vacuolar H^+ATPase in Renal Epithelia

Prolonged acid or alkali administration, mineralocorticoid administration, and sustained elevation of the P_{CO_2} are the three most important stimuli that produce chronic changes in renal acid excretion involving the kidney vacuolar H^+ATPase.

Problems in Assays Used to Assess Changes in Vacuolar H^+ATPase During Chronic Regulation

Enzymatic Assays: NEM-Sensitive ATPase Activity. Changes in Na^+-K^+-ATPase activity that occur during chronic adaptation in various physiologic settings have been studied by numerous investigators (289). In these studies, assays of whole cell Na^+-K^+-ATPase activity in different nephron segments have provided useful information because there is a specific inhibitor for the Na^+-K^+-ATPase (ouabain) which can be used in intact cells and that can provide measurements of both enzymatic activity (as ouabain-sensitive ATPase or Rb^+ uptake) and enzyme numbers (as ^{3}H-ouabain binding sites); and because nearly all of the cellular Na^+-K^+-ATPase resides on the plasma membrane.

Several studies have attempted to determine to what extent chronic changes in tubular H^+ secretion originate from the vacuolar H^+ATPase using a similar approach, but there are many problems with such studies. There is no proven specific inhibitor of the vacuolar H^+ATPases. A number of studies have used either N-ethylmaleimide (NEM)-inhibitable ATPase (290–304) or bafilomycin A_1-inhibitable ATPase (305) as assays for vacuolar H^+ATPase activity. NEM is a sulfhydryl reactive reagent that inhibits a variety of transport ATPases, and the validity of its use in assays performed on permeabilized cells or even membrane fractions remains unproven. For example, no studies have attempted to determine if immunodepletion of vacuolar H^+ATPase from these preparations removes all of the NEM-sensitive or bafilomycin-sensitive ATPase activity. In studies examining NEM-sensitive ATPase activity in different segments of the nephron in normal rats, the values for activity (expressed as pmol/hr/mm tubule length) varied more than three fold, reflecting the problems with the assay (290,295,297,306) (see Table 5).

Although bafilomycin is a high affinity inhibitor of the vacuolar H^+ATPases with an IC_{50} in the low nanomolar range, orders of magnitude below its effects on other ATPases (63,65), when used at concentrations needed to inhibit 100% of the vacuolar H^+ATPase activity, it does have effects on other enzymes. Bafilomycin has not been studied for a sufficient length of time for any other possible effects to have emerged.

A second problem in assaying vacuolar H^+ATPase microdissected tubule segments is that, in intercalated cells, most of the enzyme resides in intracellular membrane compartments instead of on the plasma membrane (26,173,248,307,308). None of the investigators using the assays of total enzyme activity (as NEM-sensitive ATPase activity) in intact cells has attempted to determine whether measured activity arises from the plasma membrane. It has been assumed that, in permeabilized cells, the activity measured represents the total enzyme content the cell (290,299,306), but some observations raise serious doubts about this assertion. For example, Khadouri et al. found that colchicine inhibited the NEM-sensitive ATPase activity in permeabilized tubules nearly completely (298). As colchicine acts, presumably, by preventing vesicular traffic of the H^+ATPase, the inhibition of ATPase activity suggests that the cellular location of the enzyme has a powerful influence on the measured activity.

Finally, measurements of total enzymatic activity in tubules provide little insight into adaptational mechanisms, since they do not divulge whether an increase in activity represents an increase in the number of H^+ATPases per cell, a kinetic activation of extant H^+ATPases, or a redistribution of preexisting-existing H^+ATPases. Some examples of problems in using whole tubule NEM-sensitive ATPase assays have been discussed previously (309).

Investigators have also attempted to quantify changes in H^+ATPase by measuring acidification kinetics in membrane fractions (305,310). Attempts to use this approach to quantify H^+ATPase are also problematic. The membrane fractions used are impure and include endosomes, lysosomes, and other acidic compartments; factors other than the H^+ATPase may affect the acidification kinetics, such as the vesicle volume, the membrane potential of the vesicle, the internal buffering capacity, and the passive proton conductance; and the experimental physiologic condition under investigation may affect the membrane fractionation procedure.

Consequently, conclusions about adaptive mechanisms used to modify renal H^+ excretion in pathophysiologic states drawn from such studies must be viewed with considerable caution.

Chronic H^+ATPase Regulation in Response to Prolonged Acid and Alkali Administration

Physiologic studies have shown that chronic acid administration increases net acid excretion in the proximal tubule (23,311–315), thick ascending limb (11,316), distal convoluted tubule (17,317,318), cortical collecting tubule (2,6,10,145,162,191,319–324), and inner medullary collecting duct (44,184,325–327). The studies discussed below indicate that the vacuolar H^+ATPase participates in this adaptational increase in H^+ secretion in the cortical and medullary collecting tubules and possibly in the proximal tubule.

Response to Prolonged Acid Administration

Cortical Collecting Tubule. The cortical collecting has the capacity to secrete protons through the luminal membrane H^+ATPase in the α intercalated cells (10,30,35,170,328) and to secrete bicarbonate (191,319,329) by chloride-bicarbonate exchange (268,279,330) in the luminal membrane of β intercalated cells (170,180,266,281) and γ intercalated cells (33).

In the cortical collecting tubule, net acid production of the animal appears to be the major determinant of whether the tubule displays net acid or bicarbonate secretion. In rabbits, chronic administration of acid in vivo suppressed bicarbonate secretion in the cortical collecting tubule (39,139,162,166,279,319,322,331,332), with little or no stimulation of H^+ secretion (bicarbonate reabsorption) (322,331,332). Bicarbonate secretion was also suppressed by incubation of rabbit cortical collecting tubules in acidic medium in vitro (324,333), without an effect on H^+ secretion (324).

Suppression of bicarbonate secretion is thought to involve inactivation or internalization of luminal Cl^-/HCO_3^- exchange (324,333), but studies in rats suggest that at least part of the response to in vivo administration of acid may result from loss of vacuolar H^+ATPase from the basolateral membrane of bicarbonate-secreting intercalated cells. In rats to which acid was administered orally for 14 days, a reduction in basolateral membrane H^+ATPase polarization and increase of cytoplasmic vesicular staining for H^+ATPase were observed in β intercalated cells of the cortical collecting tubule (179). A gradual increase in the number of intercalated cells with apical plasma membrane H^+ATPase staining was observed, suggesting that H^+ secretion increased (even though, as discussed below, no increase in H^+ secretion has been demonstrated in physiologic studies of isolated collecting ducts from the acid-loaded rabbit). No change was found in H^+ATPase content per mg of protein in cortical or medullary microsomes, determined by an anti-H^+ATPase E (31-kDa) subunit monoclonal antibody binding assay (179). The immunocytochemical changes in H^+ATPase distribution observed in the rat with chronic acid administration are in agreement with earlier morphologic findings of Dørup (334) who demonstrated that acute acid administration to rats increased the luminal membrane surface and decreased the number of intermediate size apical vesicles in intercalated cells of the cortical collecting tubule.

Three laboratories studied the effects of chronic acid administration on NEM-sensitive ATPase activity in different nephron segments (290,295,297,301). In two studies, a significant increase in NEM-sensitive ATPase activity was found in the cortical collecting tubule. It is important to note, however, that two of the same groups (297,301) found an equal or greater increase in the NEM-sensitive ATPase activity of the medullary thick limb, a segment in which the vacuolar H^+ATPase is thought to have little or no role in H^+ secretion (11).

Outer Medullary Collecting Tubule. The outer medullary collecting tubule has the highest rates of H^+ secretion in the distal nephron (39). Yet, in numerous studies, no change has been observed in in vitro tubular H^+ secretion (bicarbonate reabsorption) in outer medullary collecting tubules obtained from animals subjected to chronic acid administration (39,166,172,322). Recently, Hayashi et al. (168) measured vacuolar H^+ATPase-driven proton extrusion in individual intercalated cells (as the rate of sodium-independent pH_i recovery from NH_4Cl-induced cytosolic acidification) in outer medullary collecting tubules from rabbits subjected to 14 days of high acid intake and also found no significant change in the cells from acid-loaded rabbits.

In contrast, several studies have demonstrated marked morphologic alterations and a profound shift in the immunocytochemical distribution of H^+ATPase in the outer medullary collecting tubule in animals subjected to chronic acid administration. Madsen and Tisher (335) showed that administration of acid to rats for 15 days resulted in an increase in apical membrane area and loss of tubulovesicular structures in the apical cytoplasm of intercalated cells in the inner and outer stripe of outer medulla, changes suggesting recruitment of H^+ATPases from the tubulovesicular structures to the apical membrane. Bastani et al. (179) demonstrated directly by immunocytochemistry that chronic administration of acid to rats produced a profound redistribution of the vacuolar H^+ATPase from cytoplasmic vesicles to the plasma membrane in intercalated cells from the outer medulla. In the inner stripe only 7% of the intercalated cells exhibited plasma membrane H^+ATPase staining in control rats, whereas 63% of the cells showed plasma membrane staining after one day of acid administration, and this increased progressively to 89% after 14 days of acid intake. The outer stripe showed a similar, although slower, response. Three studies showed a modest increase in NEM-sensitive ATPase activity in outer medullary collecting tubule with chronic acid administration (Table 2), but others found that the quantity of immunoreactive H^+ATPase did not change with chronic acid administration (179).

The immunocytochemical and morphologic evidence indicates that redistribution of the H^+ATPase to the plasma membrane by vesicular traffic occurs during chronic acid administration, and suggests that an increase in H^+ secretion may occur in the outer medullary collecting tubule, though in vitro transport studies have not found any. The basis for these disparate findings is unknown at the present time. As described below, studies on the regulation of H^+ transport in response to chronic alkali administration and chronic hypercapnia have also shown that the response of the tubule in vitro differs from that in vivo.

Distal Tubule. The "distal tubule," investigated in numerous physiologic studies over several decades, consists of several distinct tubular epithelia. The distal convoluted tubule, or early distal tubule, has a single cell type (the DCT cell). The connecting tubule and initial collecting tubule, or late distal tubule, are composed of a mixture of principal cells and intercalated cells (27). Rat distal tubular transport of bicarbonate is highly variable. Various studies have shown either no bicarbonate transport (317), net bicarbonate reabsorption (336–339) or net bicarbonate secretion (284,329,338) depending on the flow rate (338,340), the luminal bicarbonate concentration (17,340), the diet of the animal (329,339), the luminal chloride concentration (17,341), and the presence or absence of potassium depletion (342).

The participation of a vacuolar H^+ATPase in distal tubular H^+ secretion was first suggested by studies demonstrating that acidification was not inhibited by amiloride, and was affected by the tubular potential difference (339). Subsequent studies indicate that a vacuolar H^+ATPase accounts for 20–35% of early distal tubular H^+ATPase H^+ secretion (bicarbonate reabsorption), and 84% or more* of late distal tubular H^+ secretion (17). Chronic acid intake (317,318,343) or an acid-ash

*Part of the H^+ secretion in the late distal tubule was attributed to an H^+,K^+-ATPase on the basis of partial inhibition by Sch28080. As discussed above however, Sch28080 also inhibits H^+ secretion by the electrogenic vacuolar H^+ATPase in intact turtle bladder (154,155), probably by an indirect mechanism.

diet (339) increases distal tubular H^+ secretion (317), but the role of the vacuolar H^+ATPase in this response is at present unknown.

Proximal Tubule. In metabolic acidosis and during chronic acid intake, proximal tubular bicarbonate reabsorption increases, originating primarily through an increase in the activity of the luminal Na^+-H^+ antiporter (23). It is unclear whether any of the acid-induced increase in proximal tubule H^+ secretion arises from an increase in vacuolar H^+ATPase activity. No change was found in the quantity of immunoreactive H^+ATPase in cortex microsomes (which contain brush border membrane) at any time point during 14 days of acid administration to rats (179). In contrast, Chambrey et al. (305) found that acid administration to rats for 4 days produced a 26% increase in NEM-sensitive ATPase activity, a 33% increase in bafilomycin-sensitive ATPase activity and a 25% higher rate of proton transport in brush border membranes from acidotic kidneys compared to membranes from control kidneys. They found no difference in either activity between the acidotic and control homogenates, and proposed that acidosis produced a redistribution of vacuolar H^+ATPase from intracellular compartments to the plasma membrane. One significant problem with the study is that the authors used 200 n*M* bafilomycin A_1, a concentration far in excess of the 15 n*M* needed to inhibit completely H^+ in cholate-treated brush border membranes (63). At this higher concentration of bafilomycin, inhibition of other ATPases has been observed (65). In two studies on intact microdissected proximal tubules from acid-loaded rats, one found no change in NEM-sensitive ATPase activity in the proximal tubule, and the other observed a decrease (Table 5).

Response to Prolonged Alkali Administration

Cortical Collecting Tubule. In most of the studies in both rat and rabbit, chronic alkali administration or induction of a sustained metabolic alkalosis increases bicarbonate secretion in the cortical collecting tubule (39,166,268,279,319,344,345).* The role of the vacuolar H^+ATPase in this response has been examined in several studies. In one investigation, the effect of chronic bicarbonate administration on the distribution of H^+ATPase in the intercalated cells of rat cortical and medullary collecting tubules (179) was examined. No change in H^+ATPase content of cortical microsomes was found, but a modest increase in the number of intercalated cells with basolateral membrane H^+ATPase staining was observed. The magnitude of the response may have been blunted as a result of the failure of the animals to develop a metabolic alkalosis (179).

More recently, Verlander et al. (346) examined the distribution of vacuolar H^+ATPase in rat intercalated cells by immunoelectron microscopy in a model of chloride depletion metabolic alkalosis induced by peritoneal dialysis of rats with 150 m*M* sodium bicarbonate (347). In α intercalated cells from the cortical and outer medullary collecting tubules of alkalotic rats, luminal membrane H^+ATPase A subunit antibody labeling was reduced, and was accompanied by an increase in the number of intracellular vacuoles labeling for H^+ATPase. H^+ATPase labeling was increased in the basolateral plasma membrane of β intercalated cells of the cortical collecting tubule.

These findings suggest that in chloride depletion alkalosis, H^+ secretion is inhibited and bicarbonate secretion is enhanced, and that both adaptational processes result, at least in part, from regulated changes in H^+ATPase distribution. In this study, done in intact rats, the change in bicarbonate secretion occurred within 45 min, and the change in H^+ATPase distribution appeared within 2 hr (345,346). In contrast, rat cortical collecting tubules that were incubated in alkaline solutions in vitro failed to exhibit an increase in bicarbonate secretion (345). This finding indicates that unidentified factors in vivo are responsible for modifying bicarbonate secretion and possibly for changing the H^+ATPase distribution. It is possible that the change in H^+ATPase distribution observed in alkalotic rats occurred as a secondary response to increased luminal Cl^-/HCO_3^- exchange. Kim et al. (249) demonstrated that chronic bumetanide administration to rats, which increases Cl^- delivery to the collecting tubule, produced nearly identical changes in H^+ATPase distribution.

Three studies have examined the effect of alkali administration on NEM-sensitive ATPase activity in cortical collecting tubule (Table 5). Two of them found no change; one found a decrease.

Distal Tubule. Numerous investigations have demonstrated that distal tubule bicarbonate secretion increases during chronic alkali administration of metabolic alkalosis (317,329,338,340, 348–350). This response is physiologically significant as distal tubule bicarbonate secretion

*Hamm et al. observed no change in bicarbonate secretion in rabbits subjected to chronic alkali administration (322).

contributes to the correction of metabolic alkalosis (350), although the collecting duct probably has a greater role (351). Bicarbonate secretion in the distal tubule is an active process (338) that is stimulated by luminal chloride (17,341,349,350). Bicarbonate secretion probably occurs in connecting tubule and initial collecting tubule β (or γ) intercalated cells by luminal Cl^-/HCO_3^- exchange (6) and a basolateral vacuolar H^+ATPase (26). The role of the basolateral vacuolar H^+ATPase in the adaptive increases in bicarbonate secretion observed in the distal nephron is unknown, but it is likely that at least part of the response involves recruitment of H^+ATPases to the basolateral membrane, as described above for the cortical collecting tubule.

Chronic metabolic alkalosis induced by diuretic administration also increases distal tubule H^+ secretion (352,353). This response may represent an effect of persistently elevated aldosterone levels (see below).

Chronic H^+ATPase Regulation from Prolonged Mineralcorticoid Administration

Chronic mineralocorticoid administration increases renal net acid excretion (354–358). The effect of chronic mineralcorticoid administration on H^+ transport in the cortical and outer medullary collecting tubules has been examined in a number of studies.

Cortical Collecting Tubule. There is some indirect evidence that mineralcorticoids stimulate H^+ secretion in the α intercalated cells in the cortical collecting tubule. Chronic administration of the mineralocorticoid deoxycorticosterone (DOC) to rabbits was found to increase the lumen-positive potential of cortical collecting tubules in the absence of luminal sodium, a response interpreted to represent an increase in apical H^+ATPase activity (164).

Accumulating evidence indicates that aldosterone does not exert a direct effect on the vacuolar H^+ATPase in β (or γ) intercalated cells (for an excellent review, see Reference 30). Recent studies by Emmons and Kurtz show that in the rabbit cortical collecting tubule, as few as 4% of cortical intercalated cell may function as α cells (33). In most of the cortical collecting tubule intercalated cells, mineralocorticoid receptor was not detectable by immunocytochemistry (359–361), probably indicating absence of the receptor in β (or γ) intercalated cells. Chronic treatment of rabbits with DOC was found to increase bicarbonate secretion in cortical collecting tubules (331) but also produced a slight alkalosis, and the increase in bicarbonate secretion was eliminated by concomitant administration of acid and DOC to the animals. This suggests that the acid-base status of the animal, rather direct effects of DOC, was the primary stimulus increasing bicarbonate secretion (331). Mineralocorticoid administration produced no change in apical or basolateral membrane surface density of cortical intercalated cells in rabbits (362) or rats (363). Yamaji et al. (269) found that the β intercalated cells in cortical collecting tubules of rabbits treated chronically with DOC had an increase in basolateral Na^+-H^+ activity but no change in the amiloride-resistant sodium-independent rate of pH_i recovery (an assay for H^+ATPase-mediated H^+ extrusion).

Outer Medullary Collecting Tubule. Several lines of evidence indicate that mineralocorticoids directly stimulate the luminal H^+ATPase in the α intercalated cells of the outer medullary collecting tubule. Prolonged administration of mineralocorticoids to rabbits increased H^+ secretion by 65–84% in outer medullary collecting tubules studied in vitro (172,265). Hays (259) found that rates sodium-independent pH_i recovery (an assay for vacuolar H^+ATPase-driven proton extrusion) increased 76% in outer medullary tubules from DOC-treated rabbits and decreased 56% in tubules from adrenalectomized animals, although no attempt was made to distinguish intercalated cells from principal cells. In studies of individual intercalated cells from outer medullary collecting tubules (outer stripe), Kuwahara et al. (145) found that the rate of sodium-independent pH_i recovery increased 111% in tubules from mineralocorticoid-treated rabbits studied in HCO_3^-/CO_2 buffers. Similarly, Weiner et al. (28) found that chronic DOC administration to rabbits increased sodium-independent pH_i recovery 306% in intercalated (minority) cells from the inner stripe studied under CO_2-free conditions. These effects probably arise from a direct increase in H^+ATPase activity induced by mineralocorticoid and not the result of cytosolic acidification, since pH_i increased. DOC had no effect on α intercalated cell basolateral Na^+-H^+ exchange but did increase concomitantly basolateral Cl^-/HCO_3^- activity (145).

Four studies have explored the effect of mineralocorticoids on NEM-sensitive ATPase activity in different nephron segments (292,293,294,304,364) (Table 5). Three of the four studies observed an increase in activity in the cortical and outer medullary collecting tubules.

Chronic H^+ATPase Regulation in Response to Prolonged Elevation of P_{CO_2}

Prolonged hypercapnia increases renal net acid excretion producing a sustained elevation in extracellular fluid bicarbonate concentration (365–367). Laski and Kurtzman (262) subjected rabbits to hypercapnia for varying lengths of time and examined rates of collecting tubule bicarbonate reabsorption in vitro. Cortical collecting tubules began to show an increase in net bicarbonate reabsorption by 6 hr, which was significant by 24 hr. After 48 hr of in vivo hypercapnia, cortical collecting tubule net bicarbonate reabsorption was 650% of control rates. Since the unidirectional rates of bicarbonate transport were not measured, it is unknown whether this response represented a suppression of bicarbonate secretion or a stimulation of H^+ secretion. However, outer medullary collecting tubules, examined in the same study, showed no change in bicarbonate reabsorption at any time point (262), suggesting that the changes in the cortex most likely resulted from suppression of bicarbonate secretion.

The basis of this adaptational increase in cortical collecting tubule bicarbonate reabsorption in response to CO_2 is presently unknown. Verlander et al. (368) found a 73–95% increase in the apical membrane surface density of α intercalated cells of the cortical collecting tubule and connecting tubule in rats after 4–5 hr of hypercapnia and no significant change in the β cells. From the time course for physiologic adaptation determined by Laski and Kurtzman, however, the length of exposure to hypercapnia studies were probably too short for the adaptive changes to have occurred.

As discussed above, Madsen and Tisher (261) found a significant increase in apical surface density of intercalated cells with a concomitant loss of apical tubulovesicles in the outer medullary collecting tubule of rats after 4–5 hr of hypercapnia. McKinney and Davidson (256) found that outer medullary collecting tubules increased H^+ secretion 146–252% in response to an in vitro elevation of P_{CO_2}; but when the same tubules were subjected to electron microscopic morphometric analysis, there was no change from controls in the apical membrane surface density or any other indices. These discrepancies between the in vitro physiologic and morphologic responses and the in vivo morphologic observations again suggest that additional unidentified factors are required for the redistribution of vacuolar H^+ATPase observed in vivo.

THE RENAL VACUOLAR H^+ATPase: SUMMARY AND CONCLUSIONS

In most eukaryotic cells, vacuolar H^+ATPases reside predominantly in intracellular compartments, where they are responsible for the acidification of the vacuolar system required for constitutive endocytic and secretory processes. In some specialized cells, such as proton-transporting renal epithelial cells, most of the vacuolar H^+ATPase resides on the plasma membrane, or in plasmalemma-associated tubulovesicles, where it functions in the bicarbonate reabsorption, regeneration, and secretion needed for acid-base homeostasis.

Acute and chronic regulation of vacuolar H^+ATPase-driven H^+ transport in renal tubular epithelial cells may occur, in principle, by any or all of the three general mechanisms shown in Figure 3: (a) kinetic regulation; (b) regulated redistribution; and (c) change in enzyme content. The experimental evidence discussed above demonstrates that both kinetic regulation and redistribution are employed by the kidney. At the present time, there is no direct evidence that changes in enzyme content have a major role in regulatory responses.

How then does the kidney achieve the physiologic regulation of plasma membrane vacuolar H^+ATPases while allowing constitutive acidification of intracellular compartments to proceed? The studies of the enzyme to date have provided a broad overview of how such regulation may occur: (a) Vacuolar H^+ATPases from different compartments of the kidney have intrinsic differences in their enzymatic properties, such as pH optima and response to changes in the lipid and ionic environment. These enzymes also appear distinct in the degree to which their activity is affected by regulatory factors. The basis for these differences in properties remains unclear. The observation that the B and E subunits are dissimilar among these enzymes provides a possible clue. (b) Renal epithelial cells have the capacity to express different structural forms of vacuolar H^+ATPase. This may provide a basis for changing the properties and regulation of the vacuolar H^+ATPase in different segments of the nephron. The cell-specific expression of different structural forms of the H^+ATPase may provide a means for sequestering the enzyme into specialized membrane compartments capable of inserting the enzyme into the plasma membrane in a regulated manner. (c) The kidney produces cytosolic regulatory proteins that interact directly with the vacuolar H^+ATPase to modify its activity. Future investigations may determine where these proteins are expressed, and whether they participate in the acute and chronic regulatory responses of renal H^+ transport discussed above.

ACKNOWLEDGMENT

This work was supported in part by NIH grants DK38848, DK09976, AR32087, and DK45181 and by a grant from the Monsanto-Washington University Biomedical Agreement. S. L. G. was a Sandoz Pharmaceutical Corporation Established Investigator of the American Heart Association. B. L. S. was supported in part by a research grant from the Arthritis Foundation.

REFERENCES

1. Rector F Jr. Renal regulation of acid-base balance. Aust N Z J Med 1981; 11:1–5.
2. Levine DZ, Jacobson HR. The regulation of renal acid secretion: New observations from studies of distal nephron segments. Kidney Int 1986; 29:1099–1109.
3. Breyer MD, Jacobson HR. Mechanisms and regulation of renal H+ and HCO_3^- transport. Am J Nephrol 1987; 7:150–161.
4. Maddox DA, Deen WM, Gennari FJ. Control of bicarbonate and fluid reabsorption in the proximal convoluted tubule. Semin Nephrol 1987; 7:72–81.
5. Paillard M, Bichara M. Recent advances in the cellular mechanisms and hormonal regulation of urine acidification. Adv Nephrol Necker Hosp 1989; 18:141–167.
6. Schuster VL. Bicarbonate reabsorption and secretion in the cortical and outer medullary collecting tubule. Semin Nephrol 1990; 10:139–147.
7. DuBose T Jr. Reclamation of filtered bicarbonate. Kidney Int 1990; 38:584–589.
8. Cogan MG. Regulation and control of bicarbonate reabsorption in the proximal tubule. Semin Nephrol 1990; 10:115–121.
9. Gluck S, Nelson R. The role of the V-ATPase in renal epithelial H+ transport. J Exp Biol 1992; 172:205–218.
10. Hamm LL, Hering-Smith KS. Acid-base transport in the collecting duct. Semin Nephrol 1993; 13:246–55.
11. Good DW. The thick ascending limb as a site of renal bicarbonate reabsorption. Semin Nephrol 1993; 13:225–235.
12. Preisig PA, Ives HE, Cragoe E Jr., et al. Role of the Na+/H+ antiporter in rat proximal tubule bicarbonate absorption. J Clin Invest 1987; 80:970–978.
13. Good DW, Knepper MA, Burg MB. Ammonia and bicarbonate transport by thick ascending limb of rat kidney. Am J Physiol 1984; 247:F35–44.
14. Good DW. Regulation of bicarbonate and ammonium absorption in the thick ascending limb of the rat. Kidney Int Suppl 1991; 33:S36–42.
15. Capasso G, Unwin R, Agulian S, Giebisch G. Bicarbonate transport along the loop of Henle: I. Microperfusion studies of load and inhibitor sensitivity. J Clin Invest 1991; 88:430–437.
16. Froissart M, Borensztein P, Houillier P, et al. Plasma membrane Na(+)-H+ antiporter and H(+)-ATPase in the medullary thick ascending limb of rat kidney. Am J Physiol 1992; 262:C963–670.
17. Wang T, Malnic G, Giebisch G, Chan YL. Renal bicarbonate reabsorption in the rat: IV. Bicarbonate transport mechanisms in the early and late distal tubule. J Clin Invest 1993; 91:2776–2784.
18. Ulate G, Fernandez R, Malnic G. Effect of bafilomycin on proximal bicarbonate absorption in the rat. Braz J Med Biol Res 26:773–777.
19. Preisig PA, Alpern RJ. Pathways for apical and basolateral membrane NH3 and NH4+ movement in rat proximal tubule. Am J Physiol 1990; 259:F587–593.
20. Zimolo Z, Montrose MH, Murer H. H+ extrusion by an apical vacuolar-type H(+)-ATPase in rat renal proximal tubules. J Membr Biol 1992; 126:19–26.
21. Hays SR, Alpern RJ. Inhibition of Na(+)-independent H+ pump by Na(+)-induced changes in cell Ca^{2+}. J Gen Physiol 1991; 98:791–813.
22. Moe OW, Preisig PA, Alpern RJ. Cellular model of proximal tubule NaCl and NaHCO3 absorption. Kidney Int 1990; 38:605–611.
23. Alpern RJ. Cell mechanisms of proximal tubule acidification. Physiol Rev 1990; 70:79–114.
24. Bank N, Aynedjian HS, Mutz BF. Proximal bicarbonate absorption independent of Na+-H+ exchange: Effect of bicarbonate load. Am J Physiol 1989; 256:F577–582.

25. Capasso G, Unwin R, Giebisch G. Role of the loop of Henle in urinary acidification. Kidney Int Suppl 1991; 33:S33–35.
26. Brown D, Hirsch S, Gluck S. Localization of a proton-pumping ATPase in rat kidney. J Clin Invest 1988; 82:2114–126.
27. Kriz W, Bankir L. A standard nomenclature for structures of the kidney: The Renal Commission of the International Union of Physiological Sciences (IUPS). Kidney Int 1988; 33:1–7.
28. Weiner ID, Wingo CS, Hamm LL. Regulation of intracellular pH in two cell populations of inner stripe of rabbit outer medullary collecting duct. Am J Physiol 1993; 265:F406–415.
29. Steinmetz PR. Cellular organization of urinary acidification. Am J Physiol 1986; 251:F173–187.
30. Schuster VL. Function and regulation of collecting duct intercalated cells. Annu Rev Physiol 1993; 55:267–288.
31. Schwartz GJ, Satlin LM, Bergmann JE. Fluorescent characterization of collecting duct cells: A second H+-secreting type. Am J Physiol 1988; 255:F1003–1014.
32. Alper SL, Natale J, Gluck S, et al. Subtypes of intercalated cells in rat kidney collecting duct defined by antibodies against erythroid band 3 and renal vacuolar H+-ATPase. Proc Natl Acad Sci USA 1989; 86:5429–5433.
33. Emmons C, Kurtz I. Functional characterization of three intercalated cell subtypes in the rabbit outer cortical collecting duct. J Clin Invest 1994; 93:417–423.
34. Gluck S, Caldwell J. Immunoaffinity purification and characterization of vacuolar H+ATPase from bovine kidney. J Biol Chem 1987; 262:15780–15789.
35. Brown D, Hirsch S, Gluck S. An H+-ATPase in opposite plasma membrane domains in kidney epithelial cell subpopulations. Nature 1988; 331:622–624.
36. Stone DK, Seldin DW, Kokko JP, Jacobson HR. Anion dependence of rabbit medullary collecting duct acidification. J Clin Invest 1983; 71:1505–1508.
37. Jacobson HR. Medullary collecting duct acidification: Effects of potassium, HCO3 concentration and pCO_2. J Clin Invest 1984; 74:2107–2114.
38. Wingo CS, Cain BD. The renal H-K-ATPase: Physiological significance and role in potassium homeostasis. Annu Rev Physiol 1993; 55:323–347.
39. Lombard WE, Kokko JP, Jacobson HR. Bicarbonate transport in cortical and outer medullary collecting tubules. Am J Physiol 1983; 244:F289–296.
40. Madsen KM, Clapp WL, Verlander JW. Structure and function of the inner medullary collecting duct. Kidney Int 1988; 34:441–454.
41. Helou CM, de Araujo M, Seguro AC. Effect of low and high potassium diets on H(+)-K(+)-ATPase and Na(+)-K(+)-ATPase activities in the rat inner medullary collecting duct cells. Renal Physiol Biochem 1994; 17:21–26.
42. Kleinman JG, Tipnis P, Pscheidt R. H(+)-K(+)-ATPase of rat inner medullary collecting duct in primary culture. Am J Physiol 1993; 265:F698–704.
43. Graber ML, Bengele HH, Schwartz JH, Alexander EA. pH and PCO_2 profiles of the rat inner medullary collecting duct. Am J Physiol 241:F659–668.
44. Graber ML, Bengele HH, Mroz E, et al. Acute metabolic acidosis augments collecting duct acidification rate in the rat. Am J Physiol 1981; 241:F669–676.
45. Bengele HH, McNamara ER, Schwartz JH, Alexander EA. Acidification adaptation along the inner medullary collecting duct. Am J Physiol 1988; 255:F1155–1159.
46. Forgac M. Structure and function of vacuolar class of ATP-driven proton pumps. Physiol Rev 1989; 69:765–796.
47. Gluck SL. The vacuolar H(+)-ATPases: Versatile proton pumps participating in constitutive and specialized functions of eukaryotic cells. Int Rev Cytol 1993; 105–137.
48. Grinstein S, Nanda A, Lukacs G, Rotstein O. V-ATPases in phagocytic cells. J Exp Biol 1992; 172:179–192.
49. Mego JL, Farb RM, Barnes J. An adenosine triphosphate-dependent stabilization of proteolytic activity in heterolysosomes: Evidence for a proton pump. Biochem J 1972; 128:763–769.
50. Phillips JH, Allison VP. Proton translocation of the bovine chromaffin-granule membrane. Biochem J 1978; 170:661–672.
51. Gluck S, Kelly S, Al-Awqati Q. The proton translocating ATPase responsible for urinary acidification. J Biol Chem 1982; 257:9230–9233.
52. Chatterjee D, Chakraborty M, Leit M, et al. Sensitivity to vanadate and isoforms of subunits A and B distinguish the osteoclast proton pump from other vacuolar H-ATPases. Proc Natl Acad Sci USA 1992; 89:6257–6261.
53. Blair HC, Teitelbaum SL, Ghiselli R, Gluck S. Osteoclastic bone resorption by a polarized vacuolar proton pump. Science 245:855–857.
54. Gluck S, Caldwell J. Proton-translocating ATPase from bovine kidney medulla: Partial purification and reconstitution. Am J Physiol 1988; 254:F71–79.

55. Sze H, Ward JM, Lai S. Vacuolar H(+)-translocating ATPases from plants: structure, function, and isoforms. J Bioenerg Biomembr 1992; 24:371–381.
56. Arai H, Pink S, Forgac M. Interaction of anions and ATP with the coated vesicle proton pump. Biochemistry 1989; 28:3075–3082.
57. Moriyama Y, Nelson N. The purified ATPase from chromaffin granule membranes is an anion-dependent proton pump. J Biol Chem 1987; 262:9175–9180.
58. Moriyama Y, Nelson N. H+-translocating ATPase in Golgi apparatus: Characterization as vacuolar H+-ATPase and its subunit structures. J Biol Chem 1989; 264:18445–18450.
59. Moriyama Y, Nelson N. Cold inactivation of vacuolar proton-ATPases. J Biol Chem 1989; 264:3577–3582.
60. Bowman BJ, Dschida WJ, Harris T, Bowman EJ. The vacuolar ATPase of Neurospora crassa contains an F1-like structure. J Biol Chem 1989; 264:15606–15612.
61. Moriyama Y, Futai M. Presence of 5-hydroxytryptamine (serotonin) transport coupled with vacuolar-type H(+)-ATPase in neurosecretory granules from bovine posterior pituitary. J Biol Chem 1990; 265:9165–9169.
62. Wang ZQ, Gluck S. Isolation and properties of bovine kidney brush border vacuolar H(+)-ATPase: A proton pump with enzymatic and structural differences from kidney microsomal H(+)-ATPase. J Biol Chem 1990; 265:21957–21965.
63. Jehmlich K, Sablotni J, Simon BJ, Burckhardt G. Biochemical aspects of H(+)-ATPase in renal proximal tubules: Inhibition by N,N′-dicyclohexylcarbodiimide, N-ethylmaleimide, and bafilomycin. Kidney Int Suppl 1991; 33:S64–70.
64. Simon BJ, Kulanthaivel P, Burckhardt G, et al. Characterization of an ATP-driven H+ pump in human placental brush-border membrane vesicles. Biochem J 1992; 287:423–430.
65. Bowman EJ, Siebers A, Altendorf K. Bafilomycins: A class of inhibitors of membrane ATPases from microorganisms, animal cells, and plant cells. Proc Natl Acad Sci 1988; 85:7972–7976.
66. Guinea R, Carrasco L. Concanamycin A: A powerful inhibitor of enveloped animal-virus entry into cells. Biochem Biophys Res Commun 1994; 201:1270–1278.
67. Muroi M, Takasu A, Yamasaki M, Takatsuki A. Folimycin (concanamycin A), an inhibitor of V-type H(+)-ATPase, blocks cell-surface expression of virus-envelope glycoproteins. Biochem Biophys Res Commun 1993; 193:999–1005.
68. Woo JT, Shinohara C, Sakai K, et al. Isolation, characterization and biological activities of concanamycins as inhibitors of lysosomal acidification. J Antibiot 1992; 45:1108–1116.
69. Nakamoto RK, Shin K, Iwamoto A, et al. Escherichia coli F0F1-ATPase. Residues involved in catalysis and coupling. Ann NY Acad Sci 1992; 671:335–3343.
70. Fillingame RH. H+ transport and coupling by the F0 sector of the ATP synthase: Insights into the molecular mechanism of function. J Bioenerg Biomembr 24:485–491.
71. Abrahams JP, Leslie AG, Lutter R, Walker JE. Structure at 2.8 A resolution of F1-ATPase from bovine heart mitochondria (see comments). Nature 1994: 370:621–628.
72. Deckers-Hebestreit G, Altendorf K. The Fo complex of the proton-translocating F-type ATPase of Escherichia coli. J Exp Biol 1992; 172:451–459.
73. Kagawa Y. Protonmotive force and secondary transport: Historical perspectives and unifying principles. Methods Enzymol 1986; 126:1–9.
74. Fillingame RH. Subunit c of F1F0 ATP synthase: structure and role in transmembrane energy transduction. Biochim Biophys Acta 1992; 1101:240–243.
75. Collinson IR, Runswick MJ, Buchanan SK, et al. Fo membrane domain of ATP synthase from bovine heart mitochondria: Purification, subunit composition, and reconstitution with F1-ATPase. Biochemistry 1994; 33:7971–7978.
76. Gresser MJ, Myers JA, Boyer PD. Catalytic site cooperativity of beef heart mitochondrial F1 adenosine triphosphatase: Correlations of initial velocity, bound intermediate, and oxygen exchange measurements with an alternating three-site model. J Biol Chem 257:12030–12038.
77. Blair DF, Berg HC. The MotA protein of E. coli is a proton-conducting component of the flagellar motor. Cell 1990; 60:439–449.
78. Nelson N. Structure and function of V-ATPases in endocytic and secretory organelles. J Exp Biol 1992; 172:149–153.
79. Nelson N. Organellar proton-ATPases. Curr Opin Cell Biol 1992; 4:654–660.
80. Arai H, Terres G, Pink S, Forgac M. Topography and subunit stoichiometry of the coated vesicle proton pump. J Biol Chem 1988; 263:8796–8802.
81. Adachi I, Puopolo K, Marquez-Sterling N, et al. Dissociation, cross-linking, and glycosylation of the coated vesicle proton pump. J Biol Chem 1990; 265:967–973.
82. Gogarten JP, Kibak H, Dittrich P, et al. Evolution of the vacuolar H+-ATPase: Implications for the origin of eukaryotes. Proc Natl Acad Sci USA 1989; 86:6661–6665.
83. Moriyama Y, Nelson N. Nucleotide binding sites and chemical modification of the chromaffin granule proton ATPase. J Biol Chem 1987; 262:14723–14729.

84. Arai H, Berne M, Terres G, et al. Subunit composition and ATP site labeling of the coated vesicle proton-translocating adenosinetriphosphatase. Biochemistry 1987; 26:6632–6638.
85. Marushack MM, Lee BS, Masood K, Gluck S. cDNA sequence and tissue expression of bovine vacuolar H(+)-ATPase M(r) 70,000 subunit. Am J Physiol 1992; 263:F171–174.
86. Saraste M, Sibbald PR, Wittinghofer A. The P-loop—A common motif in ATP- and GTP-binding proteins. Trends Biochem Sci 1990; 15:430–434.
87. Feng Y, Forgac M. Cysteine 254 of the 73-kDa subunit is responsible for inhibition of the coated vesicle (H+)-ATPase upon modification by sulfhydryl reagents. J Biol Chem 1992; 267:5817–5822.
88. Nelson RD, Guo XL, Masood K, et al. Selectively amplified expression of an isoform of the vacuolar H(+)-ATPase 56-kilodalton subunit in renal intercalated cells. Proc Natl Acad Sci USA 1992; 89:3541–3545.
89. Adachi I, Arai H, Pimental R, Forgac M. Proteolysis and orientation on reconstitution of the coated vesicle proton pump. J Biol Chem 1990; 265:960–966.
90. Pan YX, Xu J, Strasser JE, Howell M, Dean GE. Structure and expression of subunit A from the bovine chromaffin cell vacuolar ATPase. FEBS Lett 1991; 293:89–92.
91. Puopolo K, Kumamoto C, Adachi I, Forgac M. A single gene encodes the catalytic "A" subunit of the bovine vacuolar H(+)-ATPase. J Biol Chem 1991; 266:24564–24572.
92. van Hille B, Richener H, Evans DB, et al. Identification of two subunit A isoforms of the vacuolar H(+)-ATPase in human osteoclastoma. J Biol Chem 1993; 268:7075–7080.
93. Sudhof TC, Fried VA, Stone DK, et al. Human endomembrane H+ pump strongly resembles the ATP-synthetase of Archaebacteria. Proc Natl Acad Sci USA 1989; 86:6067–6071.
94. Bernasconi P, Rausch T, Struve I, et al. An mRNA from human brain encodes an isoform of the B subunit of the vacuolar H+-ATPase. J Biol Chem 1990; 17428–17431.
95. Puopolo K, Kumamoto C, Adachi I, et al. Differential expression of the "B" subunit of the vacuolar H(+)-ATPase in bovine tissues. J Biol Chem 1992; 267:3696–3706.
96. Nelson H, Mandiyan S, Noumi T, et al. Molecular cloning of cDNA encoding the C subunit of H(+)-ATPase from bovine chromaffin granules. J Biol Chem 1990; 265:20390–20393.
97. Hirsch S, Strauss A, Masood K, et al. Isolation and sequence of a cDNA clone encoding the 31-kDa subunit of bovine kidney vacuolar H+-ATPase. Proc Natl Acad Sci USA 1990; 85:3004–3008.
98. Hemken P, Guo XL, Wang ZQ, et al. Immunologic evidence that vacuolar H+ ATPases with heterogeneous forms of Mr = 31,000 subunit have different membrane distributions in mammalian kidney. J Biol Chem 1992; 267:9948–9957.
99. van Hille B, Vanek M, Richener H, et al. Cloning and tissue distribution of subunits C, D, and E of the human vacuolar H(+)-ATPase. Biochem Biophys Res Commun 1993; 197:15–21.
100. Wang SY, Moriyama Y, Mandel M, et al. Cloning of cDNA encoding a 32-kDa protein: An accessory polypeptide of the H+-ATPase from chromaffin granules. J Biol Chem 1988; 263:17638–17642.
101. Arai H, Berne M, Forgac M. Inhibition of the coated vesicle proton pump and labeling of a 17,000-dalton polypeptide by N,N′-dicyclohexylcarbodiimide. J Biol Chem 1987; 262:11006–11011.
102. Noumi T, Beltran C, Nelson H, Nelson N. Mutational analysis of yeast vacuolar H(+)-ATPase. Proc Natl Acad Sci USA 88:1938–1942.
103. Zhang J, Feng Y, Forgac M. Proton conduction and bafilomycin binding by the V0 domain of the coated vesicle V-ATPase. J Biol Chem 1994; 269:23518–23523.
104. Cross RL, Taiz L. Gene duplication as a means for altering H+/ATP ratios during the evolution of FoF1 ATPases and synthases. FEBS Lett 1990; 259:227–229.
105. Mandel M, Moriyama Y, Hulmes JD, et al. cDNA sequence encoding the 16-kDa proteolipid of chromaffin granules implies gene duplication in the evolution of H+-ATPases. Proc Natl Acad Sci USA 85:5521–5524.
106. Steinmetz PR, Husted RF, Mueller A, Beauwens R. Coupling between H+ transport and anaerobic glycolysis in turtle urinary bladder: Effect of inhibitors of H+ ATPase. J Membr Biol 1981; 59:27–34.
107. Zhang J, Myers M, Forgac M. Characterization of the V0 domain of the coated vesicle (H+)-ATPase. J Biol Chem 267:9773–9778.
108. Crider BP, Xie XS, Stone DK. Bafilomycin inhibits proton flow through the H+ channel of vacuolar proton pumps. J Biol Chem 1994; 269:17379–17381.
109. Nelson N. Structure and pharmacology of the proton-ATPases. Trends Pharmacol Sci 12:71–75.
110. Xie XS, Stone DK. Isolation and reconstitution of the clathrin-coated vesicle proton translocating complex. J Biol Chem 1986; 2492–2495.
111. Perin MS, Fried VA, Stone DK, et al. Structure of the 116-kDa polypeptide of the clathrin-coated vesicle/synaptic vesicle proton pump. J Biol Chem 1991; 266:3877–3881.
112. Green P, Lipman D, Hillier L, et al. Ancient conserved regions in new gene sequences and the protein databases. Science 1993; 259:1711–1716.
113. Peng SB, Crider BP, Xie XS, Stone DK. Alternative mRNA splicing generates tissue-specific isoforms of 116-kDa polypeptide of vacuolar proton pump. J Biol Chem 1994; 269:17262–17266.

114. Mellman I, Fuchs R, Helenius A. Acidification of the endocytic and exocytic pathways. Annu Rev Biochem 1986; 55:663–700.
115. Yamashiro DJ, Maxfield FR. Regulation of endocytic processes by pH. Trends Pharmacol Sci 1988; 9:190–193.
116. Mellman I. The importance of being acid: The role of acidification in intracellular membrane traffic. J Exp Biol 1992; 172:39–45.
117. Fuchs R, Schmid S, Mellman I. A possible role for Na+,K+-ATPase in regulating ATP-dependent endosome acidification. Proc Natl Acad Sci USA 1989; 86:539–542.
118. Cain CC, Sipe DM, Murphy RF. Regulation of endocytic pH by the Na+,K+-ATPase in living cells. Proc Natl Acad Sci USA 1989; 86:544–548.
119. Brown D, Gluck S, Hartwig J. Structure of the novel membrane-coating material in proton-secreting epithelial cells and identification as an H+ATPase. J Cell Biol 1987; 105:1637–1648.
120. Steinmetz PR, Andersen OS. Electrogenic proton transport in epithelial membranes. J Membr Biol 1982; 65:155–174.
121. Steinmetz PR. Cellular mechanisms of urinary acidification. Physiol Rev 1974; 54:890–956.
122. Youmans SJ, Worman HJ, Brodsky WA. ATPase activity and ATP-dependent proton translocation in plasma membrane vesicles of turtle bladder epithelial cells. Biochim Biophys Acta 1983; 730:173–177.
123. Dixon TE, Al-Awqati Q. H+/ATP stoichiometry of proton pump of turtle urinary bladder. J Biol Chem 1980; 255:3237–3239.
124. Andersen OS, Silveira JE, Steinmetz PR. Intrinsic characteristics of the proton pump in the luminal membrane of a tight urinary epithelium. The relation between transport rate and delta mu H. J Gen Physiol 1985; 86:215–234.
125. Gluck S, Al-Awqati Q. An electrogenic proton-translocating adenosine triphosphatase from bovine kidney medulla. J Clin Invest 1984; 73:1704–1710.
126. Kaunitz JD, Gunther RD, Sachs G. Characterization of an electrogenic ATP and chloride-dependent proton translocating pump from rat renal medulla. J Biol Chem 1985; 260:11567–11573.
127. Diaz-Diaz FD, LaBelle EF, Eaton DC, DuBose T Jr. ATP-dependent proton transport in human renal medulla. Am J Physiol 1986; 251:F297–302.
128. Sabolic I, Haase W, Burckhardt G. ATP-dependent H+ pump in membrane vesicles from rat kidney cortex. Am J Physiol 1985; 248:F835–844.
129. Sabolic I, Burckhardt G. Characteristics of the proton pump in rat renal cortical endocytolic vesicles. Am J Physiol 1986; 250:F817–826.
130. Sabolic I, Burckhardt G. Proton ATPase in rat renal cortical endocytotic vesicles. Biochem Biophys Acta 1988; 937:398–410.
131. Hilden SA, Johns CA, Madias NE. CI(⁻)-dependent ATP-driven H+ transport in rabbit renal cortical endosomes. Am J Physiol 1988; 255:F885–897.
132. Kinne-Saffran E, Beauwens R, Kinne R. An ATP-driven proton pump in brush-border membranes from rat renal cortex. J Membr Biol 1982; 64:67–76.
133. Kinne-Saffran E, Kinne R. Proton pump activity and Mg-ATPase activity in rat kidney cortex brushborder membranes: Effect of "proton ATPase" inhibitors. Pflugers Arch 1986; 407:S180–185.
134. Turrini F, Sabolic I, Zimolo Z, et al. Relation of ATPases in rat renal brush-border membranes to ATP-driven H+ secretion. J Membr Biol 1989; 107:1–12.
135. Simon BJ, Burckhardt G. Characterization of inside-out oriented H(+)-ATPases in cholate-pretreated renal brush-border membrane vesicles. J Membr Biol 1990; 117:141–151.
136. Yurko MA, Gluck S. Production and characterization of a monoclonal antibody to vacuolar H+ATPase of renal epithelia. J Biol Chem 1987; 262:15770–15779.
137. Gluck SL, Wang Z-Q, Zhang K. Properties of the lysosomal vacuolar H^+ATPase isolated from bovine kidney cortex. In preparation.
138. Nelson N. Structural conservation and functional diversity of V-ATPases. J Bioenerg Biomembr 1992; 24:407–417.
139. Schwartz GJ, Barasch J, Al-Awqati Q. Plasticity of functional epithelial polarity. Nature 1985; 318:368–371.
140. Satlin LM, Schwartz GJ. Postnatal maturation of rabbit renal collecting duct: intercalated cell function. Am J Physiol 1987; 253:F622–635.
141. Breyer MD, Jacobson HR. Regulation of rabbit medullary collecting duct cell pH by basolateral Na+/H+ and Cl-/base exchange. J Clin Invest 1989; 84:996–1004.
142. Hays SR, Alpern RJ. Apical and basolateral membrane H+ extrusion mechanisms in inner stripe of rabbit outer medullary collecting duct. Am J Physiol 1990; 259:F628–635.
143. Hays SR, Alpern RJ. Basolateral membrane Na(+)-independent Cl-HCO_3^- exchange in the inner stripe of the rabbit outer medullary collecting tubule. J Gen Physiol 1990; 95:347–367.
144. Kuwahara M, Sasaki S, Marumo F. Cell pH regulation in rabbit outer medullary collecting duct cells: Mechanisms of HCO_3(–)-independent processes. Am J Physiol 1990; 259:F902–909.

145. Kuwahara M, Sasaki S, Marumo F. Mineralocorticoids and acidosis regulate H+/HCO_3^- transport of intercalated cells. J Clin Invest 1992; 89:1388–1394.
146. Furuya H, Jacobson HR, Breyer MD. Evidence for basolateral membrane Ca2+/H+ exchange in outer medullary collecting duct. Am J Physiol 1993; 264:F88–93.
147. van Meer G, Simons K. Lipid polarity and sorting in epithelial cells. J Cell Biochem 1988; 36:51–58.
148. Simons K, Wandinger-Ness A. Polarized sorting in epithelia. Cell 1990; 62:207–210.
149. Simons K, Dupree P, Fiedler K, et al. Biogenesis of cell-surface polarity in epithelial cells and neurons. Cold Spring Harb Symp Quant Biol 1992; 57:611–619.
150. Im WB, Sih JC, Blakeman DP, McGrath JP. Omeprazole, a specific inhibitor of gastric (H+ -K+)-ATPase, is a H+ -activated oxidizing agent of sulfhydryl groups. J Biol Chem 1985; 260:4591–4597.
151. Moriyama Y, Patel V, Ueda I and Futai M. Evidence for a common binding site for omeprazole and N-ethylmaleimide in subunit A of chromaffin granule vacuolar-type H(+)-ATPase. Biochem Biophys Res Commun 1993; 196:699–706.
152. Sachs G, Besancon M, Shin JM, et al. Structural aspects of the gastric H,K-ATPase. J Bioenerg Biomembr 1992; 24:301–308.
153. Sabolic I, Brown D, Verbavatz JM, Kleinman J. H(+)-ATPases of renal cortical and medullary endosomes are differentially sensitive to Sch-28080 and omeprazole. Am J Physiol 1994; 266:F868–877.
154. Kohn OF, Mitchell PP, Steinmetz PR. Sch-28080 inhibits bafilomycin-sensitive H+ secretion in turtle bladder independently of luminal [K+]. Am J Physiol 1993; 265:F174–179.
155. Graber ML, Devine P. Omeprazole and SCH 28080 inhibit acid secretion by the turtle urinary bladder. Renal Physiol Biochem 1993; 16:257–267.
156. Sander I, Lottspeich F, Appelhans H, et al. Sequence analysis of the catalytic subunit of H(+)-ATPase from porcine renal brush-border membranes. Biochim Biophys Acta 1992; 1112:129–141.
157. Kurtz I. Apical Na+/H+ antiporter and glycolysis-dependent H+-ATPase regulate intracellular pH in the rabbit S3 proximal tubule. J Clin Invest 1987; 80:928–935.
158. Preisig PA. Luminal flow rate regulates proximal tubule H-HCO_3 transporters. Am J Physiol 1992; 262:F47–54.
159. Chan YL, Giebisch G. Relationship between sodium and bicarbonate transport in the rat proximal convoluted tubule. Am J Physiol 1981; 240:F222–230.
160. Nakhoul NL, Chen LK, Boron WF. Effect of basolateral CO2/HCO_3^- on intracellular pH regulation in the rabbit S3 proximal tubule. J Gen Physiol 1993; 102:1171–1205.
161. Stoner LC, Burg MB, Orloff J. Ion transport in cortical collecting tubule; effect of amiloride. Am J Physiol 1974; 227:453–459.
162. McKinney TD, Burg MB. Bicarbonate absorption by rabbit cortical collecting tubules in vitro. Am J Physiol 1978; 234:F141–145.
163. Hanley MJ, Kokko JP, Gross JB, Jacobson HR. Electrophysiologic study of the cortical collecting tubule of the rabbit. Kidney Int 1980; 17:74–81.
164. Koeppen BM, Helman SI. Acidification of luminal fluid by the rabbit cortical collecting tubule perfused in vitro. Am J Physiol 1982; 242:F521–531.
165. Laski ME, Kurtzman NA. Characterization of acidification in the cortical and medullary collecting tubule of the rabbit. J Clin Invest 1983; 72:2050–2059.
166. Atkins JL, Burg MB. Bicarbonate transport by isolated perfused rat collecting ducts. Am J Physiol 1985; 249:F485–489.
167. Roos A, Boron WF. Intracellular pH. Physiol Rev 1981; 61:296–434.
168. Hayashi M, Iyori M, Yamaji Y, Saruta T. Effects of in vivo and in vitro alkali treatment on intracellular pH regulation of OMCDis cells. Am J Physiol 1993; 265:F729–735.
169. Weiner ID, Hamm LL. Use of fluorescent dye BCECF to measure intracellular pH in cortical collecting tubule. Am J Physiol 1989; 256:F957–964.
170. Furuya H, Breyer MD, Jacobson HR. Functional characterization of alpha- and beta-intercalated cell types in rabbit cortical collecting duct. Am J Physiol 1991; 261:F377–385.
171. Muto S, Yasoshima K, Yoshitomi K, et al. Electrophysiological identification of alpha- and beta-intercalated cells and their distribution along the rabbit distal nephron segments. J Clin Invest 1990; 86: 1829–1839.
172. McKinney TD, Davidson KK. Bicarbonate transport in collecting tubules from outer stripe of outer medulla of rabbit kidneys. Am J Physiol 1987; 253:F816–822.
173. Verlander JW, Madsen KM, Tisher CC. Structural and functional features of proton and bicarbonate transport in the rat collecting duct. Semin Nephrol 1991; 11:465–477.
174. Koeppen BM. Conductive properties of the rabbit outer medullary collecting duct: Inner stripe. Am J Physiol 1985; 248:F500–506.
175. Ridderstrale Y, Kashgarian M, Koeppen B, et al. Morphological heterogeneity of the rabbit collecting duct. Kidney Int 1988; 34:655–670.

176. Schuster VL, Bonsib SM, Jennings ML. Two types of collecting duct mitochondria-rich (intercalated) cells: lectin and band 3 cytochemistry. Am J Physiol 1986; 251:C347–355.
177. Burnatowska-Hledin MA, Spielman WS. Immunodissection of mitochondria-rich cells from rabbit outer medullary collecting tubule. Am J Physiol 1988; 254:F907–911.
178. Schuster VL, Fejes-Toth G, Naray-Fejes-Toth A, Gluck S. Colocalization of H(+)-ATPase and band 3 anion exchanger in rabbit collecting duct intercalated cells. Am J Physiol 1991; 260:F506–517.
179. Bastani B, Purcell H, Hemken P, et al. Expression and distribution of renal vacuolar proton-translocating adenosine triphosphatase in response to chronic acid and alkali loads in the rat. J Clin Invest 1991; 88:126–136.
180. Weiner ID, Hamm LL. Regulation of intracellular pH in the rabbit cortical collecting tubule. J Clin Invest 1990; 85:274–281.
181. Sabolic I, Wuarin F, Shi LB, et al. Apical endosomes isolated from kidney collecting duct principal cells lack subunits of the proton pumping ATPase. J Cell Biol 1992; 119:111–122.
182. Rodman JS, Stahl PD, Gluck S. Distribution and structure of the vacuolar H+ ATPase in endosomes and lysosomes from LLC-PK1 cells. Exp Cell Res 1991; 192:445–452.
183. Schmidt W, Winkler H, Plattner H. Adrenal chromaffin granules: Evidence for an ultrastructural equivalent of the proton-pumping ATPase. Eur J Cell Biol 1982; 27:96–104.
184. Wall SM, Knepper MA. Acid-base transport in the inner medullary collecting duct. Semin Nephrol 1990; 10:148–158.
185. Nelson RD, Underhill DM, Hmiel SP, et al. Cell-specific amplification of vacuolar H^+ATPase B subunit expression in mammalian kidney. Submitted.
186. Zhang K, Wang ZQ, Gluck S. Identification and partial purification of a cytosolic activator of vacuolar H(+)-ATPases from mammalian kidney. J Biol Chem 267:9701–9705.
187. Zhang K, Wang ZQ, Gluck S. A cytosolic inhibitor of vacuolar H(+)-ATPases from mammalian kidney. J Biol Chem 1992; 267:14539–14542.
188. Gurich RW, DuBose T Jr. Heterogeneity of cAMP effect on endosomal proton transport. Am J Physiol 1989; 257:F777–784.
189. Mulberg AE, Tulk BM, Forgac M. Modulation of coated vesicle chloride channel activity and acidification by reversible protein kinase A-dependent phosphorylation. J Biol Chem 1991; 266:20590–20593.
190. Gurich RW, Codina J, DuBose T Jr. A potential role for guanine nucleotide-binding protein in the regulation of endosomal proton transport. J Clin Invest 1991; 87:1547–1552.
191. Schuster VL. Cortical collecting duct bicarbonate secretion. Kidney Int Suppl 1991; 33:S47–50.
192. Schuster VL. Organization of collecting duct intercalated cells. Kidney Int 1990; 38:668–672.
193. Schuster VL. Physiology and cell biology update: Control mechanisms for bicarbonate secretion. Am J Kidney Dis 1989; 13:348–352.
194. Stetson DL, Beauwens R, Palmisano J, et al. A double-membrane model for urinary bicarbonate secretion. Am J Physiol 249:F546–552.
195. Al-Awqati Q. Proton-translocating ATPases. Annu Rev Cell Biol 1986; 2:179–199.
196. Cohen LH, Mueller A, Steinmetz PR. Inhibition of the bicarbonate exit step in urinary acidification by a disulfonic stilbene. J Clin Invest 1978; 61:981–986.
197. Husted RF, Cohen LH, Steinmetz PR. Pathways for bicarbonate transfer across the serosal membrane of turtle urinary bladder: Studies with a disulfonic stilbene. J Membr Biol 1979; 47:27–37.
198. Fischer JL, Husted RF, Steinmetz PR. Chloride dependence of the HCO_3 exit step in urinary acidification by the turtle bladder. Am J Physiol 1983; 245:F564–568.
199. Drenckhahn D, Oelmann M, Schaaf P, et al. Band 3 is the basolateral anion exchanger of dark epithelial cells of turtle urinary bladder. Am J Physiol 252:C570–574.
200. Oliver JA, Himmelstein S, Steinmetz PR. Energy dependence of urinary bicarbonate secretion in turtle bladder. J Clin Invest 1975; 55:1003–1008.
201. Fritsche C, Schwartz JH, Heinen RR, et al. HCO_3^- secretion in mitochondria-rich cells is linked to an H+-ATPase. Am J Physiol 1989; 256:F869–874.
202. Leslie BR, Schwartz JH, Steinmetz PR. Coupling between Cl- absorption and HCO_3^- secretion in turtle urinary bladder. Am J Physiol 1973; 225:610–617.
203. Kohn OF, Mitchell PP, Steinmetz PR. Characteristics of apical Cl-HCO^3 exchanger of bicarbonate-secreting cells in turtle bladder. Am J Physiol 1990; 258:F9–14.
204. Husted RF, Steinmetz PR. Potassium absorptive pump at the luminal membrane of turtle urinary bladder. Am J Physiol 1981; 241:F315–321.
205. Steinmetz PR, Omachi RS, Frazier HS. Independence of hydrogen ion secretion and transport of other electrolytes in turtle bladder. J Clin Invest 1967; 46:1541–1548.
206. Al-awqati Q, Mueller A, Steinmetz PR. Transport of H+ against electrochemical gradients in turtle urinary bladder. Am J Physiol 1977; 233:F502–508.
207. Ludens JH, Fanestil DD. Acidification of urine by the isolated urinary bladder of the toad. Am J Physiol 1972; 223:1338–1344.

208. Husted RF, Steinmetz PR. The effects of amiloride and ouabain on urinary acidification by turtle bladder. J Pharmacol Exp Ther 1979; 210:264–268.
209. Beauwens R, Al-Awqati Q. Active H+ transport in the turtle urinary bladder: Coupling of transport to glucose oxidation. J Gen Physiol 1976; 68:421–439.
210. Ziegler TW, Fanestil DD, Ludens JH. Influence of transepithelial potential difference on acidification in the toad urinary bladder. Kidney Int 1976; 10:279–286.
210a. Schultz SG. Homocellular regulatory mechanisms in sodium-transporting epithelia: Avoidance of extinction by "flush-through." Am J Physiol 1981; 241:F579–590.
211. Steinmetz PR. Acid-base relations in epithelium of turtle bladder: Site of active step in acidification and role of metabolic CO_2. J Clin Invest 1969; 48:1258–1265.
212. Schwartz JH, Steinmetz PR. CO_2 requirements for H+ secretion by the isolated turtle bladder. Am J Physiol 1971; 220:2051–2057.
213. Gluck S, Cannon C, Al-Awqati Q. Exocytosis regulates urinary acidification in turtle bladder by rapid insertion of H+ pumps into the luminal membrane. Proc Natl Acad Sci USA 1982; 79:4327–4331.
214. Stetson DL, Steinmetz PR. Role of membrane fusion in CO_2 stimulation of proton secretion by turtle bladder. Am J Physiol 1983; 245:C113–120.
215. Cohen LH, Steinmetz PR. Control of active proton transport in turtle urinary bladder by cell pH. J Gen Physiol 1980; 76:381–393.
216. Husted RF, Mueller AL, Kessel RG, Steinmetz PR. Surface characteristics of carbonic-anhydrase-rich cells in turtle urinary bladder. Kidney Int 1981; 19:491–502.
217. Stetson DL, Steinmetz PR. Correlation between apical intramembrane particles and H+ secretion rates during CO2 stimulation in turtle bladder. Pflugers Arch 1986; 407:S80–84.
218. Clausen C, Dixon TE. Membrane electrical parameters in turtle bladder measured using impedance-analysis techniques. J Membr Biol 1986; 92:9–19.
219. Dixon TE, Clausen C, Coachman D, Lane B. Proton transport and membrane shuttling in turtle bladder epithelium. J Membr Biol 1986; 94:233–243.
220. Dixon TE, Clausen C, Coachman D. Constitutive and transport-related endocytotic pathways in turtle bladder epithelium. J Membr Biol 1988; 102:49–58.
221. Waddell WJ, Butler TC. Calculation of intracellular pH from the distribution of 5,5′-dimethyl-2,4-oxazolidinedione (DMO): Application to skeletal muscle of the dog. J Clin Invest 1959; 38:720–729.
222. Cannon C, van Adelsberg J, Kelly S, Al-Awqati Q. Carbon-dioxide-induced exocytotic insertion of H+ pumps in turtle-bladder luminal membrane: Role of cell pH and calcium. Nature 1985; 314:443–446.
223. van Adelsberg J, Al-Awqati Q. Regulation of cell pH by Ca^{+2}-mediated exocytotic insertion of H+-ATPases. J Cell Biol 1986; 102:1638–1645.
224. Graber ML, Dixon TE, Coachman D, et al. Fluorescence identifies an alkaline cell in turtle urinary bladder. Am J Physiol 1986; 250:F159–168.
225. Graber M, Dixon T, Coachman D, Devine P. Acetazolamide inhibits acidification by the turtle bladder independent of cell pH. Am J Physiol 1989; 256:F923–931.
226. Arruda JA, Talor Z, Dytko C. Effect of agents that alter cell calcium and microfilaments on CO_2 stimulated H+ secretion in the turtle bladder. Arch Int Pharmacodyn Ther 1988; 293:273–283.
227. Arruda JA, Dytko G, Talor Z. Stimulation of H+ secretion by CO_2 in turtle bladder: Role of intracellular pH, exocytosis, and calcium. Am J Physiol 1990; 258:R222–231.
228. Arruda JA. Calcium inhibits urinary acidification: Effect of the ionophore A23187 on the turtle bladder. Pflugers Arch 1979; 381:107–111.
229. Ehrenspeck G. Effect of calcium ionophore A23187 on electrogenic acid-base transport in turtle bladder: Inhibition of acidification and stimulation of alkalinization. Biochim Biophys Acta 1983; 732:146–153.
230. Al-Awqati Q. Effect of aldosterone on the coupling between H+ transport and glucose oxidation. J Clin Invest 1977; 60:1240–1247.
231. Schwartz JH, Steinmetz PR. Metabolic energy and PCO_2 as determinants of H+ secretion by turtle urinary bladder. Am J Physiol 1977; 233:F145–149.
232. Kelly S, Dixon TE, Al-Awqati Q. Metabolic pathways coupled to H+ transport in turtle urinary bladder. J Membr Biol 1980; 54:237–243.
233. Choate GL, Lan L, Mansour TE. Heart 6-phosphofructo-1-kinase: Subcellular distribution and binding to myofibrils. J Biol Chem 1985; 260:4815–4822.
234. Harrison ML, Rathinavelu P, Arese P, et al. Role of band 3 tyrosine phosphorylation in the regulation of erythrocyte glycolysis. J Biol Chem 1991; 266:4106–4111.
235. Beitner R. Control of glycolytic enzymes through binding to cell structures and by glucose-1,6-bisphosphate under different conditions: The role of Ca^{2+} and calmodulin. Int J Biochem 1993; 25:297–305.
236. Low PS, Rathinavelu P, Harrison ML. Regulation of glycolysis via reversible enzyme binding to the membrane protein, band 3. J Biol Chem 1993; 268:14627–14631.

237. Ludens JH, Fanestil DD. Aldosterone stimulation of acidification of urine by isolated urinary bladder of the Colombian toad. Am J Physiol 1974; 226:1321–1326.
238. Ludens JH, Vaughn DA, Fanestil DD. Stimulation of urinary acidification by aldosterone and inhibitors of RNA and protein synthesis. J Membr Biol 1978; 40 (Spec No):199–211.
239. Al-Awqati Q, Norby LH, Mueller A, Steinmetz PR. Characteristics of stimulation of H+ transport by aldosterone in turtle urinary bladder. J Clin Invest 1976; 58:351–358.
240. Ehrenspeck G. Effect of 3-isobutyl-1-methylxanthine on HCO3- transport in turtle bladder: Evidence for electrogenic HCO3- secretion. Biochim Biophys Acta 1982; 684:219–227.
241. Satake N, Durham JH, Ehrenspeck G, Brodsky WA. Active electrogenic mechanisms for alkali and acid transport in turtle bladders. Am J Physiol 1983; 244:C259–269.
242. Arruda JA, Sabatini S. Cholinergic inhibition of urinary acidification by the turtle bladder. Kidney Int 1980; 17:622–630.
243. Schneider ES, Durham JH, Matons C, Brodsky WA. Alkali secretion in the turtle bladder: Up-regulation by the phospho-inositol cascade and inhibition by diphenylamine carboxylate (DPC). Prog Clin Biol Res 1988; 258:81–92.
244. Stetson DL, Steinmetz PR. Alpha and beta types of carbonic anhydrase-rich cells in turtle bladder. Am J Physiol 1985; 249:F553–565.
245. Rich A, Dixon TE, Clausen C. Changes in membrane conductances and areas associated with bicarbonate secretion in turtle bladder. J Membr Biol 1990; 113:211–219.
246. Rich A, Dixon TE, Clausen C. Electrogenic bicarbonate secretion in the turtle bladder: apical membrane conductance characteristics. J Membr Biol 1991; 119:241–252.
247. Brown D, Lui B, Gluck S, Sabolic I. A plasma membrane proton ATPase in specialized cells of rat epididymis. Am J Physiol 1992; 263:C913–916.
248. Madsen KM, Verlander JW, Kim J, Tisher CC. Morphological adaptation of the collecting duct to acid-base disturbances. Kidney Int Suppl 33:S57–63.
249. Kim J, Welch WJ, Cannon JK, et al. Immunocytochemical response of type A and type B intercalated cells to increased sodium chloride delivery. Am J Physiol 1992; 262:F288–302.
250. Wingo CS, Armitage FE. Potassium transport in the kidney: Regulation and physiological relevance of H+, K(+)-ATPase. Semin Nephrol 1993; 13:213–224.
251. Zhou X, Wingo CS. Stimulation of total CO_2 flux by 10% CO_2 in rabbit CCD: Role of an apical Sch-28080- and Ba-sensitive mechanism. Am J Physiol 1994; 267:F114–120.
252. Armitage FE, Wingo CS. Luminal acidification in K-replete OMCDi: Contributions of H-K-ATPase and bafilomycin-A1-sensitive H-ATPase. Am J Physiol 1994; 267:F450–458.
253. Zhou X, Wingo CS. Mechanisms of rubidium permeation by rabbit cortical collecting duct during potassium restriction. Am J Physiol 1992; 263:F1134–1141.
254. Alpern RJ, Cogan MG, Rector F Jr. Effect of luminal bicarbonate concentration on proximal acidification in the rat. Am J Physiol 1982; 243:F53–59.
255. Alpern RJ, Chambers M. Cell pH in the rat proximal convoluted tubule: Regulation by luminal and peritubular pH and sodium concentration. J Clin Invest 1986; 78:502–510.
256. McKinney TD, Davidson KK. Effects of respiratory acidosis on HCO_3^- transport by rabbit collecting tubules. Am J Physiol 1988; 255:F656–665.
257. Drenckhahn D, Schluter K, Allen DP, Bennett V. Colocalization of band 3 with ankyrin and spectrin at the basal membrane of intercalated cells in the rat kidney. Science 1985; 230:1287–1289.
258. Verlander JW, Madsen KM, Low PS, et al. Immunocytochemical localization of band 3 protein in the rat collecting duct. Am J Physiol 1988; 255:F115–125.
259. Hays SR. Mineralocorticoid modulation of apical and basolateral membrane H+/OH-/HCO_3^- transport processes in the rabbit inner stripe of outer medullary collecting duct. J Clin Invest 1992; 90:180–187.
260. Koeppen BM. Electrophysiological identification of principal and intercalated cells in the rabbit outer medullary collecting duct. Pflugers Arch 1987; 409:138–141.
261. Madsen KM, Tisher CC. Cellular response to acute respiratory acidosis in rat medullary collecting duct. Am J Physiol 1983; 245:F670–679.
262. Laski ME, Kurtzman NA. Collecting tubule adaptation to respiratory acidosis induced in vivo. Am J Physiol 1990; 258:F15–20.
263. Schwartz GJ, Al-Alwqati Q. Carbon dioxide causes exocytosis of vesicles containing H+ pumps in isolated perfused proximal and collecting tubules. J Clin Invest 1985; 75:1638–1644.
264. Kuwahara M, Sasaki S, Marumo F. Cl-HCO_3 exchange and Na-HCO_3 symport in rabbit outer medullary collecting duct cells. Am J Physiol 1991; 260:F635–642.
265. Stone DK, Seldin DW, Kokko JP, Jacobson HR. Mineralocorticoid modulation of rabbit medullary collecting duct acidification: A sodium-independent effect. J Clin Invest 1983; 72:77–83.
266. Weiner ID, Hamm LL. Regulation of Cl-/HCO_3^- exchange in the rabbit cortical collecting tubule. J Clin Invest 1991; 87:1553–1558.

267. Breyer MD, Kikko JP, Jacobson HR. Regulation of net bicarbonate transport in rabbit cortical collecting tubule by pertibular pH, carbon dioxide tension, and bicarbonate concentration. J Clin Invest 1986; 77:1650–1660.
268. Star RA, Burg MB, Knepper MA. Bicarbonate secretion and chloride absorption by rabbit cortical collecting ducts: Role of chloride/bicarbonate exchange. J Clin Invest 1985; 76:1123–1130.
268a. Verlander JW, Madsen KM, Tisher CC. Effect of acute respiratory acidosis on two populations of intercalculated cells in rat cortical collecting duct. Am J Physiol 1987; 253:F1142–1156.
269. Yamaji Y, Hayashi M, Iyori M, et al. Chronic DOC treatment enhances Na(+)-H+ exchanger activity of beta-intercalated cells in rabbit CCD. Am J Physiol 1992; 262:F712–17.
270. Brown D, Sabolic I, Gluck S. Colchicine-induced redistribution of proton pumps in kidney epithelial cells. Kidney Int Suppl 1991; 33:S79–83.
271. Noel J, Vinay P, Tejedor A, et al. Metabolic cost of bafilomycin-sensitive H+ pump in intact dog, rabbit, and hamster proximal tubules. Am J Physiol 1993; 264:F655–661.
272. Dickman KG, Mandel LJ. Relationship between HCO_3^- transport and oxidative metabolism in rabbit proximal tubule. Am J Physiol 1992; 263:F342–351.
273. Paillard M. Effects of aldosterone on renal handling of sodium, potassium and hydrogen ions. Adv Nephrol Necker Hosp 1977; 7:83–104.
274. Gross JB and Kokko JP. Effects of aldosterone and potassium-sparing diuretics on electrical potential differences across the distal nephron. J Clin Invest 1977; 59:82–89.
275. Bastani B, Kalkbrenner M, Gluck S. Chronic DOCA administration increases polarization of H$^+$ATPase in medullary intercalated cells (abstr). J Am Soc Nephrol 1991; 2:694.
276. Fejes-Toth G, Naray-Fejes-Toth A. Isolated principal and intercalated cells: Hormone responsiveness and Na+-K+-ATPase activity. Am J Physiol 1989; 256:F742–50.
277. Koseki C, Yamaguchi Y, Furusawa M, Endou H. Isolation by monoclonal antibody of intercalated cells of rabbit kidney. Kidney Int 1988; 33:543–544.
278. Star RA, Nonoguchi H, Balaban R, Knepper MA. Calcium and cyclic adenosine monophosphate as second messengers for vasopressin in the rat inner medullary collecting duct. J Clin Invest 1988; 81: 1879–1888.
279. Schuster VL. Cyclic adenosine monophosphate-stimulated bicarbonate secretion in rabbit cortical collecting tubules. J Clin Invest 1985; 75:2056–2064.
280. Schuster VL. Cyclic adenosine monophosphate-stimulated anion transport in rabbit cortical collecting duct: Kinetics, stoichiometry, and conductive pathways. J Clin Invest 1986; 78:1621–1630.
281. Hayashi M, Yamaji Y, Iyori M, et al. Effect of isoproterenol on intracellular pH of the intercalated cells in the rabbit cortical collecting ducts. J Clin Invest 1991; 87:1153–1157.
282. Hays S, Kokko JP, Jacobson HR. Hormonal regulation of proton secretion in rabbit medullary collecting duct. J Clin Invest 1986; 78:1279–1286.
283. Tomita K, Pisano JJ, Burg MB, Knepper MA. Effects of vasopressin and bradykinin on anion transport by the rat cortical collecting duct: Evidence for an electroneutral sodium chloride transport pathway. J Clin Invest 1986; 77:136–141.
284. Bichara M, Mercier O, Houillier P, et al. Effects of antidiuretic hormone on urinary acidification and on tubular handling of bicarbonate in the rat. J Clin Invest 1987; 80:621–630.
285. Delahousse M, Mercier O, Bichara M, et al. Glucagon inhibits urinary acidification in the rat. Am J Physiol 1988; 254:F762–769.
286. Mercier O, Bichara M, Delahousse M, et al. Effects of glucagon on H(+)-HCO_3^- transport in Henle's loop, distal tubule, and collecting ducts in the rat. Am J Physiol 1989; 257:F1003–1014.
287. Siga E, Mandon B, Roinel N, de Rouffignac C. Effects of calcitonin on function of intercalated cells of rat cortical collecting duct. Am J Physiol 1993; 264:F221–227.
288. Hays SR, Baum M, Kokko JP. Effects of protein kinase C activation on sodium, potassium, chloride, and total CO_2 transport in the rabbit cortical collecting tubule. J Clin Invest 1987; 80:1561–1570.
289. Bertorello AM, Katz AI. Short-term regulation of renal Na-K-ATPase activity: Physiological relevance and cellular mechanisms. Am J Physiol 1993; 265:F743–755.
290. Garg LC, Narang N. Stimulation of an N-ethylmaleimide-sensitive ATPase in the collecting duct segments of the rat nephron by metabolic acidosis. Can J Physiol Pharmacol 1985; 63:1291–1296.
291. Khadouri C, Marsy S, Barlet-Bas C, Doucet A. Effect of adrenalectomy on NEM-sensitive ATPase along rat nephron and on urinary acidification. Am J Physiol 1987; 253:F495–499.
292. Garg LC, Narang N. Effects of potassium bicarbonate on distal nephron Na-K-ATPase in adrenalectomized rabbits. Pflugers Arch 1987; 409:126–131.
293. Garg LC, Narang N. Effects of aldosterone on NEM-sensitive ATPase in rabbit nephron segments. Kidney Int 1988; 34:13–17.
294. Khadouri C, Marsy S, Barlet-Bas C, Doucet A. Short-term effect of aldosterone on NEM-sensitive ATPase in rat collecting tubule. Am J Physiol 1989; 257:F177–181.

295. Garg LC, Narang N. Decrease in N-ethylmaleimide-sensitive ATPase activity in collecting duct by metabolic alkalosis. Can J Physiol Pharmacol 1990; 68:1119–1123.
296. Garg LC, Narang N. Effects of low-potassium diet on N-ethylmaleimide-sensitive ATPase in the distal nephron segments. Renal Physiol Biochem 1990; 13:129–136.
297. Sabatini S, Laski ME, Kurtzman NA. NEM-sensitive ATPase activity in rat nephron: effect of metabolic acidosis and alkalosis. Am J Physiol 1990; 258:F297–304.
298. Khadouri C, Cheval L, Marsy S, et al. Characterization and control of proton-ATPase along the nephron. Kidney Int Suppl 1991; 33:S71–78.
299. Sabatini S, Laski ME, Spohn M, Kurtzman NA. Characterization of the N-ethylmaleimide-sensitive ATPase in rat cortical and medullary collecting tubule. Min Electrolyte Metab 1991; 17:324–330.
300. Garg LC, Narang N. Changes in H-ATPase activity in the distal nephron segments of the rat during metabolic acidosis and alkalosis. Contrib Nephrol 1991; 92:39–45.
301. Khadouri C, Marsy S, Barlet-Bas C, et al. Effect of metabolic acidosis and alkalosis on NEM-sensitive ATPase in rat nephron segments. Am J Physiol 1992; 262:F583–590.
302. Eiam-Ong S, Lonis B, Kurtzman NA, Sabatini S. The biochemical basis of hypokalemic metabolic alkalosis. Trans Assoc Am Phys 1992; 105:157–164.
303. Eiam-Ong S, Dafnis E, Spohn M, et al. H-K-ATPase in distal renal tubular acidosis: urinary tract obstruction, lithium, and amiloride. Am J Physiol 1993; 265:F875–880.
304. Eiam-Ong S, Kurtzman NA, Sabatini S. Regulation of collecting tubule adenosine triphosphatases by aldosterone and potassium. J Clin Invest 1993; 91:2385–2392.
305. Chambrey R, Paillard M, Podevin RA. Enzymatic and functional evidence for adaptation of the vacuolar H(+)-ATPase in proximal tubule apical membranes from rats with chronic metabolic acidosis. J Biol Chem 1994; 269:3243–3250.
306. Ait-Mohamed AK, Marsy S, Barlet C, et al. Characterization of N-ethylmaleimide-sensitive proton pump in the rat kidney. Localization along the nephron. J Biol Chem 1986; 261:12526–12533.
307. Verlander JW, Madsen KM, Larsson L, et al. Immunocytochemical localization of intracellular acidic compartments: rat proximal nephron. Am J Physiol 1989; 257:F454–462.
308. Tisher CC, Madsen KM, Verlander JW. Structural adaptation of the collecting duct to acid-base disturbances. Contrib Nephrol 1991; 95:168–177.
309. Gluck SL, Nelson RD, Lee BS. Properties and regulation of the renal vacuolar H+-ATPase and H+-K+-ATPase. Curr Opin Nephrol Hypertens 1993; 2:715–725.
310. Chang CS, Talor Z, Arruda JA. Effect of metabolic or respiratory acidosis on rabbit renal medullary proton-ATPase. Biochem Cell Biol 1988; 66:20–24.
311. Glassman VP, Safirstein R, DiScala VA. Effects of metabolic acidosis on proximal tubule ion reabsorption in dog kidney. Am J Physiol 1974; 227:759–765.
312. Cogan MG, Maddox DA, Lucci MS, Rector F Jr. Control of proximal bicarbonate reabsorption in normal and acidotic rats. J Clin Invest 1979; 64:1168–1180.
313. Kunau R Jr., Hart JI, Walker KA. Effect of metabolic acidosis on proximal tubular total CO_2 absorption. Am J Physiol 1985; 249:F62–68.
314. Preisig PA, Alpern RJ. Chronic metabolic acidosis causes an adaptation in the apical membrane Na/H antiporter and basolateral membrane $Na(HCO_3)3$ symporter in the rat proximal convoluted tubule. J Clin Invest 1988; 82:1445–1453.
315. Santella RN, Gennari FJ, Maddox DA. Metabolic acidosis stimulates bicarbonate reabsorption in the early proximal tubule. Am J Physiol 1989; 257:F35–42.
316. Good DW. Adaptation of HCO_3^- and NH+4 transport in rat MTAL: Effects of chronic metabolic acidosis and Na+ intake. Am J Physiol 1990; 258:F1345–1353.
317. Lucci MS, Pucacco LR, Carter NW, DuBose T Jr. Evaluation of bicarbonate transport in rat distal tubule: effects of acid-base status. Am J Physiol 1982; 243:F335–341.
318. Vandorpe DH, Levine DZ. Distal tubule bicarbonate reabsorption in NH4Cl acidotic rats. Clin Invest Med 1989; 12:224–229.
319. McKinney TD, Burg MB. Bicarbonate transport by rabbit cortical collecting tubules: Effect of acid and alkali loads in vivo on transport in vitro. J Clin Invest 1977; 60:766–768.
320. McKinney TD, Burg MB. Bicarbonate secretion by rabbit cortical collecting tubules in vitro. J Clin Invest 1978; 61:1421–1427.
321. Hamm LL, Gillespie C, Klahr S. NH4Cl inhibition of transport in the rabbit cortical collecting tubule. Am J Physiol 248:F631–637.
322. Hamm LL, Hering-Smith KS, Vehaskari VM. Control of bicarbonate transport in collecting tubules from normal and remnant kidneys. Am J Physiol 1989; 256:F680–687.
323. Hamm LL, Weiner ID, Vehaskari VM. Structural-functional characteristics of acid-base transport in the rabbit collecting duct. Semin Nephrol 1991; 11:453–464.

324. Yasoshima K, Satlin LM, Schwartz GJ. Adaptation of rabbit cortical collecting duct to in vitro acid incubation. Am J Physiol 1992; 263:F749–456.
325. Bengele HH, Schwartz JH, McNamara ER, Alexander EA. Chronic metabolic acidosis augments acidification along the inner medullary collecting duct. Am J Physiol 1986; 250:F690–694.
326. Bengele HH, McNamara ER, Schwartz JH, Alexander EA. Inner medullary collecting duct function during rebound alkalemia. Am J Physiol 1987; 252:F712–716.
327. Alexander EA, Schwartz JH. Regulation of acidification in the rat inner medullary collecting duct. Am J Kidney Dis 1991; 18:612–618.
328. Jacobson HR, Furuya H, Breyer MD. Mechanism and regulation of proton transport in the outer medullary collecting duct. Kidney Int Suppl 1991; 33:S51–56.
329. Levine DZ, Iacovitti M, Nash L, Vandorpe D. Secretion of bicarbonate by rat distal tubules in vivo: Modulation by overnight fasting. J Clin Invest 1988; 81:1873–1878.
330. Tago K, Warden DH, Schuster VL, Stokes JB. Effects of inhibitors of Cl conductance on Cl self-exchange in rabbit cortical collecting tubule. Am J Physiol 1986; 251:F1009–1017.
331. Garcia-Austt J, Good DW, Burg MB Knepper MA. Deoxycorticosterone-stimulated bicarbonate secretion in rabbit cortical collecting ducts: effects of luminal chloride removal and in vivo acid loading. Am J Physiol 1985; 249:F205–212.
332. Satlin LM, Schwartz GJ. Cellular remodeling of HCO3($^-$)-secreting cells in rabbit renal collecting duct in response to an acidic environment. J Cell Biol 1989; 109:1279–1288.
333. Satlin LM, Matsumoto T, Schwartz GJ. Postnatal maturation of rabbit renal collecting duct: III. Peanut lectin-binding intercalated cells. Am J Physiol 1992; 262:F199–208.
334. Dorup J. Structural adaptation of intercalated cells in rat renal cortex to acute metabolic acidosis and alkalosis. J Ultrastruct Res 1985; 92:119–131.
335. Madsen KM, Tisher CC. Response of intercalated cells of rat outer medullary collecting duct to chronic metabolic acidosis. Lab Invest 1984; 51:268–276.
336. Malnic G, De Mello Aires M, Giebisch G. Micropuncture study of renal tubular hydrogen ion transport in the rat. Am J Physiol 1972; 222:147–158.
337. Capasso G, Kinne R, Malnic G, Giebisch G. Renal bicarbonate reabsorption in the rat: I. Effects of hypokalemia and carbonic anhydrase. J Clin Invest 1986; 78:1558–1567.
338. Iacovitti M, Nash L, Peterson LN, et al. Distal tubule bicarbonate accumulation in vivo: Effect of flow and transtubular bicarbonate gradients. J Clin Invest 1986; 78:1658–1665.
339. Kunau R Jr, Walker KA. Total CO_2 absorption in the distal tubule of the rat. Am J Physiol 1987; 252:F468–473.
340. Chan YL, Malnic G, Giebisch G. Renal bicarbonate reabsorption in the rat: III. Distal tubule perfusion study of load dependence and bicarbonate permeability. J Clin Invest 1989; 84:931–938.
341. Levine DZ, Vandorpe D, Iacovitti M. Luminal chloride modulates rat distal tubule bidirectional bicarbonate flux in vivo. J Clin Invest 1990; 85:1793–1798.
342. Capasso G, Jaeger P, Giebisch G, et al. Renal bicarbonate reabsorption in the rat: II. Distal tubule load dependence and effect of hypokalemia. J Clin Invest 1987; 80:409–414.
343. Levine DZ. An in vivo microperfusion study of distal tubule bicarbonate reabsorption in normal and ammonium chloride rats. J Clin Invest 1985; 75:588–595.
344. Gifford JD, Sharkins K, Work J, et al. Total CO_2 transport in rat cortical collecting duct in chloride-depletion alkalosis. Am J Physiol 1990; 258:F848–853.
345. Gifford JD, Ware MW, Luke RG, Galla JH. HCO_3^- transport in rat CCD: Rapid adaptation by in vivo but not in vitro alkalosis. Am J Physiol 1993; 264:F435–440.
346. Verlander JW, Madsen KM, Galla JH, et al. Response of intercalated cells to chloride depletion metabolic alkalosis. Am J Physiol 1992; 262:F309–319.
347. Galla JH, Bonduris DN, Dumbauld SL, Luke RG. Segmental chloride and fluid handling during correction of chloride-depletion alkalosis without volume expansion in the rat. J Clin Invest 1984; 73: 96–106.
348. Wesson DE, Dolson GM. Augmented bidirectional HCO_3 transport by rat distal tubules in chronic alkalosis. Am J Physiol 1991; 261:F308–317.
349. Levine DZ, Iacovitti M, Harrison V. Bicarbonate secretion in vivo by rat distal tubules during alkalosis induced by dietary chloride restriction and alkali loading. J Clin Invest 1991; 87:1513–1518.
350. Wesson DE, Dolson GM. Enhanced HCO_3 secretion by distal tubule contributes to NaCl-induced correction of chronic alkalosis. Am J Physiol 1993; 264:F899–906.
351. Galla JH, Bonduris DN, Luke RG. Superficial distal and deep nephrons in correction of metabolic alkalosis. Am J Physiol 1989; 257:F107–113.
352. Wesson DE. Augmented bicarbonate reabsorption by both the proximal and distal nephron maintains chloride-deplete metabolic alkalosis in rats. J Clin Invest 1989; 84:1460–1469.

353. Wesson DE, Dolson GM. Maximal proton secretory rate of rat distal tubules is higher during chronic metabolic alkalosis. Am J Physiol 1991; 261:F753–759.
354. Mills JN, Thomas S, Williamson KS. The acute effect of hydrocortisone, deoxycorticosterone, and aldosterone upon the excretion of sodium, potassium, and acid by the human kidney. J Physiol (Lond) 1960; 151:312–331.
355. Hulter HN, Ilnicki LP, Harbottle JA, Sebastian A. Impaired renal H+ secretion and NH3 production in mineralocorticoid-deficient glucocorticoid-replete dogs. Am J Physiol 1977; 232:F136–146.
356. Sebastian A, Sutton JM, Hulter HN, et al. Effect of mineralocorticoid replacement therapy on renal acid-base homeostasis in adrenalectomized patients. Kidney Int 1980; 18:762–773.
357. Dubrovsky AH, Nair RC, Byers MK, Levine DZ. Renal net acid excretion in the adrenalectomized rat. Kidney Int 1981; 19:516–528.
358. Wilcox CS, Cemerikic DA, Giebisch G. Differential effects of acute mineralo- and glucocorticosteroid administration on renal acid elimination. Kidney Int 1982; 21:546–556.
359. Lombes M, Farman N, Oblin ME, et al. Immunohistochemical localization of renal mineralocorticoid receptor by using an anti-idiotypic antibody that is an internal image of aldosterone. Proc Natl Acad Sci USA 1990; 87:1086–1088.
360. Farman N, Oblin ME, Lombes M, et al. Immunolocalization of gluco- and mineralocorticoid receptors in rabbit kidney. Am J Physiol 1991; 260:C226–233.
361. Farman N. Steroid receptors: distribution along the nephron. Semin Nephrol 1992; 12:12–17.
362. Wade JB, O'Neil RG, Pryor JL, Boulpaep EL. Modulation of cell membrane area in renal collecting tubules by corticosteroid hormones. J Cell Biol 1979; 81:439–445.
363. Stanton B, Janzen A, Klein-Robbenhaar G, et al. Ultrastructure of rat initial collecting tubule. Effect of adrenal corticosteroid treatment. J Clin Invest 1985; 75:1327–1334.
364. Mujais SK. Effects of aldosterone on rat collecting tubule N-ethylmaleimide-sensitive adenosine triphosphatase. J Lab Clin Med 1987; 109:34–39.
365. Relman AS, Esten B, Schwartz WB. The regulation of renal bicarbonate reabsorption by plasma carbon dioxide. J Clin Invest 1953; 32:972–978.
366. Polak A, Haynie GD, Hays RM, Schwartz WB. Effects of chronic hypercapnia on electrolyte and acid-base equilibrium: 1. Adaptation. J Clin Invest 1961; 40:1223–1237.
367. Schwartz WB, Cohen JJ. The nature of the renal response to chronic disorders of acid-base equilibrium. Am J Med 1978; 64:417–428.
368. Verlander JW, Madsen KM, Tisher CC. Effect of acute respiratory acidosis on two populations of intercalated cells in rat cortical collecting duct. Am J Physiol 1987; 253:F1142–1156.
369. Graf R, Lepier A, Harvey WR, Wieczorek H. A novel 14-kDa V-ATPase subunit in the tobacco hornworm midgut. J Biol Chem 1994; 269:3767–374.

28

Na^+/H^+ Exchangers: Structure, Function, and Regulation

Laurence Bianchini and Jacques Pouysségur
Nice-Sophia Antipolis University, Nice, France

INTRODUCTION

It was as much as 45 years ago that exchange of Na^+ for H^+ was first proposed as a mechanism for renal acidification (1). However, it was only in 1976 that the Na^+/H^+ antiport was directly demonstrated to function in vesicles from brush border membranes of kidney tubules (2). Since that time, the presence of the transporter has been identified in the plasma membrane of virtually all eukaryotic cells. Initially biochemical studies and more recently molecular cloning have provided increasing amounts of information about the structure, functional features, and regulation of the Na^+/H^+ exchangers—referred to as NHE (for recent reviews, see Refs. 3 and 4). Na^+/H^+ exchangers are integral plasma membrane proteins that catalyze the electroneutral exchange of extracellular Na^+ for intracellular H^+ with a stoichiometry of one for one. An essential feature of these exchangers is their allosteric activation by intracellular protons, which are presumed to interact at a "modifier" site that is separate from the sites involved in Na^+ and H^+ transport. The activity and expression level of the exchangers can be modulated by a remarkably wide variety of stimuli, including growth factors, tumor promoters, hormones (for review, see Ref. 5), chronic extracellular acidification (6), as well as physical factors such as changes in cell volume (7–9) or cell spreading (10). The most widely studied NHE isoform, NHE1, is ubiquitously expressed and is involved in a variety of cellular functions by virtue of its ability to govern intracellular pH. It is inhibited by the diuretic compound amiloride and its 5-amino–substituted derivatives. Besides NHE1, several other isoforms—initially characterized by their lower sensitivity to amiloride—have been identified principally in epithelia, where they perform more specialized ion transport. Five subtypes of Na^+/H^+ exchangers have been cloned and characterized to date; they define a new gene family of vertebrate transporters. These isoforms share the same structure but exhibit differences with respect to amiloride sensitivity, cellular localization, kinetic parameters, regulation by various stimuli, and plasma membrane targeting in polarized epithelial cells. Renal epithelial cells constitute a particularly relevant illustration of the latter feature. In proximal tubule cells, the polarized expression of Na^+/H^+ exchanger in either the apical or the basolateral membrane is crucial for tubular function: Na^+/H^+ exchange in the basolateral membrane performs the housekeeping functions, such as pH_i homeostasis, whereas the Na^+/H^+ exchanger present in the apical membrane is responsible for Na^+ influx into the proximal tubule cell and proton secretion into the tubular lumen necessary for HCO_3^- reabsorption (for review, see Ref. 11).

In this chapter, we offer an overview of the main features of the Na^+/H^+ antiporters, with emphasis on recent progress in understanding the structure-function relationship and the regulation of the different transporter isoforms.

MOLECULAR IDENTIFICATION OF THE Na^+/H^+ EXCHANGERS

Using a genetic strategy, Sardet and colleagues (12) were the first to fully identify a Na^+/H^+ exchanger isoform by cloning a human cDNA encoding the amiloride-sensitive, growth factor–

activatable Na^+/H^+ antiporter. The first step toward the molecular cloning of the exchanger consisted of selection of a stable exchanger-deficient mouse fibroblast cell line, which was accomplished by the proton suicide method based on the reversibility of the antiporter (13). This antiporter-deficient mutant cell line was then transfected with human genomic DNA and cells overexpressing the human exchanger were selected. From these transformants, an exon-containing genomic probe was isolated and used for the cloning of a human cDNA, which was shown to fully restore the biochemical and physiological features of the transporter, namely pH_i regulation, when transfected in antiporter-deficient cells. This human exchanger cDNA, now referred to as NHE1, is ubiquitously expressed in tissues and cells and, in polarized epithelial cells, generally resides in the basolateral membrane, although exceptions have been reported (14,15) (Roux D., Noël J., and Pouysségur J.; in preparation). Pharmacological, kinetic, and regulatory properties of Na^+/H^+ exchangers in various cell types, tissues, and species had predicted the existence of multiple isoforms of Na^+/H^+ exchangers (for review, see Ref. 16). Recent molecular cloning studies—using the 1.9-kb BamH1-BamH1 fragment of the human NHE1 cDNA as a probe to screen cDNA libraries—have confirmed that indeed Na^+/H^+ exchangers constitute a gene family. So far, five vertebrate isoforms—NHE1 (12,17–22), βNHE (23), NHE2 (24–26), NHE3 (20,27), and NHE4 (20) have been cloned and sequenced. NHE1, βNHE, NHE2, and NHE3 but not NHE4 have been shown to function as Na^+/H^+ exchangers based on functional complementation in antiporter-deficient cells: PS120 fibroblasts (21–23,25–27) or Chinese hamster ovary cells (24,28).

TISSUE DISTRIBUTION

Based on Northern blotting analysis and ribonuclease protection assay, NHE1 message was detected in all mammalian cells examined to date with two exceptions: the OK (opossum kidney) renal proximal tubule cell line (29) and rat proximal tubule S1 and S2 segments of superficial and of a majority of midcortical nephrons (30). It is noteworthy that these cells are known to lack basolateral Na^+/H^+ exchanger. The other isoforms appear to have a more specialized distribution (Table 1). NHE2 is an isoform predominantly expressed in epithelia (24,25), whereas NHE3 appears to be specifically expressed in a subset of epithelia: namely, in intestine, kidney, and stomach (20,27). In rabbit, NHE2 message is present in kidney (medulla>cortex), large intestine, adrenal gland, and small intestine and in small amount in trachea and skeletal muscle (25). In rat, NHE2 message was predominantly found in small intestine, colon, and stomach, with much lower levels present in skeletal muscle, brain, kidney, testis, uterus, heart, and lung (24). In rabbit, NHE3 message is found exclusively in kidney (cortex>medulla), intestine and stomach (27). In rat, NHE3 message was

Table 1 Tissue Distribution of the mRNAs of the Cloned Isoforms NHE1, NHE2, NHE3, and NHE4 as Determined by Northern Blotting Analysis and RNAse Protection Assays

Isoform	Tissue distribution
NHE1	Ubiquitous
NHE2	*Rabbit*: kidney medulla>intestine>kidney cortex>adrenal gland>trachea>skeletal muscle (25) *Rat*: small intestine-colon-stomach>>skeletal muscle>brain>kidney>testis>uterus>heart-lung (24)
NHE3	*Rabbit*: kidney cortex>intestine>kidney medulla>stomach (27) *Rat*: large intestine>small intestine>kidney>stomach (20)
NHE4	*Rat*: stomach>small and large intestine>>uterus-brain-kidney-skeletal muscle (20)

detected in large intestine>small intestine>kidney>stomach (20). NHE4 message (rat) is highest in stomach>small and large intestine>uterus, brain, kidney, and skeletal muscle (20).

At the protein level, only the NHE1 and NHE3 isoforms have been immunolocalized so far (Aronson et al., personal communication). Pharmacological studies had initially identified amiloride-"insensitive" NHE isoforms on the apical membranes of polarized intestinal and renal epithelial cells (reviewed in Ref. 16). To analyze further the targeting specificity of the different isoforms, Roux et al., in our group, expressed in the renal epithelial cell lines OK and MDCK either NHE1 or an epitope-tagged NHE3. The use of two approaches—immunodetection by confocal microscopy and pharmacological analysis of amiloride-sensitive ^{22}Na uptake made it possible to demonstrate that, in these two cell systems, the NHE1 isoform is expressed both apically and basolaterally, whereas NHE3 is specifically targeted to the apical membrane (Roux D., Noël J., and Pouysségur J.; in preparation). It is presently impossible to determine whether the lack of specificity of NHE1 expression observed in OK and MDCK cells is physiological or corresponds to a loss of functions of the protein trafficking machinery of these cell lines. Nevertheless, these results clearly show that the NHE3 isoform possesses all the information to be expressed specifically at the apical face of epithelial cells.

STRUCTURAL FEATURES

Based on their hydropathy profiles, Na^+/H^+ exchangers exhibit similar topologies. The molecule has two parts: the N-terminal domain (made up of 10 to 12 membrane-spanning domains), with approximately 500 amino acids, and the C-terminal domain, with 300 amino acids. The isoforms of Na^+/H^+ exchangers cloned so far are homologous (reviewed in Refs. 3 and 4). NHE1, NHE2, NHE3, and NHE4 share 40–60% overall amino acid identity: the membrane-spanning domains constitute the most highly conserved portions of the molecule and exhibit 50–60% amino acid identity; it is noteworthy that among them, the two segments M5a and M5b appear to be almost identical in all the cloned isoforms, suggesting that this part of the exchanger should play a crucial role in the structure of the molecule and/or in the ion transport mechanism (3,4,31). In addition, all the isoforms possess a first putative transmembrane segment which displays the features of a cleavable signal peptide (Counillon L., Pouysségur J., and Reithmeier R.; in preparation). The cytoplasmic domains share only 30–40% homology; all of them contain variable putative protein kinase consensus sequences. The family members identified to date exhibit little divergence among species, suggesting the conserved evolution of this gene family. For example, NHE1 has been cloned from human, rabbit, rat, pig, and hamster and shows more than 90% amino acid identity. The βNHE isoform, cloned from trout red blood cells, exhibits a large degree of homology with NHE1: 74% homology for the transmembrane domain and 48% for the cytoplasmic domain (23).

NHE1 is glycosylated. The NHE1 sequence possesses three consensus sites for N-linked glycosylation at asparagine residues 75, 370, and 410. Indeed, treatment of NHE1 with neuraminidase and endoglycosidase F but not endoglycosidase H was found to reduce the apparent size of NHE1 from 110 to 90 kDa, indicating that NHE1 is a glycoprotein (32). To analyze the potential functional consequences of deglycosylation, site-directed mutagenesis at the individual N-glycosylation consensus sites (Asn to Asp) was performed and the cDNAs containing combinations of these three mutations generated (Counillon L., Pouysségur J., and Reithmeier R.; in preparation). Expression of the mutated cDNAs in antiporter-deficient PS120 fibroblasts showed that all constructs produced functional transporters that had transport rates and pharmacological profiles similar to the wild-type molecule, indicating that the glycosylation of NHE1 is completely dispensable for its expression and function. A role for glycosylation in regulation of the Na^+/H^+ antiporter had been postulated by Yusufi and colleagues (33), who reported that enzymatic deglycosylation of rat renal brush border membrane vesicles resulted in a 50% decrease in the V_{max} of the exchanger without effect on K_m. These results should, however, be interpreted with caution, since the enzymatic treatment results in global deglycosylation of multiple membrane components that could indirectly affect transport. Counillon et al. also demonstrated that only the first glycosylation site (Asn 75) is used in NHE1. Interestingly, among the three putative N-linked glycosylation consensus sites present in NHE1 (and βNHE), it is not this site but only the second one that is conserved in the other isoforms (12,20,24,25,27), indicating the possibility that these isoforms might be lacking N-linked carbohydrates. In any case, it appears to be the case for NHE3: this isoform was indeed found to run in SDS-PAGE as a 75- to 80-kDa protein, an apparent molecular weight close to that deduced from its amino acid sequence, and its mobility did not change upon enzymatic deglycosylation (Counillon L., Pouysségur J., and Reithmeier R.; in preparation; Aronson et al., personal communication). A similar result was obtained recently for NHE2 that possesses however, like NHE1, O-linked sugars (Tse C. M., Levine S. A., Khurana S., and Donowitz M.; in preparation).

NHE1 and NHE3 form stable homodimers in intact cells. A recent study (34) demonstrated that both NHE1 and NHE3 exist as stable dimers in the membrane, suggesting that oligomerization might be a common feature of Na^+/H^+ exchange transporters. Importantly for membrane sorting, coexpression of NHE1 and NHE3 in the same cells did not lead to the formation of heterodimers, demonstrating an isoform specificity for the subunit interaction. In addition, this study showed that, despite the formation of oligomers as the basic structural unit, the monomer seems to represent the minimal functional unit for NHE1. However, further work is required before a definitive conclusion can be reached.

FUNCTIONAL STUDIES

Kinetics

NHE1, NHE2, and NHE3 kinetics properties have been studied when stably transfected in antiporter-deficient cells: PS120 fibroblasts (19,32,35,36), or Chinese hamster ovary cells (28). For all the expressed exchangers, the dependence of the rate of transport on the extracellular Na^+ concentration follows Michaelis-Menten kinetics, consistent with one single binding site with an apparent K_m value in the millimolar range: 15 to 18 m*M* for rabbit NHE1, NHE2, and NHE3; 5 to 10 m*M* for rat NHE1 and NHE3. In contrast, the dependence of forward Na_o^+/H_i^+ transport on $[H^+]_i$ is considerably steeper. Such behaviour is not predicted for a simple, saturable, one-for-one exchanger and has been attributed to the existence of a second cytoplasmic H^+-binding site, which allosterically controls the activity of the antiporter (37). The existence of a modifier site is essential for understanding how the exchanger exerts its physiological function. Despite the large inward Na^+ gradient, the antiporter is almost quiescent at physiological intracellular pH (38–41) but becomes markedly activated as the cell interior acidifies. This peculiar behavior has been attributed to the protonation of an allosteric H^+ binding site (modifier site) on the internal surface of the exchanger. When protonated, the modifier site is thought to activate Na^+/H^+ exchange, thereby counteracting the acidification of the cytosol. Once the physiological "set point" pH is attained, the allosteric site terminates exchange, preventing excessive cytoplasmic alkalinization (42). H^+ kinetic data show similar cooperativity by intracellular H^+ for the three isoforms (28,36), confirming that the presence of a modifier site is a common feature of the Na^+/H^+ exchangers.

Identification of Distinct Functional Domains

In order to study the structure-function relationship of the Na^+/H^+ antiporter, Wakabayashi et al. (35) generated a set of cDNA deletion mutants within the C-terminal cytoplasmic domain of the human antiporter and expressed them in the antiporter-deficient fibroblast cell line PS120. This study led to the following important conclusions. Deletion of the entire cytoplasmic domain (a) preserves amiloride-sensitive Na^+/H^+ exchange activity indicating that the N-terminal domain is sufficient both for insertion of the exchanger into the plasma membrane and to carry out the transport; (b) markedly shifts the pK value for intracellular H^+ to the acidic range but preserves the allosteric activation of the exchanger by the internal H^+ indicating that the H^+ modifier site must be located within the N-terminal domain; (c) abolishes growth factor–induced cytosolic alkalinization, demonstrating that the cytoplasmic domain is crucial for growth factor activation; (d) does not prevent the formation of homodimers, indicating that the transmembrane domain is sufficient for dimerization (34). From these studies can be extrapolated a model where the antiporter can be separated into two distinct functional domains: the NH2 terminal transmembrane domain, which possesses all the information to catalyze the ion exchange, and the cytoplasmic C-terminal domain, which determines the pH set point of the exchanger and mediates the activation of the exchange by growth factors. Consistent with this functional model, a study on the trout red cell exchanger βNHE, which is activated by cAMP, demonstrated that deletion of the C-terminal region of the cytoplasmic loop containing the cAMP-dependent consensus sites preserves both the ability of the exchanger to catalyze amiloride-sensitive Na^+/H^+ exchange activity and the characteristics of the H^+ modifier site while abolishing activation by cAMP (23).

Pharmacology and Identification of Amiloride Binding Site

Amiloride Sensitivity of the Different NHE Isoforms

While all Na^+/H^+ exchangers are inhibited by amiloride and its 5-amino substituted analogues, they exhibit a wide range of sensitivities to these drugs depending on the cell type but also within the same cell on the plasma membrane domains: apical vs. basolateral in polarized epithelial cells. The porcine kidney LLC-PK1 cell line provides a good illustration of this feature, since this cell line was demonstrated to display pharmacologically distinguishable Na^+/H^+ exchange activities on its apical and basolateral surfaces when grown on permeable filters to promote polarization (43). The apical Na^+/H^+ exchange activity has an apparent inhibitory constant ($K_{0.5}$) for the amiloride analog EIPA (ethylisopropylamiloride) of 10 μM, compared to a value of 20 nM for its basolateral counterpart. The $K_{0.5}$ value for amiloride for the Na^+/H^+ exchanger present in nonepithelial cells or in the basolateral membrane of polarized epithelial cells has been reported to be in the low micromolar range; this value is one to two orders of magnitude greater for the Na^+/H^+ exchanger on the apical membrane of polarized epithelial cells from kidney and intestine (reviewed in Ref. 16). Pharmacological studies on expressed cDNAs of the recently cloned isoforms NHE2 and NHE3 have shown that NHE3 is highly resistant to amiloride and its derivatives, whereas NHE2 exhibits the same sensitivity to amiloride as NHE1 but a decrease (25-fold) in affinity for EIPA (28,44,45) (Table 2). It is noteworthy that, on the basis of the amiloride sensitivity, additional members of the Na^+/H^+ exchanger gene family most probably remain to be identified, since in hippocampal neurons a Na^+/H^+ exchanger totally resistant to amiloride and its analogues has been characterized (46).

Amiloride Binding Site

Amiloride and its 5-amino substituted derivatives are reported to inhibit the transporter by competing with Na^+ on its external binding site (see Ref. 47 for review). The amiloride binding site appears to be located in the N-terminal domain of the exchanger, since NHE1, after removal of the entire cytoplasmic domain, remains sensitive to amiloride (35). NHE1 is the most sensitive isoform to amiloride and its analogues (3,4,47,48) (Table 2). Identification of the amiloride binding site of NHE1 was pursued in our group by Counillon, Franchi, and Pouysségur using the following approach: by selecting mutant cells expressing the exchanger resistant to amiloride or its analogues (49) and subsequently cloning and sequencing their exchanger cDNAs, a one point mutation was identified:

Table 2 Comparison of the Inhibition Constants $K_{0.5}$ of the Cloned Isoforms NHE1, NHE2 and NHE3 for Amiloride and Amiloride Derivatives

Isoform	$K_{0.5}$ amiloride, μM	$K_{0.5}$ DMA, μM	$K_{0.5}$ MPA, μM	$K_{0.5}$ EIPA, μM
NHE1, human	3 (44)	0.1 (44)	0.08 (44)	0.020 (25)
NHE1, rat	1.6 (28)	0.023 (28)		0.015 (28)
NHE2, rabbit	3 (44)	0.7 (44)	0.5 (44)	
	1 (25)			0.50 (25)
NHE3, rat	100 (44)	11 (44)	10 (44)	
	100 (28)	14 (28)		2.4 (28)
NHE3, rabbit	39 (45)			8 (45)

DMA, dimethylamiloride; MPA, methylpropylamiloride; EIPA, ethylisopropylamiloride. The $K_{0.5}$ values were determined by inhibition of $^{22}Na^+$ uptake initial rates measured at external Na^+ concentrations not exceeding 2 mM.

leucine to phenylalanine at position 167 (hamster amino acid sequence), which is responsible for the decreased affinity for 5-amino substitutives of amiloride observed in the selected cells (50). It is noteworthy that this residue is located within a highly conserved part of the fourth putative transmembrane domain of the antiporter. In addition, mutation of a close residue in this fourth transmembrane domain Phe 165 to Tyr was shown to generate mutants exhibiting a three- to fourfold decrease in transport rate for Na^+ and a 40-fold increased $K_{0.5}$ for amiloride (50). Interestingly, the Leu 167 to Phe substitution was found to occur naturally in the sequence of NHE3, which displays an amiloride-resistant phenotype. These results, therefore, strongly suggest that the fourth transmembrane segment is part of the amiloride-binding domain.

REGULATION

Protein kinases appear to play a predominant role in the regulation of the Na^+/H^+ exchangers, but the mechanisms of regulation at a molecular level are not fully elucidated yet. In this context, the isoform that has been best studied is the ubiquitous form NHE1.

Molecular Mechanism of Activation of NHE1

Most mitogens activate the NHE1 isoform, leading to an intracellular alkalinization (reviewed in Ref. 5) mostly detectable in the absence of bicarbonate (51,52). At least three groups have reported that mitogenic agents activate the antiporter by shifting the pH-dependence of the modifier site, adjusting the set point upward by 0.15 to 0.30 pH units, which is the magnitude of the alkalosis recorded in most cases (37,40,53,54). As a result, the exchanger is activated, but only temporarily, returning to near quiescence when pH_i attains the new set-point value. It had been speculated repeatedly that the alteration in the set point was mediated by phosphorylation of the antiporter itself or of an ancillary protein. This speculation was based on the following observations: first, the biological effects of most, if not all, of the mitogens known to activate the antiporter are believed to be mediated by protein kinases; second, in the cases where the metabolic dependence of the response was studied (55,56), the stimulation of the antiporter was shown to depend on the availability of cellular ATP, the putative substrate of the kinases; finally, in the cases of agents thought to act via stimulation of protein kinase C, depletion of this enzyme prior to addition of the stimulus precluded the activation of the antiport (57,58). Indeed, immunoprecipitation of NHE1 in ^{32}P-labeled fibroblasts demonstrated that "resting" NHE1 is phosphorylated and that mitogenic stimulation is accompanied by an increase in phosphorylation of NHE1, with a time course similar to the rise in intracellular pH (32). Moreover, okadaic acid, a serine/threonine protein phosphatase inhibitor, can by itself trigger activation of NHE1 in correlation with stimulation of its phosphorylation (56,59). Phosphorylation of NHE1 was demonstrated to occur exclusively on serine residues, whatever the stimulus used (32). This is the case for stimulation by EGF and thrombin, which are known to activate distinct transmembrane signaling pathways (receptor tyrosine kinase in the case of EGF; G protein–coupled activation of phospholipase C, followed by stimulation of protein kinase C for thrombin). Moreover, tryptic phosphopeptide maps of NHE1 immunoprecipitated from cells treated with EGF or thrombin showed a common pattern of phosphorylation (59). Taken together, these results are consistent with the notion that direct phosphorylation of the exchanger is the triggering mechanism that controls its set point. They also suggest that the final step in Na^+/H^+ exchange activation is mediated by an as yet unidentified serine protein kinase that can integrate signals from receptor tyrosine kinases and G protein–coupled receptors. Recent evidence, however, shows that the situation is more complex. Recently, Wakabayashi et al. (60), pursued their investigations on the role of phosphorylation in the activation of NHE1 by growth factors. Using a set of deletion and point mutants, they showed that while the cytoplasmic region between amino acid 567 and 635 is crucial for high pH_i-sensitivity and growth factor activation, all major phosphorylation sites are located in the cytoplasmic tail between amino acid 636 and 815. Deletion of this 636-to-815 region was shown to preserve high pHi sensitivity and part of the growth factor response, supporting the existence of an additional mechanism not requiring direct phosphorylation of the antiporter for mediating growth factor signal. The authors therefore postulate the existence of a regulatory factor that would control NHE1 activation either through interaction with the critical cytoplasmic 567-to-635 region or another part of the cytoplasmic domain. It is noteworthy that the existence of an alternative mode of activation of the antiporter not requiring its direct phosphorylation had been previously postulated by Grinstein et al. (61) in the context of their study of the activation of NHE1 during volume regulation. Like growth factors, hyperosmotic stress has been shown to activate the antiporter by increasing its sensitivity to intracellular H^+ (55). However, the shift in pH sensitivity induced by the osmotic shock is not associated with increased phosphorylation of the exchanger. Recent results demonstrate that in cultured fibroblasts, NHE1 preferentially accumulates at focal adhesions, where it is likely to interact with cytoskeletal proteins (62). This interaction might be involved in the activation of the antiporter by osmotic shrinking or during cell spreading.

Hormonal Regulation of the Different Exchanger Isoforms

The analysis of the hormonal regulation of the different exchangers is particularly complex because, in a variety of tissues, different isoforms are coexpressed and exhibit different pathways of regulation (for review, see Ref. 16). A strategy to overcome these difficulties consists in studying the regulation of the cloned exchangers by expressing single isoforms in NHE-deficient cell lines like PS120 cells. Such studies have demonstrated that modulation of the three stably expressed isoforms by external signals and second messengers is mediated by different mechanisms (4). Whereas growth factors activate NHE1 by increasing its affinity for internal protons with no change in V_{max}, NHE2 is also stimulated by growth factors, thrombin, and phorbol esters, but these agents do not appear to modify the affinity of the exchanger for H^+ and instead induce an increase in V_{max} (36). NHE3 is stimulated by serum growth factors and thrombin but is inhibited by phorbol esters (45). The effect of these agents on NHE3 is mediated by a change in V_{max}, with no apparent change in affinity for H^+. These results are interesting, but their limitation is the fact that they do not take into account the effects on regulation of the exchangers inherent to the cell type and to the polarity of epithelial cells. Indeed, the effect of protein kinases on the regulation of Na^+/H^+ exchangers differs depending on the cell type but also, within the same cell, on the membrane domain: i.e., apical vs. basolateral domain (4). Studies examining differential regulation of amiloride-sensitive and amiloride-resistant Na^+/H^+ antiporters in cultured epithelial cells (LLC-PK1) have shown that whereas cAMP-dependent protein kinase inhibits both types of antiporters, protein kinase C stimulates the amiloride-sensitive form (NHE1) but inhibits the amiloride-resistant (apical) form (63). Interestingly, studies on the apical membrane Na^+/H^+ antiporter in brush border membrane vesicles have provided different results, since this exchanger was found to be inhibited by cAMP-dependent protein kinase and calcium/calmodulin–dependent protein kinase but stimulated by protein kinase C (64–66). Modulation of Na^+/H^+ exchange activity by various hormones is likely to be mediated by these protein kinase effects. For instance, the inhibitory effects of the parathyroid hormone on Na^+/H^+ exchange and consequently on sodium and bicarbonate reabsorption in the kidney and gut most likely result from its activation of cAMP-dependent protein kinase (67–69). Similarly, stimulation of angiotensin II and alpha-2 catecholamine receptors increases Na^+/H^+ exchange, and this effect can possibly be attributed to inhibition of adenyl cyclase and resulting inhibition of cAMP-dependent protein kinase (70–71). In mesangial cells, stimulation of Na^+/H^+ exchange by serotonin and arginine vasopressin requires protein kinase C activation (72). In the context of activation of NHE by cAMP, the βNHE isoform isolated from trout red cells is interesting because it has two clustered cAMP-dependent protein kinase consensus sites (23) located in the cytoplasmic domain. βNHE is activated by an increase in cAMP (73). When expressed in PS120 fibroblasts, βNHE displayed cAMP sensitivity (23), whereas there was no effect of cAMP on the activity of any of the isoforms NHE1, NHE2, or NHE3 transfected in the same cells (23,36). The deletion or point mutation of the two protein kinase A consensus sites of βNHE strongly reduced its response to cAMP (23). Interestingly, replacing the human NHE1 cytoplasmic tail by the βNHE corresponding one conferred cAMP-sensitivity to the chimeric NHE1 isoform (Borgese F. and Pouysségur J.; personal communication). These results reinforce the notion that the cytoplasmic domain mediates and dictates the nature of the hormonal response. However, another level of regulation can be demonstrated. Indeed, NHE1, which is insensitive to variations in cAMP when expressed in fibroblasts, becomes inhibited by agents that raise cAMP when expressed in the epithelial cell line OK (74). It is noteworthy that this inhibition by cAMP is the typical response of the endogenous apically expressed "amiloride-resistant" isoform in these cells (74). These findings are important because they illustrate that the nature of the hormonal response relies not only on the sequence of the cytoplasmic domain but also on the nature of the cell expressing the NHE isoform.

In addition to the short-term regulations described above, Na^+/H^+ exchangers can also be regulated on a long-term basis. In the proximal tubule, a number of situations have been shown to chronically increase the activity of apical Na^+/H^+ exchanger (for review, see Ref. 11). In particular, chronic acidosis in vivo was demonstrated to induce an increase in proximal tubule activity that persists when the transporter is studied out of the acidotic environment, indicating an intrinsic adaptation of the transporter (6). Recently, the same group demonstrated that chronic acidosis of cultured tubular cells leads to an increase in Na^+/H^+ antiporter activity that is dependent on protein synthesis and is associated with an increase in NHE mRNA. In addition, they demonstrated that this acid-induced activation of NHE requires protein kinase C and is associated with an increase in the AP1 transcription factor activity (75).

CONCLUDING REMARKS

Identification of the primary structure of the Na^+/H^+ exchangers by cloning their cDNAs represented a major advance in the biology of these widespread transporters. Now, with the generation of specific molecular tools and the advance of molecular genetics, future work will describe the complete "anatomy" of the NHE isoforms in the nephron and other organs. Experiments exploiting the combination of site-directed mutagenesis, random mutagenesis with powerful genetic screen, will help considerably in the identification of the key residues of the NHE molecules involved in ion catalysis, H^+ sensing, and apical targeting in epithelial cells. Finally, alteration of NHE gene expression in transgenic animals or gene knockout of each isoform is another area of considerable interest to approach the physiological role of these exchangers' isoforms and their possible implication in human diseases.

ACKNOWLEDGMENTS

We are grateful to Drs. P. Aronson, C. M. Tse, F. Borgese, L. Counillon, J. Noël, and D. Roux for providing us with unpublished results. We thank Dr. J. Noël for critical reading of the manuscript. We thank all the colleagues from our laboratory for fruitful discussions. Research in the authors' laboratory is supported by the Centre National de la Recherche Scientifique (CNRS UMR 134), the Institut National de la Santé et de la Recherche Médicale (INSERM), the Fondation pour la Recherche Médicale, and the Association pour la Recherche sur le Cancer (ARC).

REFERENCES

1. Pitts RF, Ayer JL, Schiess WA. J Clin Invest 1949; 28:35–44.
2. Murer H, Hopfer U, Kinne R. Sodium/proton antiport in brush border-membrane vesicles isolated from rat small intestine and kidney. Biochem J 1976; 154:597–604.
3. Counillon L, Pouysségur J. Structure, function and regulation of vertebrate Na^+/H^+ exchangers (NHE). Current Opinion in Nephrology and Hypertension 1993; 2:708–714.
4. Tse M, Levine S, Yun C, Brant S, Counillon L, Pouysségur J, Donowitz M. Structure/function studies of the epithelial isoforms of the mammalian Na^+/H^+ exchanger gene family. J Membr Biol 1993; 135:93–108.
5. Grinstein S, Rotin D, Mason MJ. Na^+/H^+ exchange and growth factor-induced cytosolic pH changes. Role in cellular proliferation. Biochim Biophys Acta 1989; 988:73–97.
6. Horie S, Moe O, Tejedor A, Alpern RJ. Preincubation in acid medium increases Na/H antiporter activity in cultured renal proximal tubule cells. Proc Natl Acad Sci USA 1990; 87:4742–4745.
7. Cala PM. Volume regulation by Amphiuma red cells. The membrane potential and its implications regarding the nature of the ion flux pathways. J Gen Physiol 1980; 76:683–708.
8. Green J, Yamaguchi DT, Kleeman CR, Muallem S. Selective modification of the kinetic properties of Na^+/H^+ exchanger by cell shrinkage and swelling. J Biol Chem 1988; 263:5012–5015.
9. Grinstein S, Foskett JK. Ionic mechanisms of cell volume regulation in leukocytes. Annu Rev Physiol 1990; 52:399–414.
10. Schwartz MA, Both G, Lechene C. Effect of cell spreading on cytoplasmic pH in normal and transformed fibroblasts. Proc Natl Acad Sci USA 1989; 86:4525–4529.

11. Krapf R, Alpern RJ. Cell pH and transepithelial H/HCO3 transport in the renal proximal tubule. J Membr Biol 1993; 131:1–10.
12. Sardet C, Franchi A, Pouysségur J. Molecular cloning, primary structure, and expression of the human growth factor-activatable Na^+/H^+ antiporter. Cell 1989; 56:271–280.
13. Pouysségur J, Sardet C, Franchi A, et al. A specific mutation abolishing Na^+/H^+ antiport activity in hamster fibroblasts precludes growth at neutral and acidic pH. Proc Natl Acad Sci USA 1984; 81:4833–4837.
14. Kulanthaivel P, Leibach FH, Mahesh VB, et al. The Na^+/H^+ exchanger of the placental brush-border membrane is pharmacologically distinct from that of the renal brush-border membrane. J Membr Biol 1990; 265:1249–1252.
15. Kulanthaivel P, Furesz TC, Moe AJ, et al. Human placental syncytiotrophoblast expresses two pharmacologically distinguishable types of Na^+/H^+ exchangers, NHE-1 in the maternal-facing (brush border) membrane and NHE-2 in the fetal-facing (basal) membrane. Biochem J 1992; 284:33–38.
16. Clark JD, Limbird LL. Na^+/H^+ exchanger subtypes, a predictive review. Am J Physiol 1991; 261: G945–G953.
17. Hildebrandt F, Pizzona JH, Reilly RF, et al. Cloning of cDNA encoding a rabbit renal Na^+/H^+ exchanger-tissue distribution and comparison to the human sequence. Biochim Biophys Acta 1991; 1129:105–108.
18. Reilly RF, Hildebrandt F, Biemesderfer D, et al. cDNA cloning and immunolocalization of a Na^+/H^+ exchange in LLC-PK1 renal epithelial cells. Am J Physiol 1991; 261:F1088–F1094.
19. Tse CM, Ma AI, Yang VW, et al. Molecular cloning and expression of a cDNA encoding the rabbit ileal villus cell basolateral membrane Na^+/H^+ exchanger. EMBO J 1991; 10:1957–1967.
20. Orlowski, J, Kandasamy RA, Shull GE. Molecular cloning of putative members of the Na^+/H^+ exchanger gene family. J Biol Chem 1992; 267:9331–9339.
21. Takaichi K, Wang D, Blakovets DF, Warnock DG. Cloning, sequencing, and expression of Na^+/H^+ antiporters cDNAs from human tissues. Am J Physiol 1992; 262:C1069–C1076.
22. Counillon L, Pouysségur J. Nucleotide sequence of the Chinese hamster Na^+/H^+ exchanger NHE1. Biochim Biophys Acta 1993; 1172:343–345.
23. Borgese F, Sardet C, Cappadoro M, et al. Cloning and expression of a cAMP-activatable Na^+/H^+ exchanger: Evidence that the cytoplasmic domain mediates hormonal regulation. Proc Natl Acad Sci USA 1992; 89:6765–6769.
24. Wang Z, Orlowski J, Shull GE. Primary structure and functional expression of a novel gastrointestinal isoform of the rat Na^+/H^+ exchanger. J Biol Chem 1993; 268:11925–11928.
25. Tse CM, Levine SA, Yun CHC, et al. Cloning and expression of a rabbit cDNA encoding a serum-activated ethyl isopropylamiloride-resistant epithelial Na^+/H^+ exchanger isoform (NHE-2). J Biol Chem 1993; 268:11917–11924.
26. Collins JF, Honda T, Knobel S, et al. Molecular cloning, sequencing, tissue distribution, and functional expression of a Na^+/H^+ exchanger (NHE-2). Proc Natl Acad Sci USA 1993; 90:3938–3942.
27. Tse CM, Brant SR, Walker S, et al. Cloning and sequencing of a rabbit cDNA encoding an intestinal and kidney-specific Na^+/H^+ exchanger isoform (NHE-3). J Biol Chem 1992; 267:9340–9346.
28. Orlowski J. Heterologous expression and functional properties of amiloride high affinity (NHE-1) and low affinity (NHE-3) isoforms of the rat Na/H exchanger. J Biol Chem 1993; 268:16369–16377.
29. Montrose MH, Murer H. Polarity and kinetics of Na^+/H^+ exchange in cultured opossum kidney cells. Am J Physiol 1990; 259:C121–C133.
30. Krapf G, Solioz M. Na^+/H^+ antiporter in RNA expression in single nephron segments of rat kidney cortex. J Clin Invest 1991; 88:783–788.
31. Counillon L, Pouysségur J. Structure-function and growth factor activation of the Na^+/H^+ exchanger (NHE1). Cell Physiol Biochem 1992; 2:138–149.
32. Sardet C, Counillon L, Franchi A, Pouysségur J. Growth factors induce the phosphorylation of the Na^+/H^+ antiporter, a glycoprotein of 110 kDa. Science 1990; 247:723–726.
33. Yusufi ANK, Szczeparska-Konkel M, Dousa TP. Role of N-linked oligosaccharides in the transport activity of the Na^+/H^+ antiporter in rat renal brush border membrane. J Biol Chem 1988; 263:13683–13691.
34. Fafournoux P, Noël J, Pouysségur J. Evidence that Na^+/H^+ exchanger isoforms NHE1 and NHE3 exist as stable dimers in membranes with a high degree of specificity for homodimers. J Biol Chem 1994; 269:2589–2596.
35. Wakabayashi S, Fafournoux P, Sardet C, Pouysségur J. The Na^+/H^+ antiporter cytoplasmic domain mediates growth factor signals and controls "H^+ sensing." Proc Natl Acad Sci USA 1992; 89:2424–2428.
36. Levine SA, Montrose MH, Tse CM, Donowitz M. Kinetics and regulation of three cloned mammalian Na^+/H^+ exchangers stably expressed in a fibroblast cell line. J Biol Chem 1993; 268:25527–25535.
37. Aronson PS, Nee J, Suhm NA. Modifier role of internal H^+ in activating the Na^+/H^+ exchanger in renal microvillus membrane vesicles. Nature 1982; 299:161–163.

38. Grinstein S, Cohen S, Rothstein A. Cytoplasmic pH regulation in thymic lymphocytes by an amiloride-sensitive Na^+/H^+ antiport. J Gen Physiol 1984; 83:341–369.
39. Paris S, Pouysségur J. Biochemical characterization of the amiloride-sensitive Na^+/H^+ antiport in Chinese hamster lung fibroblasts. J Biol Chem 1983; 258:3503–3508.
40. Moolenaar WH, Tsien RY, van der Saag PT, de Laat SW. Na^+/H^+ exchange and cytoplasmic pH in the action of growth factors in human fibroblasts. Nature 1983; 304:645–648.
41. Moolenaar WH, Tertoolen LGJ, de Laat SW. The regulation of cytoplasmic pH in human fibroblasts. J Biol Chem 1984; 259:7563–7569.
42. Aronson PS. Kinetic properties of the plasma membrane Na^+-H^+ exchanger. Annu Rev Physiol 1985; 47:545–560.
43. Haggerty JG, Agarwal N, Reilly RF, et al. Pharmacologically different Na/H antiporters on the apical and basolateral surfaces of cultured porcine kidney cells (LLC-PK1). Proc Natl Acad Sci USA 1988; 85:6797–6801.
44. Counillon L, Scholz W, Lang HJ, Pouysségur J. Pharmacological characterization of stably transfected Na^+/H^+ antiporter isoforms using amiloride analogs and a new inhibitor exhibiting anti-ischemic properties. Mol Pharmacol 1993; 44:1041–1045.
45. Tse CM, Levine SA, Yun CHC, et al. Functional characteristics of a cloned epithelial Na^+/H^+ exchanger (NHE3): Resistance to amiloride and inhibition by protein kinase C. Proc Natl Acad Sci USA 1993; 90:9110–9114.
46. Raley-Susman KM, Cragoe E Jr, Sapolsky RM, Kopito RR. Regulation of intracellular pH in cultured hippocampal neurones by an amiloride-insensitive Na^+/H^+ exchanger. J Biol Chem 1991; 266:2739–2745.
47. Benos DJ. Amiloride: chemistry, kinetics, and structure-activity relationships. In: Grinstein S, ed. Na^+/H^+ Exchange. Boca Raton, FL: CRC Press, 1988:121–136.
48. L'Allemain G, Franchi A, Cragoe E Jr. Blockade of the Na^+/H^+ antiport abolishes growth factor-induced DNA synthesis in fibroblasts. J Biol Chem 1984; 259:4313–4319.
49. Franchi A, Cragoe J, Pouysségur J. Isolation and properties of fibroblast mutants overexpressing an altered Na^+/H^+ antiporter. J Biol Chem 1986; 261:14614–14620.
50. Counillon L, Franchi A, Pouysségur J. A point mutation of the Na^+/H^+ exchanger gene (NHE1) confers amiloride resistance upon chronic acidosis. Proc Natl Acad Sci USA 1993; 90:4508–4512.
51. L'Allemain G, Paris S, Pouysségur J. Role of Na^+-dependent Cl-HCO_3^- exchange in regulation of intracellular pH in fibroblasts. J Biol Chem 1985; 260:4877–4883.
52. Ganz MB, Boyarsky G, Sterzel RB, Boron WF. Arginine vasopressin enhances pH_i regulation in the presence of HCO_3^- by stimulating three acid-base transport systems. Nature 1989; 337:648–651.
53. Paris S, Pouysségur J. Growth factors activate the Na^+/H^+ antiporter in quiescent fibroblasts by increasing its affinity for intracellular H^+. J Biol Chem 1984; 259:10989–10994.
54. Grinstein S, Cohen S, Goetz JD, et al. Characterization of the activation of Na^+/H^+ exchange in lymphocytes by phorbol esters: Change in cytoplasmic dependence of the antiport. Proc Natl Acad Sci USA 1985; 82:1429–1433.
55. Grinstein S, Cohen S, Goetz JD, Rothstein A. Osmotic and phorbol ester-induced activation of Na^+/H^+ exchange: Possible role of protein phosphorylation in lymphocyte volume regulation. J Cell Biol 1985; 101:269–276.
56. Bianchini L, Woodside M, Sardet C, et al. Okadaic acid, a phosphatase inhibitor induces activation and phosphorylation of the Na^+/H^+ antiport. J Biol Chem 1991; 266:15406–15413.
57. Grinstein S, Mack E, Mills GB. Osmotic activation of the Na^+/H^+ antiport in protein kinase C-depleted lymphocytes. Biochem Biophys Res Commun 1986; 134:8–13.
58. Daniel TO, Ives HE. Cyclosporin A inhibits kinase C-independent activation of the Na^+/H^+ exchanger by PDGF and vanadate. Biochem Biophys Res Commun 1987; 145:111–117.
59. Sardet C, Fafournoux P, Pouysségur J. Alpha-thrombin, EGF and okadaic acid activate the Na^+/H^+ exchanger, NHE1 by phosphorylating a set of common sites. J Biol Chem 1991; 266:19166–19171.
60. Wakabayashi S, Bertrand B, Shigekawa M, et al. Growth factor activation and "H^+-sensing" of the Na^+/H^+ exchanger isoform 1 (NHE1): Evidence in favor of a regulatory "accessory" factor. J Biol Chem 1994; 269:5583–5588.
61. Grinstein S, Woodside M, Sardet C, et al. Activation of Na^+/H^+ antiporter during cell volume regulation: Evidence for a phosphorylation-independent mechanism. J Biol Chem 1992; 267:23823–23828.
62. Grinstein S, Woodside M, Waddell TK, et al. Focal localization of the NHE-1 isoform of the Na^+/H^+ antiport: Assessment of effects on intracellular pH. EMBO J 1993; 12:5209–5218.
63. Casavola V, Reshkin SJ, Murer H, Helmle-Kolb C. Polarized expression of Na^+/H^+ exchange activity in LLC-PK1/PKE20 cells: II. Hormonal regulation. Pflugers Arch 1992; 420:282–289.
64. Weinman EJ, Shenolikar S. Protein kinase C activates the renal apical membrane Na^+/H^+ exchanger. J Membr Biol 1986; 93:133–139.

65. Weinman EJ, Shenolikar S, Kahn AM. cAMP-associated inhibition of Na^+-H^+ exchanger in rabbit kidney brush-border membranes. Am J Physiol 1987; 252:F19–F25.
66. Weinman EJ, Shenolikar S, Cragoe EJ Jr, Dubinsky WP. Solubilization and reconstitution of renal brush border Na^+/H^+ exchanger. J Membr Biol 1988; 101:1–9.
67. Kahn AM, Dolson GM, Hise MK, et al. Parathyroid hormone and dibuyryl cyclic AMP inhibit Na^+/H^+ countertransport in brush border membrane vesicles isolate from a suspension of rabbit proximal tubules. Am J Physiol 1985; 248:F212–F281.
68. Pollock AS, Warnock DG, Strewler GJ. Parathyroid hormone inhibition of Na^+-H^+ antiporter activity in cultured renal cell line. Am J Physiol 1986; 250:F217–F225.
69. Felder CC, Campbell T, Albrecht F, Jose P. Dopamine inhibits Na^+/H^+ exchanger activity in renal BBM by stimulation of adenylate cyclase. Am J Physiol 1990; 259:F297–F303.
70. Nord EP, Howard MJ, Hufezi A, et al. Alpha-2 adrenergic agonists stimulate Na^+-H^+ antiport activity in the rabbit renal proximal tubule. J Clin Invest 1987; 80:1755–1762.
71. Liu F, Cogan MG. Angiotensin II stimulates early proximal bicarbonate reabsorption in the rat by decreasing cyclic adenosine monophosphate. J Clin Invest 1989; 84:83–91.
72. Saxena R, Saksa BA, Fields AP, Ganz MB. Activation of Na/H exchanger in mesangial cells is associated with translocation of PKC isoforms. Am J Physiol 1993; 265:F53–F60.
73. Motais R, Garcia-Romeu F. Effects of catecholamines and cyclic nucleotides on Na^+/H^+ exchange. In: Grinstein S, ed. Na^+/H^+ Exchange. Boca Raton, FL: CRC Press, 1988:255–270.
74. Helmle-Kolb C, Counillon L, Roux D, et al. Na/H exchange activities in NHE-1-transfected OK-cells: cell polarity and regulation. Pflugers Arch 1993; 184:1–18.
75. Horie S, Moe O, Yamaji Y, et al. Role of protein kinase C and transcription factor AP-1 in the acid-induced increase in Na/H antiporter activity. Proc Natl Acad Sci USA 1992; 89:5236–5240.

29
Calcium Channels

Alan S. L. Yu
Brigham and Women's Hospital and Harvard Medical School, Boston, Massachusetts

INTRODUCTION

Polarized epithelial cells are unique in their ability to mediate vectorial transport of ions such as calcium between apical and basolateral surfaces, but the underlying molecular mechanisms are poorly understood. The distal nephron of the kidney serves as a paradigm for calcium-absorptive epithelia. Although calcium filtered at the glomerulus is reabsorbed along the whole length of the nephron, active, and by inference transcellular, transport has been demonstrated primarily in the distal tubule (1,2) and specifically the distal convoluted tubule (DCT) (3), connecting tubule (CNT) (4), and, perhaps under certain conditions, the cortical thick ascending limb (CTAL) (4,5). Furthermore, the action of parathyroid hormone (PTH) to enhance calcium reabsorption in the CNT (3) and CTAL (5) is responsible for its hypocalciuric effect. The mechanism and regulation of calcium reabsorption at the cellular level have recently been reviewed (6). Figure 1 illustrates a model for transcellular calcium transport in a distal tubule epithelial cell, based on current knowledge. Cytosolic calcium is translocated from the apical surface to the basolateral membrane, where it is actively extruded by a calcium pump (7–10) or sodium-calcium exchanger (7,8,11–13). Until recently, however, little was known about how calcium entered these cells at the apical surface except that it must pass down a steep concentration gradient, from millimolar concentrations in the tubular fluid (1) to submicromolar concentrations within the cytosol (14), and also down a transmembrane electrical gradient of between –35 mV and –87 mV (15,16), arguing on purely teleological grounds for a passive transport mechanism. In this article, we review recent evidence favoring a role for calcium channels in this pathway and discuss the molecular genetic approaches that have been used to identify and characterize these channels.

PHYSIOLOGICAL EVIDENCE FOR RENAL CALCIUM CHANNELS

Bacskai and Friedman (17) immunodissected distal tubule epithelial cells from mouse kidney using an antibody to the Tamm-Horsfall protein, a method that purifies cells of both DCT and CTAL origin (18); they measured the cells' intracellular calcium level with the fluorescent indicator dye fura-2. Administration of PTH induced a rise in intracellular calcium after a 10- to 12-min latency, which was dependent on the presence of extracellular calcium. This suggests that PTH can activate a plasma membrane calcium entry pathway and that this pathway is the rate-limiting step in calcium traffic in these cells. Furthermore, this calcium entry was inhibited by the dihydropyridine (DHP) antagonist nifedipine and stimulated by the DHP agonist Bay K8644 at concentrations (50 μM of each), 10^2- to 10^5-times the half-maximal effective concentration for modulation of the activity of DHP-sensitive calcium channels in other tissues, such as cardiac and vascular smooth muscle (19). However, no distinction could be made in this study between apical and basolateral membrane calcium fluxes.

Brunette et al. (20,21) used isopycnic centrifugation on a Percoll gradient to separate distal tubules from rabbit kidney cortex, followed by $MgCl_2$ precipitation to isolate putative apical membrane

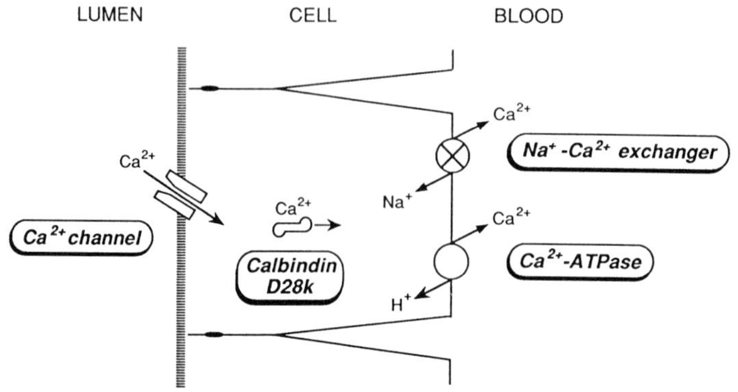

Figure 1 Model of a distal convoluted or connecting tubule epithelial cell depicting possible mechanisms involved in calcium reabsorption.

vesicles. Although the purity of their preparation could not be directly assessed, the relative exclusion of enzyme markers for other membrane fractions and the presence of thiazide-inhibitable sodium uptake suggests that some degree of enrichment was achieved. In these vesicles, a high-affinity, low-velocity calcium uptake system was observed that, like calcium entry in mouse distal tubule cells, could be activated by PTH and inhibited by the DHP antagonist nitrendipine (22). Taken together, these studies suggest that apical calcium entry may be mediated by DHP-sensitive calcium channels.

To further characterize the electrophysiological properties of these distal tubule ion channels, several investigators used single-channel patch-clamp analysis. In an SV40-transformed mouse epithelial cell line (MDCT) with an ostensibly DCT phenotype, a divalent cation-selective channel was observed that was activated by PTH in the cell-attached mode, was equally permeable to barium and calcium, and estimated to be 16-fold less permeable to sodium (23). Its single-channel slope conductance was 2 pS with 110 m*M* barium as the charge carrier. Consistent with previous observations, Bay K8644 increased and nifedipine decreased its open probability. Interestingly, the channel was unaffected by depolarization, but its open probability appeared to progressively increase with hyperpolarization beyond –20 mV. Similarly, in primary cultured epithelial cells isolated by Tamm-Horsfall antibody immunodissection from pig kidney and presumed to contain CTAL and DCT cells, a calcium-permeable channel was observed that was DHP-sensitive, and activated by 8-Br-cAMP, or by hyperpolarization (24). However, this channel had a quite different conductance of 22 to 24 pS in 50 m*M* barium. Finally, in an extensive study of rabbit DCT ("bright" distal tubule) primary cultured cells, the results of recordings from 93 active patches were reported (25). A divalent cation-selective channel with a conductance of 8 pS for 100 m*M* calcium and 13 to 15 pS for 100 m*M* barium was observed. Lanthanum, a nonspecific calcium channel blocker, reversibly abolished channel openings, while verapamil and nifedipine did so irreversibly. In the cell-attached mode, this channel exhibited rapid rundown, but the effect of PTH or cAMP analogues was not determined. The authors stated that channel activity was voltage-independent, but no formal evaluation was reported.

The conflicting results of these three studies probably reflect differences in the species of animal studied, the exact epithelial cell type from which cultures were derived, and the unpredictable alterations in cell phenotype imposed by various culture conditions, particularly by oncogenic transformation. None of the renal channels observed fit neatly into the current electrophysiological and pharmacological classification of calcium channels that are described below. Nevertheless, three characteristics were consistently observed, namely that these channels are divalent cation–selective, are sensitive to DHPs, and are not activated by membrane depolarization (and indeed may be opened by hyperpolarization).

CLASSIFICATION AND PROPERTIES OF CALCIUM CHANNELS

Calcium channels can be crudely classified on the basis of the primary mechanism for activating channel openings into voltage-dependent, receptor-operated, second-messenger–operated, and background channels. Voltage-dependent calcium channels are activated by membrane depolarization and can be subclassified on the basis of their electrophysiological and pharmacological properties into L, N, T, and P-channels (reviewed in Refs. 26 and 27). High-affinity DHP binding and sensitivity is characteristic of L-type voltage-dependent calcium channels. These are classically described as having a large single channel conductance, usually about 25 pS with ~100 m*M* barium as the charge carrier, a relatively positive voltage threshold for activation, and slow inactivation kinetics (28–30). They are activated by conventional DHP agonists such as Bay K8644 and usually inhibited by DHP antagonists such as nifedipine and nitrendipine, although under certain conditions these "antagonists" may also exhibit partial agonist effects (31,32). In addition, L channels are sensitive to inhibition by benzothiazepines such as diltiazem and by phenylalkylamines such as verapamil. Table 1 summarizes the typical properties of L, N, and T channels as exemplified by those found in chick dorsal root ganglion cells, where all three coexist (29,30), and of P channels based on in situ (33) and protein reconstitution studies (34) of channels in adult guinea pig cerebellar Purkinje cells. It has, however, become increasingly clear that there is considerable overlap in the properties of these channels as well as marked tissue- and cell type-specific differences that are incompletely described by the conventional classification (26).

DHP sensitivity has also been described in some members of a poorly defined family of calcium channels known as background, or leak, channels that share the common characteristics of having a finite open probability at resting membrane potential. Since they were originally described by Benham and Tsien (35) in rabbit vascular smooth muscle cells, the single channel properties of similar channels in rat ventricular myocytes (36), bovine sarcolemmal membranes incorporated into planar lipid bilayers (37), and human and mouse myotubes (38) have been reported. The heterogeneity of this group of channels is its most striking feature. Single channel conductances for barium vary from 7–10 pS (37,38) to 16–20 pS (35,36). Open probability was observed, in one study, to increase progressively with depolarization from –120 mV (36), while in another it exhibited a bell-shaped voltage dependence curve with maximal opening at –70 mV (37). Lack of sensitivity to the intracellular second messengers ATP, cAMP, IP_3, and calcium, was documented in only one study (36). Furthermore, in skeletal muscle myotubes and in ventricular myocytes, background channels can be activated by micromolar concentrations of either nitrendipine or Bay K8644 (36,38). Thus, there is significant overlap in the properties of this group with those of voltage-dependent channels,

Table 1 Typical Electrical and Pharmacological Properties of Voltage-Dependent Calcium Channels

	L	N	T	P
Single-channel conductance in ~100 mM Ba^{2+}	25 pS	13 pS	8 pS	9–19 pS
Single-channel kinetics	Almost no inactivation	Long burst, inactivation	Late opening, brief burst inactivation	Almost no inactivation
Relative conductance	$Ba^{2+} > Ca^{2+}$	$Ba^{2+} > Ca^{2+}$	$Ba^{2+} = Ca^{2+}$	?
Inorganic ion block	$Cd^{2+} > Ni^{2+}$	$Cd^{2+} > Ni^{2+}$	$Ni^{2+} > Cd^{2+}$	?
Threshold for activation	–10 mV	–20 mV	–70 mV	–60 to –15 mV
Inactivation range	–60 to –10 mV	–120 to –30 mV	–100 to –60 mV	Positive to +40
Decay rate (0 mV)	Slow ($\tau > 500$ ms)	Moderate ($\tau \sim 50$–80 ms)	Rapid ($\tau \sim 20$–50 ms)	Very slow ($\tau > 1100$ ms)
Dihydropyridines	Sensitive	Resistant	Resistant	Resistant
ω-Conotoxin GVIA	Resistant	Inhibited	Resistant	Resistant
ω-Conotoxin MVIIC	Resistant	Inhibited	Resistant	Inhibited
Funnel web spider toxin[a]	Resistant	Resistant	Resistant	Inhibited

[a]Including crude venom of *Agelenopsis aperta* as well as a low-molecular-weight polyamine derived from it by cation exchange chromatography (FTX) and a 48–amino acid polypeptide derived by reversed-phase HPLC (ω-agatoxin IVA).
Source: Modified from Tsien et al. (95) to accommodate recent observations of P and N channels (33,34,96,97).

while additional overlap with other classes of channels such as second-messenger–operated channels remains to be explored. Given our current difficulty in differentiating and classifying calcium channels, the recent use of biochemical and molecular cloning techniques to characterize calcium channels at the molecular level offers a more rational approach to classification based on channel structure.

MOLECULAR STRUCTURE OF VOLTAGE-DEPENDENT CALCIUM CHANNELS

Calcium channels are multisubunit proteins. This has been best characterized for the L-type voltage-dependent channel of skeletal muscle, which was first purified by digitonin solubilization and lectin affinity chromatography by Curtis and Caterall (39), and by CHAPS solubilization by Borsotto et al. (40). The results of extensive biochemical analyses, summarized in Ref. 41, demonstrate the presence of five different subunits, designated α_1 (165 to 170 kDa), α_2 (135 to 150 kDa), β (~50 kDa), γ (~30 kDa), and δ (24 to 30 kDa). The α_2 and δ subunits are linked by disulfide bonds under nonreducing conditions. Hydrophobic labels stain α_1 and γ strongly, α_2 and δ weakly, and β not at all; α_2, γ, and δ are glycosylated; and α_1 and β subunits are phosphorylated by cyclic AMP-dependent protein kinase (42). Furthermore, the receptor site for DHPs (42–44) and for phenylalkylamines (44,45), as determined by photoaffinity labeling studies, is on the α_1 subunit. Based on these observations, Takahashi et al. (42) proposed the model for the subunit structure of the skeletal muscle L-type calcium channel shown in Fig. 2, in which the α_1 subunit was postulated to form the ion pore. Recent studies of the ω-conotoxin–sensitive N-type channel suggest a similar though distinct subunit structure (46,47).

The first primary structure to be elucidated was that of the rabbit skeletal muscle α_1 subunit (48). A degenerate oligonucleotide designed from the partial amino acid sequence of a tryptic fragment of the purified α_1-subunit polypeptide was used as a probe to screen a cDNA library and thereby isolate a cDNA clone for sequencing. Since then, it has become apparent that calcium channel α_1 subunits are encoded by a family of homologous genes, of which six have been identified to date and named CaCh1 to CaCh6, according to the order in which they were first reported (Table 2). All of them share a high degree of amino acid identity and their predicted secondary structures are highly conserved and strikingly similar to those of other voltage-dependent cation channels (49). Sodium and calcium channel α_1 subunits all have four internally repeated hydrophobic motifs (I to IV), each consisting of six potential transmembrane segments (S1 to 6). Potassium channels have only one such motif but probably associate to form a tetramer (50). On the basis of recent site-directed mutagenesis studies, specific functions can now be assigned to certain structural domains (51). Thus, the fourth transmembrane region of each motif (S4), which contains a highly conserved pattern of

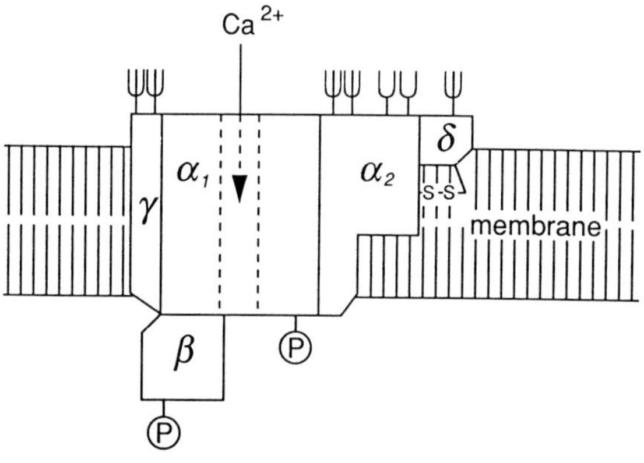

Figure 2 Proposed model for the quaternary structure of the skeletal muscle L-type voltage-dependent calcium channel. (From Ref. 42.)

Table 2 Calcium Channel α_1-Subunit Genes

α_1-subunit gene[a] (Refs.)	Snutch class[b]	Putative channel type	Tissue distribution	Human chromosomal assignment (Ref.)
CaCh1 (48)	—	L	Skeletal muscle	1q31–32 (98)
CaCh2 (67,99–101)	C	L	Heart, vascular smooth muscle, brain, lung	12p13.3 (102–104)
CaCh3 (68,105,106)	D	L	Brain, pancreas	3p14.3 (107,108)
CaCh4 (91,109)	A	P	Brain	19[c]
CaCh5 (70,110,111)	B	N	Brain	—
CaCh6 (71,112)	E	T	Brain	—

[a]Nomenclature based on Perez-Reyes et al. (113). References reporting cDNA cloning and sequencing are cited in parentheses.
[b]Alternative nomenclature in use for brain α_1-subunit isoforms (114).
[c]Unpublished observations.

positively charged residues at every third or fourth position, has been shown to play a key role in voltage sensing in potassium (52,53) and sodium (54,55) channels; by extrapolation, it probably functions in a similar capacity in calcium channels. Furthermore, mutations within the region between S5 and S6 in the potassium channel alter its single-channel conductance (56,57), ion selectivity (58), and sensitivity to both internal and external channel blockade by tetraethylammonium (56,57,59). Mutations of residues within the corresponding region of the sodium channel can confer a calcium channel–like ion selectivity (60). Thus, this so-called P region is believed to traverse the membrane, possibly in the form of a β-pleated sheet (61), and to form the lining of the ion pore.

The $\alpha_2\delta$ (which are encoded by one transcript to form a single polypeptide that is posttranslationally cleaved) (62), β (63), and γ (64,65) subunits have also been cloned and sequenced. The β subunit is encoded by a family of homologous genes, designated $\beta 1$ to $\beta 4$ (Table 3). The predicted polypeptides are generally hydrophilic, with four potential α-helical domains, each containing a similar 8–amino acid repeat that starts and ends with leucine or isoleucine. Each α_1 and β subunit isoform exhibits a distinct tissue-specific pattern of expression, but how this correlates with its physiological role is largely unknown.

Functional expression of α_1 subunits, whether alone or in combination with one or more of the other subunits, yield calcium channels, thus confirming that α_1 subunits form the ion pore. They all share the property of activation by membrane depolarization but otherwise differ in their electrophysiological and pharmacological characteristics (66–71). Attempts have been made to classify α_1 subunit isoforms according to the channel subtype profile (L, T, N, or P) that they most closely resemble (Table 2). However, the final properties of the channel protein expressed are highly dependent on the accessory subunits that are coexpressed. For instance, depending on the expression system used, β subunits have variously been reported to increase surface expression of functional α_1

Table 3 Calcium Channel β-Subunit Genes

β-subunit gene (Refs.)	Tissue distribution	Human chromosomal assignment (Ref.)
$\beta 1$ (63,115–117)	Skeletal muscle, brain, heart	17q11.2–22 (118)
$\beta 2$ (119,120	Heart, lung, brain	—
$\beta 3$ (120,121)	Brain, heart, lung	—
$\beta 4$ (92,122)	Brain, kidney	—

subunits (72,73), probably by helping α_1 to fold into its correct conformation (74), as well as increase the peak current amplitude (75), accelerate activation (72,73,75) or decay of current (75), alter the voltage threshold for activation (75), confer sensitivity to cAMP regulation (76), and even abolish sensitivity to a ligand such as Bay K8644 (74). The role of the α_2-δ and γ subunits have not been clearly defined.

Also shown in Table 2 and 3 are the human chromosomal assignments for those α_1- and β-subunit genes that have been mapped. So far, no human diseases have been linked to an abnormality of a plasma membrane calcium channel gene, but muscular dysgenesis in mice is caused by a single nucleotide deletion in CaCh1 that causes premature termination of translation (77,78).

cDNA CLONING OF RENAL CALCIUM CHANNELS

To further understand the nature of the apical calcium channel of distal tubule, we undertook to isolate the gene encoding its pore-forming ("α_1") subunit by cDNA cloning, using a homology-based approach.

Rationale and Pitfalls of a Homology-Based Approach to Cloning

Genes that share sequence similarity (are "homologous") often encode proteins with similar overall function. To take an example from the expansive potassium channel literature, multiple *Drosophila* and mammalian genes belonging to the so-called *Shaker* family have now been sequenced (79). They share from 55% to 82% amino acid identity to each other and all encode rapidly inactivating (A-type), voltage-dependent, highly potassium-selective channels. Lesser degrees of structural similarity correlate with greater functional divergence. Thus, the more distantly related *Shab* and *Shaw* families also encode voltage-dependent potassium channels, but of the delayed rectifier-type (79). Furthermore, well-circumscribed regions of structural conservation within genes may predict isolated, specific functions that are conserved. For instance, the 17-amino-acid putative pore (P) region is conserved not only within the voltage-dependent potassium channel family but also between channels as diverse as the ATP-sensitive, inward-rectifier (80), and calcium-activated channels (81), whose only common feature is a high selectivity for potassium permeation at the ion pore.*

Could one then infer that the converse might be true, namely that proteins with similar ("analogous") functions might have homologous sequences? This notion forms the theoretical basis for homology-based cloning. However, it cannot be universally true, since more than one structural solution may have evolved in parallel to tackle the same functional problem. For example, the ability to form channels that selectively allow potassium permeation can be found not only in proteins encoded by those homologous genes that contain some form of P region but also by a completely structurally unrelated gene known as minK (83), which bears no resemblance to any of the other potassium channel genes mentioned previously.

Certain functional characteristics might be expected to be better predictors of structure because they confer no evolutionary advantage and therefore would be unlikely to have arisen by convergent evolution. For example, there is no known endogenous ligand for the DHP receptor; the ability of certain calcium channels to bind exogenous DHPs with high affinity probably arose fortuitously rather than through selective pressure. Hence, all such channels might be expected to be homologous.

Multiple α_1 Subunit Transcripts Are Expressed in Kidney

As the distal tubule calcium channel appeared to be divalent cation–selective and DHP-sensitive, we hypothesized that it might be homologous to CaCh1, –2, and –3 (which also encode pore-forming

---

*On the other hand, it has also become increasingly clear that the functional properties of a protein can be significantly altered by a change in a single amino acid. For example, a sodium channel can be altered to become calcium-selective simply by a single nucleotide substitution within its gene (60). The corollary of this is that a protein bearing an apparently familiar structure may function in unexpected ways due to subtle amino acid differences, acquired presumably during divergent evolution. An example of just such a pitfall might be the cyclic nucleotide-gated cation channel, which bears a sequence with remarkable resemblance to the S4 region that is postulated to act as a voltage sensor in voltage-dependent channels. Despite this structure, the channel exhibits minimal voltage dependence (82).

subunits of DHP-sensitive channels) and, by inference, to other members of the calcium channel α_1-subunit gene family. Based on this, a homology-based PCR strategy was devised to isolate calcium channel α_1-subunit transcripts expressed in rat kidney (84). Nondegenerate oligonucleotide primers, each consisting of a single "optimal" nucleotide sequence based on a best guess of the likely target sequence (85), were designed using regions of highly conserved nucleotide sequence between the known isoforms and taking into account preferred codon usage patterns (86). To allow for some mismatch to the cognate target, annealing was performed under lowered stringency conditions. The products amplified by PCR were size fractionated by gel electrophoresis, subcloned, and sequenced. A corollary of the homology-based approach is that simultaneous amplification of multiple different but homologous isoforms may occur, yielding several similar or identical-sized products. Thus, the maximum number of different amplified species cannot be determined from the gel electrophoretic pattern. A restriction digestion-based technique was therefore devised to screen a large number of cloned PCR products rapidly without the need to sequence each individually. Forty-six clones were screened in this way, and eight different species were identified, corresponding to alternatively-spliced variants of four of the known α_1 subunit genes, CaCh1, –2, –3, and –4 (84).

Calcium channel gene expression in the kidney may originate not only from tubule epithelial cells involved in active calcium reabsorption but also form various other cell types. For instance, there is some evidence for the existence of L-type calcium channels in whole glomeruli and in mesangial cells (87,88) and of both L- and T-type channels in vascular smooth muscle cells of intralobar and arcuate arteries of the kidney (89,90). Table 4 summarizes the regional and nephron segment distribution of expression of renal α_1 subunit genes, determined by Northern blot and microdissected tubule-PCR analysis, respectively. The localization of expression of CaCh4 to the renal cortex, and more specifically to an actively calcium-reabsorbing segment such as the distal tubule, is circumstantial evidence for a potential role in transepithelial calcium reabsorption.

What functional properties can be expected of the calcium channel encoded by the renal CaCh4 transcript? The rat brain CaCh4 α_1 subunit transcript, when coexpressed with α_2 and β subunits from skeletal muscle in a *Xenopus* oocyte expression system, encodes a voltage-activated, DHP-insensitive channel that is inhibited by funnel web spider toxin, and therefore resembles most closely the P channel (69,91). However, these properties cannot necessarily be extrapolated to the CaCh4-containing channel in the kidney for two reasons. First, the renal CaCh4 transcript may differ from that expressed in the brain due to alternative splicing. Preliminary analysis of a partial-length renal CaCh4 cDNA encompassing approximately 65% of the coding region indicates two sites that differ from the rat brain transcript and could indeed represent alternative splicing (unpublished observations).

Table 4 Distribution of Calcium Channel α_1- and β-Subunit mRNA Within Rat Kidney

	CaCh1	CaCh2	CaCh3	CaCh4	β2	β3	β4
CORTEX	—	+/–	+	+	+/–	+/–	++
GLOM	—	—		+/–			
PCT	—	—		+/–			
CTAL	—	—		—			
DT	—	—		+			
CCD	—	—		+/–			
OUTER MEDULLA	—	+	++	—	+/–	+	+/–
PSL	—	—		—			
MTAL	+/–	—		—			
INNER MEDULLA	+	++	+	—	+/–	++	—

GLOM, glomerulus; PCT, proximal convoluted tubule; PST, medullary proximal straight tubule; MTAL, medullary thick ascending limb; CTAL, cortical thick ascending limb; DT, distal convoluted tubule/connecting tubule; CCD, cortical collecting duct.

Source: Compiled from Refs. 84 and 92.

Second, the properties of the renal channel also depend on the accessory subunits with which it associates. Of these, the most important in functional terms appears to be the β subunit.

Characterization of Renal Calcium Channel β Subunits

Degenerate primers, based on the amino-acid sequences of the rat $\beta 1$ and $\beta 2$ genes, were used to amplify rat kidney cDNA by PCR (92). As was found with the α_1 subunit, a complex mixture of eight different amplified products was observed, representing the alternatively-spliced transcripts of three different genes, $\beta 2$, $\beta 3$, and $\beta 4$. By Northern blot analysis, $\beta 4$ is preferentially expressed in the renal cortex (Table 4) and is therefore a candidate for the β subunit of the distal tubule calcium channel.

FUTURE DIRECTIONS: DETERMINING THE PHYSIOLOGICAL SIGNIFICANCE OF CaCh4 AND $\beta 4$

In summary, studies to date have identified multiple genes for the pore-forming and accessory subunits of renal calcium channels and identified those that, on the basis of intrarenal distribution, might be considered most likely to play a role in transepithelial calcium transport. Future studies to investigate the physiological significance of these species are now needed. Two areas in particular will be of great interest. First, regulation of the expression of any of these genes by calcium, or calciotropic hormones such as PTH or vitamin D, would support the idea that they play a physiologically relevant role. Second, the participation of a gene product in calcium reabsorption might be directly demonstrable by inhibiting its transcription with a specific antisense construct. A recent preliminary report illustrates this approach (93). CaCh2 (but not CaCh4) is normally expressed in the MDCT cell line. Introduction of an antisense oligodeoxynucleotide to CaCh2 into these cells inhibited chlorothiazide-induced calcium entry. However, the physiological relevance of this particular model to vectorial calcium transport is unclear. Primary cultured monolayers of immuno-dissected rabbit kidney cortical collecting duct and CNT cells, which exhibit vitamin D- and PTH-regulated, active, transepithelial absorption of calcium (94), may prove to be a more promising model in which to study the physiological role of calcium channels.

ACKNOWLEDGMENTS

The author thanks Jonathan Lytton for his support and advice and for critical reading of the manuscript. Work performed by the author and cited in this chapter was made possible by a fellowship from the National Kidney Foundation.

REFERENCES

1. Costanzo LS, Windhager EE. Calcium and sodium transport by the distal convoluted tubule of the rat. Am J Physiol (Renal Fluid Electrolyte Physiol) 1978; 235:F492–F506.
2. Shareghi GR, Stoner LC. Calcium transport across segments of the rabbit distal nephron in vitro. Am J Physiol 1978; 235:F367–F375.
3. Shimizu T, Yoshitomi K, Nakamura M, Imai M. Effects of PTH, calcitonin, and cAMP on calcium transport in rabbit distal nephron segments. Am J Physiol 1990; 259(3 pt 2):F408–F414.
4. Imai M. Effects of parathyroid hormone and N^6, $O^{2'}$-dibutyryl cyclic AMP on Ca^{2+} transport across the rabbit distal nephron segments perfused in vitro. Pflugers Arch 1981; 390:145–151.
5. Friedman PA. Basal and hormone-activated calcium absorption in mouse renal thick ascending limbs. Am J Physiol 1988; 254:F62–F70.
6. Friedman PA, Gesek FA. Calcium transport in renal epithelial cells. Am J Physiol 1993; 264:F181–F198.
7. Gmaj P, Murer H, Kinne R. Calcium ion transport across plasma membranes isolated from rat kidney cortex. Biochem J 1979; 178:549–557.
8. Ramachandran C, Brunette MG. The renal Na^+/Ca^{2+} exchange system is located exclusively in the distal tubule. Biochem J 1989; 257:259–264.
9. Borke JL, Caride A, Verma A, et al. Plasma membrane calcium pump and 28-kDa calcium binding protein in cells of rat kidney distal tubules. Am J Physiol 1989; 257:F842–F849.

10. Magocsi M, Yamaki M, Penniston JT, Dousa TP. Localization of mRNA coding isozymes of plasma membrane Ca^{2+}-ATPase pump in rat kidney. Am J Physiol 1992; 263:F7–F14.
11. Yu ASL, Hebert SC, Lee S-L, et al. Identification and localization of the renal Na^{+}-Ca^{2+} exchanger by the polymerase chain reaction. Am J Physiol 1992; 263:F680–F685.
12. Reilly RF, Shugrue CA. cDNA cloning of a renal Na^{+}-Ca^{2+} exchanger. Am J Physiol 1992; 262:F1105–F1109.
13. Bourdeau JE, Taylor AN, Iacopino AM. Immunocytochemical localization of sodium-calcium exchanger in canine nephron. J Am Soc Nephrol 1993; 4:105–110.
14. Bourdeau JE, Lau K. Effects of parathyroid hormone on cytosolic free calcium concentration in individual rabbit connecting tubules. J Clin Invest 1989; 83:373–379.
15. Yoshitomi K, Shimizu T, Taniguchi J, Imai M. Electrophysiological characterization of rabbit distal convoluted tubule cell. Pflugers Arch. 1989; 414:457–463.
16. Muto S, Yasoshima K, Yoshitomi K, et al. Electrophysiological identification of α- and β-intercalated cells and their distribution along the rabbit distal nephron segments. J Clin Invest 1990; 86:1829–1839.
17. Bacskai BJ, Friedman PA. Activation of latent Ca^{2+} channels in renal epithelial cells by parathyroid hormone. Nature (London) 1990; 347:388–391.
18. Pizzonia JH, Gesek FA, Kennedy SM, et al. Immunomagnetic separation, primary culture and characterization of thick ascending limb and distal convoluted tubule cells from mouse kidney. In Vitro Cell Dev Biol 1991; 27A:409–416.
19. Janis RA, Triggle DJ. 1,4-dihydropyridine Ca^{2+} channel antagonists and activators: A comparison of binding characteristics with pharmacology. Drug Dev Res 1984; 4:257–274.
20. Brunette MG, Mailloux J, Lajeunesse D. Calcium transport through the luminal membrane of the distal tubule; I. Interrelationship with sodium. Kidney Int 1992; 41:281–288.
21. Brunette MG, Mailloux J, Lajeunesse D. Calcium transport through the luminal membrane of the distal tubule: II. Effect of pH, electrical potential and calcium channel inhibitors. Kidney Int 1992; 41:289–296.
22. Lajeunesse D, Bouhtiauy I, Mailloux J, Brunette MG. Parathyroid hormone (PTH) opens calcium (Ca^{2+}) channels in the luminal membrane (LUM) from rabbit distal tubule (DT) (abstr). J Am Soc Nephrol 1991; 2:638.
23. Matsunaga H, Friedman PA, Kizer N, Stanton BA. Calcium channels in apical membranes of distal convoluted tubule cells (abstr). J Am Soc Nephrol 1991; 2:627.
24. Lau K, Quamme GST. Patch-clamp evidence for a Ca channel in apical membrane of cortical thick ascending limb (cTAL) and distal tubule (DT) cells (abstr). J Am Soc Nephrol 1991; 2:775.
25. Poncet V, Merot J, Poujeol P. A calcium-permeable channel in the apical membrane of primary cultures of the rabbit distal bright convoluted tubule. Pflugers Arch. 1992; 422:112–119.
26. Bean BP. Classes of calcium channels in vertebrate cells. Annu Rev Physiol 1989; 51:367–384.
27. Hess P. Calcium channels in vertebrate cells. Annu Rev Neurosci 1990; 13:337–356.
28. Reuter H, Stevens CF, Tsien RW, Yellen G. Properties of single calcium channels in cardiac cell culture. Nature 1982; 297:501–504.
29. Fox AP, Nowycky MC, Tsien TW. Kinetic and pharmacological properties distinguishing three types of calcium currents in chick sensory neurones. J Physiol 1987; 394:149–172.
30. Fox AP, Nowycky MC, Tsien RW. Single-channel recordings of three types of calcium channels in chick sensory neurones. J Physiol 1987; 394:173–200.
31. Thomas G, Gross R, Schramm M. Calcium channel modulation: Ability to inhibit or promote calcium influx residues in the same dihydropyridine molecule. J Cardiovasc Pharmacol 1984; 6:1170–1176.
32. Scott RH, Dolphin AC. Activation of a G protein promotes agonist response to calcium channel ligands. Nature 1987; 330:760–762.
33. Usowicz MM, Sugimori M, Cherksey B, Llinàs R. P-type calcium channels in the somata and dendrites of adult cerebellar Purkinje cells. Neuron 1992; 9:1185–1199.
34. Llinàs R, Sugimori M, Lin J-W, Cherksey B. Blocking and isolation of a calcium channel from neurons in mammals and cephalopods utilizing a toxin fraction (FTX) from funnel-web spider poison. Proc Natl Acad Sci USA 1989; 86:1689–1693.
35. Benham CD, Tsien RW. Calcium-permeable channels in vascular smooth muscle: Voltage-activated, receptor-operated, and leak channels. Soc Gen Physiol Symp 1987; 42:45–64.
36. Coulombe A, Lefèvre IA, Baro I, Coraboeuf E. Barium- and calcium-permeable channels open at negative membrane potentials in rat ventricular myocytes. J Memb Biol 1989; 111:57–67.
37. Rosenberg RL, Hess P, Tsien RW. L-type channels and calcium-permeable channels open at negative membrane potentials. J Gen Physiol 1988; 92:27–54.
38. Fong P, Turner PR, Denetclaw WF, Steinhardt RA. Increased activity of calcium leak channels in myotubes of Duchenne human and *mdx* mouse origin. Science 1990; 250:673–676.
39. Curtis BM, Caterall WA. Purification of the calcium antagonist receptor of the voltage-sensitive calcium channel from skeletal muscle transverse tubules. Biochemistry 1984; 23:2113–2118.

40. Borsotto M, Barhanin J, Fosset M, Lazdunski M. The 1,4-dihydropyridine receptor associated with the skeletal muscle voltage-dependent Ca^{2+} channel. J Biol Chem 1985; 260:14255–14263.
41. Caterall WA, Seagar MJ, Takahashi M. Molecular properties of dihydropyridine-sensitive calcium channels in skeletal muscle. J Biol Chem 1988; 263:3535–3538.
42. Takahashi M, Seager MJ, Jones JF, et al. Subunit structure of dihydropyridine-sensitive calcium channels from skeletal muscle. Proc Natl Acad Sci USA 1987; 84:5478–5482.
43. Sharp AH, Imagawa T, Leung AT, Campbell KP. Identification and characterization of the dihydropyridine-binding subunit of the skeletal muscle dihydropyridine receptor. J Biol Chem 1987; 262:12309–12315.
44. Vaghy PL, Streissnig J, Miwa K, et al. Identification of a novel 1,4-dihydropyridine- and phenylalkylamine-binding polypeptide in calcium channel preparations. J Biol Chem 1987; 262:14337–14342.
45. Streissnig J, Knaus H-G, Grabner M, et al. Photoaffinity labelling of the phenylalkylamine receptor of the skeletal muscle transverse-tubule calcium channel. FEBS Lett 1987; 212:247–253.
46. McEnery MW, Snowman AM, Sharp AH, et al. Purified ω-conotoxin GVIA receptor of rat brain resembles a dihydropyridine-sensitive L-type calcium channel. Proc Natl Acad Sci USA 1991; 88:11095–11099.
47. Witcher DR, De Waard M, Sakamoto J, et al. Subunit identification and reconstitution of the N-type Ca^{2+} channel complex purified from brain. Science 1993; 261:486–489.
48. Tanabe T, Takeshima H, Mikami A, et al. Primary structure of the receptor for calcium channel blockers from skeletal muscle. Nature (London) 1987; 328:313–318.
49. Stühmer W. Structure-function studies of voltage-gated ion channels. Annu Rev Biophys Chem 1991; 20:65–78.
50. MacKinnon R. Determination of the subunit stoichiometry of a voltage-activated potassium channel. Nature 1991; 350:232–235.
51. Miller C. Ion channel structure and function. Science 1992; 258:240–241.
52. Liman ER, Hess P, Weaver F, Koren G. Voltage-sensing residues in the S4 region of a mammalian K^+ channel. Nature 1991; 353:752–756.
53. Papazian DM, Timpe LC, Jan YN, Jan LY. Alteration of voltage-dependence of *Shaker* potassium channel by mutations in the S4 sequence. Nature 1991; 349:305–310.
54. Stühmer W, Conti F, Suzuki H, et al. Structural parts involved in activation and inactivation of the sodium channel. Nature 1989; 339:597–603.
55. Auld VJ, Goldin AL, Krafte DS, et al. A neutral amino acid change in segment IIS4 dramatically alters the gating properties of the voltage-dependent sodium channel. Proc Natl Acad Sci 1990; 87:323–327.
56. MacKinnon R, Yellen G. Mutations affecting TEA blockade and ion permeation in voltage-activated K^+ channels. Science 1990; 250:276–279.
57. Hartmann HA, Kirsch GE, Drewe JA, et al. Exchange of conduction pathways between two related K^+ channels. Science 1991; 251:942–944.
58. Yool AJ, Schwartz TL. Alteration of ionic selectivity of a K^+ channel by mutation of the H5 region. Nature 1991; 349:700–704.
59. Yellen G, Jurman ME, Abramson T, MacKinnon R. Mutations affecting internal TEA blockade identify the probable pore-forming region of a K^+ channel. Science 1991; 251:939–942.
60. Heinemann SH, Terlau H, Stühmer W, et al. Calcium channel characteristics conferred on the sodium channel by single mutations. Nature 1992; 356:441–443.
61. Durell SR, Guy HR. Atomic scale structure and functional models of voltage-gated potassium channels. Biophys J 1992; 62:238–250.
62. Ellis SB, Williams ME, Ways NR, et al. Sequence and expression of mRNAs encoding the α_1 and α_2 subunits of a DHP-sensitive calcium channel. Science 1988; 241:1661–1664.
63. Ruth P. Röhrkasten A, Biel M, et al. Primary structure of the β subunit of the DHP-sensitive calcium channel from skeletal muscle. Science 1989; 245:1115–1118.
64. Bosse E, Regulla S, Biel M, et al. The cDNA and deduced amino acid sequence of the γ subunit of the L-type calcium channel from rabbit skeletal muscle. FEBS Lett 1990; 267:153–156.
65. Jay SD, Ellis SB, McCue A, et al. Primary structure of the γ subunit of the DHP-sensitive calcium channel from skeletal muscle. Science 1990; 248:490–492.
66. Perez-Reyes E, Kim HS, Lacerda AE, et al. Induction of calcium currents by the expression of the α_1-subunit of the dihydropyridine receptor from skeletal muscle. Nature (London) 1989; 340:233–236.
67. Mikami A, Imoto K, Tanabe T, et al. Primary structure and functional expression of the cardiac dihydropyridine-sensitive calcium channel. Nature (London) 1989; 340:230–233.
68. Williams ME, Feldman DH, NcCue AF, et al. Structure and functional expression of α_1, α_2, and β subunits of a novel human neuronal calcium channel subtype. Neuron 1992; 8:71–84.
69. Sather WA, Tanabe T, Zhang J-F, et al. Distinctive biophysical and pharmacological properties of class A (BI) calcium channel α_1 subunits. Neuron 1993; 11:291–303.
70. Williams ME, Brust PF, Feldman DH, et al. Structure and functional expression of an ω-conotoxin-sensitive human N-type calcium channel. Science 1992; 257:389–395.

71. Soong TW, Stea A, Hodson CD, et al. Structure and functional expression of a member of the low voltage-activated calcium channel family. Science 1993; 260:1133–1136.
72. Lacerda AE, Kim HS, Ruth P, et al. Normalization of current kinetics by interaction between the α_1 and β subunits of the skeletal muscle dihydropyridine-sensitive Ca^{2+} channel. Nature 1991; 352:527–530.
73. Varadi G, Lory P, Schultz D, et al. Acceleration of activation and inactivation by the β subunit of the skeletal muscle calcium channel. Nature 1991; 352:159–162.
74. Nishimura S, Takeshima H, Hofmann F, et al. Requirement of the calcium channel β subunit for functional conformation. FEBS Lett 1993; 324:283–286.
75. Singer D, Biel M, Lotan I, et al. The roles of the subunits in the function of the calcium channel. Science 1991; 253:1553–1557.
76. Klöckner U, Itagaki K, Bodi I, Schwartz A. β-subunit expression is required for cAMP-dependent increase of cloned cardiac and vascular calcium channel current. Pflugers Arch 1992; 420:413–415.
77. Knudson CM, Chaudhari N, Sharp AH, et al. Specific absence of the alpha 1 subunit of the dihydropyridine receptor in mice with muscular dysgenesis. J Biol Chem 1989; 264:1345–1348.
78. Chaudhari N. A single nucleotide deletion in the skeletal muscle-specific calcium channel transcript of muscular dysgenesis (mdg) mice. J Biol Chem 1992; 267:25636–25639.
79. Salkoff L, Baker K, Butler A, et al. An essential "set" of K^+ channels conserved in flies, mice and humans. Trends Neurosci 1992; 15:161–166.
80. Ho K, Nichols CG, Lederer WJ, et al. Cloning and expression of an inwardly rectifying ATP-regulated potassium channel. Nature 1993; 362:31–38.
81. Atkinson NS, Robertson GA, Ganetzky B. A component of calcium-activated potassium channels encoded by the *Drosophila slo* locus Science 1991; 253:551–555.
82. Jan LY, Jan YN. A superfamily of ion channels. Nature 1990; 345:672.
83. Takumi T, Ohkubo H, Nakanishi S. Cloning of a membrane protein that induces a slow voltage-gated potassium current. Science 1988; 242:1042–1045.
84. Yu ASL, Hebert SC, Brenner BM, Lytton J. Molecular characterization and nephron distribution of a family of transcripts encoding the pore-forming subunit of Ca2+ channels in the kidney. Proc Natl Acad Sci USA 1992; 89:10494–10498.
85. Lathe R. Synthetic oligonucleotide probes deduced from amino acid sequence data: Theoretical and practical considerations. J Mol Biol 1985; 183:1–12.
86. Wada K, Aota S, Tsuchiya R, et al. Codon usage tabulated from the GenBank genetic sequence data. Nucleic Acids Res 1990; 18(suppl):2367–2403.
87. Iijima K, Moore LC, Goligorsky MS. Syncytial organization of cultured rat mesangial cells. Am J Physiol 1991; 260:F848–F855.
88. McDermott GF, Hurst RD, Whiteside CI. Isolated rat glomerular cells demonstrate L-type Ca^{2+}-channel activity. Cell Calcium 1993; 14:387–396.
89. Gordienko D, Goligorsky M. Voltage-operated and calcium-activated channels in renal microvascular smooth muscle cells (abstr). J Am Soc Nephrol 1992; 3:562.
90. Goligorsky MS, Colflesh D, Gordienko D, Moore LC. Functional analysis of branching points (BP) in renal microvasculature (abstr). J Am Soc Nephrol 1993; 4:579.
91. Mori Y, Friedrich T, Kim M-S, et al. Primary structure and functional expression from complementary DNA of a brain calcium channel. Nature (London) 1991; 350:398–402.
92. Yu ASL, Castellano A, Perez-Reyes E, Lytton J. Molecular cloning of the β subunit of a renal Ca^{2+} channel (abstr). J Am Soc Nephrol 1993; 4:717.
93. Barry ELR, Gesek FA, Friedman PA. Antisense inhibition of a calcium channel in distal convoluted tubule cells (abstr). J Am Soc Nephrol 1993; 4:862.
94. Bindels RJM, Hartog A, Timmermans J, Van Os CH. Active Ca^{2+} transport in primary cultures of rabbit kidney CCD: Stimulation by 1,25-dihydroxyvitamin D_3 and PTH. Am J Physiol 1991; 261:F779–F807.
95. Tsien RW, Lipscombe D, Madison DV, et al. Multiple types of neuronal calcium channels and their selective modulation. Trends Neurosci 1988; 11:431–438.
96. Mintz IM, Venema VJ, Swiderek KM, et al. P-type calcium channels blocked by the spider toxin ω-Aga-IVA. Nature 1992; 355:827–829.
97. Hillyard DR, Monje VD, Mintz IM, et al. A new Conus peptide ligand for mammalian presynaptic Ca^{2+} channels. Neuron 1992; 9:69–77.
98. Gregg RG, Couch F, Hogan K, Powers PA. Assignment of the human gene for the alpha 1 subunit of the skeletal muscle DHP-sensitive Ca2+ channel (CACNL1A3) to chromosome 1q31-q32. Genomics 1993; 15:107–112.
99. Koch WJ, Ellinor PT, Schwartz A. cDNA cloning of a dihydropyridine-sensitive calcium channel from rat aorta. J Biol Chem 1990; 265:17786–17791.
100. Snutch TP, Tomlinson WJ, Leonard JP, Gilbert MM. Distinct calcium channels are generated by alternative splicing and are differentially expressed in the mammalian CNS. Neuron 1991; 7:45–57.

101. Biel M, Ruth P, Bosse E, et al. Primary structure and functional expression of a high voltage activated calcium channel from rabbit lung. FEBS Lett 1990; 269:409–412.
102. Schultz D, Mikala G, Yatani A, et al. Cloning, chromosomal localization, and functional expression of the alpha 1 subunit of the L-type voltage-dependent calcium channel from normal human heart. Proc Natl Acad Sci USA 1993; 90:6228–6232.
103. Powers PA, Gregg RG, Hogan K. Linkage mapping of the human gene for the alpha 1 subunit of the cardiac DHP-sensitive Ca2+ channel (CACNL1A1) to chromosome 12p13.2-pter using a dinucleotide repeat. Genomics 1992; 14:206–207.
104. Sun W, McPherson JD, Hoang DQ, et al. Mapping of a human brain voltage-gated calcium channel to human chromosome 12p13-pter. Genomics 1992; 14:1092–1094.
105. Hui A, Ellinor PT, Krizanova O, et al. Molecular cloning of multiple subtypes of a novel rat brain isoform of the α_1 subunit of the voltage-dependent calcium channel. Neuron 1991; 7:35–44.
106. Seino S, Chen L, Seino M, et al. Cloning of the α_1 subunit of a voltage-dependent calcium channel expressed in pancreatic β cells. Proc Natl Acad Sci USA 1992; 89:584–588.
107. Seino S, Yamada Y, Espinosa 3rd R, et al. Assignment of the gene encoding the alpha 1 subunit of the neuroendocrine/brain-type calcium channel (CACNL1A2) to human chromosome 3, band p14.3. Genomics 1992; 13:1375–1377.
108. Chin H, Kozak CA, Kim H-L, et al. A brain L-type calcium channel α1 subunit gene (CCHL1A2) maps to mouse chromosome 14 and human chromosome 3. Genomics 1991; 11:914–919.
109. Starr TVB, Prystay W, Snutch TP. Primary structure of a calcium channel that is highly expressed in rat cerebellum. Proc Nat Acad Sci USA 1991; 88:5621–5625.
110. Dubel SJ, Starr TVB, Hell J, et al. Molecular cloning of the α-1 subunit of an ω-conotoxin-sensitive calcium channel. Proc Natl Acad Sci USA 1992; 89:5058–5062.
111. Fujita Y, Mynlieff M, Dirksen RT, et al. Primary structure and functional expression of the ω-conotoxin-sensitive N-type calcium channel from rabbit brain. Neuron 1993; 10:585–598.
112. Niidome T, Kim M-S, Friedrich T, Mori Y. Molecular cloning and characterization of a novel calcium channel from rabbit brain. FEBS Lett 1992; 308:7–13.
113. Perez-Reyes E, Wei X, Castellano A, Birnbaumer L. Molecular diversity of L-type calcium channels. J Biol Chem 1990; 265:20430–20436.
114. Snutch TP, Leonard JP, Gilbert MM, et al. Rat brain expresses a heterogeneous family of calcium channels. Proc Natl Acad Sci USA 1990; 87:3391–3395.
115. Pragnell M, Sakamoto J, Jay SD, Campbell KP. Cloning and tissue-specific expression of the brain calcium channel β-subunit. FEBS Lett 1991; 291:253–258.
116. Powers PA, Liu S, Hogan K, Gregg RG. Skeletal muscle and brain isoforms of a β-subunit of human voltage-dependent calcium channels are encoded by a single gene. J Biol Chem 1992; 267:22967–22972.
117. Collin T, Wang J-J, Nargeot J, Schwartz A. Molecular cloning of three isoforms of the L-type voltage-dependent calcium channel β subunit from normal human heart. Circ Res 1993; 72:1337–1344.
118. Gregg RG, Powers PA, Hogan K. Assignment of the human gene for the beta subunit of the voltage-dependent calcium channel (CACNLB1) to chromosome 17 using somatic cell hybrids and linkage mapping. Genomics 1993; 15:185–187.
119. Perez-Reyes E, Castellano A, Kim HS, et al. Cloning and expression of a cardiac/brain β subunit of the L-type calcium channel. J Biol Chem 1992; 267:1792–1797.
120. Hullin R, Singer-Lahat D, Freichel M, et al. Calcium channel β subunit heterogeneity: Functional expression of cloned cDNA from heart, aorta and brain. EMBO J 1992; 11:885–890.
121. Castellano A, Wei X, Birnbaumer L, Perez-Reyes E. Cloning and expression of a third calcium channel β subunit. J Biol Chem 1993; 268:3450–3455.
122. Castellano A, Wei X, Birnbaumer L, Perez-Reyes E. Cloning and expression of a neuronal calcium channel beta subunit. J Biol Chem 1993; 268:12359–12366.

30
Glucose Transporter Expression in the Kidney

Frank C. Brosius III
University of Michigan Medical School, Ann Arbor, Michigan

INTRODUCTION

Kidney cells may synthesize glucose for systemic utilization, reabsorb glucose across the cell body, or utilize glucose for energy needs. Each of these diverse processes requires the transport of glucose across the plasma membrane. The proteins mediating this transport have been identified over the past several years and the regulation of renal glucose transporter expression is being explored currently. In many cell types, the molecular expression of these transporters largely determines the cellular response to exogenous glucose and in certain cases may determine the metabolic consequences of conditions such as diabetes mellitus, which alter extracellular glucose concentrations.

Two families of glucose transport proteins are expressed in renal and other mammalian cells. The transporters most familiar to renal physiologists are the sodium-glucose cotransporters, which mediate the reabsorption of glucose from the tubular lumen across the apical membrane of proximal tubular and intestinal epithelial cells. Because transport is driven by the inward electrochemical gradient for sodium, sodium-glucose cotransporters are able to transport glucose against its chemical gradient. The second family of transporters is made up of the facilitative glucose transporters, which promote net transport of glucose down its chemical gradient, usually into cells. These transporters are probably expressed in all mammalian cells; this chapter concentrates on their regulation.

In the following subsections a synopsis of the current status of molecular research on glucose transporters is offered and related to glucose transport expression in renal tissues. This is followed by a discussion of the role of glucose transporters and transport in diabetes mellitus and diabetic nephropathy.

MOLECULAR CLONING OF GLUCOSE TRANSPORTERS

Sodium-Glucose Cotransporters

An epithelial sodium-glucose cotransporter, SGLT1, was initially cloned from a rabbit intestinal cDNA library (1). The hydropathy profile of its primary sequence predicts a membrane-associated protein with 11 membrane spans (Fig. 1). The molecular cloning of several related cDNAs has been accomplished based on sequence similarity with SGLT1. These include: (a) a cDNA which induces Na-coupled methyl-glucose uptake twofold when its cRNA is expressed in *Xenopus* oocytes and therefore may encode the low-affinity sodium-glucose cotransporter. This transporter has now been termed SGLT2 (2); (b) a sodium-nucleoside cotransporter (3); and (c) a Na^+-dependent neutral amino acid transporter (4). Although cloned via an expression cloning system, the cDNA sequence of the sodium-coupled myoinositol transporter (5), which helps to maintain cell volume in response to osmotic stress, is also similar to SGLT1 and the other members of this growing family of sodium-coupled transporters.

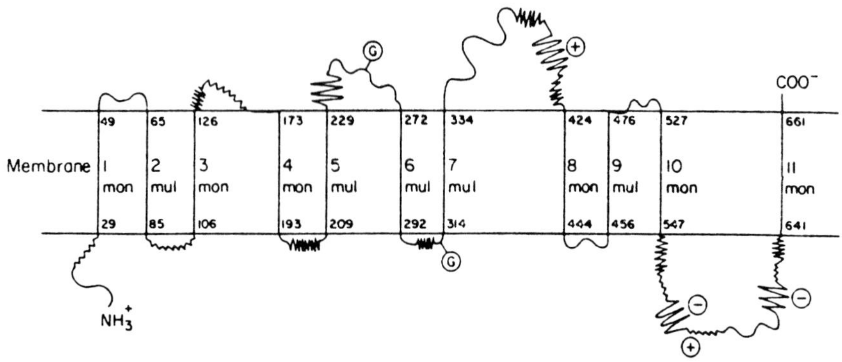

Figure 1 Proposed secondary structure for the Na^+-glucose cotransporter, SGLT1, showing 11 transmembrane spans, one potential N-linked glycosylation site (G), and clusters of negative (–) and positive (+) charges. (From Ref. 1.)

Facilitative Glucose Transporters

In contrast to the SGLT1 family or sodium-dependent cotransporters, all the members of the facilitative glucose transporter family have been shown to transport glucose (6,7), and all (except possibly GLUT7) are expressed to some degree in human and rodent kidney (Table 1) (6,8–18). The primary amino acid sequence of GLUT1, the prototypical member of the family, predicts the presence of 12 membrane spans with an extracellular loop between spans 1 and 2 and a larger intracellular loop between spans 6 and 7 (Fig. 2). The major sequence differences between GLUT1 and the other five GLUT isoforms are in these two loops and at the carboxyl and amino termini. Thus, most of the antisera that discriminate between these transporters have been directed at these areas of divergence, especially the carboxyl terminus. Many of the GLUT isoforms have been cloned from several species, including humans, and there is very high (usually >90%) sequence simularity in the same isoform from different species with the exception of GLUT3, in which rodent and human sequences diverge significantly, including at the carboxyl terminus (19,20).

RENAL EXPRESSION OF GLUCOSE TRANSPORTER ISOFORMS

SGLT1

Functional data have suggested the presence of two different sodium-glucose cotransport activities in the proximal tubule, one that has low affinity, transports one sodium molecule for every glucose molecule, and is concentrated in the S1 and S2 regions, and the another that has high affinity, transports two sodium molecules for each glucose molecule, and is concentrated in the S3 segment (21,22). Although there remains some controversy, it appears that the molecules responsible for these two activities have been identified. SGLT1 is highly expressed in the apical brush border of epithelia of the the proximal tubule, and kinetic analysis has shown it to be a high-affinity transporter (23). Although initial immunolocalization studies detected SGLT1 throughout the proximal tubule (15,24), more recent in situ hybridization analysis has shown that SGLT1 mRNA is confined to S3-segment epithelia in rat (25). SGLT2 [Hu14 in the original cloning paper (2)] has not been as well characterized but appears to be a low-affinity transporter (2,26). These studies have led to the following schema of transepithelial glucose transport in the proximal tubule. In the S1 (and possibly S2 segments) SGLT2 on the apical membrane is coupled with the low-affinity/high capacitance-facilitative transporter GLUT2, on the basolateral surface of the cells, whereas in the S3 segment, SGLT1 is coupled with the high-affinity facilitative transporter GLUT1. Together these representatives of the two glucose transport families effect transepithelial glucose reabsorption (Fig. 3).

Table 1 Properties of the Cloned Facilitative Glucose Transporters

Transporter designation	Tissue distribution	Renal distribution	Km (m*M*)	Functional features
GLUT1	Brain and nerve endothelia (blood-brain barrier), erythrocytes, placenta, kidney, most tissues	Connecting segment, CCD, MCD > MTAL > PST (S3). Low-level expression in glomerulus	2–20 (Probably on low end of scale in most native cells)	Expression in all cultured cells; may be higher in glycolytically active cells. Present in GLUT4–containing cells
GLUT2	Liver, pancreatic β cell, kidney, small intestine	PCT cells (S1)	20–66	Low-affinity transporter. In gluconeogenic cells. Part of β-cell glucose sensor.
GLUT3	Brain, testis > heart, placenta, liver > kidney	Glomerulus, TAL, MCD	Probably very low (<1) in native tissues	Major neuronal transporter.
GLUT4	Fat; skeletal, cardiac and vascular smooth muscle	Glomerular mesangial and epithelial cells, microvascular smooth muscle cells, MTAL	3–7	Insulin-responsive transporter. In intracellular vesicles in unstimulated cells, translocated to cell surface with insulin and other stimuli.
GLUT5	Intestine, testis > fat, skeletal and heart muscle, kidney, blood-brain barrier	PST	(See next column)	Functions primarily as fructose carrier. Apical transporter in intestine.
GLUT6	Pseudogene	—	—	—
GLUT7	Liver, (?) other tissues	?	?	Enodplasmic reticulum (ER) transporter, (?) transports glucose produced by glucose-6-phosphatase from ER lumen.

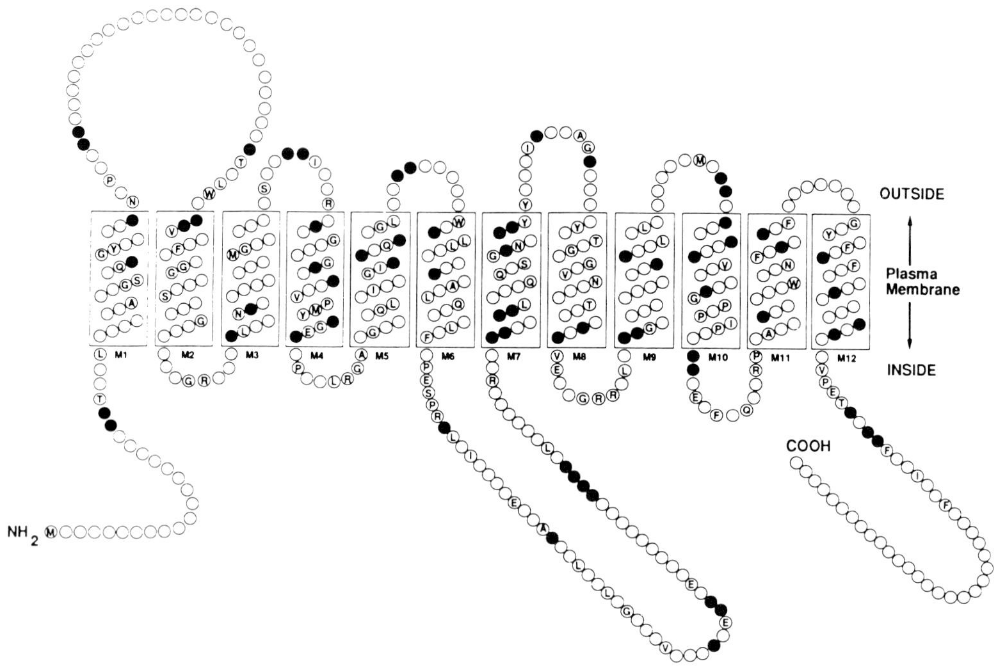

Figure 2 Proposed secondary structure for the members of the facilitative glucose transporter family. The 12 putative transmembrane spans are shown as boxes and are numbered 1 to 12. There is a potential N-linked glycosylation site in the extracellular loop between spans 1 and 2 in all members of the family. Identical amino acids in GLUT1-GLUT5 are indicated by their single-letter abbreviations, and chemically similar residues are denoted by black circles. (From Ref. 70.)

GLUT1

In contrast to the sodium-glucose cotransporters, which are confined to the apical membrane of proximal tubular cells, facilitative glucose transporters are expressed in every renal cell where their expression has been investigated and are probably present in all mammalian cells. The presence of multiple facilitative glucose transporter isoforms in kidney and other tissues implies that functional distinctions exist between the different transporters. Indeed, the pattern of isoform expression in a cell type often reflects its pattern of glucose metabolism (Table 1). For example, GLUT1 is a high-affinity transporter which is expressed on the basolateral membrane of proximal tubular cells in the S3 segment, where a higher-affinity transporter is needed given the low concentrations of luminal (and hence intracellular) glucose. It is also expressed in the thick ascending limb cells and, at highest levels, in cortical and medullary collecting tubular cells (14). These latter cell types do not participate significantly in transepithelial glucose reabsorption but are characterized by high energy needs and high glycolytic activity (14). GLUT1 may be expressed in virtually all cells at lower levels, and reports have identified this transporter in cultured vascular smooth muscle cells (27,28) and renal mesangial cells (29–30). However, given the universal induction of GLUT1 expression in culture (31), the identification of GLUT1 as a major transporter in cultured vascular smooth muscle and mesangial cells is not surprising, nor does it shed light on the expression of GLUT1 in these cells in vivo.

GLUT2

GLUT2, which is a low-affinity transporter (K_m of GLUT2 for glucose is >20 mM), is expressed on the basolateral membrane of S1 proximal tubular and intestinal epithelial cells (14,15), which reabsorb large amounts of glucose, and in hepatocytes (10). Pancreatic β cells also express GLUT2 in tandem with the low-affinity hexokinase hexokinase IV or glucokinase (the K_m for glucokinase

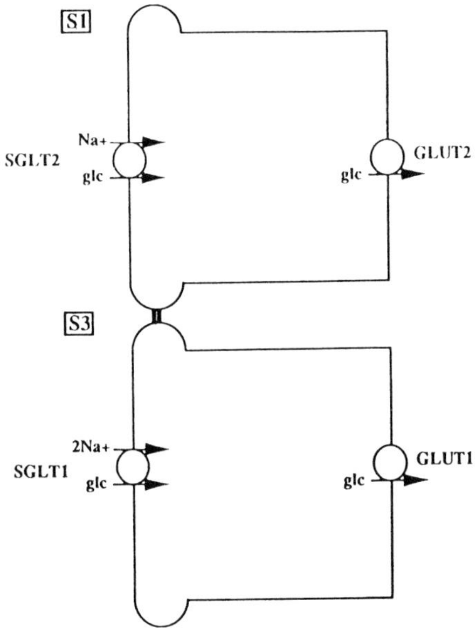

Figure 3 Schematic model of transepithelial glucose transport in the proximal tubule, showing apical SGLT2 and basolateral GLUT2 mediating transport in the S1 segment, and SGLT2 and GLUT1 performing analogous roles in the S3 segment.

is approximately 6 m*M*). Together these two molecules make up the rate-limiting steps in the glucose sensing system of the cell. Only a low-affinity system can respond significantly to physiological changes in extracellular glucose concentration (32). The other GLUTs and hexokinases have low K_ms, which are generally below the physiological range of extracellular glucose.

GLUT4

GLUT4 is the insulin-responsive transporter and is expressed at high levels in skeletal and cardiac muscle and in fat (6). In contrast to the other transporters, GLUT4 molecules are largely confined to an intracellular vesicular compartment except when cells are subjected to an appropriate stimulus such as insulin exposure. With such stimuli, GLUT4 molecules are translocated to the plasma membrane of the cell, where they participate in glucose uptake (Fig. 4). Thus, GLUT4 molecules are largely responsible for insulin-stimulated glucose uptake. Somewhat surprisingly, GLUT4 molecules are also expressed in several kidney regions that are not known to have insulin-responsive glucose uptake. It appears that GLUT4 is most highly expressed in vascular smooth muscle cells of the afferent microvasculature and in glomerular mesangial and epithelial cells (12). GLUT4 protein can easily be detected in these regions by multiple techniques (12), including immunoblotting of vascular preparations (55). It is unknown whether GLUT4 in these cells is translocated to the cell surface in response to insulin, as it is in muscle and fat tissues. However, preliminary immunoelectronmicroscopic studies of glomerular podocytes suggest that these cells may contain GLUT4 in intracellular vesicles (C. Heilig; personal communication). GLUT4 mRNA and protein were also recently localized to thick ascending limb cells (16). It was speculated that GLUT4 expression there may contribute to the elevated requirements for glucose as a fuel in this metabolically active segment and that insulin-like growth factor 1 (IGF-1) may regulate plasma membrane expression in those cells (16).

Other Transporters

Little is known about GLUT3, GLUT5, or GLUT7 expression in kidney. In preliminary studies, GLUT3 mRNA has been detected in rat glomerulus, proximal convuluted tubule, thick ascending limb, and collecting duct cells (13,33), as well as in preglomerular vessels. However, there appears

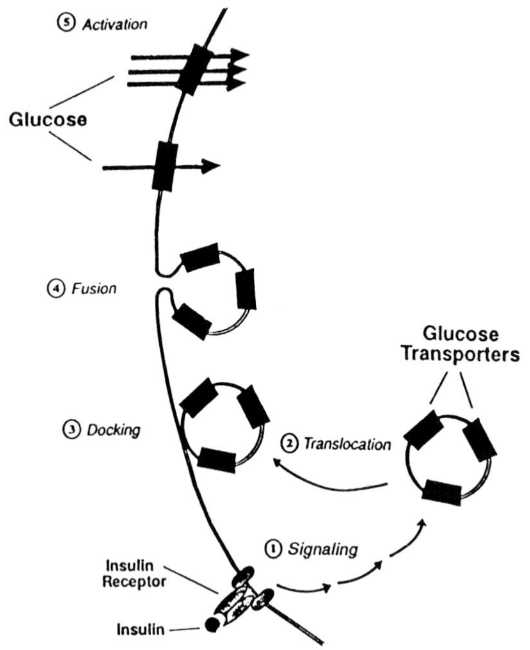

Figure 4 Representation of insulin-stimulated glucose uptake in insulin-sensitive cells. After insulin binds to its receptor, a signal transduction cascade occurs (1), which stimulates translocation of intracellular vesicles containing the insulin-responsive transporter GLUT4 to the cell surface (2). Docking (3) and fusion (4) of the vesicles with the cell membrane place a large number of GLUT4 molecules on the cell surface, where they rapidly transport glucose into the cell. There is also an activation step in which the maximal rate of transport by each individual GLUT4 molecule is increased (5). Dysregulation of any of these events will render the cell insulin-resistant. (From Ref. 34.)

to be discordance between GLUT3 mRNA and protein expression, as GLUT3 polypeptide appears to be confined to thick ascending limb cells and inner medullary collecting duct cells (C. Heilig et al., personal communication). The renal expression of GLUT3 may differ between rodent and human kidney (19,20). GLUT5 appears to function primarily as a fructose carrier (34), and its mRNA is expressed in the S3 region of the proximal tubule (16).

REGULATION OF GLUCOSE TRANSPORTER EXPRESSION

Glucose transporter expression and activity can be regulated at the transcriptional, translational, or posttranslational levels (6,34). Furthermore, for at least several of the isoforms, the subcellular distribution of the transporter is a critical determinant of cellular glucose uptake (34). Obviously, only plasma membrane transporters can function in cellular glucose uptake. In general, GLUT protein levels and functional activity (i.e., glucose uptake) parallel GLUT transcript levels, but multiple exceptions to this rule have been reported (34), so that no safe conclusions can be derived from measurements of mRNA expression alone. Also, regulation of expression of any one GLUT isoform is tissue-specific and, in certain cases, factors that increase expression and activity in one cell type cause the opposite response in another cell type (34). In the subsections below, general aspects of GLUT isoform regulation are considered. Effects of diabetes mellitus and altered extracellular glucose levels are then described in the following section.

GLUT1

GLUT1 and GLUT4 are the only isoforms for which transcriptional regulation has been studied to any significant extent. GLUT1 transcription is rapidly induced by oncogenic transformation or exposure to serum, growth factors, and various cytokines (35–39). This induction requires no new protein synthesis, thus identifying GLUT1 as an immediate early response gene (37). The GLUT1 enhancer regions in the mouse are characterized by a number of specific response elements, including serum response elements (SREs), cyclic AMP response elements (CREs), and TPA response elements (TREs) (40). Thus, any stimulus that induces binding of these elements by transcription factors also increases transcription and steady-state levels of GLUT1 mRNA. For example, cAMP and its analogues have been shown to increase GLUT1 mRNA levels in mouse granular cells from the juxtaglomerular apparatus (41) as well as in other cells, such as 3T3-L1 cells, a differentiating adipocyte cell line which has been heavily investigated as a model for insulin action on insulin-sensitive tissues (42). The promoter/enhancer elements of the GLUT1 gene account in part for the induction of GLUT1 mRNA and protein in virtually all cultured cells. Indeed, GLUT1 is frequently the predominant transporter even in cell lines that derive from tissue in which another transporter is dominant (8,31,43). Thus the study of glucose transporter expression in cultured cells has to be tempered by the realization that GLUT1 expression is likely to be mich higher in vitro than in vivo (31). It has been speculated that GLUT1 induction is necessary for oncogenic transformation; in this regard, it is interesting that several revertants from NIH 3T3 cells that had been transformed with a c-H-*ras* oncogne had GLUT1 levels which were significantly lower than those of the transformed cells and which were equivalent to GLUT1 levels in nontransformed 3T3 cells (44). However, there is evidence that oncogenic transformation in vivo does not require GLUT1 induction or activation (31), and cells from some malignant tumors have little or no GLUT1 expression (31).

Final GLUT1 expression is also determined by regulation of mRNA stability, at least in part through interaction of the 3′ untranslated region with the adenosine-uridine binding factor (45). Degrees of GLUT1 translocation can also vary, at least in isolated adipocytes and cultured cell lines (46,47), and activity of individual GLUT1 molecules may be affected by other posttranslational steps (48,49). An individual stimulus can affect GLUT1 expression at several levels. For example, TNF-α increases GLUT1 mRNA stability, GLUT1 translocation, and activity of individual GLUT1 molecules in 3T3-L1 preadipocytes (38,45,50).

Several studies have examined the effects of diabetes mellitus and extracellular glucose on glucose transporter expression in kidney. These reports are considered in the next section. Otherwise, very few studies have specifically looked at renal GLUT1 expression. In one study, isoproteronol and cyclic AMP analogues caused increased GLUT1 mRNA expression in cultured granular cells from mouse afferent arterioles. This regulation appeared to be due to an increase in transcriptional activity (41).

GLUT4

In many ways, GLUT4 expression is regulated oppositely to that of GLUT1. For example, cAMP and its analogues and TNF-α decrease GLUT4 mRNA levels and transcriptional rates in 3T3-L1 cells. Also as opposed to effects on GLUT1, cell culture appears to downregulate GLUT4 levels. Within 24 hr of growth in primary culture, the GLUT4 mRNA level in rat adipocytes decreases approximately 20-fold, whereas GLUT1 mRNA levels increase 70-fold (51). GLUT4 and GLUT1 are also dichotomous in their subcellular distribution. Under basal condition in insulin-responsive cells, virtually all GLUT1 molecules are on the plasma membrane, whereas GLUT4 is mostly confined to an intracellular vesicular compartment (Fig. 4). The signals that direct each transporter to its respective membrane compartment appear to be largely confined to the carboxyl terminal sequence of each isoform (71), with amino-terminal sequences playing a secondary signaling role (52,71).

EFFECTS OF DIABETES MELLITUS, INSULIN AND EXTRACELLULAR GLUCOSE ON GLUCOSE TRANSPORTER EXPRESSION

Diabetes has multiple effects on glucose uptake and metabolism, and many of these effects are mediated or counteracted by changes in glucose transporter activity or expression. Multiple factors play a role in modulating glucose transporter function in diabetes, the best-studied of which are extracellular glucose and insulin concentrations.

Effects of Experimental and Clinical Diabetes

Streptozotocin-diabetes in rats and diabetes (NIDDM and IDDM) in humans is associated with a dramatic decrease in GLUT4 mRNA and protein expression in adipose tissue (see Ref. 34 for references). GLUT4 expression is returned toward normal with insulin treatment (34). It was expected that similar decreases in GLUT4 expression would be seen in skeletal muscle, the major site of insulin-stimulated glucose uptake, and therefore provide a mechanism for the abnormally low insulin-stimulated glucose uptake in diabetic muscle, which characterizes both experimental and clinical diabetic states (i.e., insulin resistance). However, GLUT4 levels in diabetic skeletal muscle are modestly depressed (46,53) or unchanged (34), implying that the defect in glucose uptake is due to other causes [e.g., most likely abnormal fusion with the plasma membrane or decreased activation (Fig. 4)]. In kidney, GLUT4 mRNA and protein levels are decreased to approximately 30% and 50%, respectively, of control values in glomeruli and vascular smooth muscle cells of the preglomerular vasculature of streptozotocin-diabetic rats (54,55). Total glucose uptake is also similarly reduced in those tissues (55). However, based on in situ hybridization studies, GLUT4 mRNA in thick ascending limb epithelia does not appear to change (16). Thus, effects of diabetes on glucose transporter expression are clearly tissue-specific.

The effects of diabetes on other transporters have not been as extensively studied. GLUT1 mRNA and protein levels in adipose cells of diabetic animals are relatively normal (46), but GLUT1 levels in muscle appear to be increased in streptozotocin diabetes (53). GLUT1 mRNA and protein levels were found to decrease in proximal tubules of streptozotocin rats (56). In contrast, SGLT1 mRNA and protein was not affected, and GLUT2 mRNA and protein levels were increased in proximal tubules of diabetic animals (56).

Effects of Extracellular Glucose and Insulin: Dissecting Their Regulatory Role in Diabetes

In most cultured cells, GLUT1 plasma membrane protein expression is depressed by exposure to increased extracellular glucose (see Ref. 57 for references). This response may have protective effects on cells by helping to prevent intracellular glucose accumulation and its metabolic sequela, known as glucose toxicity (57). However, hyperglycemia appears to increase GLUT1 plasma membrane levels in skeletal muscle and in red blood cells in vivo (53,58,59). More universal is the response to lowered extracellular glucose levels or any maneuver that interrupts normal glycolysis or oxidative metabolism. Under these conditions, GLUT1 plasma membrane expression and activity are induced (e.g., Refs. 47 and 60), presumably as a compensation for deprivation of cellular fuel.

GLUT4 molecules on the plasma membrane of skeletal muscle are modestly reduced by hyperglycemia, and normalization of hyperglycemia returns GLUT4 plasma membrane levels to normal (53,58). These results may explain the effect of diabetes on muscle GLUT4 expression. In diabetic fat cells, on the other hand, GLUT4 expression remains depressed even after blood glucose levels are returned to normal with phlorizin (34,61). Because insulin treatment normalizes fat GLUT4 level, this suggests that insulin rather than extracellular glucose is the predominant regulatory factor in this tissue. Interestingly, glucose transport in fat is normalized by phlorizin treatment, demonstrating increased activation of individual GLUT4 molecules (34,61). At present, the studies on control of glucose transporter expression in diabetic kidney are limited to those described above, but it is clear from the reports of GLUT expression in other tissues that multiple factors, including extracellular glucose and insulin levels, can regulate GLUT expression and activity. The complexity of their interactions in diabetic patients is just beginning to be unraveled.

GLUCOSE TRANSPORTERS AND DIABETIC NEPHROPATHY: POTENTIAL ROLE IN DIABETIC HYPERFILTRATION

One of the initial renal effects of diabetes is an increase in renal glomerular filtration and pressure, largely due to afferent arteriolar vasodilation. A large number of animal and human studies have suggested that hyperfiltration is a necessary if not sufficient cause of nephropathy in diabetes (62,63). Despite this conclusion, there is little consensus about the cellular and molecular causes of hyperfiltration. Although many causes have been proposed to explain this phenomenon, none fully account for the the observed increase in glomerular filtration rate (64).

Altered glucose transporter expression and activity in the afferent arteriole could provide a metabolic mechanism for hyperfiltration. As noted above, GLUT4 expression and glucose uptake are decreased in preglomerular vascular smooth muscle cells from diabetic animals (55). Because glucose transport is rate-limiting for glucose metabolism in vascular smooth muscle (65), decreased glucose transport into vascular smooth muscle cells will lead to decreased glycolysis and diminished ATP generation. This, in turn, will lead to increased activity of a type of potassium channel present in vascular smooth muscle cells known as the ATP-sensitive potassium channel (K_{ATP}) (Fig. 5). Increased K_{ATP} activity causes increased K^+ efflux, leading to hyperpolarization of the cells. Hyperpolarization of smooth muscle cells causes relaxation (66) and therefore leads to afferent arteriolar vasodilation and glomerular hyperfiltration. Thus, decreased expression of GLUT4 in the vascular smooth muscle cells of afferent renal microvasculature of diabetic animals and humans could lead directly to glomerular hyperfiltration.

There are several lines of evidence that support this hypothesis. First, a similar system is present in another cell type, the pancreatic β cell, in which glucose uptake and metabolism (via GLUT2 and glucokinase as mentioned above) directly inhibit K_{ATP} activity, which, in turn, depolarizes the β cell, causing calcium influx and insulin secretion (67). Second, the activity of K_{ATP}s in cardiac muscle cells (68) and of sodium-potassium ATPase molecules in vascular smooth muscle cells (69), which are also affected by intracellular ATP concentrations, are regulated by the ATP derived from the glycolysis of exogenous (i.e., transported) glucose. Conversely, their activities are relatively independent of other cellular ATP-generating processes, such as glycogenolysis and oxidative phosphorylation (Fig. 5). Third, K_{ATP}s are present in the vascular smooth muscle cells of the preglomerular vasculature (12), and decreased glucose transport and metabolism have been shown to activate K_{ATP}s in these renal afferent arteriolar smooth muscle cells (69). Finally, activation of

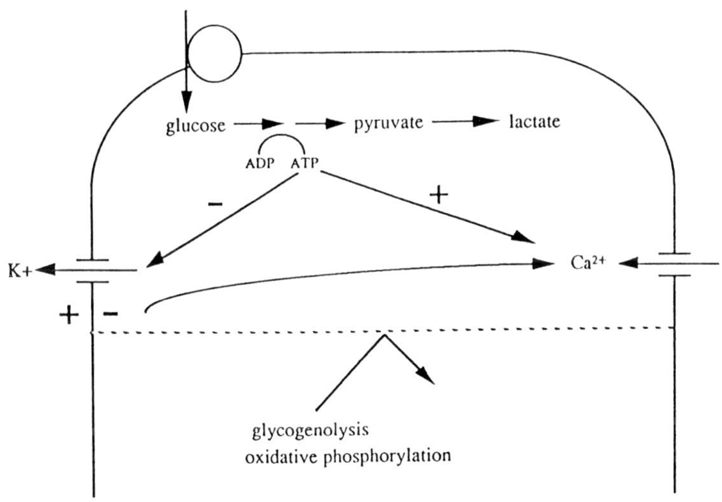

Figure 5 Schematic representation of vascular smooth muscle glucose metabolism and potential regulation of ATP-sensitive K^+ channels (K_{ATP}s) and voltage-sensitive Ca^{2+} channels by glucose uptake. Glucose uptake is rate-limiting for glucose metabolism in these cells, and ATP generated by glycogenolysis or oxidative metabolism does not impact significantly on plasma membrane ATP-sensitive activities. Therefore, metabolism of exogenous glucose appears to be critical in determining the activity of K_{ATP}s. Decreased glucose uptake and metabolism would lead to opening of K_{ATP}s, hyperpolarization of the cell, decreased activity of voltage-sensitive Ca^{2+} channels, smooth muscle relaxation, and vasodilation. This chain of events may explain afferent arteriolar vasodilation in early diabetes mellitus.

these channels causes vasodilation in isolated perfused afferent arteriole samples (69). Thus, the components of a system by which glucose transport could regulate ion transport and vascular tone are present in vascular smooth muscle cells of the preglomerular microvasculature as well as in other vessels.

SUMMARY AND CONCLUSIONS

Both facilitative and sodium-coupled glucose transporters play an important role in renal physiology and may also be important in the cellular response to diabetes mellitus and other pathological conditions. Whereas the sodium-glucose cotransporters, SGLT1 and SGLT2, are confined to epithelia participating in tubular glucose reabsorption, facilitative glucose transporters are expressed in all renal cells. The expression and function of these facilitative transporters are regulated at multiple transcriptional, translational, and posttranslational levels in a cell-specific manner, and the effect of pathological conditions on these transporters differs among different renal cells. Therefore the uptake and metabolism of glucose in conditions such as diabetes will vary markedly among renal cells. For example, proximal tubular epithelial cells expressing GLUT2 increase their plasma membrane transporters under hyperglycemic conditions. This response will increase glucose flux, and these cells will likely have glucose concentrations very close to ambient extracellular levels. Such high levels may lead to sorbitol accumulation, nonenzymatic glycosylation, and other forms of glucose toxicity. Other turbular cells and glomerular and vascular cells that contain GLUT1 and/or GLUT4 appear to decrease their plasma membrane transporter number in diabetes. This may decrease glucose uptake despite high extracellular glucose levels and may also decrease the likelihood of glucose toxicity. However, decreased glucose metabolism may have other effects, including the activation of ATP-sensitive potassium channels in vascular smooth muscle cells. This activation would lead to vasodilation and may explain renal afferent arteriolar vasodilation, hyperfiltration, and the generalized vasodilation that occurs early in diabetes.

REFERENCES

1. Hediger MH, Coady MJ, Ikeda TS, Wright EM. Expression cloning and cDNA sequencing of the Na^+/glucose cotransporter. Nature 1987; 330:379–381.
2. Wells RG, Pajor AM, Kanai Y, et al. Cloning of a human kidney cDNA with similarity to the sodium-glucose cotransporter. Am J Physiol 1992; 263:F459–F465.
3. Pajor AM, Wright EM. Cloning and functional expression of a mammalian Na^+/nucleoside cotransporter. J Biol Chem 1992; 3557–3560.
4. Kong C-T, Yei S-F, Lever JE. Cloning and expression of a mammalian Na^+/amino acid cotransporter with sequence similarity to Na^+/glucose cotransporters. J Biol Chem 1992; 268:1509–1512.
5. Kwon HM, Yamauchi A, Uchida S, et al. Cloning of the cDNA for a Na^+/*myo*-inositol cotransporter, a hypertonicity stress protein. J Biol Chem 1992; 267:6297–6301.
6. Pessin JE. Mammalian facilitative glucose transporter family: Structure and molecular regulation. Annu Rev. Physiol 1992; 54:911–930.
7. Waddell ID, Zomerschoe AG, Voice MW, Burchell A. Cloning and expression of a hepatic microsomal glucose transport protein. Biochem J 1992; 286:173–177.
8. Mueckler M, Caruso C, Baldwin SA, et al. Sequence and structure of a human glucose transporter. Science 1985; 229:941–945.
9. Birnbaum MJ, Haspel HC, Rosen OM. Cloning and characterization of a cDNA encoding the rat brain glucose-transporter protein. Proc Natl Acad Sci USA 1986; 83:5784–5788.
10. Thorens B, Sarkar HK, Kaback HR, Lodish HF Cloning and functional expression in bacteria of a novel glucose transporter present in liver, intestine, kidney, and β-pancreatic islet cells. Cell 1988; 55:281–290.
11. Kayano T, Fukumoto H, Eddy RL, et al. Evidence for a family of human glucose transporter-like proteins. J Biol Chem 1988; 263:15245–15248.
12. Brosius FC III, Briggs JP, Marcus RG, et al. Expression of the insulin-responsive glucose transporter (GLUT4) in renal microvessels and glomeruli. Kidney Int 1992; 42:1086–1092.
13. Shogren K, Goel K, Sun E, Brosius FC III. Cloning, sequencing and glomerular localization of the rat fetal muscle glucose transporter (abstr). J Am Soc Nephrol 1990; 1:744.

14. Thorens B, Lodish HF, Brown D. Differential localization of two glucose transporter isoforms in rat kidney. Am J Physiol 1990; 259:C286–C-294.
15. Dominguez JH, Camp K, Maianu L, Garvey WT. Glucose transporters of rat proximal tubule: differential expression and subcellular distribution. Am J Physiol 1992; 262:F807–F812.
16. Chin E, Zhou J, Bondy C. Anatomical and developmental patterns of facilitative glucose transporter gene expression in the rat kidney. J Clin Invest 1993; 91:1810–1815.
17. Shepherd PR, Gould GW, Colville CA, et al. Distribution of human GLUT3 glucose transporter protein in human tissues. Biochem Biophys Res Commun 1992; 188:149–154.
18. Shogren K, Goel K, Sun E, Brosius FC III. Cloning, sequencing and glomerular localization of the rat fetal muscle glucose transporter (abstr.). J Am Soc Nephrol 1990; 1:744.
19. Kayano T, Fukumoto H, Eddy RL, et al. Evidence for a family of human glucose transporter-like proteins. J Biol Chem 1988; 263:15245–15248.
20. Nagamatsu S, Kornhauser JM, Burant CF, et al. Glucose transporters in the brain. J Biol Chem 1992; 267:467–472.
21. Barfuss DW, Schafer J. Differences in active and passive glucose transport along the proximal nephron. Am J Physiol 1981; 240:F322–F332.
22. Turner RJ, Moran A. Further studies of proximal tubular brush border membrane D-glucose transport heterogeneity. J Membr Biol 1982; 70:37–45.
23. Ikeda TS, Hwang ES, Coady MJ, et al. Characterization of a Na^+/glucose cotransporter cloned from rabbit small intestine. J Membr Biol 1989; 110:87–95.
24. Takata K, Kasahara T, Kasahara et al. Localization of Na^+-dependent active type and erythrocyte/HepG2-type glucose transporters in rat kidney: Immunofluorescence and immunogold study. J Histochem Cytochem 1991; 39:287–298.
25. Lee WS, Kanai Y, Wells RG, Hediger MA. The high affinity Na^+/glucose cotransporter. Re-evaluation of function and distribution of expression. J Biol Chem 1994; 269:12032–12039.
26. Lee W-S, Hediger MA. Structure and function of the human kidney low affinity Na^+/glucose cotransporter (SGLT2). J Am Soc Nephrol 1992; 3:830.
27. Low BC, Ros IK, Grigor MR. Angiotensin II stimulates glucose transport activity in cultured vascular smooth muscle cells. J Biol Chem 1992; 267:20740–20745.
28. Kaiser N, Sasson S, Feener EP, et al. Differential regulation of glucose transport and transporters by glucose in vascular endothelial and smooth muscle cells. Diabetes 1993; 42:80–89.
29. Heilig CW, Riser B, Sastry S, Cortes P. Identification of facilitative glucose transporters in mesangial cells (abstr). J Am Soc Nephrol 1992; 3:758.
30. Kikkawa R, Kajiwara N, Haneda M, et al. GLUT1 is a main glucose transporter in rat mesangial cells (abstr). J Am Soc Nephrol 1992 3:830.
31. Tal M, Thorens B, Surana M, et al. Glucose transporter isotypes switch in T-antigen-transformed pancreatic β cells growing in culture and in mice. Mol Cell Biol 1992; 12:422–432.
32. Thorens B. Molecular and cellular physiology of GLUT-2, a high-K_m, facilitated diffusion glucose transporter. Int Rev Cytol 1992; 137A:209–239.
33. Brosius FC III, Nguyen K, England RL, et al. GLUT3 glucose transporter expression in the kidney (abstr). J Am Soc Nephrol 1993; 4:885.
34. Kahn BB. Facilitative glucose transporters: Regulatory mechanisms and dysregulation in diabetes. J Clin Invest 1992; 89:1367–1374.
35. Flier JS, Mueckler MM, Usher P, Lodish HF. Elevated levels of glucose transport and transporter messenger RNA are induced by *ras* or *src* oncogenes. Science 1987; 235:1492–1495.
36. Birnbaum MJ, Haspel HC, Rosen OM. Transformation of rat fibroblasts by FSV rapidly increases glucose transporter gene transcription. Science 1987; 235:1495–1498.
37. Hiraki Y, Rosen OM, Birnbaum MJ. Growth factors rapidly induce expression of the glucose transporter gene. J Biol Chem 1988; 263:13655–13662.
38. Cornelius P, Marlowe M, Lee MD, Pekala PH. The growth factor-like effects of tumor necrosis factor-α. J Biol Chem 1990; 265:105606–20516.
39. Hiraki Y, McMorrow IM, Birnbaum MJ. Expression of a glucose transporter gene cloned from brain in cellular models of insulin resistance: Dexamethasone decreases transporter mRNA in primary cultured adipocytes. Mol Endocrinol 1989; 3:1470–1476.
40. Murakami T, Nishiyama T, Shirotani T, et al. Identification of two enhancer elements in the gene encoding the type 1 glucose transporter from the mouse which are responsive to serum, growth factor, and oncogenes. J Biol Chem 1992; 267:9300–9306.
41. Chen M, Schnermann J, Smart AM, et al. Cyclic AMP selectively increases renin mRNA stability in cultured juxtaglomerular granular cells. J Biol Chem 1993; 268:24138–24144.
42. Cornelius P, Marlowe M, Call K, Pekala PH. Regulation of glucose transport as well as glucose transporter

and immediate early gene expression in 3T3-L1 preadipocytes by 8-bromo-cAMP. J Cell Physiol 1991; 146:298–308.
43. Rhoads DB, Takano M, Gattoni CS, et al. Evidence for expression of the facilitated glucose transporter in rat hepatocytes. Proc Natl Acad Sci USA 1988; 85:9042–9046.
44. Yamada H, Omata-Yamada T, Lengyel P. Characterization of recessive (mediator) revertants from NIH 3T3 cells transformed with a c-H-*ras* oncogene. J Biol Chem 1991; 266:4002–4009.
45. Stephens JM, Carter BZ, Pekala PH, Malter JS. Tumor necrosis factor α-induced glucose transporter (GLUT-1) mRNA stabilization in 3T3-L1 preadipocytes. J Biol Chem 1992; 267:8336–8341.
46. Garvey WT, Hueckstead TP, Birnbaum MJ. Pretranslational suppression of an insulin-responsive glucose transporter in rats with diabetes mellitus. Science 1989; 245:60–63.
47. Haspel HC, Mynarcik DC, Ortiz PA, et al. Glucose deprivation induces the selective accumulation of hexose transporter protein GLUT-1 in the plasma membrane of normal rat kidney cells. Mol Endocrinol 1991; 5:61–72.
48. Harrison SA, Buxton JM, Czech MP. Suppressed intrinsic catalytic activity of GLUT1 glucose transporters in insulin-sensitive 3T3-L1 adipocytes. Proc Natl Acad Sci USA 1991; 88:7839–7843.
49. Piper RC, James DE, Slot JW, Puri C, et al. GLUT4 phosphorylation and inhibition of glucose transport by dibutyryl cAMP. J Biol Chem 1991; 268:16557–16563.
50. Cornelius P, Marlowe M, Lee MD, Pekala PH. The growth factor like effects of tumor necrosis factor-α: Stimulation of glucose transport activity and induction of glucose transporter and immediate early gene expression in 3T3-L1 preadipocytes. J Biol Chem 1990; 265:20506–20516.
51. Gerrits PM, Olson AL, Pessin JE. Regulation of the GLUT4/muscle-fat glucose transporter mRNA in adipose tissue of insulin-deficient diabetic rats. J Biol Chem 1993; 266:640–644.
52. Piper RC, Tai C, Slot KW, et al. The efficient intracellular sequestration of the insulin-regulatable glucose transporter (GLUT-4) is conferred by the NH2 terminus. J Cell Biol 1992; 117:729–743.
53. Dimitrakoudis D, Vranic M, Klip A. Effects of hyperglycemia on glucose transporters of the muscle: Use of the renal glucose reabsorption inhibitor phlorizin to control glycemia. J Am Soc Nephrol 1992; 3:1078–1091.
54. Marcus RG, Briggs JP, Killen PD, Brosius FC. Quantitation of GLUT4 cDNA from microdissected afferent arterioles by the polymerase chain reaction (PCR) (abstr). J Am Soc Nephrol 1991; 2:523.
55. Marcus RG, England R, Nguyen K, Charron MJ, Briggs JP, Brosius FC III. Altered renal expression of the insulin-responsive glucose transporter GLUT4 in experimental diabetes mellitus. Am J Phsyiol 1994; 267:F816–F824.
56. Dominguez JH, Camp K, Maianu L, Feister H, Garvey WT. Molecular adaptations of GLUT1 and GLUT2 in renal proximal tubules of diabetic rats. Am J Physiol, 1994; 266:F283–F290.
57. Garvey WT. Glucose transport and NIDDM. Diabetes Care 1992; 15:396–417.
58. Dimitrakoudis D, Ramlal T, Rastogi S, et al. Glycaemia regulates the glucose transporter number in the plasma membrane of rat skeletal muscle. Biochem J 1992; 284:341–345.
59. Harik SI, Behmand RA, Arafah BM. Chronic hyperglycemia increases the density of glucose transporters in human erythrocyte membranes. J Clin Endocrinol Metab 1991; 72:814–818.
60. Shetty M, Loeb JN, Vikstrom K, Ismail-Beigi F. Rapid activation of GLUT-1 glucose transporter following inhibition of oxidative phosphorylation in clone 9 cells. J Biol Chem 1993; 268:17225–17232.
61. Kahn BB, Shulman GI, DeFronzo RA, et al. Normalization of blood glucose in diabetic rats with phlorizin treatment reverses insulin resistant glucose transport in adipose cells without restoring glucose transporter gene expression. J Clin Invest 1991; 87:561–570.
62. Hofstetter TH, Rennke HG, Brenner BM. Glomerular hemodynamics in experimental diabetes mellitus. Kidney Int 1981; 19:410–415.
63. Hostetter TH. Diabetic nephropathy: Metabolic versus hemodynamic considerations. Diabetes Care 1992; 15:1205–1215.
64. Bank N. Mechanisms of diabetic hyperfiltration. Kidney Int 1991; 40:792–807.
65. Lynch RM, Pail RJ. Glucose uptake in porcine carotid artery: Relation to alterations in active Na^+-K^+ transport. Am J Physiol 1984; 2457:C433–C440.
66. Nelson MT, Patlak JB, Worley JF, Standen NB. Calcium channels, potassium channels, and voltage dependence of arterial smooth muscle tone. Am J Physiol 1990; 259:C3–C18.
67. Smith PA, Rorsman P, Ashcroft FM. Modulation of dihydropyridine-sensitive Ca^{2+} channels by glucose metabolism in mouse pancreatic β-cells. Nature 1989; 342:550–553.
68. Weiss JN, Lamp ST. Glycolysis preferentially inhibits ATP-sensitive K^+ channels in isolated guinea pig cardiac myocytes. Science 1987; 238:67–69.
69. Lynch RM, Paul RJ. Compartmentation of glycolytic and glycogenolytic metabolism in vascular smooth muscle. Science 1983; 238:67–69.
70. Gould GW, Bell GI. Facilitative glucose transporters: An expanding family. TIBS 1990; 15:18–23.
71. Verhey KJ, Hausdorff SF, Birnbaum MJ. Identification of the carboxy terminus as important for the isoform-specific subcellular targeting of glucose transporter proteins. J Cell Biol 1993; 123:137–147.

31

Molecular Regulation of Organic Osmolytes in Renal Cells

Arlyn García-Pérez
National Heart, Lung, and Blood Institute, National Institutes of Health, Bethesda, Maryland

INTRODUCTION

As a consequence of the urinary concentrating mechanism, the cells of the mammalian renal medulla are routinely exposed to a greatly hyperosmotic and highly variable extracellular environment. These cells tolerate the long-term osmotic stress by accumulating osmotically active organic solutes, an adaptation mechanism that has been used by diverse organisms throughout the evolutionary chain (1–3). These solutes, denominated organic osmolytes, are accumulated preferably over inorganic ions by cells under hyperosmotic stress because they are not perturbing to cellular macromolecules; that is, they are "compatible" even at the high concentrations necessary to compensate for the extracellular hyperosmolality (1,3). The renal medulla cells are also exposed to high concentrations of urea, a perturbing solute that easily enters the cells. Therefore, some of the organic osmolytes must also act as "counteracting" solutes that oppose the harmful effects of urea (1,3).

Compatible organic osmolytes fall into three general chemical categories: sugar alcohols or polyols, amino acids or their derivatives, and methylamines. The methylamines are also counteracting osmolytes (1–3). The five predominant organic osmolytes in the mammalian kidney are sorbitol (a sugar alcohol), glycerophosphocholine (GPC, a phopholipid-derived methylamine), betaine (an amino acid–derived methylamine), *myo*-inositol (inositol, a sugar alcohol), and taurine (an amino acid derivative) (2,4). This chapter is a brief review of the mechanisms involved in the accumulation and dissipation of organic osmolytes in renal cells.

RENAL CELL LINES AS MODEL SYSTEMS

Isolated renal medullary cells and other renal cells in tissue culture have made a major contribution to the unraveling of the mechanisms that control organic osmolyte accumulation and dissipation. Unlike in vivo, the control of single experimental variables, as well as biochemical and molecular biological manipulations and measurements, are much easier in these systems. As the principles of organic osmolyte regulation have been discovered in vitro, investigators have been able to design experiments to test them better in vivo, based on a more basic understanding of the mechanisms involved.

Two principal renal cell lines were originally used to study the regulation of organic osmolytes. PAP-HT25 is derived from rabbit papillary epithelium. This cell line is adapted to grow in medium made hyperosmotic (500 mosmol/kg H_2O) by the addition of NaCl (5). Using PAP-HT25 cells, sorbitol was the first organic osmolyte shown to accumulate in cells in tissue culture under hyperosmotic conditions (6). A survey of other renal cell lines available at the time revealed that Madin-Darby canine kidney (MDCK) cells accumulate GPC, betaine, and inositol but not sorbitol under hyperosmotic conditions (7). Later, under conditions that were modified based on the results of the MDCK cell studies, PAP-HT25 cells were shown to also accumulate GPC, betaine, and inositol (8). Most recently, it has been demonstrated that MDCK cells also accumulate taurine (9). Most of what is known to date about the regulation of renal medullary organic osmolytes was first demonstrated in these two cell lines (2). An osmotically tolerant cell line from inner medullary collecting ducts of SV40 transgenic mice that accumulates all the five principal renal medullary organic osmolytes has been recently developed and may become another useful cell culture model for studying the molecular regulation of organic osmolytes in the kidney (10).

Figure 1 summarizes the mechanisms of accumulation and dissipation of compatible organic osmolytes as determined in PAP-HT25 and MDCK cells in culture (11). Some of these mechanisms have been or are presently being confirmed in the kidney in vivo (2,12–15). Accumulation of organic osmolytes is controlled through their metabolism (intracellular synthesis of sorbitol and intracellular degradation of GPC) or their transport (uptake of betaine, inositol, and taurine from the extracellular medium). Dissipation is mediated by rapid efflux of the osmolytes from the cells when the extracellular osmolality decreases (8).

MECHANISMS OF ORGANIC OSMOLYTE ACCUMULATION

Regulation of Osmolyte Metabolism

Sorbitol

Sorbitol is synthesized from glucose in a reaction catalyzed by aldose reductase (EC 1.1.1.21). Catabolism of sorbitol to fructose is catalyzed by sorbitol dehydrogenase (EC 1.1.1.14). Sorbitol, a sugar alcohol, was the first organic osmolyte to be found to accumulate in renal medullary cells in culture (PAP-HT25) exposed to medium made hypertonic (500 mosmol/kg H_2O) by addition of NaCl (5,6). After 24 hr in hypertonic medium, aldose reductase activity in the cells significantly increases and continues to increase gradually for 2 to 3 days as sorbitol accumulation follows (Fig. 2) (16). Sorbitol dehydrogenase activity is undetectable in PAP-HT25 cells in hypertonic medium and does not increase in isotonic (300 mosmol/kg H_2O) medium (17). In addition, no fructose (the product of sorbitol catabolism) is detectable in the cells in either medium. Therefore, sorbitol degradation does not appear to contribute to the osmotic regulation of sorbitol accumulation in PAP-HT25 cells. However, it may contribute in vivo, since a small but significant increase in sorbitol

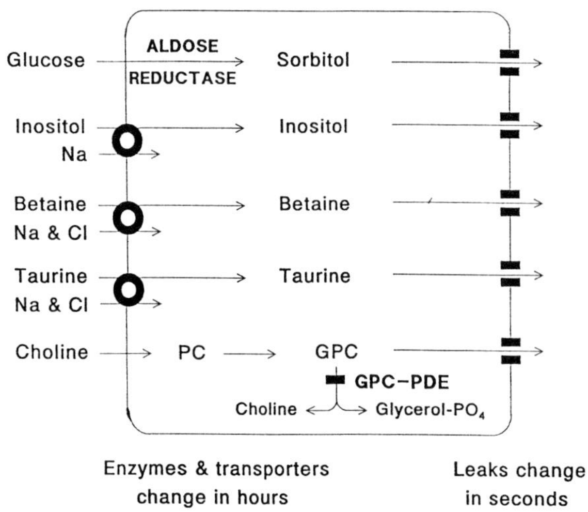

Figure 1 Mechanisms of organic osmolyte accumulation and dissipation in renal medullary cells. (From Ref. 11.)

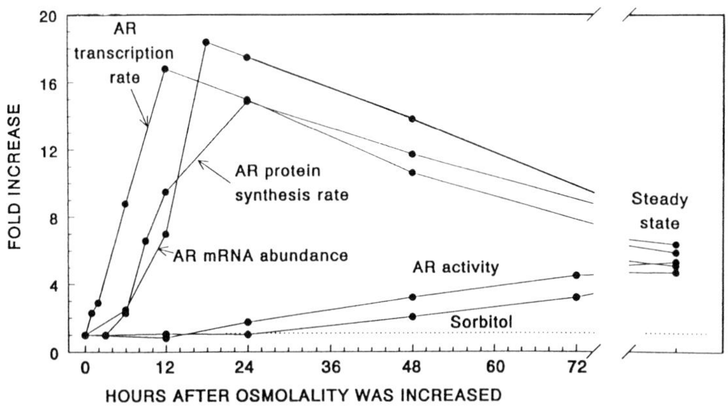

Figure 2 Effect on PAP-HT25 cells of increasing medium osmolality from isoosmotic (300 mosmol/kg H_2O) to hyperosmotic (500 mosmol/kg H_2O) by adding NaCl. The dotted line represents the levels in cells maintained in isoosmotic medium. Hyperosmotic steady-state levels were measured in cells maintained and passaged in hyperosmotic medium. (From Ref. 23.)

dehydrogenase activity is observed in terminal inner medullary collecting ducts of rats after 3 days of diuresis (2,15,18).

The increase in aldose reductase activity in PAP-HT25 cells under hypertonic conditions is due to a rise in the amount of the enzyme protein, which rises because its synthesis rate is accelerated (19–21). Aldose reductase synthesis and degradation were measured by pulse chase with ^{35}S-methionine, followed by immunoprecipitation with an aldose reductase-specific antibody (20). As shown in Fig. 2, synthesis rate increases to two times the level in isotonic medium after 6 hr of exposure to hypertonic medium. It peaks by 24 hr at approximately 15 times, then it decreases to a steady-state level that is approximately 6 times greater than that of cells in isotonic medium. The degradation of aldose reductase protein is slow (half-life is about 6 days) and does not differ between PAP-HT25 cells in isotonic and hypertonic medium (20). Therefore, the rise in the amount of aldose reductase protein in hypertonic medium is entirely due to increased rate of its synthesis.

In order to determine how medium hypertonicity increases aldose reductase protein synthesis, aldose reductase cDNA was cloned from PAP-HT25 cells, and the cloned cDNA was used as a probe to measure mRNA abundance (22). As expected for the situation in vivo, aldose reductase mRNA is highly abundant in the inner medulla, where the cells are routinely exposed to extracellular hyperosmolality, and undetectable in the cortex (22). When the PAP-HT25 cells are exposed to hypertonic medium, aldose reductase mRNA increases. The time course and magnitude of the increase closely resemble that of aldose reductase protein synthesis rate (Fig. 2). Therefore, the increased translation of enzyme protein is due to a rise in its mRNA abundance.

The rise in aldose reductase mRNA levels is a result of increased aldose reductase gene transcription rather than increased stability of the mRNA (23,24). Nuclear run-on assays were used to assess the changes in aldose reductase transcription rate after PAP-HT25 cells in isotonic medium were switched to hypertonic medium. Figure 2 shows that aldose reductase gene transcription begins to rise within 1 hr, reaches a peak increase of approximately 15-fold by 12 to 24 hr, and then decreases to a steady state of fivefold within a few days. Transcription precedes by a few hours the increases in aldose reductase mRNA abundance and protein synthesis and is large enough to entirely explain their induction. Further, the measured half-lives of aldose reductase mRNA in cells in isotonic vs. hypertonic medium are not significantly different (23). Therefore, aldose reductase mRNA is osmotically regulated through changes in its transcription (24).

In early studies on PAP-HT25 cells, the intracellular signal for induction of aldose reductase activity and subsequent sorbitol accumulation was examined by comparing the effects of raising medium osmolality with different solutes (16). As already mentioned, high extracellular NaCl increases aldose reductase activity. Raffinose, a trisaccharide that does not enter cells readily, is as effective as NaCl, indicating that neither extracellular Na nor Cl is necessary. In contrast, raising the osmolality with either urea or glycerol, which penetrate these cells readily, fails to increase aldose reductase activity. Therefore, increased osmolality per se is not sufficient. When osmolality is increased by adding raffinose, cell water decreases, and cell sodium and potassium concentrations increase. The changes persist for at least 24 hr until sorbitol content begins to rise and consequently cell volume is restored. Addition of urea, on the other hand, does not cause any significant change in cell water or electrolyte concentration, just as it fails to induce increased aldose reductase activity. Based on these correlations, the trigger for induction of aldose reductase appears to be prolonged extracellular hypertonicity.

It was postulated that the mechanism by which prolonged extracellular hypertonicity increases intracellular aldose reductase activity might involve either the reduction in cell volume or the increase in intracellular Na or K, both of which precede the rise in enzyme activity (16). To distinguish between these possibilities, ouabain was used. Ouabain generally decreases cell potassium and increases cell sodium and volume. Medium osmolality was increased by adding NaCl either without ouabain or with different concentrations of the drug. Aldose reductase activity did not correlate significantly with cell volume or sodium. It did correlate, however, with cell potassium concentration and even better with the sum of cell potassium plus sodium concentration. Thus, the hypothesis was postulated that the signal that ultimately induces sorbitol accumulation during prolonged extracellular hypertonicity is a rise in the total concentration of sodium plus potassium salts (or ionic strength) inside the cells (16).

Inherent in this hypothesis is the prediction that a reduction of the intracellular signal should decrease the response. The results of recent experiments are consistent with the hypothesis (20,23). As notable in Fig. 2, when PAP-HT25 cells are switched from isotonic to hypertonic medium, aldose reductase transcription rises slowly for 12 hr and then begins to fall. A similar but somewhat delayed time course is seen for aldose reductase mRNA abundance and translation. The decline in aldose reductase transcription and translation has been shown to coincide with increased sorbitol accumulation (20,23). When sorbitol accumulation is blocked with the aldose reductase inhibitor Tolrestat (N-methyl-5-trifluoromethyl-6-methoxy-naphthoyglycine), aldose reductase transcription and translation continue to increase past 24 hr. Presumably, sorbitol accumulation decreases the intracellular sodium plus potassium concentration through the restoration of cell volume, and this decrease in the intracellular signal then reduces aldose reductase transcription. Further support for this explanation comes from experiments in which the cells switched to hypertonic medium were allowed to accumulate large amounts of another compatible organic osmolyte, betaine (23). The usual increase in aldose reductase gene transcription was markedly inhibited, as expected if betaine, like sorbitol, lowers the intracellular signal (ionic strength) by restoring cell volume. Recent in vivo experiments also support the hypothesis that increased intracellular ionic strength is the signal for increased accumulation of at least some of the renal-compatible organic osmolytes (25).

To determine how the intracellular signal ultimately induces the transcription of the aldose reductase gene, it is necessary to clone the gene and characterize any regulatory regions in it that are necessary for the osmotic response (24). The aldose reductase gene has been cloned from human, rat, and rabbit (26–28). The gene is organized into 10 exons and 9 introns that occur in the same positions, relative to the mRNA sequence, in all three species (26–28). Both a TATA box and a CAAT box are found in the aldose reductase gene promoter (24,28,29), and both *cis* control elements are required for full basal promoter activity (29). Most recently, a DNA fragment containing approximately 3.5 kb of the 5′ flanking region of the rabbit aldose reductase gene was examined for its ability to confer hyperosmotic response capability to a reporter gene downstream (28). The reporter gene constructs were first transfected into PAP-HT25 cells and the transient transfectants were analyzed for reporter gene expression when in hyperosmotic medium or isoosmotic medium. The transient transfectants in hyperosmotic medium showed a higher than 40-fold induction of reporter gene expression compared to those in isoosmotic medium. This result suggests the existence of putative osmotic response element(s) (OREs) within the aldose reductase gene fragment tested (28). Identification and characterization of OREs and their associated *trans*-acting factors should begin to reveal the molecular mechanisms involved in osmotic regulation of gene activation (24).

Glycerophosphocholine

Glycerophosphocholine (GPC) is synthesized from phophatidylcholine (PC) by the removal of fatty acids in a reaction catalyzed by phospholipase A_1 (EC 3.1.1.32), phospholipase A_2 (EC

3.1.1.4), and lysophospholipase (EC 3.1.1.5) (2). The GPC is catabolized by hydrolysis to glycerol-3-phosphate and choline in a reaction catalyzed by GPC:choline phosphodiesterase (EC 3.1.4.2) (2).

PAP-HT25 cells and MDCK cells accumulate GPC in medium made hyperosmotic to 700 mosmol/kg H_2O with NaCl plus urea. In MDCK cells, where osmotically induced GPC accumulation has been best characterized, GPC rises slowly over $\geq$1 week when cells grown in isosmotic medium (300 mosmol/kg H_2O) are switched to hyperosmotic medium (700 mosmol/kg H_2O with NaCl plus urea) (30). Intracellular GPC rises regardless of whether the osmolality is increased with NaCl alone, NaCl plus urea, or urea alone (7,30). This effect is also seen in PAP-HT25 cells (8). If, as has been proposed, GPC acts to counteract the damaging effects of high intracellular urea, then it is reasonable that GPC accumulation should increase with high urea, even in the absence of high extracellular NaCl. In this respect, the signal that triggers GPC accumulation must differ from that for sorbitol. Elevated urea concentration does not increase the intracellular ionic strength (30,31). Thus, although high intracellular ionic strength apparently can induce both sorbitol and GPC accumulation, it is not necessary for the latter.

Phosphatidylcholine (PC), the immediate precursor for GPC formation, is synthesized from choline through the Kennedy pathway (2,32). Tissue culture medium normally contains choline, which was present in the above experiments. If the medium choline is removed at the same time that the osmolality is increased, cell GPC still rises slightly by the second day (presumably because of available intracellular PC or choline), but it then falls back to the baseline level (30). In contrast, if choline is present, the level of GPC continues to rise. Choline is taken up into MDCK cells and isolated rat inner medullary collecting duct cells by sodium-independent transport, but this transport is not affected by medium osmolality (30,33). Therefore, osmoregulation of GPC accumulation does not involve changes in choline transport capacity. It is also unlikely that GPC transport accounts for its accumulation in MDCK cells, since GPC uptake from medium containing ^{14}C-GPC is insignificant (34).

The remaining possibilities for increased GPC accumulation, namely a rise in GPC synthesis or a fall in GPC degradation, were examined (34). The rate of incorporation of ^{14}C from ^{14}C-choline into GPC, the steady-state GPC synthesis rate, and the activity of phospholipase A_2 are not increased by high NaCl and urea. In fact, all are decreased by approximately one-third. Therefore, there is no evidence that medium hyperosmolality increases the GPC synthesis rate. On the other hand, the rate coefficient for cellular GPC disappearance and the activity of GPC:choline phosphodiesterase are decreased by approximately two-thirds by high NaCl and urea. Thus, high NaCl and urea increase GPC accumulation by inhibiting its enzymatic degradation (Fig. 1). The individual effects of high extracellular NaCl vs. high extracellular urea on GPC synthesis and degradation remain to be examined.

Regulation of Osmolyte Transport

Betaine, Inositol, and Taurine

The mechanisms involved in osmotically regulated accumulation of betaine, inositol, and taurine were discovered in MDCK cells. When in hypertonic medium, these cells accumulate these compatible organic osmolytes only if they are present in the medium, indicating that uptake is the mechanism (9,35–40). Increased uptake of betaine and inositol is also the mechanism by which PAP-HT25 cells accumulate these osmolytes when switched to hypertonic medium (8). Specific transporters mediate the osmoregulated uptake of betaine, inositol, and taurine in MDCK cells (Fig. 1). The betaine and taurine transporters are Na^+ and Cl^- -dependent. The inositol transporter is Na^+-dependent (9,38–40). The betaine and inositol cotransporters are localized exclusively to the basolateral membrane in MDCK cells (39). The taurine cotransporter is in both the basolateral and apical membranes (9). However, apical taurine transport is much less than that of the basolateral membrane and is not osmotically regulated (9,40).

Because all three transport processes are sodium-dependent, most investigations of the mechanism by which medium hypertonicity increases osmolyte uptake were performed in medium made hypertonic with raffinose instead of NaCl (41,42). When mRNA isolated from MDCK cells exposed to hypertonic medium is microinjected into *Xenopus* oocytes, this mRNA induces characteristic uptakes of radiolabeled betaine, inositol, or taurine, whereas mRNA from cells in isotonic medium do not (38,41,42). These results suggested that increased uptake is due to an increase in the number of functioning transporters, probably through increased abundance of their respective mRNAs, as had been shown for aldose reductase (22).

In order to directly determine whether medium hypertonicity increases the mRNA abundance of betaine, inositol, and taurine cotransporters, their respective cDNAs were cloned (43–46). The primary structure of the cotransporter was defined from the cDNA-derived protein sequence: 614 amino acids in the betaine cotransporter (43), 718 in the inositol contransporter (44), and 655 in the taurine cotransporter (45,46). Hydropathy analysis predicted that all three cotransporters contain 12 to 13 membrane-spanning domains. Sequence homology suggested that the betaine and taurine cotransporters belong to a gene family of neurotransmitter cotransporters that includes GABA cotransporters (50–60% identity) (40). The inositol cotransporter demonstrated sequence homology to Na^+/glucose and Na^+/nucleoside cotransporters (40–60% identity) (44,47,48).

The cDNAs were then used as specific probes to measure mRNA abundance. In vivo, betaine cotransporter mRNA is clearly expressed in renal medulla but undetectable in the cortex, inositol cotransporter mRNA is more abundant in renal medulla but is present in cortex, and taurine cotransporter mRNA was equally abundant in renal medulla and cortex (43–46). As expected, the abundance of all three mRNAs rises in MDCK cells in hypertonic medium (43–46,49,50). The time course of osmotically induced increases in mRNA abundance has been examined for the betaine and inositol cotransporters (49,50). The pattern of induction is virtually identical to that of the aldose reductase mRNA in PAP-HT25 cells (22). Both betaine and inositol cotransporter mRNAs reach a peak of abundance at 16 to 24 hr after switching the MDCK cells to hypertonic medium. The peak represents a 15- to 20-fold increase over the mRNA levels in cells in isotonic medium (49,50). After the peak, the abundance of the betaine and inositol cotransporters falls somewhat (40,49,50), but not as much as that observed for aldose reductase mRNA in PAP-HT25 cells (22). As for aldose reductase, the increases in the cotransporters' mRNAs precedes the corresponding changes in the protein product function (transport rates).

The mechanisms responsible for increased mRNA abundance have been studied for the betaine and inositol transporters (40,49,50). As with aldose reductase mRNA, gene transcription of these transporters is increased in MDCK cells switched to hypertonic medium. Although the stability of the mRNAs has not been determined, the time course and magnitude of the rise in transcription can easily justify the increases in mRNA abundance (40,49,50). Whether the rise in mRNA abundance results in an increase in transporter protein synthesis rate remains to be determined.

MECHANISMS OF ORGANIC OSMOLYTE DISSIPATION

In contrast to the slow process required for osmotically induced sorbitol accumulation, sorbitol dissipation is fast (Fig. 1). PAP-HT25 cells maintained at a constant osmolality in either isotonic or hypertonic medium have a very low permeability to sorbitol (51). However, sudden decreases in extracellular NaCl concentration cause rapid, transient increases in sorbitol permeability that result in sorbitol efflux from the cells (2,8,15,51–53). One or more arachidonic acid metabolites in the cytochrome P-450 pathway may be involved in activating the sorbitol efflux (2,15,53). A similar increase in permeability to sorbitol after a fall in medium osmolality has been observed in isolated rat inner medullary collecting duct cells (54). In these cells, increased intracellular calcium may mediate the rapid efflux of sorbitol.

Although, as with sorbitol, GPC dissipation is faster than accumulation, the efflux of GPC is relatively small compared with efflux of the other organic osmolytes (8). The loss of GPC apparently occurs because of an increase in permeability (34,55).

As with sorbitol, dissipation of betaine, inositol, and taurine is much more rapid than accumulation (Fig. 1). The principal mechanism for dissipation is rapid efflux from the cells, although a decrease in their active uptake also contributes in betaine and inositol dissipation (2,8,15,36,39,40). In MDCK cells, betaine, inositol, and taurine exit through the basolateral side (40).

REFERENCES

1. Yancey P, Clark M, Hand S, et al. Living with water stress: Evolution of osmolyte systems. Science 1982; 217:1214–1222.
2. Garcia-Perez A, Burg MB. Renal medullary organic osmolytes. Physiol Rev 1991; 71:1081–1115.
3. Yancey PH. Compatible and counteracting solutes. In: Stange K, ed. Cellular and Molecular Physiology of Cell Volume Regulation. Boca Raton, FL: CRC Press, 1994:81–109.
4. Bagnasco, S, Balaban R, Fales H, et al. Predominant osmotically active organic solutes in rat and rabbit renal medullas. J Biol Chem 1986; 261:5872–5877.
5. Uchida S, Green N, Coon H, et al. High NaCl induces stable changes in phenotype and karyotype of renal cells in culture. Am J Physiol 1987; 253:C230–C242.
6. Bagnasco S, Uchida S, Balaban R, et al. Induction of aldose reductase and sorbitol in renal inner medullary cells by elevated extracellular NaCl. Proc Nat Acad Sci USA 1987; 84:1718–1720.
7. Nakanishi T, Balaban RS, Burg MB. Survey of osmolytes in renal cell lines. Am J Physiol 1988; 255:C181–C191.
8. Moriyama T, Garcia-Perez A, Burg MB. Factors affecting the ratio of the different organic osmolytes in renal medullary cells. Am J Physiol 1990; 259:F847–F858.
9. Uchida S, Nakanishi T, Kwon H, et al. Taurine behaves as an osmolyte in MDCK cells: Protection by polarized, regulated transport of taurine. J Clin Invest 1991; 88:656–662.
10. Rauchman MI, Nigam SK, Delpire E, et al. An osmotically tolerant inner medullary collecting duct cell line from an SV40 transgenic mouse. Am J Physiol 1993; 265:F416–F424.
11. Burg MB, Garcia-Perez A. How tonicity regulates gene expression. J Am Soc Nephrol 1992; 3:121–127.
12. Cowley BD, Jr., Ferraris JD, Carper D, et al. In vivo osmoregulation of aldose reductase mRNA, protein and sorbitol in renal medulla. Am J Physiol 1990; 258:F154–F161.
13. Nakanishi T, Uyama O, Sugita M. Osmotically regulated taurine content in rat renal inner medulla. Am J Physiol 1991; 261:F957–F962.
14. Nakanishi T, Uyama O, Takamitsu Y, et al. Determinants of relative amounts of medullary organic osmolytes: Effects of NaCl and urea differ. Am J Physiol 1993; 264:F472–F479.
15. Sands JM. Regulation of intracellular polyols and sugars in response to osmotic stress. In: Strange K, ed. Cellular and Molecular Physiology of Cell Volume Regulation. Boca Raton, FL: CRC Press, 1994:133–144.
16. Uchida S, Garcia-Perez A, Murphy H, et al. Signal for induction of aldose reductase in renal medullary cells by high external NaCl. Am J Physiol 1989; 256:C614–C620.
17. Bagnasco SM, Murphy HR, Bedford JJ, et al. Osmoregulation by slow changes in aldose reductase and rapid changes in sorbitol flux. Am J Physiol 1988; 254:C788–C792.
18. Sands JM, Schrader DC. Coordinated response of renal medullary enzymes regulating net sorbitol production in diuresis and antidiuresis. J Am Soc Nephrol 1990; 1:58–65.
19. Bedford JJ, Bagnasco SM, Kador PF, et al. Characterization and purification of a mammalian osmoregulatory protein, aldose reductase, induced in renal medullary cells by high extracellular NaCl. J Biol Chem 1987; 262:14255–14259.
20. Moriyama T, Garcia-Perez A, Burg MB. Osmotic regulation of aldose reductase protein synthesis in renal medullary cells. J Biol Chem 1989; 264:16810–16814.
21. Garcia-Perez A, Ferraris JD. Aldose reductase gene expression and osmoregulation in mammalian renal cells. In: Strange K, ed. Cellular and Molecular Physiology of Cell Volume Regulation. Boca Raton, FL: CRC Press, 1994:373–381.
22. Garcia-Perez A, Martin B, Murphy HR, et al. Molecular cloning of cDNA coding for kidney aldose reductase: Regulation of specific mRNA accumulation by NaCl-mediated osmotic stress. J Biol Chem 1989; 264:16815–16821.
23. Smardo F, Burg M, Garcia-Perez A. Kidney aldose reductase gene transcription is osmotically regulated. Am J Physiol 1992; 262:C776–C782.
24. Garcia-Perez A. Regulation of eukaryotic gene expression, In: Strange K, ed. Cellular and Molecular Physiology of Cell Volume Regulation. Boca Raton, FL: CRC Press, 1994:325–334.
25. Beck FX, Schmolke M, Guder WG, et al. Osmolytes in renal medulla during rapid changes in papillary tonicity. Am J Physiol 1992; 262:F849–F856.
26. Graham A, Brown L, Hedge P, et al. Structure of the human aldose reductase gene. J Biol Chem 1991; 266:6872–6877.
27. Graham C, Szpirer C, Levan G, et al. Characterization of the aldose reductase-encoding gene family in rat. Gene 1991; 107:259–267.
28. Ferraris JD, Williams CK, Martin BM, et al. Cloning, genomic organization, and osmotic response of the aldose reductase gene. Proc Natl Acad Sci USA 1994; 91:10742–10746.
29. Wang K, Bohren K, Gabbay K. Characterization of the human aldose reductase gene promoter. J Biol Chem. 1993; 268:16052–16058.

30. Nakanishi T, Burg MB. Osmoregulation of glycerophosphorylcholine content of mammalian renal cells. Am J Physiol 1989; 257:C795–C801.
31. Heilig CW, Brenner RM, Yu ASL, et al. Modulation of osmolytes in MDCK cells by solutes, inhibitors, and vasopressin. Am J Physiol 1990; 259:F653–F659.
32. Wilgram GF, Kennedy EP. Intracellular distribution of some enzymes catalyzing reactions in the biosynthesis of complex lipids. J Biol Chem 1963; 238:2615–2619.
33. Bevan C, Kinne R. Choline transport in collecting ducts isolated from the rat renal inner medulla. Pflugers Arch 1990; 417:324–328.
34. Zablocki K, Miller S, Garcia-Perez A, et al. Accumulation of glycerophosphorylcholine by renal cells: Osmotic regulation of GPC:choline phosphodiesterase. Proc Natl Acad Sci USA 1991; 88:7820–7824.
35. Nakanishi T, Burg MB. Osmoregulatory fluxes of myo-inositol and betaine in renal cells. Am J Physiol 1989; 257:C964–C970.
36. Nakanishi T, Turner RJ, Burg MB. Osmoregulatory changes in myo-inositol transport by renal cells. Proc Natl Acad Sci USA 1989; 86:6002–6006.
37. Nakanishi T, Turner RJ, Burg MB. Osmoregulation of betaine transport in mammalian renal medullary cells. Am J Physiol 1990; 258:F1061–F1067.
38. Uchida S, Kwon H. Preston A, et al. Expression of MDCK cell Na^+ and Cl^--dependent taurine transporter in Xenopus laevis oocytes. J Biol Chem 1991; 266:9605–9609.
39. Yamauchi A, Kwon H, Uchida S, et al. Myo-inositol and betaine transporters regulated by tonicity are basolateral in MDCK cells. Am J Physiol 1991; 261:F197–F202.
40. Kwon HM. Molecular regulation of mammalian osmolyte transporters, In: Strange K, ed. Cellular and Molecular Physiology of Cell Volume Regulation. Boca Raton, FL: CRC Press, 1994:383–394.
41. Kwon HM, Yamauchi A, Uchida S, et al. Renal Na-myo-inositol cotransporter mRNA expression in Xenopus oocytes: Regulation by hypertonicity. Am J Physiol 1991; 260:F258–F263.
42. Robey RB, Kwon HM, Handler JS, et al. Induction of glycinebetaine uptake in Xenopus oocytes by infection of poly(A) RNA from renal cells exposed to high extracellular NaCl. J Biol Chem 1991; 266:10400–10405.
43. Yamauchi A, Uchida S, Kwon H, et al. Cloning of a Na+ and Cl– dependent betaine transporter that is regulated by hypertonicity. J Biol Chem 1992; 267:649–652.
44. Kwon HM, Yamauchi A, Uchida S, et al. Cloning of the cDNA for a Na^+/myo-inositol cotransporter, a hypertonicity stress protein. J Biol Chem 1992; 267:6297–6301.
45. Uchida S, Kwon H, Yamauchi A, et al. Molecular cloning of the cDNA for an MDCK cell Na^+ and Cl^--dependent taurine transporter that is regulated by hypertonicity. Proc Natl Acad Sci USA 1992; 89:8230–8234.
46. Uchida S, Kwon HM, Yamauchi A, et al. Molecular cloning of the cDNA for an MDCK cell Na(+)- and Cl(–)-dependent taurine transporter that is regulated by hypertonicity (erratum). Proc Natl Acad Sci USA 1993; 90:7424.
47. Hediger MA, Coady MJ, Ikeda TS, et al. Expression cloning and cDNA sequencing of the Na+/glucose co-transporter. Nature 1987; 330:379–381.
48. Pajor AM, Wright EM. Cloning and functional expression of a mammalian NA+/nucleoside cotransporter, a member of the SGLT family. J Biol Chem 1992; 267:3557–3560.
49. Uchida S, Yamauchi A, Preston A, et al. Medium tonicity regulates expression of the Na+- and Cl-dependent betaine transporter in Madin-Darby canine kidney cells by increasing transcription of the transporter gene. J Clin Invest 1993; 91:1604–1607.
50. Yamauchi A, Uchida S, Preston AS, et al. Hypertonicity stimulates transcription of the gene for the Na+/myo-inositol cotransporter in MDCK cells. Am J Physiol 1993; 264:F20–F23.
51. Siebens A, Spring KR. A novel sorbitol transport mechanism in cultured renal papillary epithelial cells. Am J Physiol 1989; 257:F937–F946.
52. Garty H, Furlong TJ, Ellis DE, et al. The sorbitol permease: An apical membrane transporter in cultured renal papillary epithelial cells. Am J Physiol 1991; 260:F650–F656.
53. Furlong TJ, Moriyama T, Spring KR. Activation of osmolyte efflux from cultured renal papillary epithelial cells. J Membr Biol 1991; 123:269–277.
54. Bevan C, Theiss C, Kinne RKF. Role of Ca2+ in sorbitol release from rat inner medullary collecting duct (IMCD) cells under hypoosmotic stress. Biochem Biophys Res Commun 1990; 170:563–568.
55. Beck F, Dorge A, Rick R, et al. Osmoregulation of renal papillary cells. Pflugers Arch 1985; 405 (suppl 1):S28–S35.

32
Molecular Biophysics of Kidney Water Channels

A. S. Verkman
University of California, San Francisco, San Francisco, California

HISTORICAL OVERVIEW

Although a substantial body of information at the molecular level has been available for years on the structure and function of a number of ion channels and solute transporters, little information has been available about pathways for water movement until recently. The existence of "water pores" in membranes was proposed as early as 1877 by Pfeffer (1); however, controversy remained as to whether water moved across biological membranes through specialized lipid or protein/lipid assemblies, through existing ion/solute transporting proteins, or through selective water channels. It is now clear that selective water channels exist and play an important physiological role in the kidney and other organs.

In the 1950s and 1960s, it was demonstrated that certain cell plasma membranes were highly water-permeable. The erythrocyte was found to have high water permeability that was reversibly inhibited by >90% by mercurial compounds. Biophysical measurements showing a weakly temperature-dependent water permeability and a ratio of osmotic-to-diffusional water permeability of >1 suggested the existence of a continuous aqueous pore or channel that traversed the bilayer. In mammalian kidney, constitutively high water permeability was measured in the proximal tubule, whereas collecting duct water permeability was regulated by vasopressin (antidiuretic hormone, ADH). The amphibian urinary bladder was found to be a useful nonmammalian model for vasopressin-regulated water permeability. Based on morphological and functional studies, a "membrane shuttle" hypothesis was developed for vasopressin-regulated water permeability. According to this hypothesis, vasopressin induces the movement of subcellular vesicles containing functional water channels between an intracellular compartment and the cell apical plasma membrane. Additional details about the observations leading to the present understanding of water transport biology are documented in several books (2–4) and recent reviews (5–7).

THE IDENTIFICATION OF WATER CHANNELS

Biophysical Characterization of Kidney Water Channels

Water permeability measurements on dissected perfused tubules, suspended tubule epithelial cells, and purified membrane vesicles demonstrated considerable heterogeneity in water transporting characteristics along the length of the mammalian nephron. Transepithelial osmotic water permeability (P_f) in proximal tubule is high (0.1–0.5 cm/sec) and inhibited by mercurials (8). Vesicle studies indicate that both apical and basolateral membranes have a high P_f that is weakly temperature-dependent and inhibited by mercurials (9). Although endosomes and clathrin-coated vesicles from proximal tubule epithelial cells also have high P_f (10,11), it is generally believed that transepithelial water permeability in proximal tubule is constitutively high and not subject to physiological regulation. P_f is also high in the thin descending limb of Henle but very low in the ascending limb. The collecting duct has low P_f throughout its length in the absence of vasopressin but becomes water-permeable rapidly in response to vasopressin binding to V2 receptor at the basolateral membrane of principal (and inner medullary collecting duct) cells (6,7,12). High P_f was also demonstrated in a subpopulation of apical endosomes from collecting duct principal cells that participate in the vesicle shuttling mechanism (13). Taken together, these functional studies suggested the existence of water channels in epithelial cell plasma membranes in proximal tubule, thin descending limb of Henle and collecting duct, as well as in certain subcellular vesicles; in addition, rapid water movement across endothelial cells in vasa recta raised the possibility that certain endothelia may also contain water channels.

Evidence that Water Channels Are Distinct Proteins

Labeling Studies

A variety of approaches have been utilized to identify putative water transporting proteins. In erythrocyte membranes labeled with the non-specific water channel inhibitor ^{203}Hg-p-chloromercuribenzene sulfonate (pCMBS), band 3 and several other proteins were labeled (14); however, subsequent studies showed that band 3 was not involved in erythrocyte water transport (15). In toad urinary bladder, a variety of chemical and antibody-labeling studies suggested that proteins of 53 and 55 kDa may be components of the vasopressin-sensitive water channel (16,17); however, direct functional evidence that these proteins are involved in water permeability has not been obtained. In general, biochemical identification of water channels has been difficult because of the lack of specific water-channel inhibitors and of simple functional assays in fractionation/purification procedures.

Target Analysis

Radiation inactivation studies provided evidence that the erythrocyte and proximal tubule water transporters were proteins of functional size ~30 kDa (18). Frozen samples were irradiated, thawed and assayed for water transport. The target size, determined from the slope of a ln P_f vs. radiation dose plot, represents the effective size of the functional unit for water transport. The simplest interpretation of the 30-kDa target size is that the water transporter is a single subunit of 30-kDa size, although other conclusions are possible if multiple identical or different subunits form a multimeric complex in membranes.

Expression in Xenopus Oocytes

The functional expression of water transporters in *Xenopus* oocytes provided strong evidence that the water channel is a protein. Water permeability was increased by three- to fivefold in oocytes expressing mRNA from tissues believed to contain water channels, including kidney, reticulocytes, and toad bladder; the incremental oocyte P_f was weakly temperature-dependent and inhibited by $HgCl_2$ (19,20). Size fractionation studies indicated that a 2 to 3-kb mRNA encoded erythrocyte and kidney water channels (15,21). The oocyte assay system was used to demonstrate that the erythrocyte water transporter was distinct from band 3 and the glucose transporter (15). It was also demonstrated that certain proteins, including CFTR (22) and the Na-independent glucose transporter (15,23), were water-permeable; however, these proteins probably do not provide a quantitatively significant route for water transport in cells because of their low single-channel water permeabilities and/or abundances (24).

Molecular Identification of Kidney Water Channels

The water-transporting proteins identified to date are homologous to members of the MIP (major intrinsic protein of lens fiber) family of proteins, which include small channel-forming proteins from mammals, plants, bacteria, and yeast (25). The first water transporter to be identified, CHIP28 (channel forming intrinsic protein of 28 kDa), was purified from human erythrocytes and cloned from sequence information as a putative Rh factor (26,27); subsequent expression studies of human and rat CHIP28 in *Xenopus* oocytes (21,28), reconstituted proteoliposomes (29,30), and transfected CHO cells (31) indicated that CHIP28 is a water channel. As described below, CHIP28 is a major water channel in kidney proximal tubule and thin descending limb of Henle. A second water channel localized to collecting duct apical membrane (WCH-CD) was cloned by homology to CHIP28 (32,33) and may represent the vasopressin-regulated water channel (see below). Several homologous proteins from kidney and extrarenal tissues have been cloned recently (see below). It was found that a plant member of the MIP family (γ-TIP) also functions as a water channel when expressed in *Xenopus* oocytes (34), whereas MIP does not appear to transport water (35).

WATER CHANNEL STRUCTURE AND FUNCTION

Superfamily of Water Channels

The water-transporting proteins identified to date are homologous to the MIP protein and contain a number of conserved sequences. Figure 1 presents an amino acid sequence alignment for several water channels, showing many regions of identity after sequence alignment. There are several absolutely conserved sequences including two "NPA boxes." Hydropathy analysis for each of the predicted amino acid sequences indicates high hydrophobicity with multiple possible membrane-spanning domains and short extramembrane connecting segments (see below). Based on the conserved NPA sequences that are 350 to 400 bp apart in the cDNA sequence in various MIP family members, a PCR cloning strategy has been utilized to identify other putative water channels using degenerate oligonucleotide primers (32,33). The 350 to 400-bp sequences with homology to MIP produced by PCR were used to screen cDNA libraries to obtain full-length coding sequences. By this PCR cloning approach or conventional homology cloning methods, at least three additional water channels from kidney (36,37) and one from lung (38) have been identified to date, and it is likely that the water channel superfamily will grow considerably.

Expression and Functional Analysis

Oocyte Expression

Oocyte expression studies provided initial evidence that CHIP28 functions as a water channel. Human and rat CHIP28 share 94% amino acid identity and are encoded by mRNAs with an 807-bp open reading frame (21,27) and ~2.8-kb size in kidney. The 17-kb human CHIP28 gene is located on chromosome 7p14 and contains four exons (39). The water permeability in oocytes injected with transcribed cRNA encoding CHIP28 was increased >10-fold over that in water-injected (control) oocytes (21,28); the increased water permeability was inhibited by $HgCl_2$ and was weakly temperature-dependent. Two-electrode voltage-clamp studies indicated that CHIP28 was not ion-permeable. The increased water permeability in oocytes expressing heterologous mRNA from rat kidney cortex was blocked by coinjection with antisense CHIP28 cRNA (21,40). Oocytes injected with cRNA encoding WCH-CD also demonstrated a mercury-sensitive increase in water permeability (32,33).

Protein Reconstitution

Functional studies on reconstituted proteoliposomes provided direct evidence that CHIP28 is a water channel (29,30,35). CHIP28 was purified by stripping erythrocyte or renal vesicles with N-lauroylsarcosine, followed by solubilization in octylglucoside, anion-exchange chromatography, and size-exclusion high-performance liquid chromatography (35); solubilized CHIP28 was reconstituted in liposomes by detergent dilution. Figure 2 shows a stopped-flow light-scattering experiment in which proteoliposomes reconstituted with CHIP28 had very high water permeability that was >98% inhibited by $HgCl_2$. These water-permeable lipsomes had low urea permeability, indicating that urea does not pass through the CHIP28 water channel. It was also found that CHIP28 is not permeable to protons. These functional studies indicate that CHIP28 is a selective water channel which may contain a narrow aqueous pore of ~0.2-nm diameter (21).

Mammalian Cell Expression

CHO cells were stably transfected with cDNA encoding rat kidney CHIP28 using mammalian expression vectors containing CMV and RSV promoters (31). Clonal cell populations expressed CHIP28 protein strongly (up to 10^7 CHIP28 copies per cell) without cell toxicity. Functional measurements on intact cells and fractionated subcellular vesicles indicated high and mercury-sen-

```
   1-86    ----------MASEFKKKLFWRAVVAEFLATTLFVFISIGSALGFKYPVGNNQTAVQDNVKVSLAFGLSIATLAQSVGHISGAHLNPAVTLGLLLS
:  1-86    ----------MASEFKKKLFWRAVVAEFLATTLFVFISIGSALGFNYPLERNQTLVQDNVKVSLAFGLSIATLAQSVGHISGAHLNPAVTLGLLLS
   1-78    -----------MWELRSIAFSRAVLAEFLATLLFVFFGLGSALQ-------WASSPPSVLQIAVAFGLGIGILVQALGHVSGAHINPAVTVACLVG
   1-95    -MATRRYSFGRTDEATHPDSMRASLAEFASTFIFVFAGEGSGLALVKIYQDSAFSAGELLALALAHAFALFAAVSASMHVSGGHVNPAVSFGALIG
   1-89    MEPGLCNRAYLLVGGLWTAISKALFAEFLATGLYVFFGVGSVLP-------WPVALPSVLQVAITFNLATATAVQISWKTSGAHANPAVTLAYLVG

  87-181   CQISIFRALMYIIAQCVGAIVATAILSGITSSLTGSNLGRNDLADGVNSGQGLGIEIIGTLQLVLCVLAT-TDRRRRDLGGSAPLAIGLSVALGHL
: 87-181   CQISILRAVMYIIAQCVGAIVASAILSGITSSLLENSLGRNDLARGVNSGQGLGIEIIGTLQLVLCVLAT-TDRRRRDLGGSAPLAIGLSVALGHL
  79-173   CHVSFLRAAFYVAAQLLGAVAGAAILHEITPVEIRGDLAVNALHNNATAGQAVTVELFLTMQLVLCIFAS-TDERRGDNLGSPALSIGFSVTLGHL
  96-188   GRISVIRAVYYWIAQLLGSIVAALVLRLVTNNMRPSGFH---VSPGVGVGHMFILEVVMTFGLMYTVYGTAIDPKRGAVSNIAPLAIGLIVGANIL
  90-182   SHISLPRAVAYIAAQLAGATVGAALLYGVTPGGVRETLGVNVVHNSTSTGQAVAVELVLTLQLVLCVFAS-MDSRQ--TLGSPASMIGTSVALGHL

 182-269   LAIDYTGCGINPARSFGSAVITHNFSNHWIFWVGPFIGGALAVLIYDFILAPRSSDLTDRVKVWTSGQVEEYDLDADDINSRVEMKPK----------
:182-269   LAIDYTGCGINPARSFGSAVLTRNFSNHWIFWVGPFIGSALAVLIYDFILAPRSSDFTDRMKVWTSGQVEEYDLDADDINSRVEMKPK----------
 174-271   LGIYFTGCSMNPARSLAPAVVTGKFDDHWVFWIGPLVGAIIGSLLYNYLLFPSAKSLQERLAVLKGLEPDTDWEEREVRRRQSVELHSPQSLPRGSKA
 189-256   VGGPFDGACMNPALAFGPSLVGWQWHQHWIFWVGPLLGAALAALVYEYAVIPIEPPPHHHQPLATEDY------------------------------
 183-276   IGIYFTGCSMNPARSFGPAVIVGKFAVHWIFWVGPLTGAVLASLIYNFILFPDTKTVAQRLAILVGTTKVEKVVDLEPQKKESQTNSEDTEVSV----
```

Figure 1 Amino acid sequence alignment of water channels CHIP28, CHIP28k, WCH-CD, γ-TIP, and WCH3. Sequences were obtained from Refs. 21, 32, 34, and 36. Conserved sequences are enclosed by boxes.

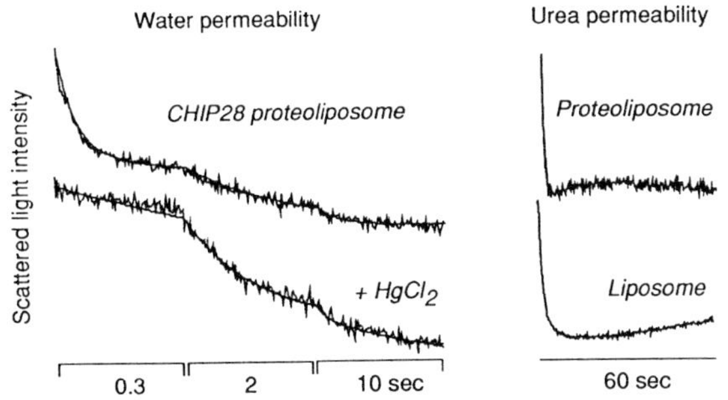

Figure 2 Osmotic water and urea permeability in proteoliposomes reconstituted with purified CHIP28 protein. Proteoliposomes were subjected to an inwardly directed gradient of sucrose (left) or urea (right) in a stopped-flow apparatus at 10°C. The time course of liposome volume was followed by 90° scattered light intensity at 520 nm. Water permeability (downward deflection) was strongly inhibited by $HgCl_2$. Urea permeability in CHIP28 proteoliposomes (upward deflection) was low and not different from that in protein-free liposomes.

sitive water permeability in plasma membrane, Golgi, and endosomes. Immunogold localization and Western analysis confirmed the presence of CHIP28 protein in these compartments.

Structure and Transporting Mechanisms

Tetrameric Subunit Association

Recent data suggests that CHIP28 molecules are assembled in membranes as tetramers in which each monomer functions independently. Initial evidence that CHIP28 may form oligomers was obtained by cross-linking and sedimentation analysis of solubilized protein (41,42). Recent freeze-fracture electron microscopy measurements showed that CHIP28 was visible as distinct intramembrane particles (IMPs) in membranes (43). In reconstituted proteoliposomes, IMPs with four distinct subunits were visualized. Freeze-fracture electron micrographs of CHIP28-expressing CHO cells and native membranes (thin descending limb of Henle) also showed a tetrameric arrangement of CHIP28 subunits with a greatest IMP diameter of 8.5 nm. Taken together with correlating IMP density with water permeability, it was concluded that CHIP28 forms tetramers in artificial and native membranes.

Functional Independence of Monomers

There is good evidence that CHIP28 monomers within the tetramer function independently. As described above, radiation inactivation studies gave a 30-kDa target size for water transport in erythrocytes and apical vesicles from rat kidney cortex (18). The simplest interpretation of this result is that the functional unit of CHIP28 is the monomer. Subsequent studies in oocytes expressing combinations of wild-type and mutant CHIP28 cDNAs supported the conclusion that CHIP28 monomers function independently (44,45). Nonfunctional CHIP28 mutants did not alter the function of wild-type CHIP28, and coexpression of a mercury-insensitive CHIP28 mutant (C189S) with wild-type CHIP28 yielded oocytes with partial mercury sensitivity. However, the functional independence of CHIP28 monomers was not proved because the presence that heterotetramers containing both mutant and wild-type monomers could not be demonstrated. To force the formation of heterodimers, chimeric CHIP28 cDNA dimers were constructed and expressed in *Xenopus* oocytes (46). The wild-type dimers were correctly processed and functionally targeted to the oocyte plasma membrane. Oocytes expressing dimers with one wild-type CHIP28 unit coupled with a nonfunctional CHIP28 mutant (C189W) had water permeability proportional to the number of wild-type dimers. Oocytes expressing a wild-type-C189S mutant showed mercury inhibition intermediate to that of wild-type CHIP28 and the C189S mutant. These results provide strong evidence that CHIP28 monomers are functionally independent.

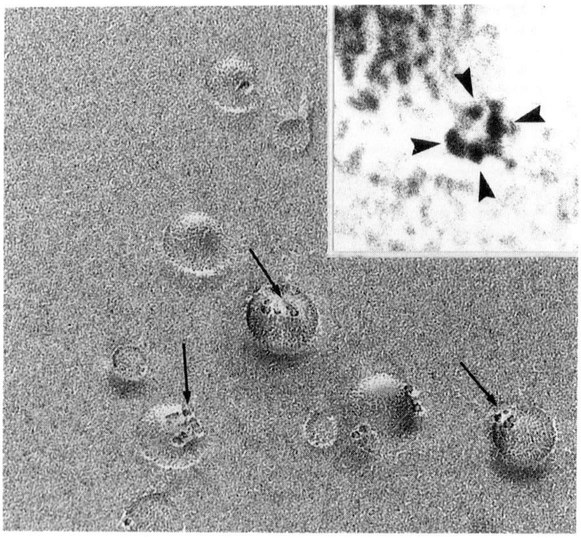

Figure 3 Freeze-fracture rotary shadowed electron micrograph of proteoliposomes containing purified CHIP28. Note the substructure of intramembrane particles showing a symmetrical arrangement of four smaller subunits. (Figure prepared by J. M. Verbavatz and D. Brown based on the study reported in Ref. 43.)

Topology of CHIP28 Monomers

Hydropathy analysis of CHIP28 suggested the presence of multiple membrane-spanning α-helical domains (Fig. 4A). Residue asparagine 42 is glycosylated in ~50% of CHIP28 monomers, although glycosylation is not important for CHIP28 function (35,45). Site-directed mutagenesis studies indicated that residue C189 is the site of action of mercury transport inhibitors (44,45) and that glycosylation was not required for CHIP28 function (45). To determine the secondary structure of CHIP28, spectroscopic studies were performed by circular dichroism and Fourier transform infrared spectroscopy (35). In detergent-solubilized and membrane-associated CHIP28, there was ~40% α-helix, ~40% β-(sheet+turn), and ~20% unordered structure. Analysis of intrinsic tryptophan fluorescence indicated that the four tryptophans in CHIP28 were located in a nonpolar environment within the confines of the bilayer (47). Analysis of CHIP28 membrane topology at the endoplasmic reticulum was performed by translation of chimeras containing truncated fragments of CHIP28 in series with a reporter domain (48). It was concluded that CHIP28 spans the membrane four times at the endoplasmic reticulum (Fig. 4B). As proposed for the structure of some ion channels, CHIP28 may contain β-sheet domains that loop into the membrane and make up part of the aqueous pathway. Crystallization and diffraction analysis will be required for high-resolution definition of CHIP28 structure and identification of the water transporting pathway. Preliminary studies showed that CHIP28 can form two-dimensional crystalline patches in membranes that diffracted electrons to 12-Å resolution (49).

PHYSIOLOGY OF WATER CHANNELS

Tissue Distribution

CHIP28

A series of studies have been performed to determine the tissue distribution of CHIP28 water channels in renal and extrarenal tissues (21,50–55). In kidney, in situ hybridization showed expression of mRNA encoding CHIP28 in proximal tubule and thin descending limb of Henle without expression in glomerulus, collecting duct, and other cell types (21). There was increased hybridization in the

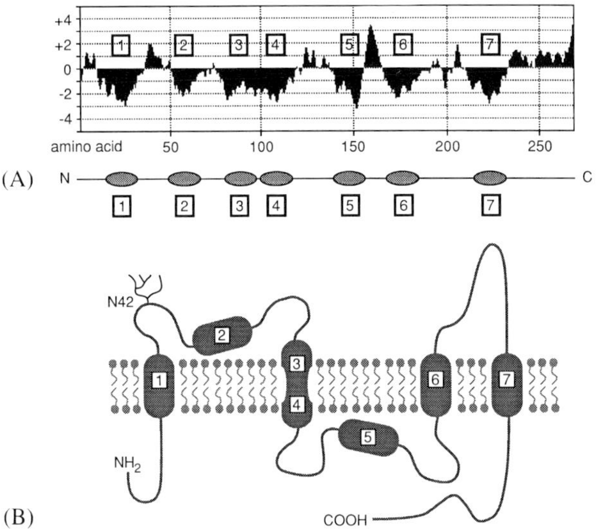

Figure 4 Kyte-Doolittle hydropathy plot (A) and proposed transmembrane topology (B) of the CHIP28 water channel at the endoplasmic reticulum showing four membrane-spanning helical domains.

deeper (S3) portions of proximal tubule. Immunofluorescence and immunogold localization studies showed strong CHIP28 protein expression in apical membrane of proximal tubule and apical and basolateral membranes of thin descending limb of Henle (52,53). There was less though detectable CHIP28 expression on basolateral membrane and endosomes in proximal tubule and in some vascular endothelia. Initial in situ hybridization studies in extrarenal tissues showed expression of mRNA encoding CHIP28 in colonic crypt, ciliary body, and alveolar epithelial cells, corneal endothelium, and red splenic pulp (50). Subsequent in situ hybridization and/or immunolocalization studies showed CHIP28 expression in epithelial cells in choroid plexus, iris, trachea, bronchial gland, pancreatic acini, sweat gland, gallbladder, placental synctiotrophoblast, and in various vascular endothelial cells (51,54,55). Where studied, the identity of mRNA encoding CHIP28 and CHIP28 protein was confirmed by Northern and immunoblot analysis.

Other Water Channels

The WCH-CD water channel was expressed only in kidney. In situ hybridization showed localization to cortical and medullary collecting duct (33) and staining with a peptide-derived polyclonal antibody showed protein expression on apical membrane of collecting duct (32). These results, taken together with data showing WCH-CD mRNA and protein upregulation with dehydration, suggested that WCH-CD represents the vasopressin-sensitive water channel (32). Other putative water channels which have been cloned from kidney include a protein that is expressed only in kidney and is upregulated by dehydration (36) and a protein expressed in kidney and small intestine (37). A mercury-insensitive water channel was cloned recently from lung and is also expressed in kidney papilla, brain, and eye (38). It is likely that distinct water channels will be identified on plasma membranes in epithelial and nonepithelial cells involved in fluid transport.

Physiological Functions

Water movement across cell membranes occurs passively in response to osmotic gradients produced by primary and secondary active ion and solute transport. High membrane water permeability is thus predicted to exist in membranes that transport water rapidly in response to relatively small osmotic gradients. The localization of CHIP28 water channels to plasma membranes in epithelial and endothelial cells in specific tissue fits nicely with its role in fluid transport. A role for intracellular water channels is less clear. Although osmotic swelling in subcellular vesicles has been proposed to be of importance in fusion events, the lack of effect of CHIP28 expression on vesicular trafficking in transfected CHO cells (31) argues against a role for intracellular water channels.

The role of water channels in osmotically induced movement of water between the blood and air-space compartments was studied directly in an in situ perfused sheep lung model (56). An autologous blood-Ringer's solution (300 mOsm) was circulated continuously through the pulmonary vasculature. The time course of blood-to-airspace water movement was measured after instillation of hypertonic saline (900 mOsm) containing radioiodinated-albumin into the air spaces. It was found that the transalveolar osmotic gradient was dissipated in <1 min and the rate of osmotic water movement was reversibly inhibited by $\sim 60\%$ by $HgCl_2$. These results provided evidence for transcellular movement of water through mercury-sensitive water channels in alveolus. The high water permeability in lung epithelial cells may be important to offset water loss accompanying respiration and for the resolution of alveolar edema.

FUTURE DIRECTIONS

Until recently, studies on water transport were directed to the phenomenological characterization of water permeability in various cell membranes. The new molecular information available about water transporters raises many new questions. The molecular mechanism by which water moves through water channels will require high-resolution structural analysis by diffraction methods. The number of water-channel family members is likely to grow and include proteins with novel structure, function, and/or tissue distribution. Modulation of the activity of specific water transporters may offer novel pharmacotherapy to a variety of clinical problems involving abnormal fluid homeostasis.

NOTE ADDED IN PROOF

A number of advances in the field have occurred since this chapter was written in September 1993. Two new members of the water channel (aquaporin) family expressed in kidney were reported: a mercurial-insensitive water channel (MIWC; ref. 38) and a glycerol intrinsic peptide (GLIP or AQP-3; Ma et al, JBC 1994; 269:21845; Ishibashi et al, PNAS 1994; 91:6269; Echevarria et al, PNAS 1994; 91:10997). By immunostaining, MIWC is expressed in basolateral membrane of kidney collecting-duct principal cells, airways, colonic villi, and cells lining the aquaductal system in brain (Frigeri et al, PNAS 1995; 92, in press). GLIP is also expressed in basolateral membrane of kidney-collecting duct as well as in several nonrenal tissues. The WCH-CD (also called AQP-CD and AQP-2) protein was proven to be the vasopressin-sensitive water channel by its mutation in non-X-linked congenital nephrogenic diabetes insipidus (Deen et al, Science 1994; 155:92) and its vasopressin-regulated trafficking (DiGiovanni et al, PNAS 1994; 91:8984). The physiological significance of CHIP28 water channels was questioned based on the observation that several humans with mutations in CHIP28 had ostensibly normal phenotypes (Preston et al, Science 1994; 265:1585). A topology study by Preston et al (JBC 1994; 269:1668) reported six membrane-spanning segments for CHIP28; an extension of the initial study by Skach et al. (48), which reported four membrane-spanning segments in the endoplasmic reticulum, showed maturation of CHIP28 topology between the endoplasmic reticulum and plasma membrane (Skach and Verkman, Biophys J 1995;68:A344). Negative-staining electron microscopy studies by Mitra et al. (49) and Walz et al. (1994; JBC 269:1583, Embo J 13:2985) provided data on CHIP28 structure in membranes, a recent projection structure at 6 Angstrom resolution by cryoelectron crystallography (Mitra et al, Clin Invest, 1995, abstr, in press) indicated that CHIP28 forms tetramers in which each monomer contains six apparent helical domains with a central cavity, possibly representing the water-transporting pathway.

REFERENCES

1. Pfeffer W. Osmotische Untersuchungen. Leipzig: Verlag von Wilhelm Engelmann, 1877.
2. House CR. Water Transport in Cells and Tissues. Baltimore, MD: Williams & Wilkins, 1974.
3. Finkelstein A. Water Movement through Lipid Bilayers, Pores, and Plasma Membranes: Theory and Reality. New York: Wiley, 1987.
4. Verkman AS. Water Channels. Austin, TX: Landes, 1993.

5. Verkman AS. Water channels in cell membranes. Annu Rev Physiol 1992; 54:97–108.
6. Harris HW, Strange K, Zeidel M. Current understanding of the cellular biology and molecular structure of the antidiuretic hormone-stimulated water transport pathway. J Clin Invest 1991; 91:1–8.
7. Brown D. Membrane recycling and epithelial cell function. Am J Physiol 1989; 256:F1–F12.
8. Berry CA, Verkman AS. Osmotic gradient dependence of osmotic water permeability in the rabbit proximal convoluted tubule. J Membr Biol 1988; 105:33–43.
9. Verkman AS. Mechanisms and regulation of water permeability in renal epithelia. Am J Physiol 1989; 257:C837–C850.
10. Verkman AS, Weyer P, Brown D, Ausiello DA. Functional water channels are present in clathrin coated vesicles from bovine kidney but not from brain. J Biol Chem 1989; 264:20608–20613.
11. Ye R, Shi LB, Lencer W, Verkman AS. Functional colocalization of water channels and proton pumps on endocytic vesicles from proximal tubule. J Gen Physiol 1989; 93:885–902.
12. Kuwahara M, Shi L-B, Marumo F, Verkman AS. Transcellular water flow modulates water channel exocytosis and endocytosis in kidney collecting tubule. J Clin Invest 1991; 88:423–429.
13. Verkman AS, Lencer W, Brown D, Ausiello DA. Endosomes from kidney collecting tubule contain the vasopressin-sensitive water channel. Nature 1988; 333:268–269.
14. Benga G, Popescu O, Borza V, et al. Water permeability in human erythrocytes: Identification of membrane proteins involved in water transport. J Cell Biol 1986; 41:252–262.
15. Zhang R, Alper S, Thorens B, Verkman AS. Evidence from oocyte expression that the erythrocyte water channel is distinct from band 3 and the glucose transporter. J Clin Invest 1991; 88;1553–1558.
16. Harris HW, Hosselet C, Guaywoodford L, Zeidel ML. Purification and partial characterization of candidate antidiuretic hormone water channel proteins of M(r) 55,000 and 53,000 from toad urinary bladder. J Biol Chem 1992; 267:22115–22121.
17. Verbavatz JM, Thoumine O, Bourguet J. Identification of apical proteins involved in the antidiuretic response of the frog urinary bladder. In: Jard S, Jamison R, eds. Vasopressin. Colleque INSERM 1991; 208:105–115.
18. Van Hoek AN, Hom ML, Luthjens LH, et al. Functional unit of 30 kDa for proximal tubule water channels as revealed by radiation inactivation. J Biol Chem 1991; 226:16633–16635.
19. Zhang R, Logee K, Verkman AS. Expression of mRNA coding for kidney and red cell water channels in Xenopus oocytes. J Biol Chem 1990; 265:15375–15378.
20. Zhang R, Verkman AS. Water and urea transport in Xenopus oocytes: Expression of mRNA from toad urinary bladder. Am J Physiol 1991; 260:C26–C34.
21. Zhang R, Skach W, Hasegawa H, et al. Cloning, functional analysis and cell localization of a kidney proximal tubule water transporter homologous to CHIP28. J Cell Biol 1993; 120:359–369.
22. Hasegawa H, Skach W, Baker O, et al. A multi-functional aqueous channel formed by CFTR. Science 1992; 258:1477–1479.
23. Fischbarg J, Kunyan K, Vera JC, et al. Glucose transporters serve as water channels. Proc Natl Acad Sci USA 1990; 87:3244–3247.
24. Echevarria M, Verkman AS. Optical measurement of osmotic water transport in cultured cells: Evaluation of the role of glucose transporters. J Gen Physiol 1992; 99:573–589.
25. Wistow GJ, Pisano MM, Chepelinski AB. Tandem sequence repeats in transmembrane channel proteins. TIBS 1991; 16:170–171.
26. Denker BM, Smith BL, Kuhajda FP, Agre P. Identification, purification, and partial characterization of a novel Mr 28,000 integral membrane protein from erythrocytes and renal tubules. J Biol Chem 1988; 263:15634–15642.
27. Preston GM, Agre P. Isolation of the cDNA for erythrocyte integral membrane protein of 28-kilodaltons: Member of an ancient channel family. Proc Natl Acad Sci USA 1991; 88:11110–11114.
28. Preston BM, Carroll TP, Guggino WB, Agre P. Appearance of water channels in Xenopus oocytes expressing red cell CHIP28 protein. Science 1992; 256:385–387.
29. Van Hoek AN, Verkman AS. Functional reconstitution of the isolated erythrocyte water channel CHIP28. J Biol Chem 1992; 267:18267–18269.
30. Zeidel ML, Ambudkar, SV, Smith BL, Agre P. Reconstitution of functional water channels in liposomes containing purified red cell CHIP28 protein. Biochemistry 1992; 31:7436–7440.
31. Ma T, Frigeri A, Tsai S-T, et al. Localization and functional analysis of CHIP28k water channels in stably transfected CHO cells. J Biol Chem 1993; 268:22756–22764.
32. Fushimi K, Uchida S, Hara Y, et al. Cloning and expression of apical membrane water channel of rat kidney collecting tubule. Nature 1993; 361:549–552.
33. Ma T, Hasegawa H, Skach W, et al. Expression, functional analysis and in situ hybridization of a cloned rat kidney collecting duct water channel. Am J Physiol 1994; 266:C189–C197.
34. Maurel C, Reizer J, Schoeder JI, Chrispeels MJ. The vacuolar membrane protein gamma-TIP creates water specific channels in Xenopus oocytes. EMBO J 1993; 12:2241–2247.

35. Van Hoek AN, Wiener M, Bicknese S, et al. Secondary structure analysis of purified CHIP28 water channels by CD and FTIR spectroscopy. Biochemistry 1993; 32:11847–11856.
36. Ma T, Frigeri A, Skach W, Verkman AS. Cloning of a cDNA from rat kidney with homology to CHIP28 and WCH-CD water channels. Biochem Biophys Res Commun 1993; 197:654–659.
37. Ishibashi K, Sasaki S, Fushimi K, et al. Molecular cloning and expressing of new water channel (WCH-3) expressed selectively in kidney and GI tract. JASN 1993; 4:855.
38. Hasegawa H, Ma T, Skach W, et al. Molecular cloning of a mercurial-insensitive water channel expressed in selected water transporting epithelia. J Biol Chem 1994; 269:5497–5500.
39. Moon C, Preston GM, Griffin CA, et al. The human aquaporin-CHIP gene: Structure, organization and chromosomal localization. J Biol Chem 1993; 268:15772–15778.
40. Echevarria M, Frindt G, Preston GM, et al. Expression of multiple water channel activities in Xenopus oocytes injected with messenger RNA from rat kidney. J Gen Physiol 1993; 101:827–841.
41. Smith BL, Agre P. Erythrocyte M_r 28,000 transmembrane protein exists as a multisubunit oligomer similar to channel proteins. J Biol Chem 1991; 266:6407–6415.
42. Van Hoek AN, Wiener MC, Lipniunas P, et al. Biochemical analysis of CHIP28 structure. JASN 1993; 4:861.
43. Verbavatz JM, Brown D, Sabolic I, et al. Tetrameric assembly of CHIP28 water channels in liposomes and cell membranes. A freeze-fracture study. J Cell Biol. 1993; 123:605–618.
44. Preston GM, Jung JS, Guggino WB, Agre P. The mercury-sensitive residue at cysteine 189 in the CHIP28 water channel. J Biol Chem 1993; 268:17–20.
45. Zhang R, van Hoek AN, Biwersi J, Verkman AS. A point mutation at cysteine 189 blocks the water permeability of rat kidney water channel CHIP28k. Biochemistry 1993; 32:2938–2941.
46. Shi LB, Skach W, Verkman AS. Functional independence of monomeric CHIP28 water channels revealed by expression of wild type-mutant heterodimers. J Biol Chem 1994; 269:10417–10422.
47. Farinas J, van Hoek AN, Shi L-B, et al. Non-polar environment of tryptophans in erythrocyte water channel CHIP28 determined by fluorescence quenching. Biochemistry 1993; 32:11857–11864.
48. Skach W, Shi LB, Calayag MC, et al. Topology and biogenesis of the CHIP28 water channel at the endoplasmic reticulum. J Cell Biol 1994; 125:803–816.
49. Mitra AK, Yaeger M, van Hoek AN, et al. Projection structure of the CHIP28 water channel at 12Å resolution. Biochemistry 1994; 33:12735–12740.
50. Hasegawa H, Zhang R, Dohrman A, Verkman AS. Tissue-specific expression of mRNA encoding rat kidney water channel CHIP28k by in situ hybridization. Am J Physiol 1993; 264:C237–C245.
51. Hasegawa H, Lian SC, Finkbeiner WE, Verkman AS. Extrarenal tissue distribution of CHIP28 water channels by in situ hybridization and antibody staining. Am J Physiol 1994; 266:C189–C197.
52. Sabolic I, Valenti G, Verbavatz JM, et al. Localization of the CHIP28 water channel in rat kidney. Am J Physiol 1992; 263:C1225–C1233.
53. Nielsen S, Smith BL, Christensen EI, et al. CHIP28 water channels are localized in constitutively water-permeable segments of the nephron. J Cell Biol 1993; 120:371–383.
54. Bondy C, Chin E, Smith BL, et al. Developmental gene expression and tissue distribution of the CHIP28 water-channel protein. Proc Natl Acad Sci USA 1993; 90:450–4504.
55. Nielsen S, Smith BL, Christensen EI, Agre P. Distribution of the aquaporin CHIP in secretory and resorptive epithelia and capillary endothelia. Proc Natl Acad Sci USA 1993; 90:7275–7279.
56. Folkesson HG, Matthay M, Hasegawa H, et al. Transcellular water transport in lung alveolar epithelium through mercurial sensitive water channels. Proc Natl Acad Sci USA 1994; 91:4970–4974.

33

Mitogen-Activated Protein Kinase Signaling Cascades

John M. Kyriakis

Massachusetts General Hospital East and Harvard Medical School, Charlestown, Massachusetts

INTRODUCTION

The characterization of the cellular signal transduction pathways mediated by the mitogen-activated protein kinases (MAPKs) has recently undergone breathtaking progress. These studies have revealed that insulin, mitogens, agents that act through heterotrimeric G proteins, as well as cellular trauma such as heat shock and even radiation-induced DNA damage all recruit a common (or at least a very similar) set of molecular players acting to mount the cell's response to these diverse stimuli. From the point of view of renal physiology, these discoveries mean that understanding phenomena as divergent as cancer, diabetic nephropathy, inflammation, and vascular regulation requires a grasp of the surprising similarities shared by different signaling mechanisms. This chapter focuses primarily on the mechanisms by which extracellular agonists, acting through receptor tyrosine kinases and heterotrimeric G proteins, as well as "intracellular" agonists such as heat shock and DNA damage, can influence gene expression and cellular physiology—primarily through activation of the MAPK family of serine/threonine protein kinases.

THE MAP KINASES

Early Studies

The discovery and early characterization of the MAPKs was somewhat apocryphal and forms the basis of the rather arcane nomenclature of this large family of protein kinases. Sturgill and Ray were exploring the mechanism by which insulin could stimulate the phosphorylation of some proteins (e.g., ribosomal S6) while stimulating the dephosphorylation of others (e.g., glycogen synthase). They hypothesized that this paradoxical phenomenon could be explained by a mechanism whereby the heat-stable inhibitor of protein phosphatase-1, inhibitor-2 (I-2), was itself inhibited by a phosphorylation event catalyzed by an insulin-stimulated protein kinase (1). Accordingly, they undertook an exploration for an insulin-stimulated 3T3-L1 cell I-2 kinase. No such kinase was found, but an insulin-stimulated kinase was observed that phosphorylated a high-molecular-weight contaminant of the I-2 preparation. The high-molecular-weight (>250 kDa) as well as the heat stability of the contaminant was reminiscent of microtubule-associated protein-2 (MAP2) and, indeed, purified MAP2 was phosphorylated very efficiently by this kinase. The kinase was named, therefore, MAP2 kinase (1). This MAP2 kinase eluted from gel filtration at a molecular weight of ≈35 to 40 kDa (2) and displayed a number of features that attracted wide interest. First, the MAP2 kinase was activated more rapidly and was quite chromatographically distinct from the insulin-stimulated ribosomal S6 kineases (3). This result suggested that the MAP2 kinase occupied a more proximal position in the signaling cascade. It was subsequently shown that MAP2 kinase could phosphorylate and activate one of these S6 kinases, the p85 Rsk (ribosomal S6 kinase) after the Rsk was dephosphorylated and inactivated with protein phosphatase (4). Second, the MAP2 kinase copurified with and was ultimately found to correspond to a 42-kDa species which became phosphorylated on tyrosine as well as threonine in response to insulin (5,6). This 42-kDa polypeptide was found to be identical to pp42, a previously uncharacterized species which is phosphorylated at tyrosine and threonine in response to a wide array of extracellular stimuli, including growth factors and phorbol esters (6). As we shall see, it was later demonstrated that MAP2 kinase requires both tyrosine and threonine phosphorylation for activity (7) and can be activated by all mitogenic stimuli, including insulin and growth factors as well as agonists acting through heterotrimeric G proteins (8–16). Accordingly, MAP2 kinase was renamed mitogen-activated protein (MAP) kinase.

Structural Features of the MAPKs: A Large Family of Protein Kinases

The Yeast Connection

Molecular cloning of the earliest known members of the MAPK family was achieved by Boulton et al. who initially isolated a partial cDNA corresponding to a 44-kDa insulin-stimulated MAP2 kinase (17). This was accomplished using a probe derived from a peptide sequence obtained from the purified polypeptide. They named this clone *erk-1* (extracellular signal regulated kinase-1). The clone showed a striking homology (56%) to *FUS3* and *KSS1*, two genes from *Saccharomyces cerevisiae*, which encode protein kinases that function to arrest the cell cycle at G1 in response to mating factor (17–19). *erk-1* was also shown to be homologous to *spk1*$^+$ from *Schizosaccharomyces pombe* (17,20). *Spk1*$^+$, when overexpressed, can confer resistance to staurosporine, implicating it in the fission yeast protein kinase C pathways (20). More recently, two additional yeast MAPK homologues have been identified: MPK1, which regulates cell wall synthesis, and HOG1, which appears to lie on an osmoregulation pathway (21,22). Thus yeast MAPKs appear to function not only in cell cycle regulation in response to extracellular stimulus but also in the regulation of a number of other cellular functions. As we shall see, the degree of conservation between mammalian and yeast signaling is quite remarkable, extending well upstream of the MAPKs.

MAPK homologues are also present in the oocytes of amphibians, marine molluscs, and echinoderms, where they are activated not only in response to stimuli which elicit oocyte maturation but also during progression through mitosis (23–29). In this capacity, MAPKs are activated at the G2/M boundary of the cell cycle, just following activation of the M-phase cyclin-dependent kinase cdc2 (23,25). Studies from Sakai and colleagues indicate that MAPK activation at G2/M mediates in part the cytoskeletal reorganization characteristic of mitosis (25). Addition of active, purified *Xenopus* or mammalian p42 MAPK to interphase extracts of *Xenopus* oocytes decreases the apparent growing speed and steady-state length of mucrotubules to that reminiscent of metaphase extracts (25).

Additional Mammalian MAPKs

Using low-stringency screening, Boulton et al. were able to isolate two additional *erk* clones, *erk-2* and *erk-3* (30). *erk-2* corresponds to the 42-kDa MAPK originally identified and subsequently cloned by Sturgill and colleagues (30,31). *erk-3* encodes a 62-kDa polypeptide which had not been detected biochemically (30). While *erk-1* and *erk-2* share 83% identity, *erk-3* is more distantly related (43% identity to *erk-1* and *erk-2*). While the *erks* are expressed ubiquitously, highest expression is observed in the brain (30).

The p54 MAPKs make up a discrete MARK subfamily. The p54 MAPK was originally purified from rat liver as the dominant MAP2 kinase activated in situ by cycloheximide (32,33). Tryptic peptide sequences of purified rat liver p54 MAPK were used to generate a CDNA probe by polymerase chain reaction (PCR) (34). This probe was used, in turn, to screen a rat brain cDNA library from which four independent clones were isolated: αI, αII, β, and γ. Sequence analysis revealed a greater than 90% homology among the p54 isoforms, with αI and αII representing mRNA splice variants. Like the *erks*, the p54 MAPKs, although essentially ubiquitous, are expressed most highly in brain (34). In addition, like the *erks*, the p54 MAPKs are strikingly homologous to the yeast MAPK homologues (55% identity to *FUS3* and *KSS1*). The p54 MAPKs share $\approx$55% identity with *erk-1* and *erk-2* and 29% identity with *erk-3* (34). Thus, based on sequence similarities, the mammalian

MAPKs can be grouped together into subfamilies, with *erk-1* and *erk-2* making up one subfamily, the p54 MAPKs another, and *erk-3* a third. It is highly likely that additional members of each MAPK subfamily remain to be discovered.

MAPK SUBSTRATES AND FUNCTIONS

The MAPKs Are Proline-Directed Protein Kinases

Erickson et al. were able to identify threonine 97 as the site on myelin basic protein (MBP), which is phosphorylated by p42 MAPK (35). This site lies within the motif VIPRTPPP and is similar in sequence to the site on the EGF receptor phosphorylated by MAPK (VEPLTPSG) in that the site of phosphorylation is followed immediately by proline (36,37). This observation raised the possibility that the MAPKs, like the cyclin-dependent kinases, were proline directed—i.e., that they required a proline immediately carboxyl terminal to the site of phosphorylation for substrate recognition. The proline-directed substrate specificity of the MAPKs was established using EGF receptor- and MBP-derived synthetic peptide substrates containing systematic sequence variations around the site of phosphorylation (37,38). These studies determined that, in addition to the C-terminal proline, the proline two residues N terminal to the phosphorylation site was also required for p42/p44 MAPK but not p54 MAPK phosphorylation, suggesting the consensus P-X-S/T-P as a common MAPK phosphorylation motif (37,38). The N-terminal proline, however, is not present in many physiological substrates and the apparent requirement for it is probably an artifact of using peptide substrates instead of bona fide protein substrates.

The MAPKs Phosphorylate and Activate the High-Molecular-Weight Cytosolic Phospholipase-A_2 ($cPLA_2$)—Implications for the Regulation of the Inflammatory Response

The phospholipase $cPLA_2$ is a member of a large family of enzymes which hydrolyze membrane phospholipids at the *sn*-2 position. It is an 85-kDa enzyme which regulates hormone-stimulated arachidonic acid release, the rate-limiting step in subsequent prostaglandin biosynthesis (39,40). In addition, the other product of $cPLA_2$ action, lysophospatidic acid, can be converted into platelet activating factor (PAF) (41). $cPLA_2$ is dramatically and stably activated in renal mesangial cells in response to a diverse array of extracellular stimuli including EGF, arginine vasopressin, and active phorbol ester. While the PMA-stimulation of $cPLA_2$ proceeds through a protein kinase C–dependent pathway, activation of $cPLA_2$ by EGF proceeds through a PKC–independent pathway inasmuch as $cPLA_2$ is activated by EGF in PKC down regulated cells (42). Recently, Nemenoff et al. demonstrated that $cPLA_2$ can be phosphorylated and activated by both purified PKC and p42 MAPK, thus providing a mechanism whereby $cPLA_2$ could be activated by PKC-dependent and independent pathways (43). While PKC phosphorylates $cPLA_2$ at sites which have been mapped to several domains [termed A (residues 1-216), B (residues 215–556), C (residues 545–749) and B′ (residues 424-556)], MAPK phosphorylation of $cPLA_2$ occurs only at domains B and B′. While domain B is phosphorylated by both PKC and MAPK, phosphorylation occurs at different tryptic peptides (43). Lin et al. reported similar results and identified the site of MAPK phosphorylation on $cPLA_2$ as Ser-505. Lin et al. also demonstrated that Ser-505 is essential for $cPLA_2$ regulation. Mutation of this Ser to Ala abolishes MAPK phosphorylation of $cPLA_2$. Moreover, the Ser-505 → Ala mutant, when expressed transiently, cannot be activated by extracellular stimuli to catalyze agonist-stimulated arachidonic acid release (44). Thus MAPKs likely play a role in agonist-stimulation of phospholipid hydrolysis, arachidonic acid release and, by implication, prostaglandin and PAF synthesis. Insofar as prostaglandins and PAF are potent vasoactive compounds and inflammatory mediators, p42/p44 MAPKs are, therefore, likely to be important regulators of the inflammatory response.

The MAPKs Phosphorylate and Activate Other Protein Kinases Involved in Signal Transduction

Consistent with the role of MAPKs as prominent signal transduction compoments is the observation that numerous other mitogen-activated Ser/Thr protein kinases are themselves MAPK substrates.

Often this MAPK-catalyzed phosphorylation is regulatory. Sturgill and colleagues observed that the insulin-stimulated 85-kDa S6 kinase from *Xenopus* oocytes (Rsk), after dephosphorylation and deactivation with phosphatase 2A, could be phosphorylated and reactivated by the p42 MAPK from insulin-stimulated 3T3-L1 cells (4). The reactivation in vitro was partial, likely due to the instability of the S6 kinase, but it is clear from subsequent studies that the p42 and p44 MAPKs are the only kinases which phosphorylate Rsk (45). Purified p54 MAPK does not phosphorylate or reactivate phosphatase-inactivated Rsk (32). This result was the first to link two consecutive Ser/Thr kinases in a mitogen signaling cascade (4).

The activation of Rsk by MAPKs is particularly important in the regulation by insulin of glycogen synthesis. Activated Rsk phosphorylates the skeletal muscle glycogen binding subunit of protein phosphatase-1 (PP1G), enhancing the binding of the phosphatase to glycogen granules. By this process, insulin promotes the dephosphorylation and activation of glycogen synthase (46,47). Thus, insulin is able to activate both protein phosphorylation (Rsk) and dephosphorylation (PP-1G) via a MAPK-dependent process (46,47).

Recently, another insulin-activated Ser/Thr kinase, termed mitogen-activated protein kinase-activated protein kinase-2 (MAPKAP kinase-2) was also shown to be regulated by the p42/p44 MAPKs (48). MAPKAP kinase-2 is of unknown function but was originally purified from insulin-stimulated rabbit skeletal muscle as a kinase capable of phosphorylating glycogen synthase at Ser-7, the same site phosphorylated in vitro by Rsk (48). Although MAPKAP kinase-2 is isolated from insulin-treated animals in an active form, there is no direct evidence as yet that it is activated by insulin. Nevertheless, purified MAPKAP kinase-2 can be deactivated with phosphatase-2A and its activity completely restored with purified p42/p44 MAPK (48). Clues as to the possible function of MAPKAP-kinase-2 come from the results of Stokoe et al. (49), who demonstrated that the low-molecular-weight heat shock proteins hsp25 and hsp27 are major MAPKAP-kinase-2 substrates. Inasmuch as both the p42/p44 MAPKs (50) and, to a much greater extent (see below) the p54 MAPKs (34), are activated by heat shock, MAPK activation of MAPKAP-kinase-2 may be one of the cell's responses to heat shock.

The MAPKs have also been shown to phosphorylate other protein kinases involved in mitogen signal transduction, most notably the Raf-1 kinase and the p70 S6 kinase (38,51–53). In the case of Raf-1, this phosphorylation can be catalyzed in vitro by the p42/p44 MAPKs but not by p54 MAPKs (53). The sites phosphorylated on Raf-1 by MAPKs comigrate on two-dimensional tryptic phosphopeptide maps, with most of the sites phosphorylated on Raf-1 in situ in response to mitogen. Yet MAPK phosphorylation of Raf-1 has no apparent effect on Raf-1 activity (53), and, as we shall see, the role of phosphorylation in the regulation of Raf-1 is moot. The p70 S6 kinase, on the other hand, clearly requires Ser/Thr phosphorylation for activity, and the phosphorylation of p70 by MAPKs (both p42/44 and p54 MAPKs) occurs at a region of the p70 polypeptide, which acts as a pseudosubstrate autoinhibitory domain (38). It seems, however, that this phosphorylation is insufficient per se to activate p70 (38). The identity of the other kinases required for p70 activation remains unknown.

Phosphorylation of Transcription Factors by MAPKs

The idea that MAPKs could phosphorylate transcription factors at first seemed counterintuitive, inasmuch as the MAPKs have been traditionally purified from cytosolic extracts. Much recent data from the laboratories of Blenis, Pouysségur, and Davis now demonstrate clearly that a portion of the cellular MAPK pool translocates to the nucleus upon stimulation with mitogens (54–56). Interestingly, Lenormand et al. demonstrated that nonmitogenic stimulation of cells with agents such as thrombin does not result in MAPK nuclear translocation (55). These workers observed that the persistent activation of MAPKs by mitogens, rather than the transient activation of MAPKs by agents acting at heptahelical receptors coupled to heterotrimeric G proteins, correlates with MAPK translocation (55,57). These cell biological data now complement a wealth of data implicating MAPKs in the regulation of nuclear transcription factors.

c-Jun Is a MAPK Substrate: Implications for the Regulation of the AP-1 Transcription Factor

The product of the protooncogene c-*jun* is a component of the AP-1 transcription factor. Typically, AP-1 consists of a heterodimer of c-Jun and a member of the *fos* protooncogene family. AP-1 binds, in a mitogen-dependent manner, to a *cis*-acting element, the TPA response element (TRE), whose minimal sequence has been defined by the palindromic motif TGA C/G TCA. Much of the regulation of AP-1 activity is mediated by c-Jun, which contains several functionally independent domains. The carboxyl terminal region contains a basically charged DNA binding domain followed by a leucine zipper–type dimerization motif. The amino terminal region of the molecule contains the *trans* activation domain (58,59). DNA binding and *trans* activation are each regulated by phosphorylation in a coordinate yet independent manner. Phosphorylation at sites just amino terminal the DNA binding domain (Thr 231, Thr 239, Ser 243, and Ser 249) inhibits c-Jun DNA binding. Phosphorylation of the C-terminal sites is catalyzed in vitro by glycogen synthase kinase-3 (GSK-3) or casein kinase-2 (60,61). In resting cells, these sites are usually phosphorylated. Phorbol ester or mitogen stimulation results in the dephosphorylation of the C-terminal sites, thereby enhancing c-Jun DNA binding (60). The mechanism by which this dephosphorylation is regulated is not clear, although it has been shown that GSK-3 is Tyr phosphorylated in resting cells (62). Mutation to Phe of the Tyr residue which undergoes phosphorylation abolishes GSK-3 activity (62). Mitogens might stimulate the Tyr dephosphorylaton and inactivation of GSK-3. Alternatively, PMA or mitogen stimulation of cells could result in the direct activation of a phosphatase which could target the c-Jun C-terminal phosphorylation sites (59). More compelling results have come from the laboratory of Cohen and colleagues, who recently demonstrated that the activity of GSK-3 could be completely inhibited by the p70 S6 kinase and, to a lesser extent by the p85 Rsk S6 kinase (63). Thus MAPKs, by activating Rsk and, possibly, p70 S6 kinases may also regulate c-Jun dephosphorylation.

In several cell types, phorbol esters, growth factors, ectopically expressed oncogenes (*ras*, *raf*, *sis*), ultraviolet radiation, or heat shock can stimulate the phosphorylation of c-Jun in the *trans* activation domain in correlation with enhanced c-Jun *trans* activation (34,64–70). The UV response is apparently mediated by Src, and, like the mitogen pathway, by Ras and Raf-1; in addition, it involves an increase in cellular oxidation, inasmuch as UV induction of AP-1 can be blocked by dominant-negative *src ras* or *raf-1* or by N-acetyl cysteine (69,70).

The phosphorylation sites at the c-Jun amino terminus have been mapped to Ser 73 and 63 which reside in two tryptic phosphopeptides termed "X" and "Y", respectively (64,65). These serines are critical to c-Jun transactivation function insofar as mutagenesis of either site to Leu severely compromises c-Jun *trans* activation of a cotransfected TRE-CAT reporter construct (64,66). Recombinant c-Jun is phosphorylated at Ser 63 and 73 by the MAPKs with p54 MAPKs phosphorylating c-Jun five-to-sevenfold more rapidly than a mixture of p42 and p44 MAPKs, when the MAPK preparations are employed at equal MAP2 phosphorylating activity (64).

The assignment of MAPKs as c-Jun N-terminal kinases has been controversial, however. Much of the controversy revolves around the observed phosphorylation of Ser 243 by p42/44 MAPKs in vitro (37). We have observed that this phosphorylation is quantitatively less prominent than the phosphorylation at Ser 63 and 73 (J. Kyriakis; unpublished) if the assays employ a bacterially expressed c-Jun polypeptide which has not undergone irreversible denaturation and retains normal DNA binding. Moreover, MAPK phosphorylation of Ser 243 would not be expected to occur physiologically inasmuch as conditions which activate MAPKs in situ (e.g., PMA) result in dephosphorylation of Ser 243 (60,61). In addition, p54 MAPKs phosphorylate c-Jun exclusively at Ser 63 and 73 in vitro (64). Moreover, mutagenesis of c-Jun at Ser 63 and 73 dramatically reduces c-Jun phosphorylation by MAPKs in vitro and in response to PMA, in vivo: while mutagenesis of both sites to Leu essentially abolishes c-Jun phosphorylation (64). In addition, the major c-Jun kinases of PMA-stimulated U937 cells copurify over several chromatographic steps with p42 and p44 MAPKs (71).

As for the role of the p54 MAPKs, As discussed below, the p54 MAPKs are activated by heat stress, the presence of misfolded proteins in the cell, and by tumor necrosis factor α (TNF-α) (34). Insofar as the p42/p44 MAPKs are activated only very weakly under these conditions, it is likely that the p54 MAPKs are major c-Jun kinases recruited as a consequence of environmental or cellular/physiological stress (34).

Interestingly, neither the p54 nor p42/p44 MAPKs can phosphorylate v-Jun despite the presence of serines analogous to 63 and 73. It has been proposed that v-Jun, which is constitutively active transcriptionally due to deletion of residues corresponding to c-Jun residues 31–57 (the delta deletion), may have lost its ability to serve as a MAPK substrate, presumably due to loss of a MAPK binding site within the delta domain (68,71,72). The regulation of c-Jun function is, then, exquisitely complex and involves coordinate (de)phosphorylation at functionally distinct domains. Dephosphorylation at the C terminus in response to agonist results in enhanced DNA binding, while phosphorylation at the amino terminal *trans* activation domain, catalyzed by MAPKs, results in enhanced *trans* activation.

p62^{TCF} and Elk-1 Are MAPK Substrates: Implications for Regulation of Transcription at the Serum Response Element

Full induction of AP-1 activity by extracellular stimuli requires not only the posttranslational modifications of c-Jun described above but also the expression of sufficient amounts of c-Fos to allow for effective Fos-Jun dimer formation (58). *c-fos* is an immediate early gene and, accordingly, is expressed very rapidly and transiently in response to mitogen. Transcription of the *c-fos* gene is under the regulation of the serum-response element (SRE), a *cis*-acting element required for the growth factor-induced transient expression of many immediate early genes (73). Activity at the SRE is dependent on the binding of two polypeptides: the serum response factor (SRF) and the ternary complex factor (p62^{TCF}) (73–75). p62^{TCF} cannot bind to the SRE itself but is apparently required for full SRE function (75). A cDNA for p62^{TCF} has not been cloned per se. However, two cDNAs encoding Ets domain proteins with p62^{TCF}-like DNA binding properties and immunoreactivity have been isolated: *sap-1* and *elk-1*.

Both Elk-1 and Sap-1 contain three homologous domains: two N-terminal domains, which mediate DNA contact and ternary complex formation, respectively, and a third C-terminal domain. The C-terminal domains of both Sap-1 and Elk-1 contain several S/T-P MAPK consensus phosphorylation sites, and this suggested that Elk-1 could be a MAPK target (76–78).

Shaw and colleagues were able to show that purified p62^{TCF} was a substrate for the p42/p44 MAPKs (78). In gel shift assays using an SRE probe, treatment of p62^{TCF} with these MAPKs led to enhanced ternary complex formation (78). Subsequent phosphatase treatment abolished complex formation. p67^{SRF} was not a MAPK substrate (78). In elegant experiments, Treisman and colleagues demonstrated that Elk-1 was a p42/p44 MAPK substrate (79). Ternary complex formation was enhanced upon treatment of recombinant Elk-1 with MAPKs (79). Tryptic phosphopeptide mapping demonstrated that p42/p44 MAPKs phosphorylate Elk-1 at the same sites that undergo phosphorylation in situ. Moreover, if the consensus C-terminal MAPK phosphorylation sites were mutated, the mutant Elk polypeptide, expressed transiently, no longer underwent serum-stimulated phosphorylation and could not *trans* activate a cotransfected SRE-CAT construct (79). Similarly, in an in vitro assay using purified polypeptides, the mutant Elk-1 proteins were no longer phosphorylated by MAPKs (79). These results demonstrate that the C-terminal domain of Elk-1 serves as a growth factor-regulated transcriptional activation domain, and that this domain is directly regulated by MAPKs, thereby linking activation of the SRE to the p42/p44 MAPK pathway. The C-terminal sites on Elk-1 are excellent potential p54 MAPK sites. Insofar as "superinduction" of *fos* can be stimulated by cycloheximide, an activator of the p54 MAPKs, it would be of considerable interest to determine if p54 MAPKs can also phosphorylate Elk-1, and if Elk-1 phosphorylation is stimulated by heat stress, tunicamycin or TNF-α (see below) (34).

c-Myc, Another Immediate Early Gene, Is Also a MAPK Substrate

c-Myc is a rapid-turnover helix-loop-helix (HLH) type nuclear protein which, like c-Fos, is the product of an immediate early gene. Transcription of c-*myc* is induced rapidly upon mitogenic stimulation, whereupon the c-Myc polypeptide forms a dimer with Max, another HLH protein, through their respective leucine zipper domains (80). The c-Myc/Max heterodimer then binds DNA in a sequence-specific manner and functions as a transcriptional regulator (80,81). The amino terminus of c-Myc contains a *trans* activation domain which is distinct from the HLH domain and the leucine zipper (82). A Ser residue in this domain (Ser 62) becomes phosphorylated upon mitogenic stimulation. This residue is also phosphorylated in vitro by a 41-kDa MAPK which is homologous to p42 MAPK (83,84). Fusion proteins containing the c-Myc *trans* activation domain and the GAL-4 DNA binding domain, when expressed transiently, can *trans* activate cotransfected GAL-4-CAT reporter constructs (84). Mutation of c-Myc Ser-62 to Ala abolishes the *trans* activating activity of these fusion proteins, attesting to the requirement for Ser-62 for c-Myc *trans* activating activity (83,84). Cotransfection of the 41-kDa MAPK cDNA with the c-Myc-GAL-4 fusion construct and the GAL-4-CAT construct enhances transactivation of the reporter gene (83,84). Taken together, these results suggest that MAPKs mediate activation of c-Myc *trans* activation through phosphorylation of Ser-62 of the c-Myc polypeptide; a result which is analogus to the regulation of c-Jun by MAPKs (83,84).

The p54 MAPKs Are on a Signaling Pathway Activated by Heat Stress and TNF-α and May Be Recruited as Part of a Sphingomyelin Signaling Pathway

The responses of cells to heat stress have been extensively characterized (reviewed in refs 85–87). These responses entail some of the most highly conserved pathways of regulated gene expression known. Many of the proteins induced by the heat-stress response bind to other cellular proteins and prevent their denaturation (85–87). There is even evidence that some stress proteins can, in an ATP-dependent manner, refold heat-denatured proteins, restoring them to their native conformations (86). In addition, heat stress activates protein translation (85–87). It is likely that much of the heat-shock signaling response is initiated by the accumulation of misfolded proteins in the cell (85–87). For example, the heat stress response transcription factor HSF (heat-shock factor), which regulates the expression of the heat-shock protein hsp70, is normally bound to hsp70 and is thereby held in an inactive state. Accumulating heat-denatured proteins compete with HSF for hsp70 binding (87). Eventually enough hsp70 is sequestered by the denatured proteins that sufficient free HSF can aggregate into the active, trimeric state and bind to its cognate *cis*-acting element, resulting in elevated hsp70 transcription (87). By this process hsp70 regulates its own synthesis. A similar regulatory mechanism was described by Matts et al. for the regulation, by heat stress, of the heme-regulated eIF-2α kinase. In this instance, denatured protein, added to crude cell extracts activates the kinase (88). This activation is prevented by the addition of excess hsp70 (89). In addition, tunicamycin, an inhibitor of N-linked protein glycosylation, also induces many genes normally activated by heat stress (86,88,90). Presumably, nonglycosylated proteins do not fold properly and their presence in the lumen of the endoplasmic reticulum (ER) signals activation of a response similar to that induced by the heat denaturation of cellular polypeptides (86,88,90).

The role of protein kinases and signaling cascades in the heat-stress response has not been clearly determined. Blenis and colleagues have demonstrated that heat stress leads to the activation of the p70 and Rsk S6 kinases (91). In addition, many cytosolic heat-shock proteins and heat-shock transcription factors become phosphorylated during the heat-stress response (48,49,91,92). Enhanced protein-tyrosine phosphorylation has also been observed in response to heat stress (93). Perhaps the most intriguing evidence for a stress-regulated signaling cascade comes from the work of Sambrook and colleagues. In these studies, it was shown that tunicamycin and heat stress can activate the transcription of reporter genes driven by a *cis* acting element, the unfolded protein response element (UPRE) (89,94). This process is mediated by *trans* acting factors, the unfolded protein response factors (UPRFs). Mutants of *S. cerevesiae* were isolated that were deficient in this response. One such mutant, *ern-1*, was found to encode a receptor-like Ser/Thr protein kinase homologous to the cyclin-dependent protein kinases (90). It has been proposed that Ern-1 binds misfolded proteins present in the lumen of the ER, thereby initiating a signaling cascade culminating in UPRE *trans* activation (90).

In our studies of the p54 MAPKs, we have observed that these kinases are not activated by insulin, mitogens, or phorbol esters. Instead, the p54 MAPKs are potently activated by heat stress and tunicamycin (34). These stimuli only weakly activate the p42/p44 MAPKs (34). We also observe that heat stress is a potent activator of c-Jun phosphorylation; and that this phosphorylation occurs in the c-Jun transactivation domain at peptides X and Y. Thus, in mammalian cells, a heat and tunicamycin-activated signaling cascade exists, which utilizes the p54 MAPKs to phosphorylate c-Jun, probably in response to the presence of misfolded proteins in the cell (34). It would be of considerable interest to determine if a mammalian *ern-1* homologue exists which couples to the p54 MAPKs.

Integration of the physiological interorgan response to external stress stimuli, in particular septic infection, is mediated in part by a number of inflammatory cytokines. An example is TNF-α, which was originally isolated from the serum of mice undergoing septic shock induced by bacille

Calmette-Guérin (BCG). Early experiments demonstrated that TNF-α could itself induce the hemorrhagic necrosis of certain transplantable tumors in inbred mice (95,96). The cellular actions of TNF-α are quite multifarious and include antagonism of insulin-stimulated lipogenesis, activation of the hepatic acute-phase response, enhanced neutrophil superoxide radical production and cytotoxic efficacy, and stimulation of T-cell cytokine secretion (95,96). These diverse cellular functions are due in part to TNF-α-induced programs of gene expression (95–98). Notably, TNF-α is one of the most potent inducers of c-Jun *trans* activation activity (97). In addition, TNF-α can strongly stimulate the activity of NF-κB (98).

This profile of stress-related cellular responses led us to ask if TNF-α could activate the p54 MAPKs. We observe a striking activation of CCD-18Co cell, primary hepatocyte and HepG2 cell p54 MAPKs by TNF-α (34). In all cases, when compared to epidermal growth factor (EGF) and PMA (which act through Ras and Raf-1, see below), TNF-α is a more potent p54 MAPK agonist (34). By contrast, EGF and PMA are much more potent inducers of p42/p44 MAPK activity (34). Thus although both classes of MAPK are activated by TNF-α, EGF and PMA, there is a dramatic difference in the relative activation of each pathway by these different stimuli. This differential activation of the p42/p44 MAPKs vs the p54 MAPKs pertains directly to a central issue in the field of signal transduction: signaling specificity. EGF and TNF-α, which each elicit widely divergent responses, may do so in part via the differential recruitment of distinct MAPK pathways.

Little is known of the mechanisms of TNF-α signaling. TNF-α binds to either of two receptors, of 50 kDa and 70 kDa, whose intracellular extensions bear no similarity to those of receptors whose signaling mechanisms are better understood (99,100). Work primarily from the laboratories of Hannun and colleagues and Kolesnick and colleagues demonstrates that the initial actions of TNF-α are mediated at least in part by the activation of a neutral sphingomyelinase, which acts to hydrolyze membrane sphingomyelins thereby generating ceramide (101,102). These studies suggest that ceramide acts as a second messenger for TNF-α insofar as addition of ceramide derivatives or bacterial sphingomyelinases to intact or permeabilized cells can elicit several of the known responses to TNF-α including activation of a heterotrimeric type 2A protein phosphatase, activation of a ceramide-dependent membrane-associated protein kinase, and possibly activation of NF-κB (101,102). We observe substantial activation of the p54 MAPKs upon addition of *Staphylococcus aureus* sphingomyelinase to intact HepG2 cells, suggesting that the p54 MAPKs lie on a sphingomyelin pathway. The sphingomyelin pathway is in no way restricted to the action of TNF-α. Stimulation of sphingomyelin hydrolysis occurs in response to numerous other stimuli including IL-1β, dihydroxy vitamin D3, interferon γ, and ischemia (101,102). It is of considerable interest to determine if the p54 MAPKs are also activated preferentially by these stimuli.

REGULATION OF THE p42/p44 MAPKs: REQUIREMENT FOR THR AND TYR PHOSPHORYLATION CATALYZED BY A NOVEL, DUAL-SPECIFICITY KINASE, MAPK OR ERK-KINASE (MEK)

All MAPKs Examined thus Far Require Tyr and Ser/Thr Phosphorylation for Activity

The ability of tyrosine phosphatases or Ser/Thr phosphatases to selectively deactivate p42/p44 MAPKs as well as p54 MAPKs established the requirement for dual Tyr and Thr phosphorylation for maintenance of MAPKs in the active state (7,33). This requirement for Tyr and Thr phosphorylation typifies the activation state of MAPKs regardless of the type of extracellular activation pathway, be it via Tyr kinases, Ca^{2+} entry, heterotrimeric G protein–coupled agonists, PKC-dependent or PKC-independent pathways (5,6,8–16).

Payne et al. identified the sites on p42 MAPK which become phosphorylated in response to agonist as Thr-183 and Tyr-185 in subdomain VIII of the catalytic domain (103). These residues lie within a domain that is highly conserved among the *erk*s, *FUS3*, and *KSS1*; a rough consensus has been described: GFΦ<u>T</u>E<u>Y</u>VATR (Φ is a hydrophobic residue and the phosphorylated residues are underlined) (103). The sequence in this region is slightly different for the p54 MAPKs, FMMTPYVVTR, and is invariant among the four known p54 MAPK subfamily members (34).

p42/p44 MAPKs Are Phosphorylated and Activated by MEK, a Novel Dual-specificity Protein Kinase

Although the initial finding that MAPKs required Tyr as well as Thr phosphorylation for activity suggested that they may be direct substrates of Tyr kinases, it is now known, at least for the p42/p44 MAPKs, that the activation is much more indirect. Ahn et al. were the first to identify a MAPK "activator" present in extracts of EGF-treated Swiss 3T3 cells (104). This activator could reactivate phosphatase-inactivated p42/p44 MAPKs back to the levels observed prior to phosphatase treatment (104). The activator exhibited dual specificity and could reactivate MAPKs whether they had been inactivated with Tyr or Ser/Thr phosphatase (104). This MAPK activator was entirely cytosolic and was easily distinguished from the MAPKs on Mono-Q anion exchange columns (104). The dual specificity MAPK reactivating activity copurified through Mono-Q, Mono-S, and gel filtration, indicating that it was a single entity or two very tightly associated activities (104). Gómez and Cohen reported similar results and were able to demonstrate that the MAPK activator was itself regulated by Ser/Thr phosphorylation, inasmuch as it could be inactivated completely with Ser/Thr phosphatase but not Tyr phosphatase (105).

The biochemical nature of the MAPK activator was initially unclear, insofar as earlier studies had shown that bacterially expressed recombinant p42 MAPK could slowly autophosphorylate at the regulatory Tyr and Thr and autoactivate (106–108). This finding suggested that the MAPK activator was not a protein kinase but instead was an allosteric regulatory protein which accelerated the rate of MAPK autoactivation. Definitive evidence that the MAPK activator was, in fact a protein kinase of dual specificity came from a number of laboratories. Adams and Parker used fluorosulfonyl benzoyl adenosine (FSBA) to chemically inactivate purified MAPK by covalent modification of the ATP binding site. This FSBA-inactivated MAPK was still phosphorylated at Tyr and Thr by partially purified MAPK activator (109). Several laboratories used site-directed mutagenesis to generate inactive recombinant MAPKs in which the invariant Lys in the ATP binding site was changed to Arg (110–114). Partially purified preparations of MAPK activator were able to phosphorylate these mutant MAPKs at Tyr and Thr. Posada and Cooper mutated the regulatory Thr or Tyr of recombinant *Xenopus* p42 MAPK to Ala or Phe, respectively. These mutants, although inactive, were phosphorylated at the remaining wild-type residue when expressed in vitro (24). Similar patterns of dual specificity have now been observed using homogeneously pure preparations of MAPK activator and recombinant MAPKs bearing the inactivating Lys → Arg mutation along with either the Thr → Ala or Tyr → Phe mutations in the phosphorylation domain (110–114). Accordingly, MAPK "activator" was renamed MAPK kinase or MAPKK.

At least two distinct MAPKK clones have now been isolated. Crews et al. were first to report a MAPKK clone and gave their clone the more ecumenical name MAPK or ERK kinase (*mek*) (115). Identical clones were isolated by Seger et al. (116) and Ashworth et al. (117) Wu and colleagues isolated a cDNA identical to *mek* (118) as well as a second distinct yet highly similar clone that they refer to as *mkk2* (119). As with the *erks*, the *meks* are strikingly homologous to elements involved in yeast signal transduction: STE7 from the *S. cerevesiae* mating factor pathway and $byr1^+$ from *S. pombe* (115–120). Consistent with the biochemical data from vertebrate systems placing Meks upstream of MAPKs, genetic studies place *STE7* upstream of *FUS3/KSS1*, the *S. cerevesiae* MAPK homologues (121,122), while the relationship between $byr1^+$, originally isolated as a supressor of *ras1* mutations, and $spk1^+$ is unknown. Inspection of the *mek* amino acid sequences places them among the Ser/Thr kinases with no indication as to the basis for dual specificity.

It is important to note that the Meks isolated thus far are entirely specific for the p42/p44 MAPKs and cannot (re)activate p54 MAPKs whether the substrate used is purified rat liver p54 MAPK inactivated with phosphatase or bacterially expressed, recombinant p54 MAPKs (J. Kyriakis; unpublished). Thus, the p54 MAPK activator is an entirely different species yet to be identified.

MEK IS A SIGNAL-INTEGRATING PROTEIN KINASE ACTIVATED BY DISTINCT PROTEIN KINASES: RAF-1 AND MEK-KINASE (MEKK)

Activation of MEK by Raf-1

The MEK purified from stimulated ^{32}P-labeled cells is phosphorylated at Ser/Thr or Thr only (111). Treatment of MEK with Ser/Thr phosphatase but not Tyr phosphatase can completely inactivate MEK activity (105,110–112). These results suggested that one or more Ser/Thr kinases couple MEK to upstream signaling elements. In attempts to identify kinases upstream of MEK, we and others observed that p42/p44 MAPKs and MEK were constitutively active in NIH3T3 cells stably transformed with v-*raf*, a viral oncogene the normal cellular homologue of which is c-*raf*-1 (123–125). c-*raf*-1 encodes a Ser/Thr kinase (126). Moreover, we observed that this constitutively active MEK could, after partial purification, be completely inactivated by phosphatase 2A (123). This observation led us to test whether or not MEK, after inactivation with phosphatase, could be reactivated in vitro with Raf-1. Initially, we used an amino terminally truncated, constitutively active form of Raf-1, BXB-Raf, and observed that this Raf-1 could phosphorylate and reactivate phosphatase-inactivated MEK to the levels of activity observed prior to phosphatase treatment (123). This result was subsequently confirmed by others (124,125). We have since shown that MEK activation is part of the normal program of agonist-stimulated Raf-1 activity (53). Notably, the ability of endogenous c-Raf-1 to phosphorylate and activate MEK is activated by insulin, mitogens, phorbol esters, thrombin, and endothelin (53). In addition, mitogen activation of Raf-1 occurs more rapidly than activation of MEK, consistent with the idea that Raf-1 lies upstream of MEK in the mitogen signaling cascade (53). Biochemical analysis of purified Raf-1 polypeptide, produced in Sf9 cells infected with recombinant baculoviruses encoding v-*ras*, c-*raf*-1 and v-*src*, indicates that MEK is a high-affinity Raf-1 subtsrate (K_m 0.8 μM) (127). Moreover, Raf-1 has an apparently very narrow substrate specificity, inasmuch as no model substrate (histones, casein, syntide, etc.) is phosphorylated at >20% of the rate of MEK phosphorylation, and heat-denatured MEK is not a Raf-1 substrate (127). These results clearly identify Raf-1 as a MEK kinase and identify the first known physiological substrate of Raf-1.

MEK-Kinase (MEKK), an Additional MEK activator: The Heterotrimeric G-Protein Connection

Several studies indicate that Raf-1 is not the only MEK-activating species. While Johnson and colleagues also observed that *raf* (and *ras*) transformation of NIH3T3 cells led to constitutive p42/p44 MAPK activity, Rat-1a cells expressing these oncogenes showed no constitutive MAPKs (128,129). Instead, transformation of Rat-1a cells with *gip2*, a constitutively active, oncogenic heterotrimeric G protein α subunit of the $G_{\alpha i2}$ type, resulted in MAPK activation (128,129). In NIH3T3 cells, however, *gip2* was without effect on MAPKs (129). In addition, Wood et al. observed that expression of v-*raf* does not result in MAPK activation in PC-12 cells (130). Finally, although there has been an astonishing conservation among the various signaling components of vertebrates and yeast (*erk*s, *FUS3*, *KSS1* and *spk1*$^+$; *mek*s, *STE7*, and *byr1*$^+$, for example), no yeast analogues of Raf-1 are known. Instead, genetic studies place *STE11* upstream of *STE7* in *S. cerevesiae* (131,132). *STE11* encodes a homologous protein Ser/Thr kinase with a similar domain topology to that of Raf-1, but aside from this similarity and the elements shared by all protein kinases, there are no significant homologies between Raf-1 and *STE11* (133).

Recently, Lange-Carter et al. used degenerate oligonucleotides based on conserved catalytic domain regions of *STE11* to isolate a murine *STE11* homologue which they have named MEK-kinase (*mekk*) (134). MEKK, when immunoprecipitated from overexpressing cells, can phosphorylate and activate MEK in vitro (134). MEKK overexpression does not activate Raf-1, indicating that the two kinases operate in parallel (134). The mechanism of activation of MEKK in situ is, however, unclear. While overexpression of MEKK in COS cells results in a dramatic increase in resting cell p42/p44 MAPK and MEK activity, this activity is not further stimulated by EGF. In fact, the Raf-1 endogenous to COS cells displays more MEK activating activity upon EGF stimulation than does the overexpressed MEKK from EGF-treated COS cells (134). While a high basal activity of overexpressed MEKK may result in full activation of endogenous MAPKs, the relatively modest activation of MEKK by EGF has been interpreted to mean that Raf-1 and MEKK lie on distinct signaling pathways subject to activation by different extracellular ligands (134). In this regard, it should be noted that, in contrast with the apparently high basal activity of MEKK when transfected transiently into COS cells, analogous overexpression of c-*raf*-1 does not result in constitutive MAPK activation (53,134). COS cells, which are SV40 transformed, may possess a constitutively active MEKK activation system which is distinct from that regulating Raf-1. On the other hand, the high basal activity of MEKK upon transfection and overexpression may be indicative of negative regulation. In other words, MEKK may be constitutively active, when assayed as a purified polypeptide in vitro. In situ, however, the enzyme may be rendered inactive via the binding of an inhibitory subunit. Overexpressed, transfected MEKK may act as a sink, absorbing out all available endogenous inhibitory subunit. Thus excess MEKK polypeptide would appear constitutively active. One candidate for such a negative regulator would be a mammalian homologue of *STE5* which is situated upstream of *STE11* in the yeast mating factor pathway (21; see Fig. 3).

If the astonishing conservation among yeast and vertebrate signaling pathways is extended, one would expect MEKK to lie on a pathway activated by ligands whose effects are mediated by heterotrimeric G proteins. Activation of the *STE11* → *STE7* → *FUS3/KSS1* pathway in *S. cerevesiae*, for example, is engendered by mating factors that interact with serpentine receptors coupled to heterotrimeric G proteins. There are data, however, indicating that divergence in the signaling mechanisms recruited by mitogens vs. those recruited by agents acting through heterotrimeric G proteins may not be so clear-cut. In spite of their data indicating that Rat-1a cells transformed with *ras* or *raf* show no constitutive MAPK activation while *gip*2 expression does result in MAPK activation, Johnson and colleagues recently demonstrated that stable expression of the m1 muscarinic receptor, which acts through a $G_{\alpha i2}$-dependent mechanism, activates both Raf-1-dependent MEK phosphorylation as well as enhanced GTP loading of Ras (135). Moreover, as mentioned above, we have observed activation of NIH3T3 cell Raf-1 by endothelin and thrombin (53). In addition, in a remarkable series of experiments, Samuels et al. (136) used hraf ER, a chimeric protein consisting of the Raf-1 catalytic domain fused to the estrogen-binding domain of the estrogen receptor. This molecule could induce the estrogen-dependent transformation of both NIH3T3 and Rat-1a cells. In an analogous observation to that of Johnson and colleagues (128,129), Rat-1a cells expressing hraf ER displayed no in situ estrogen-dependent MAPK activation (136). Surprisingly, however, estrogen did activate MEK (136). These apparently paradoxical results were reconciled when it was observed that preincubation of Rat-1a cells with okadaic acid (an inhibitor of type 2A Ser/Thr phosphatases) or sodium vanadate (a Tyr-phosphatase inhibitor) resulted in restoration of estrogen-stimulated MAPK activation (136). Thus, the simplest explanation for the lack of MAPK activation in *raf*-transformed Rat-1a cells is that Rat-1a cells possess greater endogenous levels of phosphatase activity, which act to decrease MAPK activity to unrecoverable levels. It remains to be determined whether or nor MEKK is activated under conditions in which Raf-1 activation of the MAPK pathway is not apparent as in Rat-1a cells treated with agonists such as thrombin or endothelin, or in PC-12 cells treated with NGF, or if MEKK is activated at all by extracellular stimuli. Still, MEKK represents the most proximal member of an ancient signaling cascade highly conserved among eukaryotic species. Raf-1 and Tyr kinases, for which no yeast homologues have been identified, may represent adaptations to the unique exigencies of growth control and cellular regulation resulting from multicellularity.

cAMP Agonists Inhibit Activation of the MAP Kinase Pathway via Inhibition of Raf-1

For a long time it has been known that agonists which stimulate the appearance of cAMP and the activation of the cAMP-dependent protein kinase (PKA) can antagonize the effects of insulin and mitogens. The molecular nature of this inhibition, however, remained unclear. Recently, however, Sturgill and colleagues and McCormick and colleagues demonstrated that cAMP agonists directly inhibit mitogen activation of the MAP kinase pathway (137,138). Wu et al. demonstrated that this process proceeds via PKA-catalyzed phosphorylation of Raf-1 at Ser 43 (137). This phosphorylation occurs in vitro and in situ in response to forskolin (137). In both cases, this phosphorylation inhibits the interaction of the Raf-1 amino terminus with GTP-Ras (137,138). As we shall see, this interaction is a major component of the Raf-1 activation process. These results provide a molecular basis for cross-talk between the cAMP-dependent and mitogen-activated protein phosphorylation pathways.

UPSTREAM OF RAF-1: THE CONNECTION TO RAS AND THE MEMBRANE

Raf-1 Binds Directly to Ras

While the upstream regulators of MEKK are as yet unknown, an explosion of new results has identified most of the components which couple Raf-1 to receptor and non-receptor Tyr kinases. The essential role of the products of the *ras* protooncogenes in mitogenic signaling was established several years ago when Stacey and colleagues microinjected anti-Ras antibodies into cultured mammalian cells and observed an inhibition of mitogen responsiveness and transformation by some but not all oncogenes (139). The Ras polypeptides are low-molecular-weight GTP-binding proteins. In their GTP-bound state, Ras proteins are active signal transducers, while GDP-bound Ras proteins are inactive. All Ras proteins possess a slow intrinsic autoinactivating GTPase activity, which is greatly enhanced by GTPase-activating proteins (GAPs) (140). The $p120^{GAP}$ and neurofibromin, the product of the von Reklinghausen neurofibromatosis gene comprise the major known GAPs (140,141). Ras polypeptides are activated upon dissociation of GDP in exchange for GTP, which is in excess in the cell (142). GDP dissociation is stimulated by guanine nucleotide exchange factors (142). The best understood of these is mSOS, the mammalian homolog of the *Drosophila son of sevenless* (*SOS*) gene (143). The *SOS* product is a component of the *sevenless* tyrosine kinase signaling pathway which governs the development of *Drosophila* ommatidia (See below) (144).

Implication of Ras in the activation of MAPKs has come from several lines of study. Leevers and Marshall scrape-loaded oncogenic Ras protein into Rat-1a cells and showed that this resulted in activation of p42/p44 MAPKs (145). Additional compelling evidence for a role for Ras in the activation of MAPKs came from the use of dominant negative *ras* mutants such as the N17-*ras*. These functionally impaired Ras proteins are believed to bind guanine nucleotide exchange proteins without undergoing accelerated guanine nucleotide release. As such, the dominant negatives competitively inhibit endogenous Ras guanine nucleotide exchange, thereby preventing activation of the endogenous Ras. Overexpression of these dominant negatives inhibits activation of MAPKs, Rsk, and Raf-1 by NGF, PDGF, and insulin almost completely (130,148,149). Finally, several groups have demonstrated that active Ras polypeptides can activate MAPKs in crude systems. Addition of GTP-Ras to cytosolic extracts of *Xenopus* oocytes, or Triton-disrupted NIH3T3 cells results in activation of endogenous p42/p44 MAPKs (150–154).

Ras polypeptides undergo extensive posttranslational modification, including farnesylation and palmitoylation (155). The fully processed Ras protein is then inserted in the membrane, presumably via the palmitoyl group (155). The farnesyl group is essential for Ras transforming potential, and it is interesting to note that, in addition to GTP loading, farnesylation of Ras is essential for this observed in vitro activation of MAPKs by added Ras (152).

Given, then, that Ras is upstream of Raf-1, MEK, and p42/p44 MAPKs, how does Ras activate the MAPK pathway? Either several intermediates could lie between Ras and Raf-1, or Ras and Raf-1 could interact directly, thereby eliciting Raf-1 activation. Indeed, there is some evidence that Raf-1 from insulin-stimulated cells is activated by Ser/Thr phosphorylation (156). Rapp and colleagues and others have recently shown that Raf-1 can be phosphorylated and activated by protein kinase-Cα (157,158). Still, Raf-1 constructs in which the sites of PKC phosphorylation have been mutated to alanine can still be activated by Ras and Src when all three are expressed simultaneously in Sf9 cells triple-infected with the cognate recombinant baculoviruses (157). Thus, a PKC-independent Raf-1 activation pathway must exist (157).

c-Raf-1 is one of three members of the *raf* gene family: A-*raf*, B-*raf*, and c-*raf*-1 (117). All three *raf* family members share a similar domain structure consisting of a carboxyl-terminal catalytic domain, referred to as CR-3, and two amino-terminal domains, CR-1 and CR-2 (126,159,160). CR-1 (possibly in conjunction with CR-2) probably serves as a negative regulatory domain. The best evidence for this comes from analysis of naturally occurring oncogenic *raf* mutants as well as from systematic truncations of c-*raf*-1. Specifically, v-*raf*, the viral oncogenic counterpart of c-*raf*-1, is deleted at CR-1 and CR-2, with insertion of *gag* sequences amino terminal to the CR-3 domain (126). Oncogenic B-*raf* derived from human Ewing sarcoma tumors has undergone a translocation of sequences, displacing the CR-1 and CR-2 domains and replacing them with irrelevant sequences (161). The resulting B-*raf* gene is highly transforming when expressed in NIH3T3 cells (161). By the same token, systematic deletion of the Raf-1 amino terminus increases Raf-1 transforming potential, and the highly oncogenic mutant BXB-*raf*-1 construct described above is essentially a free CR-3 domain (159,160,162). The CR-2 domain is believed to serve as a hinge region joining CR-1 and CR-2 (159,160). The effect of CR-2 deletion per se on Raf-1 transforming potential has not been determined, but this region probably contains some of the potential MAPK phosphorylation sites of the Raf-1 polypeptide (see above) (126).

It has been inferred that the CR-1 domain is largely responsible for binding upstream Raf-1–activating components. Evidence for this comes from the use of a dominant negative *raf* construct consisting of CR-1 only (162). When expressed transiently, this construct blocks *trans* activation of AP-1 or Ets-driven promoters as well as activation of p44 MAPKs by mitogens, phorbol esters, and ectopically expressed, proximal signaling oncogenes, (*ras*, *src*, *abl*, etc.) (162,163). The dominant negative construct binds available upstream components, rendering them unavailable to the endogenous Raf-1. CR-1 contains a motif (residues 139 to 184) reminiscent of the zinc-finger region of protein kinase C (126,162). Substitution of one of the critical Cys residues in this region (Cys-168) with Ser abolishes the dominant negative phenotype of the mutant CR-1 when employed in the sort of expression studies described above (162). Thus this zinc-finger region may play a role in the binding of upstream components (162).

Using direct biochemical assays, as well as a novel two-hybrid screening assay for detecting protein-protein interactions, a number of laboratories have now demonstrated that the Ha-Ras polypeptide binds directly to the Raf-1 amino terminal CR-1 domain. Moodie et al. used immobilized, bacterially expressed, unprocessed Ras, bound covalently to silica beads, to probe brain extracts for proteins which could bind Ras. With this system, Raf-1, as well as MEK and MAPK were detected in complex with the immobilized Ras (164). Incubation of the complex with ATP resulted in release of the now activated MEK and MAPK, while the Raf-1 was retained on the beads (164). Kaziro and colleagues obtained similar results by adding excess GTP-Ras to cell extracts and immunoprecipitating the Ras/Raf-1 complexes with anti-Ras antibodies (165). While these results indicated that Raf-1 could be isolated on immobilized Ras, they did not reveal whether or not the Ras/Raf-1 interaction was direct or mediated by a third protein. To demonstrate a direct Ras/Raf-1 interaction, we and others used recombinant proteins consisting of CR-1 or the cognate CR-1 Cys-168 → Ser fused to glutathione S-transferase (GST) or maltose-binding protein (166–168). These polypeptides were incubated with different preparations of purified baculoviral Ras proteins. Ras/Raf-1 complexes were then collected on glutathione agarose and bound Ras was detected by anti-Ras immunoblot. These studies demonstrated a direct Ras/Raf-1 interaction provided that two conditions were met. First, binding was most optimal if the Ras was charged with GTP (166–168). GDP loaded Ras was much less effective at binding Raf-1. Second, an intact Raf-1 zinc finger appeared necessary (although not absolutely required) for a strong Ras/Raf-1-CR-1 interaction. The Cys-168 → Ser mutant CR-1 was much less effective than wild-type CR-1 (166–168). Interestingly, however, Ras purified from cytosolic extracts, which is largely devoid of posttranslational modifications, was just as effective at binding CR-1 as was Ras purified from membrane extracts, which has undergone farnesylation and palmitoylation (166).

This result is in stark contrast with the results cited above, in which only fully processed Ras was capable of activating MAPKs upon addition to crude cell extracts (152). In this regard, it is noteworthy that purified full-length Raf-1 apparently interacts with Ras poorly if at all in this in vitro system or in the two hybrid system described below (166,168). Furthermore, coimmunoprecipitation or copurification from crude extracts of Ras, processed or not, and holo-Raf-1 has not been demonstrated unless a large excess of Ras polypeptide is added to the system (164,165). Taken together, these results suggest that the farnesyl group on Ras may increase the affinity of the Ras polypeptide for holo-Raf-1 and that additional species may be necessary, in concert with Ras, for Ras/holo-Raf-1 binding and Raf-1 activation. It should be noted, however, that activation of Raf-1 by Ras alone has not been demonstrated even under conditions in which Ras and holo Raf-1 can interact (166) (J. Kyriakis; unpublished).

Still, surprisingly, the interaction of Ras and Raf-1 CR-1 is of sufficient affinity to compete effectively with both p120^{GAP} (166,167) and neurofibromin (167) for binding to Ras. Thus the activity of these GAPs is inhibited in the presence of equimolar Raf-1 CR-1 (166,167). As expected, the Cys-168 → Ser mutant CR-1 is much less effective as a GAP inhibitor than the wild type (166). The GAPs interact with Ras at the Ras effector domain (140). This region of the Ras polypeptide is generally defined as residues 32 to 40. The region is essential for Ras transformation, but mutations in the effector domain do not alter guanine nucleotide binding or hydrolysis, nor do they affect Ras posttranslational modification or membrane localization (169). Inasmuch as Raf-1 inhibits the action of GAPs (presumably at the level of their interaction with Ras), it was of interest to determine the region of the Ras polypeptide which was necessary for Raf-1 binding.

The two-hybrid screening system was employed to map the domains of Ras which interact with Raf-1. This system detects protein-protein interactions as a result of their ability to reconstitute the *trans* activating function of the GAL-4 protein (170). cDNA sequences encoding the c-*raf*-1 CR-1 domain (residues 1 to 257) or the corresponding Cys-168 → Ser mutant CR-1 domain were fused, in frame, to sequences encoding the GAL-4 DNA binding domain. Various *ras* constructs were fused, in frame, to the GAS-4 *trans* activation domain II. These constructs were then transfected into yeast carrying a plasmid containing a GAL-4 promoter driving expression of a *lacZ* reporter. Reconstitution of GAL-4 *trans* activation, resulting from interaction between the Ras and Raf-1-containing GAL-4 fusion proteins, was then assayed using X-gal–containing plates. The results of these studies indicate that the Ras effector domain is essential for the Ras/Raf-1 interaction (166,171). The two-hybrid screen indicated that mutations in and around the effector domain compromise the Ras/Raf interaction in direct correlation with the ability of these mutations to inhibit the transforming potential of Ras (166,171). Specifically, effector mutants, corresponding to Asp-38 → Asn, and Δ 34/Asp-38 → Ala, both of which are known to abrogate GAP binding and Ras transformation (167), showed a dramatic inhibition of Raf-1 binding (166). Mutation of Ras residues around the effector domain—at residues 26, 27, 30, 31, and 45—impair Ras transforming activity with little or no effect on GAP binding (169). The Asp-45 → Glu mutation, which results in a striking loss of Ras transforming potential (169), was severely compromised in its interaction with Raf-1 in spite of a modest enhancement in GAP and neurofibromin binding (166). Asn 26/His27 → Gly/Ile mutation substantially decreases Ras transformation and also impairs Raf-1 binding while sparing the interaction with GAPs (169). Asp30/Glu31 → Glu/Lys only modestly impairs the Ras/Raf-1 interaction in correlation with a modest inhibition of Ras transforming potential (166).

The two-hybrid screen also detected an interaction between Raf-1 and Rap-1b (166). *rap*-1b encodes a small GTP-binding protein in the Ras superfamily, which was originally isolated as a supressor of *ras* transformation (172). The interaction of Raf-1 and Rap-1b, taken together with the observation that Rap-1b supresses the *ras*-transformed phenotype, provides the basis for a plausible mechanism for Raf-1 inhibition mediated by Rap-1b binding in competition with Ras.

Inasmuch as mutations which inhibit Ras binding to Raf-1 also inhibit Ras transformation and the C-168 → S mutant Raf-1 CR-1 can no longer serve as a dominant negative, it can be concluded that the Ras/Raf-1 interaction is required for the activation of Raf-1 kinase activity. This result sheds light on the results of the experiments, described above, which have utilized the dominant-negative *raf* CR-1 construct to inhibit agonist activation of MAPKs and AP-1 (162,163). These results, taken together with the results demonstrating a Ras/Raf-1 interaction, implicate the dominant negative *raf* CR-1 construct as a probe for Ras-dependent signaling. An important caveat of this result is that as a competitor for Ras binding, the dominant negative *raf* is not necessarily a tool for identifying Raf-1–dependent signaling. Indeed, other Ras targets may be competitively inhibited by the CR-1 construct. With this in mind, it is interesting to note that Wigler and colleagues, using the two-hybrid screen, observed not only a Ras/Raf-1 interaction but also an interaction between Ras and Ste-11, the *S. cerevesiae* MEKK homologue (171). Thus MEKK may also be regulated by Ras, and its activation by extracellular agonist might be inhibited by dominant negative *raf*.

Thus, it would seem that the zinc-finger region of Raf-1 binds to Ras at the Ras effector domain. This is apparently not, however, the case. Instead, it seems that the zinc-finger loop of Raf-1 CR-1, while it can influence the Ras/Raf-1 interaction (166–168), does not actually contain the Ras binding site. In their two hybrid studies of the Ras/Raf-1 interaction, Vojtek et al. employed a cDNA library engineered to contain small cDNA fragments to screen for polypeptides which could interact with Ras. Their results indicated that Ras could still interact with a Raf-1 construct consisting of only the first 81 amino acids of CR-1 (168). This region is far outside the putative zinc-finger loop of CR-1, which lies between residues 139 and 184 of the Raf-1 polypeptide (Ref. 126 and references therein). These results suggest that Ras and Raf-1 interact via the extreme N terminus of Raf-1 CR-1 and that this reaction is stabilized by the zinc-finger loop. Deletion or mutagenic compromise of the zinc-finger loop, while reducing the avidity of the Ras/Raf-1 interaction, does not eliminate it. By contrast, full length Raf-1 and Ras do not interact well—as purified polypeptides—in vitro or in the two hybrid system (166–168).

Taken together, these results suggest that a third species is required for activation. This third species may bind at the zinc-finger loop and facilitate the interaction between Ras and holo-Raf-1. Ras and the third species may then work in concert to activate Raf-1. This activation clearly takes place as a mechanism of disinhibition insofar as the CR-1 region, when deleted, results in constitutive activation of Raf (159,160).

Activation of Ras Involves the Formation of Protein Complexes Containing mSOS and Proteins with SH2 and SH3 Domains

Ras polypeptides are activated when they exchange GDP for GTP. The rate-limiting step in this process is GDP dissociation, inasmuch as GTP is in excess inside the cell (14–142, 171, 172). Ras polypeptides possess a modest intrinsic GDP dissociation activity, which is enhanced two- to fourfold by guanine nucleotide exchange factors such as mSOS (142–144, 173, 174). Ras guanine nucleotide exchange is stimulated by mitogens thereby enhancing the ratio of GTP/GDP on Ras (175–181). Presumably this increase in Ras GTP loading is due to increased exchange factor activity, as decreased GAP activity in response to mitogens has not been observed (175–181).

Recently, the amino acid sequence of mSOS was deduced from cDNA clones and was found to contain a proline-rich domain with the motif VPVPPPVPP (143). This motif closely resembles XPXXPPPΦXP (where X is any amino acid and Φ is hydrophobic), a proposed consensus-binding site for proteins containing Src homology-3 (SH3) domains (182). SH3 and SH2 domains are so named for their homology to two distinct noncatalytic portions of the Src tyrosine kinase (183). Numerous polypeptides, including phosphatidyl inositol-3 kinase (PI-3 kinase) 85-kDa subunit, phospholipase-C γ, the Tyr phosphatase SH-PTP, the actin-binding protein talin and $p120^{GAP}$ contain SH2 and/or SH3 domains. In addition, a number of proteins, some with transforming potential, are composed solely of SH2 domains or SH2 and SH3 domains (i.e., Shc, Nck, Crk, GRB-2/Sem-5, and GRB-7) (for review, see Ref. 183).

SH2 and SH3 domains mediate protein-protein binding and, in the case of signal transduction, multiprotein signaling complexes arise from these interactions. SH2 domains bind to phosphotyrosine residues, with SH2 domains from different proteins recognizing P-Tyr residues within specific motifs (PI-3 kinase 85-kDa subunit, for example, binds P-Tyr preferentially within the motif Tyr-P-Met-X-Met, where X is any amino acid) (183). Typically, mitogen receptors with intrinsic Tyr kinase activity undergo rapid autophosphorylation upon binding ligand. Receptors decorated with phosphotyrosines can then recruit SH2-containing molecules, thereby initiating a signaling cascade (183). An exception to this rule is the insulin receptor. Insulin-stimulated autophosphorylation of the insulin receptor activates its Tyr kinase activity. The receptor then phsophorylates, on Tyr residues, a 130-kDa polypeptide referred to as insulin receptor substrate-1 (IRS-1). IRS-1, rather than the receptor, then serves as an SH2 docking protein (184–188).

Using the Tyr autophosphorylated EGF receptor intracellular domain as a probe, Schlessinger and colleagues screened expression libraries for molecules that bind specifically to the Tyr-phosphorylated receptor. Among the clones that were isolated (classified as growth factor receptor binding proteins (GRBs)) was a novel protein, GRB-2, which had the structure SH3-SH2-SH3 (184). The apparent lack of a catalytic domain in GRB-2 suggested that it and other proteins consisting only of SH2/SH3 domains serve as adapter proteins, which mediate the formation of multiprotein signaling complexes. GRB-2 is homologous to *sem-5*, a gene from *C. elegans* which has been implicated as an upstream activator of *let-60*, the *C. elegans ras* homologue (189–190). It was subsequently shown that GRB-2, via its SH2 domain, binds to the Tyr phosphorylated EGF receptor in situ upon EGF stimulation (191). This binding occurs directly through EGF receptor P-Tyr residues or indirectly through a third protein, Shc. Shc, another adapter protein, consists of an SH2 domain and a Gly/Pro-rich region (191,192). Upon EGF receptor autophosphorylation, Shc binds to the receptor through its SH2 domain and is Tyr-phosphorylated by the receptor. GRB-2 presumably binds to Shc through this P-Tyr residue. In neither case does GRB-2 itself become Tyr-phosphorylated.

Using direct biochemical assays or two-hybrid screening, a number of laboratories have now shown that mSOS and GRB-2 exist as a cytosolic complex in resting cells and that this interaction requires the SH3 domain of GRB-2 and the VPVPPPVPP motif on mSOS (193–198). Upon receptor activation, the GRB-2/mSOS complex then binds to autophosphorylated Tyr kinases via an interaction between the GRB-2 SH2 domain and either the P-Tyr on Shc or the P-Tyr on the receptor itself (193–198). In the case of the insulin receptor, GRB-2 complexes with IRS-1 (199). By this process, autophosphorylated Tyr kinases can recruit the GRB-2/mSOS complex to the membrane. In vitro, formation of this complex does not activate mSOS per se (193–198). Perhaps additional species are needed. More likely, however, the purpose of forming this complex is to bring the Ras activation machinery to the membrane where Ras resides, thereby allowing for enhanced guanine nucleotide exchange without increased intrinsic mSOS activity (200).

THE KNOWN SIGNALING COMPONENTS PRESENT IN MAMMALIAN CELLS ARE CONSERVED IN *DROSOPHILA* AND *C. ELEGANS*, WHERE THEY CAN BE ANALYZED GENETICALLY

The observation that numerous developmental processes in *Drosophila* and *Caenorhabditis elegans* were controlled by genes encoding receptor Tyr kinases, Ras homologues and other key elements known to be involved in vertebrate cell growth control and signal transduction suggested not only that there was a striking conservation of signaling molecules among metazoan species but also that genetic and biochemical approaches to the study of signal transduction could be mutually beneficial. *Drosophila* is known to possess at least five receptor Tyr kinases: Torso and Sevenless as well as *Drosophila* insulin, EGF and FGF receptor homologues (reviewed in Ref. 201 and references therein). The Torso and Sevenless pathways have been studied in detail. The *torso* gene is required for the proper formation of the *Drosophila* anteroposterior axis (202,203). Perrimon showed that the *Drosophila c-raf-1* homolog (*Draf*) was required for the expression of a gain of function *torso* phenotype (204).

The *Drosophila* ommatidium consists of 8 photoreceptor cells (R1–R8) surrounded by 12 accessory cells. During development, previously determined cells instruct neighboring uncommitted cells to adopt a particular fate. In this stepwise developmental plan, the R7 photoreceptor cells is the last cell to be recruited to differentiate (205,206). The differentiation of R7 is under the control of the *sevenless* gene, which encodes a receptor Tyr kinase expressed on the R7 cell surface (207,208). The *sevenless* ligand, *bride of sevenless* (*boss*), is expressed on the R8 photoreceptor cell surface; and upon interaction of Boss with Sevenless, a signaling cascade is initiated that culminates in the differentiation of the R7 cell into a photoreceptor (204,205). The Sevenless pathway has been elucidated in good detail, and it has been shown that *ras1*, the *Drosophila ras* homologue, is required for the expression of a gain-of-function *sevenless* mutant phenotype (209). Moreover, constitutively active *Draf* mutants can rescue loss-of-function *sevenless* mutants and *ras1* mutants (210). As mentioned above, *Drosophila* Ras1 is, in turn, regulated by the *SOS* gene product, which encodes a guanine nucleotide exchange factor (144). Recently, Rubin and colleagues as well as Schlessinger, Pawson, and colleagues identified a *Drosophila* GRB-2 homolog, *drk* (*downstream of receptor kinases*) (211,212). Mutations in the *drk* SH2 domain suppress *sevenless* gain-of-function mutations, placing the *drk* product downstream of the *sevenless* product (211,212). In vitro, Drk binds to the Sevenless Tyr kinase and to the Pro-rich motif of the *SOS* product (211,212). Taken together, these data indicate that the *sevenless* pathway is essentially identical to the vertebrate Tyr kinase pathway, up to the level of Raf-1. Nishida and colleagues recently identified *Dsor1*, a *Drosophila mek* homologue, which is required for the expression of *Draf* gain-of-function mutants (213). Finally, Biggs and Zipursky identified DmERK, a *Drosophila* homologue of mammalian p42/44 MAPKs, further demonstrating the conservation of signaling components between *Drosophila* and vertebrates (214).

In the nematode worm *Caenorhabditis elegans*, induction of vulval development is mediated by a Tyr kinase signaling pathway remarkably similar to that of vertebrates (reviewed in Ref. 215). In these animals, the gonadal anchor cell induces three of six ectodermal cells to develop into vulval tissue (215). The *lin-3* gene, expressed by the anchor cell, encodes an EGF-like growth factor which probably binds to and activates the product of the *let-23* gene, which encodes a transmembrane receptor Tyr kinase of the EGF receptor family (216,217). *let-60* encodes a *ras*-like protein which is essential for *let-23* induction of the vulval cell fate (218,219). As described above, *sem-5* is homologous to GRB-2 (189,190). Loss-of-function mutants of *sem-5* were originally isolated by virtue of their ability to suppress loss-of-function *lin-15* mutants (190). *lin-15* encodes a repressor of the vulval phenotype, and loss-of-function *lin-15* mutants display excessive vulval tissue formation (the multivulval phenotype) (215). Thus, against a *lin-15* loss of function background, *sem-5* mutants appear vulvaless (190). Genetic studies indicate that, as is the case in vertebrates, *sem-5* is upstream of *let-60* insofar as loss-of-function *sem-5* mutants can be rescued by gain-of-function *let-60* mutants (190). Finally, Sternberg and colleagues identified *lin-45*, a *C. elegans c-raf-1* homologue (220). Inasmuch as loss-of-function *lin-45* mutants are vulvaless, suppress *lin-15* loss-of-function, and *let-60* gain-of-function mutants, it appears that the *C. elegans c-raf-1* homologue acts downstream of the *C. elegans ras* homologue, just as is observed in the case of vertebrates (220).

The similarities between vertebrate, *Drosophila*, and *C. elegans* signaling pathways are shown in Fig. 1. Given the body of knowledge collected thus far, the astounding similarities in signaling pathways among metazoans as well as the genetic manipulations possible in *Drosophila* and *C. elegans*, it should be possible, using these simple species, to begin to dissect genetically the development of other organ systems, including renal tissue.

CONCLUSIONS AND PERSPECTIVES

This chapter attempts to summarize recent progress in our understanding of signal transduction mediated by the MAPKs. This area has undergone astonishing advancement during the last 3 years. From these results, we can propose a general scheme for signaling from receptor Tyr kinases to the p42/p44 MAPKs and from there to the nucleus. This scheme is shown in Fig. 2. The figure also illustrates other pathways about which less is known. Figure 3 compares the metazoan and yeast (*S. cerevisiae*) mating-factor pathways, illustrating the conservation of eukaryotic signaling. Given the diversity of cellular stimuli that activate MAPKs as well as the very large and expanding number of putative MAPK substrates, it is clear that these kinases are not merely "mitogen-activated" kinases, nor are they really extracellular signal-regulated kinases, inasmuch as heat shock and DNA damage, which do not act at cell surface receptors, can activate MAPKs.

These kinases should be thought of as part of a generalized cassette of protein kinases that are recruited to regulate or respond to mitogenic stimuli (growth-factor activation of AP-1), metabolic demands (insulin activation of glycogen synthase), cell cycle (M-phase activation) embryonic development (*sevenless, torso, and lin-3*) pathways, and trauma [heat shock, ultraviolet radiation (UV)]. Other parts of this signaling cassette include MEK and Raf-1/MEKK, highly specific kinases that activate, respectively, p42/p44 MAPKs and MEK. Whether other MAPKs such as the p54 MAPKs are part of this cassette or are on a parallel pathway is unclear. We know that MEK does not activate p54 MAPKs. Data from Karin and colleagues suggest that Ras and Raf-1 are necessary for c-Jun N-terminal phosphorylation in response to UV irradiation, suggesting that certain responses

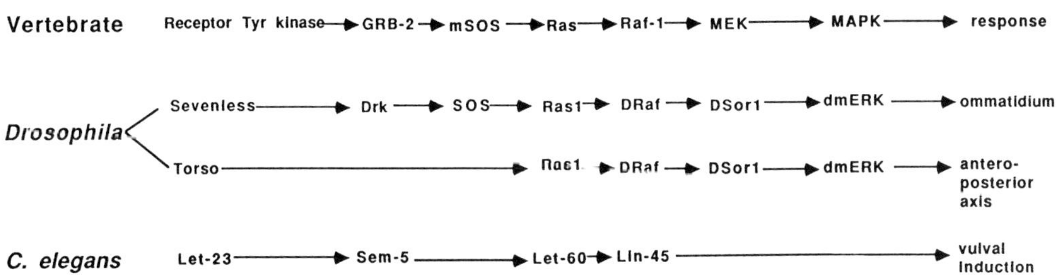

Figure 1 Similarities among metazoan Tyr kinase signaling pathways.

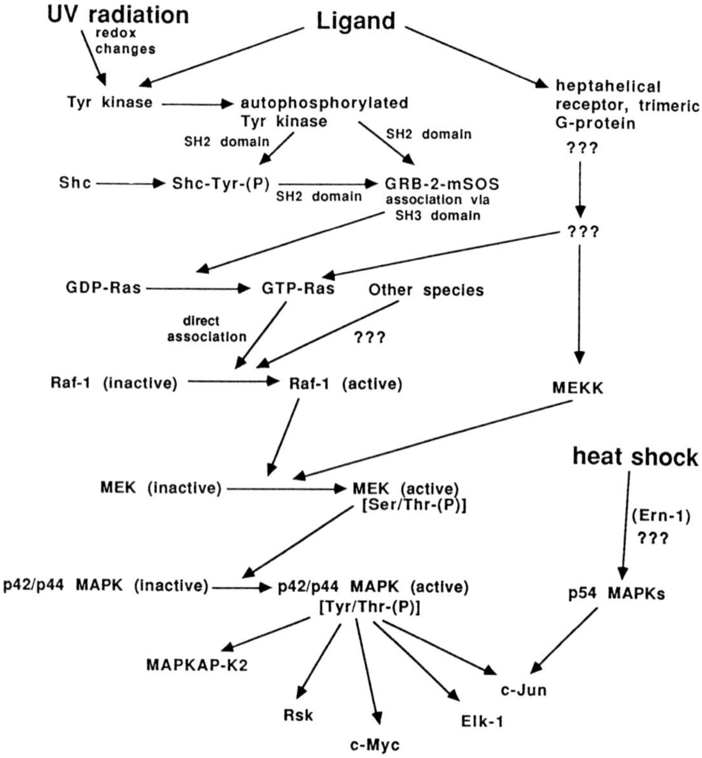

Figure 2 General scheme for signal transduction to and from MAPKs.

to trauma may employ proteins previously thought of as protooncogenes. Inasmuch as heat shock is a poor activator of the p42/p44 MAPKs and a potent p54 MAPK activator, a role for Ras and Raf-1 in heat shock is, however, doubtful, at best.

So where is the specificity? If a single group of related enzymes is used by nearly every signaling stimulus, how are different responses generated? Part of this specificity of different signaling networks may be due to recruitment of different MAPK species. We have seen that the p54 MAPKs for example, have a much different substrate specificity and cellular regulation from that of the p42/p44 MAPKs, and that the p54 MAPKs are activated preferentially in response to heat shock, the presence of misfolded proteins in the cell, or by TNF-α (possibly as part of a sphingomyelin signaling pathway), rather than by mitogenic agonists. Specificity may also be achieved by cell type and the background of MAPK downstream targets that a cell expresses. For example, MAPK activation of skeletal muscle glycogen synthase would not be expected to occur in fibroblasts where the muscle-specific phosphatase-1 glycogen-binding subunit is not present. Subcellular localization and protein-protein complexes may also provide for specific responses. Raf-1, MEK, and MAPK have been shown to exist as complexes, as do GRB-2 and mSOS. Additional complexes containing different SH3/SH2 proteins, Raf-1 targets, etc. may be prepositioned in the cell adjacent to receptors poised to respond to different stimuli. Finally, specificity of signaling may arise from the repertoire of signaling pathways recruited by a particular stimulus. This discussion has focused on the best-understood pathway—the p42/p44 MAPK pathway. Other pathways surely exist. We know, for example that the p70 S6 kinase is not activated by phosphorylation catalyzed by the p42/p44 MAPKs alone and that other input from other pathways is required for p70 activation. Different agonists may utilize other pathways in addition to or in the absence of the p42/p44 MAPK pathway. Different SH2-containing proteins bind different P-tyr residues, depending on the residues flanking the P-Tyr; and a good probe for signaling specificity might be the identification of SH2/SH3 adaptor proteins used by different signaling pathways.

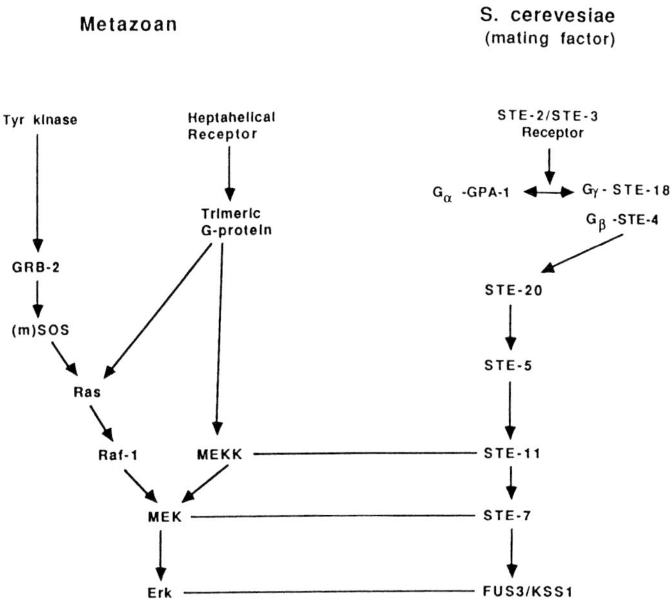

Figure 3 Comparison of metazoan and yeast MAPK signaling pathways. Horizontal lines connect homologous proteins.

We do not yet know the answers to these questions and many others, including the mechanisms by which the p54 MAPKs and Raf-1 are activated and how heterotrimeric G protein–coupled heptahelical receptors hook up to Ras. In addition, it is likely that other pathways branch from Ras and Raf-1 which account for the pleiotrophic effects of *ras* and *raf* transformation. Thus, if the current rate of progress continues, we can look forward to many more exciting advances in this field.

NOTE ADDED IN PROOF

Since completion of this manuscript, the p54-MAP kinases have been renamed stress-activated protein kinases (SAPKs). SAPK/ERK-kinase-1 (SEK1), a novel MEK homolog, was identified as an activator of the SAPKs (Sánchez I, Hughes RT, Mayer BJ, et al. Role of SAPK/ERK kinase-1 in the stress-activated pathway regulating transcription factor c-Jun. Nature 1994; 372:794–798). In addition, MEKK has been shown to preferentially activate the SAPK pathway, as compared to the MAPK pathway, and is a potent activator of SEK1 in vitro and in situ (Yan M, Dai T, Deak JC, et al. Activation of stress-activated protein kinase by MEKK1 phosphorylation of its activator SEK1. Nature 1994; 372:798–800).

ACKNOWLEDGMENTS

Work in the author's laboratory is supported by a United States Public Health Service FIRST award. I thank Thomas Force for comments on the manuscript and Martha Chambers for assistance in preparation of the manuscript. This review was completed in December 1993.

REFERENCES

1. Sturgill TW, Ray LB. Muscle proteins related to microtubule associated protein-2 are substrates for an insulin-stimulatable kinase. Biochem Biophys Res Commun 1986; 134;565–571.

2. Ray LB, Sturgill TW. Characterization of insulin-stimulated microtubule-associated protein kinase. Rapid isolation and stabilization of a novel serine/threonine kinase from 3T3-L1 cells. J Biol Chem 1988; 263:12721–12727.
3. Ray LB, Sturgill TW. Rapid stimulation by insulin of a serine/threonine kinase in 3T3–L1 adipocytes that phosphorylates microtubule-associated protein 2 in vitro. Proc Natl Acad Sci USA 1987; 84:1502–1506.
4. Sturgill TW, Ray LB, Erikson E, Maller JL. Insulin-stimulated MAP-2 kinase phosphorylates and activates ribosomal protein S6 kinase II. Nature 1988; 334:715–718.
5. Ray LB, Sturgill TW. Insulin-stimulated microtubule-associated protein kinase is phosphorylated on tyrosine and threonine in vivo. Proc Natl Acad Sci USA 1988; 85:3753–3757.
6. Rossomando AJ, Payne DM, Weber MJ, Sturgill TW. Evidence that pp42, a major tyrosine kinase target protein, is a mitogen-activated serine-threonine protein kinase. Proc Natl Acad Sci USA 1989; 86:6940–6943.
7. Anderson NG, Maller JL, Tonks NK, Sturgill TW. Requirement for integration of signals for two distinct phosphorylation pathways for activation of MAP kinase. Nature 1990; 343:651–653.
8. Ahn NG, Krebs EG. Evidence for an epidermal growth factor-stimulated protein kinase cascade in Swiss 3T3 cells: Activation of serine peptide kinase activity by myelin basic protein kinases in vitro. J Biol Chem 1990; 265:11495–11501.
9. Anderson NG, Kilgour E, Sturgill TW. Activation of mitogen-activated protein kinase by BC_3H1 myocytes by fluoroaluminate. J Biol Chem 1991; 266;10131–10135.
10. Winston LA, Bertics PJ. Growth hormone stimulates the tyrosine phosphorylation of 42- and 45-kDa ERK-related proteins. J Biol Chem 1992; 267:4747–4751.
11. Casillas A, Hanekom C, Williams K, et al. Stimulation of B-cells via the membrane immunoglobulin receptor or with phorbol myristate 13-acetate induces tyrosine phosphorylation and activation of a 42-kDa microtubule-associated protein-2 kinase. J Biol Chem 1991; 266:19088–19094.
12. Bading H, Greenberg ME. Stimulation of protein tyrosine phosphorylation by NMDA receptor activation. Science 1991; 253:912–914.
13. Wang HCR, Erikson RL. Activation of protein serine/threonine kinases p42, p63, and p87 in Rous sarcoma virus-transformed cells: Signal transduction/transformation-dependent MBP kinases. Mol Biol Cell 1992; 3:1329–1337.
14. Bird TA, Sleath PR, DeRoos PC, et al. Interleukin-1 represents a new modality for the activation of extracellular signal-regulated kinases/microtubule-associated protein-2 kinases. J Biol Chem 1991; 266:22661–22670.
15. Nel AE, Pollack S, Landreth G, et al. CD–3-mediated activation of MAP-2 kinase can be modified by ligation of the CD4 receptor. J Immunol 1990; 145:971–979.
16. Sturgill TW, Wu J. Recent progress in characterization of protein kinase cascades for phosphorylation of ribosomal protein S6. Biochim Biophys Acta 1991; 1092:351–357.
17. Boulton TG, Yancopoulos GD, Gregory GS, et al. An insulin-stimulated protein kinase similar to yeast kinases involved in cell cycle control. Science 1990; 249:64–67.
18. Elion EA, Grisafi PL, Fink GR. FUS3 encodes a $cdc2^+$/CDC28-related kinase required for the transition from mitosis into conjugation. Cell 1990; 60:649–664.
19. Courchesne WE, Kunisawa R, Thorner J. A putative protein kinase overcomes pheromone-induced arrest of cell cycling in S. cerevisiae. Cell 1989; 58:1107–1119.
20. Toda T, Shimanuki M, Yanagida M. Fission yeast genes that confer resistance to staurosporine encodes an AP-1-like transcription factor and a protein kinase related to the mammalian ERK1/MAP2 and budding yeast FUS3 and KSS1 kinases. Genes Dev 1991; 5:60–73.
21. Levin DE, Errede B. A multitude of MAP kinase activation pathways. J NIH Res 1993; 5:49–52.
22. Brewster JL, de Valoir T, Dwyer ND, et al. An osmosensing signal transduction pathway in yeast. Science 1993; 259:1760–1763.
23. Gotoh Y, Moriyama K, Matsuda S, et al. Xenopus M phase MAP kinase: Isolation of its cDNA and activation of MPF. EMBO J 1991; 10:2661–2668.
24. Posada J, Cooper JA. Requirements for phosphorylation of MAP kinase during meiosis in Xenopus oocytes. Science 1992; 255:212–215.
25. Gotoh Y, Nishida E, Matsuda S, et al. In vitro effects on microtubule dynamics of purified Xenopus M phase-activated MAP kinase. Nature 1991; 349:251–254.
26. Nishida E, Gotoh Y. The MAP kinase cascade is essential for diverse signal transducation pathways. TIBS 1993; 18:128–131.
27. Chung J, Pelech SL, Blenis J. Mitogen-activated Swiss mouse 3T3 RSK kinase I and II are related to $pp44^{mpk}$ from sea star oocytes and participate in the regulation of $pp90^{rsk}$ activity. Proc Natl Acad Sci USA 1991; 88;4981–4985.
28. Shibuya EK, Boulton TG, Cobb MH, Ruderman JV. Activation of p42 MAP kinase and the release of oocytes from cell cycle arrest. EMBO J 1992; 11:3963–3975.

29. Sanghera JA, Paddon HB, Bader SA, Pelech SL. Purification and characterization of a maturation-activated myelin basic protein kinase from sea star oocytes. J Biol Chem 1990; 265:52–57.
30. Boulton TG, Nye SH, Robbins DJ, et al. ERKs: A family of protein-serine/threonine kinases that are activated and tyrosine phosphorylated in response to insulin and NGF. Cell 1991; 65:663–675.
31. Her JH, Wu J, Rall TB, et al. Sequence of pp42/MAP kinase, a serine/threonine kinase regulated by tyrosine phosphorylation. Nucleic Acid Res 1991; 19:3743–0000.
32. Kyriakis JM, Avruch J. pp54 microtubule-associated protein 2 kinase: A novel serine/threonine protein kinase regulated by phosphorylation and stimulated by poly-L-lysine. J Biol Chem 1990; 265:17355–17363.
33. Kyriakis JM, Brautigan DL, Ingebritsen TS, Avruch J. pp54 microtubule-associated protein-2 kinase requires both tyrosine and serine/threonine phosphorylation for activity. J Biol Chem 1991; 266;10043–10046.
34. Kyriakis JM, Banerjee P, Nikolakaki E, et al. SAPKs, a MAP kinase subfamily activated by cellular stress and TNF-α. Manuscript submitted; 1994.
35. Erikson AK, Payne DM, Martino PA, et al. Identification by mass spectrometry of threonine 97 in bovine myelin basic protein as a specific phosphorylation site for mitogen-activated protein kinase. J Biol Chem 1990; 265:19728–19735.
36. Clark-Lewis I, Sanghera JS, Pelech SL. Definition of a consensus sequence for peptide substrate recognition by $p44^{mpk}$, the meiosis-activated myelin basic protein kinase. J Biol Chem 1991; 266:15180–15184.
37. Alverez E, Northwood IC, Gonzalez FA, et al. Pro–Leu-Ser/Thr is a consensus primary sequence for substrate protein phosphorylation: Characterization of the phosphorylation of c-myc and c-jun proteins by an epidermal growth factor receptor threonine 669 protein kinase. J Biol Chem 1991; 266:15277–15285.
38. Mukhopadhyay NK, Price DJ, Kyriakis JM, et al. An array of insulin-activated, proline-directed serine/threonine protein kinases phosphorylate the p70 S6 kinase. J Biol Chem 1992; 267:3325–3335.
39. Irvine RF. How is the level of free arachidonic acid controlled? Biochem J 1982; 204:3–16.
40. Samuelsson B, Dahlen SE, Lindgren JA, et al. Leukotrienes and lipoxins: Structures, biosynthesis and biological effects. Science 1987; 237:1171–1176.
41. Hanahan DJ. Platelet activating factor: A biologically active phosphoglyceride. Annu Rev Biochem 1986; 55:483–509.
42. Gronich JH, Bonventre JV, Nemenoff RA. Identification and characterization of a hormonally regulated form of phospholipase A_2 in rat renal mesangial cells. J Biol Chem 1988; 263:16645–16651.
43. Nemenoff RA, Winitz S, Qian N-X, et al. Phosphorylation and activation of a high molecular weight form of phospholipase A_2 by p42 microtubule-associated protein 2 kinase and protein kinase C. J Biol Chem 1993; 268:1960–1964.
44. Lin L-L, Wartmann M, Lin AY, et al. $cPLA_2$ is phosphorylated and activated by MAP kinase. Cell 1993; 72:269–278.
45. Grove JR, Price DJ, Banerjee P, et al. Regulation of an epitope-tagged recombinant Rsk-1 S6 kinase by phorbol ester and erk/MAP kinase. Biochemistry 1993; 32:7727–7738.
46. Dent P, Lavoinne A, Nakielny S, et al. The molecular mechanism by which insulin stimulates glycogen synthesis in mammalian skeletal muscle. Nature 1990; 348:302–308.
47. Lavoinne A, Erikson E, Maller JL, et al. Purification and characterization of the insulin-stimulated protein kinase from rabbit skeletal muscle: Close similarity to S6 kinase-II. Eur J Biochem 1991; 199:723–728.
48. Stokoe D, Campbell DG, Nakielny S, et al. MAPKAP kinase-2: A novel protein kinase activated by mitogen-activated protein kinase. EMBO J 1992; 11:3985–3994.
49. Stokoe D, Engel K, Campbell DG, et al. Identification of MAPKAP kinase 2 as a major enzyme responsible for the phosphorylation of the small mammalian heat shock proteins. FEBS Lett 1992; 313:307–313.
50. Chung J, Kuo CJ, Crabtree GR, Blenis J. Rapamycin-FKBP specificity blocks growth-dependent activation of a signalling by the 70 kd S6 protein kinases. Cell 1992; 69:1227–1236.
51. Anderson NG, Li P, Marsden LA, et al. Raf-1 is a potential substrate for mitogen-activated protein kinase in vivo. Biochem J 1991; 277:573–596.
52. Lee R-M, Rapp UR, Blackshear PJ. Evidence for one or more Raf-1 kinase kinase(s) activated by insulin and polypeptide growth factors. J Biol Chem 1991; 266;10351–10357.
53. Kyriakis JM, Force TL, Rapp UR, et al. Mitogen regulation of c-Raf-1 protein kinase activity toward mitogen-activated protein kinase-kinase. J Biol Chem 1993; 268:16009–16019.
54. Chen R-H, Sarnecki C, Blenis J. Nuclear localization and regulation of erk- and rsk-encoded protein kinases. Mol Cell Biol 1992; 12:916–927.
55. Lenormand P, Dardet C, Pagés G, et al. Growth factor induces nuclear translocation of MAP kinases ($p42^{mapk}$) but not their activator MAP kinase kinase ($p45^{mapkk}$) in fibroblasts. J Cell Biol 1993; 122:1079–1988.
56. Gomzaley FA, Seth A, Raden DL, et al. Serum-induced translocation of mitogen-activated protein kinase to the cell surface ruffling membrane and the nucleus. J Cell Biol 1993; 122:1089–1101.
57. Méloche S, Pagés G, Pouysségur J. Biphasic and synergistic activator of $p44^{mapk}$ (ERK1) by growth factors: Correlation between late phase activation and mitogenicity. Mol Endocrinol 1992; 6:845–854.

58. Woodgett JR. Fos and jun: Two into one will go. Cancer Biol 1990; 1:389–397.
59. Hunter T, Karin M. The regulation and transcription by phosphorylation. Cell 1992; 70:375–387.
60. Boyle WJ, Smeal T, Defize LHK, et al. Activation of protein kinase C decreases phosphorylation of c-jun at sites that negatively regulate its DNA-binding activity. Cell 1991; 64:573–584.
61. Li A, Frost J, Deng T, et al. Casein kinase II is a negative regulatory of c-Jun DNA binding and AP-1 activity. Cell 1992; 70:777–789.
62. Hughes K, Nikolakaki E, Plyte DE, et al. Modulation of the glycogen synthase kinase-3 by tyrosine phosphorylation. EMBO J 1993; 12:803–808.
63. Sutherland C, Leighton IA, Cohen P. Inactivation of glycogen synthase kinase-3β by phosphorylation: New kinase connections in insulin and growth factor signalling. Biochem J 1993; 296:15–19.
64. Pulverer BJ, Kyriakis JM, Avruch J, et al. Phosphorylation of c-jun mediated by MAP kinases. Nature 1992; 353:670–673.
65. Binetruy B, Smeal T, Karin M. Ha-Ras augments c-Jun activity and stimulates phosphorylation of its activation domain. Nature 1991; 351:122–127.
66. Smeal T, Binetruy B, Mercola DA, et al. Oncogenic and transcriptional cooperation with Ha-Ras requires phosphorylation of c-Jun on serines 63 and 73. Nature 1991; 354:494–496.
67. Smeal T, Binetruy B, Mercola D, et al. Oncoprotein-mediated signalling cascade stimulates c-Jun activity by phosphorylation of serines 63 and 73. Mol Cell Biol 1992; 12:3507–3513.
68. Baichwal VR, Park A, Tjian R. v-Src and EJ Ras alleviate repression of c-Jun by a cell-specific inhibitor. Nature 1991; 352:165–168.
69. Devary Y, Gottlieb R, Smeal T, Karin M. The mammalian ultraviolet response is triggered by activation of Src tyrosine kinases. Cell 1992; 71:1081–1091.
70. Radler-Pohl A, Sachsenmaier C, Gebel S, et al. UV-induced activation of AP-1 involves obligatory extranuclear steps including Raf-1 kinase. EMBO J 1993; 12:1005–1012.
71. Pulverer BJ, Hughes K, Franklin CC, et al. Co-purification of mitogen-activated protein kinases with phorbol ester-induced c-Jun kinase activity in U937 leukaemic cells. Oncogene 1993; 8:407–415.
72. Adler V, Franklin CC, Kraft AS. Phorbol esters stimulate the phosphorylation of c-Jun but not v-Jun: Regulation by the N-terminal δ domain. Proc Natl Acad Sci USA 1992; 89:5341–5343.
73. Treisman R. The SRE: A growth factor-responsive transcriptional regulator. Semin Cancer Biol 1990; 1:47–58.
74. Norman C, Runswick M, Pollock R, Treisman R. Isolation and properties of cDNA clones encoding SRF, a transcription factor that binds to the c-fos serum response element. Cell 1988; 55:989–1003.
75. Shaw PE, Shröter H, Nordheim A. The ability of a ternary complex to form over the serum response element correlates with serum inducibility of the human c-fos promoter. Cell 1989; 56:563–572.
76. Dalton S, Treismann R. Characterization of SAP-1, a protein recruited by serum response factor of the c-fos serum response element. Cell 1992; 68:597–562.
77. Hipskind RA, Rao VN, Mueller CG, et al. Ets-related protein Elk-1 is homologous to the c-fos regulatory factor $p62^{TCF}$. Nature 1991; 354:531–534.
78. Gille H, Scharrocks AD, Shaw PE. Phosphorylation of transcription factor $p62^{TCF}$ by MAP kinase stimulates ternary complex formation at c-fos promoter. Nature 1992; 358:414–417.
79. Marais R, Wynne J, Treisman R. The SRF accessory protein Elk-1 contains a growth factor-regulated transcriptional activation domain. Cell 1993; 73:381–393.
80. Blackwood EM, Eisenmann RM. Max: A helix loop-zipper protein that forms a sequence-specific DNA binding complex with Myc. Science 1991; 251:1211–1217.
81. Blackwell K, Ktriynrt L, Blackwood RM, et al. Sequence-specific DNA binding by the c-Myc protein. Science 1990; 250:1149–1151.
82. Kato GJ, Barrett J, VillaGarcia M, Dang CV. An amino-terminal c-Myc domain required for neoplastic transformation activates transcription. Mol Cell Biol 1990; 10:5914–5924.
83. Seth A, Gonzalez FA, Gupta S, et al. Signal transduction within the nucleus by mitogen-activated protein kinase. J Biol Chem 1992; 267:24796–24804.
84. Seth A, Alverez E, Gupta S, Davis RJ. A phosphorylation site located in the NH_2-terminal domain of c-Myc increases transactivation of gene expression. J Biol Chem 1991; 266:23521–23524.
85. Schlesinger MJ. Heat shock proteins. J Biol Chem 1990; 265:12111–12114.
86. Gething M-J, Sambrook J. Protein folding in the cell. Nature 1992; 33–45.
87. Morimoto RI. Cells in stress: Transcriptional activation of heat shock genes. Science 1993; 259:1409–1410.
88. Normington K, Kohno K, Kozutsumi Y, et al. S. cerevisiae encodes an essential protein homologous in sequence and function to mammalian BiP. Cell 1989; 57:1223–1236.
89. Matts RL, Hurst R, Xu Z. Denatured proteins inhibit translation in hemin-supplemented rabbit reticulocyte lysate by inducing the activation of the heme-regulated eIF-2α kinase. Biochemistry 1993; 32:7322–7328.
90. Mori K, Ma W, Gething M-J, Sambrook J. A transmembrane protein with a $cdc2^{+}$/CDC28-related kinase activity is required for signaling from the ER to the nucleus. Cell 1993; 74:743–756.

91. Jurivich DA, Chung J, Blenis J. Heat shock induces two distinct S6 protein kinase activates in quiescent mammalian fibroblasts. J Cell Physiol 1991; 148:252–259.
92. Zhou M, Lambert H, Landry J. Transient activation of a distinct serine protein kinase is responsible for 27-kDa heat shock protein phosphorylation in mitogen-stimulated and heat-shocked cells. J Biol Chem 1993; 268:35–43.
93. Xu Y, Lindquist S. Heat-shock protein hsp90 governs the activity of $pp60^{v\text{-}src}$ kinase. Proc Natl Acad Sci USA 1993; 90:7074–7078.
94. Kohno K, Normington K, Sambrook J, et al. The promoter region of the yeast KAR2 (BiP) gene contains a regulatory domain that responds to the presence of unfolded proteins in the endoplasmic reticulum. Mol Cell Biol 1993; 13:877–890.
95. Beutler B, Cerami A. Tumor necrosis cachexia, shock and inflammation: A common mediator. Annu Rev Biochem 1988; 57:505–518.
96. Goeddel DV, Aggarwal BB, Gray PW, et al. Tumor necrosis factors: Gene structure and biological activities. Cold Spring Harbor Symp Quant Biol 1986; 51:597–609.
97. Brenner DA, O'Hara M, Angel P, et al. Prolonged activation of jun and collagenase genes by tumour necrosis factor-α. Nature 1989; 337:661–663.
98. Osborn L, Kunkel S, Nabel GJ. Tumor necrosis factor α and interleukin 1 stimulate the human immunodeficiency virus enhancer by activation of the nuclear factor κB. Proc Natl Acad Sci USA 1989; 86:2336–2340.
99. Loetscher H, Pan Y-CE, Lahm H-W, et al. Molecular cloning and expression of the human 55 kd tumor necrosis factor receptor. Cell 1990; 61:351–359.
100. Heller RA, Song K, Onasch MA, et al. Complementary DNA cloning of a receptor for tumor necrosis factor and demonstration of a shed form of the receptor. Proc Natl Acad Sci USA 1990; 87:6151–6155.
101. Hannun YA. The sphingomyelin cycle and the second messenger function of ceramide. J Biol Chem. In press.
102. Kolesnick RN. Sphingomyelin and derivatives as cellular signals. Prog Lipid Res 1991; 30:1–38.
103. Payne DM, Rossomando AJ, Martino P, et al. Identification of the regulatory phosphorylation sites in pp42/mitogen-activated protein kinase (MAP kinase). EMBO J 1991; 10:885–892.
104. Ahn NG, Seger R, Bratlien RL, et al. Multiple components in an epidermal growth factor-stimulated protein kinase cascade: In vitro activation of a myelin basic protein/microtubule-associated protein 2 kinase. J Biol Chem 1991; 266;4220–4227.
105. Gómez N, Cohen P. Dissection of the protein kinase cascade by which nerve growth factor activates MAP kinases. Nature 1991; 253:170–173.
106. Seger R, Ahn NG, Boulton TG, et al. Microtubule-associated protein 2 kinases, ERK1 and ERK2, undergoes autophosphorylation on both tyrosine and threonine residues: Implications for their mechanism of activation. Proc Natl Acad Sci USA 1991; 88:6142–6146.
107. Crews CM, Allessandrini AA, Erikson RL. Mouse Erk-1 gene product is a serine/threonine protein kinase that has the potential to phosphorylate tyrosine. Proc Natl Acad Sci USA 1991; 88:8845–8849.
108. Wu J, Rossomando AJ, Her J-H, et al. Autophosphorylation in vitro of recombinant 42-kilodalton mitogen-activated protein kinase on tyrosine. Proc Natl Acad Sci USA 1991; 88:9508–9512.
109. Adams PD, Parker PJ. Activation of mitogen-activated protein (MAP) kinase by a MAP kinase-kinase. J Biol Chem 1992; 267:13135–13137.
110. Nakielny S, Cohen P, Wu J, Sturgill T. MAP kinase activator from insulin-stimulated skeletal muscle is a protein threonine/tyrosine kinase. EMBO J 1992; 11:2123–2129.
111. Kosako H, Gotoh Y, Matsuda S, et al. Xenopus MAP kinase activator is a serine/threonine/tyrosine kinase activated by threonine phosphorylation. EMBO J 1992; 11:2903–2908.
112. Seger R, Ahn NG, Posada J, et al. Purification and characterization of mitogen-activated protein kinase activator(s) from epidermal growth factor-stimulated A431 cells. J Biol Chem 1992; 267:14373–14381.
113. Crews CM, Erikson RL. Purification of a murine protein-tyrosine/threonine kinase that phosphorylates and activates Erk-1 gene product: Relationship to the fission yeast byr1 gene product. Proc Natl Acad Sci USA 1992; 89:8205–8209.
114. Alessandrini A, Crews CM, Erikson RL. Phorbol ester stimulates a protein-tyrosine/threonine kinase that phosphorylates and activates the Erk-1 gene product. Proc Natl Acad Sci USA 1992; 89:8200–8204.
115. Crews CM, Alessandrini A, Erikson RL. The primary structure of MEK, a protein kinase that phosphorylates the Erk gene product. Science 1992; 258:478–480.
116. Seger R, Seger D, Lozeman FJ, et al. Human T-cell mitogen-activated protein kinase kinases are related to yeast signal transduction kinases. J Biol Chem 1992; 267:25628–25631.
117. Ashworth A, Nakielny S, Cohen P, Marshall C. The amino acid sequence of a mammalian MAP kinase kinase. Oncogene 1992; 7:2555–2556.
118. Wu J, Harrisøn JK, Vincent LA, et al. Molecular structure of a protein-tyrosine/threonine kinase activating p42 mitogen-activated protein (MAP) kinase: MAP kinase kinase. Proc Natl Acad Sci USA 1993; 90:173–177.

119. Wu J, Harrison JK, Dent P, et al. Identification and characterization of a new mammalian mitogen-activated protein kinase kinase, MKK2. Mol Cell Biol 1993; 13:4539–4548.
120. Teague MA, Chaleff DT, Errede B. Nucleotide sequence of the yeast regulatory gene STE7 predicts a protein homologous to protein kinases. Proc Natl Acad Sci USA 1986; 83:7371–7375.
121. Gartner A, Nasmyth K, Ammerer G. Signal transduction in Saccharomyces cerevisiae requires tyrosine and threonine phosphorylation of FUS3 and KSS1. Genes Dev 1992; 6:1280–1292.
122. Errede B, Gartner A, Zhou Z, et al. MAP kinase-related FUS3 from S. cerevisiae is activated by STE7 in vitro. Nature 1993; 362:261–264.
123. Kyriakis JM, App H, Zhang X-F, et al. Raf-1 activates MAP kinase-kinase. Nature 1992; 358:417–421.
124. Dent P, Hasear W, Haysted TAJ, et al. Activation of mitogen-activated protein kinase kinase by v-Raf in NIH 3T3 cells and in vitro. Science 1992; 257:1404–1407.
125. Howe LR, Leevers SJ, Gómez N, et al. Activation of the MAP kinase pathway by the protein kinase raf. Cell 1992; 71:335–342.
126. Rapp UR. Role of Raf-1 serine/threonine protein kinase in growth factor signal transduction. Oncogene 1991; 6:495–500.
127. Force T, Bonventre JV, Heidecker G, et al. Enzymatic characteristics of the c-Raf-1 protein kinase. Proc Natl Acad Sci USA. In press.
128. Gupta SK, Gallego C, Johnson GL, Heasley LE. MAP kinase is constitutively activated in gip2 and src transformed rat 1a fibroblasts. J Biol Chem 1992; 267:7987–7990.
129. Gallego C, Gupta SK, Heasley LE, et al. Mitogen-activated protein kinase activation resulting from selective oncogene expression in NIH 3T3 and Rat 1a cells. Proc Natl Acad Sci USA 1992; 89:7355–7359.
130. Wood KW, Sarnecki C, Roberts TM, Blenis J. ras mediates nerve growth factor receptor modulation of three signal-transducing protein kinases: MAP kinase, Raf-1 and RSK. Cell 1992; 68:1041–1050.
131. Cairns BR, Ramer SW, Kornberg RD. Order of action of components in the yeast pheromone response pathway revealed with a dominant allele of the STE11 kinase and the multiple phosphorylation of STE7 kinase. Genes Dev 1992; 6:1305–1318.
132. Stevenson BJ, Rhodes N, Errede B, Sprague GE Jr. Constitutive mutants of the protein kinase STE11 activate the yeast pheromone response pathway in the absence of the G protein. Genes Dev 1992; 6:1293–1304.
133. Rhodes N, Connell L, Errede B. STE11 is a protein kinase required for cell-type-specific transcription and signal transduction in yeast. Genes Dev 1990; 4:1862–1874.
134. Lange-Carter CA, Pleiman CM, Gardner AM, et al. A divergence in the MAP kinase regulatory network defined by MEK kinase and Raf. Science 1993; 260:315–319.
135. Winitz S, Russell M, Qian N-X, et al. Involvement of Ras and Raf in the G_i-coupled acetylcholine muscarinic m2 receptor activation of mitogen-activated protein (MAP) kinase kinase and MAP kinase. J Biol Chem 1993; 268:19196–19199.
136. Samuels ML, Weber MJ, Bishop M, McMahon M. Conditional transformation of cells and rapid activation of the mitogen-activated protein kinase cascade by an estradiol-dependent human Raf-1 protein kinase. Mol Cell Biol 1993; 13:6241–6252.
137. Wu J, Dent P, Jelinek T, et al. Inhibition of the EGF-activated MAP kinase pathway by adenosine 3′,5′-monophosphate. Science 1993; 262:1065–1069.
138. Cook SJ, McCormick F. Inhibition by cAMP of Ras-dependent activation of Raf. Science 1993; 262:1069–1072.
139. Smith MR, DeGudicibus SJ, Stacey DW. Requirement for c-ras proteins during viral oncogene transformation. Nature 1986; 320:540–543.
140. McCormick F. ras GTPase-activating protein: signal transmitter and signal terminator. Cell 1989; 56:5–8.
141. DeClue JE, Papageorge AG, Fletcher JA, et al. Abnormal regulation of mammalian $p21^{ras}$ contributes to malignant tumor growth in von Recklinghausen (type I) neurofibromatosis. Cell 1992; 61:265–273.
142. Wolfman A, Macara IG. A cytosolic protein catalyzes the release of GDP from $p21^{ras}$. Science 1990; 248:67–69.
143. Botwell D, Fu P, Simon M, Senior P. Identification of murine homologues of the Drosophila son of sevenless gene: Potential activators of ras. Proc Natl Acad Sci USA 1992; 89:6511–6515.
144. Bonfini L, Karlovich CA, Dasgupta C, Banerjee U. The son of sevenless gene product: A putative activator of Ras. Science 1992; 255:603–606.
145. Leevers SJ, Marshall CJ. Activation of extracellular signal-regulated kinase, ERK2, by p21ras oncoprotein. EMBO J 1992; 11:569–574.
146. Thomas SM, DeMarco M, D'Arcangelo G, et al. Ras is essential for nerve growth factor- and phorbol ester-induced tyrosine phosphorylation of MAP kinases. Cell 1992; 68:1031–1040.
147. Troppmair J, Bruder JT, App H, et al. Ras controls coupling of growth factor receptors and protein kinase C in the membrane to Raf-1 and B-Raf protein serine kinases in the cytosol. Oncogene 1992; 7:1867–1873.
148. de Vries-Smiths AMM, Burgering AMTh, Leevers SJ, et al. Involvement of $p21^{ras}$ in activation of extracellular signal-regulated kinase 2. Nature 1992; 357:602–604.

149. Robbins DJ, Cheng M, Zhen E, et al. Evidence for a Ras-dependent extracellular signal-regulated protein kinase (ERK) cascade. Proc Natl Acad Sci USA 1992; 89:6924–6928.
150. Hattori S, Fukuda M, Yamashita T, et al. Activation of mitogen-activated protein kinase and its activator by ras in intact cells and in a cell-free system. J Biol Chem 1992; 267:20346–20351.
151. Shibuya EK, Polverino AJ, Chang E, et al. Oncogenic Ras triggers the activation of 42-kDa mitogen-activated protein kinase in extacts of quiescent Xenopus oocytes. Proc Natl Acad Sci USA 1992; 89:9831–9835.
152. Itoh T, Kaibuchi K, Masuda T, et al. The post-translational processing of ras p21 is critical for its stimulation of mitogen-activated protein kinase. J Biol Chem 1993; 268:3025–3028.
153. Dent P, Wu J, Romero G, et al. Activation of the mitogen-activated protein kinase pathway in Triton X-100 disrupted NIH-3T3 cells by p21 ras and in vitro by plasma membranes from NIH 3T3 cells. Mol Biol Cell 1993; 4:483–493.
154. VanRenterghem B, Gibbs JB, Maller JL. Reconstitution of $p21^{ras}$-dependent and -independent mitogen-activated protein kinase activation in a cell-free system. J Biol Chem 1993; 268:19935–19938.
155. Marshall CJ. Protein prenylation: A mediator of protein-protein interactions. Science 1993; 259:1865–1866.
156. Kovacina KS, Yonezawa K, Brautigan DL, et al. Insulin activates the kinase activity of the Raf-1 proto-oncogene by increasing its serine phosphorylation. J Biol Chem 1990; 265:12115–12118.
157. Kolch W, Heidecker G, Kochs G, et al. Protein kinase Cα activates RAF-1 by direct phosphorylation. Nature 1993; 364:249–252.
158. Sözeri O, Vollmer K, Kiyanage M, et al. Activation of the c-Raf protein kinase by protein kinase C phosphorylation. Oncogene 1992; 7:2259–2262.
159. Heidecker G, Huleihel M, Cleveland JL, et al. Mutational activation of c-raf-1 and definition of the minimal transforming sequence. Mol Cell Biol 1990; 10:2503–2512.
160. Stanton VP Jr, Nichols DW, Laudano AP, Cooper GM. Definition of the human raf amino-terminal regulatory region by deletion mutagenesis. Mol Cell Biol 1989; 9:639–647.
161. Ikawa S, Fukui M, Ueyama Y, et al. B-raf, a new member of the raf family, is activated by DNA rearrangement. Mol Cell Biol 1988; 8:2651–2654.
162. Bruder JT, Heidecker G, Rapp UR. Serum-, TPA-, and Ras-induced expression from Ap-1/Ets-driven promoters requires Raf-1 kinase. Genes Dev 1992; 6:545–556.
163. Troppmair J, Bruder JT, Muñoz H, et al. MAP kinase activation by oncogenes, serum and TPA requires Raf and is necessary for transformation. J Biol Chem. In press.
164. Moodie SA, Willumsen BM, Weber MJ, Wolfman A. Complexes of Ras·GTP with Raf-1 and mitogen-activated protein kinase kinase. Science 1993; 260:1158–1161.
165. Koide H, Satoh T, Nakafuku M, Kaziro Y. GTP-dependent association of Raf-1 with Ha-Ras: Identification of Raf as a target downstream of Ras in mammalian cells. Proc Natl Acad Sci USA 1993; 90:8683–8686.
166. Zhang XF, Settleman J, Kyriakis JM, et al. Normal and oncogenic $p21^{ras}$ proteins bind to the amino-terminal regulatory domain of c-Raf-1. Nature 1993; 364:308–313.
167. Warne PH, Viciana PR, Downward J. Direct interaction of Ras and the amino-terminal region of Raf-1 in vitro. Nature 1993; 364:352–355.
168. Vojtek AB, Hollenberg SM, Cooper JA. Mammalian Ras interacts directly with the serine/threonine kinase Raf. Cell 1993; 74:205–214.
169. Marshall MS, Davis LJ, Keys RD, et al. Identification of amino acid residues required for Ras p21 target activation. Mol Cell Biol 1991; 11:3997–4004.
170. Fields S, Song O-K. A novel genetic system to detect protein-protein interactions. Nature 1989; 340:245–246.
171. Van Aelst L, Barr M, Marcus S, et al. Complex formation between RAS and RAF and other protein kinases. Proc Natl Acad Sci USA 1993; 90:6213–6217.
172. Kitayama H, Sugimoto Y, Matsuzaki T, et al. A ras-related gene with transformation suppressor activity. Cell 1989; 56:77–84.
173. Downward J. Ras regulation: putting back the GTP. Curr Biol 1992; 2:329–331.
174. Satoh T, Nakafuku M, Kaziro Y. Function of Ras as a molecular switch in signal transduction. J Biol Chem 1992; 267:24149–24152.
175. Downward J, Graves JD, Warne PH, et al. Stimulation of $p21^{ras}$ upon T-cell activation. Nature 1990; 346:719–723.
176. Zhang K, Papageorge AG, Lowy DR. Mechanistic aspects of signaling through Ras in NIH 3T3 cells. Science 1992; 257:671–674.
177. Satoh T, Endo M, Nakafuku M, et al. Platelet-derived growth factor stimulates formation of active $p21^{ras}$-GTP complex in Swiss mouse 3T3 cells. Proc Natl Acad Sci USA 1990; 87:5993–5997.
178. Satoh T, Nakafuku M, Miyajima A, Kaziro Y. Involvement of ras p21 protein in signal-transduction pathways from interleukin 2, interleukin 3, and granulocyte/macrophage colony-stimulating factor, but not from interleukin 4. Proc Natl Acad Sci USA 1991; 88:3314–3318.

179. Medema RH, de Vries-Smits AMM, van der Zon GCM, et al. Ras activation by insulin and epidermal growth factor through enhanced exchange of guanine nucleotides on $p21^{ras}$. Mol Cell Biol 1993; 13:155–162.
180. Li B-Q, Kaplan D, King H-F, Kamata T. Nerve growth factor stimulation of the Ras-guanine nucleotide exchange factor and GAP activities. Science 1992; 256:1456–1459.
181. Buday L, Downward J. Epidermal growth factor regulates the exchange rate of guanine nucleotides of $p21^{ras}$ in fibroblasts. Mol Cell Biol 1993; 13:1903–1910.
182. Ren R, Mayer BJ, Cicchetti P, Baltimore D. Identification of a ten-amino acid proline-rich SH3 binding site. Science 259:1157–1161.
183. Pawson T, Gish GD. SH2 and SH3 domains: From structure to function. Cell 1992; 71:359–362.
184. White MF, Maron R, Kahn CR. Insulin rapidly stimulates tyrosine phosphorylation of a M_r-185,000 protein in intact cells. Nature 1985; 318:183–186.
185. Sun XJ, Rothenberg P, Kahn CR, et al. Structure of the insulin receptor substrate IRS-1 defines a unique signal transduction protein. Nature 1991; 352:73–77.
186. Sun XJ, Miralpeix M, Myers MG Jr, et al. Expression and function of IRS-1 in insulin signal transmission. J Biol Chem 1992; 267:22662–22672.
187. Shoelson SE, Chatterjee S, Chaudhuri M, White MF. YMXM motifs of IRS-1 define substrate specificity of the insulin receptor kinase. Proc Natl Acad Sci USA 1992; 89:2027–2031.
188. Kuhné M, Pawson T, Lienhard GE, Feng G-S. The insulin receptor substrate 1 associates with the SH2-containing phosphotyrosine phosphatase Syp. J Biol Chem 1993; 268:11479–11481.
189. Lowenstein EJ, Daly RJ, Batzer AG, et al. The SH2 and SH3 domain-containing protein GRB2 links receptor tyrosine kinases to ras signaling. Cell 1992; 70:431–442.
190. Clark SG, Stern MJ, Horvitz HR. C. elegans cell-signalling gene sem-5 encodes a protein with SH2 and SH3 domains. Nature 1992; 356:340–344.
191. Rozakis-Adcock M, McGlade J, Mbamalu G, et al. Association of the Shc and Grb2/Sem5 SH2-containing proteins is implicated in activation of the Ras pathway by tyrosine kinases. Nature 1992; 360:5689–5692.
192. Pelicci G, Lanfrancone L, Grignani F, et al. A novel transforming protein (SHC) with an SH2 domain is implicated in mitogenic signal transduction. Cell 1992; 70:92–104.
193. Egan SE, Giddings BW, Brooks MW, et al. Association of Sos Ras exchange protein with Grb2 is implicated in tyrosine kinase signal transduction and transformation. Nature 1993; 363:45–51.
194. Rozakis-Adcock M, Fernley R, Wade J, et al. The SH2 and SH3 domains of mammalian Grb2 couple the EGF receptor to the Ras activator of mSos1. Nature 1993; 363:83–85.
195. Li N, Batzer A, Daly R, et al. Guanine-nucleotide–releasing factor hSos1 binds to Grb2 and links receptor tyrosine kinases to Ras signaling. Nature 1993; 363:85–88.
196. Gale NW, Kaplan S, Lowenstein EJ, et al. Grb2 mediates the EGF-dependent activation of guanine nucleotide exchange on Ras. Nature 1993; 363:88–92.
197. Buday L, Downward J. Epidermal growth factor regulates $p21^{ras}$ through the formation of a complex of receptor, Grb2 adapter protein, the Sos nucleotide exchange factor. Cell 1993; 73:611–620.
198. Chardin P, Camonis JH, Gale NW, et al. Human Sos1: A guanine nucleotide exchange factor for Ras that binds to GRB2. Science 1993; 260:1338–1343.
199. Skolnik EY, Lee C-H, Vicentini LM, et al. The SH2/SH3 domain-containing protein GRB2 interacts with tyrosine-phosphorylated IRS1 and Shc: implications for insulin control of ras signalling. EMBO J 1993; 12:1929–1936.
200. McCormick F. How receptors turn Ras on. Nature 1993; 363:15–16.
201. Pazin MJ, Williams LT. Triggering signaling cascades by receptor tyrosine kinases. TIBS 1992; 17:374–378.
202. Sprenger F, Stevens LM, Nüsslein-Volhard C. The Drosophila gene torso encodes a putative receptor tyrosine kinase. Nature 1989; 338:478–483.
203. Perrimon N. The torso receptor protein-tyrosine kinase signaling pathway: An endless story. Cell 1993; 74:219–222.
204. Ambrosio L, Mahowald AP, Perrimon N. Requirement of the Drosophila raf homologue for torso function. Nature 1989; 342:288–291.
205. Tomlinson A. Cellular interactions in the developing Drosophila eye. Development 1986; 104:183–193.
206. Banerjee U, Zipusky SL. The role of cell-cell interaction in the development of the Drosophila visual system. Neurons 1990; 4:177–187.
207. Hafen E, Basler K, Edstroems JE, Rubin GM. Sevenless, a cell-specific homeotic gene of Drosophila, encodes a putative transmembrane receptor with a tyrosine kinase domain. Science 1987; 236:55–63.
208. Tomlinson A, Reddy DF. Sevenless: A cell specific homeotic mutation of the Drosophila eye. Science 1986; 231:400–402.
209. Fortini ME, Simon MA, Rubin CM. Signalling by the sevenless protein tyrosine kinase is mimicked by Ras1 activation. Nature 1992; 355:559–561.

210. Dickson B, Sprenger F, Morrison D, Hafen E. Raf functions downstream of Ras1 in the sevenless signal transduction pathway. Nature 1992; 360:600–603.
211. Simon MA, Dodson GS, Rubin GM. An SH3-SH2-SH3 protein is required for $p21^{Ras1}$ activation and binds to sevenless and Sos proteins in vitro. Cell 1993; 73:169–177.
212. Olivier JP, Raabe T, Henkemeyer M, et al. A Drosophila SH2/SH3 adapter protein implicated in coupling the sevenless tyrosine kinase to an activator of Ras guanine nucleotide exchange, Sos. Cell 1993; 73:179–191.
213. Tsuda L, Inøue YH, Yo M-A, et al. A protein kinase similar to MAP kinase activator acts downstream of the Raf kinase in Drosophila. Cell 1993; 72:407–414.
214. Biggs WH, Zipursky SL. Primary structure, expression and signal-dependent tyrosine phosphorylation of a Drosophila homolog of extracellular signal-regulated kinase. Proc Natl Acad Sci USA 1992; 89:6295–6299.
215. Horvitz HR, Sternberg PW, Multiple intercellular signalling systems control the development of the Caenorhabiditis. Nature 1991; 351:535–341.
216. Hill RJ, Sternberg PW. The gene lin-3 encodes an inductive signal for vulval development in C. elegans. Nature 1992; 358:470–476.
217. Aroian RV, Koga M, Mendel JE, et al. The let-23 gene necessary for Caenorhabditis elegans vulval induction encodes a tyrosine kinase of the EGF receptor subfamily. Nature 1990; 348:693–699.
218. Han M, Sternberg PW. Let-60, a gene that specifies cell fates during C. elegans vulval induction, encodes a ras protein. Cell 1990; 63:921–931.
219. Beitel GJ, Clark SG, Horvitz HR. Caenorhabditis elegans ras gene let-60 acts as a switch in the pathway of vulval induction. Nature 1990; 348:503–509.
220. Han M, Golden A, Han Y, Sternberg PW. C. elegans lin-45 raf gene participates in let-60 ras-stimulated vulval differentiation. Nature 1993; 363:133–140.

34
Heterotrimeric Guanine Nucleotide Binding Proteins

Louis Ercolani
Massachusetts General Hospital, Charlestown, Massachusetts

INTRODUCTION

The successful adaptation of eukaryotic cells to diverse environments has depended on their ability to recognize and respond to external signals. Several successful mechanisms for the detection and unidirectional transmission of external signals across impermeant hydrophobic membranes developed early in evolution. One tripartite mechanism that has been highly conserved from yeast to mammals includes the coupling of receptor, transducer, and effector molecules. In this method of signal transduction, the membrane-spanning receptor is first modified upon detection of the extracellular signal. The modified receptor can then interact with the trigger the modification of a transducer, which is an intermediary guanine nucleotide binding protein (G protein) positioned at the cytoplasmic face of the plasma membrane. The modified G protein then couples to and influences (either positively or negatively) a proximate effector molecule such as an enzyme or ion channel, which alters the cell's internal environment (see Figure 1).

G proteins represent a family of guanine nucleotide binding regulatory proteins that have been conserved in all eukaryotes, including yeast and *Dictyostelium* (1–7). Two classes of G proteins distinguished by molecular weight and subunit structure have been characterized. High-molecular-weight G-proteins are heterotrimers composed of α (M_r 39000–52000), β (M_r 35000–36000), and γ (M_r 8000–10000) subunits that couple a variety of enzyme and ion transport transmembrane signaling processes in mammalian cells (reviewed in Refs. 1–4). Each subunit is encoded by a supergene family that has been conserved by eukaryotes throughout evolution. Low-molecular-weight G proteins are single subunits (M_r 19000–25000) that include the Ha-ras, Ki-ras, N-ras, $rho_{a,b,c}$, ral, R-ras, $rap_{1a,1b,2}$, $SMG_{1,2,3}$, and ypt1 families of proteins, which are implicated in a variety of oncogenic, vesicle, and ion transport functions (8–13).

RECEPTOR-DEPENDENT ACTIVATION OF G PROTEINS

All heterotrimeric G proteins are postulated to unidirectionally transduce signals from receptors to effectors through a cyclic change in the G protein holoenzyme conformation (1). One simplified model for G protein action is seen in Figure 2. The hormone-activated receptor (HR) complexes with the inactive GDP-protein holenzyme ($\beta\gamma$ α -GDP) to form HR-$\beta\gamma$ α -GDP which results in a change in the conformation of the α subunit's gunanine nucleotide binding pocket. The conformational change lowers the affinity for GDP and allows its egress. A GTP-for -GDP exchange reaction can then occur in the α subunit nucleotide binding pocket because the concentration of GTP is normally higher than GDP in the cell. A transiently stable HR-$\beta\gamma$ α-GTP complex immediately dissociates in the presence of Mg^{+2} into HR (14,15) (which can then amplify the signal by associating with another inactive $\beta\gamma$ α -GDP holoenzyme) (16) and $\beta\gamma$ α-GTP. The latter complex then dissociates into $\beta\gamma$

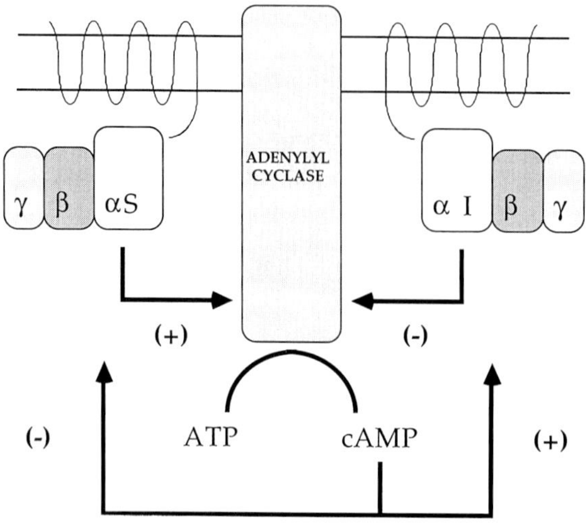

Figure 1 Schematic view of the organization of receptors, G proteins, and effectors in the plasma membrane, α_S $\beta\gamma$; the subunits of the heterotrimeric stimulatory guanine nucleotide binding protein, Gs, coupled to adenylyl cyclase; α_i $\beta\gamma$, the heterotrimeric pertussis-toxin sensitive guanine nucleotide-binding protein; G_i, which inhibits adenylyl cyclase.

and α-GTP subunits. It is notable than in this model, amplification by HR is limited by a reduced affinity of H for R in the absence of the GDP-holenzyme, which favors dissociation of the HR complex (17). The α-GTP subunit then combines with a proximate effector molecule (E) such as an enzyme or ion channel to form an α-GTP-E complex that activates E. The intrinsic GTPase activity of the α subunit converts the GTP in its binding pocket to GDP + PO_4^{-2}, which halts the cycle of effector activation and allows the subsequent dissociation of the α-GDP subunit from the effector molecule and its reassociation with the $\beta\gamma$ subunit complex to reform the inactive holoenzyme complex $\beta\gamma$ α-GDP. Therefore, in this model of G protein action, the GTPase activity of the α-GTP subunit functions as a "timer" for the activation of E. The entire process remains unidirectional because the α-GDP subunit cannot enzymatically convert GDP for GTP and intrinsically has a low basal exchange rate of GDP for GTP in the absence of HR or $\beta\gamma$. It is also evident from this model of G-protein action that the dissociated $\beta\gamma$ subunit complex may play a potential direct or indirect

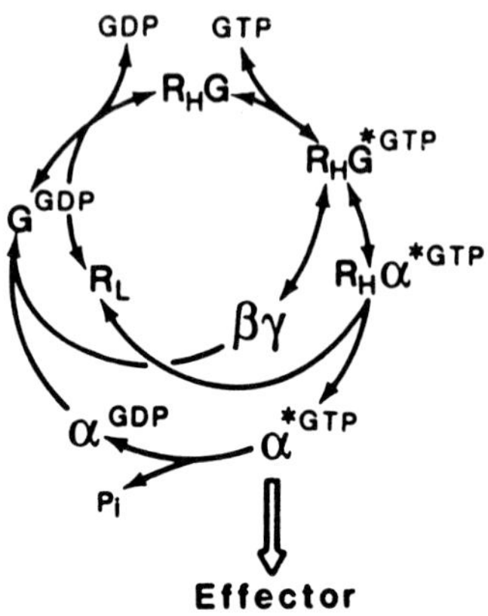

Figure 2 Simplifed model of the mechanism by which a receptor (R) catalyzes the activation of a G protein by GTP and the possible reaction sequences in which a receptor causes release of bound GDP from the α subunit of a G protein. (From Ref. 3.)

role in signal transduction. Indeed in more primitive eukaryotes such as yeast, the $\beta\gamma$ subunit complex can directly stimulate effectors such as adenylyl cyclase (18–20). Indirect "mass action" effects of the $\beta\gamma$ subunit complex in molar excess have been shown to be inhibitory for both adenylyl cyclase activation in native membranes or reconstituted phospholipid vesicles and during muscarinic activation of potassium channels in guinea pig atrial heart cells (1,21–23). Indirect inhibition occurs by a mass-action effect in which (a) excess $\beta\gamma$ prevents the normal dissociation of the $\beta\gamma$ α-GTP complex and (b) excess $\beta\gamma$ reassociates with free α-GTP to form an inactive complex. In these studies, $\beta\gamma$ effects are more effective in the absence of agonist which indicates that the affinity of $\beta\gamma$ is greatest for the free α-GTP complex. Such $\beta\gamma$ effects are postulated to improve the signal-to-noise ratio for agonists by reducing agonist-independent background activation of effectors through the low but basal GDP for GTP exchange reaction that converts α-GDP into α-GTP (22). Recent studies suggest a direct role for $\beta\gamma$ in the modulation of phospholipase C and isoforms of adenylyl cyclase (24). As more effectors are found to be influenced by G protein–coupled pathways, it would not be suprising to find additional roles for $\beta\gamma$ in cell signaling. Indeed, it has recently been found that $\beta\gamma$ can also stimulate the mitogen activate protein kinase pathway in COS-7 cells (25).

The effects of guanine nucleotide analogues and AlF_4^- on G-protein function can readily be understood based on a change in G-protein conformation. GTPγS (a nonhydrolyzable analogue of GTP) can maintain the active conformation of α, which allows a "non-timed" interaction with E because the α subunit GTPase "timer" cannot hydrolyze GTP to GDP + PO_4^{-2}. Conversely GDPβS is not readily displaced for GTP following HR-$\beta\gamma$ α -GDP complex formation, thereby preventing a conformational change that would allow the interaction of α with E (26). The AlF_4^- ion is an analogue of the γ phosphoryl of GTP. The introduction of AlF_4^- into the inactive GDP-protein holoenzyme causes a conformational activation in the absence of HR or the need for guanine nucleotide exchange (27,28). It has recently been proposed that intermediary enzymes, such as nucleoside diphosphate kinases, may also play a role in G-protein holoenzyme activation, as these enzymes are associated with cell membranes and can convert GDP to GTP by the transfer of a γ phosphate (29,30).

MOLECULAR DIVERSITY OF G PROTEINS

High-molecular-weight G proteins are highly homologous structures. Thus far distinct genes for seventeen G-protein α subunits (α_s, α_{olf}, α_{gust}, $\alpha_{i\text{-}1}$, $\alpha_{i\text{-}2}$, $\alpha_{i\text{-}3}$, α_o, α_z, $\alpha_{t\text{-}c}$, $\alpha_{t\text{-}r}$, α_{11}, α_{12}, α_{13}, α_{14}, α_{15}, α_{16}, α_q) (7,31–35), four G-protein β subunits (7,36); and seven G-protein γ subunits (7,37) have been identified by molecular cloning (38). Further diversity can be generated within certain G-protein α subunits genes by alternative splicing of their mRNAs. Thus there are five variant subunits of the α_s gene (39,40,41), two of the α_o gene (42,43), two of the $\alpha_{i\text{-}2}$ gene (44), and two of the $\alpha_{i\text{-}1}$ gene (45).

The high-molecular-weight G-protein holoenzymes are principally distinguished by their α subunits, which exhibit only minor structural diversity but nevertheless still vary: (a) as GTPases [α_z has low activity (46)] (b) in their ability to exchange GDP for GTP [α_t has no basal exchange (47,48), α_{11} and α_q exchange at a very low rate (33), whereas the exchange rate is much higher for $\alpha_{i\text{-}2} >> \alpha_{i\text{-}3} > \alpha_{i\text{-}1}$ (49) and $\alpha_{s45kd} >> \alpha_{s52kd}$ (50)], (c) in their affinities for $\beta\gamma$ [$\alpha_s > \alpha_i > \alpha_o$ (51,52)], (d) as substrates for cholera toxin [only α_s, α_{olf}, and $\alpha_{t\text{-}c}$, $\alpha_{t\text{-}r}$ (1,53) subunits are ADP-ribosylated on an internal arginine residue, which decreases their affinity for $\beta\gamma$ and reduces their GTPase activity] and pertussis toxin [only holoenzymes $G_{i\text{-}1,2,3}$, G_o, and G_t proteins are uncoupled from their receptors following ADP-ribosylation of a terminal carboxy cysteine residue (54–56], (e) as substrates for conformation-dependent inhibitory phosphorylation of α-GDP by protein kinase C [α_t, $\alpha_{i\text{-}1,2,3}$, and α_z can be phosphorylated (57–61)], and (f) as substrates for modification by lipid acylation which may potentiate hydrophobic interactions with $\beta\gamma$ subunits and/or membranes [α_o, $\alpha_{i\text{-}1,2,3}$, and α_z are myristolated (62–64)].

STRUCTURAL CONSERVATION AMONG GTP–BINDING PROTEINS

The amino terminus of all α subunits is the site for binding to the $\beta\gamma$ complex as determined by α subunit N-terminal cleavage (65–68). Figure 3 compares the amino acid sequences among known

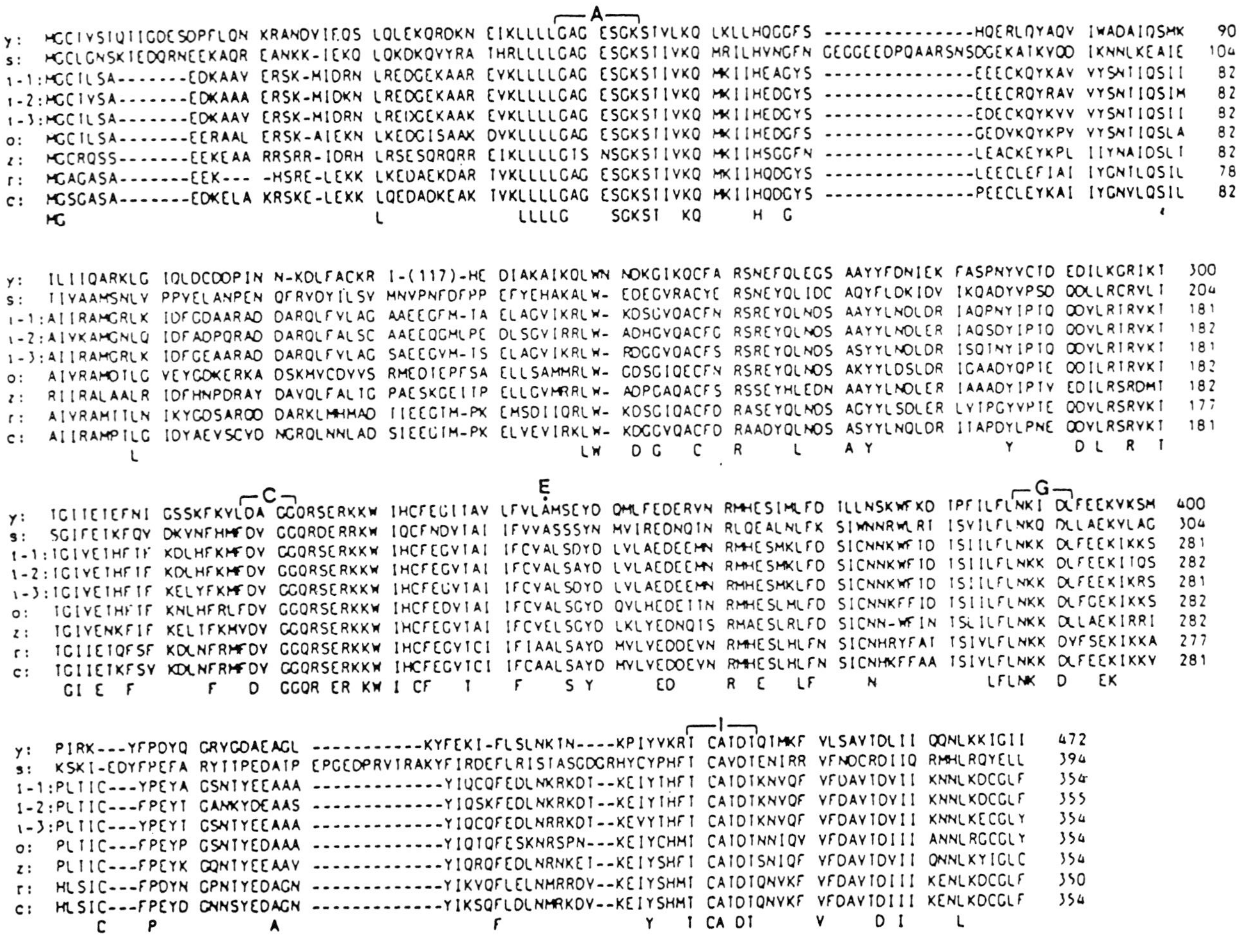

Figure 3 Comparison of the amino acid sequence homologies by single letter code among G protein alpha subunits. Abbreviations: A, C, E, G, and I represent Halliday regions; yeast GP1, (y); rat Gs, (s); $G_{i1\text{-}3}$, (i-1, i-2, i-3); human Go (o); Gz, (z); and bovine transducin Gr, (r), Gc(c). (From Ref. 4.)

G-protein α subunits. Not suprisingly, the amino terminus among all G-protein α subunits is highly conserved. Other areas in that are highly conserved among α subunits occur in domains that are postulated to be involved with guanine nucleotide exchange and GTPase activity. Similar domains are found in other guanine nucleotide binding molecules such as the c-Ha-*ras* proto-oncogene ($p21^{RAS}$) and bacterial elongation factor EF-Tu. Importantly the orientation of these domains is virtually identical in both molecules' tertiary structures (69,70). The four Halliday regions designated A, C, E, and G in Figure 3 represent areas in G-protein α subunits that are corresponding turns following β strands in EF-Tu (71).

A tertiary structure-function model for G-protein α subunits is seen in Figure 4, which is based on comparison of conserved amino acid areas between the $p21^{RAS}$ to G protein $\alpha_{i\text{-}2}$, α_o, $\alpha_{t\text{-}r}$, and $\alpha_{t\text{-}c}$; mutagenesis studies; antibody recognition and blocking studies; partial proteolysis analysis; and toxin effects on these and other G-protein α subunits (72). This model predicts that amino acid residues 57 to 152, which are the least conserved between G-protein α subunits, correspond to replacement of the short loop 27–39 of $p21^{RAS}$ (L2, Figure 4), with a much larger domain R2 in G-protein α subunits. L2 of $p21^{RAS}$ has been proposed as the "effector binding region" in $p21^{RAS}$ that can also bind a GTP-ase activating protein (GAP) (73,74). Hence R2 in G-protein α subunits may confer specificity for interaction with effectors or for differential spatial distribution in polarized cells. The binding sites for guanine nucleotides have been conserved in a noncontiguous region of amino acids in G-protein α subunits called the *G-box*. These amino acids correspond to residues Asn-270 and Asp-273 bind the guanine base, residues Asp-59 and Lys-271 bind to the ribose of GDP, and Cys-326 forms a hydrogen bond to the guanine base. The phosphate binding consensus in mononucleotide binding proteins, Gly-$(Xaa)_4$-Gly-Lys (75), corresponds to residues 35–37 and has been designated the *PO_4-box*. The *G-Box* and *PO_4-box* are predicted to be the areas of GDP/GTP binding in G-protein α subunits. Invariant residues 207–217 involved in possible conformation change have been designated the conformational switch box or *S-Box*. The corresponding residues in G-protein α subunits are Gly-203, Gln-205, and Ser-207. A mutation of Gln-205 to Leu produces a G-α_s that constitutively activates adenylyl cyclase, presumably by locking the structure into a specific activating conformation (76). Conversely, a mutation of Gly-204 to Ala blocks conformational change normally induced by GTP or analogue binding with resultant inability of the complex to dissociate from $\beta\gamma$ (77). Interaction with receptors is likely to be contained in corresponding terminal carboxy amino residues from 315–355. Supporting data include the block of interaction of G-α_{t1} with photorhodopsin

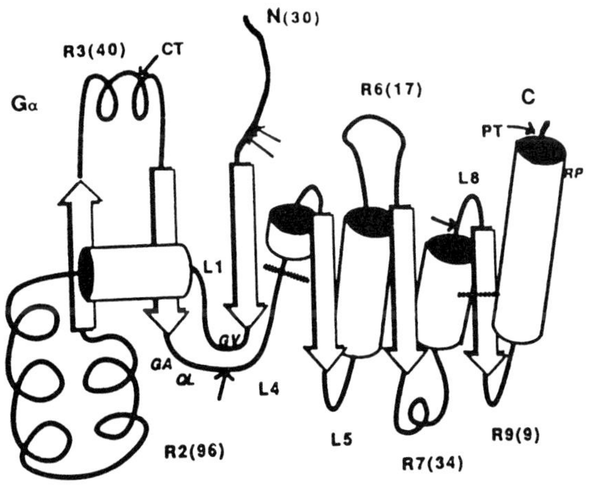

Figure 4 Schematic (topological) diagram of the model for G protein alpha subunits. Beta strands are indicated by thick arrows, alpha helices are indicated by cylinders, and the loop regions are indicated by black lines connecting the secondary structural elements. Loop regions in p21 *ras* are designated L, whereas longer loop regions in G alpha are designated as R. Parentheses indicate the number of residues. CT indicates the cholera toxin site, PT indicates the pertussis toxin site, C indicates the carboxyl terminus, N indicates the amino terminus. (From Ref. 72.)

following ribosylation of Cys-352 with pertusis toxin (78) and the ability of two synthetic peptides corresponding to 316–334 and 345–355 to compete with G-α_t for interaction with photorhodopsin that is dependent in the first peptide on Cys-326 (79). Additionally, a mutation of Arg-350 to Pro prevents activation of G-α_s by hormones (80) and a G-$\alpha_{i\text{-}2}/\alpha_s$ hybrid composed of G-$\alpha_{i\text{-}2}$ (N terminal, 60%) and G-α_s (C terminal, 40%) is comparable to G-α_s in receptor mediated stimulation of adenylyl cyclase (81). Recent studies have confirmed tertiary structure of the GTP binding pocket in both $p21^{RAS}$ and transducin has been conserved (Figure 5). Despite only an ~18% identity in primary structure between these proteins, their GTPase core domains are strikingly conserved in three dimensions, the β sheet and α helices are arranged identically and the contacts with the bound GTP analogue GTPγS are similar (82). An unexpected activity of the R2 loop region in G proteins as an intrinsic GTPase region has also been confirmed by Bourne and coworkers (83). This stretch of 113 amino acids contains a second domain composed of α helices that is inserted into the core GTP binding domain. This structural arrangement strongly suggests that the R2 loop region is centrally involved in turning the Gα switch on and off.

G-PROTEIN SIGNALING NETWORKS

Determining the roles of G proteins in cell signaling is becoming increasingly complex. Molecular cloning has revealed that these highly conserved protein structures have a wide but variable tissue distribution. Some are highly tissue specific, such as α_{olf}, which is only found in the neuroolfactory bulb, where it couples odorant modulation of adenylyl cyclase. $\alpha_{t\text{-}c}$ is found only in retinal cones,

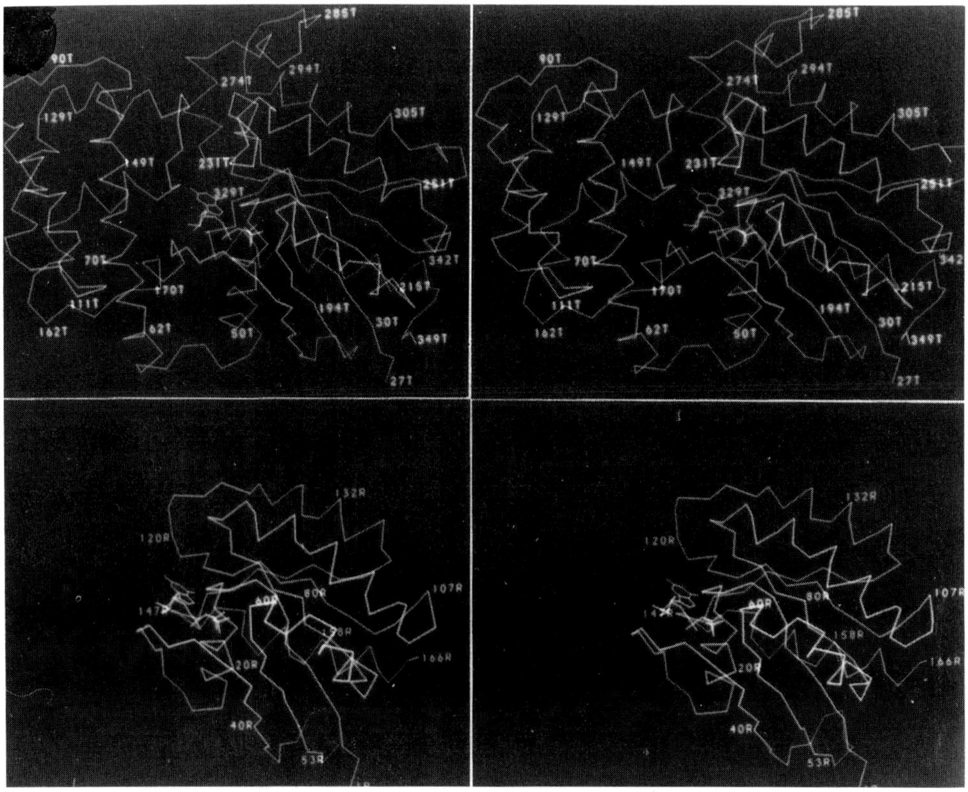

Figure 5 Stereoview of the carbon trace and bound nucleotides for G alpha transducin GTPγS (upper panel) and Ras GMP PNP (lower panel) demonstrating tertiary conservation of the GTP-binding pocket in both proteins. (From Ref. 82.)

in contrast to $\alpha_{t\text{-}r}$, which is found only in retinal rods, where it regulates cGMP phosphodiesterase. However, the other α subunits can be found in many different tissues, where they are often present in varying ratios. One of the original criteria for recognizing a G protein–mediated function was its modulation by guanine nucleotides, their analogues, and/or by AlF_4^-, subsequently distinguishing it from other processes by its sensitivity to cholera or pertussis toxins. However, the recently described G_z, G_{11-16}, and G_q are among a potentially growing family of G proteins that are insensitive to both toxins. These proteins are candidates for modulation of ion channel regulation (84) and modulation of phospholipase C in hepatocytes (85), cardiac myocytes (86), astrocytoma cells (87), or fibroblasts (88). Hence, responses to cholera or pertussis toxin may not distinguish G protein–mediated processes from others or necessarily identify the G protein responsible for transducing a specific signal. Even greater complexity has arisen because individual α subunits were each postulated to activate a *single effector* such as an enzyme or an ion channel, but reconstitution and membrane experiments demonstrated that this assumption is not always true, for α_s can modulate three effectors in the heart: voltage-dependent sodium channels, calcium channels, and adenylyl cyclase (89).

G_i was originally thought to be a single protein that mediated hormone-dependent inhibition of adenylyl cyclase by hormones, such as α_2 agonists, whose function could be specifically blocked by pertussis toxin. That pertussis toxin blocked G-mediated inhibition of adenylyl cyclase suggested that other processes blocked by pertussis toxin—including stimulation of PLC, PLA_2, and modulation of potassium and calcium channels—were also mediated by the same protein. However, in tissues where G_i was present, activation of all of the potential effectors could not been demonstrated (see Refs. 1 to 3). The apparent diversity of G_i function was subsequently revealed by molecular cloning. There are at least three α_i subunits corresponding to peptides from 41 kDa for $\alpha_{i\text{-}1}$ and $\alpha_{i\text{-}3}$ to 40 kDa for $\alpha_{i\text{-}2}$ that are the products of separate genes (human chromosome: 7 for $\alpha_{i\text{-}1}$; 3 or 12 for $\alpha_{i\text{-}2}$; and 1 for $\alpha_{i\text{-}3}$) and another pertussis toxin substrate α_o (human chromosome 2) that encodes a 39-kDa peptide. In many cells, more than one α_i can be detected in addition to α_o. This has made it difficult to assign receptor coupling and effector activation functions to any particular G_i protein. The unexpected similarity of function for the three α_i subunits has been demonstrated by the molecular cloning of $\alpha_{i\text{-}3}$. $\alpha_{i\text{-}3}$ was thought to be solely responsible for increasing the frequency of openings for voltage-sensitive potassium channels in heart muscle patches and hence was tentatively named α_k (90). However, subsequent studies demonstrated that the addition of $\alpha_{i\text{-}1}$ or $\alpha_{i\text{-}2}$ to these patches was as effective as $\alpha_{i\text{-}3}$ for opening these channels (91). The number of effectors, particularly ion channels, that G proteins can couple to is accumulating rapidly (92–95). G proteins have been implicated in the regulation of cardiac pacemaker channels ($G_o > G_i$ is inhibitory, G_s is stimulatory) (96) and are themselves subject to neuronal regulation by GAP-43 protein (G_o) (97).

Selectivity of α-subunit function for modulaton of effector function can be demonstrated during in vitro reconstitution studies in which α subunits are first preactivated by incubation with GTPγS and then directly added to excised membrane patches (98) or phospholipid vesicles (99). The former approach has allowed the identification of transduction pathways that modulate an amiloride-sensitive sodium channel (100,101), a chloride channel by $\alpha_{i\text{-}3}$ in renal epithelial cells (102), and adenylyl cyclase by $\alpha_{i\text{-}2}$ (103). Similarly selectivity of isoforms of G proteins for membrane receptors have also been demonstrated: αi-3 for the adenosine A1 (104), α2-adrenergic (105) and serotenergic 5-HT1a (106) receptors, and αo for the muscarinic M2 (107) receptor. Such coupling may be cell-specific, as the release of endothelium-derived relaxing factor via α2-adrenergic receptors in mediated by αi-2.

Experimentally, many G proteins are potentially capable of coupling the same effector as well as other defined and still undefined effectors in reconstituted artificial systems. If the known G-protein α, β, and γ subunits were combined independently, the resultant holoenzymes would represent an astronomically high number of unique G proteins available for cell signaling. Hence, it is likely that in vivo, there are constraints on the expression and coupling of discrete G protein to both receptors and effectors to maintain an ordered pattern of intracellular signaling. What is the evidence for such a premise? It is now clear that the dispersal of unique G-protein α subunit genes to different chromosomes following the duplication of an earlier progenitor α gene must have occurred very early in evolution. Evolutionary selection pressures can be correlated with the functional importance of tertiary protein structures (108). Over millions of years, all DNA is subject to nucleotide replacement, insertions, or deletions that result from recombinant events or mutagenizing background irradiation. Should these alterations occur in critical areas encoding proteins, they can result in the alteration of protein function (e.g., sickle cell disease or lethality for the organism). Hemoglobin is a protein critical for the survival of all vertebrates. Over a 500-million-year span from the amphibians to humans, the genes for this molecule have undergone nucleotide alterations that have allowed the primary protein sequence of the amphibian to vary by 60% from that of the human (109). By contrast, the genes encoding the G-protein α_o, $\alpha_{i\text{-}1}$, $\alpha_{i\text{-}3}$, and α_s subunits have also undergone nucleotide alterations over this time frame but have only allowed their primary protein sequences to vary by 3% in similarity (110,111). This would argue strongly that in vivo, the minor amino acid differences between all G-protein α subunits is critical for discrete rather than promiscuous signaling activities between receptors and effectors. This argument is supported by two independent cross-species experiments. It has recently been demonstrated that only a human $\alpha_{i\text{-}3}$ subunit added to excised membrane patches of amphibian A6 renal cells can activate an apically located amiloride-sensitive sodium via a PLA_2/cyclooxygenase pathway (112). Only the injection of a human α_o subunit to amphibian *Xenopus laevis* oocytes can activate a membrane associated phosphatidyl inositol pathway (113).

G-PROTEIN NETWORKS: REGULATION BY SPATIAL ORIENTATION

Specificity of G-protein function can be accomplished by targeting of α subunit isoforms to distinct membranes where their coupled receptors and effectors reside. Such specificity can be conferred by the physical segregation of the receptor/G-protein/effector complex to a distinct cellular membrane or membrane microdomain. Evidence supporting this premise is accumulating. G-protein $\alpha_{i\text{-}1,2,3}$ subunits are found in platelet membranes and are all potentially capable of inhibiting adenylyl cyclase. Nevertheless, only antiserum for $\alpha_{i\text{-}2}$ is effective in blocking inhibition by α_i in platelet membranes (114). As these subunits have been shown to be equally efficacious in activating other effectors such as ion channels. It is therefore likely that only $\alpha_{i\text{-}2}$ is translocated to its effector adenylyl cyclase. How might this occur? It is known that epineprine induces platelet aggregation by mechanisms independent of thrombin action. Epinephrine but not thrombin stimulates the translocation of G-protein $\alpha_{i\text{-}2}$ subunits from a Triton-soluble to a Triton-insoluble membrane compartment. These findings suggest that the association of $\alpha_{i\text{-}2}$ proteins with the membrane skeleton may be involved in hormone-induced translocation processes (115). Direct evidence for the segregation of G-protein α subunits has been found in polarized renal epithelial cells (LLC-PK1) using specific α_i antibodies and immunofluorescence. The $\alpha_{i\text{-}2}$ subunit was localized to basolateral membranes, whereas the $\alpha_{i\text{-}3}$ subunit was concentrated in the Golgi and was also detected at low levels on the apical membrane of some cells. Induction of a chimeric mouse metallothionein-I rat or canine $\alpha_{i\text{-}2}$ gene stably transfected into the LLC-PK_1 cells produced an increase in the content of the $\alpha_{i\text{-}2}$ subunit, which was targeted only to the basolateral membrane (see Figure 6). This finding demonstrates that one mechanism by which α_i subunit specificity for effectors may be achieved in polarized renal epithelial cells is by their geographic segregation to different cellular membranes (116). As might be expected, geographic diversity of these subunit isoforms can also be found in rat kidney (117). The presence of Gαi-3 on Golgi membranes appears to function in a signaling cascade that retards movement of heparan sulfate proteoglycans through the Golgi stack (118). In addition to its role in transcytosis, Gαi-3 has since been implicated in the activation of exocytosis as well (119). In addition to Gαi-3, Gs (120,121), and Go (122) may also participate in cellular pathways necessary for transcytosis and exocytosis.

Recent studies have extended these findings. It is now clear that the carboxyl terminus of αi-2 and αi-3 confers the necessary structural information for selected targeting to distinct membranes. Chimeric Gαi2/3 and Gαi3/2 subunit cDNAs were constructed and then stably integrated in LLC-PK1 cells under the control of a mouse metallothionein-I promoter-enhancer. Following transactivation of these genes with 5 μM cadmium chloride, Gαi2/3 subunit proteins were detected in the Golgi complex, whereas Gαi3/2 subunit proteins were detected in a subdomain of the lateral membrane of LLC-PK1 cells (123). As previously noted, the Gαi-2 gene product can be alternatively spliced, producing a second isoform with a carboxyl terminal region that is more similar to Gαi-3. Like Gαi-3, the resultant Gαi-2 subunit isoform is targeted to the Golgi complex.

G-PROTEIN NETWORKS: REGULATION BY EXPRESSION

The importance of temporally regulated G-protein α subunit expression during differentiation has been convincingly demonstrated in lower eukaryotes. In *Dictyostelium*, differentiation is triggered

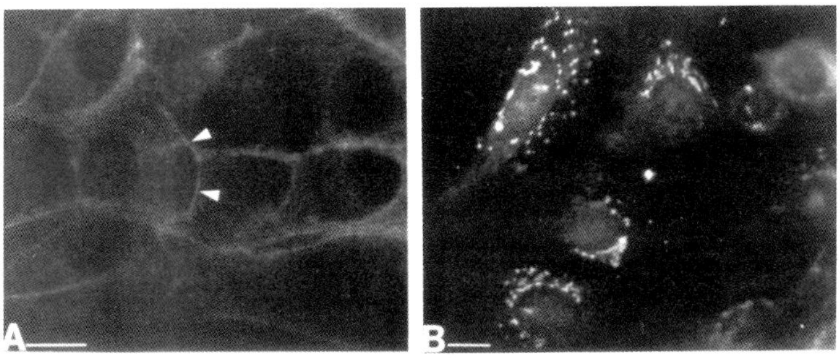

Figure 6 Confluent monolayers of LLC-PK$_1$ cells showing immunolocalization of α_{i-2} and α_{i-3} subuits on cellular membranes. Cell monolayers were fixed in paraformaldehyde, permeabilized with Triton X100, and reacted with the antibodies as described in the text. (A) Cells were reacted with AS7 antibody which is specific for the α_{i-2} subunit in these cells. There is some diffuse cytoplasmic staining, but most of the α_{i-2} is found in a typical cobblestone-like pattern representing staining of the basolateral membranes of these polarized cells (arrowheads). When viewing a monolayer of closely apposed cells, staining on the basolateral membrane is most concentrated at the perimeters of the cells and appears as a single line around each cell border. (B) Permeabilized cells were reacted with the EC antibody which is specific for the α_{i-3} subunit. No staining of the cell membranes in these cells was detected, the staining is concentrated in the perinuclear region of the cytoplasm in a Golgi-like distribution. (Bars = 10 mm.)

by a cyclic AMP-dependent increase in the transcription of α subunit genes (124). Gα4 null mutants created by gene disruption have aberrant morphological differentiation, reduced levels of prespore gene expression, and are unable to produce spores[125]. In *Drosophila*, gastrulation is impaired for homozygotes, with mutations of the concertina gene, which encodes a Gα protein (126). These studies strongly suggest that G proteins are participatory in temporally regulated signal transduction pathways requisite for differentiation and growth.

As the gene family encoding Gα subunits is highly conserved in all eukaryotes, it is likely that mechanisms for their regulation have also been conserved. Indeed, functional studies have suggested that there is a selective alteration of Gi subunit levels during differentiation of LLC-PK$_1$ cells. Following synchronization of these cells with 5-fluoruridine deoxyriboside, calcitonin receptors couple to Gi during the S phase, whereas this coupling could not be demonstrated in quiescent cells during G2 phase, implying a selective loss or modification of Gi subunits in these cells (127). After prolonged incubation of quiescent LLC-PK$_1$ cells, intracellular cAMP levels rise in these cells, which also suggests an adaptive loss of inhibitory Gi input on adenylyl cyclase (128). During culture, LLC-PK$_1$ renal cells differentiate from a rounded cell type to a fully polarized epithelium. Differential expression of the mRNAs for α_s and α_{i-2} occurs during the development of epithelial cell polarity (129). Similar changes in α_i and α_s protein and mRNA levels occur in 3T3-L1 fibroblasts (130), U-937, and HL-60 monocytes (131) following their treatment by hormones and second messengers to induce differentiation. Alteration of G-protein isoforms during differentiation and during embryonic cardiac development are accompanied by concomitant changes in hormone responsiveness (132–134). Hormones and lymphokines that modulate transcription in target genes—such as corticosterone, thyroxine, and interleukin 1-β—also differentially alter α_i and α_s subunit mRNA levels in rat cerebral cortex, rat fat, rat cardiac heart, and human endothelial cells respectively (135–138). There is considerable evidence that individual α-subunit genes are expressed variably in different tissues (139). Similar differences in tissue expression are found for another pertussis toxin–sensitive α isoform α_o, which is highly expressed in neural but not peripheral tissues (140). Furthermore, its differing content in rat cardiocytes and rat pituitary GH4 cells results from a differential regulation of α_o protein translation in these cells (141). Recent studies have confirmed the importance of temporal G-protein α subunit expression during development and differentiation. Inhibition of αs expression by antisense oligonucleotides accelerates differentiation of 3T3-L1 fibroblasts into adipocytes (142). Similar inhibition of αi-2 expression potentiates the conversion of F9 teratocarcinoma cells into primitive endoderm (143). In transgenic mice, inhibition of αi-2 expression by expression of a chimeric antisense Gαi-2/phosphoenolpyruvate carboxykinase gene inhibited growth, was associated with elevated cAMP levels, fat, and morphological kidney abnormalities including absence of development and prominent vacuolation localized to the proximal tubule (144).

There is also growing evidence that, like cell surface receptors, G-protein transducers are subject to in vivo compensatory mechanisms such as "downregulation" and "desensitization," which modulate cellular responses to hormones. Parathyroid hormone (PTH)-stimulated Na/Ca exchange and adenylyl cyclase activity is blunted in renal cortical cells from aged rats with chronically elevated PTH levels. These cells had decreased Gs-α and Gi-α proteins, which is consistent with a PTH hormone–induced heterologous desensitization involving G proteins. These effects could be reversed by parathyroidectomy in these animals (145). Prostaglandin E1 mediates a cAMP–independent downregulation of Gs but not of other Gi or Go isoforms in neroblastomaxglioma hybrid cells (146). In S49 mouse lymphoma cells, chronic activation of the stimulatory pathway of adenylyl cyclase by β-adrenergic agents reduced Gs levels of protein and mRNA. By contrast, Gi-2 protein and mRNA levels increased three- to fourfold, which indicated that there is hormonal cross-regulation between the inhibitory and stimulatory pathways of adenylyl cyclase at the level of G-proteins (147). Prolonged incubation of rat adipocytes with (–)-N6-phenylisopropyl adenosine (PIA) (an A1 adenosine receptor agonist) downregulates A1 adenosine receptors. Following their incubation for up to 7 days with 0 to 1000 n*M* PIA, there was almost complete loss of $\alpha_{i\text{-}1,3}$ and about 50% loss of $\alpha_{i\text{-}2}$ subunits from PIA-treated cells. The loss of each α_i was detectable after 24 hr with 300 n*M* PIA and maximal by 4 days. After 4 days, downregulation was detectable with 3 n*M* and maximal with 100 n*M* PIA. There was approximately 50% loss of G-protein β subunits in cells treated with 300 n*M* PIA for 4 days. When cells were incubated for 4 days with 300 n*M* PIA and then washed to remove PIA, $\alpha_{i\text{-}1,2,3}$ and β subunits returned to control levels within 5 days. By contrast 43- and 47-kDa forms of α_s subunits in PIA-treated cells were unchanged. These findings support the above observations that G-protein α-subunit isoforms are specifically downregulated along with their coupled receptor in response to prolonged hormonal stimulation (148). These findings have direct relevance to disease states such as diabetes mellitus, where hepatic adenylyl cyclase activity is consistently and chronically increased. Recent observations suggest that this metabolic alteration, which increases intracellular cAMP levels, may arise from increased G-protein α_s and/or α_i subunits that are inactivated by phosphorylation (149).

G PROTEINS ARE PROTOONCOGENES

It is now apparent that even a subtle alterations in the conformation of a G-protein α subunit or the over or underexpression of normal α subunits can have profound effects on cellular physiology. Mutations in pituitary tumors of only one allele of the α_s gene from Arg-201 to Cys/His or Gln-227 to Arg resulted in decreased GTPase activity of the expressed protein and correlated well with the tumor's phenotype (a high basal adenylyl cyclase activity and that responds poorly to stimulatory agents). The transfection and expression of the 227-Arg protein into Swiss 3T3 cells, increases their cyclic AMP levels and augments their DNA synthesis in serum-depleted medium (150). These mutations transform a normal G protein–transducing protein into the putative oncogene *gsp* (151). Somatic mutations have also been found in tumors of the adrenal cortex and ovary in one allele of the $\alpha_{i\text{-}2}$ gene from Arg-179 to Cys/His (predicted to decrease GTPase activity) tranform this gene into the putative oncogene *gip2* (152). Recently it has been demonstrated that GTPase deficient αq (153), αo (154), and α12 (155,156) can also induce transformation in NIH 3T3 cells.

The nonregulated overexpression of normal α subunits has been shown to affect cellular metabolism and growth. A murine adrenal cell line (Y1) retrovirally transfected with a rat α_o cDNA expressed large amounts of α_o subunit. The transfected Y1 cell had an altered cellular morphology and a reduced rate of cell division. In addition, the GTP-γS stimulated release of arachidonic acid from these cells was significantly increased compared to control cells (157). These findings are consistent with the unpublished observations of many laboratories attempting to constitutively overexpress α subunits in other cell types. Furthermore, it has recently be demonstrated that in autonomous thyroid adenoma, continued cell proliferation in this tumor is attributable in part to the unregulated overexpression of Gαi-1 (158).

The underexpression of normal α subunits may also have significant effects on cellular physiology. It has recently been documented that a mutation in one allele of the α_s gene in its translation initiator from Met-ATG to Val-GTG can cause the autosomal dominant disorder. Albright's hereditary osteodystrophy. This proband produces a truncated α_s polpeptide. The phenotype is characterized by a short stocky build, round facies, brachydactyly, and subcutaneous ossifications. There are alterations in metabolism, which is characterized by widespread resistance of target organs to parathyroid hormone and other hormones that act by stimulating adenylyl cyclase activity. This point mutation is not found in all patients. However, most patients studied have decreased level of α_s mRNA, which suggest that alterations in normal α_s gene expression are causal in producing the disorder. It is intriguing that these patients have a normal α_s gene on their unaffected chromosome that appears to be incapable of producing sufficient peptide to offset the metabolic alterations incurred in this disease (159).

G PROTEINS: GENOMIC REGULATION IN RENAL CELLS

The cloning of chromosomal genes for $\alpha_{i\text{-}1,2,3}$, α_s, α_t, and α_z offers potential insights into the genetic regulation of their products (160–163). Thus far the regulatory promoter-enhancer regions of two G-protein α subunit genes *Gαi-2* and *Gαi-3* have been characterized. As described earlier, both genes are expressed in porcine renal LLC-PK1 cells in a manner that suggested potential genomic regulation during culture. The porcine and human $\alpha_{i\text{-}2}$ subunit genes share a 78% sequence identity in their 5′ flanks, which suggested an evolutionary conservation of *cis* elements required to influence their transcription. The porcine $\alpha_{i\text{-}2}$ gene promoter lacks typical "TATA-like" sequences but does contain a "GC" box and a "TGTGG" sequence. The porcine gene promoter shares a 76% sequence identity with the promoter of another GTP-binding protein, the human c-Ha-*ras* protooncogene which would imply possible coordination of the expression of each gene product. By contrast, the porcine $G\alpha_{i\text{-}3}$ gene minimal promoter lacks "TATAAA" and "GC" boxes but does contain a sequence GGAAGTG conserved in both the human and porcine gene that could potentially bind an adenovirus E4TF1 transcription factor. In cells stably transfected with $G\alpha_{i\text{-}2}$ or $G\alpha_{i\text{-}3}$ gene 5′ flanking sequences fused to firefly luciferase cDNA reporter, temporal 10- to 15-fold transcriptional activation of both genes occurred before cellular polarization (see Figure 7). Utilizing mobility shift assays that compared nuclear extracts from cells before and after cell polarization, a motif in the 5′ region of the $G\alpha_{i\text{-}3}$ minimal promoter "GTACTTCCGCT" identifies an induced nuclear protein complex during trancriptional activation.

In polarized cells complemented with the human glucocorticoid receptor, dexamethasone respectively decreased $G\alpha_{i\text{-}2}$ by 50% but increased $G\alpha_{i\text{-}3}$ basal transcription and mRNA content threefold (see Figure 8). These studies demonstrated that both $G\alpha_i$ genes are dynamically regulated in LLC-PK$_1$ cells. Furthermore, these studies suggest the $G\alpha_{i\text{-}3}$ gene as a likely participant in the renal adaptive response to mineralocorticoids, which increases vectorial salt and water transport in the kidney (164).

In LLC-PK$_1$ renal cells, vasopressin-stimulated adenylyl cyclase (AC) activity is regulated in part by the counterbalancing activity of stimulatory G proteins (Gs) and inhibitory pertussis toxin-sensitive G proteins (Gi). After stimulating polarized LLC-PK1 cells with forskolin, which raises intracellular cAMP levels 50-fold, $G\alpha_{i\text{-}2}$ but not *Gαi-3* protein is increased threefold at 12 hr and remains elevated above control values by 24 hr. In cells stably transfected with $G\alpha_{i\text{-}2}$ or $G\alpha_{i\text{-}3}$ gene 5′ flanking sequences fused to firefly luciferase cDNA reporter gene, forskolin treatment increases *Gαi-2* transcription threefold but inhibits *Gαi-3* transcription by 50% at 12 hr. In vivo footprinting of forskolin-treated cells demonstrates protected guanosines in a 135-bp area previously associated with enhancer activity of this gene in nonpolarized cells. This DNA segment does not contain a classical cAMP response element (CRE). Utilizing discrete segments of this 135-bp area as a probe in mobility shift assays, a "CCAAT" box motif was found which detects an induced nuclear protein complex during forskolin-induced *Gαi-2* gene transcriptional activation. Importantly, the "CCAAT" box motif is functionally active as an enhancer in forskolin-treated cells. Chronic cAMP elevation initiates a counterregulatory response in renal cells, which includes increased transcription of the *Gαi-2* gene. In contrast to other cAMP-responsive genes, increased *Gαi-2* gene transcription is mediated by a cAMP pathway that requires either modification or induction of a member of the "CCAAT" box family of DNA binding proteins (165).

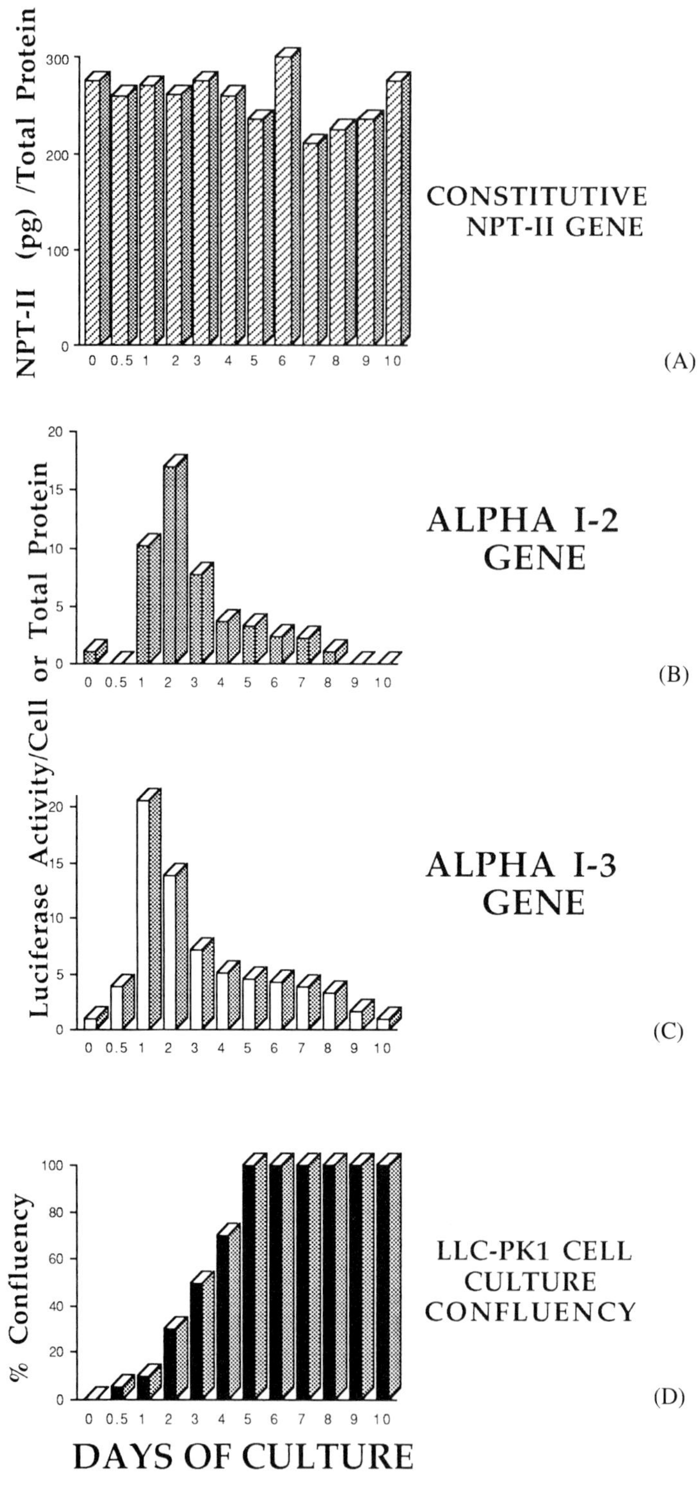

Figure 7 Transcription of *NPT II*, $G\alpha_{i\text{-}2}$, and $G\alpha_{i\text{-}3}$ genes in LLC-PK_1 cells during culture. Quiescent LLC-PK_1 cells stably transfected with pRMH140 and either SacII[LUC] or 13-2 LUC from day 10 of culture were trypsinized (day 0) and cultured for successive days. Panel D depicts confluency of these cells on culture days following trypsinization. Luciferase activity of these clonal cells stably transfected with $G\alpha_{i\text{-}3}$ Sac II [LUC] or $G\alpha_{i\text{-}2}$ 13-2 LUC is depicted in Panels B and C, respectively. Panel A depicts average NPT-II activity of clonal cells from Panels B and C.

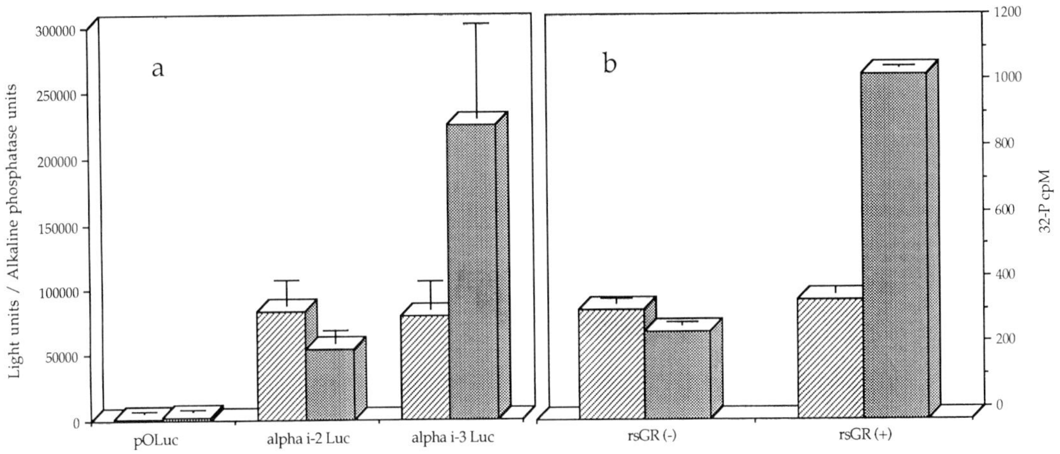

Figure 8 Dexamethasone alters transcription of Gα_i luciferase plasmids and G$\alpha_{i\text{-}3}$ mRNA content in renal epithelial cells. (a) poLUC, 13-2 LUC (G$\alpha_{i\text{-}2}$),or Sac II [Luc] ($G\alpha_{i\text{-}3}$) were cotransfected with pRShGRα into LLC-PK$_1$ cells and examined for luciferase activity 16 hr after treatment without (striped bars) or with (solid bars) dexamethasone 10^{-8} *M*. Luciferase activity results are expressed as mean light units ± S.E.M., normalized for human placental alkaline phosphatase activity in each of six individual experiments. (b) LLC-PK$_1$ cells were transfected with or without pRShGRα and examined 16 hr after treatment without (striped bars) or with (solid bars) dexamethasone 10^{-8} *M* for $G\alpha_{i\text{-}3}$ mRNA content. $G\alpha_{i\text{-}3}$ mRNA was determined by S$_1$ nuclease analysis. Mean corrected ^{32}P counts/minute from excised bands corresponding to these protected fragments are displayed in the right hand axis of panel b from three experiments.

Gαi-2 expression in polarized LLC-PK1 renal cells coincides the pertussis toxin–sensitive inhibition of adenlyl cyclase. It was initially surprising that the content of *Gαi-2* was as much as tenfold greater in nonpolarized cells without an appreciable inhibitory effect on adenylyl cyclase activity. This finding could be attributed to failure of the nonpolarized cell to deliver *Gαi-2* to a microdomain membrane site containing adenylyl cyclase and/or that *Gαi-2* might be functioning in another capacity as a protooncogene to influence effectors necessary for growth and differentiation.

The early-growth-response zinc-finger transcription factor (*EGR-1*) plays a pivotal role in signaling pathways that control cell growth and differentiation. Interestingly, the *Gαi-2* gene 5′ flanking region contains a putative binding site (5′-CGCCCCCGC-3′) for EGR-1 that may allow it to be a target gene for *EGR-1* mitogenic signaling. In LLC-PK1 renal cells, there is a temporal expression of *EGR-1* protein by immunoblotting and immuncytochemistry coincident with the maximal activation of the *Gαi-2* gene during cell growth. Overexpression of either *Gαi-2* or *EGR-1* with plasmids encoding cDNAs for *Gαi-2* (pRSV *Gαi-2*) or EGR-1 (pRSV EGR-1) driven by a viral Rous sarcoma promoter-enhancer increased epithelial cell growth in LLC-PK1 cells. Furthermore, a 320% enhancement of *Gαi-2* transcription was found only in LLC-PK1 cells following their transfection with plasmids that contained both the *EGR-1* binding site and overexpressed *EGR-1* protein. Utilizing mobility shift assays that compared nuclear extracts from cells before and after cell polarization, a probe containing the *EGR-1* motif detected induced nuclear protein complexes during transcriptional activiation of the *Gαi-2* gene. An anti-*EGR-1* antibody specifically retarded the mobility of the induced nuclear complexes, indicating that the *EGR-1* protein was a component of these complexes (see Figure 9). These findings indicate that renal cells have a novel mitogenic signaling pathway coupling proximal signaling events that activate *EGR-1* gene expression to a target protooncogene *Gαi-2* that is participatory for renal growth and differentiation (166).

These studies emphasize that G proteins couple a variety signaling pathways necessary for signal transduction, growth, ion transport, and protein transport. In turn, G proteins are themselves subject to regulatory processes that are essential for normal and developmental renal physiology.

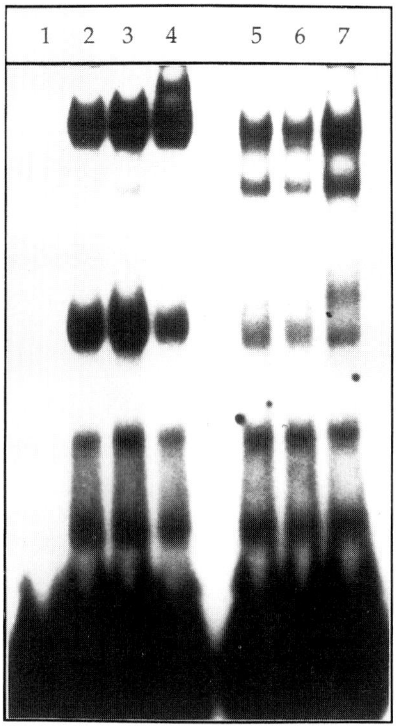

Figure 9 Mobility shift assays with the 23-bp DNA segment of the *Gαi-2* gene containing the EGR-1 binding site identify EGR-1 as a component of an induced nuclear complex in dividing LLC-PK1 cells. Nuclear extracts were prepared from LLC-PK1 cells 24 or 144 hr after trysinization and culture. A 23-bp DNA segment containing the EGR-1 consensus sequence (5′-ATCCGCC*CGCCCCCGC*CGTCGGG-3′) was used as a probe in mobility shift assays. Lane 1: probe alone. Lane 2: probe with 24-hr nuclear extracts. Lane 3: probe with 24-hr nuclear extracts preincubated with preimmune rabbit IgG. Lane 4: probe with 24-hr nuclear extracts preincubated with immune rabbit IgG anti EGR-1 Wi 21 (alpha 1). Lane 5: probe with 144-hr nuclear extracts. Lane 6: probe with 144-hr nuclear extracts preincubated with preimmune rabbit IgG. Lane 7: probe with 144-hr nuclear extracts preincubated with immune rabbit IgG anti EGR-1 Wi 21 (alpha 1).

REFERENCES

1. Gilman AG. G proteins: Transducers of receptor-generated signals. Annu Rev Biochem 1987; 56:615–649.
2. Stryer L, Bourne, H-R. G proteins: A family of signal transducers. Annu Rev Cell Biol 1986; 2:391–419.
3. Birnbaumer L, Codina J, Mattera R, et al. Brown AM. Signal transduction by G proteins. *Kidney Int Suppl* 1987; 23:S14–42.
4. Lochrie MA, Simon MI. G protein mutiplicity in eukaryotic signal transduction systems. Biochemistry 1988; 27:4957–4965.
5. Nakafuku M, Itoh H, Nakamura S, Kaziro Y. Occurrence in Saccharomyces cerevisiae of a gene homologous to the cDNA coding for the alpha subunit of mammalian G proteins. Proc Natl Acad Sci USA 1987; 84:2140–2144.
6. Nakafuku M, Obara T, Kaibuchi K, et al. Isolation of a second yeast Saccharomyces cerevisiae gene (GPA2) coding for guanine nucleotide-binding regulatory protein: Studies on its structure and possible functions. Proc Natl Acad Sci USA 1988; 85:1374–1378.
7. Kumagai A, Pupillo M, Gundersen R, et al. Regulation and function of G alpha protein subunits in Dictyostelium. Cell 1989; 57:265–275.
8. Barbacid M. ras genes. Annu Rev Biochem 1987; 56:779–827.
9. Paterson H, Reeves B, Brown R, et al. Activated N-ras controls the transformed phenotype of HT1080 human fibrosarcoma cells. Cell 1987; 51:803–812.

10. Matsui Y, Kikuchi A, Kondo J, et al. Nucleotide and deduced amino acid sequences of a GTP-binding protein family with molecular weights of 25,000 from bovine brain. J Biol Chem 1988; 263:11071–11074.
11. Bourne HR, Sanders DA, McCormick F. The GTPase superfamily: A conservered switch for diverse cell functions. Nature 1990; 348:125–132.
12. Yatani A, Okabe K, Polakis P, et al. ras p21 and GAP inhibit coupling of muscarinic receptors to atrial K+ channels. Cell 1990; 61:769–766.
13. Collin C, Papageorge AG, Lowy DR, Akon DL. Early enhancement of calcium currents by H-ras oncoproteins injected into hermissenda neurons. Science 1990; 250:1743–1745.
14. Higashijima T. Ferguson KM, Sternweis PC, et al. Effects of Mg2+ and the beta gamma-subunit complex on the interactions of guanine nucleotides with G proteins. J Biol Chem 1987; 262:762–766.
15. Iyengar R, Rich KA, Herberg JT, et al. Glucagon receptor-mediated activation of Gs is accompanied by subunit dissociation. J Biol Chem 1988; 263:15348–15353.
16. Ransnas LA, Insel PA. Subunit dissociation is the mechanism for hormonal activation of the Gs protein in native membranes. J Biol Chem 1988; 263:17239–17242.
17. Rojas FJ, Birnbaumer L. Regulation of glucagon receptor binding: Lack of effect of Mg and preferential role for GDP. J Biol Chem 1985; 260:7829–7835.
18. Dietzel C, Kurjan J. The yeast SCG1 gene: a G alpha-like protein implicated in the alpha- and alpha-factor response pathway. Cell 1987; 50:1001–1010.
19. Miyajima I, Nakafuku M, Nakayama N, et al. GPA1, a haploid-specific essential gene, encodes a yeast homolog of mammalian G protein which may be involved in mating factor signal transduction. Cell 1987; 50:1011–1019.
20. Whiteway M, Hougan L, Dignard D, et al. The STE4 and STE18 genes of yeast encode potential beta and gamma subunits of the mating factor receptor-coupled G protein. Cell 1989; 56:467–477.
21. Katada T, Bokoch GM, Northup JK, et al. The inhibitory guanine nucleotide-binding regulatory component of adenylate cyclase: Properties and function of the purified protein. J Biol Chem 1984; 259:3568–3577.
22. Okabe K, Yatani A, Evans T, et al. Beta gamma dimers of G proteins inhibit atrial muscarinic K+ channels. J Biol Chem 1990; 265:12854–12858.
23. Hildebrandt JD, Kohnken RE. Hormone inhibition of adenylyl cyclase: Differences in the mechanisms for inhibition by hormones and G protein beta gamma. J Biol Chem 1990; 265:9825–9830.
24. Birnbaumer L. Receptor to effector signaling through G proteins: Roles for beta gamma dimers as well as alpha subunits. Cell 1992; 71:1069–1072.
25. Faure M, Voyno-Ysentskaya TA, Bourne HR. cAMP and beta gamma subunits of heterotrimeric G proteins stimulate the mitogen-activated protein kinase pathway in COS-7 cells. J Biol Chem 1994; 269:7851–7854.
26. Eckstein F. Nucleoside phosphorothioates. Annu Rev Biochem 1985; 54:367–402.
27. Bigay J, Deterre P, Pfister C, Chabre M. Fluoride complexes of aluminium or beryllium act on G-proteins as reversibly bound analogues of the gamma phosphate of GTP. EMBO J 1987; 6:2907–2913.
28. Chabre, M. Aluminofluoride and beryllofluoride complexes: New phosphate analogs in enzymology. Trends Biochem Sci 1990; 15:6–10.
29. Kimura N, Shimada N. Evidence for complex formation between GTP binding protein(Gs) and membrane-associated nucleoside diphosphate kinase. Biochem Biophys Res Commun 1990; 168:99–106.
30. Kikkawa S, Takahashi K, Takahashi K, et al. Conversion of GDP into GTP by nucleoside diphosphate kinase on the GTP-binding proteins. J Biol Chem 1990; 265:21536–21540.
31. Jones D-T, Reed R-R. Golf: An olfactory neuron specific-G protein involved in odorant signal transduction. Science 1989; 244:790–795.
32. Fong H-K, Yoshimoto KK, Eversole et al. Identification of a GTP-binding protein alpha subunit that lacks an apparent ADP-ribosylation site for pertussis toxin. Proc Natl Acad Sci USA 1988; 85:3066–3070.
33. Matsuoka M, Itoh H, Kozasa T, Kaziro Y. Sequence analysis of cDNA and genomic DNA for a putative pertussis toxin-insensitive guanine nucleotide-binding regulatory protein alpha subunit. Proc Natl Acad Sci USA 1988; 85:5384–5388.
34. Stathmann M, Wilkie TM, Simon MI. Diversity of the G-protein family: sequences from five additional alpha subunits in the mouse. Proc Natl Acad Sci USA 1989; 86:7407–7409.
35. Pang IH, Sternweiss PC. Purification of unique alpha subunits of GTP-binding regulatory proteins (G proteins) by affinity chromatography with immobilized beta gamma subunits. J Biol Chem 1990; 265:18707–18712.
36. Simon MI. Personal communication.
37. Simon MI. Personal communication.
38. Hepler JR, Gilman AG. G proteins. Trends Biochem 1992; 17:383–387.
39. Bray P, Carter A, Simons C, et al. Human cDNA clones for four species of G alpha s signal transduction protein. Proc Natl Acad Sci USA 1986; 83:8893–8897.
40. Kozasa T, Itoh H, Tsukamoto T, Kaziro Y. Isolation and characterization of the human Gs alpha gene. Proc Natl Acad Sci USA 1988; 85:2081–2085.

41. Ishikawa Y, Bianchi C, Nadal-Ginard B, Homcy CJ. Alternative promoter and 5′ exon generate a novel Gs alpha mRNA. J Biol Chem 1990; 265:8458–8462.
42. Hsu WH, Rudolph U, Sanford J, et al. Molecular cloning of a novel splice variant of the alpha subunit of the mammalian Go protein. J Biol Chem 1990; 265:11220–11226.
43. Strathmann M, Wilkie TM, Simon MI. Alternative splicing produces transcripts encoding two forms of the alpha subunit of GTP-binding protein Go. Proc Natl Acad Sci USA 1990; 87:6477–6481.
44. Montmayeur JP, Borrelli E. Targeting of G alpha i2 to the Gogi by alternative spliced carboxy-terminal region. Science 1984; 263:95–98.
45. West K, Holtzman E, Kinane B, Ercolani L. Unpublished observation.
46. Casey PJ, Fong HK, Simon MI, Gilman AG. Gz, a guanine nucleotide-binding protein with unique biochemical properties. J Biol Chem 1990; 265:2383–2390.
47. Stryer L. Cyclic GMP cascade of vision. Annu Rev Neurosci 1986; 9:87–119.
48. Fawzi AB, Northup JK. Guanine nucleotide binding characteristics of transducin: Essential role of rhodopsin for rapid exchange of guanine nucleotides. Biochemistry 1990; 29:3804–3812.
49. Carty DJ, Padrell E, Codina J, et al. Distinct guanine nucleotide binding and release properties of the three Gi proteins. J Biol Chem 1990; 265:6268–6273.
50. Graziano MP, Freissmuth M, Gilman AG. Expression of Gs alpha in Escherichia coli: Purification and properties of two forms of the protein. J Biol Chem 1989; 264:409–418.
51. Pang IH, Sternweis PC. Isolation of the alpha subunits of GTP-binding regulatory proteins by affinity chromatography with immobilized beta gamma subunits. Proc Natl Acad Sci USA 1989; 86:7814–7818.
52. Marbach I, Bar-Sinai A, Minich M, Levitzki A. Beta subunit copurifies with GppNHp-activated adenylyl cyclase. J Biol Chem 1990; 265:9999–10004.
53. Jones DT, Masters SB, Bourne HR, Reed RR. Biochemical characterization of three stimulatory GTP-binding proteins: The large and small forms of Gs and the olfactory-specific G-protein, Golf. J Biol Chem 1990; 265:2671–2676.
54. Moss J, Vaughan M. ADP-ribosylation of guanyl nucleotide-binding regulatory proteins by bacterial toxins. Adv. Enzymol 1988; 61:303–379.
55. Sunyer T, Monastirsky B, Codina J, Birnbaumer L. Studies on nucleotide and receptor regulation of Gi proteins: Effects of pertussis toxin. Mol Endocrinol 1989; 3:1115–1124.
56. Ribeiro-Neto F-A, Rodbell M. Pertussis toxin induces structural changes in G alpha proteins independently of ADP-ribosylation. Proc Natl Acad Sci USA 1989; 86:2577–2581.
57. Katada T, Gilman AG, Watanabe Y, et al. Protein kinase C phosphorylates the inhibitory guanine-nucleotide-binding regulatory component and apparently suppresses its function in hormonal inhibition of adenylate cyclase. Eur J Biochem 1985; 151:431–437.
58. Zick Y, Sagi-Eisenberg R, Pines M, et al. Miltisite phosphorylation of the alpha subunit of transducin by the insulin receptor kinase and protein kinase C. Proc Natl Acad Sci USA 1986; 83:9294–9297.
59. Pyne NJ, Murphy GJ, Milligan G, Houslay MD. Treatment of intact hepatocytes with either the phorbol ester TPA or glucagon elicits the phosphorylation and functional inactivation of the inhibitory guanine nucleotide regulatory protein Gi. FEBS Lett 1989; 243:77–82.
60. Crouch MF, Lapetina EG. A role for Gi in control of thrombin receptor-phospholipase C coupling in human platelets. J Biol Chem 1988; 263:3363–3371.
61. Carlson KE, Brass LF, Manning DR. Thrombin and phorbol esters cause the selective phosphorylation of a G protein other than Gi in human platelets. J Biol Chem 1989; 264:13298–13305.
62. Buss JE, Mumby SM, Casey PJ. Myristoylated alpha subunits of guanine nucleotide-binding regulatory proteins. Proc Natl Acad Sci USA 1987; 84:7493–7497.
63. Jones TL, Simonds WF, Merendino JJ. Myristoylation of an inhibitory GTP-binding protein alpha subunit is essential for its membrane attachment. Proc Natl Acad Sci USA 1990; 87:568–572.
64. Mumby SM, Heukeroth RO, Gordon JI, Gilman AG. G-protein alpha-subunit expression, myristoylation, and membrane association in COS cells. Proc Natl Acad Sci USA 1990; 87:728–732.
65. Hurley JB, Simon MI, Teplow DB. Homologies between signal transducing G proteins and ras gene products. Science 1984; 226:860–862.
66. Neer EJ, Pulsifer L, Wolf LG. The amino terminus of G protein alpha subunits is required for interaction with beta gamma. J Biol Chem 1988; 263:8996–9000.
67. Fung BK, Nash CR. Characterization of transducin from bovine retinal rod outer segments: II. Evidence for distinct binding sites and conformational changes revealed by limited proteolysis with trypsin. J Biol Chem 1983; 258:10503–10510.
68. Navon SE, Fung, BK. Characterization of transducin from bovine retinal rod outer segments: J Biol Chem 1987; 262:15746–15751.
69. Jurnak F. Structure of the GDP domain of EF-Tu and location of the amino acids homologous to ras oncogene proteins. Science 1985; 230:32–36.
70. Tong L. Milburn MV. deVos AM, Kim SH. Structure of ras proteins (letter). Science 1989; 245:244.

71. Masters SB, Stroud RM, Bourne HR. Family of G protein alpha chains: Amphipathic analysis and predicted structure of functional domains. Protein Eng 1986; 1:47–54.
72. Holbrook SR, Kim SH. Molecular model of the G protein alpha subunit based on the crystal structure of the hRAS protein. Proc Natl Acad Sci USA 1989; 86:1751–1755.
73. Cales C, Hancock JF, Marshall CJ, Hall A. The cytoplasmic protein GAP is implicated as the target for regulation by the ras gene product. Nature 1988; 332:548–551.
74. Adari H, Lowy DR, Willumsen BM. Guanosine triphosphatase activating protein (GAP) interacts with the p21 ras effector binding domain. Science 1988; 240:518–521.
75. Moller W, Amons R. Phosphate-binding sequences in nucleotide-binding proteins. FEBS Lett 1985; 186:1–7.
76. Bourne HR, Masters SB, Miller RT. Mutations probe structure and function of G-protein alpha chains. Cold Spring Harbor Symp Quant Biol 1988; 53:221–228.
77. Miller RT, Masters SB, Sullivan KA, et al. A mutation that prevents GTP-dependent activation of the alpha chain of Gs. Nature 1988; 334:712–715.
78. Van Dop C, Yamanaka G. Steinberg F, et al. ADP-ribosylation of transducin by pertussis toxin blocks the light-stimulated hydrolysis of GTP and cGMP in retinal photoreceptors. J Biol Chem 1984; 259:23–26.
79. Hamm HE, Deretic D, Arendt A. Site of G protein binding to rhodopsin mapped with synthetic peptides from the alpha subunit. Science 1988; 241:832–835.
80. Sullivan KA, Miller RT, Masters SB, et al. Identification of receptor contact site involved in receptor-G protein coupling. Nature 1987; 330:758–760.
81. Masters SB, Sullivan KA, Miller RT, et al. Carboxyl terminal domain of Gs alpha specifies coupling of receptors to stimulation of adenylyl cyclase. Science 1988; 241:448–451.
82. Noel JP, Hamm HE, Sigler PB. The 2.2 A crystal structure of transducin-a complexed with GTPgS. Nature 1993; 366:654–663.
83. Markby DW, Onrust R, Bourne HR. Separate GTP binding and GTPase activating domains of a G alpha subunit. Science 1993; 262:1895–1901.
84. Nakajima Y, Nakajima S, Inoue M. Pertussis toxin-insensitive G protein mediates substance P-induced inhibition of potassium channels in brain neurons. Proc Natl Acad Sci USA 1988; 85:3643–3647.
85. Uhing RJ, Prpic V, Jiang H, Exton JH. Hormone-stimulated polyphosphoinositide breakdown in rat liver plasma membranes: Roles of guanine nucleotides and calcium. J Biol Chem 1986; 261:2140–2146.
86. Masters SB, Martin MW, Harden TK, Brown JH. Pertussis toxin does not inhibit muscarinic-receptor-mediated phosphoinositide hydrolysis or calcium mobilization. Biochem J 1985; 227:933–937.
87. Murayama T, Ui M. Receptor-mediated inhibition of adenylate cyclase and stimulation of arachidonic acid release in 3T3 fibroblasts: Selective susceptibility to islet-activating protein, pertussis toxin. J Biol Chem 1985; 260:7226–7233.
88. Cockcroft S. Phosphoinositide phophodiesteras: Regulation by a novel guanine nucleotide binding protein Gp. Trends. Biochem Sci 1987; 12:75–78.
89. Schubert B, VanDongen AM, Kirsch GE, Brown AM. Beta-adrenergic inhibition of cardiac sodium channels by dual G-protein pathways. Science 245:516–519.
90. Codina J, Olate J, Abramowitz J, et al. Alpha i-3 cDNA encodes the alpha subunit of Gk, the stimulatory G protein of receptor-regulated K+ channels. J Biol Chem 1988; 263:6746–6750.
91. Yatani A, Mattera R, Codina J. et al. The G protein-gated atrial K+ channel is stimulated by three distinct Gi alpha-subunits. Nature 1988; 336:680–682.
92. Brown AM, Yatani A, VanDongen AM, et al. Networking ionic channels by G proteins. Soc Gen Physiol Ser 1990; 45:1–9.
93. Birnbaumer L, Yatani A, VanDongen AMJ, et al. G protein coupling of receptors to ionic channels and other effector systems. Soc Gen Physiol 1990; 45:169–183.
94. Yatani A, Birnbaumer L, Brown AM. Direct coupling of the somatostatin receptor to potassium channels by a G protein. Metabolism 1990; 39:91–95.
95. Kirsch GE, Codina J, Birnhaumer L, Brown AM. Coupling of ATP-sensitive K+ channels to A1 receptors by G proteins in rat ventricular myocytes. Am J Physiol 1990; 259:H820–H826.
96. Yatani A, Okabe K, Codina J, et al. Heart rate regulation by G proteins acting on the cardiac pacemaker channel. Science 1990; 249:1163–1166.
97. Strittmatter SM, Valenzuela D, Kennedy TE, et al. GO is a major growth cone protein subject to regulation by GAP-43. Nature 1990; 344:836–841.
98. VanDongen AM, Codina J, Olate J, et al. Newly identified brain potassium channels gated by the guanine nucleotide binding protein Go. Science 1988; 242:1433–1437.
99. Senogles SE, Spiegel AM, Padrell E. Specificity of receptor-G protein interactions. Discrimination of Gi subtypes by the D2 dopamine receptor in a reconstituted system. J Biol Chem 1990; 265:4507–4514.
100. Cantiello HF, Patenaude CR, Ausiello DA. G protein subunit, alpha i-3, activates a pertussis toxin-sensitive Na+ channel from the epithelial cell line, A6. J Biol Chem 1989; 264:20867–20870.

101. Light DB, Ausiello DA, Stanton BA. Guanine nucleotide-binding protein, alpha i-3, directly activates a cation channel in rat renal inner medullary collecting duct cells. J Clin Invest 1989; 84:352–356.
102. Schwiebert EM, Light DB, Fejes-Toth G, et al. A GTP-binding protein activates chloride channels in a renal epithelium. J Biol Chem 1990; 265:7725–7728.
103. Tausig R, Iniguez-Lluhi JA, Gilman AG. Inhibition of adenylyl cyclase by Gi alpha. Science 1993; 261:218–221.
104. Friessmuth M, Schutz Linder ME. Interactions of the bovine brain A1 adenosine receptor with recombinant G protein alpha subunits. Selectivity for Gi alpha 3. J Biol Chem 1991; 266:17778–17783.
105. Kurose H, Regan JW, Cafon MG, Lefkowitz RJ. Functional interactions of recombinant alpha 2 adrenergic receptor subtypes and G-proteins in reconstituted phospholipid vesicles. Biochem 1990; 30:3335–3342.
106. Bertin B, Freissmuth M, Breyer RM, et al. Functional expression of the human serotonin 5-HT1A receptor in Escherichia coli. J Biol Chem 1992; 267:8200–8206.
107. Parker, EM, Kameyama, K, Higashijima T, Ross EM. Reconstitutively active G protein coupled receptors purified from baculovirus infected calls. J Biol Chem 1991; 266:519–527.
108. Ercolani L, Florence B, Denaro M, Alexander M. Isolation and complete sequence of a functional human glyceraldehyde-3-phosphate dehydrogenase gene. J Biol Chem 1988; 263:15335–15341.
109. Wilson AC, Carlson SS, White TJ. Biochemical evolution. Annu Rev Biochem 1977; 46:573–639.
110. late J, Jorquera H, Purcell P. Molecular cloning and sequence determination of a cDNA coding for the alpha-subunit of a Go-type protein of Xenopus laevis oocytes. FEBS Lett 1989; 244:188–192.
111. Olate J, Martinez S, Purcell P. Molecular cloning and sequence determination of four different cDNA species coding for alpha-subunits of G proteins from Xenopus laevis oocytes. FEBS Lett 1990; 268:27–31.
112. Cantiello HF, Patenaude CR, Codina J. Galphai-3 regulates epthithelial sodium channels by activation of phospholipase A2 and lipoxygenase pathways. J Biol Chem 1990; 265:21624–21628.
113. Moriarty TM, Padrell E, Carty DJ. Go protein as signal transducer in the pertussis toxin-sensitive phosphatidylinositol pathway. Nature 1990; 343:79–82.
114. Simonds WF, Goldsmith PK, Codina J. Gi2 mediates alpha 2-adrenergic inhibition of adenylyl cyclase in platelet membranes: in situ identification with G alpha C-terminal antibodies. Proc Natl Acad Sci USA 1989; 86:7809–7813.
115. Crouch MF, Winegar DA, Lapetina EG. Epinephrine induces changes in the subcellular distribution of the inhibitory GTP-binding protein Gi alpha-2 and a 38-kDa phosphorylated protein in the human platelet. Proc Natl Acad Sci USA 1989; 86:1776–1780.
116. Ercolani L, Stow JL, Boyle JF. Membrane localization of the pertussis toxin-sensitive G-protein subunits alpha i-2 and alpha i-3 and expression of a metallothionein-alpha i-2 fusion gene in LLC-PK1 cells. Proc Natl Acad Sci USA 1990; 87:4635–4639.
117. Stow JL, Sabolic I, Brown D. Heteogenous localization of G protein alpha subunits in rat kidney. Am J Physiol 1991; 261:F831–F840.
118. Stow JL, de Almeida JB, Narula N. A heterotrimeric G protein, Galpha i-3 on Golgi membrances regulate the secretion of a heparan sulfate proteoglycan in LLC-PK1 epithelial cells. J Cell Biol 1991; 114:1113–1124.
119. Aridor M, Rajmilevich G, Beaven MA, Sagi-Eisenberg R. Activation of exocytosis by the heterotrimeric G protein Gi3. Science 1993; 262:1569–1572.
120. Bomsel M, Mostov KE. Possible role of both the alpha and beta gamma subunits of the heterotrimeric G protein, Gs in transcytosis of the polymeric immunoglobulin receptor. J Biol Chem 1993; 268:25824–25835.
121. Piplikar SW, Simons K. Regulation of apical transport in epithelial cells by a Gs of heterotrimeric G protein. Nature 1993; 362:456–458.
122. Vitale N, Mukai H, Rouot B. Exocytosis in chromaffin cells: Possible involvement of the heterotrimeric GTP-binding protein Go. J Biol Chem. 1993; 268:14715–14723.
123. deAlmeida JB, Holtzman EJ, Peter P. Targeting of chimeric Galphai proteins to specific membrane domains. J Cell Sci 1994; 107:507–515.
124. Firtel RA, van Haastert PJ, Kimmel AR, Devreotes PN. G protein linked signal transduction pathways in development: Dictyostelium as an experimental system. Cell 1989; 58:235–239.
125. Hadwiger JA, Firtel RA. Analysis of Galpha4, a G-protein subunit required for multicellular development in Dictyostelium. Genes Dev 1992; 6:38–49.
126. Parks S, Wieschaus E. The drosophila gastulation gene concertina encodes a G alpha like protein. Cell 1991; 64:447–458.
127. Chakraborty MD, Chatterjee S, Kellokumpu H. Cell cycle dependent coupling of the calcitonin receptor to different G-proteins. Science 1991; 251:1078–1082.
128. Weiss ER, Amsler K, Dawson WD, Cook JS. Ann NY Acad Sci 1985; 456:420–435.
129. Holtzman EJ, Soper B, Stow JL, et al. Regulation of the G-protein alpha i-2 subunit gene in LLC-PK1 cells and isolation of porcien genomic clones encoding the gene promoter. J Biol Chem 1991; 266:1763–1771.

130. Watkins DC, Rapiejko PJ, Ros M, et al. G-protein mRNA levels during adipocyte differentiation. Biochem Biophys Res Commun 1989; 165:929–934.
131. Murphy PM, Eide B, Goldsmith P, et al. Detection of multiple forms of Gi alpha in HL60 cells. FEBS Lett 1987; 221:81–86.
132. Watkins DC, Northup JK, Malbon CC. Regulation of G-proteins in differentiation. Altered ratio of alpha- to beta-subunits in 3T3-L1 cells. J Biol Chem 1987; 262:10651–10657.
133. Liang BT, Hellmich MR, Neer EJ, Galper JB. Development of muscarinic cholinergic inhibition of adenylate cyclase in embryonic chick heart: Its relationship to changes in the inhibitory guanine nucleotide regulatory protein. J Biol Chem 1986; 261:9011–9021.
134. Luetje CW, Tietje KM, Christian JL, Nathanson NM. Differential tissue expression and developmental regulation of guanine nucleotide binding regulatory proteins and their messenger RNAs in rat heart. J Biol Chem 1988; 263:13357–13365.
135. Saito N, Guitart X, Hayward M, et al. Corticosterone differentially regulates the expression of Gs alpha and Gi alpha messenger RNA and protein in rat cerebral cortex. Proc Natl Acad Sci USA 1989; 86:3906–3910.
136. Ros M, Northup JK, Malbon CC. Steady-state levels of G-proteins and beta-adrenergic receptors in rat fat cells: Permissive effects of thyroid hormones. J Biol Chem 1988; 263:4362–4368.
137. Levine MA, Feldman AM, Robishaw JD, et al. Influence of thyroid hormone status on expression of genes encoding G protein subunits in the rat heart. J Biol Chem 1900; 265:3553–3560.
138. Lee RT, Brock TA, Tolman C, et al. Subtype-specific increase in G-protein alpha-subunit mRNA by interleukin 1 beta. FEBS Lett 1989; 249:139–142.
139. Jones DT, Reed RR. Molecular cloning of five GTP-binding protein cDNA species from rat olfactory neuroepithelium. J Biol Chem 1987; 262:14241–14249.
140. Huff RM, Axton JM, Neer EJ. Physical and immunological characterization of a guanine nucleotide-binding protein purified from bovine cerebral cortex. J Biol Chem 1985; 260:10864–19871.
141. Silbert S, Michel T, Lee R, Neer EJ. Differential degradation rates of the G protein alpha o in cultured cardiac and pituitary cells. J Biol Chem 265:3102–3105.
142. Wang Hy. Y, Watkins DC, Malbon CC. Nature 1992; 358:334.
143. Watkins DC, Johnson GL, Malbon CC. Regulation of the differentiation of teratocarcinoma cells into primitive endoderm by Galpha i2. Science 1992; 258:1373–1375.
144. Moxham CM, Hod Y, Malbon CC. Induction of Galphai-2 specific antisense RNA in vivo inhibits neonatal growth. Science 1993; 260:991–995.
145. Hanai H, Liang CT, Cheng L, Sacktor B. Desensitization to parathyroid hormone in renal cells from aged rats is associated with alterations in G-protein activity. J Clin Invest 1989; 83:268–277.
146. McKenzie FR, Milligan G. Prostaglandin E1-mediated, cyclic AMP-independent, down-regulation of Gsalpha in neuroblastoma x glioma hybrid cells. J Biol Chem 1990; 265:17084–17093.
147. Hadcock JR, Ros M, Watkins DC, Malbon CC. Cross-regulation between G-protein-mediated pathways: Stimulation of adenylyl cyclase increases expression of the inhibitory G-protein, Gi alpha 2. J Biol Chem 1990; 265:14784–14790.
148. Green A, Johnson JL, Milligan G. Down-regulation of Gi subtypes by prolonged incubation of adipocytes with an A1 adenosine receptor agonist. J Biol Chem 1990; 265:5206–5210.
149. Lynch CJ, Blackmore PF, Johnson EH, et al. Guanine nucleotide binding regulatory proteins and adenylate cyclase in livers of streptozotocin- and BB/Wor-diabetic rats: Immunodetection of Gs and Gi with antisera prepared against synthetic peptides. J Clin Invest 1989; 83:2050–2062.
150. Zachary I, Masters SB, Bourne HR. Increased mitogenic responsiveness of Swiss 3T3 cells expressing constitutively active Gs alpha. Biochem Biophys Res Commun 1990; 168:1184–1193.
151. Landis CA, Masters SB, Spada A. GTPase inhibiting mutations activate the alpha chain of Gs and stimulate adenylyl cyclase in human pituitary tumours. Nature 1989; 340:692–696.
152. Lyons J, Landis CA, Harsh G, et al. Two G protein oncogenes in human endocrine tumors. Science 1990; 249:655–659.
153. Kalenec G, Nazaarali AJ, Hermouet S, et al. Mutated alpha subunit of the Gq protein induces malignant transformation in NIH 3T3 cells. Mol Cell Biol 1992; 12:4687–4693.
154. Kroll SD, Chen J, De Vivo M, et al. The Q205:Go alpha subunit expressed in NIH-3t3 cells induces transformation. J Biol Chem 1992; 267:23183–23188.
155. Xu N, Bradley L, Ambdukar I, Gutkind JS. A mutant alpha subunit of G12 potentiates the eicosanoid pathway and is highly oncogenic in NIH 3T3 cells. Proc Natl Acad Sci USA 1993; 90:6741–6745.
156. Jiang H, Wu D, Simon MI. The transforming activity of activated G alpha 12. FEBS Lett 1993; 330:319–322.
157. Bloch DB, Bonventre JV, Neer EJ, Seidman JG. The G protein alpha o subunit alters morphology, growth kinetics, and phospholipid metabolism of somatic cells. Mol Cell Biol 1989; 12:5434–5439.
158. Selzer E, Wilfing A, Schiferer A, et al. Stimulation of human thyroid growth via the inhibitory guanine

nucleotide binding (G) protein Gi: Constitutive expression of the G-protein alpha subunit Gi alpha –1 in autonomous adenoma. Proc Natl Acad Sci USA 1993; 90:1609–1613.
159. Patten JL, Johns DR, Valle D, et al. Mutation in the gene encoding the stimulatory G protein of adenylate cyclase in Albright's hereditary osteodystrophy. N Engl J Med 1990; 322:1412–1419.
160. Itoh H, Toyama R, Kozasa T, et al. Presence of three distinct molecular species of Gi protein alpha subunit. Structure of rat cDNAs and human genomic DNAs. J Biol Chem 1988; 263:6656–6664.
161. Weinstein LS, Spiegel AM, Carter AD. Cloning and characterization of the human gene for the alpha-subunit of Gi2, a GTP-binding signal transduction protein. FEBS Lett 1988; 232:333–340.
162. Raport CJ, Dere B, Hurley JB. Characterization of the mouse rod transducin alpha subunit gene. J Biol Chem 1989; 264:7122–7128.
163. Matsuoka M, Itoh H, Kaziro Y. Characterization of the human gene for Gx alpha, a pertussis toxin-insensitive regulatory GTP-binding protein. J Biol Chem 1990; 265:13215–13220.
164. Holtzman EJ, Kinane TB, West K, et al. Transcriptional regulation of G-protein alpha i subunit genes in LLC-PK1 renal cells and characterization of the porcine Galphai-3 promoter. J Biol Chem 1993; 268:3964–3975.
165. Kinane TB, Shang C, Finder JD, Ercolani L. cAMP regulates G-protein alphai-2 subunit gene transcription in polarized LLC-PK1 cells by induction of a CCAAT box nuclear binding factor. J Biol Chem 1993; 268:24669–24676.
166. Kinane TB, Finder JD, Kawashima, et al. Growth of LLC-PK1 renal cells is mediated by EGR-1 upregulation of G-protein αi-2 protooncogene transcription. J Biol Chem (in press).

35
ADH Receptors: Molecular Biology and Signal Transduction

Mariel Birnbaumer
UCLA School of Medicine, Los Angeles, California

G PROTEIN–COUPLED RECEPTORS

The antidiuretic hormone (ADH) receptor belongs to the large structurally related superfamily of proteins referred to as *G protein–coupled receptors*, which relates to their mode of action, or as *seven transmembrane–spanning or heptahelical receptors*, which relates to their common structure. Cloning of the cDNAs encoding the ADH receptors opened the possibility to learn through mutagenesis about the regions of the protein involved in ligand binding and in coupling to the G protein G_s (1–3). Prior to random mutagenesis, the identification of mutations in the coding region that reduce or abolish receptor activity in individuals affected with X-linked nephrogenic diabetes insipidus had already identified regions of the receptor that must remain unchanged to sustain function (4–8). The disease and the underlying mutations are treated in another chapter, but there is reference to the mutations in this chapter because they are helpful in identifying some functional features of the receptor protein.

G Proteins

G proteins are heterotrimeric components of the cell plasma membrane composed of α, β, and γ subunits anchored to the plasma membrane through the γ subunit, which is either farnesylated or geranylgeranylated, and variously through the α subunit derivatized by myristic and/or palmitic acid. The α subunit binds guanosine triphosphate (GTP) and guanosine diphosphate (GDP) and has intrinsic GTPase activity; in the resting state, the α subunit has GDP bound rather than GTP. Interaction of the G protein with agonist occupied receptors promotes the exchange of GDP for GTP, followed by dissociation of α-GTP from $\beta\gamma$. The free α-GTP and often but not always the $\beta\gamma$ dimers regulate the specific effectors through which receptors signal. Among the effectors regulated by G proteins one finds adenylyl cyclase, phospholipases of the type C and Ca^{2+}, and K^+ ion channels. After GTP hydrolysis, the newly formed α-GDP complex loses its affinity for the effectors and regains its affinity for the $\beta\gamma$ subunits. The $\beta\gamma$ subunits are involved in signal transduction, acting both as primary regulators and coregulators with the α subunits (for a comprehensive review see Reference 9).

Receptor-stimulated G proteins link hormone-activated receptors to cellular effectors and thus transduce the signal across the plasma membrane to the interior of the cell. Their enzymatic activity makes them amplifiers of the receptor signal; they are independent of receptor interaction once they have been activated by GTP. The magnitude of amplification of the signal depends on how many G proteins are activated by a receptor before it becomes desensitized or loses bound hormone and on whether the signal is only α-GTP or whether $\beta\gamma$ also participates. The number of effectors stimulated by α-GTP before its activity decays due to hydrolysis is another key step determining the extent of signal amplification. The receptors are intrinsic membrane proteins, and the transducing

G proteins are membrane-bound; as a consequence, signal transduction is a process localized to the cytoplasmic face of the plasma membrane, where effector-generated second messengers such as cAMP and inositol phosphates are synthesized and from where they diffuse into the cytoplasm.

Specificity of Receptor–G Protein Interaction

There is a high degree of specificity in the interaction between a receptor and a G protein. There is also a high degree of specificity in the interaction between G proteins and effectors. This dual selectivity determines the identity of the effectors that will respond to receptor activation. The ADH receptor has been known for a long time to mediate its antidiuretic activity by activating G_s, which, in turn, stimulates adenylyl cyclase activity, thus increasing the levels of cAMP in the principal cells of the collecting duct. The experiments of Orloff and Handler established cAMP as the intracellular effector (10). Recent data confirmed the role of protein kinase A, and hence the requirement for phosphorylation (11), in the pathway that connects receptor activation by ADH and the increase in water permeability of the apical membrane of the collecting duct cells caused by the translocation of water pores.

With the proliferation of studies carried out in transfected cells, it is worth noting that specificity of interaction with a particular G protein may no longer be true when receptors are expressed at very high levels. High receptor abundance generates conditions in which G protein specificity is blurred. Conditions of this kind are often found in stably or transiently transfected cells that are made to express G protein–coupled receptors. The ADH receptor can be used to illustrate this point. Expression cloning of the human ADH receptor gave rise to several cell lines expressing the receptor at different levels: from 5000 to 500,000 molecules/cell (1); all these values represent significantly higher abundance than the one believed to be present in kidney cells. When cells containing up to 100,000 receptors/cell were loaded with the fluorescent dye Fura II and challenged with a very high dose of vasopressin, no Ca^{2+} mobilization was observed (12,13). But when the experiment was repeated with cells expressing 500,000 sites/cell, a discreet measurable response in terms of Ca^{2+} mobilization and inositol phosphate production was detected (14). These results suggest caution when one is interpreting studies of receptor coupling in transiently transfected cells that typically synthesize receptors in excess of 10^5 per cell.

In addition to their role in signal transduction G proteins, guanine nucleotides and magnesium modify the affinity of interaction of some receptors with their agonists. This interaction results in tight control of ligand-binding affinity by ions and nucleotides and has been documented extensively for the β_2-adrenergic receptor (15). Although it has been assayed for proof that modulation of affinity by G_s/GTP occurs in the case of the ADH receptor is still lacking (M. Birnbaumer, unpublished). The recent cloning of prostaglandin E_1 receptors identified two forms that arise as a consequence of alternative splicing and have their affinities either increased or decreased by interactions with G proteins (16)—an unexpected finding for a receptor of this family and another reason to refrain from generalizing the effects observed with adrenergic receptors to all G protein–coupled receptors without experimental verification.

COMPOSITION OF ADH RECEPTORS FROM DIFFERENT SPECIES

The human, rat and mouse arginine vasopressin (AVP) (17) receptor proteins consist of 371 amino acids, while the pig LVP receptor has 370 amino acids. The amino acid sequence of the receptors of different species is highly conserved, around 85% overall, with the mouse and rat receptors showing 96% identity. Figure 1 shows the amino acid sequence alignment of the ADH receptors of the four species mentioned deduced from their cloned genes and cDNAs. As illustrated in Figure 2 the differences in composition among these receptors are clustered at the amino- and the carboxyl-terminal segments of the protein, with a few other differences scattered throughout.

THE ADH RECEPTOR PROTEIN

The ADH Receptor and the Cell Membrane

As mentioned in the introduction, the G protein–coupled receptors are predicted by Kyte Doolittle analysis of the amino acid sequence to traverse the cell membrane seven times. The arrangement of these putative seven-transmembrane segments (TMs) in relation to each other was initially inferred

```
                                 **********I*********
MLRA-TTSAVPRALSWPAAPGNGSEREPLDDRDPLLARVELALLSTVFVAVALS  53  pV2
MLMASTTSAVPGHPSLPSLPSNSSQERPLDTRDPLLARAELALLSIVFVAVALS  54  hV2
MLLVSTVSAVPGLFSPPSSPSNSSQEELLDDRDPLLVRAELALLSTIFVAVALS  54  rV2
MILVSTTSAVPGALSSPSSPSNSSQEELLDDRDPLLVRAELALLSTIFVAVALS  54  mV2

*********            ********II**********                  ******III**
NGLVLGALVRRGRRGRWAPMHVFIGHLCLADLAVALFQVLPQLAWDATYRFRGPDALCRAVKYLQMVGMY 123 pV2
NGLVLAALARRGRRGHWAPIHVFIGHLCLADLAVALFQVLPQLAWKATDRFRGPDALCRAVKYLQMVGMY 124 hV2
NGLVLGALIRRGRRGRWAPMHVFISHLCLADLAVALFQVLPQLAWDATDRFHGPDALCRAVKYLQMVGMY 124 rV2
NGLVLGALIRRGRRGRWAPMHVFISHLCLADLAVALFQVLPQLAWDATDRFHGPDALCRAVKYLQMVGMY 124 mV2

**********                         *********IV**********
ASSYMILAMTLDRHRAICRPMLAYRHGGGARWNRPVLVAWAFSLLLSLPQLFIFAQRDVGDGSGVLD  190  pV2
ASSYMILAMTLDRHRAICRPMLAYRHGSGAHWNRPVLVAWAFSLLLSLPQLFIFAQRNVEGGSGVTD  191  hV2
ASSYMILAMTLDRHRAICRPMLAYRHGGGARWNRPVLVAWAFSLLLSLPQLFIFAQRDVGNGSGVFD  191  rV2
ASSYMILAMTLDRHRAICRPMLAYRHGGGARWNRPVLVAWAFSLLLSLPQLFIFAQRDVGNGSGVFD  191  mV2

               *********V**********
CWASFAEPWGLRAYVTWIALMVFVAPALGIAACQVLIFREIHTSLVPGPAERAGG  245  pV2
CWACFAEPWGRRTYVTWIALMVFVAPTLGIAACQVLIFREIHASLVPGPSERPGG  246  hV2
CWARFAEPWGLRAYVTWIALMVFVAPALGIAACQVLIFREIHASLVPGPSERAGR  246  rV2
CWARFAEPWGLRAYVTWIALMVFVAPALGIAACQVLIFREIHASLVPGPSERAGR  246  mV2

                         ***********VI*************          ****
HRGGRRAGSPREGARVSAAMAKTARMTLVIVAVYVLCWAPFFLVQLWSVWDPKAPREGPPFVLLM  310  pV2
RRRGRRTGSPGEGAHVSAAVAKTVRMTLVIVVVYVLCWAPFFLVQLWAAWDPEAPLEGAPFVLLM  311  hV2
RRRGRRTGSPSEGAHVSAAMAKTVRMTLVIVIVYVLCWAPFFLVQLWAAWDPEAPLERPPFVLLM  310  rV2
RRRGHRTGSPSEGAHVSAAMAKTVRMTLVIVIVYVLCWAPFFLVQLWAAWDPEAPLERPPFVLLM  311  mV2

**VII***********
LLASLNSCTNPWIYASFSSSISSELRSLLCCPRRRTPPSLRPQEESCATASSFSARDTSS@  370  pV2
LLASLNSCTNPWIYASFSSSVSSELRSLLCCARGRTPPSLGPQDESCTTASSSLAKDTSS@  371  hV2
LLASLNSCTNPWIYASFSSSVSSELRSLLCCAQRHTTHSLGPQDESCATASSSLMKDTPS@  371  rV2
LLASLNSCTNTWIYASFSSSVSSELRSLLCCAQRHTTHSLGPQDESCATASSSLMKDTPS@  371  mV2
```

Figure 1 Amino acid composition of the V2 vasopressin receptor from pig, human, rat, and mouse. The composition of the human protein is shown in bold letters.

from the structural homology of rhodopsin to bacteriorhodopsin, for which it has been possible to obtain a three-dimensional structure by electron microscopy with a resolution between 3.5 and 7 Å and which showed the TMs to be perpendicular to the plane of the membrane enclosing a central space (18,19). A similar picture was obtained for rhodopsin on the basis of electron diffraction projection maps derived from two-dimensional crystals that formed upon reconstitution of the purified protein into phospholipid vesicles (20,21). Figure 2 shows a scheme in which the receptor has been flattened to simplify description of its primary features.

The seven-transmembrane domains define an extracellular N-terminal domain, three intra- and three extracellular loops, and an intracellular C-terminal tail. Similar to what has been found for other members of the receptor family, the ADH receptor has a cysteine about 13 amino acids from the end of TM-VII that appears to be palmitoylated, providing what is assumed to be another membrane anchor and the formation of a fourth intracellular loop. A mutation that results in the truncation of the receptor protein four amino acids prior to this location has been identified in a patient suffering from diabetes insipidus, suggesting that this truncated form of ADH receptor is not biologically active (8). While removal by mutagenesis of the palmitoylation site does not affect function in some receptors (rhodopsin, α_2-adrenergic) (22), it impairs function in others. For example, a β_2-adrenergic receptor mutant (Cys-341 to Gly) is hyperphosphorylated and largely uncoupled from the G_s/adenylyl cyclase system (23). For the ADH receptor, mutagenesis of the cysteines will be necessary to determine whether the loss of activity is due to the missing anchor that interferes with protein conformation and coupling or to the missing portion of the carboxyl-terminal segment.

The Extracellular Segment of the ADH Receptor

Examination of the amino acid alignment shown in Figure 1 reveals that the amino-terminal portion of the protein varies significantly among species, even among the AVP-binding receptors. One may

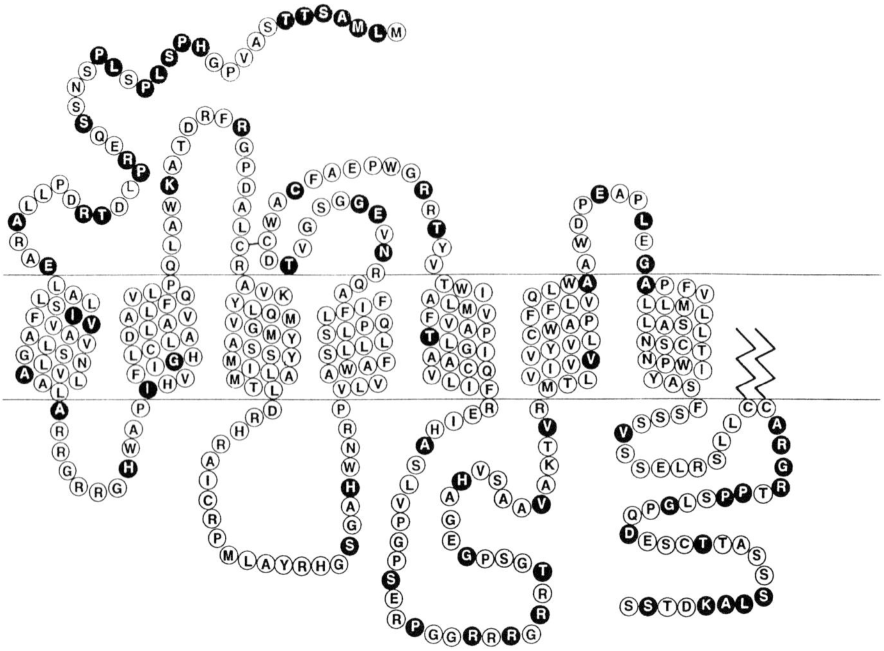

Figure 2 Predicted structure of ADH receptors. The diagram shows the predicted arrangement of the amino acids across the plasma membrane according to Kyte and Doolittle and highlights the regions of greatest similarity among the receptors shown in Figure 1. Backbone is human V2R. Dark beads identify nonidentities.

conclude that this portion of the molecule does not contribute to form the binding site that accommodates the hormone. It is possible that the amino-terminal region plays a role in the binding of synthetic ligands known to behave differently toward ADH receptors from different species (24). The amino acid sequence predicts a single N-glycosylation site at Asn^{22}. While not required for function once assembled, for some receptors removal of the glycosylation sites impairs their proper assembly and/or membrane insertion resulting in defective cell surface expression. The predicted molecular weight of the human receptor protein is 41,400 Da, and only recently has information been published showing that the glycosylated receptor migrates in SDS-polyacrylamide gels with an apparent molecular weight of 69,000 (25).

The remainder of the extracellular portion of the protein deserves close scrutiny since it has been assumed to play an important role in forming the binding site for AVP. Of the two variable amino acids in the first extracellular loop, neither Lys^{100} nor Arg^{106} present in the human receptor are conserved in the other species (Figure 2), although their location suggests that they will be displayed prominently in a putative binding site. Direct proof of the contribution of this region to the hormone-binding region was provided recently by Kojro et al. (26). These authors were able to covalently link a photoactive tritiated vasopressin probe to the receptor and identified the radioactivity as covalently attached to Arg^{106} of extracellular loop I. They obtained a photolabeled protein with an apparent Mr of 30,000 which by amino acid sequence analysis had Val^{93} at the amino terminus. The existence of a protease-sensitive link between Gln^{92} and Val^{93} was proposed (26). These results explain the discrepancies between the molecular mass predicted from the cDNA sequence, the M_r values of the native receptor reported by Guillon et al. (about 80,000 Da) (27), and the values obtained from photoaffinity labeling studies (around 30,000) (28).

Most receptors of this superfamily have cysteines in the first and second extracellular loops, which in rhodopsin, and by inference in other receptors, may form a disulfide bridge that contributes to the stability of the seven-transmembrane structure. In the second extracellular loop of the ADH receptor, the preservation of Cys^{192} in all four species suggests that this is the amino acid pairing with Cys^{112} from the first extracellular loop to help acquire and preserve the protein structure. Several of the published mutations associated with diabetes insipidus consist in the appearance of a third cysteine in the second extracellular loop; this is not surprising, since extracellular loops I and II seem to be key contributors to the formation of the hormone-binding site. Any structural alteration in this region would be expected to significantly reduce hormone binding. The availability of the new nonpeptidic antagonist to the V2 receptor will undoubtedly facilitate the characterization of other segments of receptor important for the binding of agonists and antagonists.

Transmembrane and Intracellular Segments of the ADH Receptor

The transmembrane and intracellular segments of the protein contribute to the overall structure and are responsible for signal transduction. As mentioned earlier, all vasopressin type 2 receptors lack a canonical R-R/K-X-S/T consensus site for phosphorylation by cAMP-dependent protein kinase (29).

Two consensus sites for protein kinase C phosphorylation were identified in the human ADH receptor, and the receptor of the MDCK cells derived from dog kidney has been reported to be desensitized following treatment with phorbol esters (30). Such effect can not be obtained with the human receptor expressed in L cells. Rather than a reduction in activity, a significant stimulation of adenylyl cyclase activity after the treatment was detected in these cells (Birnbaumer M., unpublished). These findings suggest that there is no direct PKC effect on the ADH receptor and that the reported effects of PKC activation on ADH receptor may be downstream from the receptor affecting a subsequent step in the signaling cascade; for example, adenylyl cyclase. The differences in composition found in the third intracellular loop and the carboxyl-terminal segment of receptors from different species might be related to different coupling efficiencies.

Conserved Amino Acids Among G Protein–Coupled Receptors

Analysis of sequence alignments has defined the existence of at least three distinct subfamilies of G protein–coupled receptors. One of these subfamilies has as a structural signature a DRY-motif and encompasses the vast majority of the >200 G protein–coupled receptors cloned so far, including the ADH receptor. These proteins have about 12 highly conserved amino acids in their TMs—3–4 in TM-II, 2 in TM-VI, and 2–3 in TM-VII, and, at the interface between the membrane and the cytoplasm, at the end of TM-III, the so-called DRY consensus motif (Asp-Arg-Tyr). The R is absolutely conserved in all receptors of this subfamily, the D is mostly D but can also be E (rhodopsin), and the Y, while present in about 100 members, varies in the others, the most frequent replacements being F, H, and C, DRY-motif–containing receptors do not show a G protein preference, or preference for neurotransmitter (small) vs. peptide hormone (large). As mentioned in detail below, an Arg^{137}His mutation was identified in an NDI patient and the impact of the single amino acid change in receptor function was characterized (31).

Another highly conserved amino acid among members of this subfamily is the Asp^{85} present in transmembrane region II of the ADH receptor. A significant role for this amino acid was identified by Limbird and collaborators in the α_2-adrenergic receptor. They demonstrated that replacing Asp^{85} with Asn^{85} caused loss of the ion flux response to agonist without loss of adenylyl cyclase inhibition, a G protein–coupled response (32). In similar experiments, we examined whether sodium plays a role in the coupling properties of the V2 receptor to G_s. We modeled our experiments on those reported for the adrenergic receptor and sought to determine whether replacing sodium by glucamine in phosphate buffered saline modified the dose-response curve of cAMP accumulation in cells bearing the receptor when challenged with AVP (33). We found that in the presence of 140 m*M* Na or 140 m*M* glucamine, the maximal stimulation of cAMP levels remained unchanged and there was no alteration of the E_{50} for receptor activation, as shown in Figure 3. This experiment implies that features conserved among proteins of this family do not serve similar functions.

BIOCHEMICAL CHARACTERIZATION OF ADH RECEPTOR MUTATIONS

Among the mutations described for the ADH receptor, two have been characterized functionally. Both are due to single amino acid changes and frame transmembrane domain III.

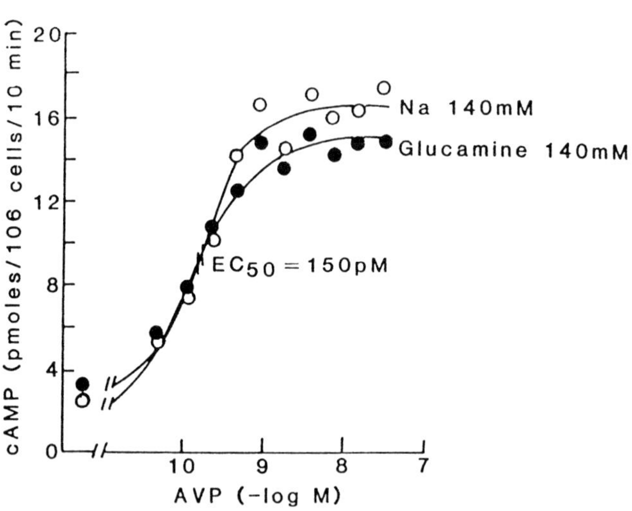

Figure 3 Analysis of ADH receptor sensitivity to Na^+. Vasopressin stimulation of cAMP accumulation in HTB-2 cells (1) was examined in the presence of phosphate buffer containing either 140 m*M* Na^+ or 140 m*M* Glucamine in the presence of 1 m*M* IBMX following published protocols. (From Ref. 35.)

1. The Arg-137 to His (Q2 allele) mutation is located immediately after TM-III at the center of the DRY motif—which is DRH for wild-type ADH receptor. This mutation completely uncouples the receptor from G_s, while other agonist-dependent functions (binding and receptor sequestration) remain unaltered, and it is discussed above. This confirmed the role of the DRH motif in G protein–receptor coupling (9,30).

2. The other mutation, Arg-113 to Trp (Q3 allele), just prior to TM-III, is located in the putative first extracellular loop of the receptor next to Cys^{112}, thought to be part of the extracellular disulfide bridge. This mutation lowers the receptor binding affinity for AVP by a factor of 20, interferes with its maturation/transport to the cell surface by a factor of 5 or so, and as a consequence diminishes the efficacy of the receptor, so that at equal receptor density threefold higher concentrations of AVP are required for adenylyl cyclase stimulation when compared to the wild-type receptor (34). The extracellular location of the mutation predicted the reduction in ligand-binding affinity and the interference with protein maturation, but the reduction in signal transduction was an unexpected consequence. These results confirmed the importance of TM-III in the transmission of the hormone binding signal, perhaps by modifying the location of the DRH motif. It is to be expected that further analysis of other amino acid changes will reveal new aspects of structure function relations in the ADH receptor.

SUMMARY

The primary structure of the ADH receptor encodes a hormone-binding site that, when occupied, changes receptor conformation to an active form able to stimulate G_s and an intracellular region that mediates receptor sequestration at high levels of receptor occupancy by agonist (35). The primary ligand-binding function seems to reside in the first two extracellular loops of the protein, although it may be assumed on the basis of the inactivating mutations identified in the transmembrane segments that the "activating" function of the ligand is exerted at the level of the transmembrane and extracellular aspects of the receptor. Receptor activation involves conformational changes that alter the relationship among transmembrane domains, which cause the acquisition of high affinity for the G protein. Taken together, studies of naturally occurring receptor variants and mutants, as well as man-made mutations, will help elucidate the participation of the intracellular appendages in the interaction of the ADH receptor with G proteins. Furthermore, analysis of mutations that result in diseases may highlight the importance of a particular region of these proteins not yet subjected to thorough experimental scrutiny. A case in point is the R137H mutation, which demonstrates the importance of the amino acid components of the second intracellular loop in receptor–G protein interaction. More data of this type can be expected from the analysis of disease-causing mutant receptors.

REFERENCES

1. Birnbaumer M, Seibold A, Gilbert S, et al. Molecular cloning of the receptor for human antidiuretic hormone. Nature 1992; 357:333–335.
2. Lolait SJ, O'Carroll A-M, McBride OW, et al. Cloning and characterization of a vasopressin V2 receptor and possible link to nephrogenic diabetes insipidus. Nature 1992, 357:336–339.
3. Gorbulev V, Buechner H, Akhundova A, Fahrenholz F. Molecular cloning and functional characterization of V_2 [8-lysine]vasopressin and oxytocin receptors from a pig kidney cell line. Eur J Biochem 1993; 215:1–7.
4. Rosenthal W, Seibold A, Antaramian A, et al. Molecular identification of the gene responsible for congenital nephrogenic diabetes insipidus. Nature 1992; 359:233–235.
5. Pan Y, Metzenberg A, Das S, Gitschier J. Mutations in the V2 vasopressin receptor gene are associated with X-linked nephrogenic diabetes insipidus. Nature Genetics 1992; 2:103–106.
6. Van den Ouweland AMW, Dreesen JCFM, Verdijk M, et al. Mutations in the vasopressin type 2 receptor gene AVPR2 associated with nephrogenic diabetes insipidus. Nature Genet 1992; 2:99–102.
7. Merendino JJ, Spiegel AM, Crawford JD, et al. A mutation in the vasopressin V2 receptor gene in a kindred with X-linked nephrogenic diabetes insipidus. N Engl J Med 1993; 328:1538–1541.
8. Bichet DG, Birnbaumer M, Lonergan M, et al. Nature and recurrence of AVPR2 mutations in X-linked nephrogenic diabetes insipidus. Am J Hum Genet 1994; 55:278–286.
9. Birnbaumer L, Birnbaumer M. Signal transduction by G proteins: functional considerations, primary structures of the components involved, and structure-function relations. In: Shiniztky, ed. Signal Transduction Across Membranes, Vol. 3. of Handbook of Biomembranes, Rehovoth, Israel, Balaban Publishers, 1994.
10. Orloff J, Handler JS. The role of adenosine 3′,5′-phosphate in the action of antidiuretic hormone. Am J Med 1967; 42:757–768.
11. Snyder HM, Noland TD, Breyer MD. cAMP-dependent protein kinase mediates hydrosmotic effect of vasopressin in collecting duct. Am J Physiol 1992; 263:C147–C153.
12. Birnbaumer M, Hinrichs V, Themmen APN. Development and characterization of a mouse cell line expressing the human V2 vasopressin receptor gene. Mol Endocrinol 1990; 4:245–254.
13. Gudermann T, Birnbaumer M, Birnbaumer L. Evidence for dual coupling of the murine luteinizing hormone receptor to adenylyl cyclase and phosphoinositide breakdown and Ca^{2+} mobilization: Studies with the cloned murine luteinizing hormone receptor expressed in L cells. J Biol Chem 1992; 267:4479–4488.
14. Zhu X, Gilbert S, Birnbaumer M, Birnbaumer L. Dual signaling potential is common among G_s-coupled receptors and dependent on receptor density. Mol Pharmacol 1994; 46:460–469.
15. Maguire ME, Van Arsdale PM, Gilman AG. An agonist-specific effect of guanine nucleotides on binding to the beta adrenergic receptor. Mol Pharmacol 1976; 12:335–339.
16. Sugimoto Y, Negishi M, Hayashi Y, et al. Two isoforms of the EP_3 receptor with different carboxyl-terminal domains: Identical ligand binding properties and different coupling properties with G_i proteins. J Biol Chem 1993; 268:2712–2718.
17. Seibold A, Gilbert S, Birnbaumer M. Expression and structure of the murine vasopressin type 2 receptor gene. In preparation.
18. Henderson R, Unwin PNT. Three-dimensional model of purple membrane obtained by electron microscopy. Nature 1975; 257:28–32.
19. Henderson R, Baldwin JM, Ceska TA, et al. Model for the structure of bacteriorhodopsin based in high-resolution electron cryomicroscopy. J Mol Biol 1990; 213:899–929.
20. Schertler GFX, Villa C, Henderson R. Projection structure of rhodopsin. Nature 1993; 362:770–772.
21. Baldwin J. The Probable arrangement of the helices in G-protein coupled receptors. EMBO J 1993; 12:1693–1703.
22. Kennedy ME, Limbird LE. Mutations of the α_{2A}-adrenergic receptor that eliminate detectable palmitoylation do not perturb receptor-G protein coupling. J Biol Chem 1993; 268:8003–8011.
23. Moffett SW, Mouillac B, Bonin H, Bouvier M. Altered phosphorylation and desensitization patterns of a human β_2-adrenergic receptor lacking the palmitoylated Cys341. EMBO J 1993; 12:349–356.
24. Butlen D, Guillon G, Rajerison RM, et al. Structural requirements for activation of vasopressin sensitive adenylate cyclase, hormone binding and antidiuretic action: Effects of highly potent analogues and competitive inhibitors. Mol Pharmacol 1978; 14:1006–1017.

25. Pan Y, Wilson P, Gitschier J. The effect of eight V2 vasopressin receptor mutations on stimulation of adenylyl cyclase and binding to vasopressin. J Biol Chem 1994; 269:31933–31937.
26. Kojro E, Eich P, Gimpl G, Fahrenholz F. Direct identification of an extracellular agonist binding site in the renal V2 vasopressin receptor. Biochemistry 1993; 32:13537–13544.
27. Guillon G, Couraud P-O, Butlen D, et al. Size of vasopressin receptors from rat liver and kidney. Eur J Biochem 1980; 111:287–294.
28. Fahrenholz F, Boer R, Crause P, Toth MV. Photoaffinity labeling of the renal V_2 vasopressin receptor: Identification and enrichment of a vasopressin-binding subunit. Eur J Biochem 1985; 152:589–595.
29. Kennelly PJ, Krebs EG. Consensus sequences as substrate specificity determinants for protein kinases and protein phosphatases. J Biol Chem 1991; 266:15555–15558.
30. Aiyar N, Nambi P, Crooke ST. Phorbol esters induced desensitization of the AVP stimulated adenylate cyclase in MDCK cells. Cell Sign 1990; 2:153–160.
31. Rosenthal W, Antaramian A, Gilbert S, Birnbaumer M. Nephrogenic diabetes insipidus: A V2 vasopressin receptor unable to stimulate adenylyl cyclase. J Biol Chem 1993; 268:13030–13033.
32. Surprenant A, Horstman D, Akbarali H, Limbird LE. A point mutation of cloned α-adrenoceptor that blocks coupling to potassium but not calcium currents. Science 1992; 257:977–980.
33. Horstman D, Brandon S, Wilson AL, et al. An aspartate conserved among G-protein receptors confers allosteric regulation of α_2-adrenergic receptors by sodium. J Biol Chem 1990; 265:21590–21595.
34. Birnbaumer M, Gilbert S, Rosenthal W. An extracellular CNDI mutation of the vasopressin receptor reduces cell surface expression, affinity for ligand and coupling to the G_s/adenylyl cyclase system. Mol Pharmacol 1994; 8:886–894.
35. Birnbaumer M, Antaramian A, Themmen APN, Gilbert S. Desensitization of the human V2 vasopressin receptor: Homologous effects in the absence of heterologous desensitization. J Biol Chem 1992; 267:11783–11788.
36. Kyte J, Doolittle RF. A simple method for displaying the hydropathic character of a protein. J Mol Biol 1982; 157:105–132.

36
Steroid Response Elements

David Pearce
San Francisco General Hospital and University of California, San Francisco, San Francisco, California

INTRODUCTION

Steroid hormones, particularly the mineralocorticoids and glucocorticoids, have profound effects on renal function, yet little is known about their specific mechanisms of action. Many if not all of the kidney's responses to steroids are mediated by nuclear receptors that alter cellular behavior through effects on the transcription rate of specific target genes. The DNA sequences that nuclear receptors act through to regulate transcription are referred to as hormone response elements (HREs). In this chapter the role of HREs in determining the renal response to steroid hormones and the mechanisms underlying HRE activity are reviewed. While the focus is predominantly on the HREs, discussion also necessarily includes the receptors themselves, as it is the interaction between receptors and DNA that determines the specific nature of the hormonal response. General concepts of receptor and HRE function that have been developed in model systems are reviewed first, followed by discussion of regulatory events in the kidney.

STEROID RECEPTOR AND HRE FUNCTION IN MODEL SYSTEMS

Receptors

The steroid receptors comprise the estrogen receptor (ER) and four functionally and structurally closely related receptors: the mineralocorticoid (MR), glucocorticoid (GR), androgen (AR), and progesterone (PR) receptors (1). They are members of the nuclear receptor superfamily which, in addition to the steroid receptors, includes the retinoic acid receptor (RAR), thyroid hormone receptor (TR), vitamin D receptor (VDR), and retinoid X receptor (RXR) as well as other more distantly related proteins, including several *Drosophila* developmental regulators (1). All members of the nuclear receptor superfamily are intracellular proteins that bind hormone and exert transcriptional effects directly (2,3). In some cases the receptors are localized to the nucleus and can have regulatory effects in the absence of hormone, while in others they are cytoplasmic in the absence of hormone and only translocate to the nucleus upon binding hormone, as is shown in Figure 1 for MR and GR, the two receptors most important to renal function. These two closely related proteins share many features in common. In the absence of hormone, they are inactive. Each is held within an aporeceptor complex that includes at least three distinct heat shock proteins; hsp90, hsp70, and hsp56 (4). Upon binding hormone, they undergo a conformational change, dissociate from the aporeceptor complex, translocate to the nucleus, and modulate the activity of target genes. In general, the nuclear receptors can act to increase or decrease the rate of transcription, a process—as discussed below—that involves both protein-DNA and protein-protein interactions.

The nuclear receptors share common structural features, as shown in Figure 2: an N-terminal

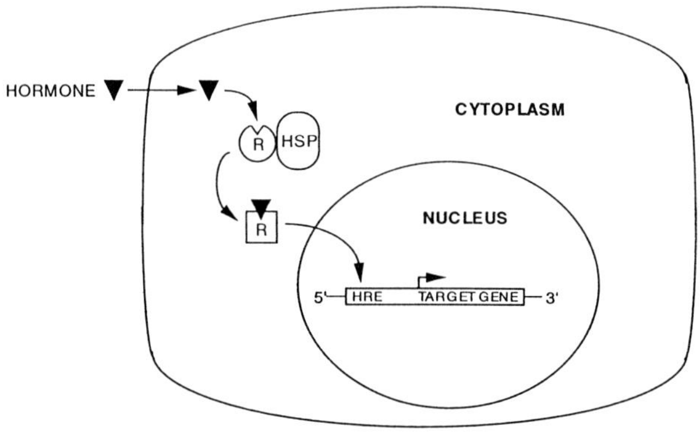

Figure 1 Steroid hormone effects are mediated by intracellular receptors that act directly to modulate transcription. Hormone (black triangle) enters the cell and binds to the aporeceptor complex, composed of a monomer of receptor (R) associated with heat-shock proteins (HSP), including hsp90. The hormone-bound receptor dissociates from the complex and translocates to the nucleus, where it acts at HREs to alter the transcription rate of linked genes.

region of variable length, a centrally located DNA-binding domain, and a C-terminal ligand-binding domain (5). None of the receptors share significant homology in the N-terminal region, which is encoded by a single exon. Significant homology is found in the ligand-binding domain (sometimes referred to as the "signaling" region) of the molecule (Figure 2). The highest degree of homology is found in the DNA-binding domain (DBD); the more closely related members of the family share more than 90% amino acid identity over 60 amino acids. This region has been shown by genetic and biochemical data to be necessary and sufficient for response element recognition and specific DNA binding. Its structure and DNA-binding properties, which constitute the defining characteristic of the nuclear receptor superfamily, are discussed further below.

Hormone Response Elements

The steroid receptors exert their regulatory effects by interacting with specific DNA sequences, the HREs. An HRE was first identified in the long terminal repeat (LTR) of murine mammary tumor virus (MMTV) DNA as a sequence that was specifically bound by the GR and was necessary for the receptor to stimulate transcription (6). Furthermore, it conferred glucocorticoid responsiveness to a heterologous promoter, functioned in either orientation, and its position relative to the transcription start site was flexible. Thus, this site filled the criteria for a hormone-inducible enhancer

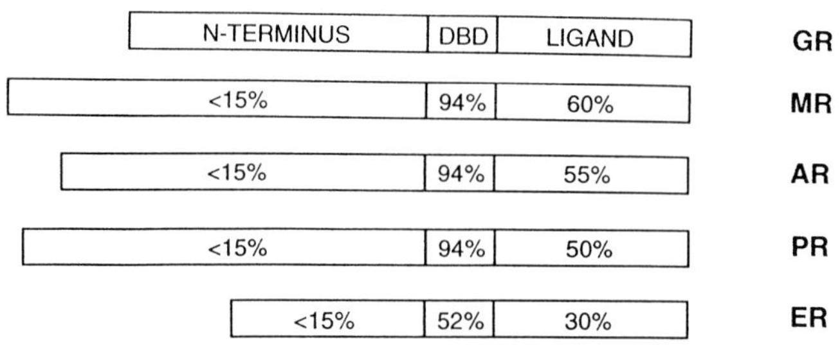

Figure 2 The steroid receptors share common structural features. See text. N terminus: a highly variable region that harbors a potent transcriptional activation domain. DBD: DNA-binding domain—also called zinc finger region to reflect the coordination of two distinct modules by Zn^+ ions (see Figure 5). Ligand: Ligand-binding domain. Homology relative to GR is shown for the different receptor domains.

GRE	AG**AA**CANNNTG**TT**CT TC**TT**GTNNNAC**AA**GA
ERE	AG**GT**CANNNTG**AC**CT TC**CA**GTNNNAC**TG**GA

Figure 3 The simple GRE and ERE are similar. Each is composed of two half-sites separated by three nucleotides. The idealized elements shown, which are based on the consensus sequences, are palindromes. The GRE half-site differs from the ERE half-site at only two out of six positions, shown in bold.

element* (7) and was termed a glucocorticoid response element (GRE). Similar elements were identified linked to other glucocorticoid-responsive genes such as tyrosine amino transferase and metallothionine IIA (see Refs. 2 and 8 for review). Sequence comparison yielded a 15-bp GRE consensus sequence. A distinct but similar "estrogen response element" (ERE) conferred specific estrogen responsiveness to several chicken and mammalian genes, including vitellogenin and lactoferrin (Figure 3 and below) (2,8).

These observations pointed initially to a simple paradigm for receptor action: the hormone-activated receptor binds to DNA sequences in the vicinity of target genes and interacts with the general transcription machinery to stimulate the rate of transcription initiation. According to this view, the HRE serves merely as an attachment site to dock the receptor in the vicinity of the target gene; the receptor's transcriptional activation domains then engage the general transcription factors (9,10), which, in turn, direct the binding of RNA polymerase II. This picture, while appealing and useful, is incomplete for several reasons. First, GR *represses* the transcriptional rate of some target genes, [including the adrenocorticotropic hormone precursor proopiomelanocortin (11) and the genes for the glycoprotein hormones prolactin (12) and proliferin (13)], an effect which is not consistent with this paradigm. Second, other transcriptional regulatory factors have been shown to bind within some HREs in conjunction with the receptors and to exert important modulatory effects (14,15). Finally, HREs have been identified that do not bind receptor; rather, the receptor acts on these elements indirectly (16,17). Thus, in general, HREs are DNA sequences that mediate receptor enhancement *or* repression of transcription; receptor activity at the HRE may require other nonreceptor regulatory factors, and the receptor may even act indirectly, *without* direct receptor DNA-binding.

Three Different Types of Hormone Response Elements

With the above considerations in mind, the HREs can be divided into three distinct classes: (a) "simple HREs" that bind steroid receptors directly, resulting in a stimulatory response, regardless of the effects of other factors bound nearby; (b) "composite HREs" that bind receptors and other protein factors, resulting in either a stimulatory or repressive response depending on the composition of the other factors; and (c) "indirect HRE's" that do not bind receptors, rather, the receptors act through protein-protein interactions with other factors bound at the site. The complete physiological response to a steroid hormone in a particular cell type may involve the coordinate regulation of any of these types of response elements. Below, each of these is discussed in greater detail.

Simple HREs. The role of the simple HRE is to position a dimer of the appropriate receptor in the vicinity of the general transcription machinery. The simple HRE can be found at a variable distance, usually but not always upstream of the transcription start site, as shown in Figure 4. A variety of genetic, biochemical and biophysical studies have contributed to characterizing the response element and to elucidating receptor-DNA interactions at a simple HRE. DNA electrophoretic mobility shift and DNase I footprinting experiments using purified receptor and response elements mutated at specific positions led to identification of the nucleotides critical for receptor binding. The idealized simple GRE and simple ERE are both 15-nucleotide palindromic DNA sequences; a six-bp "half site" is separated by three nucleotides from a second half site (Figure 3). The sequence of the

*Enhancers are DNA sequences that stimulate transcription when physically linked to a gene. Their position relative to the transcription start site is flexible and they can be present in either orientation. Enhancers serve as binding sites for protein factors that interact with the transcription machinery to increase the rate and/or extent of functional initiation complex formation.

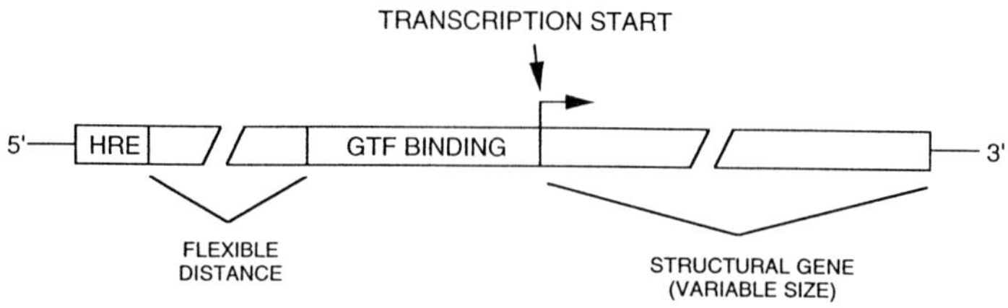

Figure 4 HREs localize steroid receptors to the vicinity of the transcription start site. Binding sites for the receptor (HRE) and the general transcription factors (GTF-binding) are shown. The GTFs include TFIID (the TATA-binding protein and its associated factors), TFIIB, other members of the TFII series, and RNA polymerase II. Steroid receptors, like other transcriptional activators, are thought to enhance transcription by helping to recruit GTFs such as TFIID and TFIIB (9,10).

intervening nucleotides is unimportant; however, the three-nucleotide spacing is required for cooperative binding of a receptor dimer. The ERE and GRE half sites differ at only two of six positions (Figure 3) and, as discussed below, the differences in amino acid–nucleotide interaction that determine the distinct DNA-binding specificities of GR and ER are surprisingly subtle (18).

The receptor features that determine DNA-binding specificity have also been explored extensively. Domain-swap experiments* between ER and GR showed that the first zinc finger of the DBD determines DNA-binding specificity (19). In fact, most of the discrimination is determined by three amino acids at the base of the first zinc finger (Figure 5) (20). The recent determination by x-ray crystallography of the structure of the GR (21) and ER (18) DBDs in complex with their response elements has provided a detailed picture of the protein-DNA interactions that lead to receptor target specificity (Figure 5). An alpha helix, beginning near the base of the first zinc finger, lies along the major groove of the DNA and provides all of the specific base contacts as well as several phosphate backbone contacts. Differential DNA-binding specificity is determined not only by differences in the residues that make specific contacts but, surprisingly, is also dependent on differences in noncontact residues that contribute to positioning of the contact residues (18).

Composite HREs. While specific protein-DNA interactions distinguish ER and GR specificities, this is not the case for distinguishing GR from the more closely related receptors, MR, PR, and AR. All four of these receptors bind to and activate transcription from a simple HRE (22–25). This similarity leads to a paradox: how can these receptors whose DNA-binding specificities are identical achieve differential regulatory effects? It is now apparent that protein-DNA interactions are inadequate for determining specificity; protein-protein interactions between the receptors and other nonreceptor transcriptional regulatory factors play a key role in determining receptor specificity (reviewed in Ref. 25). Accordingly, the role of some HREs is not merely to provide a tethering site for the receptor: composite HREs—response elements of the second type described above—often have a nonconsensus sequence and are bound by the receptor in conjunction with nonreceptor factors with which the receptor interacts (14,15,24,26,27). For example, a 25-bp composite HRE termed plfG binds both GR and members of the AP1 family of transcriptional regulatory factor (14). The AP1 family is made up of several related members, which form dimers through a leucine-rich region termed a "leucine zipper." cJun and cFos, the prototypical members of this family, form heterodimers with each other. Additionally, cJun forms homodimers while cFos does not (28). The behavior of GR at plfG is determined by the composition of AP1 bound to the element. cJun/cFos heterodimers act to stimulate transcription of plfG-linked genes while cJun/cJun homodimers, alone have little effect. Hormone-activated GR represses cJun/cFos–mediated transcription, while, interestingly, it acts synergistically with cJun to stimulate transcription of a plfG-linked gene.

The behavior of MR at plfG is quite different from that of GR. The basal level of transcription

*The domain-swap experiment consists of substituting the coding information for a particular functional domain of one protein with the corresponding information for another. This powerful technique has revealed many of the determinants of specificity in signal transduction molecules.

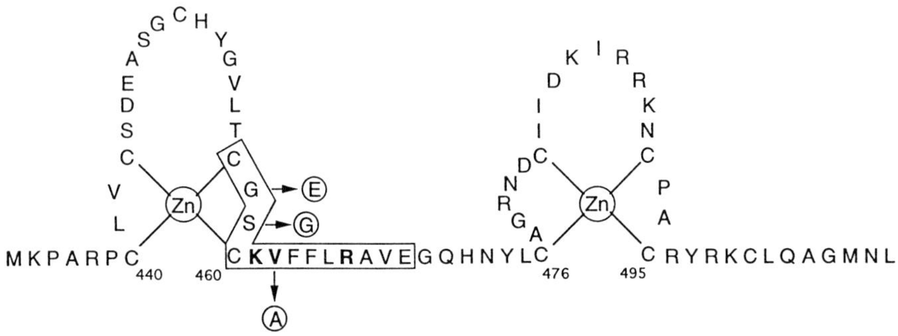

Figure 5 DNA-binding domain (DBD) or zinc-finger region (ZFR) of rat GR. The region of rat GR used for structure determination by x-ray crystallography and DNA-binding studies is shown (21). DNA recognition helix is boxed; residues that contact specific bases are shown in bold; corresponding amino acids of ER critical for response element recognition are circled next to the sequence. Note that residues that make specific base contacts (in bold) and residues that determine ER vs. GR DNA-binding specificity (circled) are not identical. Also note that GR, MR, AR, and PR all share 100% identity in their recognition helices (not shown).

induced by cJun/cFos is specifically repressed by GR through a combination of protein-DNA and protein-protein interactions. Figure 6 portrays a speculative model of the protein-protein and protien-DNA interactions that determine GR repression of AP1 mediated transcription at plfG. AP1 activity is not repressed by MR (27) because it cannot interact with cJun/cFos (although it can bind to the element) (29). Similarly, MR does not synergize with cJun homodimers (25) (not shown in the model).

Indirect HREs. At the third type of element, the indirect HRE, a steroid receptor modulates transcription without binding directly to the DNA. The receptor is believed to repress or activate transcription at this type of element through direct protein-protein interaction with other transcription factor(s) that can bind to the site (16,17,30).

MINERALOCORTICOID AND GLUCOCORTICOID EFFECTS IN THE KIDNEY

In spite of the important role that mineralocorticoids and glucocorticoids play in regulating renal function, the specific molecular mechanisms underlying MR, GR, and HRE function in the kidney are not well understood. The information and paradigms of receptor and HRE action that are described above can serve as a road map for identifying the mechanisms operating to achieve steroid responses in renal cells. In the following sections, some examples of mineralocorticoid and glucocorticoid effects and the target genes that mediate these effects are considered. Only a few of the target genes have been identified and in most cases the response elements have yet to be localized. A full understanding of the mechanisms underlying responses to steroids will require analysis of the response elements as well as isolation and characterization of the factors that the receptors interact with in achieving their transcriptional effects.

Mineralocorticoid Effects on Ion Transport in the Collecting Tubule

The effects of mineralocorticoids on ion transport in the collecting tubule have been studied extensively in a number of systems, including isolated perfused tubules, toad bladder preparations, and cultured cells (31). Sodium and potassium ion transport are stimulated and the activities of Na,K-ATPase, citrate synthase, and sodium channels are all increased. Inhibitor studies using cycloheximide and actinomycin D indicate a requirement for new protein synthesis and changes in transcription (32–34), respectively, and aldosterone stimulation of specific (as yet unidentified)

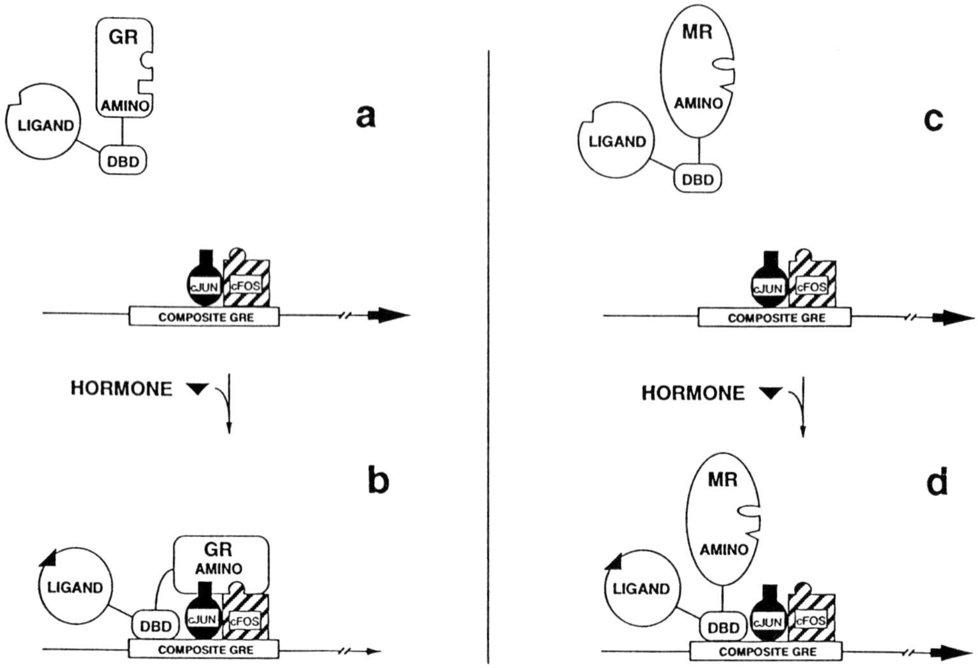

Figure 6 MR and GR behave differently at a composite HRE. Activity of a gene linked to a composite GRE in the presence of cJun, cFos, and either MR or GR is shown: in the absence of hormone a cJun/cFos heterodimer (AP1) stimulates a high level of transcription, represented by the large arrows (a and c). In a cell that expresses GR, this activity is repressed (small arrow) in a hormone-dependent fashion (b). Note that GR repression is envisioned as occurring through cooccupancy of receptor and AP1; receptor acts to block the transcriptional activation function of AP1 through direct protein-protein interaction. MR, while able to bind to the element, is not able to interact with AP1 and thus does not block its transcriptional activity (d). This type of specificity probably contributes to the distinct effects of mineralocorticoids and glucocorticoids in some target tissues.

peptides (termed "aldosterone-induced proteins") has been demonstrated by two-dimensional gel electrophoresis using ^{35}S labeled proteins from cultured cells (35). In the case of the alpha and beta subunits of the Na,K-ATPase, a direct effect of mineralocorticoids on the rate of transcription has been demonstrated using nuclear run-on assays in cultured toad kidney cells (36). Furthermore, the 5′-flanking region of the rat and human alpha subunit has a consensus "GRE," but its function has not been tested (37). Less is known about other candidate mineralocorticoid-responsive genes, which include the recently cloned alpha subunit of the epithelial sodium channel (38), the epithelial potassium channel (39), and enzymes of intermediary metabolism such as citrate synthase (40). At this time it is not clear whether MR and GR mediate distinct or disparate responses in collecting tubule cells (41,42).

Glucocorticoid Effects on Na/H Exchange in the Proximal Tubule

Glucocorticoids but not mineralocorticoids stimulate the V_{max} of proximal tubule brush border membrane Na/H exchange, an effect consistent with an increase in Na/H exchanger number in the membrane (43). There are at least four different isoforms of the Na/H exchanger (NHE1–4), at least two of which have been identified in renal cortex (44,45). mRNA levels of NHE1 have been shown to increase with metabolic acidosis (46), an effect that may be influenced or mediated by glucocorticoids (47). Glucocorticoid stimulation of NHE3 mRNA also has been reported in rat ileum (48) but not kidney. The 5′-flanking region of NHE1 has been cloned and sequenced and four partial

GREs have been identified (on the basis of sequence) (49), but functional studies have not been reported. One or more of these "partial GREs" may form part of a composite response element. Thus, it is likely that GR regulates the transcription of at least two isoforms of NHE, but, the underlying mechanisms remain unknown.

PEPCK

PEPCK controls the rate-limiting step in gluconeogenesis (50). Its activity is crucial in both kidney and liver, although it plays different roles in the two tissues. Not surprisingly, it is differentially regulated. For example, in the kidney but not the liver, extracellular pH strongly stimulates PEPCK expression (51). In both tissues, glucocorticoids but not mineralocorticoids stimulate PEPCK transcription and raise mRNA levels greater than fourfold (15,50,52). The mechanisms that control glucocorticoid effects on PEPCK expression in liver have been studied extensively (15). A complex glucocorticoid response unit (GRU) has been identified that mediates the stimulatory effects of glucocorticoids, glucagon, and retinoic acid as well as the inhibitory effects of insulin. Less is known about the regulation of PEPCK in the kidney. Renal PEPCK responds briskly to glucocorticoid treatment as well as decreased pH and is repressed by glucose administration. As in the liver, the regulation is complex; for example, the repression by glucose is not seen in the presence of acidosis (51). It is likely that a GRU similar to the one acting in the liver (perhaps the same GRU differentially employed) integrates multiple regulatory inputs in the kidney as well.

The Roles of Other Steroid Receptors

Other steroid receptors, including AR and ER, have been shown to have effects on renal development and function. However, their effects on renal physiological responses are relatively minor and are not further considered here.

CONCLUSIONS

The last decade has witnessed an enormous expansion in our understanding of the molecular mechanisms underlying steroid hormone receptor and HRE activities. A number of response elements have been identified and nucleotides important for receptor binding have been pinpointed; some of the regulatory factors that modify receptor transcriptional effects have been characterized, and high-resolution crystal structures of two receptors with their response elements have been solved. Understanding the nature of the protein-protein and protein-DNA interactions that mediate renal responses to steroids in general, and mineralocorticoids and glucocorticoids in particular, will require identification of the target genes and HREs involved as well as characterization of the nonreceptor regulatory factors that influence the tissue-specific regulatory responses.

ACKNOWLEDGMENTS

Natasha Kralli is gratefully acknowledged for helpful comments on the manuscript. Bonnie Maler, Keith Yamamoto, and members of the Yamamoto laboratory provided much support and guidance during the course of my work in the lab.

REFERENCES

1. Amero SA, Kretsinger RH, Moncrief ND, et al. The origin of nuclear receptor proteins: A single precursor distinct from other transcription factors. Mol Endocrinol 1992; 6:3–7.
2. Beato M. Gene regulation by steroid hormones. Cell 1989; 56:335–344.
3. Yamamoto KR. Steroid receptor regulated transcription of specific genes and gene networks. Annu Rev Genet 1985; 19:209–252.
4. Pratt WB. The role of heat shock proteins in regulating the function, folding, and trafficking of the glucocorticoid receptor. J Biol Chem 1993; 268:21455–21458.
5. Evans RM. The steroid and thyroid hormone receptor superfamily. Science 1988; 240:889–895.

6. Chandler VL, Maler BA, Yamamoto KR. DNA sequences bound specifically by glucocorticoid receptor in vitro render a heterologous promoter hormone responsive in vivo. Cell 1983; 33:489–499.
7. de Villiers J, Olson L, Banerji J, Schaffner W. Analysis of the transcriptional enhancer effect. Cold Spring Harbor Symp Quant Biol 1983; 2:911–919.
8. Freedman LP, Luisi BF. On the mechanism of DNA binding by nuclear hormone receptors: A structural and functional perspective. J Cell Biochem 1993; 51:140–150.
9. Ing NH, Beekman JM, Tsai SY, et al. Members of the steroid hormone receptor superfamily interact with TFIIB (S300-II). J Biol Chem. 1992; 267:17617–17623.
10. Choy B, Green MR. Eukaryotic activators function during multiple steps or prinitiation complex assembly. Nature 1993; 366: 531–536.
11. Charron J, Drouin J. Glucocorticoid inhibition of transcription from episomal proopiomelanocortin gene promoter. Proc Natl Acad Sci USA 1986; 83:8903–8907.
12. Sakai DD, Helms S, Carlstedt DJ, et al. Hormone-mediated repression: a negative glucocorticoid response element from the bovine prolactin gene. Genes Dev 1988; 2:1144–1154.
13. Mordacq JC, Linzer DI. Co-localization of elements required for phorbol ester stimulation and glucocorticoid repression of proliferin gene expression. Genes Dev 1989; 3:760–769.
14. Diamond MI, Miner JN, Yoshinaga SK, Yamamoto KR. Transcription factor interactions: Selectors of positive or negative regulation from a single DNA element. Science 1990; 249:1266–1272.
15. Granner D, O'Brien R, Imai E, et al. Complex hormone response unit regulating transcription of the phosphoenolpyruvate carboxykinase gene: From metabolic pathways to molecular biology. Recent Prog Horm Res 1991; 47:319–346; discussion, 346–348.
16. Konig H, Ponta H, Rahmsdorf HJ, Herrlich P. Interference between pathway-specific transcription factors: Glucocorticoids antagonize phorbol ester-induced AP-1 activity without altering AP-1 site occupation in vivo. EMBO J 1992; 11:2241–2246.
17. Gaub MP, Bellard M, Scheuer I, et al. Activation of the ovalbumin gene by the estrogen receptor involves the fos-jun complex. Cell 1990; 63:1267–1276.
18. Schwabe JWR, Chapman L, Finch JT, Rhodes D. The crystal structure of the estrogen receptor DNA-binding domain bound to DNA: How receptors discriminate between their response elements. Cell 1993; 75:567–578.
19. Green S, Kumar V, Theulaz I, et al. The N-terminal DNA-binding "zinc finger" of the oestrogen and glucocorticoid receptors determines target gene specificity. Embo J 1988; 7:3037–3044.
20. Mader S, Kumar V, de VH, Chambon P. Three amino acids of the oestrogen receptor are essential to its ability to distinguish an oestrogen from a glucocorticoid-responsive element. Nature 1989; 338:271–274.
21. Luisi BF, Xu WX, Otwinowski Z, et al. Crystallographic analysis of the interaction of the glucocorticoid receptor with DNA [see comments]. Nature 1991; 352:497–505.
22. Tsai MJ, Tsai SY, Klein HL, et al. Cooperative interactions of steroid hormone receptors with their cognate response elements. Cold Spring Harbor Symp Quant Biol 1988; 2:829–833.
23. Govindan MV, Leclerc S, Roy R, et al. Differential regulation of mouse mammary tumor virus-bacterial chloramphenical acetyltransferase chimeric gene by human mineralocorticoid hormone-receptor complexes. J Steroid Biochem Mol Biol 1991; 39:91–103.
24. Adler AJ, Danielsen M, Robins DM. Androgen-specific gene activation via a consensus glucocorticoid response element is determined by interaction with nonreceptor factors. Proc Nat Acad Sci USA 1992; 89:11660–11663.
25. Pearce D. A mechanistic basis for distinct mineralocorticoid and glucocorticoid receptor transcriptional specificities. Steroids 1994; 59:153–159.
26. Zhang XK, Dong JM, Chiu JF. Regulation of alpha-fetoprotein gene expression by antagonism between AP-1 and the glucocorticoid receptor at their overlapping binding site. J Biol Chem 1991; 266:8248–8254.
27. Pearce D, Yamamoto KR. Mineralocorticoid and glucocorticoid receptor activities distinguished by nonreceptor factors at a composite response element. Science 1993; 259:1161–1165.
28. Abate C, Curran T. Encounters with Fos and Jun on the road to AP-1. Semin Cancer Biol 1990; 1:19–26.
29. Yamamoto KR, Pearce D, Thomas J, Miner JN. Combinational Regulation at a Mammalian Composite Response Element. Cold Spring Harbor, NY: Cold Spring Harbor Press 1992:1169–1192.
30. Jonat C, Rahmsdorf HJ, Park KK, et al. Antitumor promotion and aniinflammation: Down-modulation of AP-1 (Fos/Jun) activity by glucocorticoid hormone. Cell 1990; 62:1189–1204.
31. Marver D. Aldosterone. Methods Enzymol 1990; 191:520–550.
32. Horisberger JD, Diezi J. Inhibition of aldosterone-induced antinatriuresis and kaliuresis by actinomycin D. Am J Physiol 1984; 246:F201–204.
33. Asher C, Garty H. Aldosterone increases the apical Na+ permeability of toad bladder by two different mechanisms. Proc Natl Acad Sci USA 1988; 85:7413–7417.
34. Girardet M, Geering K, Gaeggeler HP, Rossier BC. Control of transepithelial Na+ transport and Na-K-ATPase by oxytocin and aldosterone. Am J Physiol 1986; 251: F662–F670.

35. Szerlip HM, Weisberg L, Geering K, et al. Aldosterone-induced glycoproteins: Electrophysiological-biochemical correlation. Biochim Biophys Acta 1988; 940:1–9.
36. Verrey F, Kraehenbuhl JP, Rossier BC. Aldosterone induces a rapid increase in the rate of Na,K-ATPase gene transcription in cultured kidney cells. Mol Endocrinol 1989; 3:1369–1376.
37. Pathak BG, Pugh DG, Lingrel JB. Characterization of the 5′-flanking region of the human and rat Na,K-ATPase alpha 3 gene. Genomics 1990; 8:641–647.
38. Canessa CM, Horisberger JD, Rossier BC. Epithelial sodium channel related to proteins involved in neurodegeneration. Nature 1993; 361:467–470.
39. Desir GV, Hamlin HA, Puente E, et al. Isolation of putative voltage-gated epithelial K-channel isoforms from rabbit kidney and LLC-PK1 cells. Am J Physiol 1992; 262:F151–F157.
40. Minuth WW, Struck M, Zwanzig M, Gross P. Action of aldosterone on citrate synthase in cultured renal collecting duct cells. Renal Physiol Biochem 1989; 12:85–95.
41. Naray-Fejes-Toth A, Fejes TG. Glucocorticoid receptors mediate mineralocorticoid-like effects in cultured collecting duct cells. Am J Physiol 1990; 259:F672–F678.
42. Laplace JR, Husted RF, Stokes JB. Cellular responses to steroids in the enhancement of Na transport by rat collecting duct cells in culture: Differences between glucocorticoid and mineralocorticoid hormones. J Clin Invest 1992; 90:1370–1378.
43. Kinsella JL, Freiberg JM, Sacktor B. Glucocorticoid activation of Na+/H+ exchange in renal brush border vesicles: kinetic effects. Am J Physiol 1985; 248:F233–F239.
44. Tse M, Levine S, Yun C, et al. Structure/function studies of the epithelial isoforms of the mammalian Na+/H+ exchanger gene family. J Membr Biol 1993; 135:93–108.
45. Sardet C, Franchi A, Pouyssegur J. Molecular cloning, primary structure, and expression of the human growth factor-activatable Na+/H+ antiporter. Cell 1989; 56:271–280.
46. Krapf R, Pearce D, Lynch C, et al. Expression of rat renal Na/H antiporter mRNA levels in response to respiratory and metabolic acidosis. J Clin Invest 1991; 87:747–751.
47. Kinsella J, Cujdik T, Sacktor B. Na+-H+ exchange activity in renal brush border membrane vesicles in response to metabolic acidosis: The role of glucocorticoids. Proc Natl Acad Sci USA 1984; 81:630–634.
48. Yun CH, Gurubhagavatula S, Levine SA et al. Glucocorticoid stimulation of ileal Na+ absorptive cell brush border Na+/H+ exchange and association with an increase in message for NHE-3, an epithelial Na+/H+ exchanger isoform. J Biol Chem 1993; 268:206–211.
49. Miller RT, Counillon L, Pages G, et al. Structure of the 5′-flanking regulatory region and gene for the human growth factor-activatable Na/H exchanger NHE-1. J Biol Chem 1991; 266:10813–10819.
50. Felig P, Baxter JD, Broadus AE, Frohman LA. Endocrinology and Metabolism, 2d ed. New York: McGraw-Hill, 1987.
51. Pollock AS. Induction of renal phosphoenolpyruvate carboxykinase mRNA: Suppressive effect of glucose. Am J Physiol 1989; 257:F145–151.
52. Pollock AS, Long JA. The 5′region of the rat phosphoenolpyruvate carboxykinase gene confers pH sensitivity to chimeric genes expressed in renal and liver cell lines capable of expressing PEPCK. Biochem Biophys Res Commun 1989; 164:81–81.

37

Transcription Factors in Kidney Development and Renal Injury

Ralph Witzgall and Joseph V. Bonventre

Harvard Medical School, Massachusetts Institute of Technology, and Massachusetts General Hospital, Boston, Massachusetts

INTRODUCTION

The kidney is a very heterogeneous organ with many types of cells having different phenotypic characteristics. This complexity can be traced, at least in part, to the differential activation of various genes, resulting in the expression of some proteins primarily in the kidney. The expression of kidney-specific proteins may be determined either by kidney-specific transcription factors or by transcription factors that are expressed in more than one organ but whose coordinated expression may be unique to the kidney. Examples of proteins that are expressed predominantly or exclusively in the kidney include the V2 vasopressin receptor (1,2) a chloride channel (3), and a Na/P_i cotransporter (4). Other proteins, though not specific to the kidney, are expressed during specific times in renal development and repair and contribute to the renal phenotype. Many transcriptional regulatory proteins are synthesized in a limited number of cell types. Kid-1 (see below) is an example of such a protein whose expression occurs predominantly in the kidney (5), as is HFH-3, a member of the hepatocyte nuclear factor 3/forkhead DNA-binding-domain family (6). Transcription factors are essential for the control of renal development and differentiation. In addition, they are likely important for the regulation of processes involved in repair of the kidney after an injury. Kidney injury and repair recapitulate many aspects of development, since they involve dedifferentiation and regeneration of epithelial cells followed by differentiation (7–10). The ability to regenerate epithelial structure and restore differentiated function after an ischemic or toxic insult is an important property of the kidney, an ability not possessed by heart and brain, where myocytes or neurons cannot be replaced.

TRANSCRIPTION

The regulation of transcription in eukaryotes is much more complex and less well understood than the relatively simple switch mechanisms of prokaryotes (11). An initial step in the activation of any gene is the interaction of a set of proteins (*trans*-acting elements, or transcription factors) with "regulatory" elements in the gene (*cis*-acting elements), resulting in the initiation of a sequence of events that leads to an increase in the cellular levels of mRNA and ultimately the protein encoded by that gene (Figure 1). The proteins involved in this process must recognize DNA or recognize other proteins in a regulatory region of DNA. Interactions between these proteins and the DNA can occur within a few hundred base pairs or much further away from the site in the gene where transcription starts (the "transcriptional start site"). The more proximal region upstream of the start site is termed the "promoter" region. More distal *cis*-acting elements are referred to as "enhancers." The promoter region of most genes contains a region rich in A-T base pairs, the so-called TATA

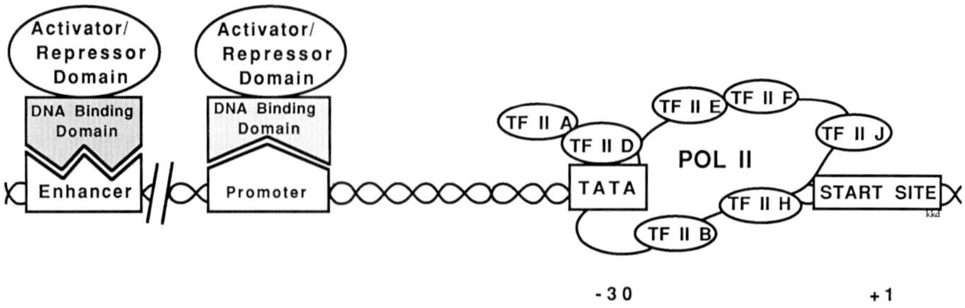

Figure 1 *Cis*- and *trans*-acting elements in the regulatory region of a gene. DNA binding proteins (the *trans*-acting components in the regulatory machinery) typically possess a DNA-binding domain and a *trans*-acting domain, which can have activator or repressor function or both. The specific DNA-binding proteins bind at particular sites in the regulatory region of the gene, the *cis*-acting elements, which can be very close ("promoter") or at a far distance ("enhancer") from the transcriptional start site. The transcriptional start site is defined as the nucleotide in the DNA that is complementary to the first nucleotide in the mRNA. After the specific transcription factors have bound to the DNA, they interact with the basal transcription factors (TFIIA, B, D, E, F, H, J) and promote their assembly together with RNA poymerase II over the TATA box. The TATA box (typically a nucleotide sequence of "TATAAA" or "TATATA") is recognized by the "TATA binding protein (TBP)," which together with the "TBP-associated factors (TAFs)" constitutes TFIID. Subsequent to the binding of TFIID, the other basal transcription factors and RNA polymerase II assemble and transcription can begin.

box, located approximately 30 bp upstream from the transcriptional start site. Transcription factors that activate gene expression, and some that serve as repressors, have two functionally distinct domains: a DNA binding domain and a *trans*-acting domain (11). Protein-DNA interactions occur via the DNA binding domain, which positions the protein on the DNA so that the *trans*-acting part of the protein can interact with other proteins such as those being assembled at the site of the TATA box (the "basal transcription factors"). The fact that DNA can fold allows for the interaction of a transcription factor that binds to DNA many kilobases upstream from the TATA box with proteins close to the site of initiation of transcription and hence allows for regulation from great distances. Other explanations for long-range interactions include the assembly of several proteins spanning the region between the distant *cis*-acting element and the transcriptional start site as well as alterations in the structural properties of the DNA.

Transcription factors can be classified into two groups. One group, general or basal transcription factors, is necessary and sufficient, at least in vitro, for transcription from a TATA box. The second group of transcription factors act only at certain promoters. It is this second type of transcription factor that is discussed in greater detail in this chapter.

STRUCTURAL MOTIFS OF EUCARYOTIC TRANSCRIPTION FACTORS

The DNA-binding regions of many eukaryotic transcription factors are built from a limited number of motifs. Many, but not all, transcription factors are members of three families: zinc-finger, leucine-zipper, and helix-turn-helix proteins. Whereas the zinc-finger and helix-turn-helix motifs are DNA-binding motifs, the leucine zipper is a domain involved in protein-protein interactions.

Zinc-Finger Proteins

The analysis of the amino acid sequence of *Xenopus laevis* TFIIIA, an abundant protein that regulates transcription of the gene for ribosomal 5S RNA, led Klug to postulate that the zinc-finger (Figures 2 and 3) represented a DNA-binding motif (12). TFIIIA has nine repeats of 30 amino acids each with two cysteine residues at one end and two histidine residues at the other. The last histidine

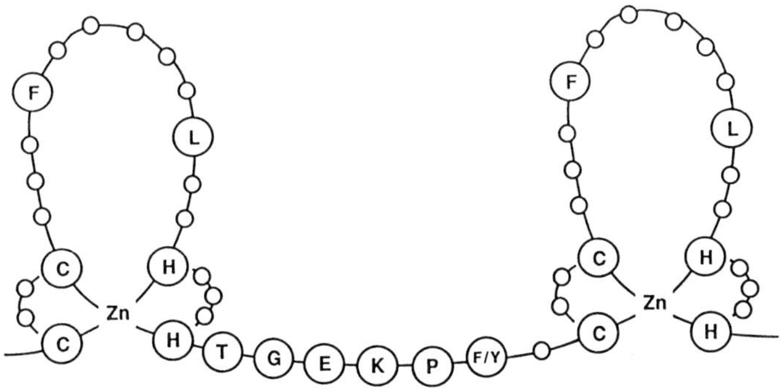

Figure 2 Schematic diagram of a zinc-finger protein of the C_2H_2 family. The members of the C_2H_2 family of zinc-finger proteins are characterized by two cysteines and two histidines, which coordinate a zinc ion at the base of a finger-like structure ("zinc finger"). "F" (phenylalanine) and "L" (leucine) are highly conserved residues in many of these proteins. The zinc finger itself constitutes the DNA-binding domain. Between the individual finger domains, immediately following the second histidine, a highly conserved structure can be found. This so-called "H/C-link" has the sequence "TGEKP(Y or F)." The function of this linker region is not fully understood.

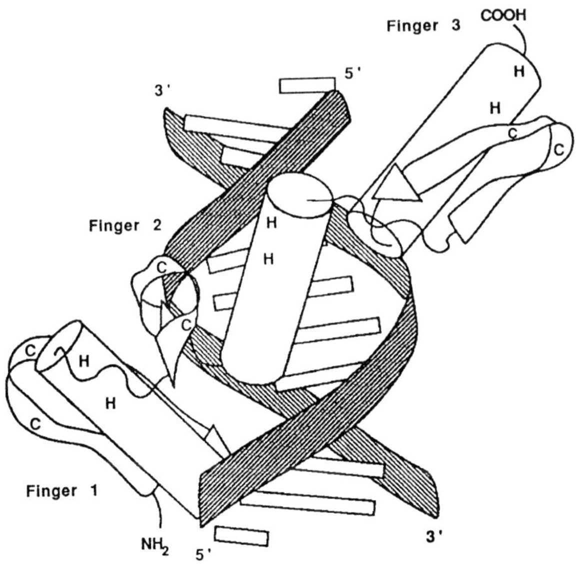

Figure 3 One model for the recognition of DNA by C_2H_2 zinc-finger proteins. The structure of a C_2H_2 zinc-finger/DNA complex was solved for the first time by the analysis of a cocrystal between the three zinc fingers of zif268/Egr-1 and their recognition sequence (92). A model was derived in which each individual finger is folded in a very similar fashion. The NH_2-terminal part of a finger consists of a two-stranded antiparallel beta sheet (depicted as ribbons) and is followed by an alpha helix (shown as a cylinder). The approximate positions of the two cysteines and two histidines in each zinc finger are shown. In the case of zif268/Egr-1, amino acids in all three zinc fingers make contacts in the major groove of the DNA. Analyses of two other crystal structures, however, indicate that alternative models are required to explain the interaction between C_2H_2 zinc fingers and DNA. (From Ref. 92.)

residue and the first cysteine residue of the next repeat are often separated by a highly conserved region of 12 amino acids. Since the protein contained zinc and the zinc was critical to the transcriptional control function of the protein, Klug proposed that the cysteines and histidines were complexed together by zinc and that the intervening amino acids then formed a finger-like structure which would fit into the major groove of the DNA double helix.

Since the original description of this motif, a very large number of proteins containing it have been identified. The number of repeats varies a great deal among this group of proteins. These Cys_2-His_2 proteins have been joined by other families of zinc-finger proteins, such as the Cys_2-Cys_2 family and the Cys-X_2-Cys-X_6-Cys-X_6-Cys-X_2-Cys-X_6-Cys family (where X is any amino acid). The glucocorticoid, thyroid hormone, retinoic acid, vitamin D_3, progesterone, estrogen, and mineralocorticoid receptors belong to the Cys_2-Cys_2 family. GAL 4 is an example of a member of the third zinc-finger family. This protein from *Saccharomyces cerevisiae* is necessary for transcription of genes encoding galactose-metabolizing enzymes. In this family, it is proposed that the six cysteine residues are held together in a cluster by zinc.

Leucine-Zipper Proteins

The leucine zipper motif was first recognized in the yeast transcription factor GCN 4, which activates transcription of the *his*3 gene (13). This motif is also found in C/EBP, fos, jun, and myc. In each of these proteins there is a region of approximately 30 amino acids where each seventh amino acid is a leucine. The leucines form a ridge on one side of an α-helix, so that the leucines from two α-helices can interact with each other. The leucines are apposed to each other, rather than interacting in a zipper-like fashion as had been originally thought. The leucine zipper therefore represents a dimerization domain (Figure 4). Dimerization is necessary for transcription factor function. A number of proteins that have this structural motif, such as GCN 4, fos, and jun, have been shown to form homo- and heterodimers with this region mediating the dimerization. The DNA-binding region of the proteins is a basic domain amino terminal to the leucine zipper.

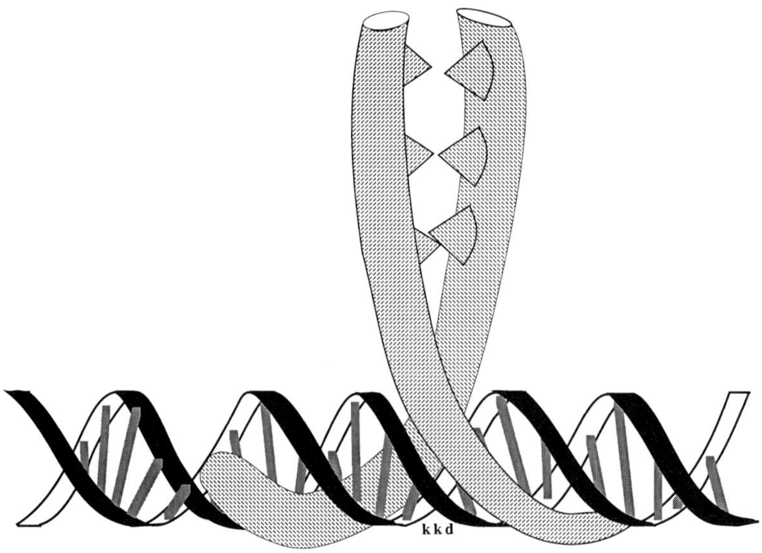

Figure 4 Leucine-zipper proteins bind to DNA as dimers. In leucine-zipper proteins, another common class of transcriptional regulatory factors, the heptad repeats of leucines (depicted as spikes in this schematic diagram) are arranged on one side of an alpha helix and serve as dimerization motifs. The term "leucine zipper" is misleading, because the leucine zipper domains from two proteins do not interdigitate but rather lie adjacent to each other. The basic domain in each protein contacts its recognition site by interacting with the DNA in the major groove. Efficient binding to the DNA requires bending of the protein and as a consequence the dimer assumes a Y-shaped structure. (Adapted from Ref. 94.)

Helix-Turn-Helix Proteins

This is a common motif in transcriptional activators and repressors in prokaryotes, where it was first described (14). Many of the proteins in this family regulate cell-specific transcription. The DNA-binding region consists of two α helices separated by a β turn. In eukaryotes the helix-turn-helix motif is used in "homeodomain" proteins. The homeodomain is a region of 60 amino acids, consisting of three α helices held together by short linker regions of amino acids. While prokaryotic helix-turn-helix proteins bind to DNA as dimers, eucaryotic homeodomain proteins bind DNA as monomers (Figure 5). These proteins are particularly important for eukaryotic development, since it has been found that the genes are tightly regulated during development and are capable of "homeotic" transformations where one structure is transformed into another (e.g., in the case of antennapedia, the transformation of antennae into an additional pair of legs).

Space constraints prevent a more detailed overview of the properties of eukaryotic transcriptional regulation. The reader is referred to various books and reviews that discuss the general aspects of the structure of transcription factors and what is known about how they interact with DNA (14–19).

RENAL DEVELOPMENT

Kidney development proceeds in three stages from the pronephros to the mesonephros and finally the metanephros. The first two stages are transitory but necessary stages in the ultimate development of the mammalian kidney, which is derived from the metanephros. At approximately the end of the second gestational week in the mouse and rat, the first steps of metanephrogenesis occur. The kidney is remarkable in that many of its epithelial structures (proximal tubules, thin limbs of Henle, and distal tubules) originate from mesenchymal precursors. The collecting duct system derives from the ureter, which invades the metanephric blastema mesenchymal cells and undergoes consecutive branching. The buds of the ureter branches interact in a very close fashion with the loose metanephrogenic mesenchyme, first resulting in an aggregation of the mesenchymal cells around

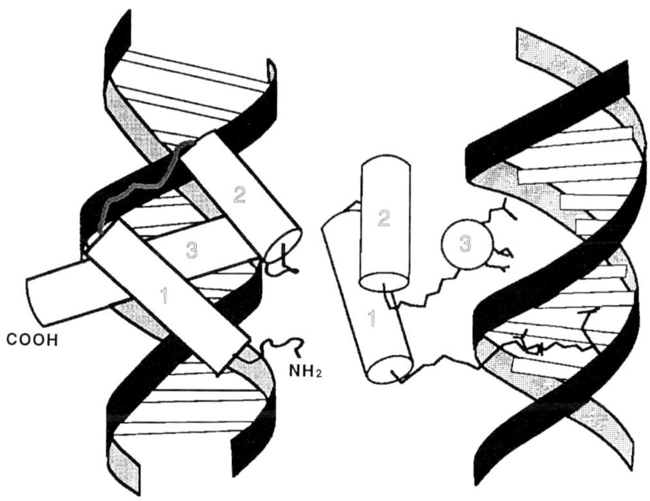

Figure 5 Interaction between a eukaryotic helix-turn-helix protein and DNA. The schematic diagram is derived from the structural analysis of a eukaryotic helix-turn-helix motif, in this case the homeodomain of the engrailed protein, and its recognition site (93). The right-hand side of the figure represents a 90° rotation of the diagram on the left. Helices 2 and 3 (shown as barrels) are separated by a beta turn and together form the conserved helix-turn-helix motif. Whereas in prokaryotes helix-turn-helix proteins bind to DNA as dimers, eukaryotic members of this family interact with DNA as monomers. Contact points are established by residues NH_2-terminal to the first helix, which reach into the minor groove of DNA, and by amino acids in the third helix, which make contact in the major groove. (From Ref. 93.)

the buds. The condensed mesenchyme undergoes several dramatic morphological changes into comma- and S-shaped bodies, a lumen forms in the cell mass, a basement membrane is established, and blood vessels grow into the proximal portion of the prospective nephron. The tubular structures will fuse at their distal ends with the collecting ducts. A continuous lumen develops, and a fully (but not terminally) differentiated nephron forms. In the rat, S-shaped bodies can be found until 4 to 5 days after birth (20), and thymidine incorporation, used as an indicator for cell proliferation, does not decline to baseline levels until 2 to 4 weeks after birth (21,22). By contrast, in humans, kidney development is complete by the time of birth. The morphological sequence of events that occurs in the developing kidney has been described in great detail. (For excellent reviews on this subject see, Refs. 23 and 24.)

Differentiation of the metanephric blastema cells into epithelial cells is a critical event in kidney morphogenesis. What makes an epithelial cell distinct from a mesenchymal cell has to lie to some extent in the induction of specific genes that will confer the phenotype. An approach to the understanding of this process is to know the genes that are induced with this transition from mesenchyme to epithelium and then trace back which *trans*-acting factors control the activation of those genes. Some of these *trans*-acting factors are likely to be "kidney-specific."

Which Genes Are Induced with Renal Development?

The dramatic morphological changes that occur as the kidney forms into a complex heterogenous structure have to be accompanied by similarly drastic changes in the genetic program of the differentiating cells. A basement membrane has to be formed, the apical surface of the newly formed epithelium has to be demarcated by different kinds of junctions, and a brush border will appear in the proximal tubule. The different tubular segments must be invested with different permeability and transport characteristics to electrolytes, water, and urea (25). In recent years evidence has accumulated for the activation and repression of certain genes that have been implicated in the transition from the mesenchymal precursor cells to the fully developed nephron. These genes encode proteins belonging to a wide variety of different families, such as extracellular matrix proteins, integral membrane proteins, cytoskeletal proteins, and nuclear proteins. Early in kidney development, cells express collagen I and III (26) as extracellular matrix proteins, N-CAM (27), syndecan (28,29), and α_1- and α_4-integrins (30) as cell surface proteins and vimentin as an intermediate filament-type cytoskeletal protein (31,32). In the differentiated tubular cells, those proteins will disappear and new proteins will emerge. The tubular epithelium now expresses collagen IV (26) and laminin A (33) as building blocks of the basement membrane; uvomorulin/E-cadherin (27); α_2-, α_3-, and α_6-integrins, which substitute for N-CAM; and α_1- and α_4-integrins (30). Vimentin is replaced by cytokeratins (31,32), and new enzymes [alkaline phosphatase, g-glutamyltransferase (21)]. Transporters such as the P-glycoprotein (34) and glucose transporters (35), and different junctional components [desmosomal as well as gap junction proteins (36,37)] are synthesized so that the renal epithelia can fulfill their characteristic functions.

The signals responsible for these changes in the genetic program have been poorly defined. TGF-α (38) and the receptor for IGF-I (39) have been shown to be necessary for metanephric development in vitro. Hepatocyte growth factor and its receptor, the c-met tyrosine kinase, are expressed transiently during metanephric development and may be of importance (40–42). (For a review on the role of growth factors in renal development see Ref. 43.) How changes in the genetic program(s) occur is not clear at present, because the *trans*-acting factors regulating the structural genes in general and how they are modulated during renal development in particular are largely unknown. This review attempts to describe different transcription factors and their potential role in the kidney. Among the genes we discuss are the *myc* family of protooncogenes, the paired box genes *Pax2* and *Pax8*, the genes encoding the homeodomain proteins LFB1 and LFB3, and the zinc finger genes *Kid-1* and *WT-1*. Other DNA-binding proteins of interest that will not be discussed further in this chapter are Hox-3.2, a homeodomain protein (44,45), and MFH-1 (46) and HFH-3 (6), two members of the HNF-3 family (also see below). Another protein that may be important for renal development but for which there is little information at present is δEF1. This transcription factor has both zinc fingers and a homeodomain. In the mesonephros δEF1 is expressed briefly. It is expressed again to a strong level in the condensed mesenchyme and early metanephric tubules, but tubule structures cease the expression of δEF1 after the tubule structures mature to the point where they connect to the Wolffian duct (47). Since entire chapters in this book are devoted to the Pax family of transcription factors and WT-1, these proteins are discussed only briefly.

THE *myc* FAMILY OF PROTOONCOGENES

The first member of the *myc* family of nuclear protoonocogenes to be isolated was c-*myc*. It represents the cellular homologue of the transforming sequence in the avian myelocytomatosis virus (AMV). Subsequently, two other members were identified in neuroblastomas and small cell lung carcinomas, N-*myc* and L-*myc*, respectively. The products of the three full-length members of the *myc* gene family—c-*myc*, L-*myc*, and N-*myc*—are among the most thoroughly investigated nuclear protooncogenes (besides those three genes, two other truncated *myc* genes have been cloned, B-*myc* and S-*myc*). (For reviews, see Refs. 48 and 49.) They can be classified as basic helix-loop-helix/leucine-zipper proteins, where a basic domain functions as the DNA-binding portion and the helix-loop-helix and leucine-zipper domains serve as dimerization motifs mediating protein-protein interactions. The c-*myc* gene has been implicated in cell proliferation, whereas the roles played by other *myc* genes are less well defined (50). High levels of N-*myc* have been found in Wilm's tumor and other tumors of embryonic and neuroendocrine origin (51–53). By employing PCR, a binding site for c-*myc* has been defined; it is the so-called E box motif "CACGTG." Despite efforts from many laboratories, no clear-cut target gene for the Myc proteins has been found, and until recently no interacting proteins were cloned. Recently identified proteins that interact with c- and N-Myc include Max (54), Mxi1 (55), and Mad (56). Like Myc itself these proteins also contain basic helix-loop-helix/leucine-zipper motifs. Through in vivo and in vitro experiments, it could be shown that Max and Mad can form homodimers and heterodimers with each other and also with Myc (54,56,57), and that Mxi heterodimerizes with Max (55). Thus there are several possibilities for interactions among the different proteins. Each of the different complexes also differs in its DNA-binding and *trans*-acting activities (58). One can therefore imagine a very complex network with varying biological activities resulting from the various interactions among these four proteins, and it is likely that as yet unknown other proteins may interact with these. In interpreting the expression pattern of the different members of the *myc*-family, this fact has to be kept in mind.

The expression patterns of c-*myc*, L-*myc*, and N-*myc* during kidney development differ strikingly from each other. The c-*myc* mRNA can be found in all proliferating cells in the developing nephron, i.e., loosely aggregated and condensed mesenchymal cells, the comma- and S-shaped bodies, and in the elongating tubule. The c-*myc* gene is not expressed in the fully developed nephron (59,60). mRNA for L-*myc*, however, can only be detected in cells with a very low mitotic rate, that is, in the cells of the ureter stems in the early stages of the developing kidney. In the collecting ducts of the adult kidney, L-*myc* can no longer be found (59,60). The N-*myc* gene, the third member of the *myc*-family, is activated a little later in development than its cousin c-*myc*. N-*myc* appears first and at its highest levels in the condensed mesenchyme. Thereafter N-*myc* expression declines, so that the latest stage at which its mRNA is present is in the S-shaped bodies (59,60).

How do these developmental findings relate to findings obtained in pathophysiological states of the kidney, such as acute renal injury, polycystic kidneys, and renal tumors? In a model of folic acid–induced acute tubular necrosis in the mouse, elevated levels of c-*myc* could be detected at 24 hr after the intraperitoneal injection of folic acid, consistent with the notion that c-*myc* is expressed in the regenerating cells that enter the cell cycle (61). In the kidneys of mice [C57BL/6J (*cpk*)] homozygous for a hereditary form of autosomal recessive polycystic kidney disease, there were elevated levels of c-*myc* expression at 2 and 3 weeks after birth as compared to expression in kidneys from normal animals (61,62). c-*myc* mRNA has been localized to the lining epithelium of collecting duct cysts as well as normal-appearing proximal tubules of mice with polycystic kidney disease (62a).

More direct insight into the roles played by the *myc* family of transcription factors comes from the establishment of transgenic mice carrying a murine c-*myc* transgene under the control of the SV40 enhancer and mice in which the N-*myc* locus has been mutated by homologous recombination. The mice carrying the c-*myc* transgene consistently developed polycystic kidney disease and died of renal failure between 6 weeks to 3 months after birth (63). This supports the hypothesis that c-*myc* plays a role in the pathogenesis of polycystic kidney disease, though as yet there are no naturally occurring mutations in any of the *myc* genes found in hereditary or spontaneous renal diseases in humans or animals. Homozygous mice with a mutated N-*myc* locus die prenatally at approximately 11.5 days of gestation (64). A number of developing organs are affected, including the mesonephros, nervous system, gut, and lung. The entire mesonephros is disorganized. Although some tubules appear to be normal, others fail to form or degenerate prematurely. There is also an abnormality of the genital ridge in these animals.

THE PAIRED BOX GENES *Pax2* AND *Pax8*

Pax2 and Pax8 belong to a subgroup of homeodomain proteins, the paired box family. This family contains another highly conserved structure in addition to the homeodomain, the paired box, which was first described in three *Drosophila* segmentation genes (65) and subsequently found in other species such as mammals, worms, fish, amphibia, and birds. Recently it was established that some members of the *Pax* family of proteins possess oncogenic potential (65a). (For a more in-depth description of the *Pax* genes, the reader is referred to Chapter 1 of this book and to recent reviews—Refs. 66 and 67.)

Pax2 and N-*myc* are very related in their expression patterns. In a manner similar to N-*myc* mRNA, *Pax2* mRNA and protein are expressed first and most highly in the condensed mesenchyme, after which their expression declines. The latest stage in which *Pax2*-positive, mesenchyme-derived cells are seen is in the "S-shaped body" stage. In striking contrast to N-*myc*, however, *Pax2* mRNA and protein are also present in the ureter buds and even beyond the S-shaped stage in the collecting ducts (68–70). In a recent report the establishment of transgenic *Pax2* mice has been described. The *Pax2* transgene was placed under the control of the cytomegalovirus (CMV) enhancer, a strong enhancer active in wide variety of different cell types. Despite the expression of the *Pax2* transgene in kidney, hindbrain, liver, lung, pancreas, heart, and gut, only kidney abnormalities and precocious opening of the eyes were reported. The anatomic abnormalities and laboratory parameters of the transgenic mice resemble features described for congenital nephrotic syndrome (71).

Like the *myc* genes, different members of the *Pax* family are expressed at different times during development. *Pax8*, like *Pax2*, appears early, its mRNA is detected first in the condensed mesenchyme. Thereafter, however, its expression increases to reach its peak at the S-shaped stage. Beyond the S-shaped bodies, *Pax8* mRNA is absent. This implies, that the *Pax8* gene is shut off abruptly and/or that the *Pax8* mRNA becomes increasingly unstable. Furthermore, at no time during renal development is *Pax8* present in the ureteral buds, thus differing from *Pax2* (72,73).

As yet, no genetic evidence exists that *Pax2* or *Pax8* are involved in the pathogenesis of spontaneous or hereditary renal disease, though overexpression of *Pax2* in transgenic mice leads to congenital nephrotic syndrome (71). Three other members of the *Pax* gene family have been implicated in hereditary disorders involving organs other than the kidneys. In the mouse, a mutant exists, called *undulated,* which is characterized by a kinky tail and vertebral malformations and is probably caused by a mutation in the *Pax1* gene (66,67). Mutations in the *Pax3* gene have been made responsible for two corresponding syndromes in mouse (*splotch*) and humans (Waardenburg syndrome) (66,67). The mouse *splotch* mutants present with abnormalities in the nervous system (exencephaly, spina bifida, meningocele, absence or reduction of dorsal root ganglia), white spotting, and heart defects. The Waardenburg syndrome in humans manifests itself as deafness, pigmentary deficiency (heterochromia irides, white forelock and eyelash), and in some cases a lateral displacement of the inner corner of the eye. Two very similar conditions are caused by mutations in the *Pax6* gene, *small eye* in the mouse and aniridia in humans (66,67). *Small eye* mice present with underdevelopment of the eye or even with complete absence of eyes and nose. Patients with aniridia show partial or complete absence of the iris, which is often accompanied by impaired vision, cataracts, and other eye defects.

LFB1 AND *LFB3*, TWO TRANSCRIPTION FACTORS INVOLVED IN THE ACTIVATION OF LIVER-SPECIFIC GENES

It is possible to learn a good deal about organ-specific gene activation by examining the genetic programs operant in the liver, where a number of proteins have been identified which are expressed predominantly in this organ. The activation of these genes is not controlled by liver-specific transcription factors but by transcription factors which can be found in many different organs, such as LFB1 (HNF-1, HNF-1α), LFB3 (vHNF-1, HNF-1β), HNF-3, HNF-4, and CCAAT-enhancer binding protein (C/EBP). They contain very diverse sequence motifs found in different families of transcription factors, such as POU domains (HNF-1), basic leucine-zipper motifs (C/EBP), forkhead domains (HNF-3), and zinc fingers (HNF-4) (for reviews see Refs. 74 and 75).

At first, the fact that these transcription factors are not exclusively expressed in the liver appears very surprising. At second glance, however, this finding also makes sense, because employing organ-specific transcription factors to regulate organ-specific genes only postpones the problem of how to establish organ specificity. In the case of the liver, it is the interaction of more or less "promiscuous" transcription factors, which regulate the genes encoding organ-specific proteins such as albumin, α1-antitrypsin, and transthyretin. Two of these transcription factors, which are involved in the expression of liver-specific proteins, are also expressed in the context of renal development; they are LFB1 and LFB3.

The expression of *LFB3* occurs with time characteristics somewhat reminiscent of those of *Pax8*. Its mRNA is first detected in the condensed mesenchymal cells and reaches its peak in the S-shaped bodies. Whereas *Pax8* cannot be found beyond this stage, however, *LFB3* mRNA remains present in the maturing and fully differentiated tubules and collecting ducts, though at lower levels than in the S-shaped bodies. The expression of *LFB3* mRNA in the ureteric buds occurs with a pattern similar to that of *Pax2* and quite distinct from that of *Pax8* (76).

LFB1 mRNA appears much later than *LFB3* mRNA and is absent in the ureter buds. It can be seen for the first time in the S-shaped bodies and is present even in the fully developed tubules (76).

THE ZINC-FINGER GENES *Kid-1* AND *WT-1*

Of all DNA-binding proteins, the zinc-finger family of transcription factors has the largest number of known members. It is estimated that there are several hundred zinc-finger genes in the mammalian genome. Two representatives of the zinc-finger family are discussed: *WT-1* and *Kid-1*.

WT-1

The *WT-1* gene was identified by positional cloning techniques as the gene responsible for a hereditary form of pediatric kidney tumors—nephroblastoma or Wilms' tumor. The gene lies on human chromosome 11p13 and is composed of 10 exons (77). It belongs to the rapidly expanding family of tumor suppressor genes, the counterpart of protooncogenes. Most tumor suppressor genes are defined on a genetic level; that is, inactivating mutations in both alleles of a certain gene are required in order to render a cell malignant (Knudson's "two-hit hypothesis" of malignant transformation)—a mechanism very different from that of protooncogenes, where one activating mutation or high expression of the protein product will transform a cell. The WT-1 protein contains four zinc fingers at its COOH-terminus, the specificity of which makes WT-1, together with Sp1 and the Egr proteins (78,79), a member of a family of transcription factors that recognize GC-rich binding sites. Alternatively spliced forms of the *WT-1* transcript are known to occur. These forms differ in their DNA-binding characteristics. Through transfection assays, it was possible to determine that the WT-1 protein acts as a transcriptional repressor, whose presumptive target genes are *IGF-II* and *PDGF-A* and potentially many more. (For reviews on *WT-1*, see Refs. 80 and 81 and Chapter 52 of this book.)

The *WT-1* transcript, like many of the other transcription factors mentioned above, appears first in the condensed mesenchyme. In the comma-shaped bodies, the steady-state level of the *WT-1* mRNA increases. At the next stage, in the S-shaped bodies, *WT-1*–expressing cells are still present. They are, however, not distributed evenly throughout the S-shaped bodies but are concentrated at the proximal end. This pattern anticipates the localization of *WT-1* in the adult kidney, where *WT-1* is expressed only in the podocytes of the glomerulus (83–85). The importance of *WT-1* is emphasized by the fact that mice in which both alleles of *WT-1* have been deleted (so-called knockout mice), no kidney development occurs. The differentiation of the metanephros in the knockout mice stops at an early stage. The ureter does not invade the metanephrogenic mesenchyme and does not branch (86).

Kid-1

In an attempt to find other transcription factors which play a role in kidney development and repair after renal injury, we screened cDNA libraries from normal and postischemic adult rat kidneys with an oligonucleotide encoding a consensus sequence present in zinc-finger proteins. It was possible to clone a novel cDNA, *Kid-1* (a gene expressed predominantly in the kidney and regulated in ischemia and renal development). *Kid-1* codes for a 66-kDa protein with 13 zinc fingers. These zinc fingers are clustered in groups of four and nine fingers and lie at the COOH-terminus of the protein. The mRNA as well as the protein contain instability motifs, suggesting a short half-life of both mRNA and protein. The protein also contains a nuclear targeting signal. At the very NH_2-terminus of the Kid-1 protein lie two highly conserved motifs, the KRAB-A and KRAB-B domains (5).

By Northern blot analysis and reverse transcriptase PCR, *Kid-1* can only be detected predominantly in the kidney. As already suggested by its acronym, *Kid-1* is regulated during renal development. As mentioned in the introduction to this review, the rat kidney has not fully matured in the newborn animal. At time of birth, the steady-state level of *Kid-1* is very low. After birth, the expression of *Kid-1* slowly increases and reaches the highest levels in the adult animal (5).

There is increasing evidence that recovery after renal injury and renal development are related in a reverse manner. In the injured organ, necrotic and apoptotic cells have to be replaced by the surviving epithelial cells. This can only be achieved if the latter leave G_0-phase and enter the cell cycle. At about the same time, the cells dedifferentiate. They now express proteins that are only present early in development or they shut off genes that are only activated late in development. Several models of acute tubular necrosis exist, such as temporary interruption of blood flow by occlusion of the renal artery and intraperitoneal injection of high concentrations of folic acid. Within 5 hr of reperfusion after renal ischemia, *Kid-1* mRNA disappears. It takes approximately 7 days after ischemia for the *Kid-1* mRNA levels in the post-ischemic kidney to return to normal. Very similar results were obtained by intraperitoneal administration of folic acid. By 3 hr after injection of folic acid, *Kid-1* mRNA levels start to decline (5).

The above findings suggest that the expression of *Kid-1* is low in cells that proliferate and are not fully differentiated. An important example of continuously dividing cells in a low-differentiation state is cancer. In the rat, a hereditary form of renal cell carcinoma has been described—the Eker tumors (87). When RNA from three samples of Eker tumors was examined, the *Kid-1* transcript was present at lower levels than in the adult normal kidney (unpublished data). Similarly, in epithelial cell lines from the rat kidney, *Kid-1* mRNA was barely detectable (unpublished results).

In mouse, rat, and human *Kid-1* is present as a single-copy gene. By linkage analysis, somatic hybrid experiments, and fluorescence in situ-hybridization, the *Kid-1* gene was localized to rat chromosome 10q21.3-q22, possibly corresponding to mouse chromosome 11 and human chromosome 5. The rat *Kid-1* gene extends over approximately 14 kbp. The protein coding region is divided into four exons and three introns, closely mirroring the domain structure of the protein. The first exon contains the 5′-untranslated region and sequence coding for the first 11 amino acids. The second exon encodes only and entirely the KRAB-A domain. The largest part of the third exon is composed of KRAB-B coding sequence. All 13 zinc fingers are encoded by exon 4 (88) (Figure 6). We recently have identified an additional 5′ exon that encodes nontranslated 5′ sequence.

The binding-site for Kid-1 is unknown. In order to establish whether Kid-1 is indeed a transcription factor, fusion proteins between the DNA-binding domain of the yeast transcription factor GAL4 and the non–zinc-finger portion of Kid-1 were employed in transient transfection experiments. The fusion protein thus has the DNA-binding properties of GAL4 and the *trans*-acting properties of Kid-1. Reporter plasmids in these experiments contained either five GAL4 binding-sites, a TATA-box, and a chloramphenicol acetyltransferase (CAT) gene (basal reporter plasmid) or five GAL4 binding-sites, the SV 40 enhancer, a TATA-box, and a CAT gene (SV 40 driven reporter plasmid). In the case of the basal reporter plasmid, the CAT gene is driven only by basal transcription factors. By contrast, in the SV 40–driven reporter plasmid, the CAT gene is under the control of a strong constitutive enhancer, which promotes the assembly of the basal transcription factors over the TATA box and thus enhances transcription of the CAT gene. In either case, cotransfection of a plasmid coding for a GAL4/Kid-1 fusion protein with CAT constructs leads to lower CAT activity, indicating that the non–zinc-finger region of Kid-1 functions as a transcriptional repressor (5) (Figure 7). Genes containing a Kid-1 binding site should therefore be repressed by Kid-1.

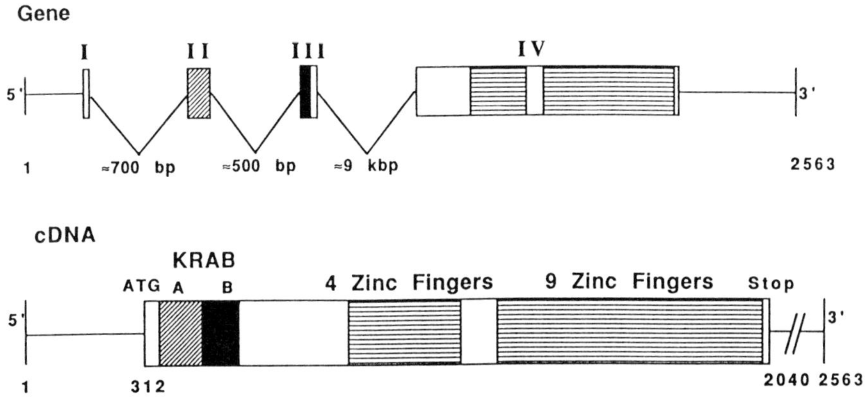

Figure 6 Comparison of the *Kid-1* mRNA and gene. Four exons in the *Kid-1* gene represent the (functional) building blocks of the protein. The main structural motifs in the Kid-1 protein are the Krüppel-associated boxes (KRAB) A and B and the two zinc-finger domains of four and nine zinc fingers each. Exon II encodes the complete KRAB-A domain. Most of exon III consists of KRAB-B encoding sequence. All 13 zinc fingers are encoded by exon IV. (From Ref. 88.)

We have mapped the transcriptional repressor activity of Kid-1 to the KRAB-A domain (89) (Figure 7). KRAB-A and B domains are present in approximately one-third of all zinc-finger proteins and consist of a highly conserved region of approximately 75 amino acids at the NH_2 terminus of these proteins (90). The evolutionary conservation, wide distribution, and genomic organization of the KRAB domain is consistent with an important role of this region in the transcriptional regulatory function of zinc-finger proteins. The KRAB-A domain of another zinc-finger protein, ZNF2, also has repressor activity. Site-directed mutagenesis of conserved amino acids in this motif results in decreased repressor activity. These findings provide a functional significance for the KRAB-A domain.

CONCLUSIONS

The development of the mammalian kidney and its repair after injury are complicated processes resulting from complex genetic programs which are poorly understood. The repair process recapitulates many aspects of the normal developmental process, and hence a better understanding of renal development will likely lead to new experimental paradigms to hasten and modulate the repair process. Developmental processes involve the transformation of a mesenchymal structure into an epithelium with highly specialized functions. Probably many genes have to be turned on or off in that process. We know only a small amount about a minority of these genes, and so far we have little insight into the regulation of these genes during the organogenesis of the kidney. In recent years, a number of transcription factors have been found to be regulated during renal development. The c-*myc* gene is present in all proliferating cells and may have nothing to do with the formation of the kidney per se. N-*myc*, *Pax2*, *Pax-8*, *LFB3*, and *WT-1* are expressed only after an induction process has occurred—that is, after the ureter has invaded the metanephrogenic mesenchyme, has branched, and has caused the condensation of the mesenchymal cells. It is in that condensed mesenchyme that N-*myc*, *Pax2*, *Pax8*, *LFB3*, and *WT-1* appear for the first time. *WT-1* can be assumed to play a necessary though probably not a sufficient role in this earliest morphological transformation. In *WT-1* "knockout mice," kidney development is arrested extremely early. The kidney does not even reach the stage of the condensed mesenchyme. In the case of N-*myc* knockout mice, the situation is less clear, because those animals die prematurely at day 11.5 in utero—that is, before the time of metanephric development. It could be demonstrated, however, that mesonephric development was delayed and disorganized (64). A rather different effect has been noticed in *bcl-2* knockout mice. Bcl-2 is a protein that can prevent apoptosis in many different circumstances. Mice in which both *bcl-2* alleles have been inactivated develop renal failure from polycystic kidney disease (91).

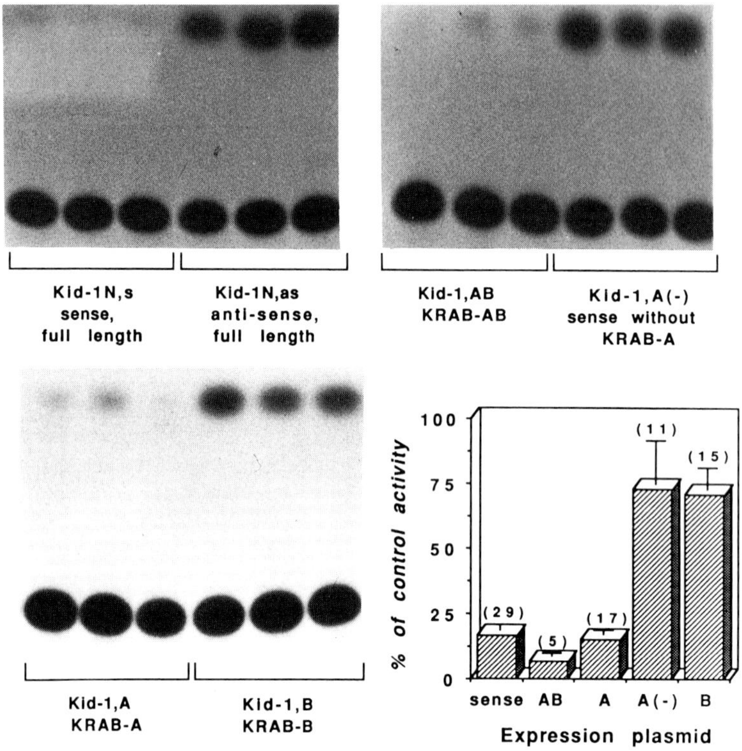

Figure 7 Kid-1 represses transcription—the KRAB-A domain as a transcriptional repressor motif. In transient transfection experiments, the NH_2-terminal, non–zinc-finger region of Kid-1 (Kid-1N,s) strongly represses transcription of a chloramphenicol acetyltransferase (CAT) gene driven by the SV40 promoter. High CAT activity results in the formation of acetylated chloramphenicol, which appears as a second, upper spot on chromatography plates. Deletion mutagenesis identifies the KRAB-A domain as the motif responsible for this repressor effect and defines a novel class of transcriptional repressors.

Expression of fusion proteins containing Kid-1N,s, Kid-1,AB, or Kid-1,A, each of which includes the KRAB-A domain, results in marked repression of CAT activity, when compared to the CAT activity observed in cells transfected with the control antisense construct (Kid-1N,as). In contrast, when the KRAB-A domain is missing from the NH_2-terminus of Kid-1 (Kid-1,A(–) or Kid-1,B), CAT-activity is similar to that of the control antisense plasmid. The graph in the lower right hand corner provides quantitative CAT activity with activity obtained with the antisense Kid-1N,as plasmid taken as 100%. The numbers above the standard error bars indicate the number of independent experiments. (From Ref. 89.)

The time of peak expression is different for each transcription factor, and this timing may provide insights into their regulatory functions. The majority of the discussed transcription factors are undetectable in the fully differentiated kidney, and it can be assumed that they only regulate genes transiently during renal development. This, however, does not necessarily mean that those target genes are not active any longer in the kidneys of the adult animal. *LFB1* and *LFB3* are still present throughout the fully developed tubules. *LFB3* and *Pax2* are expressed in the adult collecting duct system. *WT-1* is expressed in the adult kidney in the podocytes of Bowman's capsule. *Kid-1* is not expressed early in postnatal development and is maximally expressed in adult kidneys.

Though in recent years much has been learned about the genetic control of kidney development, many questions remain unanswered. Which transcription factors are necessary and/or sufficient for the kidney to develop into a functional organ? What are the target genes? What is the exact relationship between renal injury and differentiation? Do any of those transcription factors participate in the pathogenesis of renal cell carcinomas and polycystic kidney disease? Modern molecular and cell biology techniques such as knockout and transgenic animals, positional cloning, and others will hopefully shed some light on these issues and provide answers to the questions posed.

ACKNOWLEDGMENTS

The work described in this review that was performed in the authors' laboratory was supported by NIH grants DK 38452 and DK 39773.

REFERENCES

1. Birnbaumer M, Seibold A, Gilbert S, et al. Molecular cloning of the receptor for human antidiuretic hormone. Nature 1992; 357:333–335.
2. Lolait SJ, O'Carroll A-M, McBride OW, et al. Cloning and characterization of a vasopressin V2 receptor and possible link to nephrogenic diabetes insipidus. Nature 1992; 357:336–339.
3. Uchida S, Sasaki S, Furukawa T, et al. Molecular cloning of a chloride channel that is regulated by dehydration and expressed predominantly in kidney medulla. J Biol Chem 1993; 268:3821–3824.
4. Magagnin S, Werner A, Markovich D, et al. Expression cloning of human and rat renal cortex Na/P_i cotransport. Proc Natl Acad Sci USA 1993; 90:5979–5983.
5. Witzgall R, O'Leary E, Gessner R, et al. *Kid-1*, a putative renal transcription factor: Regulation during ontogeny and in response to ischemia and toxic injury Mol Cell Biol 1993; 13:1933–1942.
6. Clevidence DE, Overdier DG, Tao W, et al. Identification of nine tissue-specific transcription factors of the hepatocyte nuclear factor 3/forkhead DNA-binding-domain family. Proc Natl Acad Sci USA 1993; 90:3948–3952.
7. Bacallao R, Fine LG. Molecular events in the organization of renal tubular epithelium: From nephrogenesis to regeneration. Am J Physiol 1989; 257:F913–F924.
8. Molitoris BA, Hoilien CA, Dahl R, et al. Characterization of ischemia-induced loss of epithelial polarity. J Memb Biol 1988; 106:233–242.
9. Wallin A, Zhang G, Jones TW, et al. Mechanism of nephrogenic repair response: Studies on proliferation and vimentin expression after ^{32}S-1,2-dichlorovinyl-L-cysteine nephrotoxicity in vivo and in cultured proximal tubule epithelial cells. Lab Invest 1992; 66:474–484.
10. Witzgall R, Brown D, Schwarz C, Bonventre JV. Localization of proliferating cell nuclear antigen, vimentin, Fos, and clusterin in the post-ischemic kidneys: Evidence for a heterogeneous response among nephron segments, and a large pool of mitotically active and dedifferentiated cells. J Clin Invest 1994; 93:2175–2188.
11. Ptashne M. A Genetic Switch. Cambridge, MA: Blackwell Scientific Publications, 1992.
12. Klug A, Rhodes D. "Zinc fingers": A novel protein motif for nucleic acid recognition. Trends Biochem Sci 1987; 12:464–469.
13. Landschulz WH, Johnson PF, McKnight SL. The leucine zipper: A hypothetical structure common to a new class of DNA-binding proteins. Science 1988; 240:1759–1764.
14. Struhl, K. Helix-turn-helix, zinc-finger, and leucine-zipper motifs for eukaryotic transcriptional regulatory proteins. Trends Biochem Sci 1989; 14:137–140.
15. Ptashne M. How eukaryotic transcriptional activators work. Nature 1988; 335:683–689.
16. Struhl, K. Molecular mechanisms of transcriptional regulation in yeast. Annu Rev Biochem 1989; 58:1051–1077.
17. Renkawitz R. Transcriptional repression in eukaryotes. Trends Genet 1990; 6:192–196.
18. Branden C, Tooze J. Introduction to Protein Structure. New York: Garland, 1991.
19. Travers A. DNA-Protein Interactions. London: Chapman and Hall, 1993.
20. Larsson L. The ultrastructure of the developing proximal tubule in the rat kidney. J Ultrastruct Res 1975: 51:119–139.
21. Chailler P. Brière N. Integration of proliferation and differentiation phenomena during rodent kidney ontogeny. Growth Dev Aging 1991; 55:11–18.
22. Stöcker E, Butter D. Die DNS-Synthese in Leber und Niere junger Rattan: Autoradiographische Untersuchungen mit ^{3}H-Thymidin. Experientia 1968; 24:704–705.
23. Saxén L. Organogenesis of the Kidney. Cambridge, England: Cambridge University Press, 1987.
24. Clapp WL, Abrahamson DR. Development and gross anatomy of the kidney. In: Tisher C, Brenner BM, eds: Renal Pathology. Philadelphia: Lippincott. In press.
25. Jones DP, Chesney RW. Development of tubular function. Clin Perinatol 1992; 19:33–57.
26. Ekblom P, Lehtonen E, Saxén L, Timpl R. Shift in collagen type as an early response to induction of the metanephrogenic mesenchyme. J Cell Biol 1981; 89:276–283.

27. Nouwen EJ, Dauwe S, von der Biest I, de Broe ME. Stage- and segment-specific expression of cell-adhesion molecules N-CAM, A-CAM, and L-CAM in the kidney. Kidney Int 1993; 44:147–158.
28. Vainio S, Lehtonen E, Jalkanen M, et al. Epithelial-mesenchymal interactions regulate the stage-specific expression of a cell surface proteoglycan, syndecan, in the developing kidney. Dev Biol 1989; 134:382–391.
29. Vainio S, Jalkanen M, Bernfield M, Saxén L. Transient expression of syndecan in mesenchymal cell aggregates of the embryonic kidney. Dev. Biol. 1992; 152:221–232.
30. Korhonen M, Laitinen L, Ylänne J, Gould VE, et al. Integrins in developing, normal and malignant human kidney. Kidney Int 1992; 41:641–644.
31. Holthöfer H, Miettinen A, Lehto V-P, et al. Expression of vimentin and cytokeratin types of intermediate filament proteins in developing and adult human kidneys. Lab Invest 1984; 50:552–559.
32. Moll R, Hage C, Thoenes W. Expression of intermediate filament proteins in fetal and adult human kidney: Modulations of intermediate filament patterns during development and in damaged tissue. Lab Invest 1991; 65:74–86.
33. Ekblom M, Klein G, Mugrauer G, et al. Transient and locally restricted expression of laminin A chain mRNA by developing epithelial cells during kidney organogenesis. Cell 1990; 60:337–346.
34. Dutt A, Priebe TS, Teeter LD, et al. Postnatal development of organic cation transport and *MDR* gene expression in mouse kidney. J Pharmacol Exp Ther 1992; 261:1222–1230.
35. Chin E, Zhou J, Bondy C. Anatomical and developmental patterns of facilitative glucose transporter gene expression in the rat kidney. J Clin Invest 1993; 91:1810–1815.
36. Garrod DR, Fleming S. Early expression of desmosomal components during kidney tubule morphogenesis in human and murine embryos. Development 1990; 108:313–321.
37. Sainio K, Gilbert SF, Lehtonen E, et al. Differential expression of gap junction mRNAs and proteins in the developing murine kidney and in experimentally induced nephric mesenchyme. Development 1992; 115:827–837.
38. Rogers SA, Ryan G, Hammerman MR. Metanephric transforming growth factor-α is required for renal organogenesis in vitro. Am J Physiol 1992; 262:F533–F539.
39. Liu ZZ, Wada J, Alvares K, et al. Distribution and relevance of insulin-like growth factor-I receptor in metanephric development. Kidney Int 1993; 44:1242–1250.
40. Sonnenberg E, Gödecke A, Walter B, et al. Transient and locally restricted expression of the *ros1* protooncogene during mouse development. EMBO J 1991; 10:3693–3702.
41. Sonnenberg E, Meyer D, Weidner KM, Birchmeier C. Scatter factor/hepatocyte growth factor and its receptor, the c-met tyrosine kinase, can mediate a signal exchange between mesenchyme and epithelia during mouse development. J Cell Biol 1993; 123:223–235.
42. Tessarollo L, Nagarajan L, Parada LF. c-*ros*: The vertebrate homolog of the *sevenless* tyrosine kinase receptor is tightly regulated during organogenesis in mouse embryonic development. Development 1992; 115:11–20.
43. Hammerman MR, O'Shea M, Miller SB. Role of growth factors in regulation of renal growth. Annu Rev Physiol 1993; 55:305–321.
44. Erselius, JR, Goulding MD, Gruss P. Structure and expression pattern of the murine *Hox-3.2* gene. Development 1990; 110:629–642.
45. Kress C, Vogels R, De Graaff W, et al. Hox-2.3 upstream sequences mediated lacZ expression in intermediate mesoderm derivatives of transgenic mice. Development 1990; 109:775–786.
46. Miura, N, Wanaka A, Tohyama M, Tanaka K, MFH-1, a new member of the fork head domain family, is expressed in developing mesenchyme. FEBS Lett 1993; 1:171–176.
47. Funahashi J-i, Sekido R, Murai K, et al. δ-crystallin enhancer binding protein δEF1 is a zinc finger-homeodomain protein implicated in postgastrulation embryogenesis. Development 1993; 119:433–446.
48. Marcu KB, Bossone SA, Patel AJ. *myc* function and regulation. Annu Rev Biochem 1992; 61:809–860.
49. Prendergast GC, Ziff EB. A new bind for myc. Trends Genet. 1991; 8:91–96.
50. Cole MD. The myc oncogene: Its role in tranformation and differentiation. Annu Rev Genet 1986; 20:361–384.
51. Kohl NE, Kanda N, Schrenk RR, et al. Transposition and amplification of oncogene related sequences in human neuroblastomas. Cell. 1983; 35:3659–3673.
52. Lee WH, Murphree AL, Benedict WF. Expression and amplification of the N *myc* gene in primary retinoblastoma and related tumors. Nature 1984; 309:458–460.
53. Kohl NE, Gee CE, Alt FW. Activated expression of the N *myc* gene in human neuroblastomas and related tumors. Science 1984; 226:1335–1337.
54. Blackwood EM, Eisenman RN. Max: A helix-loop-helix zipper protein that forms a sequence-specific DNA-binding complex with myc. Science 1991; 251: 1211–1217.
55. Zervos, AS, Gyuris J, Brent R. Mxi1, a protein that specifically interacts with max to bind myc-max recognition sites. Cell 1993; 72:223–232.

56. Ayer DE, Kretzner L, Eisenman RN. Mad: A heterodimeric partner for max that antagonizes myc transcriptional activity. Cell 1993; 72:211–222.
57. Prendergast GC, Lawe D, Ziff EB. Association of Myn, the murine homology of Max, with c-Myc stimulates methylation-sensitive DNA binding and Ras cotransformation. Cell 1991; 61:395–407.
58. Kretzner L, Blackwood EM, Eisenman RN. Myc and max proteins possess distinct transcriptional activities. Nature 1992; 359:426–429.
59. Mugrauer G, Alt FW, Ekblom P. *N-myc* proto-oncogene expression during organogenesis in the developing mouse as revealed by in situ hybridization J Cell Biol 1988; 107:1325–1335.
60. Mugrauer G, Ekblom P. Contrasting expression patterns of three members of the *myc* family of protooncogenes in the developing and adult mouse kidney. J Cell Biol 1991; 112:12–25.
61. Cowley BD Jr, Smardo FL Jr, Grantham JJ, Calvet JP. Elevated c-*myc* protooncogene expression in autosomal recessive kidney disease. Proc Natl Acad Sci USA 1987; 84:8394–8398.
62. Cowley BD Jr, Chadwick LJ, Grantham JJ, Calvet JP. Elevated proto-oncogene expression in polycystic kidneys of the C57BL/6J (*cpk*) mouse. J Am Soc Nephrol 1991; 1:1048–1053.
62a. Harding MA, Gattone VH II, Grantham JJ, Calvet JP. Localization of overexpressed c-*myc* in polycystic kidneys of the *cpk* mouse. Kidney Int 1992; 41:317–325.
63. Trudel M, D'Agati V, Costantini F. c-*myc* as an inducer of polycystic kidney disease in transgenic mice. Kidney Int 1991; 39:665–671.
64. Stanton BR, Perkins AS, Tessarollo L, et al. Loss of N-*myc* function results in emryonic lethality and failure of the epithelial component of the embryo to develop. Genes Dev 1992; 6:2235–2247.
65. Bopp D, Burri M, Baumgartner S, et al. Conservation of a large protein domain in the segmentation gene *paired* and in functionally related genes of *Drosophila*. Cell 1986; 47:1033–1040.
65a. Maulbecker CC, Gruss P. The oncogenic potential of Pax genes. EMBO J 1993; 12:2361–2367.
66. Chalepakis G, Tremblay P, Gruss, P. *Pax* genes, mutants and molecular function. J Cell Sci 1992; 16: 61–67.
67. Gruss P, Walther C. Pax in development. Cell 1992; 69:719–722.
68. Dressler GR, Deutsch U, Chowdhury K, et al. *Pax2*, a new murine paired-box-containing gene and its expression in the developing excretory system. Development 1990; 109:787–795.
69. Dressler GR, Douglass EC. Pax-2 is a DNA-binding protein expressed in embryonic kidney and Wilms tumor. Proc Natl Acad Sci USA 1992; 89:1179–1183.
70. Eccles MR, Wallis LJ, Fidler AE, et al. Expression of the *Pax2* gene in human fetal kidney and Wilms' tumor. Cell Growth Diff 1992; 3:279–289.
71. Dressler GR, Wilkinsin JE, Rothenpieler UW, et al. Deregulation of *Pax-2* expression in transgenic mice generates severe kidney abnormalities. Nature 1993; 362:65–67.
72. Plachov D, Chowdhury K, Walther C, et al. *Pax8*, a murine paired box gene expressed in the developing excretory system and thyroid gland. Development 1990; 110:643–651.
73. Poleev A, Fickenscher H, Mundlos S, et al. *Pax8*, a human paired box gene: Isolation and expression in developing thyroid, kidney and Wilm's tumors. Development 1992; 116:611–623.
74. Simone Vd, Cortese R. Transcription factors and liver-specific genes. Biochim Biophys Acta 1992; 1132:119–126.
75. Xanthopoulos KG, Mirkovitch J. Gene regulation in rodent hepatocytes during development, differentiation and disease. Eur J Biochem 1993; 216:353–360.
76. Lazzaro D, Simone Vd, Magistris Ld, et al. LFB1 and LFB3 homeoproteins are sequentially expressed during kidney development. Development 1992; 114:469–479.
77. Haber DA, Sohn RL, Buckler AJ, et al. Alternative splicing and genomic structure of the Wilms tumor gene *WT1*. Proc Natl Acad Sci USA 1991; 88:9618–9622.
78. Sukhatme VP, Cao X, Chang LC, et al. A zinc finger-encoding gene coregulated with *c-fos* during growth and differentiation, and after cellular depolarization. Cell 1988; 53:37–43.
79. Christy BA, Lau LF, Nathans D. A gene activated in mouse 3T3 cells by serum growth factors encodes a protein with "zinc finger sequences. Proc Natl Acad Sci USA 1988; 85:7857–7861.
80. Coppes MJ, Campbell CE, Williams BRG. The role of *WT1* in Wilms tumorigenesis. FASEB J 1993; 7:886–895.
81. Rauscher FJ III. The WT1 Wilms tumor gene product: A developmentally regulated transcription factor in the kidney that functions as a tumor suppressor. FASEB J 1993; 7:896–903.
82. Armstrong JF, Pritchard-Jones K, Bickmore WA et al. The expression of the Wilms' tumour gene, WT1, in the developing mammalian embryo. Mech Dev 1992; 40:85–97.
83. Pelletier J, Schalling M, Buckler AJ, et al. Expression of the Wilms' tumor gene WT1 in the murine urogenital system. Genes Dev 1991; 5:1345–1356.
84. Pritchard-Jones K, Fleming S, Davidson D, et al. The candidate Wilms' tumor gene is involved in genitourinary development. Nature 1990; 346:194–197.
85. Sharma PM, Yang X, Bowman M, et al. Molecular cloning of rat Wilms' tumor complementary DNA

and a study of messenger RNA expression in the urogenital system and the brain. Cancer Res 1992; 52:6407–6412.

86. Kreidberg JA, Sariola H, Loring JM, et al. WT-1 is required for early kidney development. Cell 1993; 74:679–691.
87. Eker R, Mossige J. A dominant gene for renal adenomas in the rat. Nature. 1961; 189:858–859.
88. Witzgall R, Volk R, Yeung R, Bonventre JV. Genomic structure and chromosomal localization of the rat gene encoding the zinc finger transcription factor Kid-1. Genomics 1994; 20:203–209.
89. Witzgall R, O'Leary E, Leaf A, et al. The Krüppel-associated box-A (KRAB-A) domain of zinc finger proteins mediates transcriptional repression. Proc Natl Acad Sci USA 1994; 91:4514–4518.
90. Bellefroid EJ, Poncelet DA, Lecocq PJ, et al. An evolutionary conserved Kruppel-associated box domain defines a subfamily of eukaryotic multifingered proteins. Proc Natl Acad Sci USA 1991; 88:3608–3612.
91. Veis DJ, Sorenson CM, Shutter JR, Korsmeyer SJ. Bcl-2-deficient mice demonstrate fulminant lymphoid apoptosis, polycystic kidneys, and hypopigmented hair. Cell 1993; 75:229–240.
92. Pavletich NP, Pabo CO. Zinc finger-DNA recognition: Crystal structure of a zif268-DNA complex at 2.1 Å. Science 1991; 252:809–817.
93. Kissinger, CR, Liu B, Martin-Blanco E, Kornberg TB, et al. Crystal structure of an engrailed homeodomain-DNA complex at 2.8 Å resolution: a framework for understanding homeodomain-DNA interactions. Cell 1990; 63:579–590.
94. Vinson CR, Sigler PB, McKnight SL. Scissors-grip model for DNA recognition by a family of leucine zipper proteins. Science 1989; 246:911–916.

38
Erythropoietin and Hypoxia-Sensitive Regulation

David L. Porter and Mark A. Goldberg
Brigham and Women's Hospital and Harvard Medical School, Boston, Massachusetts

INTRODUCTION

The kidney is perhaps the most versatile organ required to maintain homeostasis in higher organisms. In addition to the more obvious role in acid-base and fluid and electrolyte balance, the kidney is crucial to the regulation of the red blood cell mass through its elaboration of the glycoprotein hormone erythropoietin (Epo). It thus plays a crucial role in ensuring adequate tissue oxygen delivery. Understanding the mechanisms that regulate the Epo gene is critically important for comprehending how appropriate oxygen supply to tissues is maintained in the face of changing environmental conditions and in physiological and pathological states. This chapter reviews current knowledge regarding regulation of Epo gene expression. With the technological explosion of molecular biology in the past decade, we are now beginning to understand some of the detailed molecular interactions involved in induction of Epo by a hypoxic stimulus. The availability of molecular probes has provided new insights into the elusive identity of the Epo-producing cell, and we can now begin to address perhaps one of the most intriguing issues related to Epo gene regulation; how does a cell sense changes in oxygen supply and what intracellular signals ultimately lead to altered expression of the Epo gene?

THE DISCOVERY OF ERYTHROPOIETIN

In 1906, Carnot and Deflandre first reported experiments demonstrating that red blood cell production is regulated via a humoral factor (1). These findings were controversial and difficult to verify for many years, but between 1943 and 1953 three independent reports ultimately established the presence of an inducible circulating plasma factor capable of stimulating erythropoiesis. Despite somewhat different experimental conditions, both Krumdieck (2) and Erslev (3) demonstrated that plasma from anemic rabbits contained erythropoietic activity when injected into normal animals. Reissman, using a parabiotic rat model, reached similar conclusions (4). By the end of 1953 it was clear that erythrocyte production was controlled by a circulating hormone (termed erythropoietin) with activity induced by anemia or hypoxia. Research over the next 20 years tended to concentrate on identifying the site of Epo production. Conclusive experiments into the detailed regulation of the hormone would wait until the future development of more sensitive assays and ultimately the availability of modern day molecular tools.

THE SITE OF ERYTHROPOIETIN PRODUCTION

It has now been well established that the kidney is the primary source of Epo production after birth, while the liver is the major source of fetal Epo synthesis. Though the association of renal disease with anemia had been well known, it was the organ ablation experiments of Jacobson and colleagues (5) that unequivocally defined the kidney as the primary source of adult Epo production. Animals subjected to bilateral nephrectomy, but not ablation of other organs, lost the erythropoietic response to severe anemia. Confirmation of these findings was provided when Epo activity was later identified in perfusates of isolated hypoxic kidneys but not other hypoxic organs (6,7,8). The subsequent availability and use of Epo cDNA as a radioactive probe permitted quantitative measurements of Epo mRNA and further confirmed that the kidney is the primary site of Epo mRNA accumulation after birth (9,10).

In the fetus, Epo production occurs primarily in the liver. This was initially defined by organ ablation experiments (11) and supported by identifying Epo activity in perfusates of isolated fetal livers. As noted below, the Epo gene was actually cloned from a human fetal liver cDNA library (12). The liver also retains at least some ability to produce Epo in the adult. Epo activity has been identified in plasma from anephric patients (13), and Epo activity from the plasma of hypoxic anephric rats could be ablated after a partial hepatectomy (14,15). Quantitation of Epo mRNA levels in animals has revealed that the liver may account for up to 30% of the Epo production during periods of hypoxic stress (16).

While it is clear that the majority of Epo is produced in the kidney, the cell type responsible for production of the hormone has been the topic of some controversy. Evidence that relied on demonstrating an association of the Epo protein with specific cell types was initially presented to implicate both the glomeruli (17–19) and tubular cells (20) as the source of Epo production. These findings have been contradicted, however, with the recent use of molecular probes that more precisely identify the site of transcription within specific cells. Most studies using in situ hybridization techniques with antisense Epo mRNA now support the hypothesis that Epo is produced in a peritubular interstitial cell located in the inner cortex and outer medulla of the kidney (21–27), perhaps of endothelial (22,23) or fibroblast (27) origin. Some evidence has been presented in favor of a tubular cell of origin, but as pointed out in a recent exchange on this topic (28,29), many technological variables can affect the interpretation of in situ hybridization experiments, and at least for now, the precise identity of the Epo-producing cell in the kidney remains elusive. It is interesting that no renal cell line has yet been reported that exhibits appropriate regulation of the Epo gene. While identification of such a cell line would be of great value, it is also possible that the cells responsible for sensing changes in oxygen supply may not necessarily be the same cells responsible for Epo synthesis. Resolution of some of these issues may depend on the development of an appropriate tissue culture system.

PHYSIOLOGICAL REGULATION OF ERYTHROPOIETIN IN HEALTH AND DISEASE

Under normal conditions, the level of circulating Epo is very low. For many years it was difficult to obtain accurate measurements of the hormone, thus limiting the ability to obtain information on Epo regulation. The development of a sensitive and accurate radioimmunoassay (30) has led to a clearer understanding of Epo biology and physiology. During periods of tissue hypoxia, as occurs with anemia, Epo is synthesized and released into the bloodstream from the Epo-producing cells of the kidney. Epo is a true hormone traveling through the blood to the bone marrow, where it stimulates erythroid progenitor cells to differentiate and proliferate. The resultant increased red cell mass improves the oxygen-carrying capacity of the blood. The enhanced oxygen delivery then serves to downregulate Epo production in the kidney, completing a classic regulatory feedback loop, as illustrated in Figure 1.

The unique physiology of the kidney makes it a logical source for the majority of Epo production. This organ may be able to appropriately sense changes in tissue oxygen supply that result specifically from diminished blood oxygen-carrying capacity (31). The majority of renal oxygen consumption provides energy for sodium reabsorption, which is determined in large part by the glomerular filtration rate and renal blood flow. A fall in renal blood flow, resulting in decreased oxygen delivery, results in a similar fall in sodium reabsorption and hence less oxygen consumption. The net result will be a relatively constant oxygen tension in the region of the kidney where the oxygen sensor appears to reside. Thus, the kidney should sense changes in the blood's oxygen-carrying capacity (i.e., red cell

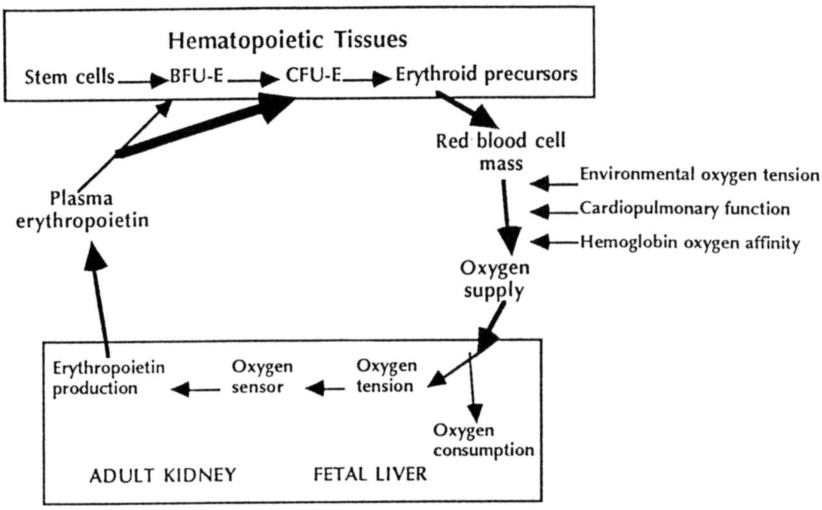

Figure 1 Feedback loop for the regulation of erythropoiesis. *Abbreviations*: BFU-E, burst forming units—erythroid; CFU-e, colony forming units—erythroid. (From Ref. 81.)

mass) independent of its own oxygen requirements (31). Interestingly, loop diuretics, which are expected to decrease sodium reabsorption and oxygen consumption and therefore result in a net increase in oxygen tension, have been shown to blunt the induction of Epo in response to a given degree of hypoxia (32).

Under normal conditions, Epo levels increase proportionally to a given degree of anemia (33) except in patients with renal failure, presumably due to loss of the cells responsible for oxygen sensing and/or Epo production. The cloning of the Epo gene in 1985 (12,34) eventually led to the availability of large quantities of recombinant human Epo (r-HuEpo) for pharmacological use. In patients with renal failure, replacement therapy with r-HuEpo has had a dramatic impact on the anemia and on the quality of life in patients with chronic renal failure. A number of other disease states have been associated with a blunted Epo response to anemia, including a variety of inflammatory disease ("anemia of chronic disease") (35,36), malignancy (37), HIV infection (38), and prematurity (39). It remains unclear why Epo levels are inappropriately low in these conditions, but several studies in vitro demonstrate that hypoxic induction of the Epo gene can be inhibited by various inflammatory cytokines, such as tumor necrosis factor and interleukin-1 (40,41), which are known to be elevated in chronic disease states. While many patients with inappropriately low Epo levels may benefit from pharmacological doses of r-HuEpo, clearly others do not.

THE Epo GENE IS TRANSCRIPTIONALLY REGULATED

A great deal is now known about the molecular mechanisms regulating expression of the Epo gene. This work was initially facilitated by three critical developments. In 1977 Miyake and coworkers purified the hormone from vast quantities of human urine (42). From the purified protein, the amino acid sequence was obtained and appropriate molecular probes were developed that led directly to the isolation of both genomic and cDNA clones of the gene (12,34). Finally, the identification of two human hepatoma cell lines (Hep3B and HepG2) that produced Epo in a regulated fashion in response to hypoxia provided an ideal model system to study the molecular regulation of the Epo gene (43).

It is now known that there is a single copy of the Epo gene that is approximately 3000 base pairs (bp) in length, consisting of 5 exons and 4 introns. A protein of 194 amino acids is initially synthesized, but cleavage of a 27–amino acid leader sequence and removal of the carboxyl-terminal arginine (44) results in a mature protein of 165 amino acids. Although the calculated molecular weight is 18,398 Da, the functional hormone requires extensive glycosylation, accounting for the observed molecular weight of 30,400 Da (45).

Epo production is increased 50- to 100-fold in the Hep3B cell line in response to hypoxia (43,46). This regulation is due largely to transcriptional activation of the gene (47,48). These in vitro findings appear to have physiological significance, as similar increases in Epo transcription have been noted in rat kidney cells after exposure to hypoxia (49). Dramatic increases in Epo mRNA levels have also been noted in murine kidney and liver in response to both hypoxia and severe anemia as detected by Northern blot analysis (9,10,50), in situ hybridization studies (21–27), and a quantitative competitive polymerase chain reaction assay (51). However, some data suggest that not all of the increase in steady-state Epo mRNA levels in response to hypoxia may be accounted for solely on the basis of an increased rate of gene transcription (48). Whether additional posttranscriptional regulatory mechanisms are significantly involved in hypoxic induction of Epo expression, for instance by affecting Epo mRNA stability (48,52), remains to be determined.

MECHANISMS OF OXYGEN SENSING

The precise mechanisms by which a cell can sense changes in oxygen tension and the subsequent second messengers that ultimately lead to increased Epo gene expression are unknown and have been difficult to define. In the Hep3B cell line, Epo production is not induced by manipulations of multiple second-messenger pathways. For instance, no increase in Epo production is noted when these cells are exposed to phorbol ester, calcium ionophore, lananthum (a potent calcium channel blocking agent), hydrogen peroxide, heat shock, forskolin, interleukin-1, alpha-interferon, or androgens (46). However, exposure to any of three transition metals—cobalt, nickel and manganese—results in stimulation of Epo production (46), though exposure to iron and cadmium has no effect. Notably, cobalt (53) and nickel (54) can both induce erythrocytosis in animal models. Goldberg et al. have presented a hypothesis consistent with these data suggesting that the oxygen sensor is a heme protein (46) whose activity would be affected by the binding of oxygen to the heme moiety (Figure 2). A shift from the inactive (oxy) to the active (deoxy) state would be anticipated during hypoxic stress. Cobalt, nickel, and manganese can all be incorporated into the porphyrin ring in place of iron, resulting in a molecule that would bind oxygen with either a low affinity or not at all. These metals would be expected to lock the putative sensor in the active, deoxy state. This hypothesis was further tested by demonstrating that carbon monoxide can block hypoxia-induced but not cobalt-induced Epo production in Hep3B cells. Carbon monoxide can bind heme in a manner analogous to oxygen, thereby locking the putative sensor in the inactive oxy state; however, it cannot bind cobalt, nickel, or manganese protoporphyrin and, as predicted, does not to block Epo induction after exposure to these metals (46). It is interesting to note that the oxygen sensor in the prokaryotic organism *Rhizobium meliloti* has been shown to be a heme protein with kinase activity that is dependent on the oxygen tension of the cells (55). It is very possible that this mechanism of oxygen sensing may be conserved through evolution.

The identity of the oxygen sensor in mammalian cells is not known. Fandrey et al. (56) have suggested that the heme proteins of the microsomal mixed-function oxidase system may be involved in oxygen sensing and regulation of Epo synthesis. Regardless of the identity of the sensor, one might anticipate that most, if not all, cells in an organism must be capable of responding to hypoxic stress for survival. After a change in oxygen tension via a common mechanism is sensed, the subsequent pattern of response of these cells may be determined by other cell-type specific factors. For instance, one response of Hep3B cells and the Epo-producing cells in the kidney to hypoxia is the induction of Epo gene transcription. A similar sensing mechanism has been implicated in other systems that result in different responses. In endothelial cells, hypoxia results in the induction of endothelin gene expression (57); hypoxic induction can also be partially inhibited by carbon monoxide (57), analogous to the Epo system. Hypoxia has been shown to induce the expression of a number of other mammalian genes in cell culture experiments, and there is some evidence that at least some of these genes are also induced by cobalt exposure, again suggesting they may share a common mechanism of oxygen sensing (See Table 1).

Other evidence for a generalized oxygen-sensing system in mammalian cells has recently been provided. Two groups have demonstrated that the 3′ enhancer element of the Epo gene confers

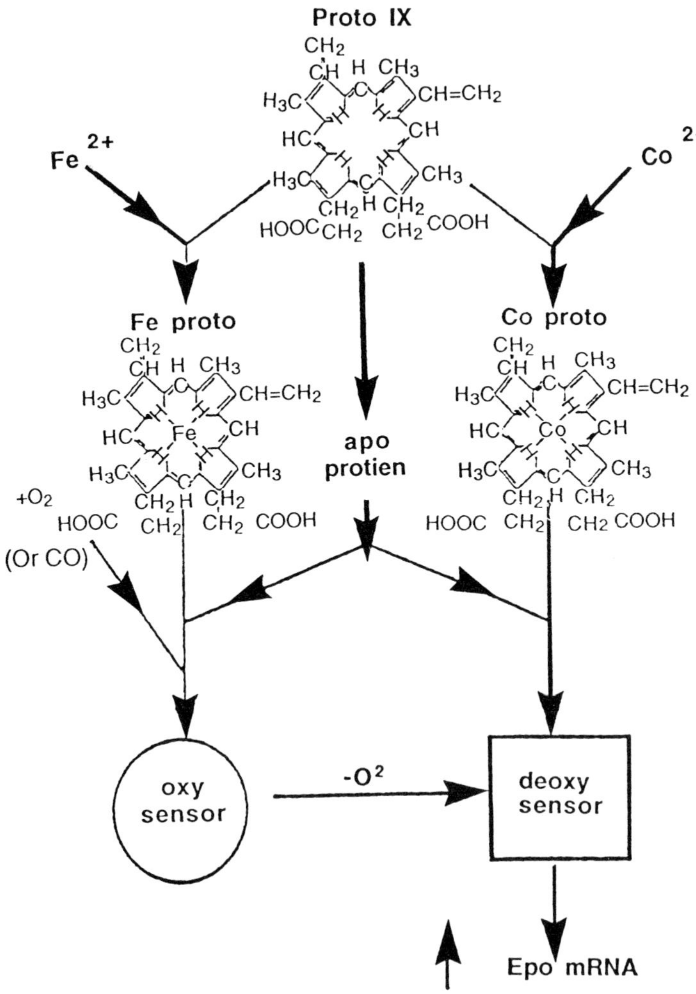

Figure 2 Proposed model for the mammalian oxygen sensor. See text for detailed description. This model suggests a mechanism by which cobalt, nickel, and manganese can mimic hypoxic stimulation of Epo production through incorporation into the porphyrin ring. *Abbreviations*: Proto, protoporphyrin; Fe^{+2}, iron; O_2, oxygen; CO, carbon monoxide; Co^{+2}, cobalt. (From Ref. 81.)

hypoxic regulation on a reporter gene construct after transfection into many different cell types, despite the restricted expression of Epo (67,68). Additionally, exposure of Hep3B cells to hypoxia results in induction of a factor, termed HIF-1 (hypoxia inducible factor-1), with DNA binding activity specific for sequences in the 3′ Epo enhancer element (69,70). HIF-1 DNA binding activity can also be detected in several non-Epo-producing cell lines after exposure to hypoxia (68,70) or cobalt (68). These data further support the notion of a generalized oxygen-sensing mechanism in mammalian cells. The identification of the oxygen sensor and the downstream signal transduction pathways remain an area of active investigation.

cis-REGULATORY ELEMENTS OF THE ERYTHROPOIETIN GENE

Important *cis*-acting regulatory elements involved in hypoxia-induced transcriptional regulation of the Epo gene have been defined by various strategies. Direct comparisons of the DNA sequence

Table 1 Mammalian Genes Induced by Hypoxia or Other Stimuli in Cell Culture

Gene	Induction stimulus	Cell type	Ref.
Erythropoietin	Hypoxia, cobalt, nickel, manganese	Hep3B HepG2	46
Endothelin	Hypoxia	Vascular endothelial cells	57
Vascular endothelial growth factor (VEGF)	Hypoxia, cobalt	C6	58
		Hep3B	59
		Cardiac myocytes	60
c-*Jun*, c-*Fos*	Hypoxia, cobalt	Hep3B	60
		Cardiac myocytes[a]	61
Interleukin-1α	Hypoxia	Human umbilical vein endothelial cells	62
Platelet-derived growth factor (PDGF)	Hypoxia	Human umbilical vein endothelial cells	63
Tumor growth factor-B1(TGF-B1)	Hypoxia	Fibroblasts	64
Tyrosine hydroxylase	Hypoxia	PC12	65
HSP70	Hypoxia	C2C12	66

[a]Cobalt chloride not tested as a stimulus in cardiac myocytes (61).

between different species have identified highly conserved sequences in the immediate 5′ and 3′ noncoding and flanking regions, suggesting the presence of potentially important regulatory elements (71–74). Unlike the case with many other mammalian genes, knowledge of the DNA sequence immediately 5′ to the gene has provided little insight as to important regulatory elements. Sequences typically associated with "promoter" activity, such as a TATA box or CAAT box, are not present. One strategy taken by a number of groups to identify important regulatory elements employs transient transfection into Hep3B cells of plasmids containing a reporter gene linked to candidate sequences. Initially it was shown that such a construct containing large segments of 5′ and 3′ flanking sequence could confer hypoxic and cobalt induction to the growth hormone gene after transfection into Hep3B cells (75). A series of reports over the next several years have demonstrated that a small segment of the 3′ flanking region of the Epo gene is sufficient to confer at least partial hypoxic regulation to various reporter genes. Semenza et al. initially identified this 3′ hypoxia responsive enhancer (HRE) as a 256-bp DNA fragment (beginning approximately 120 bases downstream from the polyadenylation site of the gene) (76). Subsequent experiments have demonstrated hypoxia-inducible enhancer activity within subsets of this 3′ element—contained in fragments of 150 bp (78), 43 bp (47), 33 bp (69), and finally a region as small as 29 bp (70)—appears to be sufficient to mediate appropriate hypoxia-inducible regulation.

Similar experiments performed by Blanchard et al. (47) defined the 117-bp of DNA sequence immediately 5′ of the transcriptional start site as the minimal promoter element necessary to confer hypoxic induction to a luciferase reporter gene. Deletion of the distal 53-bp sequence ablates the hypoxia response. However, this promoter element mediates only a 6- to 10-fold induction. A 43 bp of the 3′ enhancer can mediate a 10- to 15-fold induction in the same construct. A combination of these two elements on the same plasmid mediates up to 50-fold induction of the reporter gene, similar to the level of induction of the endogenous Epo gene. This suggests that the 5′ and 3′ regulatory sequences may function in a cooperative manner. DNA sequence comparison of the 5′ and 3′ fragments demonstrates that both contain direct repeats previously shown to function as response elements for the thyroid-steroid hormone-receptor superfamily. The significance of this finding is currently under further investigation.

An alternative strategy used by Semenza and coworkers to define important *cis*-regulatory elements of the Epo gene takes advantage of a transgenic mouse system to analyze various human Epo transgenes (21,78,79). Transgenic mice were developed that all contained the full-length gene

(~3 kb) and 0.7 kb of 3′ flanking sequences. Three strains differed in the size of 5′ flanking sequence that was included. Transgenes containing either 0.4 kb or 6 kb of 5′ flanking sequence were inducible in the liver but not the kidney of hypoxic or anemic mice. This suggests that elements required for appropriate induction in the kidney are not contained within these regions. Transgenes containing 14 kb of 5′ flanking sequence demonstrated appropriate kidney-specific, hypoxia-inducible activity, mapping kidney specific *cis*-regulatory elements to a region between 6 and 14 kb 5′ of the gene. A high level of constitutive expression of the human transgene containing only 0.4 kb of 5′ sequence was noted both in the liver and in typically non-Epo-producing organs. This suggests that negative regulatory elements, which can eliminate promiscuous expression, are contained in sequences between 0.4 kb and 6 kb 5′ of the transcriptional start site.

Trans-REGULATORY FACTORS OF THE ERYTHROPOIETIN GENE

Much less detail is known about *trans*-activating factors that are required for hypoxic regulation of the Epo gene. Although induction of Epo is primarily under transcriptional control, protein synthesis inhibitors, such as cyclohexamide, will block hypoxia-induced transcription of the gene, implying that a newly synthesized protein(s), presumably with a short half-life, is necessary for the proper response to hypoxia. Beru et al. (80) have identified four RNA species and two proteins that bind specifically to the 5′ promoter region of the mouse Epo gene. They noted that the level of two of the RNA species fell after mice were stimulated with cobalt and suggested that levels and binding of these ribonucleoproteins may regulate Epo transcription through specific interaction with the promoter. More recently, a hypoxia-inducible factor has been identified that demonstrates specific binding to sequences in the 3′ enhancer element as described above (68,70). The presence of this factor has been assayed by its ability to shift the electrophoretic mobility of a DNA fragment containing the minimal hypoxia-responsive enhancer. Initial characterization demonstrates that this factor is also induced by cobalt (68) and has a molecular weight of approximately 120 kDa. Pretreatment of cells with protein synthesis inhibitors abolishes induction of this binding activity, suggesting that this factor is either newly synthesized or that de novo protein synthesis is otherwise required for activation of its DNA-binding capacity (68,70). In addition, treatment of the protein extract prior to the electrophoretic mobility shift assay with protein phosphatases (81) or low concentrations of deoxycholate (70) abolishes DNA-binding activity, suggesting a phosphorylation event and protein-protein interactions are required for sequence-specific binding. Epo-enhancer DNA-binding activity of this protein is induced by hypoxia in multiple cell lines (68,70) that do not express Epo, suggesting that it may be involved in the cellular response to hypoxic stress in general and not be specific to Epo regulation.

CONCLUSION

Though the existence of erythropoietin has been known for almost a century, it is only in the last decade that we have begun to understand some of the molecular interactions involved in regulating expression of the gene. Investigators are now identifying important *cis*-regulatory elements and *trans*-activating factors of the Epo gene. Molecular probes have permitted visualization of individual cells that make Epo, though the histological identity of these cells remains controversial. Available evidence suggests that a heme protein may serve as the oxygen sensor that transmits the signal that ultimately leads to transcriptional activation of the Epo gene. It also appears that this mechanism of oxygen sensing may be conserved among many cell types and through evolution. Understanding the molecular regulation of the *Epo* gene may therefore provide a paradigm to understand how cells adapt to changes in oxygen availability, a response that must be crucial to the survival of all organisms.

ACKNOWLEDGMENTS

This work was supported in part by NIH grants T32HL07623 (D.L.P.) and 1RO1DK45098 (M.A.G.). We are grateful for additional support from the friends and family of Alan Johnson.

REFERENCES

1. Carnot P, Deflandre C. Sur l'activite hemopoietique du serum. Compt rend Acad d Sc 1906; 143:432–435.
2. Krumdieck N. Erythropoietic substance in the serum of anemic animals. Proc Soc Exp Biol Med 1943; 54:14–17.
3. Erslev A. Humoral regulation of red cell production. Blood 1953; 8:349–357.
4. Reissmann KR. Studies on the mechanism of erythropoietic stimulation in parabiotic rats during hypoxia. Blood 1950; 5:372–380.
5. Jacobson LO, Goldwasser E, Fried W, Plzak L. Role of the kidney in erythropoiesis. Nature 1957; 179:633–634.
6. Kuratowska Z, Lewartowski B, Michalak E. Studies on the production of erythropoietin by isolated perfused organs. Blood 1961; 18:527–534.
7. Erslev A. Renal biogenesis of erythropoietin. Am J Med 1975; 58:25–30.
8. Fisher JW, Langston JW. The influence of hypoxemia and cobalt on erythropoietin production in the isolated perfused dog kidney. Blood 1967; 29:114–125.
9. Beru S, McDonald J, Lacombe C, Goldwasser E. Expression of the rythropoietin gene. Mol Cell Biol 1986; 7:2571–2575.
10. Bondurant M, Koury M. Anemia induces accumulation of erythropoietin mRNA in the kidney and liver. Mol Cell Biol 1986; 6:2731–2733.
11. Zanjani ED, Poster J, Burlington H, et al. Liver as the primary site of erythropoietin formation in the fetus. J Lab Clin Med 1977; 69:640–644.
12. Jacobs K, Shoemaker C, Rudersdorf R, et al. Isolation and characterization of genomic and cDNA clones of human erythropoietin. Nature 1985; 313:806–810.
13. Nathan DG, Schupak E, Stohlman F Jr, Merrill JP. Erythropoiesis in anephric man. J Clin Invest 1964; 43:2158–2165.
14. Fried W. The liver as a source of extrarenal erythropoietin production. Blood 1972; 40:671–677.
15. Fried W, Kilbridge T, Krantz S, et al. Studies on extrarenal erythropoietin. J Lab Clin Med 1969; 73:244–248.
16. Tan CC, Eckardt KU, Firth JD, Ratcliffe PJ. Feedback modulation of renal and hepatic erythropoietin mRNA in response to graded anemia and hypoxia. Am J Physiol 1992; 263:F474–F481.
17. Burlington H, Cronkite EP, Reincke U, Zanjani ED. Erythropoietin production in cultures of goat renal glomeruli. Proc Natl Acad Sci USA 1972; 12:3547–3550.
18. Kurtz A, Jelkmann W, Sinowatz F, Bauer C. Renal mesangial cell cultures as a model for study of erythropoietin production. Proc Natl Acad Sci USA 1983; 80:4008–4011.
19. Ueno M, Nagakura K, Chen I-L, et al. Immunocytochemical localization of erythropoietin (Ep) in the glomerular epithelial cells of the rat kidney. Blood 1986; 68:182a.
20. Caro J, Erslev AJ. Biologic and immunologic erythropoietin in extracts from hypoxic whole rat kidneys and in their glomerular and tubular fractions. J Lab Clin Med 1984; 103:9222.
21. Semenza GL, Koury ST, Nejfelt MK, et al. Cell-type specific and hypoxia-inducible expression of the human erythropoietin gene in transgenic mice. Proc Natl Acad Sci USA 1991; 88:8725–8729.
22. Lacombe C, Da Silva J, Bruneval P, et al. Peritubular cells are the site of erythropoietin synthesis in the murine hypoxic kidney. J Clin Invest 1988; 81:620–623.
23. Koury ST, Bondurant MC, Koury MJ. Localization of erythropoietin synthesizing cells in murine kidneys by in situ hybridization. Blood 1988; 71:524–527.
24. Koury ST, Koury MJ, Bondurant MC, et al. Quantitation of erythropoietin-producing cells in kidneys of mice by in situ hybridization: Correlation with hematocrit, renal erythropoietin mRNA, and serum erythropoietin concentration. Blood 1989; 74:645–651.
25. Koury ST, Bondurant MC, Koury MJ, Semenza GL. Localization of cells producing erythropoietin in murine liver by in situ hybridization. Blood 1991; 77:2497–2503.
26. Schuster SJ, Koury ST, Bohrer M, et al. Cellular sites of extarenal and renal erythropoietin production in anaemic rats. Br J Haematol 1992; 81:153–159.
27. Bachmann S, Le Hir M, Eckardt K. Co-localization of erythropoietin mRNA and ecto-5′-nucleotidase immunoreactivity in peritubular cells of rat renal cortex indicates that firbroblasts produce erythropoietin. J Histochem Cytochem 1993; 41:335–3341.
28. Rich IN. The site of erythropoietin production: Localization of erythropoietin mRNA by radioactive in situ hybridization (letter). Blood 1991; 78:1469.
29. Koury ST, Bondurant MC, Koury MJ. The site of erythropoietin production: Localization of erythropoietin mRNA by radioactive in situ hybridization (response). Blood 1991; 78:1470–1471.
30. Garcia JF, Sherwood J, Goldwasser E. Radioimmunoassay of erythropoietin. Blood Cells 1979; 5:405–419.
31. Erslev A. Erythropoietin coming of age. N Engl J Med 1987; 316:101–103.
32. Eckhardt KU, Kurtz A, Bauer C. Erythropoietin formation is related to proximal tubular function. Am J Physiol 1989; 256:F942.

33. Caro J, Brown S, Miller O, et al. Erythropoietin levels in uremic nephric and anephric patients. J Lab Clin Med 1979; 93:449–458.
34. Lin P, Suggs S, Lin C, et al. Cloning and expression of the human erythropoietin gene. Proc Natl Acad Sci USA 1985; 82:7580–7584.
35. Baer AN, Dessypris EN, Goldwasser E, Krantz SB. Blunted erythropoietin response to anaemia in rheumatoid arthritis. Br J Haematol 1987; 66:559–564.
36. Hochberg MC, Arnold CM, Hogans BB, Spivak JL. Serum immunoreactive erythropoietin in rheumatoid arthritis: Impaired response to anemia. Arthritis Rheum 1988; 31:1318–1321.
37. Miller CB, Jones RJ, Piantadosi S, et al. Decreased erythropoietin response in patients with the anemia of cancer. N Engl J Med 1990; 322:1689–1692.
38. Spivak JL, Barnes DC, Fuchs E, Quinn TC. Serum immunoreactive erythropoietin in HIV-infected patients. JAMA 1989; 261:3104–3107.
39. Brown MS, Garcia JF, Phibbs RH, Dallman PR. Decreased response of plasma immunoreactive erythropoietin to "available oxygen" in anemia of prematurity. J Pediatr 1984; 105:793–798.
40. Faquin WC, Schneider TJ, Goldberg MA. Effect of inflammatory cytokines on hypoxia-induced erythropoietin production. Blood 1992; 79:1987–1994.
41. Jelkmann W, Fandrey J, Wiedemann G. Immunoreactive erythropoietin in the anemia of non-renal chronic diseases. Biomed Biochem Acta 1990; 49:S265–S270.
42. Miyake T, Kung CK, Goldwasser E. Purification of human erythropoietin. J Biol Chem 1977; 252:5558–5564.
43. Goldberg MA, Glass GA, Cunningham JM, Bunn HF. The regulated expression of erythropoietin by two human hepatoma cell lines. Proc Natl Acad Sci USA 1987; 84:7972–7976.
44. Recny MA, Scoble HA Kim Y. Structural characterization of natural human urinary and recombinant DNA–derived erythropoietin. J Biol Chem 1987; 262:17156–17163.
45. Davis JM, Arakawa T, Strickland TW, Yphanntis DA. Characterization of recombinant human erythropoietin produced in Chinese hamster ovary cells. Biochemistry 1987; 26:2633–2638.
46. Goldberg MA, Dunning SP, Bunn HF. Regulation of the erythropoietin gene: Evidence that oxygen sensor is a heme protein. Science 1988; 242:1412–1415.
47. Blanchard KL, Acquaviva AM. Galson DL, Bunn HF. Hypoxic induction of the human erythropoietin gene: Cooperation between the promoter and enhancer, each of which contains steroid receptor response elements. Mol Cell Biol 1992; 12:5373–5385.
48. Goldberg MA, Gaut CC, Bunn HF. Erythropoietin mRNA levels are governed by both the rate of gene transcription and posttranscriptional events. Blood 1991; 7:271–277.
49. Schuster SJ, Badiavas EV, Costa-Giomi P, et al. Stimulation of erythropoietin gene transcription during hypoxia and cobalt exposure. Blood 1989; 73:13–16.
50. Schuster SJ, Wilson JH, Erslev A, Caro J. Physiologic regulation and tissue localization of renal erythropoietin messenger RNA. Blood 1987; 70:316–318.
51. Fandrey J, Bunn HF. In vivo and in vitro regulation of erythropoietin mRNA: measurement by competitive polymerase chain reaction. Blood 1993; 81:617–623.
52. Rondon IJ, MacMillan L, Beckman BS, et al. Hypoxia up-regulates the activity of a novel erythropoietin mRNA binding protein. J Biol Chem 1991; 266:16594–16598.
53. Goldwasser E, Jacobson LO, Fried W, Plzak LF. Studies on erythropoiesis: V. The effect of cobalt on the production of erythropoietin. Blood 1958; 13:55–60.
54. Morse EE, Lee T-Y, Reiss RF, Sunderman FW Jr. Dose-response and time-response study of erythrocytosis in rats after intrarenal injection of nickel subsulfide. Ann Clin Lab Sci 1977; 7:17–24.
55. Gilles-Gonzalez MA, Ditta GS, Helinski DR. A haemoprotein with kinase activity encoded by the oxygen sensory of Rhizobium meliloti. Nature 1991; 350:170–172.
56. Fandrey J, Seydel FP, Siegers CP, Jelkmann W. Role of cytochrome P_{450} in the control of the production of erythropoietin. Life Sciences 1990; 47:127–134.
57. Kourembanas S, Marsden PA, McQuillan LP, Faller DV. Hypoxia induces endothelin gene expression and secretion in cultured human endothelium. J Clin Invest 1991; 88:1054–1057.
58. Shweiki D, Itin A, Soffer D, Keshet E. Vascular endothelial growth factor induced by hypoxia may mediate hypoxia-initiated angiogenesis. Nature 1992; 359:843–845.
59. Goldberg MA, Schneider TJ. Similarities between the oxygen-sensing mechanisms regulating the expression of vascular endothelial growth factor and erythropoietin. J Biol Chem 1994; 269:4355–4359.
60. Levy AP, Levy NS, Loscalzo J, et al. Regulation of vascular endothelial growth factor in cardiac myocytes. Circ Res 1995, in press.
61. Webster KA, Discher DJ, Bishopric NH. Induction and nuclear accumulation of Fos and Jun proto-oncogenes in hypoxic cardiac myocytes. J Biol Chem 1993; 268:16852–16858.
62. Shreeniwas R, Koga S, Karakurum M, et al. Hypoxia-mediated induction of endothelial cell Interleukin-1a. J Clin Invest 1992; 90:2333–2339.

63. Kourembanas S, Hanna RL, Faller DV. Oxygen tension regulates the expression of the platelet-derived growth factor-β chain gene in human endothelial cells. J Clin Invest 1990; 86:670–674.
64. Falanga V, Qian SW, Danielpour D, et al. Hypoxia upregulates the synthesis of TGF-B1. J Invest Dermatol 1991; 97:634–637.
65. Czyzyk-Krzeska MF, Furnari BA, Lawson EE, Millhorn DE. Hypoxia increases rate of transcription and stability of tyrosine hydroxylase mRNA in pheochromocytoma (PC12) cells. J Biol Chem 1994; 268:9940–9945.
66. Benjamin IJ, Kroger B, Williams RS. Activation of the heat shock transcription factor by hypoxia in mammalian cells. Proc Natl Acad Sci USA 1990; 87:6263–6267.
67. Maxwell PH, Pugh CW, Ratcliff PJ. Inducible operation of the erythropoietin 3′ enhancer in multiple cell lines: Evidence for a widespread oxygen-sensing mechanism. Proc Natl Acad Sci USA 1993; 90:2423–2427.
68. Wang GL, Semenza GL. General involvement of hypoxia-inducible factor 1 in transcriptional response to hypoxia. Proc Natl Acad Sci USA 1993; 90:4304–4308.
69. Semenza GL, Wang GL. A nuclear factor induced by hypoxia via de novo protein synthesis binds to the human erythropoietin gene enhancer at a site required for transcriptional activation. Mol Cell Biol 1992; 12:5447–5454.
70. Beck I, Weinmann R, Caro J. Characterization of hypoxia-responsive enhancer in the human erythropoietin gene shows presence of hypoxia-inducible 120-Kd nuclear DNA-binding protein in erythropoietin-producing and nonproducing cells. Blood 1993; 82:704–711.
71. McDonald J, Lin FK, Goldwasser E. Cloning, sequencing and evolutionary analysis of the mouse erythropoietin gene. Mol Cell Biol 1986; 6:842–848.
72. Shoemaker CB, Mitsock LD. Murine erythropoietin gene: Cloning, expression and human gene homology. Mol Cell Biol 1986; 6:849–858.
73. Wen D, Boissel JR, Tracy TE, et al. Erythropoietin structure-function relationships: High degree of sequence homology among mammals. Blood 1993; 82:1507–1516.
74. Galson DL, Tan CC, Ratcliffe PJ, Bunn HF. Comparison of the human and mouse erythropoietin genes shows extensive homology in the flanking regions. Blood 1993; 82:3321–3326.
75. Imagawa S, Goldberg MA, Doweiko J, Bunn HF. Regulatory elements of the erythropoietin gene. Blood 1991; 77:278–285.
76. Semenza GL, Nejfelt MK, Chi SM, Antonarakis SE. Hypoxia-inducible nuclear factors bind to an enhancer element located 3′ to the human erythropoietin gene. Proc Natl Acad Sci USA 1991; 88:5680–5684.
77. Beck I, Ramirez S, Weinmann R, Caro J. Enhancer element at the 3′-flanking region controls transcriptional response to hypoxia in the human erythropoietin gene. J Biol Chem 1991; 266:15563–15566.
78. Semenza GL, Traystman MD, Gearhart JD, Antonarakis SE. Polycythemia in transgenic mice expressing the human erythropoietin gene. Proc Natl Acad Sci USA 1989; 86:2301–2305.
79. Semenza GL, Dureza RC, Traystman MD, et al. Human erythropoietin gene expression in transgenic mice: Multiple transcription initiation sites and cis-acting regulatory elements. Molec Cell Biol 1990; 10:930–938.
80. Beru N, Smith D, Goldwasser E. Evidence suggesting negative regulation of the erythropoietin gene by ribonucleoprotein. J Biol Chem 1990; 265:14100–14104.
81. Goldberg MA. Biology of erythropoietin. In: Garnick MB, ed. Erythropoietin in Clinical Applications: An International Perspective. New York, Marcel Dekker, 1990.

39

Insulin-like Growth Factors in Mature and Developing Kidney

Marc R. Hammerman and Steven B. Miller
Washington University School of Medicine, St. Louis, Missouri

INSULIN-LIKE GROWTH FACTORS (IGF)

IGF I is a proinsulin-like peptide 70 amino acids in length. It bears structural homology, not only to proinsulin but also to a related growth factor, insulin-like growth factor II (IGF II). IGF I acts through its own unique receptor to regulate the development, metabolism, and proliferation of a variety of tissues (1,2).

IGF I circulates in plasma at a concentration two to three orders of magnitude higher than that of insulin. Liver is the major source of circulating IGF I which serves an endocrine function. However, in addition to liver, IGF I is produced in a variety of tissues in which it serves an autocrine or paracrine growth factor. Many of the growth promoting actions of somatotropin or growth hormone (GH) are mediated by GH-enhanced synthesis of IGF I (1,2).

The genes for IGF I have been partially characterized in several species of vertebrates. The sequences of the exons encoding the mature peptide are highly conserved. An IGF I–like molecule has been characterized in the Atlantic hagfish, a chordate, and an IGF/insulin hybrid molecule has been detected in *Amphioxis*, a protochordate. Therefore the lineage of IGF I–like molecules extends backwards over 500 million years (3).

The mature IGF I peptide consists of regions designated A and B domains that correspond to the A and B insulin chains, joined by two disulfide bonds, and a C domain that corresponds to the connecting peptide of insulin. The structure of IGF I differs from insulin in that the C domain contains unique carboxyl-terminal extensions and cannot be cleaved away from the A and B domains. In addition, IGF I has a D domain at the carboxyl terminus of the A region (Figure 1) and IGF I-precursor contains an E domain (1–4).

Although IGF I is a relatively simple protein, its gene structure and pattern of expression are complicated. In the rat and human, the IGF I gene spans more than 80 kb of chromosomal DNA and consists of 6 exons and 5 introns. Exons 1 and 2 encode alternate leader sequences including 5′ untranslated regions and the amino termini of signal peptides. Exons 3 and 4 contain the mature IGF I peptide-coding sequence. Exons 5 and part of exon 6 encode alternate E peptides that are cleaved posttranslationally in mature IGF I. The bulk of exon 6 contains the 3′ untranslated region. Use of alternative promoters acting on multiple initiation sites, differential RNA splicing, and variable RNA polyadenylation are responsible for the production of multiple IGF I mRNA species in mammals and ultimately IGF IA and IGF IB proteins that differ in their E domains (1–2).

IGF II is a 67–amino acid molecule with a domain structure similar to that of IGF I. The sequence of the mature peptide is highly conserved among six mammalian species. In humans, a variant IGF II molecule has been characterized by both cDNA cloning and by protein purification and amino acid sequencing. In this protein, a serine residue is replaced by the tetrapeptide, arginine-leucine-proline-glycine. The variant growth factor makes up approximately 25% of total circulating IGF II. Other variant IGF II peptides have been described in humans (1).

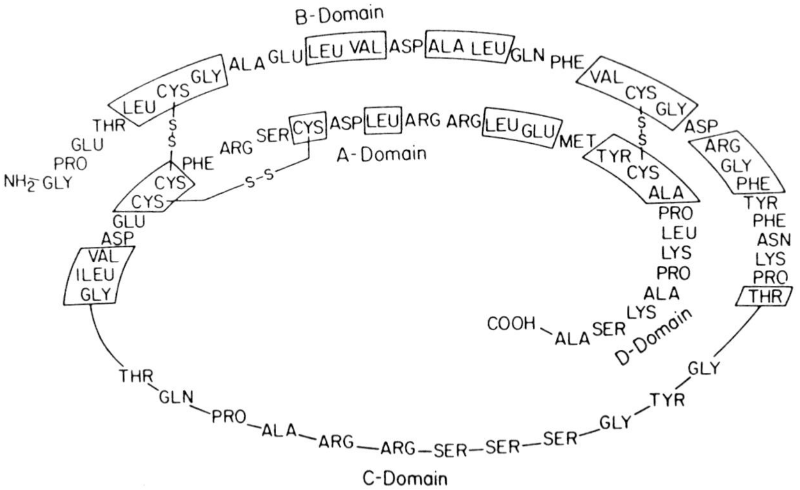

Figure 1 The primary structure of human IGF I. Areas of homology with human proinsulin are enclosed. (From Ref. 4.)

Structural information on the IGF II gene is available for several mammalian species. In humans, rat, and mouse, IGF II and insulin (insulin 2 in rodents) form a conserved linkage group, suggesting that the IGF II-insulin locus was present prior to evolution of these species. The human, rat, and mouse genes contain multiple 5′ untranslated exons. In all three genes, the coding region for prepro-IGF II is contained within the last three exons (7 to 9 in the human, 4 to 6 in rodents). Human exon 7 and rodent exon 4 encode the mature 67–amino acid IGF II molecule as well as a 24–amino acid signal peptide. Human exon 8 and rodent exon 5 encode the initial 11 amino acids of the E domain. The remaining codons of the E domain and the 3′ untranslated region of IGF II mRNA are found on human exon 9 and rodent exon 6 (1). In humans and in rodents the IGF II gene contains alternative promoters that are located adjacent to distinct 5′ noncoding exons. Alternative RNA polyadenylation also adds to a multiplicity of IGF II mRNAs (1).

The biological role of IGF II is not well defined. The fall in IGF II expression that occurs shortly following birth in rodents suggests that IGF II serves as a fetal analogue of IGF I. However, no such fall occurs in humans (1).

IGF Expression in Mature Kidney

The production of IGF I in extrahepatic tissues such as kidney supports both autocrine and paracrine functions and appears to be regulated differently from production in liver. In rat liver, transcription initiation occurs at four distinct sites in exon 1 of the IGF I gene and at a cluster of sites in exon 2. Exon 2 transcripts appear later in postnatal development than do exon 1 transcripts, coincident with the appearance of circulating IGF I. Exon 1 transcripts are present in all tissues where they show moderate GH dependence. Exon 2 transcripts are expressed in liver, testis, lung, stomach, and kidney. They appear to be more GH-dependent in liver than in nonhepatic tissues. The usage of transcription start sites is altered in kidney during postnatal development. Within exon 1, start site 3 is expressed constitutively throughout perinatal and postnatal development, whereas usage of start site 2 is not detected until weaning. In addition, exon 2 transcripts do not appear in kidney until the postnatal period. The different mRNAs produced at different times during development in kidney through the use of alternative start sites may reflect differential regulation of IGF I production for autocrine or paracrine function (5).

Most of the studies characterizing IGF I synthesis within kidney have utilized animal models, usually rat. Although the presence of IGF I mRNA in human kidney has been questioned (6), the evidence is overwhelmingly in favor of a renal localization in the human as well as in the rat. Han et al. (7) and Hill et al. (8) localized immunoreactive IGF I to human fetal kidney and Han et al. detected IGF I mRNA in human fetal kidney (9). Bell et al. detected mRNAs for both IGF I and IGF II in adult human kidney (10). Aron et al. described the presence of IGF I mRNA in glomerular mesangial cells cultured from human kidney and documented synthesis of IGF I in vitro (11). We have probed RNA originating from human liver and kidney for IGF I mRNA using a highly sensitive and specific solution-hybridization nuclease-protection assay. As shown in Figure 2, we were able to detect IGF I mRNA in adult human kidney. There is approximately as much IGF I mRNA extractable from human whole kidney relative to human whole liver as is present in rat whole kidney relative to rat whole liver (12). It is likely that the autocrine/paracrine/endocrine roles of IGF I are similar in rat and in human renal tissue.

Immunohistochemical studies have localized IGF I within kidney to cortical and medullary collecting duct, the thin limb of Henle's loop, and the distal convoluted tubule (12–15). Studies designed to detect IGF I mRNA using in situ hybridization have generated somewhat conflicting results. Matejka et al. found IGF I mRNA to be localized in medullary collecting ducts and sparsely in cortical collecting duct cells of rat kidney. In addition, IGF I mRNA was expressed in scattered proximal tubular cells in the cortex and in cells confined to the glomerular tuft (16). In contrast, Chin et al. found IGF I mRNA to be localized in the epithelial cells of medullary thick ascending limbs of Henle's loop (17). Using a solution-hybridization nuclease-protection assay, we detected relatively large quantities IGF I mRNA in medulary collecting ducts isolated from rat kidney (approximately 25% of the level in whole rat liver) and lesser quantities in proximal tubules and glomeruli. In our studies, the distribution of IGF I mRNA corresponded to the distribution of immunostainable IGF I peptide (12).

IGF I is produced at multiple sites in kidney. The collecting duct is a major source of renal IGF I production. The evidence that this is the case, in addition to that summarized above, is that collecting ducts freshly isolated from rat kidney produce IGF I in a GH-dependent manner in vitro (18) and that collecting duct cells cultured from rabbit kidney secrete immunoreactive IGF I into their media (19). As noted above, IGF I is produced by human mesangial cells in culture (11). It is also produced by mesangial cells from rat (20), consistent with a glomerular origin of the peptide. Following acute ischemic injury to rat kidneys, immunostainable IGF I (21) and IGF I mRNA (22) can be detected in cells located in the region of the proximal tubule, suggesting that under these conditions IGF I is expressed in this location. The identity of the cells is undetermined. It is possible that they are dedifferentiated proximal tubular cells or are stem cells activated by the ischemic injury or they may be nonproximal tubular cells that migrate into the area of injury. Finally, the presence of IGF I mRNA in the medullary thick ascending limb of Henle's loop in the rat and human nephron suggests that IGF I is produced here in addition (6,17).

The synthesis of IGF I in renal collecting duct is stimulated directly by GH (18) and by epidermal growth factor (EGF) (23). The effect of EGF to enhance IGF I synthesis was originally described in fibroblasts (24) and has been reported in liver (25). The fact that kidney is a major site of EGF

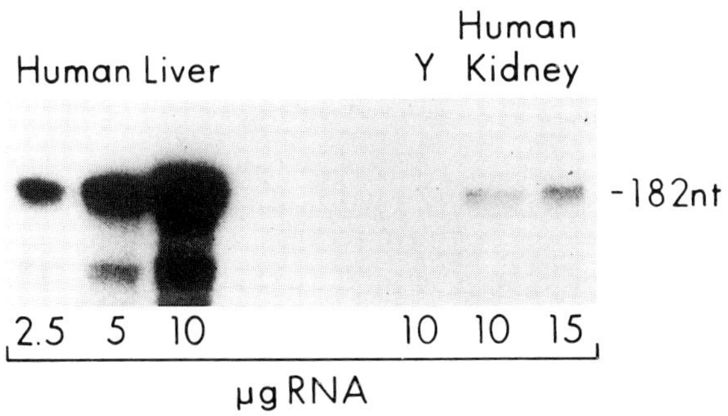

Figure 2 Autoradiogram depicting the result of a solution-hybridization nuclease-protection experiment using a ^{32}P-labeled human IGF I exon 4 antisense probe (protected fragment = 182 nucleotides). Illustrated are protected fragments originating from RNA extracted from whole human liver and whole human kidney. Y (yeast tRNA). (From Ref. 46.)

synthesis (26) establishes the potential for an EGF-IGF I axis within this organ. Expressions of EGF and IGF I in rat kidney are both enhanced in the setting of compensatory renal growth (13,27–29). It is possible, although unproven, that renal EGF induces renal IGF I expression in this setting.

In addition to compensatory hypertrophy, synthesis of IGF I in kidney is enhanced in experimental diabetes mellitus (30–37) and synthesis is increased in normal-appearing tissue adjacent to infarcted kidney (38). The identity of stimuli that promote IGF I expression under these circumstances is unknown. GH may play a role to enhance renal IGF I production in diabetes (37). However, the enhancement postinfarction cannot be explained by the presence of a circulating factor, because kidneys contralateral to infarcted kidneys do not exhibit increased IGF I synthesis (38).

Levels of IGF I mRNA in rat kidney are decreased following 48 hr of fasting. The decrease cannot be explained entirely on the basis of reduced circulating GH (39). Caloric restriction prevents the increase in renal cortical collecting duct IGF I content that is observed 2 weeks following 5/6 nephrectomy of rats fed ad libidum (40).

Hypersomatotropism (41), compensatory hypertrophy (42), and diabetes mellitus (43) are all accompanied by increases in the glomerular filtration rate. In addition, each of these conditions is characterized by growth of glomeruli and proximal convoluted tubules, structures known to have IGF I receptors (see below). Unlike the case in hypersomatotropism, in which levels of circulating IGF I are increased in addition to renal IGF I (41), elevated levels of renal IGF I in diabetes mellitus (43) and compensatory hypertrophy (28,44,45) occur in the absence of changes in circulating peptide. The temporal relationship between increases in levels of IGF I in kidney and the changes in glomerular filtration rate and renal size is an area of controversy. Some investigators demonstrate that the timing of alterations of renal IGF I is such that it can explain the enhancements of renal growth and glomerular filtration rate. Other studies show that the changes in renal size and glomerular filtration are initiated prior to alterations in IGF I synthesis (46).

In contrast to what is known about IGF I expression in mature kidney, little is known about the expression of IGF II. Very little IGF II mRNA can be detected in kidneys from adult rats (6,12). However, IGF II mRNA is present in human kidney and appears to be concentrated in the renal vascular system, including afferent arterioles and the medullary interstitium (6).

IGF BINDING PROTEINS (IGFBP)

Virtually all IGFs in circulation are in tight, noncovalent association with specific binding proteins (IGFBP). The coexpression of IGFs and IGFBPs in a number of tissues suggests that the IGF-IGFBP interaction plays an important role to modulate autocrine and paracrine actions of locally produced IGFs as well as endocrine functions of circulating IGFs. To date six IGFBPs (IGFBPs 1–6) have been cloned (47). In vitro, one or more IGFBPs have been shown to both inhibit and enhance the actions of IGFs, consistent with complex roles for these peptides in the regulation of IGF activity in vivo. Because the affinity of IGFs for their binding proteins in vitro is higher under most circumstances than the affinity of IGFs for their receptors, and the IGF-IGFBP complexes do not appear to bind to IGF receptors, it has been suggested that the IGFBPs serve to functionally inactivate IGFs through sequestration. This is undoubtedly true for circulating IGFBPs and explains why IGF I that circulates at a concentration two to three orders of magnitude higher than insulin and has approximately 6% of the hypoglycemic potency of insulin does not induce hypoglycemia in everyone. Conceivably, IGFBPs that have bound IGFs could release the IGFs at selected sites of action and through this mechanism exert control over their biological functions.

All six IGFBPs contain at least 18 cystine residues that are aligned. The functions of IGFBPs appear to be regulated by posttranslational modifications. IGFBPs 3, 4, 5, and 6 can be glycosylated. IGFBPs 2, 3, 4, and 5 are proteolytically cleaved and specific proteases have been identified for the latter 3 IGFBPs. In addition, IGFBPs 1, 2, 3, and 5 are phosphorylated. Phosphorylation of IGFBP1 results in enhancement of its affinity for IGFs I and II (47).

IGFBPs produced within a given tissue may serve to keep IGFs within tissue compartments, thereby increasing their local bioavailability. IGFBPs 1 and 2 contain arginine-glycine-aspartic acid (RGD) sequences near their carboxyl terminus consistent with their ability to bind to cell surface membrane integrin receptors (47–48). In this location they could serve to position IGFs near the

IGF receptor and either inhibit or enhance the access of IGFs to their receptors, or regulate the signal-tranducing potency of IGFs.

IGFBP Expression in Kidney

IGFBP-1 mRNA has been detected in the medullary thick ascending limbs of Henle's loop and in the straight portion of cortical distal tubules in adult rat kidney using in situ hybridization (17). Immunohistochemistry revealed IGFBP-1 to be localized predominantly in papillary collecting ducts with moderate staining in the cortical collecting ducts and medullary thick ascending limbs of Henle's loop (15). IGFBP-1 (49) and IGFBP-2 (49,50) mRNAs are present in fetal rat kidney. In fetal human kidney, IGFBP-1 mRNA has been localized by in situ hybridization to epithelial cells of the collecting ducts as well as to the cells of developing glomeruli and the subcapsular metanephric blastema. IGFBP-1 protein was detected by immunoperoxidase staining around small blood vessels, in epithelial cells of collecting ducts and in stromal connective tissue (51). The relative abundance of IGFBP-2 mRNA is eightfold higher than that of IGFBP-1 mRNA in fetal rat kidney (49). Expression of IGFBP-2 mRNA is reduced in kidney from adult rats relative to expression in fetal rats (50,52). Chin and Bondy localized IGFBP-2 mRNA to glomeruli of both adult rat and human kidneys, to the medullary interstitium of rat kidneys and to the epithelium of the distal nephron and collecting ducts of human kidneys (6). IGFBP-3 mRNA is present in adult rat kidney (53).

Liver is the major source for circulating IGFBP-3. Synthesis of this binding protein in liver is GH-dependent (53,54). It is of interest that, in rat, levels of IGFBP-3 mRNA are higher in kidney than in liver and that the production of renal IGFBP-3 is not enhanced by GH in hypophysectomized rats. The divergent responses of renal and hepatic IGFBP-3 gene expression to hypophysectomy and GH replacement indicate that this gene, like the gene for IGF I, is under tissue-specific regulation (53). The abundance of IGFBP-5 mRNA is greater in rat kidney than in any other tissue in which it was measured (55).

IGF RECEPTORS

Insulin and IGF I receptors exist as $\alpha_2\beta_2$ heterotetrameric complexes that are assembled from two identical $\alpha\beta$ heterodimeric half-receptor precursors. The α-subunits contain the high-affinity ligand-binding domains whereas the intracellular region of the β subunits contain a tyrosine-kinase domain. The receptors are autophosphorylated in response to ligand binding. Both insulin and IGF I stimulate an intramolecular *trans*-autophosphorylation reaction between two adjacent β subunits within the holoreceptors (56).

In contrast to insulin and IGF I receptors, the IGF II receptor is a monomer that is homologous to the cation-independent mannose-6 phosphate receptor (57). A role for the IGF II receptor as a signal-transducing entity is controversial (58).

IGF Receptors in Kidney

The distribution of IGF I and IGF II receptor mRNAs has been mapped in rat and human kidney using in situ hybridization. In both species each IGF receptor mRNA was found to be abundant in the tubular epithelium of the medulla and barely detectable in proximal tubules. IGF I receptor mRNA was present in glomeruli (6). Binding of ^{125}I-IGF I in rat kidney was found to be widely distributed throughout the entire kidney. Specific binding was highest in the inner medulla (22). We (57,59) and others (60) have reported previously, that ^{125}I-IGF I can be cross-linked to the α subunit of its receptor in glomeruli (60) and proximal tubules (57,59,60) from rat kidney. We have shown that the site of binding in the proximal tubule of rat and dog is the basolateral membrane of the renal proximal tubular cell (57,59). Subsequent descriptions of IGF I enhancement of gluconeogenesis (a metabolic process restricted to proximal tubule) in proximal tubule suspensions from dog kidney (61) and of IGF I stimulation of Na^+-dependent phosphate transport in isolated-perfused proximal convoluted tubules from rabbit kidney (62) provide compelling evidence for the presence of IGF I receptors in the renal proximal tubule.

IGF II receptors are localized to both apical and basolateral membranes of the renal proximal tubular cell in dog kidney (59).

NEPHROGENESIS

It is customary to distinguish between three spatially and temporally different embryonic renal excretory organs. These are the pronephros, the mesonephros, and the metanephros. The pronephros is the most primitive of these organs and it is functional during embryogenesis only in some of the lower vertebrates. The mesonephros, located further caudally, is functional during embryogenesis in higher fishes and amphibians. The metanephros, located most caudally, serves as the permanent kidney of the amniotes. The pronephros, mesonephros, and metanephros each consist of paired organs derived from the intermediate mesoderm that is located immediately lateral to the somites. Pronephric tubules empty into the primary nephric ducts. These ducts are appropriated by the developing mesonephros and, after degeneration of the pronephric tubules, are designated mesonephric ducts. These ducts empty into the cloaca. At a later stage in development, paired outgrowths develop from the mesonephric ducts near their cloacal ends. This occurs during the fifth week of gestation in humans, during day 12 of embryonic rat development, and during day 11 of embryonic mouse development (63). These so-called metanephric diverticula, or ureteric buds, collect about their distal ends intermediate mesoderm caudal to the mesonephros. This mesoderm gives rise to the excretory tubules of the metanephros, and for that reason is designated metanephrogenic mesenchyme, or metanephric blastema. Numerous outgrowths arise from the distal end of the ureteric bud which push radially into the surrounding mass of metanephric blastema. These outgrowths become hollow and give rise to the collecting ducts of the kidneys. The proximal ends of the ureteric bud give rise to the ureter and renal pelvis. The metanephric blastema differentiates into all of the tubular structures of the adult nephron with the exception of the collecting system.

Differentiation of the metanephric blastema and of the ureteric bud is dependent upon an inductive event (or events) that occur when the ureteric bud encounters the metanephric blastema. The nature of this event (these events) is unknown. There is disagreement as to whether humoral agents trigger differentiation or whether cell-cell contact is also required for this process to be initiated (63).

Following induction of the metanephros, tubulogenesis proceeds through a histologically defined sequence of stages. Initially the metanephric blastema undergoes condensation into a rounded structure the cells in which proliferate as part of a growth stage. Following the growth phase, mitotic activity decreases, and the tubular anlage assumes a comma shape. Cells farthest from the collecting duct become elongated and some become funnel shaped. This is the site of formation of a slit that represents the first sign of the glomerular crevice. While glomerulogenesis is taking place, a second slit forms at the opposite distal pole, the tubular anlage assumes an S shape and joins the collecting system (63).

Vascularization of the nephron results from the interaction of a pair of vessels arising from the dorsal aorta with the S-shaped body. These vessels invade the metanephric blastema in close association with the branching ureteric bud. The endothelial cells of the vessels migrate in apposition to the condensing metanephric blastema and into the lower crevice of the S-shaped glomerular anlage. At this point migration ceases, and the endothelial basement membrane fuses to that of epithelial podocytes to create the glomerular basement membrane (63).

The agents that control and regulate the postinductive growth and differentiation of the metanephros are unknown. It has been demonstrated that a number of cell adhesion molecules, components of the extracellular matrix and polypeptide growth factors coordinate the differentiative events (64–67).

IGF and Nephrogenesis

To examine the roles that endogenously produced IGF I and IGF II play in growth and development during renal organogenesis, we removed metanephroi from 13-day-old rat embryos and grew them in organ culture using chemically defined serum free conditions. Growth of metanephroi in vitro recapitulates many events of nephrogenesis in vivo and has provided a useful model for kidney development (65,66).

Individual metanephric kidneys were allowed to grow for up to 6 days in organ culture. Over this period of time the metanephroi increased in size and morphological complexity. The diameter of the long axis increased by approximately 50% and the renal anlage adopted a morphology that was more "kidney-like" in appearance. The ureteric bud underwent extensive arborization during 6 days in culture, and elements of the nephron became differentiated within the metanephric blastema. Metanephrogenesis proceeds in vitro through the stages described for this process in vivo (65,66). By 4 to 5 days in culture, nephrons with avascular glomeruli had differentiated within developing rat kidneys (65). Since the origin of the glomerular blood vessels is extrametanephric, vascularization of the nephron does not occur in the organ culture system (65).

Messenger RNAs for both IGFs were detected in the metanephroi by amplification of cDNA following reverse transcription of mRNA, using the polymerase chain reaction (PCR) (Figure 3). IGF I and IGF II contents of media were determined by specific radioimmunoassays following extraction and separation of IGFs by molecular weight using reverse-phase high-performance liquid chromatography (HPLC). Immunoreactive IGF I and IGF II were produced by the renal anlagen and released into culture media (Figure 4). Levels of these peptides were relatively constant during the 6 days in culture and averaged 5.5×10^{-9} *M* IGF I and 8.3×10^{-9} *M* IGF II in media removed from metanephroi after 24 hr of contact (68). Such levels exceed the K_i for binding of IGFs to most receptors including those in renal tissue (69).

IGF I produced by the metanephroi was indistinguishable from recombinant human IGF I in a radioreceptor assay that measured binding of ^{125}I-IGF I to isolated canine renal proximal tubular basolateral membranes. IGF II produced by the metanephroi was indistinguishable from human recombinant IGF II in a biological assay that measured mannose 6-phosphate activated phospholipase C activation in proximal tubular basolateral membranes (68).

Metanephric kidneys were cultured in the absence or presence of highly specific anti-IGF I or anti-IGF II antibodies or appropriate control additions. Growth and development of metanephroi as evaluated by gross visual inspection and by histological examination of tissues (54) were prevented by both anti-IGF I and anti-IGF II antibodies. Similarly, anti-IGF II receptor antibodies prevented growth and development in vitro (Figure 5). These observations demonstrate production of IGF I and IGF II by developing rat metanephroi in organ culture. Each of the peptides is necessary for growth and development of the renal anlage to take place in vitro. Our findings suggest that both IGFs are produced within the developing metanephros in vivo and promote renal organogenesis (68).

The Wilms' Tumor Gene Product IGF and Nephrogenesis

Wilms' tumor is a renal malignancy of complex pathology that manifests itself in young children, constituting 25% of the tumors found in this population. The embryonic origin of Wilms' tumor is metanephric blastema (70). Wilms' tumor cells have undergone a deletion of genes located on chromosome 11p13. Recently, mRNA transcripts that are expressed in kidney and map to the Wilms' tumor deletion region have been defined (71,72). One cDNA clone (WT1) has characteristics of a

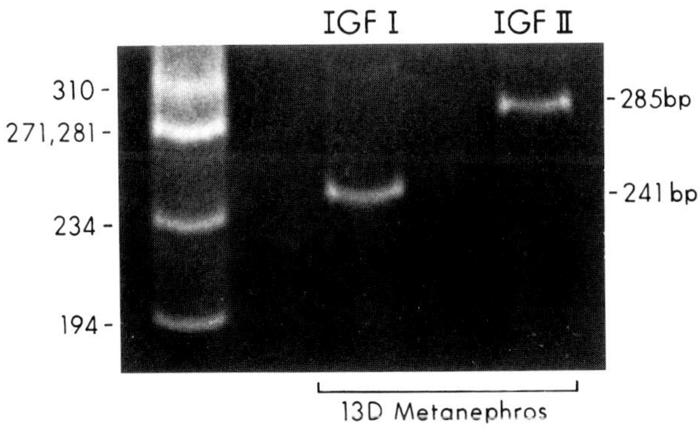

Figure 3 IGF I and IGF II mRNAs are present in the rat metanephros. Shown in a 5% polyacrylamide gel stained with ethidium bromide. On the left are molecular size markers expressed in base pairs. On the right are the sizes of IGF I (241 bp) and IGF II (285 bp) cDNAs amplified using the polymerase chain reaction. (From Ref. 68.)

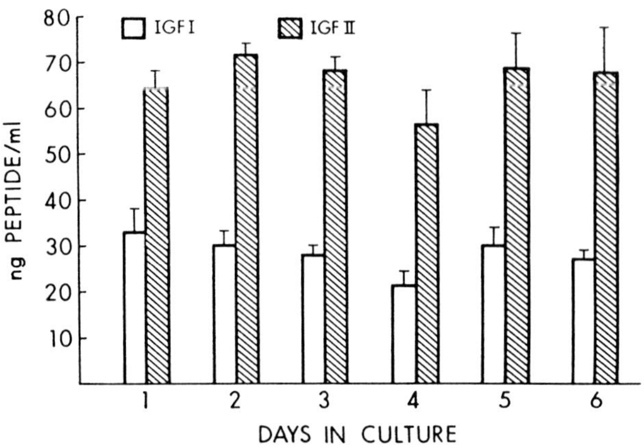

Figure 4 Levels of IGF I and IGF II in media removed from developing rat metanephroi. (From Ref. 68.)

tumor-suppressor gene and encodes a protein that contains four zinc fingers and a glutamine and proline-rich amino terminus, structural motifs associated with binding to DNA and transcriptional-regulatory functions. In fact, the Wilms' tumor gene product does repress transcription (73). The *WT1* gene is expressed in condensing mesenchyme and in tubular and glomerular epithelia of developing kidney, consistent with a function in normal kidney differentiation (74). Introduction of

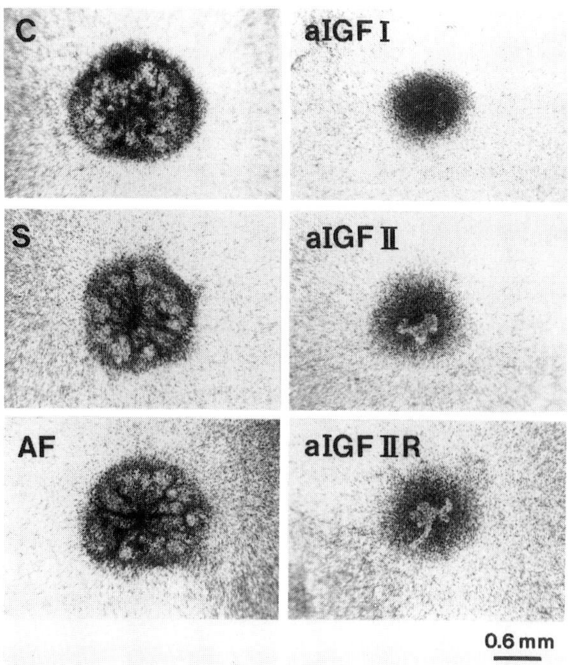

Figure 5 Photomicrographs of metanephroi. Shown are metanephroi cultured for 4 days in serum-free chemically defined media (control, C) or in media to which the following additions were made: mouse ascites fluid (AF); normal rabbit serum (S); anti-IGF I antibodies (aIGF I); anti-IGF II antibodies (aIGF II); or anti-IGF II receptor antibodies (aIGF IIR). (From Ref. 68.)

a mutation into the murine *WT1* tumor suppressor gene by means of gene targeting in embryonic stem cells is lethal in homozygotes and reveals a failure of kidney development (75).

It is possible that the zinc-finger protein encoded by the Wilms' tumor locus regulates the pattern of growth factor expression involved in kidney organogenesis. It is well documented that Wilms' tumor tissue expresses high levels of IGF II (76,77). IGF II mRNA has been localized to the most primative tumor cells. Adjacent relatively differentiated epithelial cells show a relative absence of expression (78). Recently, it has been shown that the WT1 protein effects transcriptional repression of the IGF II gene (79). Receptors for IGF I are found in Wilms' tumors (80). Antibodies to the IGF I receptor inhibit the growth of Wilms' tumor both in vitro and of tumors transplanted to athymic mice consistent with a role for IGF I in oncogenesis (81). In view of the role that IGF I and IGF II of metanephric origin play in metanephrogenesis, derangements of their expression could result in neoplastic transformation of the metanephric blastema.

THE KIDNEY IN GENETIC MODELS OF IGF EXCESS AND DEFICIENCY

Mice transgenic for IGF I develop nephromegaly. Glomerular enlargement occurs in these animals. However, it is of interest that mice transgenic for IGF I with levels of circulating IGF I no different than those in mice transgenic for GH do not develop glomerulosclerosis (82,83). This finding is consistent with the glomerulosclerotic action of GH in rodents being mediated via a mechanism other than its action to increase the synthesis and release of IGF I.

Mice homozygous for deletion of the IGF II gene are dwarfed at birth but normally developed. It is proposed that IGF II is an indispensable participant in some early crucial proliferation events but that subsequent growth becomes IGF II-independent. However, such a proposal cannot account for the pattern of IGF II expression during embryogenesis that implies a role in organogenesis. Accordingly it is suggested that there may be overlap or compensation of IGF II function by other gene products affecting growth (84).

SUMMARY AND CONCLUSIONS

It is clear that kidney is an important site for expression of all components of IGF activity, IGF peptides, receptors, and binding proteins. IGFs play important roles in kidney development, regulate metabolic events in mature kidney, and are likely to be involved in processes of renal growth and repair following renal injury. It should be noted that an extensive literature has accumulated relating to the expression of a number of growth factors in kidney in addition to IGF (85). Clearly it is important to gain an understanding of the interplay between these agents in order to fully comprehend the specific functions of IGFs.

ACKNOWLEDGMENTS

We acknowledge the administrative assistance of Ms. Lynn Wesselmann. S. B. Miller was supported by a Clinician Scientist Award from the American Heart Association and by grant DK-45181 from the NIH. M. R. Hammerman was supported by grants DK-27600, DK-45181, and DK-20579 from the NIH and by Grant-in-Aid 91006660 from the American Heart Association.

REFERENCES

1. Rotwein P. Structure, evolution, expression and regulation of insulin-like growth factors I and II. Growth Factors 1991; 5:3–18.
2. Rotwein P, Bichell DP, Kikuchi K. Multifactorial regulation of IGF-I gene expression. Mol Reprod Dev 1993; 35:358–364.
3. LeRoith D, Kavsan VM, Koval AP, Roberts CT Jr. Phylogeny of the insulin-like growth factors (IGFs) and receptors: A molecular approach. Mol Reprod Dev 1993; 35:332–338.

4. Clemmons DR. Structure and functional analysis of insulin-like growth factors. Br Med Bull 1989; 45:465–480.
5. Shemer J, Adamo ML, Roberts CT Jr, LeRoith D. Tissue-specific transcription start site usage in the leader exons of the rat insulin-like growth factor-I gene: Evidence for differential regulation in the developing kidney. Endocrinology 1992; 131:2793–2799.
6. Chin E, Bondy C. Insulin-like growth factor system gene expression in the human kidney. J Clin Endocrinol Metab 1992; 75:962–968.
7. Han VKM, Hill DJ, Strain AJ, et al. Identification of somatomedin/insulin-like growth factor immunoreactive cells in the human fetus. Pediatr Res 1987; 22:245–247.
8. Hill DJ, Clemmons DR, Wilson S, et al. Immunological distribution of one form of insulin-like growth factor (IGF)-binding protein and IGF peptides in human fetal tissues. J Mol Endocrinol 1989; 2:31–38.
9. Han VKM, Lund PK, Lee DC, D'Ercole AJ. Expression of somatomedin/insulin-like growth factor messenger ribonucleic acids in the human fetus: Identification, characterization, and tissue distribution. J Clin Endocrinol Metab 1988; 66:422–429.
10. Bell GI, Gerhard DS, Fong NM, et al. Isolation of the human insulin-like growth factor genes: Insulin-like growth factor II and insulin genes are contiguous. Proc Natl Acad Sci USA 1985; 82:6450–6454.
11. Aron DC, Rosenzweig JL, Abboud HE. Synthesis and binding of insulin-like growth factor I by human glomerular mesangial cells. J Clin Endocrinol Metab 1989; 68:585–591.
12. Bortz JD, Rotwein P, DeVol D, et al. Focal expression of insulin-like growth factor I in rat kidney collecting duct. J Cell Biol 1988; 107:811–819.
13. Anderson GL, Skottner A, Jennische E. Immunocytochemical and biochemical localization of insulin-like growth factor I in the kidney of rats before and after uninephrectomy. Acta Endocrinol 1988; 119:555–560.
14. Hansson HA, Nilsson A, Isgaard J, et al. Immunohistochemical localization of insulin-like growth factor I in the adult rat. Histochemistry 1988; 89:403–410.
15. Kobayashi S, Clemmons DR, Venkatachalam MA. Colocalization of insulin-like growth factor-binding protein with insulin-like growth factor I. Am J Physiol 1991; 261:F22–F28.
16. Matejka GL, Eriksson PE, Carlsson B, Jennische E. Distribution of IGF-I mRNA and IGF-I binding sites in the rat kidney. Histochemistry 1992; 97:173–180.
17. Chin E, Zhou J, Bondy C. Anatomical relationships in the patterns of insulin-like growth factor (IGF)-I, IGF binding protein-1, and IGF-I receptor gene expression in the rat kidney. Endocrinology 1992; 130:3237–3245.
18. Rogers SA, Miller SB, Hammerman MR. Growth hormone stimulates IGF I gene expression in isolated rat renal collecting duct. Am J Physiol 1990; 259:F474–F479.
19. Aron DC, Saadi HF, Nye CN, Douglas JG. Secretion of insulin-like growth factor I and its binding proteins by collecting duct cells. Kidney Int 1991; 39:27–32.
20. Conti FG, Striker LJ, Elliot SJ, et al. Synthesis and release of insulin like growth factor I by mesangial cells in culture. Am J Physiol 1988; 255:F1214–F1219.
21. Anderson G, Jennische E. IGF-I immunoreactivity is expressed by regenerating renal tubular cells after ischaemic injury in the rat. Acta Physiol Scand 1988; 132:453–457.
22. Matejka GL, Jennische E. IGF-I binding and IGF mRNA expression in the post-ischemic regenerating rat kidney. Kidney Int 1992; 42:1113–1123.
23. Rogers SA, Miller SB, Hammerman MR. IGF I gene expression in isolated rat renal collecting duct is stimulated by epidermal growth factor. J Clin Invest 1991; 87:347–351.
24. Clemmons DR. Multiple hormones stimulate the production of somatomedin by cultured human fibroblasts. J Clin Endocrinol Metab 1984; 58:850–856.
25. Barreca A, Voci A, Minuto F, et al. Effect of epidermal growth factor on insulin-like factor-I (IGF-I) and IGF-binding protein synthesis by adult rat hepatocytes. Mol Cell Endocrinol 1992; 84:119–126.
26. Fisher DA, Salido EC, Barajas L. Epidermal growth factor and the kidney. Annu Rev Physiol 1989; 51:67–80.
27. Jennische E, Anderson G, Hansson HA. Epidermal growth factor is expressed by cells in the distal tubules during postnephrectomy renal growth. Acta Physiol Scand 1987; 129:449–450.
28. Lajara R, Rotwein P, Bortz JD, et al. Dual regulation of insulin-like factor I expression during renal hypertrophy. Am J Physiol 1989; 257:F252–F261.
29. Miller SB, Rogers SA, Estes CE, Hammerman MR. Increased distal nephron EGF content and altered distribution of peptide in compensatory renal hypertrophy. Am J Physiol 1992; 262:F1032–F1038.
30. Bach LA, Jerums G. Effect of puberty on initial kidney growth and rise in kidney IGF-I in diabetic rats. Diabetes 1990; 39:557–562.
31. Bach LA, Stevenson JL, Allen TJ, et al. Kidney insulin-like growth factor-I mRNA levels are increased in postpubertal diabetic rats. J Endocrinol 1991; 129:5–10.
32. Catanese VM, Sciavolino PJ, Lango MN. Discordant, organ-specific regulation of insulin-like growth factor-I messenger ribonucleic acid in insulin-deficient diabetes in rats. Endocrinology 1993; 132:496–503.

33. Flyvbjerg A, Thorlacius-Ussing O, Nearaa R, et al. Kidney tissue somatomedin C and initial renal growth in diabetic and uninephrectomised rats. Diabetologia 1988; 31:310–314.
34. Flyvbjerg A, Bornfeldt KE, Marshall SM, et al. Kidney IGF-I mRNA in initia renal hypertrophy in experimental diabetes in rats. Diabetologia 1990; 33:334–338.
35. Flyvbjerg A, Jorgensen KD, Marshall SM, Orskov H. Inhibitory effect of octreotide on growth hormone-induced IGF-I generation and organ growth in hypophysectomized rats. Am J Physiol 1991; 260:E568–E574.
36. Flyvbjerg A, Kessler U, Dorka B, et al. Transient increase in renal insulin-like growth factor binding proteins during initial kidney hypertrophy in experimental diabetes in rats. Diabetologia 1992; 35:589–593.
37. Flyvbjerg A, Frystyk J, Thorlacius-Ussing O. Somatostatin analogue administration prevents increase in kidney somatomedin C and initial renal growth in diabetic and uninephrectomized rats. Diabetologia 1989; 32:261–265.
38. Rogers SA, Miller SB, Hammerman MR. Enhanced renal IGF I expression following partial kidney infarction. Am J Physiol 1993; 264:F963–F967.
39. Lowe WL Jr, Adamo M, Werner H, et al. Regulation by fasting of rat insulin-like growth factor I and its receptor. J Clin Invest 1989; 84:619–626.
40. Kobayashi S, Venkatachalam MA. Differential effects of calorie restriction on glomeruli and tubules of the remnant kidney. Kidney Int 1992; 42:710–717.
41. O'Shea MH, Layish DT. Growth hormone and the kidney: A case presentation and review of the literature. J Am Soc Nephrol 1992; 3:157–161.
42. Fine L. The biology of renal hypertrophy. Kidney Int 1986; 29:619–634.
43. Schwieger J, Fine LG. Renal hypertrophy, growth factors, and nephropathy in diabetes mellitus. Semin Nephrol 1990; 10:242–253.
44. Fagin JA, Melmed S. Relative increase in insulin-like growth factor I messenger ribonucleic acid levels in compensatory renal hypertrophy. Endocrinology 1987; 120:718–723.
45. Stiles AD, Sosenko IRS, D'Ercole AJ, Smith BT. Reaction of kidney tissue somatomedin-C/Insulin-like growth factor I to postnephrectomy renal growth in the rat. Endocrinology 1985; 117:2397–2401.
46. Hammerman MR, Miller SB. The growth hormone insulin-like growth factor axis in kidney revisted. Am J Physiol 1993; 265:F1–F14.
47. Clemmons DR. IGF binding proteins and their functions. Mol Reprod Dev 1993; 35:368–375.
48. Ruoslahti E, Pierschbacher MD. New perspectives in cell adhesion: RGD and integrins. Science 1987; 238:491–497.
49. Ooi GT, Orlowski CC, Brown AL, et al. Different tissue distribution and hormonal regulation of messenger RNAs encoding rat insulin-like growth factor-binding proteins-1 and -2. Mol Endocrinol 4:321–328.
50. Brown AL, Chiariotti L, Orlowski CC, et al. Nucleotide sequence and expression of a cDNA clone encoding a fetal rat binding protein for insulin-like growth factors. J Biol Chem 1989; 264:5148–5154.
51. Suikkari AM, Leivo I, Kamarainen M, et al. Expression of insulin-like growth factor binding protein-1 mRNA in human fetal kidney. Kidney Int 1992; 42:749–754.
52. Orlowski CC, Brown AL, Ooi GT, et al. Tissue, development, and metabolic regulation of messenger ribonucleic acid encoding a rat insulin-like growth factor-binding protein. Endocrinology 1990; 126:644–652.
53. Albiston AL, Herington AC. Tissue distribution and regulation of insulin-like growth factor (IGF)-binding protein-3 messenger ribonucleic acid (mRNA) in the rat: Comparison with IGF-I mRNA expression. Endocrinology 1992; 130:497–502.
54. Sara VR, Hall K. Insulin-like growth factors and their binding proteins. Physiol Rev 1990; 70:591–614.
55. Shimasaki S, Shimonaka M, Zhang HP, Ling N. Identification of five different insulin-like growth factor binding proteins (IGFBPs) from adult rat serum and molecular cloning of a novel IGFBP-5 in rat and human. J Biol Chem 1991; 266:10646–10653.
56. Pessin JE, Frattali AL. Molecular dynamics of insulin/IGF-I receptor transmembrane signaling. Mol Reprod Dev 1993; 35:339–345.
57. Hammerman MR. The growth hormone-insulin-like growth factor axis in kidney. Am J Physiol 1989; 257:F503–F514.
58. Nishimoto I. The IGF-II Receptor system: A G protein-linked mechanism. Mol Reprod Dev 1993; 35:339–345.
59. Hammerman MR, Rogers SA. Distribution of IGF receptors in the plasma membrane of the proximal tubular cell. Am J Physiol 1987; 253:F841–F847.
60. Pillion DJ, Haskell JF, Meezan E. Distinct receptors for insulin-like growth factor I in rat renal glomeruli and tubules. Am J Physiol 1988; 255:E504–E512.
61. Rogers SA, Karl IE, Hammerman MR. Growth hormone directly stimulates gluconeogenesis in canine renal proximal tubule. Am J Physiol 1989; 257:E751–E756.
62. Quigley R, Baum M. Effects of growth hormone and insulin-like growth factor I on rabbit proximal convoluted tubule transport. J Clin Invest 1991; 88:368–374.

63. Saxen L. Organogenesis of the Kidney. Cambridge, England: Cambridge University Press, 1987.
64. Avner E. Polypeptide growth factors and the kidney: A developmental perspective. Pediatr Nephrol 1990; 4:345–353.
65. Hammerman MR, Rogers SA, Ryan G. Growth factors and metanephrogenesis. Am J Physiol 1992; 262:F523–F532.
66. Avner ED, Sweeney WE Jr, Ellis D. Serum-free organ culture of embryonic mouse metanephros. In: Sirbasku DA, Barnes DW, Sato GH, eds. Methods of Serum-Free Culture of Epithelial and Fibroblastic Cells. New York: Liss, 1984:33–41.
67. Brenner BM. Determinants of epithelial differentiation during early nephrogenesis. J Am Soc Nephrol 1990; 1:127–139.
68. Rogers SA, Ryan G, Hammerman MR. Insulin-like growth factors I and II are produced in the metanephros and are required for growth and development in vitro. J Cell Biol 1991; 113:1447–1453.
69. Hammerman MR, Gavin JR III. Binding of insulin-like growth factor II and multiplication-stimulating activity-stimulated phosphorylation in basolateral membranes from dog kidney. J Biol Chem 1984; 259:13511–13517.
70. Murphy GP, Kawinski E, Horoszewicz JS. Cell cultures derived from Wilms' tumour animal model. Cancer Res 1987; 6:717–720.
71. Gessler M, Poustka A, Cavenee W, et al. Homozygous deletion in Wilms tumours of a zinc finger gene identified by chromosome jumping. Nature 1990; 343:774–775.
72. Huang A, Campbell CE, Bonetta L, et al. Tissue, developmental, and tumor-specific expression of divergent transcripts in Wilms' tumor. Science 1990; 250:991–992.
73. Madden SL, Cook DM, Morris JF, et al. Transcriptional repression mediated by the WT1 Wilms tumor gene product. Science 1991; 253:1550–1553.
74. Pritchard-Jones K, Fleming S, Davidson D, et al. The candidate Wilms' tumour gene is involved in genitourinary development. Nature 1990; 346:194–197.
75. Kreidberg JA, Sariola, H, Lorin ˎ JM, et al. WT-1 is required for early kidney development. Cell 1993; 74:679–691.
76. Haselbacher GK, Irminger JC, Zapf J, et al. Insulin-like growth factor II in human adrenal pheochromocytomas and Wilms' tumors: Expression at the mRNA and protein level. Proc Natl Acad Sci USA 1987; 84:1104–1106.
77. Scott J, Cowell J, Robertson ME, et al. Insulin-like growth factor-II gene expression in Wilms' tumour and embryonic tissues. Nature 1985; 317:260–262.
78. Hirvonen H, Sandberg M, Kalimo H, et al. The N-myc proto-oncogene and IGF II growth factor mRNAs are expressed by distinct cells in human fetal kidney and brain. J Cell Biol 1989; 108:1093–1104.
79. Drummond, IA, Madden, SL, Rohwer-Nutter, P, et al. Repression of the insulin-like growth factor II gene by the Wilms' tumor supressor WT1. Science 1992; 257:674–678.
80. Gansler T, Allen KD, Burant CF, et al. Detection of type I insulinlike growth factor (IGF) receptors in Wilms' tumors. Am J Pathol 1988; 130:431–435.
81. Gansler T, Furlanetto R, Gramling TS, et al. Antibody to type I insulinlike growth factor receptor inhibits growth of Wilms' tumor in culture and in athymic mice. Am J Pathol 1989; 135:961–966.
82. Doi T, Striker LJ, Gibson CC, et al. Glomerular lesions in mice transgenic for growth hormone and insulinlike growth factor-I. Am J Pathol 11990; 37:541–552.
83. Quaife CJ, Mathews, LS, Pinkert CA, et al. Histopathology associated with elevated levels of growth hormone and insulin-like growth factor I in transgenic mice. Endocrinology 1989; 124:40–48.
84. DeChiara TM, Robertson EJ, Efstratiadis A. Parental imprinting of the mouse insulin-like growth factor II gene. Cell 1991; 64:849–859.
85. Hammerman, MR, O'Shea, M, Miller, SB. Role of growth factors in regulation of renal growth. Annu Rev Physiol 1993; 55:305–321.

40

Cell Biology of Platelet-Derived Growth Factor

Hanna E. Abboud, Basant Bhandari, and Goutam Ghosh Choudhury
The University of Texas Health Science Center at San Antonio and Audie L. Murphy Department of Veterans Affairs Hospital, San Antonio, Texas

INTRODUCTION

Platelet-derived growth factor (PDGF) is one of many pleiotropic peptide mediators, referred to collectively as cytokines. Cytokines have the potential to mediate many biological responses of cells and tissue including renal glomerular, vascular, and interstitial cells (1–3). Cytokines including PDGF possess diverse biological properties highly relevant to renal pathology (4–6). Biological effects of PDGF include promotion of hypertrophy and proliferation, regulation of matrix metabolism, vasoactive properties, regulation of immune-inflammatory responses such as chemotaxis, activation or deactivation of inflammatory cells, and a role in development and differentiation (2,3). The physiological role of PDGF in the adult kidney is not known, but upregulation or overexpression of PDGF or its receptor(s) plays a role in kidney development and has pathogenic consequences in the injured kidney (2,3,7). Whether PDGF plays a constructive role in tissue remodeling that follows renal injury remains to be proven.

Extensive literature has been published in the field of PDGF biology (4,5,8–10). The role of PDGF in renal disease is discussed in an accompanying chapter by Johnson et al. In this review, we focus on the cellular and molecular mechanisms of PDGF synthesis and actions and explore its role in renal cell biology.

BIOSYNTHESIS AND RELEASE

Biologically active PDGF is a disulfide-linked dimer composed of two polypeptides designated A and B chains (5,9). The two peptide chains share 60% homology in their amino acid sequence and are encoded by two separate genes (5,11). The initial observation that PDGF-B chain was almost identical to a part of *p28 sis*, the transforming protein of simian sarcoma virus (SSV), provided the first link between growth factors and oncogenes and suggested a mechanism whereby oncogene products are involved in cell transformation and growth (10,11). PDGF exists as a heterodimer, PDGF AB, or as homodimers, PDGF-AA and PDGF-BB. Among several peptide growth factors, PDGF stands out as the most potent mitogen for mesenchymal cells. All three PDGF isoforms, promote mitogenesis in the appropriate target cells (4,5). While PDGF is biologically active as a dimer, the interchain disulfide bonds do not seem to be critical for the mitogenic effect of PDGF (12).

PDGF was first purified from human platelets by several groups (13–16) using routine chromatographic techniques that could not separate its two constituent chains. However, the introduction of high-resolution reversed-phase HPLC allowed the separation of the two chains, which were termed A and B, according to the order of their elution (17). The PDGF chains are synthesized as precursor molecules with signal sequences. The mature molecules are formed after N- and C-terminal processing (18–22). The relative expression of PDGF chains is cell-specific, with most cells expressing both chains and some cells expressing either of the two chains. PDGF purified from platelets is predominately AB heterodimer, with small percentages of BB and AA homodimers (21). The PDGF isoform secreted by renal cells have not been adequately characterized, although mesangial cells release predominantly AA homodimers while human microvascular endothelial cells secrete BB homodimer, based on predominance of the PDGF chain expressed and ligand displacement data (3,23,24). Studies in CHO cells overexpressing the two chains indicate that assembly of the two monomers into three different isoforms is a random process (i.e., dictated by the concentration of each chain) (18–22). There is good evidence for compartmentalization of PDGF homodimers. In SSV transformed cells, PDGF-BB remains cell-associated and undergoes proteolytic processing to a 24-kDa form (25,26). The retention is dependent on a stretch of amino acids in the C-terminal part of the B chain. The A chain occurs in two spliced variants. The long A chain, which also contains a motif similar to that present in the B chain, is retained, whereas the short variant of the A chain is secreted (25–27). Rains et al. (28) and Kelly et al. (29), recently reported that this sequence may also mediate interaction with heparan sulfate proteoglycans of the connective tissue matrix. Precise localization of PDGF in situ in kidney tissue and blood vessel wall may reveal interesting qualitative and quantitative distribution relevant to glomerulointerstitial pathology and pathobiology of the vessel wall.

REGULATION OF PDGF GENES

In spite of various studies related to genes of the PDGF-A and PDGF-B chains, only recently have mechanisms of their transcriptional regulation been explored. The *cis*-acting DNA elements that control transcription are yet to be fully identified and characterized. PDGF-A chain (27,30,31,37) and PDGF-B chain gene (32–36) are cloned and their gene structure is known. The PDGF-A and PDGF-B chain genes are located on human chromosomes 7 and 22 respectively (5,11). Both genes contain 7 exons and are approximately 22 to 24 kb in size (5,10). The 5′-flanking region of the PDGF-A chain gene promoter is shown in Figure 1. A "TATA box" but not "CAAT" box has been located at –31 nt from the transcription initiation site (+1). This transcription initiation site is 845 nt upstream from the translation initiation site (37). It is interesting to note that the promoter contains a "GC-rich" region, which expands from –1 to –92 nt. Sequence analysis of the A-chain promoter revealed putative binding sites for several transcription factors including *NGFIA*, *Krox 24*, *Zif268*, *Tis 8*, *Egr-1*, and *SP-1*. Wang et al. (38) performed S1-nuclease analysis of the PDGF-A chain promoter to localize possible binding sites that regulate transcription and observed two S1 nuclease-hypersensitive regions. These sites are found within the GC-rich region (38,39). Furthermore, it has been shown that the S1 nuclease-sensitive site is DNA-strand specific and is thus likely to play an important role in the regulation of PDGF-A chain gene

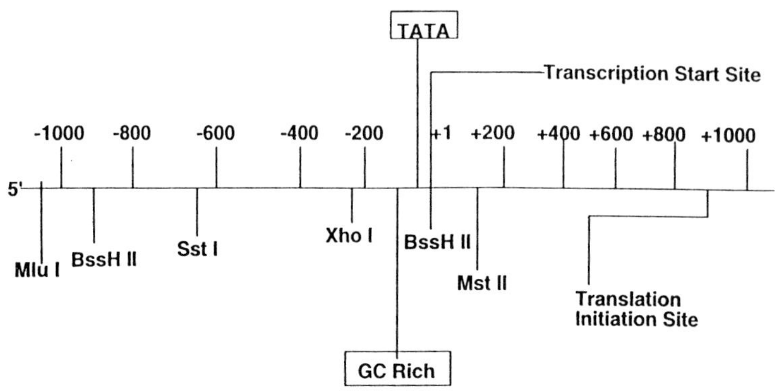

Figure 1 PDGF-A chain gene promoter. The 5′-flanking sequence of the PDGF-A chain promoter and the position of TATA box and GC-rich region is shown. Early growth response elements (EGR) and SP-1 binding sites are also present in this GC-rich region. Location of transcription start site and translation initiation site is marked.

transcription. PDGF-A chain promoter/CAT reporter fusion gene constructs have been used to identify regions of functional importance. A region that expands from –618 to +392 nt is necessary for maximum PDGF-A chain promoter activity (40). It is interesting to note that more than 80% of this activity is localized within GC-rich region that also contains three SP-1 binding sites (37–41). Furthermore, the GC-rich region is protected by DNase I digestion and is thus the binding site for transcription factors including SP-1 (40). The transcriptional control of PDGF-A chain promoter by S1-hypersensitive sequences have been confirmed using gel mobility shift analyses. Nuclear extracts prepared from human embryonal rhabdomyoscarcoma cells exhibited a nuclear protein/DNA complex in gel mobility shift assay when S1 hypersensitive region (–103 to –82) was used as a labeled DNA probe. The interaction of the protein/DNA complex likely involves a protein from the NF-κB family (39). Using other S1 hypersensitive regions (–74 to –51) in gel mobility shift assay, Wang et al. observed two different DNA/protein complexes, one of which competes with transcription factor SP-1 (39). In addition, another S1-nuclease–sensitive region +50 to +67 and –482 to –513, corresponding to the binding site for early growth response gene 1 (*Egr-1*) and enhancer, is located in the promoter region of the PDGF-A chain gene (41). A serum-responsive element located at –477 to –468 nt has also been identified in the PDGF-A chain promoter region, and it has been demonstrated that PDGF stimulates PDGF-A chain gene transcription via this element (40). A region (–98 to –49) that participates in the repressive effect of Wilms' tumor suppressor WT1 on PDGFA chain gene transcription has been demonstrated by DNase I footprint analysis (42). We have analyzed the 5′-flanking region of the PDGF-A chain promoter. Using DNA footprint analysis, we identified a region (–82 to –102) that is likely involved in the regulation of the PDGF-A chain gene (43). It is interesting to note that one of the S1 nuclease-sensitive sites demonstrated by Wang et al. is within the region identified by DNase I footprint analysis in our work (43). Thus nuclear extracts from human renal mesangial cells contain a protein (PDGF-A-BP-1) which binds to the promoter region (–82 to –102 nt) of the PDGF-A chain. We have further shown by gel mobility analysis that this nuclear protein, PDGF-A-BP-1 is a novel protein that is robustly induced by PMA (>20-fold). PDGF-A-BP-1 has homology with sequences that bind *SP1* and *Egr-1*; however, gel mobility competition data indicate that PDGF-A-BP-1 is neither SP-1 nor Egr-1. A summary of the various *cis-* and *trans*-acting factors located in the promoter regions of the PDGF-A chain gene is shown in Figure 2.

The 5′-flanking region of the PDGF-B chain gene is cloned and sequenced (5,10,32–35,44,45). The structure of this gene is shown in Figure 3. "TATA" box is located very close to the 5′ of the first exon; however, its location has been reported differently from RNA initiation site, namely –10 to –7 nt (34) and at –24 to –19 nt (44). A GC-rich region is present 80 nt upstream of the transcription start site (45). The presence of GC-rich nucleotides indicates a secondary structure. There are four ATG initiation codons, and it is speculated that translation starts at the fourth codon (45). Exon 1 of the PDGF-B chain contains 1026 bp (34) or 1022 bp (44) of 5′ untranslated sequences. In addition, a 1625-bp untranslated region has been located at 3′ of the coding region. The regions in the 5′-untranslated portion inhibit translation (45). It was shown that deletion of the 5′ untranslated region reduced the expression of the protein by at least 40-fold (46). In addition, the 5′ untranslated sequences have been shown to lower the transforming efficiency of the PDGF-B chain gene (46). A PMA-inducible element has been demonstrated by functional analysis of PDGF-B chain promoter at the location –140 to –350 nt from transcription-start site in K562 cells (47). However, this region is not effective using in vivo studies for PDGF-B chain mRNA expression (48). It is interesting to note that a PMA-responsive element responsible for PMA-mediated induction of PDGF-B chain transcription in K562 cells is located at –58 to –39 nt (49). Analysis of the PDGF-B chain promoter revealed a DNase I-hypersensitive site located at –90 to +60 from transcription start site in carcinoma-derived HeLa, T_{24}, and PC3 cell lines but not in cytotropholast-derived cell lines JEG-3, JAR, Hufi, as well as in myeloid leukemia cells K562 (49). Similar experiments in exon 1 region of the PDGF-B chain promoter indicated various cell-specific DNase I hypersensitive sites whereas functional analysis indicated negative regulatory elements in intron 1 (48,50). More recently a shear-stress responsive element at –125 to –120 nt in the PDGF-B chain promoter region has been identified (51). Comparison of the PDGF-B chain promoter sequence with several known transcription factor binding sites reveals similarities that are summarized in Figure 3. It is likely that these putative elements have a potential to regulate PDGF-B chain gene transcription.

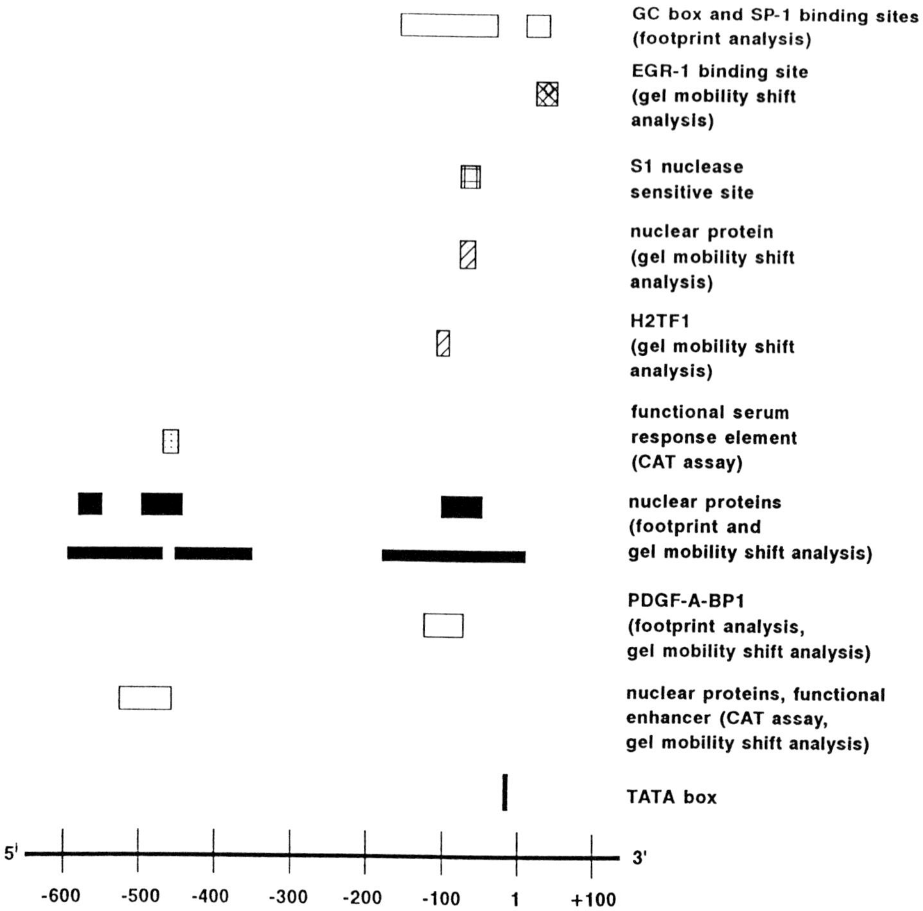

Figure 2 Summary of the *cis*-elements and *trans*-acting factors in PDGF-A chain promoter. The figure summarizes location of various *cis*-elements and *trans*-acting factors identified by gel mobility shift assays, DNA-footprint analysis, S1 nuclease analysis and chloramphenicol acetyl transferase (CAT assays). Positions of TATA and GC-box are also marked. Numbers represent nucleotide positions relative to the transcription start site.

REGULATION OF PDGF GENES IN RENAL CELLS

The factors that regulate PDGFA and B chain genes and their mechanism of action have been studied in several hematopoietic cell lines, other immortalized as well as tumor cells. In the kidney, PDGF gene regulation has been best studied in mesangial and microvascular endothelial cells (52–58) (Table 1). Immortalized monkey kidney epithelial cells of the BSC-1 line also express PDGF (59).

Three PDGF-A chain mRNA transcripts 1.9, 2.3 and 2.8 kb are expressed in most cells including mesangial cells (5–8,52–58). The size of PDGF-B chain mRNA transcript is 3.5 kb to 4.2 kb although smaller size transcripts can be expressed (3,5,6,59–63). The heterogeneity in size of the A chain mRNA is due to use of three polyadenylation signals and transcription from two different promoters. The smaller B chain mRNA transcript is also due to transcription from a different promoter (3,5). Human as well as rat mesangial cells release PDGF and express PDGF-A and PDGF-B mRNAs. The effect of several polypeptide mitogens on DNA synthesis, regulation of PDGF mRNAs and PDGF protein release in human mesangial and microvascular endothelial cells have been investigated (52–68). Growth factors including serum regulate the steady-state levels of PDGF-A and PDGF-B

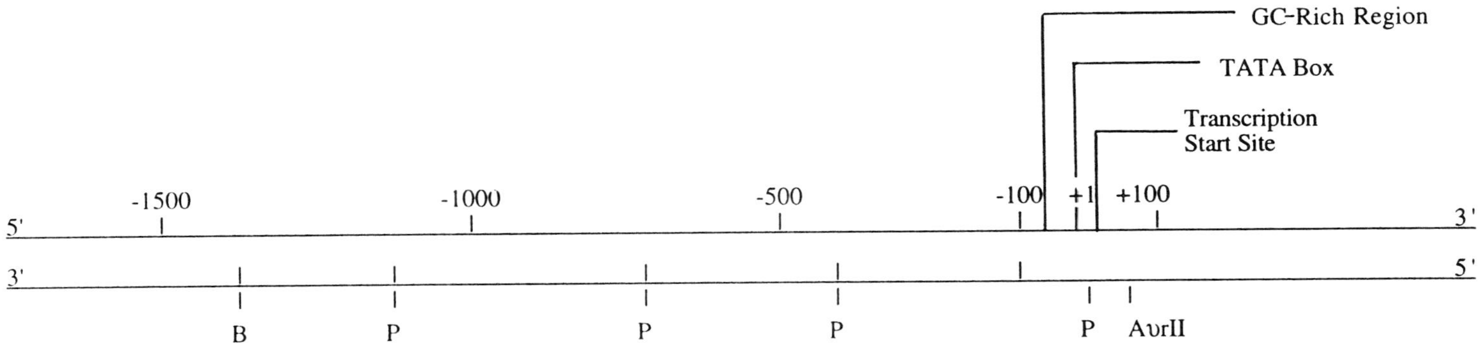

Number of putative binding sites for					
AP-1	1	4	2	3	-
AP-2	-	-	-	2	1
SP-1	-	1	-	2	4
EGR-1	-	-	-	-	4
Dexamethasone	-	10	2	6	3
MYB	3	5	4	2	4

Figure 3 Putatived DNA-binding sites in PDGF-B chain promoter. The 5′-flanking region of the PDGF-B chain promoter and the position of the transcription starting site, box, and GC-rich region is shown. Restriction sites Bam HI (B), PST I (P), and Avr II are also marked. The number of various putative DNA-binding sites in PDGF-B chain-promoter region is marked.

Table 1 Factors That Regulate PDGF Expression

Positive regulation
Cytokines: Platelet-derived growth factor (PDGF), epidermal growth factor (EGF), fibroblast growth factor (FGF), tumor necrosis factor (TNF), transforming growth factor beta (TGFβ), interleukin-1 (IL-1).
Lipids: Phosphatidic acid (PA), phosphatidyl serine (PS), low-density lipoprotein (LDL), very low density lipoprotein (VLDL), phorbal myrystate acetate (PMA).
Vasoactive hormones: Ang II, endothelin, thrombin.
Hemodynamics and other factors: shear stress, hypoxia.
Immune mediators: Immune complexes, membrane attack complex.
Negative regulation
Adenylate cyclase agonists and cAMP analogues (e.g., isoproterenol, prostacyclin, PGE_1 and analogues).
Phosphodiesterase inhibitors, glucocorticoids.

chain mRNAs and stimulate the release of PDGF (52–58). Autoinduction of PDGF and PDGF receptor (PDGFR) mRNAs occurs in response to PDGF (61–62). Cyclic AMP analogues and agents such as forskolin, which elevate the levels of cyclic AMP, have been shown to block PDGF-A and B chain mRNA induction in response to cytokines (66). Data in mesangial, smooth muscle cells and fibroblasts strongly suggest that PDGF and its product(s) constitute an important early signal common to several polypeptide growth factors and that PDGF acts in an autocrine mechanism to stimulate DNA synthesis (61,62).

Gene transcription is one of the molecular mechanisms that regulates mRNA abundance (66–74). PMA and PDGF BB or AB increase PDGF-A and PDGF-B chain gene transcription in human renal mesangial cells (71–73). These data are in contrast to those reported for microvascular endothelial cells where PMA increases mRNA levels, but does not stimulate PDGF-A chain gene transcription (67). TGF-β but not thrombin stimulates PDGF-A chain gene transcription in microvascular endothelial cells (67). In endothelial cells, human glioblastoma and in stem cell line K-562, it has been shown that the increased expression of PDGF-B chain in response to PMA, thrombin and TGF-β is at least in part due to gene transcription (63–68,69,74).

In mammalian cells, transcription as well as posttranscriptional mechanisms regulate mRNA levels (75,76). We measured the half-life of PDGF-A chain and PDGF-B chain mRNAs in response to PMA as well as PDGF BB homodimer in human renal mesangial cells. mRNA degradation was measured directly by using the pulse-chase approach. This method excludes RNA synthesis inhibitors, which are known to alter the rate of synthesis of mRNAs. The half-life of PDGF-A or PDGF-B chain mRNA is approximately 100 min in renal mesangial cells (71–73). PMA destabilizes PDGF-A or PDGF-B chain mRNA by 30% whereas PDGF-BB homodimer increases the PDGF-B chain mRNA half-life to 156 min (Table 2). It is of interest to note that mRNA degradation in different cell types as measured by methods using inhibitors varies considerably for both PDGF-A chain (102 to 240 min) or PDGF-B chain (40 to 204 min). Certain specific sequences at the 5′ and 3′ end of mRNA influence its degradation. An A-U rich region located near 3′-end in various genes is known to affect mRNA half-life (76). Comparison of PDGF-A and PDGF-B chain sequences revealed that A-U rich region is present only in PDGF-B chain sequence. The PDGF-A and PDGF-B chain mRNA half-lives are similar in human renal mesangial cells as well as in human umbilical vein endothelial cells (Table 2) suggesting that there are factors other than A-U regions which affect mRNA half-life.

PDGF RECEPTORS AND SIGNALING

The relative distribution of PDGF receptors on responsive cells is a major determinant of the biological role of specific PDGF isoforms. Two distinct types of PDGF receptors have been cloned and characterized (77–82). More recently a soluble form of the PDGF receptor has been identified (83). The signals transduced by both receptors and the biological effects are very similar. However, cell surface actin reorganization or “ruffling” is mediated solely by the β receptor (5). Identification of PDGFRs was reported as early as 1981 (84). PDGF binding to cells induced receptor internalization and down regulation (85). PDGFR stimulation follows activation of its intrinsic tyrosine kinase

Table 2 PDGF-A and PDGF-B Chain mRNA Half-Life[a]

Cell type		PDGF-A mRNA (min)	PDGF-B mRNA (min)
Human renal mesangial	Untreated	101–106	102
	PMA	74	72
	PDGF BB	111	156
Human umbilical vein endothelial	Untreated	144–168	96–108
	HBGF-1	144–150	90–108
	proliferating	102–126	84–90
Rat aortic smooth muscle	Untreated	240	40–50
Human renal microvascular endothelial	Untreated	—	70–90
Human glioma	Untreated	—	60–90
Human glioblastoma A172 and A2781	Untreated	—	156–204
	PMA	—	138
	TGF-B	—	198
Human T_{24} bladder carcinoma	Untreated	—	150

[a]See Refs. 69–73.

activity with phosphorylation of several substrate proteins in the cell. For molecular cloning, ligand-activated and tyrosine-phosphorylated PDGFR was purified from BALB/c 3T3 cells. Using degenerate oligonucleotides from proteolytically digested peptides of this receptor, the cDNA was cloned from cDNA libraries established from mouse placenta and cultured NR6 mouse fibroblasts (86). Analysis of translated cDNA revealed an open reading frame of 1098 amino acids with a 31–amino acid long signal sequence in its N terminus. The mature receptor protein has a 499–amino acid extracellular domain with a 25–amino acid transmembrane domain followed by a long 543–amino acid intracytoplasmic sequence. The extracellular domain of the PDGFR is cystein-rich and composed of five immunoglobulin-like loops. The cytoplasmic part of the receptor consists of a large tyrosine kinase domain interrupted by a sequence of about 100 amino acids. This sequence has been termed the kinase insert (KI) domain (89). A similar KI sequence of variable length is found in the tyrosine kinase domains of colony stimulating factor (CSFIR), fibroblast growth factor receptor (FGFR), and *c-kit* protein. Thus these transmembrane molecules constitute a class of receptor tyrosine kinases. The precise functional role of this KI sequence has not been elucidated; however, different substrate molecules of PDGFR have been shown to interact with this region. The more recent finding that different isoforms of PDGF are not equally mitogenic for fibroblasts lead to the identification of a second PDGFR (77–81). This new receptor termed PDGFRα interacts with both chains of PDGF isoforms, while the previously identified PDGFR was termed β. Both α and β receptors share structural features with 44% amino acid sequence homology. In vitro cross-linking experiments using PDGF BB with purified PDGFRβ indicated the formation of a receptor dimer (90). On the basis of the existing data, homo- and heterodimerization of PDGFR occurs. Thus PDGF BB can cause dimerization consisting of $\alpha\alpha$, $\alpha\beta$, and $\beta\beta$ subunits, whereas PDGF AA only interacts with $\alpha\alpha$ subunits. PDGF AB can bind to $\alpha\alpha$ or $\alpha\beta$ subunits. This ligand-induced receptor dimerization stimulates autophosphorylation of the receptor (91). Using kinase-defective PDGFRβ, in which the ATP binding site at lysine 635 was mutated to arginine (K635R), the ligand-induced autophosphorylation was shown to be intermolecular (92). The intrinsic tyrosine kinase activity of the receptor is an absolute requirement for all biological activities. Phospho-amino acid analysis of peptides derived from human PDGFRβ after ligand stimulation showed eight tyrosine phosphorylated sites. Two of these are in the juxtamembrane region of the receptor (Y579 and Y581). Three are in the KI sequence of the receptor (Y740, Y751, and Y771). One, the Y857, is in the second tyrosine kinase domain, whereas the other two are in the cytoplasmic tail downstream of the tyrosine kinase domain (93–97).

Activated PDGFR undergoes autophosphorylation at certain tyrosine residues, which serve as binding sites for several signaling proteins (Figure 4). These proteins contain an SH2 domain that physically interacts with tyrosine phosphorylated residues in the PDGFR. Some of these proteins possess enzymatic activities, while others act as adapter molecules (98). Addition of PDGF to cells stimulates phospholipase Cγl (PLCγl) which directly binds to the tyrosine phosphorylated PDGFR at 1009 and 1021 (96). Tyrosine phosphorylation of PLCγl is required for its enzymatic activity (99,100). Mutation of tyrosine residues which specifically bind PLCγl in the PDGFR results in loss of PI turnover as well as mitogenesis (101,102). Furthermore this complex formation between PDGFR and PLCγl may be permissive but not sufficient for cell growth. This conclusion was reached from the observation that mutation of tyrosine 825 in PDGFR does not stimulate mitogenesis, even though the receptor forms complexes with PLCγl and induces PI turnover (95,103). However, activation of PLCγl by PDGFR stimulates hydrolysis of PIP_2 to generate second messengers IP_3 and DAG. The former mobilizes Ca^{+2}, while both Ca^{+2} and DAG stimulate conventional PKCs (104).

The observation that the KI domain deletion mutant of PDGFR was not mitogenic suggested that this spacer sequence plays an important role in mitogenesis although this mutant receptor was capable of inducing PI turnover and Ca^{+2} transient (105). Subsequent experiments showed that this mutant receptor could not associate with an enzyme called phosphatidylinositol 3 kinase (PI 3 kinase) (105,107). This enzyme is a heterodimer of a 110-kDa catalytic subunit and 85-kDa regulatory subunit. The regulatory subunit consists of only SH2 and SH3 domains (108). It has been shown that the SH2 domain of PI 3 kinase binds to phosphorylated tyrosine 740 and 751 (95,102). Mutation

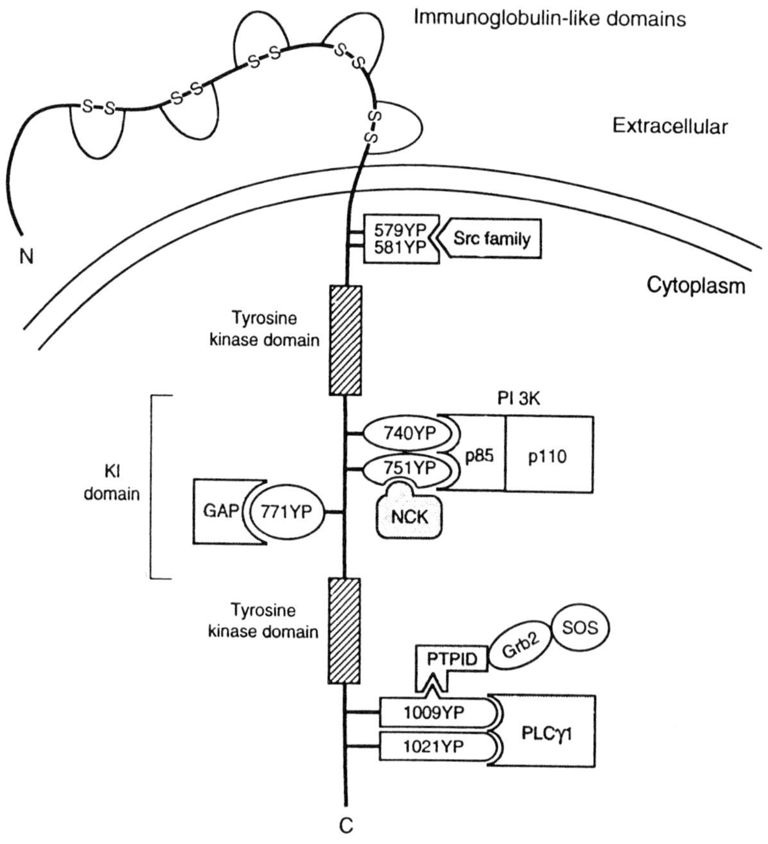

Figure 4 Structure of PDGF receptor. Extracellular domain consists of five immunoglobulin-like loops. Intracytoplasmic domain consists of juxtamembrane sequences, kinase domain split by kinase insert (KI) region, and C-terminal end. Phosphotyrosine residues responsible for binding to different signaling molecules are shown.

of these two tyrosines abolish the mitogenic potential of the PDGFR (95). Binding of the PI 3 kinase to the receptor activates its intrinsic lipid kinase activity to produce D3 phosphorylated inositides. Although the level of these phosphoinositides are very high in transformed cells, their precise biological functions in mitogenic signaling are not yet clear. However, an observation that the D3 phosphorylated inositide can stimulate the activity of the Ca^{2+} and DAG independent PKC ξ in vitro suggests that these may be the second messenger for this novel PKC (109). Using "add back" mutagenesis of an F5 mutant of PDGFR where the five autophosphorylation sites—Y740, 751, 771, 1009, and 1021—were mutated to phenylalanine, it has recently been shown that binding of PI 3 kinase to the PDGFR is necessary for its internalization (110). The receptor internalization and downregulation is thought to be a deactivation mechanism of those signals generated by the ligand binding. However, this is the first demonstration that a mitogenic signal transducer enzyme also plays an unequivocal role in receptor internalization. One of the other most important biological function of PDGF is its potent chemotactic activity. Using the same F5 mutant, Kundra et al. recently showed that association of both PLCγ1 and PI 3 kinase with activated PDGFR positively regulates the directed migration of cells towards PDGF BB (111).

PDGF also stimulates *p21ras* (112,113). This low-molecular-weight GTP binding protein is involved in producing mitogenic signals induced by PDGF, since microinjection of *Ras* antibodies blocks the mitogenic effect of PDGF (114). Addition of PDGF stimulates the conversion of RasGTP to the inactive RasGDP form. The GTPase activity of Ras protein is facilitated by another enzyme called GAP. This SH2 domain-containing molecule is tyrosine phosphorylated and physically associates with the KI region of PDGFR in response to PDGF (115–117). Mutation of Y771 of PDGFR showed that this is the binding site of GAP. GAP stimulates the RasGTPase activity after ligand stimulation to convert RasGTP to inactive RasGDP. Thus GAP is thought to be a negative regulator of Ras function. Using the same "add back" mutagenesis of F5 mutant receptor, it has recently been shown that along with positive regulation of both PLCY1 and PI 3 kinase, GAP negatively regulates the chemotactic property of the PDGFR (111). These data suggest that after ligand activation, PDGFR can recruit both migration-promoting and migration-suppressing activities to drive chemotaxis in response to PDGF BB.

Two other functionally opposite enzymes with SH2 domains are also associated with activated PDGFR. They are tyrosine kinases and tyrosine phosphatase. The former group includes $p60^{c\text{-}src}$, $p59^{fyn}$, and p62*c-yes* (118). Although the activation of c-src was reported earlier (119), the documentation of its physical association was not shown until recently (120). The autophosphorylation sites Y579 and Y581 in the juxtamembrane domain of PDGFRβ have been identified as the binding sites of src family tyrosine kinases (97). A protein tyrosine phosphatase called PTP1D (Syp) has recently been shown to be associated with activated EGFR and PDGFR (121,122). The tyrosine autophosphorylation site in the C terminus of PDGFR β (Y1009) is the binding site of PTP1D. This enzyme is tyrosine phosphorylated in response to PDGF (121). This posttranslational modification correlates with an increase in its catalytic activity (122). However, tyrosine phosphorylated PDGFR is not a substrate for PTP1D (122). This suggests that PTP1D is not involved in direct inactivation of the signals generated by the autophosphorylated PDGFR.

Besides these enzymes, PDGFR can also associate with other SH2 domain-containing molecules that do not possess any enzymatic activity. These are known as adapters (123). One such protein is growth factor receptor bound protein, Grb-2 (124). This protein, containing one SH2 domain flanked by two SH3 domains, was discovered by its ability to associate with EGFR. In PDGF-stimulated cells, Grb-2 associates with the PDGFR via its SH2 domain. Tyrosine 1009 of PDGFR is the binding site of Grb-2. A phosphopeptide containing YXNX motif inhibits this binding. Several of this sequence motif are present in PTP1D. Furthermore, the tyrosine phosphatase PTP1D also binds to tyrosine 1009 of PDGFR. Recently, it has been shown that Grb-2 is bound to PTP1D in a PDGF-dependent manner and that Grb-2 also binds to the tyrosine phosphorylated PDGFR in vitro (125). From these data, it was concluded that Grb-2 does not directly bind to PDGFR at Y1009. Rather, it binds to tyrosine phosphorylated PTP1D, which is directly bound to autophosphorylated PDGFR at Y1009 (125). Thus at least one biological function of the tyrosine phosphatase PTP1D in PDGFRβ signal transduction is to act as a docking molecule to associate the further downstream adapter molecule Grb-2 to PDGFR. This binding of Grb-2 to PDGFR recruits a recently identified molecule called SOS, which is the mammalian homologue of *Drosophila* "son of sevenless" gene product (126). The SH3 domain of Grb-2 binds to a proline-rich region of SOS (127). The amino acid residues from 641 to 1066 of human SOS protein have significant sequence homology with the C-terminal region of CDC25 protein, a guanine nucleotide exchange factor for Ras from yeast (126). In fact SOS is a guanine nucleotide exchange factor in mammalian cells and can substitute GTP for GDP onto inactive GDP bound Ras protein (126). Thus recruitment of SOS to the PDGFR-PTP1D-Grb-2 complex stimulates RasGTP to physically bind a serine/threonine kinase Raf1 (127), the enzymatic activity of which has previously been shown to be increased in response to PDGF (128,129). Activated Raf1 then phosphorylates MAP kinase kinase (MEK), which is a dual specific kinase (both tyrosine and threonine) and a candidate signal amplifier in the cascade of MAP kinase activation, which has been shown to be the target of mitogenic pathway induced by a whole array of mitogens (130,131). Thus, after ligand activation of PDGFR Grb-2, binding through PTP1D stimulates the kinase cascade in which activated GTP-bound Ras is the upstream regulator.

Nck is another adapter molecule like Grb-2. It also contains SH2 and SH3 domains and does not have any intrinsic enzymatic activity (132). Activated growth factor receptors, including PDGFR, phosphorylate Nck at tyrosine residues, which then coimmunoprecipitate with PDGFR (133). Overexpression of Nck in fibroblasts leads to cell transformation and tumor formation in nude mice (134). Mutation of Y751 in the KI domain of PDGFRβ abolishes the binding of Nck in vivo and in vitro, resulting in inhibition of tyrosine phosphorylation of this protein (133). As described above, Y751 shares the binding site for PI 3 kinase 85 kDa regulatory subunit (95,102). Using PDGFR-derived phosphopeptides in competition experiments, it was recently suggested that different amino acid residues around the Y751 influence the binding of Nck and p85 (133). However, the nonmitogenic mutants of PDGFR lacking a PI 3 kinase binding site also lack Nck binding to the receptor. As a corollary, the requirement of PI 3 kinase binding to the receptor for DNA synthesis can also be attributed to Nck binding to PDGFR. Similarly, two other recently identified biological functions of PI 3 kinase in PDGF signal transduction, chemotaxis and receptor internalization, can also result partly from the loss of Nck binding to the PDGFR. However, precise biological role of this small nonenzyme adapter molecule is yet to be established.

The final pathways that link these signaling mechanisms to the biological effect of PDGF remain to be identified. In addition to the ras MAP kinase pathway, a more direct pathway that involves tyrosine phosphorylation of cytoplasmic proteins that translocate to the nucleus may also be involved (134).

PDGF RECEPTOR SIGNALING IN MESANGIAL CELLS

Few studies have explored signal transduction mechanisms induced by PDGF in mesangial cells. Cells from different tissues, when activated by the same agent, elicit different biological activities. Mesangial cells exposed to PDGF may transduce qualitatively or quantitatively specific signaling proteins that ultimately mediate the biological response. Recently characterized cytoplasmic or nuclear transcription factors are likely candidates that may explain convergent or divergent mechanisms of actions of cytokines in cells and tissue, including mesangial cells (135,136).

Ligand-binding studies demonstrate specific binding of labeled recombinant PDGF BB and AB and, to a lower extent, AA to human mesangial cells consistent with predominant expression of PDGF beta receptor in these cells (23). In vitro, PDGF receptors can be regulated by matrix components and other cytokines (137,138). PDGF purified from human platelets and recombinant PDGF BB have been used as agonists to explore the mitogenic and other signals transduced by PDGF in these cells. Activation of phospholipase C γ 1 and PI 3 kinase by PDGF has been demonstrated in mesangial cells (105,139,140). Induction of PDGF A and B chain genes also occurs when mesangial cells are treated with PDGF (54). Preliminary studies indicate that the potency of the PDGF isoforms to stimulate signal transduction proteins in most but not all instances correlates with their mitogenic potency (141). The precise role of each mechanism in mediating the biological role for PDGF remains to be determined. While H_7, a serine threonine kinase inhibitor, blocked PDGF-induced DNA synthesis, downregulation of protein kinase C or use of more specific inhibitors of PKC demonstrates that PDGF-induced DNA synthesis is not mediated solely by the PMA-sensitive PKC pathway (142). The role of D-3 phosphorylated inositides in mediating the biological effects of PDGF in mesangial cells also remains to be defined. We find that the PI 3 kinase pathway is insensitive to H_7, which inhibits DNA synthesis and PKC activation, indicating that PI 3 kinase is insensitive to PKC. PDGF-induced DNA synthesis but not activation of PI 3 kinase appears to be dependent at least partially on pertussis-sensitive G protein (105). HMGCoA inhibitors such as simvastatin block PDGF-induced DNA synthesis in mesangial cells without interfering with PKC activation (143). Inhibition of PI 3 kinase by simvastatin may be the underlying mechanism of DNA synthesis inhibition (144).

It should be emphasized that elucidation of the signal transduction pathway that mediates the biological effects of PDGF in renal cells is important for therapeutic purposes. The in vitro observations should be followed by in vivo experiments to establish temporal relationships between the expression of signaling proteins and glomerular pathology as a prerequisite for the therapeutic efficacy of signal transduction inhibitors.

SOURCES AND BIOLOGICAL EFFECTS OF PDGF IN THE KIDNEY

The half-life of PDGF administered into the systemic circulation is very short (145). Circulating PDGF is sequestered in platelet alpha granules, and any amount released immediately binds to α_2-macroglobulin. PDGF therefore acts in an autocrine or paracrine fashion. In the normal adult kidney, there is very little expression of PDGF or PDGF receptors. However, the peptide is upregulated in renal disease and during mammalian renal development (2,3). The first evidence that PDGF is produced in the kidney was reported in cultured rat mesangial and human renal microvascular endothelial cells (1,3). In addition, inner medullary collecting duct (146), vascular smooth muscle, and glomerular epithelial in culture also produce PDGF (2,147). Activated fibroblasts also produce PDGF (5). Mesangial cells, interstitial fibroblasts, and smooth muscle cells express PDGF receptors (7,8,148). In disease states, platelets and infiltrating inflammatory cells including monocytes and lymphocytes are a major source of cytokines, including PDGF (1–4). PDGF, like many other cytokines, is subject to regulation by many biologically active agents. Exposure of mesangial cells in vitro to several cytokines, products of inflammatory cells and platelets, results in a coordinate induction of PDGF A and B chain mRNAs and release of the protein (52–54). Vasoactive compounds such as Ang II have recently been shown to induce PDGF in smooth muscle cells. In mesangial cells, endothelin and Ang II stimulate PDGF expression (7,56). Lipid mediators and lipoproteins also stimulate PDGF expression in mesangial cells (58,149). Ang II synergizes with lipid mediators to promote DNA synthesis and PDGF gene induction (149). Changes in local hemodynamics may also influence PDGF production. High shear stress has been reported to induce PDGF in endothelial cells via a specific response element in PDGF β chain gene (150). These in vitro observations may have correlates in vivo. The protective effect of Ang II receptor(s) blockade or angiotensin converting enzyme inhibition against progression of renal injury may be mediated at least in part by decrement in the expression of PDGF and other cytokines.

Both PDGF-A and B chains are also induced in human renal microvascular endothelial cells by exposure to thrombin and transforming growth factor beta (3). Bovine glomerular endothelial cells respond to thrombin with increase in PDGF-B but not A chain mRNA levels. On the other hand, EGF and TGF-α increase PDGF-A chain levels in these cells (Grandaliano et al., unpublished observations). The recent observation that components of the immune system and in particular the membrane attack complex stimulate production of PDGF and other cytokines in endothelial cells is highly relevant to enhanced PDGF expression in immune-mediated glomerular disease (151,152). Cultured glomerular epithelial as well as bovine glomerular and human renal microvascular endothelial cells do not express PDGF receptors and therefore are not responsive to any of the PDGF isoforms, unlike endothelial cells from other microvascular beds (153,154). The data indicate that somatic parenchymal renal cells respond to various forms of injury by releasing PDGF. Since PDGF induces its own expression in responsive cells, an amplification loop is created that helps sustain PDGF expression. PDGF released at sites of tissue injury acts via autocrine or paracrine mechanisms on somatic renal cells or adherent and infiltrating monocyte/macrophages. Matrix glycoproteins and perhaps other mechanisms operate to limit the availability or interfere with the biological activity of PDGF (155,156).

PDGF exerts multiple biological effects in target cells. In addition to its mitogenic effect, it is a chemoattractant for mesangial cells (157), smooth muscle cells, and fibroblasts (148). Rat mesangial cells migrate in response to PDGF purified from human platelets, which is predominantly an AB heterodimer (157). Mesenchymal cell migration in response to PDGF appears to be essential for proper development of the glomerular structure in the mammalian kidney. PDGF also elicits a contractile response in vascular smooth muscle cells (158) and has been demonstrated to elicit contraction or relaxation in different vascular beds (1), depending on whether the endothelial cells lining such vessels express receptors for PDGF and release endothelium-derived relaxing factors. Mene et al. (139) reported that PDGF contracts mesangial cells and therefore may influence glomerular hemodynamics. The ultimate effect of PDGF on determinants of glomerular filtration rate, however, has to take into consideration its effect on afferent and efferent arteriolar tones. Infusion of PDGF into the isolated microperfused glomerulus results in marked increase in intraglomerular capillary pressure associated with decrease in flow rate and marked increase in resistance (Osgood and Abboud, unpublished observations). PDGF may regulate matrix metabolism in mesangial cells either directly or through release of other growth factors (159). Advanced glycosylation products stimulate collagen synthesis in mesangial cells, an effect inhibited by an antibody to PDGF (160). We have recently found that PDGF stimulates release of TGF-β by mesangial cells (161). Increased expression of PDGF and PDGF receptors in renal tissue has been demonstrated in experimental animals with proliferative glomerular diseases as well as in human kidney biopsies obtained from patients with a variety of proliferative lesions. PDGF and PDGF receptors localize primarily within mesangial areas of glomeruli and to some extent in the interstitium and correlate with the degree of hypercellularity and interstitial fibrosis (1–3).

Several observations suggest that PDGF may also be involved in mediating vascular and interstitial injury. Vascular endothelial and smooth muscle cells are potential sources of PDGF, and injury to the endothelium may result in an increased production of PDGF that stimulates smooth muscle cell proliferation (3,148). It is also known that proliferating smooth muscle cells produce large amounts of PDGF. Antibody to PDGF when infused into the rat decreases intimal hyperplasia in a rat model of vascular stenosis (162). Therefore local release of PDGF by these cells as well as by infiltrating monocytes or macrophages may result in the progression of arterial and arteriolar lesions within the renal vasculature. An additional mechanism by which PDGF contributes to interstitial fibrosis is through its ability to stimulate fibroblast proliferation. In addition to infiltrating monocytes in the interstitium, inner medullary collecting duct cells appears to be an important source of PDGF (146). Inner medullary collecting duct epithelial cells or conditioned medium from these cells stimulate DNA synthesis in isolated papillary fibroblasts. This effect was specific for this cell type, since proximal tubular epithelial cells had no effect on the proliferation of fibroblasts. Inner medullary collecting duct cells also produced PDGF, and the effect of these cells on DNA synthesis in papillary fibroblasts was inhibited by an antibody to PDGF. Of interest in this study is that the papillary fibroblasts were more responsive than cortical fibroblasts to PDGF. This paracrine system may be important in the pathogenesis of interstitial fibrosis of the kidney.

SUMMARY AND CONCLUSION

PDGF exerts multiple biological effects highly relevant to renal development and the pathogenesis of renal disease. Mitogenesis, chemotaxis, vasoactive effects, and effects on matrix metabolism are among the known biological effects of PDGF. Studies in cultured cells expressing α- or β-type receptors and using highly purified recombinant PDGF isoforms provided fundamental concepts relevant to regulation of cell growth. Moreover, these studies provided an impetus to study PDGF expression in disease. The biological relevance of other actions of PDGF (e.g., inhibition of nitric oxide synthesis and phospholipase A_2 stimulated by other cytokines) remains to be determined (163,164). Structure/function studies of PDGF and its receptors may yield to a discovery of specific antagonists of PDGF or its receptors. In spite of the similarities in signaling molecules between various cytokines, the recent development of potent and specific EGF receptor kinase antagonists suggest that sufficient structural diversity exists to discriminate between signaling proteins (165). The identification of key intermediates in growth factor–dependent transcription will allow us to target overlapping or unique sets of genes and proteins that are regulated by specific cytokines (134,136). Understanding the mechanism of action of PDGF alone or in concert with other cytokines is essential for the development and application of practical tools to protect the function and structure of diseased kidneys.

REFERENCES

1. Abboud HE. Growth factors in glomerulonephritis. Kidney Int 1993; 43:252–257.
2. Johnson RJ, Floege J, Couser WG, Alpers CE. Role of platelet-derived growth factor in glomerular disease. J Am Soc Nephrol 1991; 2:434.
3. Daniel TO, Kumjian DA. Platelet-derived growth factor in renal development and disease. Semin Nephrol 1993; 13:87–95.
4. Ross R, Raines EW, Bowen-Pope DF. The biology of platelet-derived growth factor. Cell 1986; 46:155–169.
5. Heldin CH. Structural and functional studies on platelet-derived growth factor. EMBO J 1992; 11:4251–4259.
6. Westermark B, Helden C-H. Platelet-derived growth factor in autocrine transformation. Cancer Res 1991; 51:5087–5092.
7. Abboud HE. Role of platelet-derived growth factor in renal injury. Annu Rev Physiol 1995; 57:297–309.
8. Abboud HE. Growth factors and the mesangium. J Am Soc Nephrol 1992; 2:S1185–S189.
9. Hannink M, Donog DJ. Structure and function of platelet-derived growth factor (PDGF) and related proteins. Biochim Biophys Acta 1989; 989:1–10.
10. Westermark B. The molecular and cellular biology of platelet-derived growth factor. Acta Endocrinol 1990; 123:131–142.
11. Betscholtz C, Johnsson A, Heldin CH, et al. cDNA sequence and chromosomal localization of human platelet-derived-growth factor A-chain and its expression in tumour cell lines. Nature 1986; 320:695–699.
12. Kenney WC, Haniu M, Herman AC, et al. Formation of mitogenically active PDGF-B dimer does not require interchain disulfide bonds. J Biol Chem 1994; 269:12351–12359.
13. Heldin CH, Westermark B, Wasteson A. Platelet-derived growth factor: Purification and partial characterization. Proc Natl Acad Sci USA 1979; 76:3722–3726.
14. Antoniades HN, Scher CD, Stiles CD. Purification of human platelet-derived growth factor. Proc Natl Acad Sci USA 1979; 76:1809–1812.
15. Rains EW, Russell R. Platelet-derived growth factor, high yield purification and evidence for multiple forms. J Biol Chem 1982; 257 9:5154–5160.
16. Deuel TF, Huang JS, Proffitt RT, et al. Human platelet-derived growth factor, purification and resolution into active protein fraction. J Biol Chem 1981; 256, 17:8896–8899.
17. Heldin C-H, Johnsson A, Wennergren S, et al. A human osteosarcoma cell line secretes a growth factor structurally related to a homodimer of PDGF A chains. Nature 1986; 3:19:511–515.
18. Ostman A, Rall L, Hammacher A, et al. Synthesis and assembly of a functionally active recombinant PDGF-AB heterodimer. J Biol Chem 1988; 263:1602–1608.
19. Ostman A, Thyberg J, Westermark B, Heldin C-H. PDGF-AA and PDGF-BB biosynthesis: Proprotein processing in the golgi complex and lysosomal degradation of PDGF-BB retained intracellularly. J Cell Biol 1992; 118:509–519.
20. Ostman A, Andersson M, Betsholtz C, et al. Identification of a cell retention signal in the B-chain of platelet-derived growth factor and in the long splice version of the A-chain. Cell Reg 1991; 2:503–512.
21. Hammacher A, Hellman U, Johnsson A, et al. A major part of PDGF purified from human platelets is a heterodimer of one A chain and one B chain. J Biol Chem 1988; 263:16493–16498.
22. Bywater M, Rorsman F, Bongcam-Rudloff E, et al. Expression of recombinant platelet-derived growth factor A- and B-chain homodimers in rat-1 cells and human fibroblasts reveals differences in proteins processing and autocrine effects. Mol Cell Biol 1988; 8:2753–2762.
23. Abboud HE, Pinzani M, Knauss T, et al. Actions of platelet-derived growth factor isoforms in mesangial cells. J Cell Physiol 1994; 158:140–150.
24. Pfeilschifter J, Hosang M. Effects of homo- and heterodimeric isoforms of PDGF on signaling events in rat renal mesangial cells. Cell Sign 1991; 3:413–424.
25. Heldin C-H, Westermark B. Growth factors as transforming proteins. Eur J Biochem 1989; 184:487–496.
26. Tong BD, Auer DE, Jaye M, et al. cDNA clones reveal differences between human glial and endothelial cell platelet-derived growth factor A-chain. Nature 1987; 328:619–621.
27. Bonthron DT, Morton CC, Orkin SH, Collins T. Platelet-derived growth factor A chain: Gene structure, chromosomal location, and basis for alternative mRNA splicing. Proc Natl Acad Sci USA 1988; 85:1492–1496.
28. Raines EW, Ross R. Compartmentalization of PDGF on extracellular binding sites dependent on exon-6-encoded sequences. J Cell Biol 1992; 116:533–543.
29. Kelly JL, Sanchez A, Brown GS, et al. Accumulation of PDGF B and cell-binding forms of PDGF A in the extracellular matrix. J Cell Biol 1993; 121:1153–1163.
30. Rorsman F, Bywater M, Knott TJ, et al. Structural characterization of the human platelet-derived growth factor A-chain cDNA and gene: Alternative exon usage predicts two different precursor proteins. Mol Cell Biol 1988; 8:571–577.

31. Collins T, Bonthron DT, Orkin SH. Alternative RNA splicing affects function of encoded platelet-derived growth factor A chain. Nature 1987; 328:621–624.
32. Chiu IM, Reddy EP, Givol D, et al. Nucleotide sequence analysis identifies the human c-sis proto-oncogene as a structural gene for platelet-derived growth factor. Cell 1984; 37:123–129.
33. Ratner L, Josephs SF, Jarrett R, et al. Nucleotide sequence of transforming human c-sis cDNA clones with homology to platelet-derived growth factor. Nucl Acid Res 1985; 13:5007–5018.
34. Ratner L, Thielan B, Collins T. Sequences of the 5′ portion of the human c-sis gene: Characterization of the transcriptional promoter and regulation of expression of the protein product by 5′ untranslated mRNA sequences. Nucleic Acids Res 1987; 15:6017–6036.
35. Collins T, Ginsburg D, Boss JM, et al. Cultured human endothelial cells express platelet-derived growth factor B chain. cDNA cloning and structural analysis. Nature 1985; 316:748–750.
36. Josephs SF, Guo C, Ratner L, Wong-Staal F. Human proto-oncogene sequences corresponding to the transforming region of simian sarcoma virus. Science 1984; 223:487–490.
37. Takimoto Y, Wang Z-Y, Kobler K, Deuel TF. Promoter region of the human platelet-derived growth factor A-chain gene. Proc Natl Acad Sci USA 1991; 88:1686–1690.
38. Wang Z, Lin X-H, Nobyuoshi M, et al. Binding of single-stranded oligonucleotides to a non-B-form DNA structure results in loss of promoter activity of the platelet-derived growth factor A-chain gene. J Biol Chem 1992; 267:13669–13674.
39. Wang Z-Y, Lin X-H, Qui Q-Q, Deuel TF. Modulation of transcription of the platelet-derived growth factor A-chain gene by a promoter region sensitive to S1 nuclease. J Biol Chem 1992; 267:17022–17031.
40. Lin X, Wang Z, Gu L, Deuel TF. Functional analysis of the human platelet-derived growth factor A-chain promoter region. J Biol Chem 1992; 267:25614–25619.
41. Wang Z-Y, Qiu Q-Q, Deuel TF. An S1 nuclease sensitive region in the PDGFA-chain gene promoter contains a postive transcriptional regulatory element. Biochem Biophys Res Commun 1994, 198:103–110.
42. Gashler AL, Bonthron DT, Madden SL, et al. Human platelet-derived growth factor A chain is transcriptionally repressed by the Wilms' tumor suppressor WT1. Proc Natl Acad Sci USA 1992; 89:10984–10988.
43. Bhandari B, Wenzel UO, Marra F, Abboud HE. A nuclear protein in mesangial cells that binds to promoter region of the PDGF A chain gene: Induction by phorbol ester. J Biol Chem 1995. In press.
44. Rao CD, Igarashi H, Chiu IM, et al. Structure and sequence of the human c-sis/platelet-derived growth factor 2(SIS/PDGF2) transcriptional unit. Proc Natl Acad Sci USA 1986; 83:2392–2396.
45. Van den Ouweland MW, Roebroek AJM, Schalken JA, et al. Structure and nucleotide sequence of the 5′ region of the human and feline c-sis proto-oncogene. Nucleic Acids Res 1986; 14:765–778.
46. Rao CD, Pech M, Robbins KC, Aaronson SA. The 5′ untranslated sequence of the c-sis/platelet-derived growth factor 2 transcript is a potent translational inhibitor. Mol Cell Biol 1988; 8:284–292.
47. Pech M, Rao CD, Robbins KC, Aaronson SA. Functional identification of regulatory elements within the promoter region of PDGF2. Mol Cell Biol 1989; 9:396–405.
48. Dirks RPH, Jansen HJ, Gerritsma J, et al. Localization and functional analysis of DNase-I-hypersensitive sites in the human c-sis/PDGF-β gene transcription unit and its flanking regions. Eur J Biochem 1993; 11:509–519.
49. Jin HM, Brady ML, Fahl WE. Identification and characterization of an essential, activating regulatory element of the human SIS/PDGFB promoter in human megakaryocytes. Proc Natl Acad Sci USA 1993; 90:7563–7567.
50. Franklin GC, Donovan M, Adam GIR, et al. Expression of the human PDGF-B gene is regulated by both positively and negatively acting cell type-specific regulatory element located in the first intron. EMBO J 1991; 10:1365–1373.
51. Resnick N, Collins T, Atkinson W, et al. Platelet-derived growth factor B chain promoter contains a cis-acting fluid shear-stress element. Proc Natl Acad Sci USA 1993; 90:4591–4595.
52. Abboud HE, Poptic E, DiCorleto P. Production of platelet derived growth factor-like protein by rat mesangial cells in culture. J Clin Invest 1987; 80:675–683.
53. Shultz PJ, DiCorleto PE, Silver BJ, Abboud HE. Mesangial cells express PDGF mRNAs and proliferate in response to PDGF. Am J Physiol 1988; 255:F674–F684.
54. Silver BJ, Jaffer FE, Abboud HE. Platelet-derived growth factor (PDGF) synthesis in mesangial cells: Induction by multiple peptide mitogens. Proc Natl Acad Sci USA 1989; 86:1056–1060.
55. Shultz PJ, Knauss TC, Mene P, Abboud HE. Mitogenic signals for thrombin in mesangial cells: Regulation of phospholipase C and PDGF genes. Am J Physiol 1989; 257:F366–F374.
56. Jaffer FE, Knauss TC, Poptic E, Abboud HE. Endothelin stimulates PDGF secretion in cultured human mesangial cells. Kidney Int 1990; 38:1193–1198.
57. Jaffer F, Saunders C, Shultz P, et al. Regulation of mesangial cell growth by polypeptide mitogens. Am J Pathol 1989; 135:261–269.

58. Knauss TC, Jaffer FE, Abboud HE. Phosphatidic acid modulates DNA synthesis, phospholipase C and PDGF mRNAs in mesangial cells. J Biol Chem 1990; 265:14457–14463.
59. Kartha S, Bradham DM, Grotendorst GR, Toback FG. Kidney epithelial cells express c-sis protooncogene and secrete PDGF-like protein. Am J Physiol 1988; 255:F800–F806.
60. Heldin C-R, Westermark B. Platelet-derived growth factor: Mechanism of action and possible in vivo function. Cell Reg 1990; 1:555–566.
61. Eriksson A, Nister M, Leveen P, et al. Induction of platelet-derived growth factor α- and β-receptor mRNA and protein by platelet-derived growth factor BB. J Biol Chem 1991; 266:21138–21144.
62. Raines EW, Dower SK, Ross R. Interleukin-1 mitogenic activity for fibroblasts and smooth muscle cells is due to PDGF-AA. Science 1989; 243:393–396.
63. Fen Z, Daniel TO. 5′ untranslated sequences determine degradative pathway for alternate PDGF B/c-sis mRNAs. Oncogene 1991; 6:953–959.
64. Daniel TO, Gibbs VC, Milfay DF, Williams LT. Agents that increase cAMP accumulation block endothelial c-sis induction by thrombin and transforming growth factor-β. J Biol Chem 1987; 262:11893–11896.
65. Daniel TO, Gibbs VC, Milfay DE, et al. Thrombin stimulates c-sis gene expression in microvascular endothelial cells. J Biol Chem 1986; 261:9579–9582.
66. Daniel TO, and Fen Z. Distinct pathways mediate transcriptional regulation of platelet derived growth factor B/c-sis expression. J Biol Chem 1988; 263:19815–19820.
67. Kavanaugh WM, Harsh GR, Starksen NF, et al. Transcriptional regulation of the A and B chain genes of platelet-derived growth factor in microvascular endothelial cells. J Biol Chem 1988; 263:8470–8472.
68. Starksen NF, Harsh GR, Gibbs VC, Williams LT. Regulated expression of the platelet-derived growth factor A chain gene in microvascular endothelial cells. J Biol Chem 1987; 260:14381–14384.
69. Press RD, Misra A, Gillaspy G, et al. Control of the expression of c-sis mRNA in human glioblastoma cells by phorbol ester and transforming growth factor β1. Cancer Res 1989; 49:2914–2920.
70. Marra F, Ghosh Choudhury G, Bhandari B, Abboud HE. Biology and regulation of platelet-derived growth factor. In: Surrenti C, Casini A, Milani S, Pinzani M, eds. Falk Symposium 71; Fat-Storing Cells and Liver Fibrosis. Hingham, MA: Kluwer, 1994:209–221.
71. Bhandari B, Abboud HE. Platelet-derived growth factor A-chain gene expression in cultured mesangial cells: Regulation by phorbol ester at the level of mRNA abundance, transcription and mRNA stability. Mol Cell Endocrinol 1993; 91:185–191.
72. Bhandari B, Grandaliano G, Abboud HE. Platelet-derived growth factor (PDGF) BB homodimer regulates PDGF A and PDGF B-chain gene transcription in human mesangial cells. Biochem J 1994; 297:385–388.
73. Bhandari B, Woodruff K, Abboud HE. Platelet-derived growth factor B-chain gene expression in mesangial cells: Effect of phorbol ester on gene transcription and mRNA stability. Mol Cell Biochem 1994; 140:31–36.
74. Colamonici OR, Trepel JB, Vidal CA, Neckers LM. Phorbol ester induces c-sis gene transcription in stem cell line K-562. Mol Cell Biol 1986; 6:1847–1850.
75. Cavalieri RL, Havell EA, Vilcek J, Pestka S. Induction and decay of human fibroblast interferon mRNA. Proc Natl Acad Sci USA 1977; 74:4415–4419.
76. Shaw G, Kamen R. A conserved AU sequence from the 3′ untranslated region of GM-CSF m RNA mediates selective mRNA degradation. Cell 1986; 46:659–667.
77. Claesson-Welsh L, Eriksson A, Westermark B, Heldin CH. cDNA cloning of the human A type receptor establishes structural similarity to the B type receptor. Proc Natl Acad Sci USA 1989; 86:491721.
78. Hart CE, Forstrom JW, Kelly JD, et al. Two classes of PDGF receptors recognize different isoforms of PDGF. Science 1988; 240:1529–1531.
79. Bowen-Pope DF, Hart CE, Seifert RA. Sera and conditioned media contain different isoforms of platelet-derived growth factor (PDGF) which bind to different classes of PDGF receptor. J Biol Chem 1989; 264:2502–2508.
80. Heldin CH, Backström G, Ostman A, et al. Binding of different dimeric forms of PDGF to human fibroblasts: Evidence for two separate receptor types. EMBO J 1988; 7:1387–1393.
81. Matsui T, Heidaran M, Miki T, et al. Isolation of a novel receptor cDNA establishes the existence of two PDGF receptor genes. Science 1989; 243:800–804.
82. Heidaran MA, Beeler JF, Yu J-C, et al. Differences in substrate specificities of α and β platelet-derived growth factor (PDGF) receptors. J Biol Chem 1993; 268:9287–9295.
83. Tiesman J, Hart CE. Identification of a soluble receptor for platelet-derived growth factor in cell-conditioned medium and human plasma. J Biol Chem 1993; 268:9621–9628.
84. Heldin CH, Westermark B, Wasteson A. Specific receptors for platelet-derived growth factor on cells derived from connective tissue and glia. Proc Natl Acad Sci USA 1981; 78:3664–3668.
85. Heldin C-H, Wasteson A, Westermark B. Interaction of platelet-derived growth factor with its fibroblast receptor: Demonstration of ligand degradation and receptor modulation. J Biol Chem 1982; 257:4216–4221.
86. Yarden Y, Escobedo JA, Kuang W-J, et al. Structure of the receptor for platelet-derived growth factor helps define a family of closely related growth factor receptors. Nature 1986; 323:226–232.

87. Hammacher A, Mellstrom K, Heldin C-H, Westermark B. Isoform-specific induction of actin reorganization by platelet-derived growth factor suggests that the functionally active receptor is a dimer. EMBO J 1989; 8:2489–2495.
88. Ueno H, Colbert H, Escobedo, Williams L. Inhibition of PDGF β receptor signal transduction by coexpression of truncated receptor. Science 1991; 252:844–848.
89. Williams LT. Signal transduction by the platelet-derived growth factor receptor. Science 1989; 243:1564–1570.
90. Bishayee S, Majumdar S, Khire J, Das M. Ligand-induced dimerization of the platelet-derived growth factor receptor. J Biol Chem 1989; 264:11699–11705.
91. Heldin C-H, Ernlund A, Rorsman C, Ronnstrand L. Dimerization of B type receptors occurs after ligand binding and is closely associated with receptor kinase activation. J Biol Chem 1989; 264:8905–8912.
92. Kelly JD, Haldeman BA, Frant FJ, et al. Platelet-derived growth factor (PDGF) stimulates PDGF receptor subunit dimerization and intersubunit transphosphorylation. J Biol Chem 1991; 266:8987–8992.
93. Fantl WJ, Escobedo JA, Martin GA, et al. Distinct phosphotyrosines on a growth factor receptor bind to specific molecules that mediate signaling pathways. Cell 1992; 69:413–423.
94. Kashishian A, Kazlauskas A, Cooper JA. Phosphorylation sites in the PDGF receptors with different specificities for binding GAP and PI 3 kinase in vivo. EMBO J 1992; 11:1373–1382.
95. Kazlauskas A, Cooper JA. Autophosphorylation of the PDGF receptor in the kinase insert region regulates interaction with cell proteins. Cell 1989; 58:1121–1133.
96. Ronnstrand L, Mori S, Jonsson A-K, et al. Identification of two C-terminal autophosphorylation sites in the PDGFβ receptor: Involvement in the interaction of phospholipase Cγ. EMBO J 1992; 11:3911–3919.
97. Mori S, Rönnstrand L, Koutari Y, et al. Identification of two juxtamembrane autophosphorylation sites in the PDGF β-receptor: Involvement in the interaction with src family tyrosine kinases. EMBO J 1993; 12:2257–2264.
98. Koch CA, Anderson D, Moran MF, et al. SH2 and SH3 domains: Elements that control interactions of cytoplasmic signaling proteins. Science 1991; 252:668–674.
99. Kim HK, Kim JW, Zilberstein A, et al. PDGF stimulation of inositol phospholopid hydrolysis requires PLCγ1 phosphorylation on tyrosine residues 783 and 1254. Cell 1991; 65:435–441.
100. Nishibe S, Wahl MW, Hernandes-Sotomayor SMT, et al. Increase in the catalytic activity of phospholipase C-γ1 by tyrosine phosphorylation. Science 1990; 250:1253–1256.
101. Valius M, Bazenet C, Kazlauskas A. Tyrosines 1021 and 1009 are phosphorylation sites in the carboxy terminus of the platelet-derived growth factor receptor—subunit and are required for binding of phospholipase Cγ and a 65 kD protein, respectively. Mol Cell Biol 1993; 13:7266–7277.
102. Valius M, Kazlauskas A. Phospholipase C-γ1 and phosphatidylinositol 3 kinase are the downstream mediators of the PDGF receptor's mitogenic signal. Cell 1993; 73:321–334.
103. Morrison DK, Kaplan DR, Rhee SG, Williams LT. Platelet-derived growth factor (PDGF)-dependent association of phospholipase C-γ with the PDGF receptor signaling complex. Mol Cell Biol 1990; 10:2359–2366.
104. Niskizuka Y. Intracellular signaling by hydrolysis of phospholipids and activation of protein kinase C. Science 1992; 258:607–614.
105. Escobedo JA, Williams LT. A PDGF receptor domain essential for mitogenesis but not for many other responses to PDGF. Nature 1988; 335:85–87.
106. Ghosh Choudhury G, Biswas P, et al. PDGF-mediated activation of phosphatidylinositol 3 kinase in human mesangial cells. Kidney Int 1994; 46:37–47.
107. Coughlin SN, Escobedo JA, Williams LT. Role of phosphatidylinositol kinase in PDGF receptor signal transduction. Science 1989; 243:1191–1194.
108. Skolnik EY, Margolis B, Mohammadi M, et al. Cloning of PI 3 kinase associated p85 utilizing a novel method for expression/cloning of target proteins for receptor tyrosine kinases. Cell 1991; 65:83–90.
109. Nakanishi H, Brewer KA, Exton JH. Activation of the ζ isoenzyme of protein kinase C by phosphatidylinositol 3,4,5 trisphosphate. J Biol Chem 1993; 268:13–16.
110. Joly M, Kazlauskas A, Fay FS, Corvera S. Disruption of PDGF receptor trafficking by mutation of its PI-3 kinase binding sites. Science 1994; 263:684–687.
111. Kundra V, Escobedo JA, Kazlauskas A, et al. Regulation of chemotaxis by the platelet-derived growth factor receptor-β. Nature 1994; 367:474–476.
112. Satoh T, Endo M, Nakafuku M, et al. Platelet-derived growth factor stimulates formation of active $p21^{ras}$: GTP complex in Swiss mouse 3T3 cells. Proc Natl Acad Sci USA 1990; 87:5993–5997.
113. Gibbs JB, Marshall MS, Scolnick EM, et al. Modulation of guanine nucleotide bound to Ras in NIH 3T3 cells by oncogenes, growth factors and the GTPase activating protein (GAP). J Biol Chem 1990; 265:20437–20442.
114. Mulcahy LS, Smith MP, Stacey DW. Requirement for ras proto-oncogene function during serum-stimulated growth in NIH-3T3 cells. Nature 1985; 313:241–243.

115. Molloy CJ, Bottaro DP, Fleming RP, et al. PDGF induction of tyrosine phosphorylation of GTPase activating protein. Nature 1989; 342:711–714.
116. Kazlauskas A, Ellis C, Pawson T, Cooper JA. Binding of GAP to activated PDGF receptors. Science 1990; 247:1578–1581.
117. Kaplan DR, Morrison DK, Wong G, et al. PDGFβ-receptor stimulates tyrosine phosphorylation of GAP and association of signaling complex. Cell 1990; 61:125–133.
118. Kypta RM, Goldberg Y, Ulug ET, Courtneidge SA. Association between PDGF receptor and members of the src family of tyrosine kinases. Cell 1990; 62:481–492.
119. Ralston R, Bishop JM. The product of the protooncogene c-src is modified during the cellular response to platelet-derived growth factor. Proc Natl Acad Sci USA 1985; 82:7845–7849.
120. Courtneidge SA, Kyptas RM, Cooper JA, Kazlauskas A. Platelet-derived growth factor receptor sequences important for binding of src family tyrosine kinases. Cell Growth Diff 1991; 2:483–486.
121. Feng GS, Hui C-C, Pawson T. SH2-containing phosphotyrosine phosphatase as a target protein tyrosine kinases. Science 1993; 259:1607–1611.
122. Vogel W, Lammers JR, Huang J, Ullrich A. Activation of phosphotyrosine phosphatase by tyrosine phosphorylation. Science 1993; 259:1611–1614.
123. Pawson T, Gish GD. SH2 and SH3 domains: From structure to function. Cell 1992; 71:359–362.
124. Lowenstein EJ, Daly RJ, Batzer AG, et al. The SH2 and SH3 containing protein Grb-2 links receptor tyrosine kinases to Ras signaling. Cell 1992; 70:431–442.
125. Li W, Nishimure R, Kashiahian A, et al. A new function for a phosphotyrosine phosphatase: Linking Grb2-SOS to a receptor tyrosine kinase. Mol Cell Biol 1994; 14:509–517.
126. Chardin P, Camonis JH, Gale NW, et al. Human Sos 1: A guanine nucleotide exchange factor for Ras that binds to Grb2, Science 1993; 260:1338–1343.
127. Moodi SA, Williamson BM, Weber MJ, Wolfman A. Complexes of Ras-GTP with Raf-1 and mitogen-activated protein kinase. Science 1993; 260:1658.
128. Morrison DK, Kaplan DR, Escobedo JA, et al. Direct activation of the serine/threonine kinase activity of Raf-1 through tyrosine phosphorylation of the PDGFβ-receptor. Cell 1989; 58:649–657.
129. Morrison DK, Kaplan DR, Rapp UR, Roberts TM. Signal transduction from membrane to cytoplasm: Growth factors and membrane-bound oncogene products increase raf-1 phosphorylation and associated protein kinase activity. Proc Natl Acad Sci USA 1988; 85:8855–8859.
130. David RJ. The mitogen-activated protein kinase signal transduction pathway. J Biol Chem 1993; 268:14553–14556.
131. Blenis J. Signal transduction via MAP kinases: Proceed at your own RSK. Proc Natl Acad Sci USA 1993; 90:5889–5892.
132. Lehmann JM, Reithmuller G, Johnson JP. Nck, a melanoma cDNA encoding a cytoplasmic protein consisting of the src homology units SH2 and SH3. Nucleic Acids Res 1990; 18:1048.
133. Nishimura R, Li W, Kashishian A, et al. Two signaling molecules share a phosphotyrosine-containing binding site in the platelet-derived growth factor receptor. Mol Cell Biol 1993; 11:6889–6896.
134. Silvennoinen O, Schindler C, Schlessinger J, Levy DE. Ras-independent growth factor signaling by transcription factor tyrosine phosphorylation. Science 1993; 261:1736–1746.
135. Darnell JE, Kerr IM, Stark GR. Jak-STAT pathways and transcriptional activation in response to IFNs and other extracellular signaling proteins. Science 1994; 264:1415–1421.
136. Montminy M. Trying on a new pair of SH2s. Science 1993; 261:1694–1695.
137. Marx M, Daniel TO, Kashgarian M, Madri JA. Spatial organization of the extracellular matrix modulates the expression of PDGF-receptor subunits in mesangial cells. Kidney Int 1993; 43:1027–1041.
138. Haberstroh U, Zahner G, Disser M, et al. TGF-beta stimulates rat mesangial cell proliferation in culture: Role of PDGF beta-receptor expression. Am J Physiol 1993; 264:F199–205.
139. Mene P, Abboud, HE, Dubyak GR, Scarpa A, Dunn MJ. Effect of platelet-derived growth factor on inositol phosphates, cytosolic calcium and contraction of mesangial cells. Am J Physiol 1987; 253:F458–F463.
140. Bonaventure JV, Weber PC, Gronich JH. Paf and PDGF increase cytosolic (Ca^{2+}) and phospholipase activity in mesangial cells. Am J Physiol 1988; 254:F87–F94.
141. Choudhury G, Grandaliano G, Abboud HE. Differential activation of PDGF-receptor subunits by homo- and heterdineric forms of PDGF. J Am Soc Nephrol 1993; 4:463.
142. Ghosh Choudhury G, Biswas P, et al. Involvement of PKC-α in PDGF-mediated mitogenic signaling in human mesangial cells. Am J Physiol 1993; 265:F631–F642.
143. Grandaliano G, Biswas P, Ghosh Choudhury G, Abboud HE. Simvastatin inhibits PDGF-induced DNA synthesis in human mesangial cells. Kidney Int 1993; 44:503–508.
144. McGuire TF, Corey SJ, Sebi SM. Lovastatin inhibits platelet-derived growth factor (PDGF) stimulation of phosphatidylinositol 3-kinase activity as well as association of p85 subunit to tyrosine-phosphorylated PDGF Receptor. J Biol Chem 1993; 268(30):22227–22230.

145. Bowen-Pope DF, Malpass TW, Foster DM, Ross R. Platelet-derived growth factor in vivo: Levels, activity, and rate of clearance. Blood 1984; 64:458–469.
146. Knecht A, Fine LG, Kleinman KS, et al. Fibroblasts of rabbit kidney in culture. II. Paracrine stimulation of papillary fibroblasts of PDGF. Am J Physiol 21991; 61:F292–299.
147. Couser WG, Johnson RJ. Mechanisms of progressive renal disease in glomerulonephritis. Am J Kidney Dis 1994; 23:193–198.
148. Ross R. The pathogenesis of atherosclerosis: A perspective for the 1990s. Nature 1993; 362:801–809.
149. Gröne HJ, Abboud HE, Höhne M, et al. Action of lipoproteins in culture human mesangial cells: Modulation by mitogenic vasoconstrictors. Am J Physiol 1992; 263:F686–F696.
150. Malek AM, Gibbons GH, Dzau VJ, Izumo S. Fluid shear stress differentially modulates expression of genes encoding basic fibroblast growth factor and platelet-derived growth factor B chain in vascular endothelium. J Clin Invest 1993; 92:2013–2021.
151. Benzaquen LR, Nicholson-Weller A, Halperin JA. Terminal complement proteins C5b-9 release basic fibroblast growth factor and platelet-derived growth factor from endothelial cells. J Exp Med 1994; 179:985–992.
152. Schönermark M, Deppisch R, Riedasch G, et al. Induction of mediator release from human glomerular mesangial cells by the terminal complement components C5b-9. Int Arch Allergy Appl Immunol 1991; 96:331–337.
153. Bar RS, Boes M, Booth BA, et al. The effects of platelet-derived growth factor in cultured microvessel endothelial cells. Endocrinology 124:1841–1848.
154. Beitz JG, Kim IS, Calabresi P, Frackelton AR. Human microvascular endothelial cells express receptors for platelet-derived growth factor. Proc Natl Acad Sci USA 1991; 88:2021–2025.
155. Raines EW, Lane TF, Iruela-Arispe L, et al. The extracellular glycoprotein SPARC interacts with platelet-derived growth factor (PDGF)-AB and B and inhibits the binding of PDGF to its receptors. Proc Natl Acad Sci USA 1992; 89:1281–1285.
156. Johnson RJ. The glomerular response to injury: Progression or resolution? gkidney Int 1994; 45:1769–1782.
157. Barnes JL, Hevey KA. Glomerular mesangial migration in response to platelet-derived growth factor. Lab Invest 1990; 62:379–382.
158. Berk BC, Alexander RW, Brock TA, et al. Vasoconstriction: A new activity for platelet-derived growth factor. Science 1986; 232:87–90.
159. Pierce GF, Vande-Berg J, Rudolf R et al. Platelet-derived growth factor-BB and transforming growth factor beta 1 selectively modulate glycosaminoglycans, collagen, and myofibroblasts in excisional wounds. Am J Pathol 1991; 138:639–646.
160. Doi T, Vlassara H, Kirstein M, Yamada Y, Striker GE, Striker LJ. Receptor-specific increase in extracellular matrix production in mouse mesangial cells by advanced glycosylation end products is mediated via platelet-derived growth factor. Proc Natl Acad Sci USA 1992; 89:2873–2877.
161. Marra F, Bonewald L, Park I, Park-Snyder S, Woodruff K, Abboud HE. Secretion of multiple forms of latent transforming growth factor-β by human mesangial cells. J Am Soc Nephrol 1994; 5:697.
162. Ferns GAS, Raines EW, Sprugel KH, et al. Inhibition of neointimal smooth muscle accumulation after angioplasty by an antibody to PDGF. Science 1991; 253:1129–1132.
163. Pfeilschifter J. Platelet-derived growth factor inhibits cytokine induction of nitric oxide synthase in rat renal mesangial cells. Eur J Pharmacol 1991; 208:339–340.
164. Mühl H, Geiger T, Pignat W, et al. PDGF suppresses the activation of group II phospholipase A_2 gene expression by interleukin 1 and forskolin in mesangial cells. FEBS Lett 1991; 291:249–252.
165. Fry DW, Kraker AJ, McMichael A, et al. A specific inhibitor of the epidermal growth factor receptor tyrosine kinase. Science 1994; 265:1093–1098.

41
TGF-β in Renal Pathophysiology

Markus Ketteler, Nancy A. Noble, and Wayne A. Border
University of Utah Health Sciences Center, Salt Lake City, Utah

INTRODUCTION

Progression to renal failure in kidney diseases is characteristically associated with increasing glomerular and tubulointerstitial fibrosis (1). This process occurs uniformly and independently of the primary nature of the underlying disorder (1). Glomerular hypertension, sustained immunological injury, metabolic abnormalities, or altered cytokine expression are potential mechanisms involved in the development of chronic renal failure (1). In recent years, we have focused studies on the role of transforming growth factor-β (TGF-β), a multifunctional cytokine with major profibrotic properties (2–4). TGF-β contributes to fibrosis by three distinct mechanisms: (a) induction of synthesis of extracellular matrix proteins such as fibronectin, collagens, and proteoglycans; (b) decreased matrix degradation by suppression of proteases and by induction of protease inhibitors; and (c) modulation of expression of the integrin class of cell adhesion receptors, which participate in matrix assembly (2–4). Whereas these properties may be beneficial in wound healing or in development, they may be deleterious where progressive sclerosis is a pathophysiological feature. TGF-β is capable of autoinducing its own production (5–7), which appears to be a key factor causing sustained TGF-β expression in chronic sclerosis. However, events leading to TGF-β autoinduction and sustained overexpression in vivo are poorly understood. This review will give an overview of the possible role of TGF-β in renal pathophysiology and will attempt to develop future perspectives for research and therapeutic strategies.

TGF-β BIOLOGY

General Aspects

TGF-β is a dimeric protein with a molecular weight of 25 kDa (3,4,8). In mammalian species, three isoforms (TGF-β1, 2, and 3) have been identified, which usually appear as homodimers, though heterodimers have also been found (3,4,8). The three genes are located on different chromosomes (3). TGF-βs are secreted as latent high-molecular-weight proteins and must be activated to exert their biological effects (3,8). The first step involves proteolytic processing, leading to cleavage of the TGF-β signal peptide from the TGF-β precursor at specific positions (3). Then, activation is achieved by dissociation of the dimeric, mature TGF-β protein from latency-associated peptides, which are remainders of the TGF-β precursor (3). Activation does not result in structural changes of subunits but represents weakening of noncovalent, stabilizing binding (3).

In vitro, activation can be achieved by plasmin, cathepsin D or glycosidase treatment, acidification, and heating (3,8). There are also soluble TGF-β binding proteins that can bind to active TGF-β (3,8). Binding to α_2-macroglobulin and to the proteoglycan decorin inactivates TGF-β (3,8,9). The in vivo mechanisms for TGF-β activation remain unclear (3,8).

The TGF-β Gene

The human TGF-β1 precursor gene is encoded by seven defined exons (3,10). The size of the introns is not known (3). The gene is estimated to be more than 100 kb (3,10) in length. The three TGF-β isoforms share all intron/exon junctions except the first, although the mRNA species range from 1.7 to 6.5 kb and the noncoding regions differ greatly among the TGF-β isoforms (3,10).

Two major promoter regions for the human TGF-β1 gene have been characterized (3,11). The positive regulatory region of the upstream promoter contains binding sites for transcription factors including nuclear factor 1 (NF-1), SP-1 and AP-1, the latter of which is thought to be involved in the regulation of TGF-β's ability to autoinduce its own expression (3,6,11). The second promoter region is localized between the two start sites (3,11). Whether there are species differences in the promoter regions or whether the other TGF-β genes differ from the TGF-β1 gene in this respect is uncertain.

TGF-β Isoform Interaction

The functional interrelationship of the three mammalian TGF-β isoforms remains to be determined. TGF-β1 and 2 have been detected in different ratios in different cell types. In platelets, the most concentrated natural source of TGF-β1, the ratio is 4:1 (3). The isoforms appear to share comparable biological properties, as they react interchangeably in most biological assays (3). However, it has been suggested that TGF-β1 is most important in regulating extracellular matrix synthesis and cell-matrix interactions, whereas TGF-β2 is more important in morphogenetic processes (12). There is also a differential activation of TGF-β isoforms by proinflammatory cytokines. IL-1β selectively suppresses TGF-β1 but induces TGF-β3 expression in chondrocytes (13).

TGF-β Receptors

TGF-βs exert their biological effects by binding to specific cell surface receptors (3,8,14–17). Three different receptors have been defined to date and can be found in most cells, but there are other, less well characterized membrane-bound proteins capable of binding TGF-β (3,8,14–17). The TGF-β receptors have been cloned and termed type I (53 kDa), type II (70 to 80 kDa), and type III (300 kDa) (3,8,14–17).

The type III receptor (betaglycan) possesses a proteoglycan-like structure and its function is not entirely clear (14,15). It is probably not directly involved in signal transduction (8,14,15). The type II receptor has a characteristic serine/threonine kinase domain in its cytoplasmic portion (16). Study of the function of the type I receptor supports the concept that the presence and interaction of both type I and type II receptors are needed for TGF-β action (8,17). Both receptors have higher affinity for TGF-β1 than for TGF-β2 and 3 in most, but not all, cell types (3,8).

Biological Action of TGF-βs

TGF-βs play a major role in the control of development, inflammation, and repair in most organisms (3,8). They have a pivotal influence on the following biological events: (a) cell proliferation (growth can be inhibited or induced in different cell types); (b) angiogenesis; (c) chemoattraction; (d) induction of other cytokines or cytokine receptors; and (e) extracellular matrix synthesis (2–4,8). As mentioned above, TGF-β increases overall extracellular matrix accumulation by distinct mechanisms (2–4). Taken with the ability of TGF-β to autoinduce its own synthesis (5–7), it has been suggested that TGF-β expression starts a vicious cycle leading finally to self-perpetuating accumulation of extracellular matrix in vital tissues (2).

Studies on wound healing have shown that TGF-β is needed for scar formation and that topically or systemically applied TGF-β enhances wound healing effectively even in healing-impaired experimental models (18–21). However, in chronic inflammatory fibrotic disorders, the potential of TGF-β to induce and increase deposition of extracellular matrix proteins like collagens and proteoglycans in tissues may lead to scar formation within vital organs and thereby to loss of organ function (2,18). Our studies on experimental glomerulonephritis and diabetic nephropathy as well as studies on liver cirrhosis and pulmonary fibrosis strongly suggest that TGF-β plays a major pathophysiological role in promoting chronic progressive sclerosis in these diseases (2,18,22–28).

INDUCTION OF EXTRACELLULAR MATRIX SYNTHESIS IN GLOMERULAR CELLS

Effects of TGF-β on Glomerular Cells in Vitro

We performed in vitro experiments to determine whether TGF-β induces synthesis of specialized matrix proteins (collagens I, III, IV, and V; tenascin; fibronectin; and chondroitin/dermatan sulfate proteoglycans) by glomerular cells, as it was known to do in many different cell types (3,4). Cultured mesangial cells responded to stimulation by TGF-β with increased synthesis of proteoglycans (29). This effect was specific for TGF-β and could not be observed with other cytokines; PDGF, TNF-α, and IL-2 (29).

Glomerular epithelial cells in culture showed increased protein synthesis of collagen IV, fibronectin, laminin, and biglycan following stimulation with TGF-β (30). Thus, both glomerular cell types responded to TGF-β stimulation in vitro with significantly enhanced production of extracellular matrix components (30).

TGF-β Expression in Acute Mesangioproliferative Glomerulonephritis in the Rat

To investigate and prove the significance of the in vitro findings, in vivo studies were performed in a well-defined model of experimental glomerulonephritis induced by antithymocyte antibodies in the rat (ATS-GN). Injection of antithymocyte serum leads to an initial, complement-dependent mesangial cell injury followed by characteristic accumulation of extracellular matrix within the glomerulus (22). In ATS-GN, TGF-β1-mRNA expression was increased from day 4 to day 14 after ATS injection, and this increase preceded increased extracellular matrix synthesis (Figure 1A–C) (22). Cultured glomeruli obtained from glomerulonephritic animals on days 4, 7, and 14 after ATS injection demonstrated significantly increased proteoglycan synthesis compared to controls (22). Conditioned medium from these glomeruli applied to cultured mesangial cells also induced increased proteoglycan synthesis in these cells, and this effect could be specifically blocked with a TGF-β neutralizing antibody (22).

These results were then confirmed by administration of a TGF-β neutralizing antibody in vivo in ATS-GN (31). This maneuver specifically suppressed extracellular matrix accumulation and proteinuria in this model without affecting increased TGF-β gene expression (Fig. 1D,E) (31). In conclusion, extracellular matrix accumulation in ATS-GN was proven to be TGF-β-dependent and prevention of matrix expansion abolished proteinuria, indicating a major pathophysiological role of TGF-β in this model.

In the same glomerulonephritis model, studies confirmed that PDGF is a key mitogenic cytokine inducing mesangial cell proliferation, which can be observed starting at about day 3 after ATS induction (32,33). Interestingly, TGF-β is a potential regulator of PDGF in tissues by inducing PDGF-mRNA and PDGF-β-receptor-mRNA expression (34,35). Thus, interaction of these two cytokines may coordinate proliferative and fibrotic changes in glomerular diseases, as is discussed in more detail below.

Inhibition of the Plasmin Protease System in Experimental Glomerulonephritis

Another well-investigated mechanism by which TGF-β increases matrix deposition in tissues is its potential to decrease synthesis and secretion of proteases [plasminogen activator (PA), collagenase, elastase, transin/stromelysin] and to stimulate secretion of protease inhibitors [TIMP, plasminogen activator inhibitor (PAI-1)] (2–4). We have also investigated these properties in ATS-GN in vivo (36). Marked decreases in PA activity and increases in PAI-1 synthesis were seen when TGF-β was added to normal glomeruli (36). Diseased glomeruli also showed decreased PA activity, increased PAI-1 synthesis, and increased PAI-1 deposition into matrix. Administration of anti-TGF-β serum to glomerulonephritic rats blocked the expected increase in glomerular PAI-1 deposition. These changes in the PA/PAI-1 balance would favor accumulation of matrix. Thus, a TGF-β-induced decrease in matrix degradation may well be another factor contributing to the accumulation of extracellular matrix in experimental glomerulonephritis.

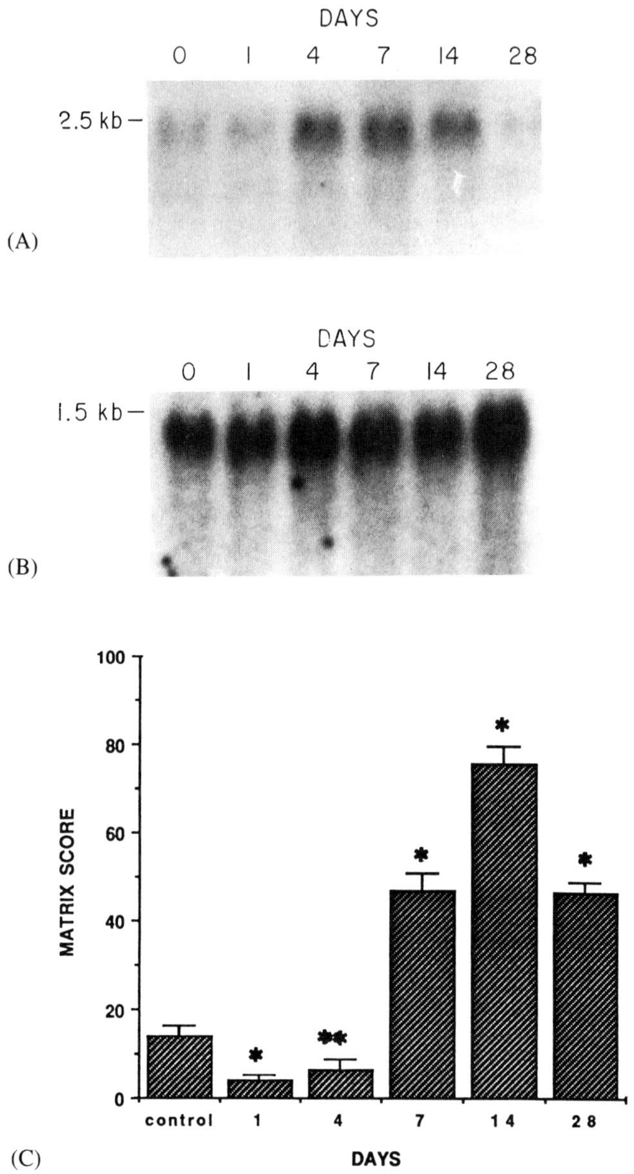

Figure 1 Northern blotting of TGF-β (A) and GAPDH-mRNA (B) in relation to extracellular matrix accumulation (C) in the time course of experimental glomerulonephritis (ATS-GN). After in vivo administration of anti-TGF-β antibody, TGF-β-mRNA expression (D) is slightly increased at day 7 compared to disease control and normal rats, whereas matrix accumulation (E) is greatly reduced by this treatment. For Northern blotting, total glomerular RNA was used, separated on an agarose gel and transferred to a nylon membrane by capillary action. Extracellular matrix accumulation was determined by scoring the percent of glomerular area occupied by extracellular matrix in periodic acid-Schiff (PAS)-stained kidney tissue slices. (From Refs. 22 and 31.)

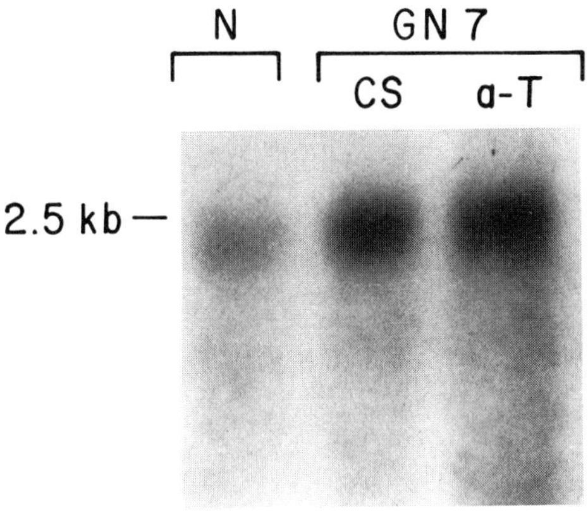

(D)

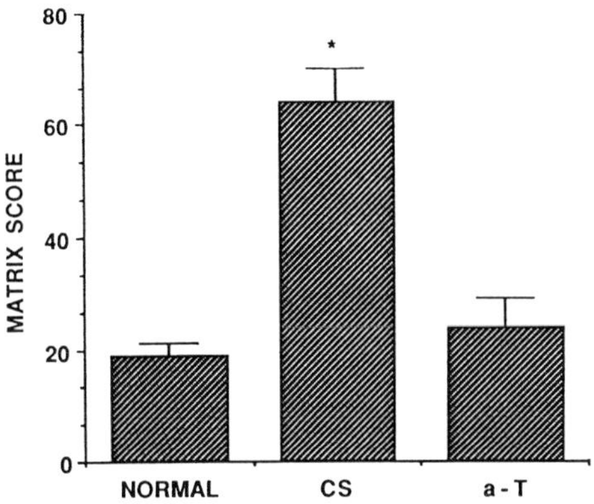

(E)

Induction of Integrin Expression by TGF-β in Vivo

The integrin class of cell adhesion receptors are transmembrane links between the extracellular matrix and the cytoskeletal elements of the cell (37). TGF-β1 and TGF-β2 induce increased expression of specific integrins necessary for extracellular matrix assembly (3,38).

In vitro, TGF-β1 stimulated β1 integrin expression in cultured, normal glomeruli (39). We then investigated expression of β1 integrins in ATS-GN using immunofluorescence and biosynthetic labeling techniques (39). In ATS-GN, we found an increase in the $\alpha 1\beta 1$ and $\alpha 5\beta 1$ integrins and a decrease in the $\alpha 3\beta 1$ integrin (39). $\alpha 5\beta 1$ is the major fibronectin receptor and is needed for matrix deposition (40,41). Its expression closely paralleled increased fibronectin accumulation (39). The $\alpha 3\beta 1$ integrin has no known role in matrix deposition. Thus, we obtained evidence that TGF-β is involved in the process of extracellular matrix accumulation in experimental glomerulonephritis by inducing (a) increased matrix protein synthesis, (b) decreased matrix protein degradation, and (c) increased and coordinated integrin expression.

TGF-β IN CHRONIC DISEASE MODELS

Diabetic Nephropathy

ATS-GN is an acute model of glomerulonephritis and disease is self-limiting. To further investigate the relevance of TGF-β expression in the process of progressive glomerular and tubulointerstitial fibrosis, we concluded studies in rat models of chronic renal disease (23,42).

In diabetes mellitus induced by injection of streptozotocin in the rat, development of nephropathy was associated with a slow, progressive increase in TGF-β-mRNA in the glomerulus (23). This was paralleled by significant increases in fibronectin and tenascin deposition within glomeruli, as shown by histological staining (23). Both increased TGF-β expression and matrix deposition was blunted but not abolished by moderate insulin treatment, correcting average blood glucose levels to 350 mg% compared to 550 mg% in non-insulin-treated diabetic rats (23). Studies on human biopsies confirmed that increased TGF-β expression was associated with diabetic nephropathy (23). Figure 2 shows immunofluorescence micrographs of human glomeruli from normal controls (A), patients with minimal change disease (B), and patients with diabetic nephropathy (C and D), all stained with an anti-TGF-β antibody.

Glomerulosclerosis Induced by Repeated ATS Injections

Another chronic disease model was developed using a second injection of ATS in the rat (42). In contrast to the single-bolus injection in acute ATS-GN, this maneuver leads to progressive glomerulosclerotic changes closely resembling glomerulosclerosis in the human (42). As in diabetic nephropathy, sustained TGF-β expression was an intriguing finding and was closely correlated with progressive glomerular and tubulointerstitial sclerosis in this model (42).

The mechanism leading to this chronic disease course remains undefined. We hypothesize that the second ATS-induced mesangial injury causes cellular events that finally lead to sustained TGF-β production. TGF-β overexpression, in turn, leads to progressive and uncontrolled synthesis and deposition of matrix molecules within glomerular and tubulointerstitial areas. Potential molecular mechanisms focusing on cell-matrix and matrix-matrix interactions are currently under investigation in our laboratory.

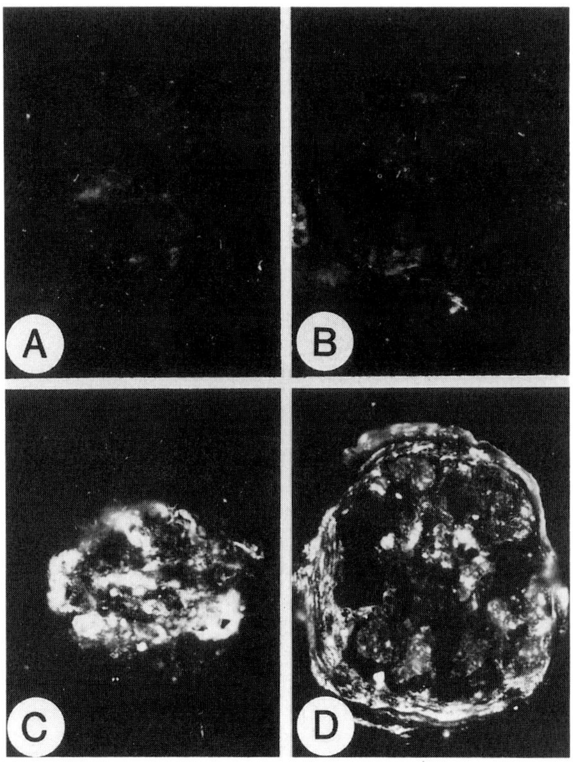

Figure 2 Immunofluorescence of human glomeruli stained with anti-TGF-β1 antibody. (A) Glomerulus from a normal kidney. (B) Glomerulus from the kidney of a patient with minimal change disease. (C and D) Glomeruli from two patients with severe matrix accumulation characteristic of diabetic glomerulosclerosis. (From Ref. 23.)

HIV Nephropathy and Other Chronic Fibrotic Diseases

Additional information supporting the importance of TGF-β as a fibrogenic cytokine in renal disease comes from the area of HIV research. In HIV-infected patients, increased systemic TGF-β production is frequently noted (43,44). It has been proposed that this finding is associated with clinical immunosuppression because of TGF-β's significant immunosuppressive properties (3,18,43,44). On the other hand, HIV-associated nephropathy is characterized by severe glomerulosclerosis (45). We recently studied human kidney biopsies by using immunofluorescence techniques and found a most striking overexpression in the glomeruli of patients with HIV-associated nephropathy closely correlated with the severity of sclerotic changes (46).

Thus, evidence that TGF-β is an important mediator of chronic fibrosis is accumulating. In addition to our studies, other investigators have obtained data showing elevated expression of TGF-β in different animal models of renal disease, including anti-GBM nephritis and puromycin aminonucleoside nephrosis (47,48). Experimental and human studies in liver cirrhosis, pulmonary fibrosis, vitreoretinopathy, and systemic sclerosis support the notion that TGF-β overexpression is significantly involved in the pathophysiology of these diseases (24–28,49,50). These findings suggest that potential therapeutic strategies targeting TGF-β overexpression may be beneficial treatments in chronic fibrotic disease.

ANTAGONISM OF TGF-β AS A THERAPEUTIC STRATEGY

Decorin: A TGF-β-Binding Proteoglycan

As shown in Figure 1C and D, in vivo administration of a TGF-β neutralizing antibody prevented extracellular matrix accumulation in ATS-GN (31). However, treatment with a foreign antibody in chronic diseases is not suitable because of its potential immunogenicity. As pointed out above, decorin, a naturally occurring proteoglycan, has the ability to bind and inactivate TGF-β (8,9). Decorin is a small dermatan sulfate proteoglycan with a molecular mass of approximately 100 kDa (a core protein and a single glycosaminoglycan chain) characterized by 10 leucine-rich repeats (8,9). Such leucine-rich sequences have been postulated to mediate protein-protein and protein-membrane interactions (8). In addition to TGF-β, decorin is also capable of binding fibronectin, collagens (type I and IV), and C1q (8,51).

Pharmacokinetic studies showed that decorin appeared to target kidney, liver, and lung of rats after intravenous injection (52). We then conducted a study in ATS-GN using intravenous administration of recombinant human decorin to observe its effect on extracellular matrix accumulation (53). Decorin was given daily beginning 1 hr after ATS (53). Injections of aggrecan (a non-TGF-β-binding proteoglycan), ovalbumin, bovine serum albumin, and PBS (vehicle) were used as control for specific decorin effects (53). Four to six daily injections of decorin reduced proteinuria and deposition of matrix proteins fibronectin and tenascin in the nephritic glomeruli compared to disease control rats (53). Interestingly, daily decorin injection for the first 3 days after ATS injection was without effect in ATS-GN, whereas two single injections on days 4 and 5 were as effective in preventing extracellular matrix accumulation as six daily injections (52,53). This suggests a differential susceptibility of the microenvironment of the glomerulus to decorin effects. It is possible that decorin's binding to collagens may somehow mediate this effect. Studies in experimental models of chronic kidney diseases are currently under way in our laboratory to test the hypothesis that decorin beneficially affects progressive glomerular and tubulointerstitial fibrosis. If this were the case, decorin might have enormous potential as a new and effective treatment of chronic fibrotic diseases in general.

Low-Protein Diet

A low-protein diet has been proven to ameliorate the course of most experimental and human chronic kidney diseases (54–57). However, the mechanism of this effect still remains to be determined. We were interested in how dietary protein restriction would affect TGF-β expression and matrix accumulation in ATS-GN.

Rats were fed normal-protein (22%) and low-protein diets (6%) starting after ATS injection (58). We observed a marked decrease in extracellular matrix accumulation at days 7, 14, and 28 after disease induction accompanied by significantly decreased proteinuria starting at day 4 compared to control animals (58). Even more striking was the observation that a low-protein diet abolished the increase of TGF-β-mRNA expression that is otherwise characteristic of ATS-GN (58). This occurred in spite of a very similar degree of initial mesangial cell injury in both groups. Thus, it is possible that part of the beneficial effects of a low-protein diet are mediated by direct suppression of growth factor expression.

TGF-β: INTERACTION WITH OTHER GROWTH FACTORS OR PEPTIDES

Platelet-Derived Growth Factor (PDGF)

PDGF is another cytokine proposed to play a pathophysiological role in the progression of chronic renal disease (1,33). PDGF is a strong mitogen and its expression is closely associated with mesangial cell proliferation in vivo and in vitro (32,33). Mesangial hypercellularity is observed in the time course of most progressive experimental and human kidney diseases and is thought to precede or possibly contribute to pronounced glomerulosclerotic changes (1,33). However, a direct effect of PDGF on glomerular or tubulointerstitial matrix accumulation has not been demonstrated.

TGF-β is antiproliferative for mesangial cells and fibroblasts (3). However, TGF-β is capable of inducing PDGF-B and PDGF-β-receptor expression in vitro (31,32). A recent study showed that the TGF-β effect on mesangial cells is biphasic: TGF-β was growth-inhibitory for the first 36 hr and growth-stimulatory in the following 36 hr (34). This observation was due at least in part to induction of PDGF-B- and PDGF-β-receptor mRNA synthesis (34). The in vivo interaction of TGF-β and PDGF in models of acute and chronic renal disease deserves further study.

In this context, a recent study of Isaka and coworkers used in vivo transfection of cytokine cDNA as a tool to investigate cytokine-specific effects on kidney tissue (59). HVJ liposomes containing TGF-β- or PDGF-B-cDNA were injected into the left renal artery of rats. Both genes were subsequently expressed in the otherwise normal left kidney. TGF-β expression caused prominent extracellular matrix accumulation within glomeruli as reflected by increased collagen I and III deposition, whereas PDGF-B expression was followed by marked mesangial hypercellularity (59).

TGF-β and Proinflammatory Cytokines

TGF-β is also known for its significant anti-inflammatory effects (3,18,60). In a TGF-β1 gene knockout model, mice die in a state of generalized inflammation (60). This finding may involve TGF-β's ability to control expression of acute-phase cytokines interleukins-1 to -3 (IL-1 to IL-3), tumor necrosis factor-α (TNF-α), and interferon-γ (IFN-γ) (3,18). TNF-α, IL-1, IL-6, and IL-8 have been implicated in immunological injury in experimental and human glomerular disease (61–64). Recent studies showed that administration of an IL-1 receptor antagonist suppressed experimental crescentic glomerulonephritis induced by anti-GBM nephrotoxic serum (62,65). Whether acute-phase cytokine-induced glomerular injury and TGF-β expression are interconnected or whether TGF-β plays a role in suppressing early inflammatory processes in vivo is still unclear. Further studies would certainly help our understanding of the complexity of immune-mediated injury in renal diseases.

Angiotensin II

Angiotensin II, a peptide hormone and a mitogen, has been implicated as a mediator of progression of renal diseases (1,66,67). Angiotensin II causes increased intraglomerular pressure and might thereby promote damage to the glomerulus (1,66,67). Angiotensin II converting enzyme inhibitors (ACE-I) ameliorate the course of chronic renal failure; their beneficial effect may be in part independent of glomerular hemodynamics, since they are superior to some other antihypertensive drugs (68,69).

Recent studies in vascular smooth muscle cells and proximal tubular cells have clearly demonstrated that angiotensin II in physiological concentrations induces TGF-β-mRNA expression and that this expression is responsible for cell hypertrophy in vitro (70,71). We have performed experiments on cultured mesangial cells and found that angiotensin II directly increases TGF-β-mRNA expression, causes activation of latent TGF-β, and that it increases the synthesis of matrix proteins collagen I and biglycan (72). TGF-β expression and matrix protein synthesis could be suppressed by an angiotensin II receptor antagonist (72). Angiotensin II–induced increases in collagen I and biglycan expression were suppressed by addition of a neutralizing TGF-β antibody (72). These findings suggest that angiotensin II, independent of glomerular hemodynamic changes, induces TGF-β expression, which, in turn, induces the synthesis and accumulation of extracellular matrix (72). Thus, the beneficial properties of ACE-I in progressive renal disease may be partly due to this mechanism. Further studies on the role of the tissue renin angiotensin system (tRAS) will be of great interest (73,74).

PERSPECTIVES

Decorin Treatment of Fibrosis

From the studies outlined above, there is significant evidence that TGF-β is an important mediator of chronic fibrotic diseases and may play a major pathophysiological role in glomerular and tubulointerstitial sclerosis. Treatments that target TGF-β-mediated fibrosis will therefore be one focus of future research. Decorin is a potential candidate for therapy (18,53).

A recent study on bleomycin-induced pulmonary fibrosis produced the interesting finding that decorin expression was greatly decreased in the initial stages of disease, later rebounding to normal in the resolution phases of the disease (26). These data suggest that decorin plays a role in the normal healing process, possibly shutting down TGF-β production. An interesting hypothesis is that local decorin deficiency contributes to chronic TGF-β overexpression during chronic fibrosis.

Decorin also binds collagens and fibronectin (3,8). The observation that decorin treatment in ATS-GN was most effective on days 4 and 5 after disease induction raises the possibility that synthesis and deposition of collagen I, not normally present within the mesangium, influences the decorin effect on TGF-β expression. Using immunohistochemistry, we recently found a significant colocalization of collagen I and exogenously injected decorin in glomeruli of nephritic animals (unpublished observation). Whether this is of functional importance remains to be determined.

Since TGF-β receptors type I, II, and III have been cloned, receptor agonists and antagonists may become available (14–17). Knowledge about complex receptor physiology is increasing; the type III receptor betaglycan probably serves as a binding reservoir of free TGF-β and might thereby regulate TGF-β release to type I and II receptors (8,14,15). Influencing this interaction may become another therapeutic approach.

Arginine Metabolism and TGF-β

Another therapeutic strategy that affected TGF-β expression in vivo was a low-protein diet (58). We hypothesized that the amino acid L-arginine might play a role in mediating the effect of a low-protein diet, because activation of the L-arginine/nitric oxide (NO) pathway had been implicated in immune-mediated tissue injury (75,76). In fact, we were able to demonstrate decreases in proteinuria, matrix accumulation, and TGF-β expression in ATS-GN with a normal-protein diet (22%) depleted of L-arginine (77). Rats fed a low-protein diet (6%) where L-arginine was supplemented in the drinking water showed no reduction in disease activity (77). We have also shown that L-arginine–restricted diets and L-NMMA, a competitive inhibitor of NO synthesis, prevents mesangial cell lysis in ATS-GN when injected 60 min prior to disease induction (78). Thus, L-arginine metabolism may be involved in renal pathophysiology.

In addition to NO, L-arginine is metabolized to L-ornithine, a substrate for L-proline and polyamine synthesis (79,80). L-Proline is a necessary substrate for the buildup of collagens (81,82). Polyamines (putrescine, spermine, spermidine) are potent inducers of DNA and RNA synthesis and regulate growth and proliferation in many tissues (83,84). Polyamine synthesis can be stimulated in mesangial cells in vitro by angiotensin II and PDGF, and it has been speculated that polyamines act as a second-messenger system for these mitogenic molecules (85,86). Thus, activation of both L-proline and polyamine synthesis could be involved in sclerotic and proliferative changes in diseased

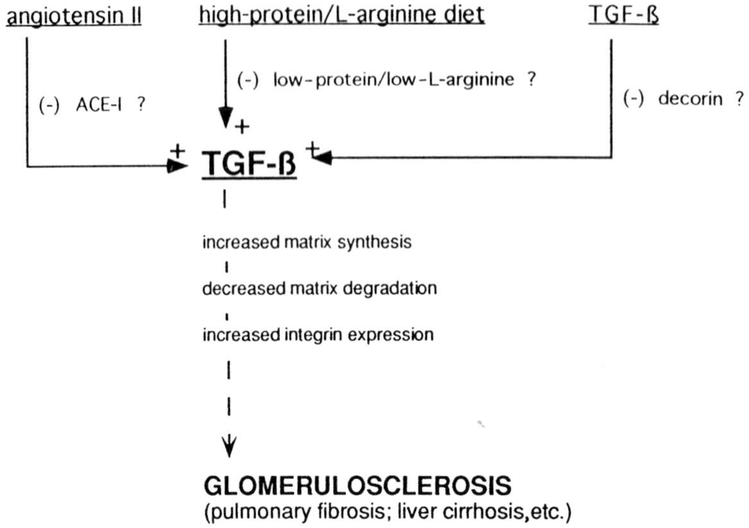

Figure 3 The suggested role of TGF-β in glomerulosclerosis and other chronic fibrotic diseases. Angiotensin II, high protein, and possibly high L-arginine intake may play a role in the induction of TGF-β expression. TGF-β may also autoinduce its own production in chronic fibrotic diseases.

kidneys. Studies addressing the regulation of L-arginine metabolism especially focusing on its influence on TGF-β expression in chronic models of kidney disease are under way.

Angiotensin II Antagonism

Finally, the observation that angiotensin II is capable of directly inducing TGF-β expression is certainly a very interesting one (70–72). Experimental studies that try to block the deleterious effects of angiotensin II on the kidney by antagonizing TGF-β action in vivo may elucidate the relevance of a TGF-β/angiotensin II interaction. The effect of angiotensin II receptor antagonists or ACE-I on TGF-β expression in vivo would be another reasonable approach. Finally, understanding of the regulation of the tissue renin angiotensin system and its connection to growth factor expression will be a very challenging project for future research.

CONCLUSION

TGF-β is a multifunctional cytokine with predominant stimulatory effects on extracellular matrix production. In renal pathophysiology, TGF-β plays a pivotal role in mediating progressive glomerular and tubulointerstitial sclerosis in chronic kidney diseases (Figure 3 presents a schematic picture). Data from experimental and human kidney diseases strongly support this concept. The mechanisms leading to sustained TGF-β overexpression are very poorly understood. Elevated angiotensin II may promote chronic induction of TGF-β in the kidney. Decorin, a TGF-β neutralizing proteoglycan, or L-arginine-restricted diets may become new and specific treatments of TGF-β-mediated chronic fibrosis, though their mechanisms are not yet entirely understood. New molecular biology techniques such as in vivo transfection of cytokine cDNA offer more powerful tools to investigate the complex interaction of growth factors and extracellular matrix synthesis.

REFERENCES

1. Klahr S, Schreiner G, Ichikawa I. The progression of renal disease. N Engl J Med 1988; 318:1657.
2. Border WA, Ruoslahti E. Transforming growth factor-β in disease: the dark side of tissue repair. J Clin Invest 1992; 90:1.

3. Roberts AB, Sporn MB. The transforming growth factor-βs. In: Sporn MB, Roberts AB, eds. Handbook of Experimental Pharmacology: Peptide Growth Factors and Their Receptors I (Vol 95/I). Springer Verlag, 1992: 419.
4. Roberts AB, McCune BK, Sporn MB. TGF-β: regulation of extracellular matrix. Kidney Int 1992; 41:557.
5. Van Obberghen-Schilling E, Roche NS, Flanders KC, et al. Transforming growth factor β1 regulates its own expression in normal and transformed cells. J Biol Chem 1987; 263:7741.
6. Kim SJ, Angel P, Lafyatis R, et al. Autoinduction of transforming growth factor β1 is mediated by the AP-1 complex. Mol Cell Biol 1990; 10:1492.
7. Kaname S, Uchida S, Ogata E, Kurokawa K. Autocrine secretion of transforming growth factor-β in cultured rat mesangial cells. Kidney Int 1992; 42:1319.
8. Miyazono K, Ichijo H, Heldin CH. Transforming growth factor-β: Latent forms, binding and receptors. Growth Factors 1993; 8:11.
9. Yamaguchi Y, Mann DM, Ruoslahti E. Negative regulation of transforming growth factor-β by the proteoglycan decorin. Nature 1990; 346:281.
10. Derynck R, Rhee L, Chen EY, Van Tilburg A. Intron-exon structure of human transforming growth factor-β precursor gene. Nucleic Acids Res 1987; 15:3188.
11. Kim SJ, Glick A, Sporn MB, Roberts AB. Characterization of the promoter region of the human transforming growth factor-β1 gene. J Biol Chem 1989; 264:402.
12. Streuli CH, Schmidhauser C, Kobrin N, et al. Extracellular matrix regulates expression of the TGF-β gene. J Cell Biol 1993; 120:253.
13. Villiger PM, Kusari AB, ten Dijke P, Lotz M. IL-1β and IL-6 induce transforming growth factor-β isoforms in human articular chondrocytes. J Immunol 1993; 151:3337.
14. Wang XF, Lin HY, Ng-Eaton E, et al. Expression cloning and characterization of the TGF-β type III receptor. Cell 1991; 67:797.
15. Lopez-Casillas F, Cheifetz S, Doody J, et al. Structure and expression of the membrane proteoglycan betaglycan, a component of the TGF-β receptor system. Cell 1991; 67:785.
16. Lin HY, Wang XF, Ng-Eaton E, et al. Expression cloning of the TGF-β type II receptor, a functional transmembrane serine/threonine kinase. Cell 1992; 68:775.
17. Ebner R, Chen RH, Shum L, et al. Cloning of a type I TGF-β receptor and its effect on TGF-β binding to the type II receptor. Science 1993; 260:1344.
18. Roberts AB, Sporn MB. Physiological actions and clinical applications of transforming growth factor-β (TGF-β). Growth Factors 1993; 8:1.
19. Beck LS, Chen TL, Mikalauski P, Ammann AJ. Recombinant human transforming growth factor-β1 (rhTGF-β1) enhances healing and strength of granulation skin wounds. Growth Factors 1990; 3:267.
20. Beck LS, DeGuzman L, Lee WP, et al. TGF-β1 accelerates wound healing: Reversal of steroid-impaired healing in rats and rabbits. Growth Factors 1991; 5:295.
21. Bernstein EF, Harisiadis L, Salomon G, et al. Transforming growth factor-β improves healing of radiation-impaired wounds. J Invest Dermatol 1991; 97:430.
22. Okuda S, Languino LR, Ruoslahti E, Border WA. Elevated expression of transforming growth factor-β and proteoglycan production in experimental glomerulonephritis. J Clin Invest 1990; 86:453.
23. Yamamoto T, Nakamura T, Noble NA, et al. Expression of transforming growth factor β is elevated in human and experimental diabetic nephropathy. Proc Natl Acad Sci USA 1993; 90:1814.
24. Broekelmann TJ, Limper AH, Colby TV, McDonald JA. Transforming growth factor-β1 is present at sites of extracellular matrix gene expression in human pulmonary fibrosis. Proc Natl Acad Sci USA 1991; 88:6642.
25. Khalil N, O'Connor RN, Unruh HW, et al. Increased production and immunohistochemical localization of transforming growth factor-β in idiopathic pulmonary fibrosis. Am J Respir Cell Mol Biol 1991; 5:155.
26. Westergren-Thorsson G, Hernnas S, Sarnstrand B, et al. Altered expression of small proteoglycans, collagen and transforming growth factor-β1 in developing bleomycin-induced pulmonary fibrosis in rats. J Clin Invest 1993; 92:632.
27. Friedmann SL. The cellular basis of hepatic fibrosis: Mechanisms and treatment strategies. N Engl J Med 1993; 328:1828.
28. Castilla A, Prieto J, Fausto N. Transforming growth factors β1 and α in chronic liver disease. N Engl J Med 1991; 324:933.
29. Border WA, Okuda S, Languino LR, Ruoslahti E. Transforming growth factor-β regulates production of proteoglycans by mesangial cells. Kidney Int 1990; 37:689.
30. Nakamura T, Miller D, Ruoslahti E, Border WA: Production of extracellular matrix by glomerular epithelial cells is regulated by transforming growth factor-β1. Kidney Int 1992; 41:1213.
31. Border WA, Okuda S, Languino LR, et al. Suppression of experimental glomerulonephritis by antiserum against transforming growth factor-β1. Nature 1990; 346:371.
32. Iida H, Seifert R, Alpers CE, et al. Platelet-derived growth factor (PDGF) and PDGF receptor are induced in mesangial proliferative nephritis in the rat. Proc Natl Acad Sci USA 1991; 88:6560.

33. Floege J, Eng E, Young BA, Johnson RJ: Factors involved in the regulation mesangial cell proliferation in vitro and in vivo. Kidney Int 1993; 43:S47.
34. Haberstroh U, Zahner G, Disser M, et al. TGF-β stimulates rat mesangial cell proliferation in culture: Role of PDGF β-receptor expression. Am J Physiol 1993; 264:F199.
35. Gronwald RGK, Seifert RA, Bowen-Pope DF: Differential regulation of two platelet-derived growth factor receptor subunits by transforming growth factor-β. J Biol Chem 1989; 264:8120.
36. Tomooka S, Border WA, Marshall BC, Noble NA: Glomerular matrix accumulation is linked to inhibition of the plasmin protease system. Kidney Int 1992; 42:1462.
37. Hynes RO: Integrins: A family of cell surface receptors. Cell 1987; 48:549.
38. Ignotz RA, Endo T, Massague J: Regulation of fibronectin and type I collagen mRNA levels by transforming growth factor-β. J Biol Chem 1987; 262:6443.
39. Kagami S, Border WA, Ruoslahti E, Noble NA. Coordinated expression of β1 integrins and TGF-β1-induced matrix proteins in glomerulonephritis. Lab Invest 1993; 69:68.
40. Roman J, LaChance RM, Broekelmann TJ, et al. The fibronectin receptor is organized by extracellular matrix fibronectin: Implications for oncogenic transformation and for cell recognition of fibronectin matrices. J Cell Biol 1989; 108:2529.
41. Akiyama SK, Yamada SSD, Chen WT, Yamada KM. Analysis of fibronectin receptor function with monoclonal antibodies: Roles in cell adhesion, migration, matrix assembly, and cytoskeletal organization. J Cell Biol 1989; 109:863.
42. Yamamoto T, Noble NA, Miller DE, Border WA. Sustained expression of transforming growth factor-β1 as a molecular mechanism of fibrotic disease. Kidney Int 1994; 45:916.
43. Kekow J, Wachsmann W, McCutchan JA, et al. Transforming growth factor-β and suppression of humoral immune responses in HIV infection. J Clin Invest 1991; 87:1010.
44. Kekow J, Wachsmann W, McCutchan JA, et al. Transforming growth factor-β and noncytophatic mechanisms of immunedeficiency in human immunedeficiency virus infection. Proc Natl Acad Sci USA 1990; 87:8321.
45. Seney FD Jr, Burns DK, Silva FG. Acquired immunedeficiency syndrome and the kidney. Am J Kidney Dis 1990; 16:1.
46. Border WA, Yamamoto T, Noble NA, et al. HIV-associated nephropathy is linked to TGF-β and matrix protein expression in human kidney (abstr). J Am Soc Nephrol 1993; 4:675.
47. Coimbra T, Wiggins R, Noh JW, et al. Transforming growth factor-β production in anti-glomerular basement membrane disease in the rabbit. Am J Pathol 1991; 138:223.
48. Jones CL, Buch S, Post M, et al. Pathogenesis of interstitial fibrosis in chronic purine aminonucleoside nephrosis. Kidney Int 1991; 40:1020.
49. Gruschwitz M, Mueller PU, Sepp N, et al. Transcription and expression of transforming growth factor type beta in the skin of progressive systemic sclerosis: A mediator of fibrosis? J Invest Dermatol 1990; 94:197.
50. Connor TJ Jr, Roberts AB, Sporn MB, et al. Correlation of fibrosis and transforming growth factor-β type 2 levels in the eye. J Clin Invest 1989; 83:1661.
51. Krumdiek R, Hook M, Rosenberg LC, Volanakis JE. The proteoglycan decorin binds C1q and inhibits the activity of the C1 complex. J Immunol 1992; 149:3695.
52. Noble NA, Harper JR, Border WA. In vivo interactions of TGF-β and extracellular matrix. Progr Growth Factor Res 1993; 4:369.
53. Border WA, Noble NA, Yamamoto T, et al. Natural inhibitor of transforming growth factor-β protects against scarring in experimental kidney disease. Nature 1992; 360:361.
54. Hostetter TH, Meyer TW, Rennke HG, Brenner BM. Chronic effect of dietary protein in the rat with intact and reduced renal mass. Kidney Int 1986; 30:509.
55. Rosman JB, Meijer S, Sluiter WJ, et al. Prospective randomized trial of early dietary protein restriction in chronic renal failure. Lancet 1984; 2:1291.
56. Brenner BM, Meyer TW, Hostetter TH. Dietary protein intake and the progressive nature of kidney disease: The role of hemodynamically mediated glomerular injury in the pathogenesis of progressive glomerular sclerosis in aging, renal ablation and intrinsic renal disease. N Engl J Med 1982; 307:652.
57. Ihle BU, Becker GJ, Whitworth JA, et al. The effect of protein restriction on the progression of renal insufficiency. N Engl J Med 1990; 321:1773.
58. Okuda S, Nakamura T, Yamamoto T, et al. Dietary protein restriction rapidly reduces transforming growth factor-β1 expression in experimental glomerulonephritis. Proc Natl Acad Sci USA 1991; 88:9765.
59. Isaka I, Fujiwara I, Ueda N, et al. Glomerulosclerosis induced by in vivo transfection of TGF-β or PDGF gene into the rat kidney. J Clin Invest 1993; 92:2597.
60. Shull MM, Ormsby I, Kier AB, et al. Targeted disruption of the mouse transforming growth factor-β1 gene results in multifocal inflammatory disease. Nature 1992; 359:693.
61. Egido J, Gomez-Chiarri M, Ortiz A, et al. Role of tumor necrosis factor-α in the pathogenesis of glomerular diseases. Kidney Int 1993; 43:S59.0

62. Lan HY, Nikolic-Paterson DJ, Zarama M, et al. Suppression of experimental crescentic glomerulonephritis by the interleukin-1 receptor antagonist. Kidney Int 1993; 43:479.
63. Horii Y, Iwano M, Hirata E, et al. Role of interleukin-6 in the progression of mesangial proliferative glomerulonephritis. Kidney Int 1993; 43:S71.
64. Sterzel RB, Schulze-Lohoff E, Marx M. Cytokines and mesangial cells. Kidney Int 1993; 43:S26.
65. Tang VW, Feng L, Vannice JL, Wilson CB. Interleukin-1 receptor antagonist ameliorates experimental anti-glomerular basement membrane antibody-associated glomerulonephritis. J Clin Invest 1994; 93:273.
66. Miller PL, Rennke HG, Meyer TW. Glomerular hypertrophy accelerates hypertensive glomerular injury in rats. Am J Physiol 1991; 261:F459.
67. Johnson RJ, Alpers CE, Yoshimura A, et al. Renal injury from angiotensin II-mediated hypertension. Hypertension 1992; 19:464.
68. Brunner HR. ACE inhibitors in renal disease. Kidney Int 1992; 42:463.
69. Diamond JR, Anderson S. Irreversible tubulointerstitial damage associated with chronic aminonucleoside nephrosis: Amelioration by angiotensin I converting enzyme inhibition. Am J Pathol 1990; 137:1323.
70. Gibbons GH, Pratt RE, Dzau VJ. Vascular smooth muscle cell hypertrophy vs. hyperplasia: Autocrine transforming growth factor-β1 expression determines growth response to angiotensin II. J Clin Invest 1992; 90:456.
71. Wolf G, Mueller E, Stahl RAK, Ziyadeh F. Angiotensin II-induced hypertrophy of cultured murine proximal tubular cells is mediated by endogenous transforming growth factor-β. J Clin Invest 1993; 92:1366.
72. Kagami S, Border WA, Miller DE, Noble NA. Angiotensin II stimulates extracellular matrix protein synthesis through induction of transforming growth factor-β expression in rat glomerular mesangial cells. J Clin Invest 1994; 93. In press.
73. Paul M, Wagner J, Dzau VJ. Gene expression of the renin-angiotensin system in human tissues. J Clin Invest 1993, 91:2058.
74. Dzau VJ, Burt DW, Pratt RE. Molecular biology of the renin-angiotensin system. Am J Physiol 1988; 255:563.
75. Mulligan MS, Hevel JM, Marletta MA, Ward PA. Tissue injury caused by deposition of immune complexes is L-arginine dependent. Proc Natl Acad Sci USA 1991; 88:6338.
76. McCartney-Francis N, Allen JB, Mizel DE, et al. Suppression of arthritis by an inhibitor of nitric oxide synthase. J Exp Med 1993; 178:749.
77. Narita I, Border WA, Ketteler M, et al. L-Arginine may mediate the therapeutic effects of low protein diets. Proc Natl Acad Sci USA. In press.
78. Narita I, Border WA, Ketteler M, Noble NA. Nitric oxide mediates immunologic injury to kidney mesangium in experimental glomerulonephritis. Lab Invest 1995; 72:17.
79. Barbul A. Arginine: Biochemistry, physiology, and therapeutic implications. J Parenter Enter Nutr 1986; 10:227.
80. Shih VE. Regulation of ornithine metabolism. Enzyme 1981; 27:254.
81. Rojkind M, deLeon D. Collagen synthesis in cirrhotic rat liver slices: A regulatory mechanism. Biochim Biophys Acta 1970; 217:512.
82. Smith RJ, Phang JM. Proline metabolism in cartilage: The importance of proline biosynthesis. Metabolism 1978; 27:685.
83. Davis RH, Morris DR, Coffino P. Sequestered end-products and enzyme regulation: The case of ornithine decarboxylase. Microbiol Rev 1992; 56:280.
84. Pegg AE. Polyamine metabolism and its importance in neoplastic growth and as a target for chemotherapy. Cancer Res 1988; 48:759.
85. Schulze-Lohoff E, Brand K, Fees H, et al. Role of ornithine decarboxylase for proliferation of mesangial cells in culture. Kidney Int 1991; 40:648.
86. Schulze-Lohoff E, Koehler M, Fees H, et al. Divergent effects of arginine vasopressin and angiotensin II on proliferation and expression of the immediate early genes c-fos, c-jun and EGR-1 in cultured rat glomerular mesangial cells. J Hypertens 1993; 11:127.

42

Molecular Regulation of the Heat-Shock/Stress Response: Nephrologists' Perspective

Kerensa Fuller and Barbara S. Polla
Laboratoire de Physiologie respiratoire, UFR Cochin Port-Royal, Université Paris V, Paris, France

INTRODUCTION

In response to adverse conditions affecting the intracellular environment, a cell initiates a number of steps including the synthesis of new proteins or the increased transcription of existing ones (reviewed in Refs. 1–3). Although historically known as the heat shock (HS) response, since it was first observed in *Drosophila* chromosomes exposed to increased temperature (4), a similar response has been shown with a diverse array of stimuli including HS, amino acid analogues, heavy metals, ionophores, glucose deprivation, oxidative injury, and—in vivo—ischemia-reperfusion. At first glance, these stimuli seem to have little in common, suggesting that HS proteins (HSP) are members of a larger family of "stress proteins."

HSP are classified on the basis of apparent molecular weight on sodium dodecylsulfate polyacrylamide gel electrophoresis (SDS-PAGE) and their response to different stimuli. Not all stress proteins respond to the same stimuli: the classic HSP are those which respond to a rise in temperature, while the glucose-regulated proteins (GRP) are induced by glucose deprivation, calcium ionophores, and anoxia. The two groups are not exclusive: transition heavy metals and amino acid analogues have been shown to induce both (5). Some HSP are expressed constitutively and play important roles in normal cell development, particularly in growth. These constitutively expressed proteins are found in certain cell compartments and at specific times in the cell cycle (2). They are associated with most aspects of protein-protein interaction, including synthesis, translocation, folding, and molecular chaperoning (1,6–8). Proteins that are not constitutively expressed show induction at the level of transcription (9) and stabilization of the mRNA transcript (10).

HSP families include the low-molecular-weight (around 20 kDa) HSP, the hsp60–65, the hsp70, and the hsp90 families (1) (Figure 1). The precise role of the low-molecular-weight proteins has remained elusive. Recently two members of this family (heme oxygenase and a 23-kDa stress protein cloned from mouse macrophages) have been implicated in protection against oxidative injury and renal ischemia (11–13). Members of the hsp60 family are located in the mitochondria and chloroplasts and serve a role as molecular chaperones within these organelles. Significantly reduced levels of hsp60 were found in a severe mitochondrial disease, showing decreased activity of mitochondrial enzymes found in the inner membrane/matrix compartment and morphological abnormalities (14). Hsp60 was the first stress protein suggested to be involved in the development of autoimmunity (15–17). The hsp70 family consists of several members, some expressed constitutively, but whose expression rises upon HS and others that are expressed only in response to HS. They have been found to be highly conserved within species and across species with *E. coli* DnaK and human HSP70 showing 50% homology (18) and the homology within a family being as high as 90% (human hsp70-1 and hsp70-Hom). They are implicated in many different forms of protein-protein interaction, including p72 (the uncoating ATPase), which releases clathrin from coated vesicles; PBP72/74, recently confirmed as a member of the HSP family (19), which is a peptide-binding protein (20); and GRP78 (BiP), which is expressed

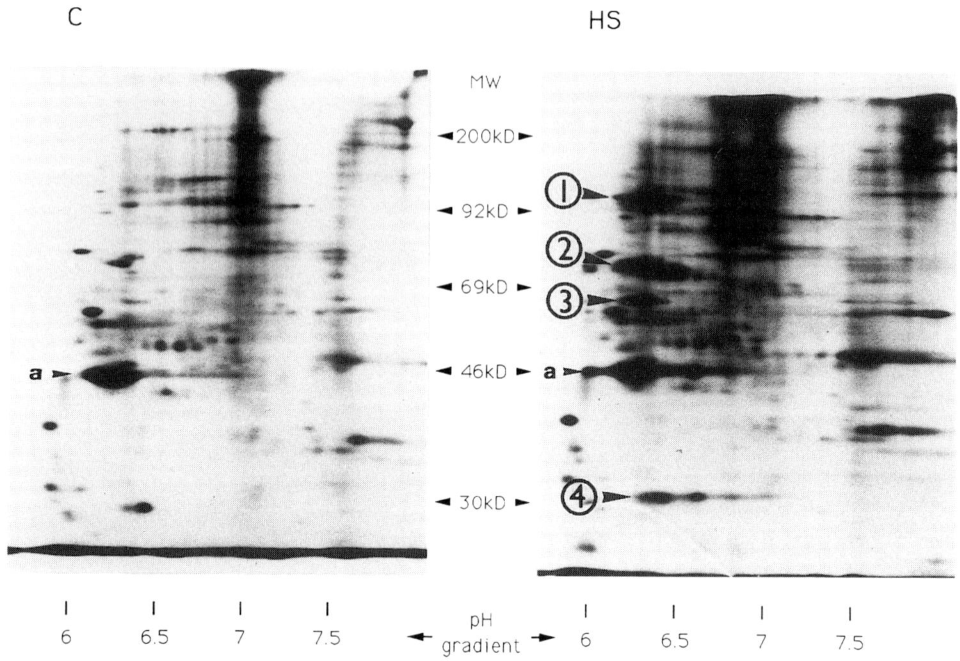

Protein	Location	Induction	Major Function	Possible involvement in disease
hsp110	cytoplasmic	heat inducible	not known	thermotolerance
① hsp90	endoplasmic reticulum, cytoplasmic	constitutive and heat inducible	associates with other proteins e.g. steroid receptors.	MHC-like role in tumor antigenicity
② hsp70	in all subcellular compartments	constitutive and heat inducible	synthesis and translocation of proteins; assembly of protein complexes; antigen processing and presentation	MHC-like role in tumor antigenicity; development of thermotolerance and drug resistance
③ hsp60	mitochondrial matrix	constitutive	correct assembly of mitochondrial proteins	autoimmune diseases; tumor antigens?
④ heme oxygenase	cytoplasmic	constitutive; heat inducible in rodents not in humans	heme oxygenase	protection from oxidative injury
hsp27*	cytoplasmic	heat inducible	unknown	tumor antigen and indicator of prognosis (phosphorylated isoforms); thermolerance and multidrug resistance

Figure 1 Major heat-shock proteins synthesized by rat mesangial cells. Upper panel: Two-dimensional gel electrophoresis of 35S-methionine–labeled proteins from control (C) and cells exposed to 44°C for 20 min (HS). Small arrows indicate major molecular weight markers (a = actin). Numbers and large arrows indicate the major heat-shock proteins whose localization and function(s) are presented in the lower panel. [a]hsp27 is induced in response to HS but does not label with methionine.

constitutively and binds to the immunoglobulin heavy chain in the absence of light chains. The hsp90 family possesses at least three subgroups of 90, 100, and 105 kDa; of these, hsp90 is the major one. Hsp90 is expressed in a tissue-dependent manner under normal conditions. Its distribution is predominantly cytoplasmic, where it interacts with many proteins including glucocorticoid receptors to repress their DNA binding activity and cytoskeletal proteins.

The study of HSP has grown rapidly over the last few years and not all aspects can be covered here. Hence this review concentrates on:

1. HS genes: characterization, location and polymorphism
2. Transcriptional control of HS genes and comparison with immediate early genes (IEG)
3. HSP: the kidney as paradigm for their localization and functions with particular reference to members of the hsp70 family
4. Protection: HS and multidrug resistance (MDR)

The involvement of HSP in immunity, a rapidly expanding topic, has recently been dealt with in detail elsewhere (21–25).

HS GENES: CHARACTERIZATION, LOCATION, AND POLYMORPHISM

The human genome is thought to contain at least eight genes that show sequence homology to the hsp70 family (26). Analysis of the genes cloned using probes from rat and *Drosophila* (26,27) has shown their localization to at least five chromosomes [chromosomes 1, 6, 14, 21, and recently chromosome 5 (28)]. Chromosome 1 is believed to contain the genes for hspA6 and hspA7, two genes which show over 95% homology to each other and sufficient homology to hsp70 to be considered HSP, although they are basic proteins and not heat-inducible (29). Localization of other HSP genes to chromosome 21 has been found in some studies (30) but not others (29).

The HSP genes found on chromosome 6 lie within the major histocompatibility complex (MHC) on the short arm of this chromosome (31). The genes for three hsp70 proteins map to the MHC class III region (31), between the MHC class I and II regions. The MHC class III region contains an hereogeneous array of genes including three for the complement system, those for tumor necrosis factors (TNF) α and β (32,33), and other genes whose functions have yet to be identified. The HS genes are found 92 kb telomeric to the C2 gene and 280 kb centromeric to the TNFα gene (34,35). Two of the HS genes are identical in amino acid sequence and code for hsp70-1 and hsp70-2. Neither gene contains introns and they differ only in their 5′ and 3′ untranslated regions. This variation, however, leads to differences in regulation: Moseley et al. (36) recently showed that HS can regulate hsp70 gene expression posttranscriptionally, through the 3′-untranslated region. Hsp70-1 is expressed constitutively and its levels rise after HS; hsp70-2 is expressed only after HS (37). The third gene, hsp70-Hom, despite 90% homology to hsp70-1, shows different regulation and is expressed both pre- and post-HS but only at low levels.

Polymorphism within the hsp70 genes may increase the susceptibility or resistance to disease as well as having a role in the correct haplotyping of transplant organs. Because of the relevance to biological function and disease of the polymorphism in class I and II genes and although there is less prominent structural polymorphism within class III genes, the investigation of polymorphism in the hsp70 genes has, up to now, been concentrated on the hsp70 genes present on chromosome 6 (38–41). Some polymorphism within a pig hsp70 gene, not present within the SLA major histocompatibility complex, has recently been reported (42), suggesting genes present on other chromosomes may also exhibit polymorphism.

Although the coding regions for hsp70-1 and hsp70-2 on chromosome 6 are identical, the differences in the 5′ and 3′ flanking regions allow them to be amplified specifically and the identification of polymorphic regions made (40). The degree of polymorphism within the hsp70 genes is low, with only silent mutations being isolated from the hsp70-1 and –2 genes. One of these mutations in hsp70-2 corresponds to a *PstI* restriction site which has been implicated in a number of diseases (43,44). The *NcoI* restriction site in the gene for hsp70-Hom may be of greater importance as it is present within the coding region and results in an amino acid substitution (Met → Thr). This occurs in the putative peptide-binding domain and may cause variations in peptide-binding specificity.

The polymorphism within the hsp70-2 gene that causes the creation or destruction of a *PstI* site seems to associate with the DR3 haplotype (45). Although an 8.5-kb allele isolated from the *PstI* digest has been implicated in insulin dependent diabetes mellitus (IDDM), Graves' disease, and celiac disease (34,46), the association with the DR3 haplotype, already known to be linked to disease, means that the involvement of the 8.5-kb allele is still a mystery. The 8.5-kb allele is more prevalent in patients suffering from hyperthyroid Graves' disease, where it is associated with a deletion of the

C4 gene (44). Even without this deletion, the 8.5-kb allele is significantly more frequent in patients than controls, suggesting that the hsp70 locus may be relevant to the development of this disease.

Increased levels of hsp70 mRNA are found in spontaneously hypertensive rats and mice (SHR and SHM) who show an increased sensitivity to elevations of temperature (43,47). These animals exhibit a higher level of hsp70 protein following HS than controls, due to increased transcription rate and mRNA stability (43). Restriction digests with *BamHI* revealed polymorphism within the hsp70 gene. A 3-kb fragment found in SHR from three different origins was associated with a blood pressure difference of 15 mmHg (38).

Careful consideration of polymorphism within the HS genes present on chromosome 6 led to an increased survival rate with bone marrow transplants (48). The study revealed polymorphism within the class III region (among the genes for C4, Bf, hsp70, and TNF) even when a DRb/DQB match had been obtained in the class II region by other methods (49,50).

TRANSCRIPTIONAL CONTROL OF HS GENES AND COMPARISON WITH IMMEDIATE EARLY GENES (IEG)

The HS genes present a unique opportunity to study transcription of a set of genes responding to known stimuli. The response occurs in conditions where most normal gene transcription and protein synthesis ceases. The induction of the stress response by a number of diverse stimuli promotes intriguing questions regarding regulation. The situation is complicated in that not all stimuli promote the same response, and within any response there may be a variation in levels of expression of particular HSP (51). Although the stimuli are diverse and include environmental, physiological, and pathophysiological perturbations (52), the majority of the activating factors would appear to cause denaturation of existing proteins or adversely affect newly synthesized proteins (51,53,54). Transcription of HSP has been more extensively studied in the hsp70 family. Here it would appear that while all species studied have a similar mechanism, each has its own refinements (55).

The complexity of the stimuli that give rise to HSP transcription, including physiological conditions supporting induction in normal cellular conditions and the exogenous stimuli promoting the stress response—are reflected in the complexity of the promoter region for the human hsp70 gene, which has two distinct functional domains (2).

The proximal domain of the hsp70 promoter is required for the basal activity of the constitutively expressed hsp70 genes. By DNA footprinting, gel mobility shift assays, and methylation studies, this region has been shown to contain binding sites for ATF and Sp1 as well as CCAAT and TATA boxes and a purine-rich region (56). Deletion experiments showed the essential binding site to be the CCAAT box (2). Methylation studies showed the same factors bound to the proximal promoter region before and after HS, indicating that induction of hsp70 by HS does not interfere with the basal promoter elements (56).

The distal promoter contains the elements responsible for the induction by HS and other physiological stresses (2). A region –66 to –47 upstream of the *Drosophila* hsp70 gene was found to be essential for heat-induced expression and was called the HS element (HSE) [first identified by Pelham (57) and Mirault et al. (58)]. The consensus sequence CTG-GAA-T-TTC-TAG-A is found upstream of *Drosophila* HS genes (59). The isolation of related sequences in the promoter region of all eukaryote HS genes has led to the definition of the HSE as inverted repeats of the pentamer NGAAN [the first N is usually an A (60)]. Multiples of this element arranged either head-to-head (NGAANNTTC) or tail-to-tail (NTTCNNGAAN) are found in all HSEs and the HS transcription factor (HSF) is able to bind both of these arrangements (59) (Figure 2).

HSF is known to bind DNA as a trimer, and evidence suggests that each monomer interacts with a pentameric unit (61,62). Two of these units are required for a stable complex, but only three units result in a functional HSF. HSFs have been cloned from a number of species (63–65), and it is interesting to note that while yeast and *Drosophila* appear to have only one gene coding for HSF, other species (chicken, tomato, human, and mouse) appear to have at least two genes coding for functional products (52). The HSFs isolated show little overall sequence homology (<40%), but they do show two highly conserved regions, both close to the amino terminal. The first is known to be a DNA-binding domain and the second is an array of hydrophobic heptads that function as the oligomerization domain.

In unstressed eukaryotic cells, HSF is present as a nonactive, non-DNA-binding monomer in both cytoplasm and nucleus (66). Induction causes oligomerization, acquisition of DNA-binding

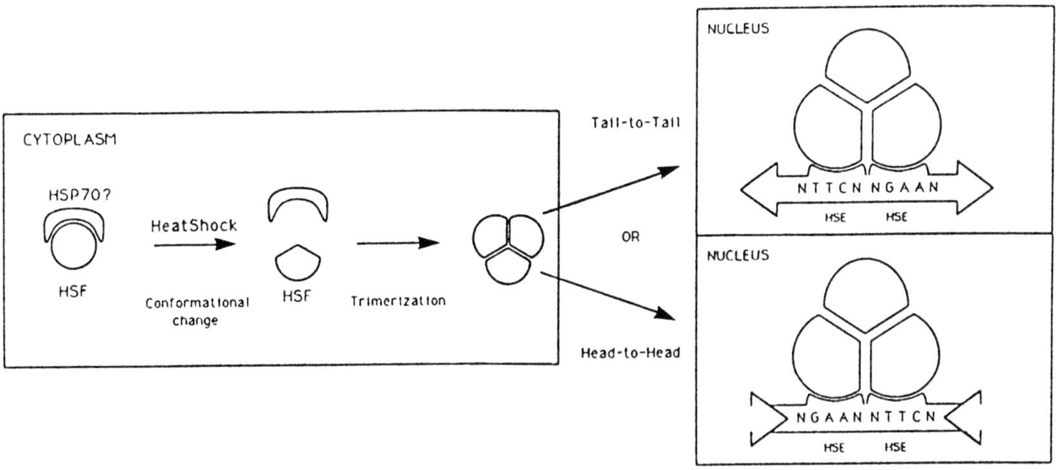

Figure 2 Regulation of heat-shock gene transcription. The heat-shock factor(s) (HSF) is present in the cytoplasm as a non-DNA-binding monomer. It may form a complex with another protein, possibly a member of the HSP70 family. Upon activation, the complex dissociates and HSF undergoes a conformational change, trimerizes, and relocates to the nucleus, where it is able to bind to the heat-shock element (HSE). Only two subunits need bind to the sequence to form a stable complex; however, the binding of three subunits is required for activation. The binding arrangement can be either tail-to-tail or head-to-head.

activity, and relocalization to the nucleus, where it binds to the HSE and initiates transcription. The response is extremely fast in eukaryotic cells, with transcription of hsp70 in *Drosophila* occurring within 1 min of induction (67). Yeast HSF is constitutively bound to HSE but activity is repressed by a conserved heptapeptide (68). *Drosophila* HSP70 genes have the RNA polymerase attached to the transcript (69,70), but this is not true of higher eukaryotes. Further modification may be required, such as phosphorylation (71). Transcription occurs at a rate of 1.2 kb/min, with the activity of other genes being repressed at a similar rate (67). Active HSF is a trimer in *Drosophila*, and this trimerization requires a conformational change that may be constrained by intramolecular coiled-coil interactions between amino and carboxyl termini in the monomer (72).

The retention of inactive HSF as a monomer in the cytoplasm of cells has attracted several theories. Many support an autoregulatory role whereby HSF is regulated by hsp70 in the cytoplasm and kept in an inactive form (73). Upon induction, hsp70 is released from HSF either because of competition for other abnormal proteins or by a conformational change. The first hypothesis has come from an observed increase in HS response to increased levels of misfolded or denatured proteins (8,52). In vitro experiments have shown that the addition of hsp70 can block the conversion of HSF to an active form (74). However, hydrodynamic studies have failed to find any evidence of an inactive HSF-hsp70 complex (72). Two subregions at the carboxyl terminal of human HSF1 have been shown to maintain it as a monomer under normal conditions (75); this is not the case in the yeast HSF, which is constitutively expressed as a trimer. Once this interaction is disrupted by HS, activation would occur.

Some species have been shown to possess more than one gene coding for a functional HSF. Two HSFs have been found in human and mouse. Mouse HSF1 and HSF2 show little overall homology (38%) but do possess strong homology in their DNA-binding and oligomerization domains (64,76). Monoclonal antibodies raised to the two mouse HSFs identified HSF1 as the mediator of the heat-shock-induced transcription of HSP (71). Stress (in the form of HS, cadmium sulfate, and the amino acid analogue L-azetidine-2-carboxylic acid) caused HSF1 to oligomerize, relocate to the nucleus, and bind to DNA. HS and cadmium sulfate also induce phosphorylation, which is not seen with the amino acid analogue, supporting the idea that phosphorylation is not essential for activity. Overexpression of HSF1 and HSF2 in transfected mouse 3T3 cells enables both factors to oligomerize, initiate transcription, and bind DNA constitutively, indicating that HSF1 can be activated in the absence of a stress response (71). The cellular locations of the overexpressed proteins are different, with HSF1 being found only in the nucleus and HSF2 in both nucleus and cytoplasm. HSF2 is not involved in the HS induction of HSP, but it does have a physiological role in the differentiation of erythrocytes and may be responsible for the response to oxidative injury. Hemin, an inducer of erythroid differentiation (shown in the human erytholeukemia cell line K562), causes the transcription of two members of the HSP70 family through interaction with the HSE (78). Activation of HSF1 by HS and HSF2 by hemin produces different patterns of expression (77), shown in Table 1. Although HSF1 and HSF2 occupy the same promoter region, they do so with nonidentical binding patterns, leading to a different rate of transcription, with HSF2 being the weaker transactivator. The differences in sequence may reflect different interactions with other transcription factors once bound to the promoter region.

The immediate early genes (IEG), like the HSP, are a diverse group of genes produced rapidly and transiently in response to several stimuli including HS. Several are known to encode transcription factors and regulate gene transcription directly (79). Many of the stimuli shown to promote HS gene expression affect the expression of c-*fos*, *Egr-1* and c-*myc*. Expression patterns of c-*fos* mRNA closely resemble those of hsp70 in response to reactive oxygen species and HS (80,81). As with hsp70 induction, not all stimuli promote the same level of expression (82). Although control of c-*fos* mRNA occurs at the posttranscriptional level by stabilization of the mRNA transcript (83), some degree of transcriptional control is indicated by the levels of response. Stabilization of c-*myc* mRNA also occurs in response to HS, but inhibition of expression causes an overall decrease in the levels of c-*myc* (84).

Induction of c-*fos*, *Egr-1* and hsp70 occurs during the immediate early and early phases of human cytomegalovirus infection (85,86). This induction does not require specific promoter elements and a minimal promoter of only 50 to 60 bp permits activation. The immediate early proteins IE1 (a 72-kDa protein) and IE2 (82 kDa) may be responsible for this upregulation, with the highest expression achieved when both were present, although they could function independently (86).

Levels of c-*fos* mRNA in Madin-Darby canine kidney (MDCK) cells are upregulated by hyperosmotic NaCl (an impermeant solute) and urea (a membrane-permeant solute) in a time- and dose-dependent manner (87,88). Unlike NaCl, urea leads to increased DNA synthesis and total cellular DNA content, has no effect on the expression of the hsp70 gene, but causes the induction of the IEG *Egr-1*. The effect of urea is tissue-dependent and only observed in renal epithelial cell lines such as MDCK and LLC-PK-1 (88).

The protooncogenes have been implicated in the regulation of hsp70 expression. In particular, c-*myc* is able to activate the *Drosophila* and human hsp70 genes (89), but in a manner distinct from basal expression or the induction by heat shock, serum, or viruses (90). Two sequences, showing considerable homology to the c-*myc* binding domain previously isolated from the upstream promoter region of c-*myc* itself, are present in the human hsp70 promoter region and specifically bind c-*myc* (91,92). This suggests that c-*myc* or a protein complex containing c-*myc* may play a role in hsp70 expression by binding directly to the promoter region (92).

Table 1 HSF-1 and -2 Are Activated by Different Stimuli and Exert Distinct Effects on Genes Transcription

HSF-1	HSF-2
Mediates induction of HSPs by heat shock and oxidative stress	Mediates induction of HSPs by hemin (cell differentiation)
Levels of HSP70 and HSP90 reach maximum after 30–45 min	Levels of HSP70 and HSP90 reach maximum after 12–24 hr
Weak inducer for BiP	Strong inducer for BiP
Negligible induction of p72 (hsc70)	2-to 3-fold induction of p72 (hsc70)
Decrease in expression of β actin	No effect on expression of β actin

HS PROTEINS: THE KIDNEY AS PARADIGM FOR THEIR LOCALIZATION AND FUNCTIONS

The expression patterns of HSP in response to stimuli vary between organs such as kidney, liver, skin, brain, and lung (93) and within different regions of a tissue (94). The localization in vivo of HSP within the kidney has not been extensively studied (95). The distribution of hsp90 in normal kidneys shows a different pattern than hsp70 (96). Constitutively expressed hsp73 is present in the epithelial cells of the Bowman's capsule, glomerular podocytes, and tubular epithelial cells of the nephron from the proximal tubule to the collecting tubule of normal kidneys. Within these cell types, hsp73 is found in both cytoplasm and nucleus—with the exception of proximal tubule, where it is found only in the nucleus (97). The distribution of hsp73 is different in rats with puromycin aminonucleoside nephrosis, with a greater accumulation in the cytoplasm; again the distribution in the proximal tubule is different, with hsp73 being found in both the nucleus and the cytoplasm. The inducible form of hsp70 is undetectable in normal rat kidney, but the rapid induction of hsp70 occurs in conditions of HS or transient renal ischemia (Figure 3) (94). When 90 min of renal ischemia is used no hsp70 is detected, reflecting the physiological situation where 90 min of ischemia results in unrecoverable renal failure. Levels of mRNA were reduced within 24 hr following stress, indicating that slow degradation of the protein, as opposed to persistent synthesis, was responsible for the presence of hsp70 protein up to 10 days following induction (98). Hsp70 was found in both soluble and microsomal fractions following ischemia, indicating a possible association with plasma membrane proteins (98). Thus, hsp72 may be implicated in the recovery of cells following ischemia.

HSP possess cytoprotective effects against many forms of injury, and their induction by reactive oxygen species may be important in protection from renal disease. Reactive oxygen species can result in severe disruption of normal kidney function by damaging membranes and causing lipid peroxidation (99,100). This oxidative injury has been implicated in several kidney diseases, including ischemic and toxin-induced renal failure, graft rejection, and acute glomerulonephritis (101). Renal ischemia is known to promote the specific induction of particular HSP (94,98), and treatment causing the induction of HSP can promote resistance to acute renal failure if the cells are rechallenged with the same agent. This may lead to a cross-resistance to other toxins and insults, but this is not always the case and a prior treatment can lead to a greater susceptibility (102). When pig kidneys were submitted to warm ischemia

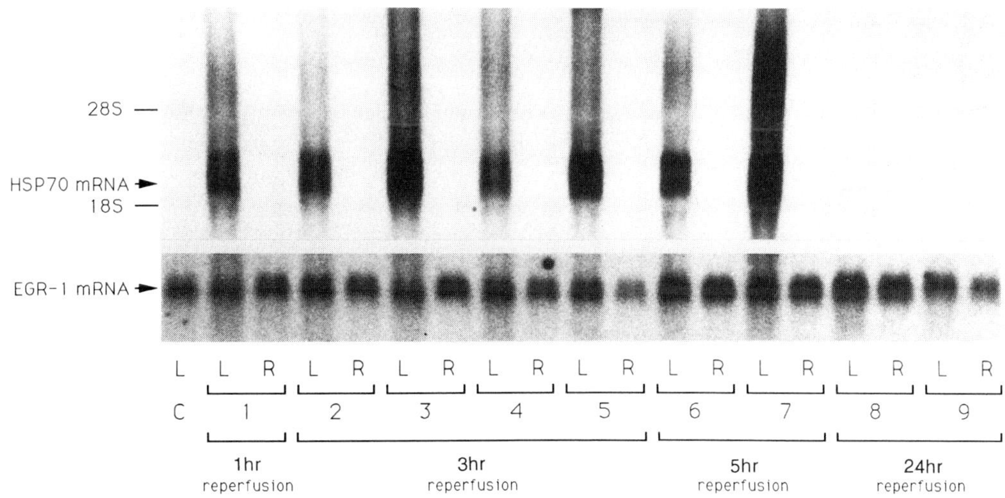

Figure 3 Ischemia induces HSP70 expression in the kidney. Kidney ischemia was imposed on anesthesized rats by clamping the left pedicle for 40 min. The clamp was then removed for reperfusion sequences of 1 hr (1), 3 hr (2–5), 5 hr (6 and 7), or 24 hr (8 and 9). Both left (L) and right (R) kidneys were removed and RNA was extracted for analysis of HSP expression by Northern blot. HSP70 mRNA accumulates in the kidney (L) during postischemic reperfusion. GAPDH was used as a housekeeping probe.

in situ (promoting the enhanced induction of HSP) and then transplanted, there was a significant increase in the survival rate of the recipient as compared with survival in pigs transplanted with nontreated kidneys (103). Other studies failed to show any protection from acute renal failure when ischemia was induced 4 to 6 hr following prior HS treatment (104).

HS AND MDR

The treatment of most cancers and tumors involves surgery, radiation, or chemotherapy. The first two are successful in only half of the cases of cancer in the United States (105), whereas the use of chemotherapy is severely hampered by the natural or acquired drug resistance exhibited by many tumors. This resistance is not only to the drug being used but often to any drugs, even if unrelated, used later. The phenomenon of multidrug resistance (MDR) has been attributed to the product of the MDR1 gene, P-plycoprotein. P-glycoprotein is an energy-dependent efflux pump which serves to prevent the accumulation of toxins within the cell by actively pumping them out (106). Another gene, MDR2, with 80% homology to MDR1 at the amino acid level, has been found close to the MDR1 gene on chromosome 7 (107). MDR2 shows a similar distribution in normal tissues as MDR1 but does not confer drug resistance and its function is unknown (109).

The P-glycoprotein is expressed in normal tissues in a cell- and tissue-specific manner. Expression has been found on kidney, adrenal, brain, colon, liver, small intestine, and testis (110,111). Lower levels of expression have been found in other organs including lung, muscle, and the endometrium of pregnant mice (107,111). Hence P-glycoprotein appears to serve a normal physiological role in the export of toxins from tissues.

An increase in MDR1 levels has been shown in cancers arising from tissue that normally express it. However, tumors from other tissues can also show high expression of MDR1; this can occur in untreated cancers or in cancers that have become resistant to chemotherapy (105). Drug resistance is exhibited by some cancers that show no increased amplification of the MDR1 gene (112), indicating that MDR1 expression is only one of several mechanisms used for drug resistance. The high level of MDR1 mRNA in tumor cell lines is not due to an increase in transcription, as nuclear runoff assays show no upregulation; instead it would appear to be a result of a posttranscriptional event such as stabilization of the mRNA (113).

It has been suggested that MDR1 is an HS gene. The promoter region of MDR has two functional domains. The downstream promoter region possesses a CAAT box and two GC box-like sequences but no TATA box (114). Transcription in normal tissues starts from this area only. MDR1 expression in a renal carcinoma cell line (HTB-46) was increased 10-fold by HS or treatment with sodium arsenite and studies isolated two HSE upstream of the basal promoter region (115). Deletion analysis showed that induction following sodium arsenite treatment was due to these elements (116,117). Treatment with quercetin, a bioflavonoid that prevents induction of HS proteins by interaction with HSF (118), inhibited the expression of the MDR1 gene (116,117). The possibility that MDR1 is an HS gene suggests that observed resistance to drugs following HS may not be as a result of classic HSP induction.

CONCLUSIONS

The role of HSP in the pathology of renal disease requires further investigation, but a number of interesting features are becoming apparent. The location, polymorphism, and regulation of HSP and related genes such as MDR1 and the IEG may be of particular importance when considering renal injury as a result of oxidative stress. If there is a protective role for the HS response, then understanding the genetic mechanisms responsible for the generation of this response may lead to the development of therapies designed to initiate or enhance the response.

ACKNOWLEDGMENTS

Work mentioned here has been supported in part by grants from the Fonds National Suisse pour la Recherche Scientifique (FNRS) #32-28645.90 and #32-37464.93 to BSP. BSP is currently supported by INSERM. The authors would like to express their thanks to Yves Donati and Joseph V. Bonventre for providing the data shown in Figure 3.

REFERENCES

1. Lindquist S, Craig EA. The heat-shock proteins. Annu Rev Genet 1988; 22:631–677.
2. Morimoto RI, Milarski KL. Expression and function of vertebrate hsp70 genes. In: Morimoto RI, Tissières A, Georgopoulos C, eds. Stress Proteins in Biology and Medicine. Cold Spring Harbor, NY: Cold Spring Harbor Laboratory Press, 1990:323–359.
3. Welch WJ. The mammalian stress response: Cell physiology and biochemistry of stress proteins. In: Morimoto RI, Tissières A, Georgopoulos C, eds. Stress Proteins in Biology and Medicine. Cold Spring Harbor, NY: Cold Spring Harbor Laboratory Press, 1990:223–279.
4. Ritossa F. A new puffing pattern induced by temperature shock and DNP in Drosophila. Experientia 1962; 18:571–573.
5. Watowich SS, Morimoto RI. Complex regulation of heat shock- and glucose-responsive genes in human cells. Mol Cell Biol 1988; 8:393–405.
6. Chirico WJ, Waters MG, Blobel G. 70K heat shock related proteins stimulate protein translocation into microsomes. Nature 1988; 332:805–810.
7. Cheng MY, Hartl FU, Martin J, et al. Mitochondrial heat-shock protein hsp60 is essential for assembly of proteins imported into yeast mitochondria. Nature 1989; 337:620–625.
8. Morimoto RI. Cells in stress: Transcriptional activation of heat shock genes. Science 1993; 259:1409–1410.
9. Mosser DD, Theodorakis NG, Morimoto RI. Coordinate changes in heat shock element-binding activity and HSP70 gene transcription rates in human cells. Mol Cell Biol 1988; 8:4736–4744.
10. Theodorakis NG, Morimoto RI. Posttranscriptional regulation of hsp70 expression in human cells: Effects of heat shock, inhibition of protein synthesis and adenovirus infection on translation and mRNA stability. Mol Cell Biol 1987; 7:4357–4368.
11. Keyse SM, Tyrrell RM. Heme oxygenase is the major 32-kDa stress protein induced in human skin fibroblasts by UVA radiation, hydrogen peroxide and sodium arsenite. Proc Natl Acad Sci USA 1989; 86:99–103.
12. Ishii T, Yamada M, Sato H, et al. Cloning and characterization of a 23-kDa stress-induced mouse peritoneal macrophage protein. J Biol Chem 1993; 268:18633–18636.
13. Maines MD, Mayer RD, Ewing JF, McCoubrey WK Jr. Induction of kidney heme oxygenase-1 (HSP32) mRNA and protein by ischemia/reperfusion: Possible role of heme as both promoter of tissue damage and regulator of hsp32. J Pharm Exp Ther 1993; 264:457–462.
14. Agsteribbe E, Huckriede A, Veenhuis M, et al. A fatal, systemic mitochondrial disease with decreased mitochondrial enzyme activities, abnormal ultrastructure of the mitochondria and deficiency of heat shock protein 60. Biochem Biophys Res Commun 1993; 193:146–154.
15. Lamb JR, Bal V, Mendez-Samperio, et al. Stress proteins may provide a link between the immune response to infection and autoimmunity. Int Immunol 1989; 1:191–196.
16. Life PF, Bassey EOE, Gaston JSH. T-Cell Recognition of bacterial heat-shock proteins in inflammatory arthritis. Immunol Rev 1991; 121:113–135.
17. Polla BS, Young D. Heat shock proteins and immunity. Immunol Today 1989; 10:393–394.
18. Hunt C, Morimoto RI. Conserved features of eukaryotic hsp70 genes revealed by comparison with the nucleotide sequence of human hsp70. Proc Natl Acad Sci USA 1985; 82:6455–6459.
19. Domanico SZ, DeNagel DC, Dahlseid JN, et al. Cloning of the gene encoding peptide-binding protein 74 shows that it is a new member of the heat shock protein 70 family. Mol Cell Biol 1993; 13:3598–3610.
20. DeNagel DC, Pierce SK. A case for chaperones in antigen processing. Immunol Today 1992; 13:86–89.
21. Young RA. Stress proteins and immunology. Annu Rev Immunol 1990; 8:401–420.
22. Healy AM., Mariéthoz E, Pizurki L, Polla BS. Heat shock proteins in cellular defense mechanisms and immunity. Ann NY Acad Sci 1992; 663:319–330.
23. Kaufmann SHE. The cellular immune response to heat shock proteins. Experientia 1992; 48:640–643.
24. Yang X-D, Feige U. Heat shock proteins in autoimmune disease: From causative antigen to specific therapy? Experientia 1992; 48:650–656.
25. Young D, Roman E, Moreno C, et al. Molecular chaperones and the immune response. Phil Trans R Soc Lond B 1993; 339:363–368.
26. Mues GI, Munn TZ, Raese JD. A human gene family with sequence homology to Drosophila melanogaster Hsp70 heat shock genes. J Biol Chem 1986; 261:874–877.
27. Wu B, Hunt C, Morimoto R. Structure and expression of the human gene encoding major heat shock protein HSP70. Mol Cell Biol 1985; 5:330–341.
28. Fathallah DM, Cherif D, Dellagi K, Arnaout MA. Molecular cloning of a novel human hsp70 from a B cell line and its assignment to chromosome 5. J Immunol 1993; 151:810–813.
29. Leung TKC, Hall C, Rajendran M, et al. The human heat-shock genes HSPA6 and HSPA7 are both expressed and localize to chromosome 1. Genomics 1992; 12:74–79.
30. Harrison GS, Drabkin HA, Kao FT, et al. Chromosomal location of human genes encoding major heat-shock protein HSP70. Somatic Cell Mol Genet 1987; 13:119–130.

31. Sargent CA, Dunham I, Trowsdale J, Campbell RD. Human major histocompatibility complex contains genes for the major heat shock protein HSP70. Proc Natl Acad Sci USA 1989; 86:1968–1972.
32. Carroll MC, Campbell RD, Bentley DR, Porter RR. A molecular map of the human major histocompatibility complex class III region, linking complement genes C4, C2 and factor B. Nature 1984; 307:237–241.
33. Dunham I, Sargent CA, Trowsdale J, Campbell RD. Molecular mapping of the human major histocompatibility complex by pulsed-field gel electrophoresis. Proc Natl Acad Sci USA 1987; 84:7237–7241.
34. Pugliese A, Awdeh ZL, Galluzzo A, et al. No independent association between HSP70 gene polymorphism and IDDM. Diabetes 1992; 41:788–791.
35. Campbell RD, Trowsdale J. Map of the human MHC. Immunol Today 1993; 14:349–352.
36. Moseley PL, Wallen ES, McCafferty JD, et al. Heat stress regulates the human 70-kDa heat-shock gene through the 3′-untranslated region. Am J Physiol 1993; 264:L533–L537.
37. Milner CM, Campbell RD. Structure and expression of the three MHC-linked HSP70 genes. Immunogenetics 1990; 32:242–251.
38. Hamet P, Kong D, Pravenec M, et al. Restriction fragment length polymorphism of hsp70 gene, localized in the RT1 complex, is associated with hypertension in spontaneously hypertensive rats. Hypertension 1992; 19:611–614.
39. Jacob CO, Hwang F. Definition of microsatellite size variants for TNFα and Hsp70 in autoimmune and nonautoimmune mouse strains. Immunogenetics 1992; 36:182–188.
40. Milner CM, Campbell RD. Polymorphic analysis of the three MHC-linked HSP70 genes. Immunogenetics 1992; 36:357–362.
41. Lanng S, Thorsteinsson B, Pociot F, et al. Diabetes mellitus in cystic fibrosis: Genetic and immunological markers. Acta Paedriatr 1993; 82:150–154.
42. Dezeure F, Vaiman M, Chardon P. Characterization of a polymorphic heat shock protein 70 gene in swine outside the SLA major histocompatibility complex. Biochim Biophys Acta 1993; 1174:17–26.
43. Hashimoto T, Mosser RD, Tremblay J, Hamet P. Increased accumulation of hsp70 messenger RNA due to enhanced activation of heat-shock transcription factor in spontaneously hypertensive rats. J Hypertens 1991; 9 (suppl 6):S170–S171.
44. Ratanachaiyavong S, Demaine AG, Campbell RD, McGregor AM. Heat shock protein 70 (HSP70) and complement C4 genotypes in patients with hyperthyroid Graves' disease. Clin Exp Immunol 1991; 84:48–52.
45. Cascino I, Sorrentino R, Tosi R. Strong genetic association between HLA-DR3 and a polymorphic variation in the regulatory region of the HSP70-1 gene. Immunogenetics 1993; 37:177–182.
46. Partanen J, Milner C, Campbell RD, et al. HLA-linked heat-shock protein 70 (HSP70-2) gene polymorphism and celiac disease. Tissue Antigens 1993; 41:15–19.
47. Lukashev ME, Klimanskaya IV, Postnov YV. Synthesis of heat shock proteins in cultured fibroblasts from normotensive and spontaneously hypertensive rat embryos. J. Hypertens 1991; 9:S182–S183.
48. Dorak MT, Chalmers EA, Sproul AM, et al. MHC Class III polymorphisms in selection of donors for BMT. Bone Marrow Transpl 1993; 11:37–41.
49. Hows JM, Bradley BA. The use of unrelated marrow donors for transplantation. Br J Haematol 1990; 76:1–6.
50. Roux E, Helg C, Chapuis B, et al. Evolution of mixed chimerism after allogenic bone marrow transplantation as determined by granulocytes and mononuclear cells by the polymerase chain reaction. Blood 1992; 79:2775–2783.
51. Anathan J, Goldberg AL, Voellmy R. Abnormal proteins serve as eukaryotic stress signals and trigger the activation of heat shock genes. Science 1986; 232:522–524.
52. Morimoto RI, Sarge KD, Abravaya K. Transcriptional regulation of heat shock genes. J Biol Chem 1992; 267:21987–21990.
53. Goff SA, Goldberg AL. Production of abnormal proteins in E coli stimulates transcription of ion and other heat shock genes. Cell 1985; 41:587–590.
54. Mosser DD, Kotzbauer PT, Sarge KD, Morimoto RI. In vitro activation of heat shock transcription factor DNA-binding by calcium and biochemical conditions that affect protein conformation. Proc Natl Acad Sci USA 1990; 87:3748–3752.
55. Sorger PK, Lewis MJ, Pelham HRB. Heat shock factor is regulated differently in yeast and HeLa cells. Nature 1987; 329:81–84.
56. Abravaya K, Sarge KD, Phillips B, et al. In vivo and in vitro studies on the activation and binding of human heat shock transcription factor. In: Maresca B, Lindquist S, eds. Heat Shock. New York: Springer-Verlag, 1991:17–34.
57. Pelham HRB. A regulatory upstream promoter element in the Drosophila Hsp70 heat-shock gene. Cell 1982; 30:517–528.
58. Mirault ME, Southgate R, Delwart E. Regulation of heat-shock genes: A DNA sequence upstream of Drosophila hsp70 genes is essential for their induction in monkey cells. EMBO J 1982; 1:1279–1285.
59. Lis JT, Xiao H, Perisic O. Modular units of heat shock regulatory regions: Structure and function: In

Morimoto RI, Tissières A, Georgopoulos C, eds. Stress Proteins in Biology and Medicine. Cold Spring Harbor, NY: Cold Spring Harbor Laboratory Press, 1990:411–428.
60. Cunniff NFA, Morgan WD. Analysis of heat shock element recognition by saturation mutagenesis of the human HSP70.1 gene promoter. J Biol Chem 1993; 268:8317–8324.
61. Jakobsen BK, Pelham HRB. Constitutive binding of yeast heat shock factor to DNA in vivo. Mol Cell Biol 1988; 8:5040–5042.
62. Perisic O, Xiao H, Lis JT. Stable binding of Drosophila heat shock factor to head-to-head and tail-to-tail repeats of a conserved 5 bp recognition unit. Cell 1989; 59:797–806.
63. Clos J, Westwood JT, Becker PB, et al. Molecular cloning and expression of a hexameric Drosophila heat shock factor subject to negative regulation. Cell 1990; 63:1085–1097.
64. Rabindran SK, Giorgi G, Clos J, Wu C. Molecular cloning and expression of a human heat shock factor, HSF1. Proc Natl Acad Sci USA 1991; 88:6906–6910.
65. Sorger PK, Pelham HRB. Yeast heat shock factor is an essential DNA-binding protein that exhibits temperature-dependent phosphorylation. Cell 1988; 54:855–864.
66. Sheldon LA, Kingston RE. Hydrophobic coiled-coil domains regulate the subcellular localization of human heat shock factor 2. Genes Dev 1993; 7:1549–1558.
67. O'Brien T, Lis JT. Rapid changes in Drosophila transcription after an instantaneous heat shock. Mol Cell Biol 1993; 13:3456–3463.
68. Jakobsen BK, Pelham HRB. A conserved heptapeptide restrains the activity of the yeast heat shock transcription factor. EMBO J 1991; 10:369–375.
69. Gilmour DS, Lis JT. RNA polymerase II interacts with the promoter region of the noninduced hsp70 gene in Drosophila melanogaster cells. Mol Cell Biol 1986; 6:3984–3989.
70. Lee HS, Kraus KW, Wolfner MF, Lis JT. DNA sequence requirements for generating paused polymerase at the start of hsp70. Genes Dev 1992; 6:284–295.
71. Sarge KD, Murphy SP, Morimoto RI. Activation of heat shock gene transcription by heat shock factor 1 involves oligomerization, acquisition of DNA-binding activity and nuclear localizaton and can occur in the absence of stress. Mol Cell Biol 1993; 13:1392–1397.
72. Westwood JT, Wu C. Activation of Drosophila heat shock factor: Conformational change associated with a monomer-to-trimer transition. Mol Cell Biol 1993; 13:3481–3486.
73. Mosser DD, Duchaine J, Massie B. The DNA-binding activity of the human heat shock transcription factor is regulated in vivo by hsp70. Mol Cell Biol 1993; 13:5427–5438.
74. Abravaya K, Myers MP, Murphy SP, Morimoto RI. The human heat shock protein hsp70 interacts with HSF, the transcription factor that regulates heat shock gene expression. Genes Dev 1992; 6:1153–1164.
75. Rabindran SK, Haroun RI, Clos J, et al. Regulation of heat shock factor trimer formation: Role of a conserved leucine zipper. Science 1993; 259:230–234.
76. Sarge KD, Zimarino V, Holm K, et al. Cloning and characterization of two mouse heat shock factors with distinct inducible and constitutive DNA-binding ability. Genes Dev 1991; 5:1902–1911.
77. Sistonen L, Sarge KD, Phillips B, et al. Activation of heat shock factor 2 during hemin-induced differentiation of human erythroleukemia cells. Mol Cell Biol 1992; 12:4104–4111.
78. Theodorakis NG, Zand DJ, Kotzbauer PT, et al. Hemin-induced transcriptional activation of the HSP70 gene during erythroid maturation in K562 cells is due to a heat shock factor-mediated stress response. Mol Cell Biol 1989; 9:3166–3173.
79. Sassone-Corsi P, Sisson JC, Verma IM. Transcriptional autoregulation of the proto-oncogene fos. Nature 1988; 334:314–319.
80. Andrews GK, Harding MA, Calvet JP, Adamson ED. The heat shock response in HeLa cells is accompanied by elevated expression of the c-fos proto-oncogene. Mol Cell Biol 1987; 7:3452–3458.
81. Crawford D, Zbinden I, Amstad P, Cerutti P. Oxidant stress induces the proto-oncogenes c-fos and c-myc in mouse epidermal cells. Oncogene 1988; 3:27–32.
82. Hollander MC, Fornace AJ Jr. Induction of fos RNA by DNA-damaging agents. Cancer Res. 1989; 49:1687–1692.
83. Colotta F, Polentarutti N, Staffico M, et al. Heat shock induces the transcriptional activation of c-fos protooncogene. Biochem Biophys Res Commun 1990; 168:1013–1019.
84. Bukh A, Martinez-Valdez H, Freedman SJ, et al. The expression of c-fos, c-jun and c-myc genes is regulated by heat shock in human lymphoid cells. J Immunol 1990; 144:4835–4840.
85. Santomenna LD, Colberg-Poley AM. Induction of cellular hsp70 expression by human cytomegalovirus. J Virol 1990; 64:2033–2040.
86. Hagemeier C, Walker SM, Sissons PJG, Sinclair JH. The 72K IE1 and 80K IE2 proteins of human cytomegalovirus independently trans-activate the c-fos, c-myc and hsp70 promoters via basal promoter elements. J Gen Virol 1992; 73:2385–2393.
87. Cohen DM, Wasserman JC, Gullans SR. Immediate early gene and HSP70 expression in hyperosmotic stress in MDCK cells. Am J Physiol 1991; 261:C594–C601.

88. Cohen DM, Gullans SR. Urea induces Egr-1 and c-fos expression in renal epithelial cells. Am J Physiol 1993; 264:F593–F600.
89. Kingston RE, Baldwin Jr AS, Sharp PA. Regulation of heat shock protein 70 gene expression by c-myc. Nature 1984; 312:280–282.
90. Kaddurah-Daouk R, Greene JM, Baldwin AS Jr, et al. Activation and repression of mammalian gene expression by the c-myc protein. Genes Dev 1987; 1:347–357.
91. Ariga H, Imamura Y, Iguchi-Ariga SMM. DNA replication origin and transcriptional enhancer in c-myc gene share the c-myc protein binding sequence. EMBO J 1989; 8:4273–4279.
92. Taira T, Negishi Y, Kihara F, et al. c-myc protein complex binds to two sites in human hsp70 promoter region. Biochim Biophys Acta 1992; 113:166–174.
93. Blake MJ, Gershon D, Fargnoli J, Holbrook NJ. Discordant expression of heat shock protein mRNAs in tissues of heat-stressed rats. J Biol Chem 1990; 265:15275–15279.
94. Emami A, Schwartz JH, Borkan SC. Transient ischemia or heat stress induces a cytoprotectant protein in rat kidney. Am J Physiol 1991; 260:F479–F485.
95. Lovis C, Mach F, Donati YRA, et al. Heat shock proteins and the kidney. Renal Failure 1994; 16:179–192.
96. Matsubara O, Kasuga T, Marumo F, et al. Localization of 90-kDa heat shock protein in the kidney. Kidney Int 1990; 38:830–834.
97. Komatsuda A, Wakui H, Imai H, et al. Renal localization of the constitutive 73-kDa heat-shock protein in normal and PAN rats. Kidney Int 1992; 41:1204–1212.
98. Van Why SK, Hildebrandt F, Ardito T, et al. Induction and intracellular localization of HSP72 after renal ischemia. Am J Physiol 1992; 263:F769–F775.
99. Bonventre JV. Mediators of ischemic renal injury. Annu Rev Med 1988; 39:531–544.
100. Bonventre JV, Weinberg JM. Kidney preservation ex vivo for transplantation. Annu Rev Med 1992; 43:523–553.
101. Baud L, Ardaillou R. Reactive oxygen species: Production and role in the kidney. Am J Physiol 1986; 251:F765–F776.
102. Honda N, Hishida A, Ikuma K, Yonemura K. Acquired resistance to acute renal failure. Kidney Int 1987; 31:1233–1238.
103. Perdrizet GA, Kaneko H, Buckley TM, et al. Heat shock and recovery protects renal allografts from warm ischemic injury and enhances HSP72 production. Transplant Proc 1993; 25:1670–1673.
104. Bonventre JV. Mechanisms of ischemic acute renal failure. Kidney Int 1993; 43:1160–1178.
105. Chin K-V, Pastan I, Gottesman MM. Function and regulation of the human multidrug resistance gene. Adv Cancer Res 1993; 60:157–180.
106. Horio M, Gottesman MM, Pastan I. ATP-dependent transport of vinblastine in vesicles from human multidrug resistant cells. Proc Natl Acad Sci USA 1988; 85:3580–3584.
107. Chin JE, Soffir R, Noonan KE, et al. Structure and expression of the human MDR (P-Glycoprotein) gene family. Mol Cell Biol. 1989; 9:3808–3820.
108. Kane SE, Pastan I, Gottesman MM. Genetic basis of multidrug resistance of tumor cells. J Bioenerg Biomembr 1990; 22:593–618.
109. Thiebaut F, Tsuro T, Hamada H, et al. Cellular localization of the multidrug-resistance gene product P-Glycoprotein in normal human tissues. Proc Natl Acad Sci USA 1987; 84:7735–7738.
110. Thiebaut F, Tsuro T, Hamada H, et al. Immunohistochemical localization in normal tissues of different epitopes in the multidrug transport protein P170: Evidence for localization in brain capillaries and crossreactivity of one antibody with a muscle protein. J Histochem Cytochem 1989; 37:159–164.
111. Arceci RJ, Croop JM, Horowitz SB, Housman D. The gene encoding multidrug resistance is induced and expressed at high levels during pregnancy in the secretory epithelium of the uterus. Proc Natl Acad Sci USA 1988; 85:4350–4354.
112. Lai SL, Goldstein LJ, Gottesman MM, et al. MDR1 gene expression in lung cancer. JNCI 1989; 81:1144–1150.
113. Marino PA, Gottesman MM, Pastan I. Regulation of the multidrug resistance gene in regenerating rat liver. Cell Growth Diff 1990; 1:57–62.
114. Ueda K, Pastan I, Gottesman MM. Isolation and sequence of the promoter region of the human multidrug-resistance (P-glycoprotein) gene. J Biol Chem 1987; 262:17432–17436.
115. Chin K-V, Tanaka S, Darlington G, et al. Heat shock and arsenite increase expression of the multidrug resistance (MDR1) gene in human renal carcinoma cells. J Biol Chem 1990; 265:221–226.
116. Kioka N, Yamano Y, Komano T, Ueda K. Heat-shock responsive elements in the induction of the multidrug resistance gene (MDR1) FEBS Lett 1992; 301:37–40.
117. Kioka N, Hosokawa N, Komano T, et al. Quercetin, a bioflavonoid, inhibits the increase of human multidrug resistance gene (MDR1) expression caused by arsenite. FEBS Lett 1992; 301:307–309.
118. Hosokawa N, Hirayoshi K, Nakai A, et al. Flavonoids inhibit the expression of heat shock proteins. Cell Structure Funct 1990; 15:393–401.

43

Interleukin-6 and Interleukin-8 as Potential Inflammatory Mediators of Injury in Renal Diseases

Carla Zoja and Giuseppe Remuzzi
Mario Negri Institute for Pharmacological Research, Bergamo, Italy

INTRODUCTION

Cytokines, including interleukin-6 (IL-6) and interleukin-8 (IL-8), mediate inflammatory responses and may contribute to the development of renal injury. IL-6 is a pleiotropic cytokine originally identified as a T-cell–derived lymphokine that induced antibody production in B cells and was originally called B-cell differentiation factor (BCDF) or B-cell stimulatory factor 2 (BSF2) (1). IL-6 regulates immune responses, acute phase reactions, and hematopoiesis, and it plays a central role in host defense mechanisms (1–3). Experimental and clinical data suggest that IL-6 may have the interesting potential of modulating glomerular injury and perhaps even disease progression. This possibility is linked to the finding of abnormally high IL-6 levels in the urine of patients with various kidney diseases, including mesangioproliferative glomerulonephritis (4) and active lupus nephritis (5). Of interest for a possible role of IL-6 in renal injury are experiments with IL-6 transgenic mice obtained with the human IL-6 gene coupled to the human Ig heavy-chain gene enhancer (6). These mice had high serum IL-6, proteinuria, and mesangioproliferative glomerulonephritis; treatment with anti-human IL-6 antibodies prevented mesangial cell proliferation (7). In vitro studies have shown that IL-6 is synthesized by glomerular mesangial cells (8–10) and that these cells proliferate in response to exogenous IL-6 (4,10). These findings have been taken to suggest that IL-6 is an autocrine growth factor for mesangial cells (10), but other experiments showing that IL-6 inhibits the growth of mesangial cells in culture (11) indicate that the issue is still far from clear.

The recent finding that IL-6 upregulates extracellular matrix protein gene expression in mesangial cells (12) suggests that it may indeed play a role in the process of extracellular matrix deposition, which leads to progressive glomerulosclerosis.

IL-8 is a chemotactic factor, initially isolated from supernatants of lipopolysaccharide (LPS)-stimulated human peripheral blood monocytes (13). Subsequent studies showed a regulated production of IL-8 in a variety of cell types (14,15), including glomerular mesangial cells (8,9,16,17). IL-8 may control the intensity of inflammatory reactions through its potent chemotactic effects toward neutrophils and lymphocytes (14,18). The demonstration that human glomerular mesangial cells in culture stimulated by interleukin-1 (IL-1) and tumor necrosis factor (TNF) or LPS expressed IL-8 mRNA and released IL-8 protein (8,9,16,17) suggests that in situ production of this chemoattractant is instrumental to the regulation of local leukocyte recruitment in glomerulonephritis.

INTERLEUKIN-6

Gene Structure and Regulation

The genes for human, mouse, and rat IL-6 have been cloned and are approximately 5, 7, and 10 kb in length, respectively (19–21). They all contain four introns and five exons and show a high degree of conservation in the 3′ and 5′ untranslated regions. Comparisons of the cDNA of the three species showed 92% homology between rat and mouse, 65% between mouse and human, and 68% between rat and human. The gene for human IL-6 has been mapped to chromosome 7 (22) and was recently localized to 7p21 (23); the murine gene has been mapped to chromosome 5 (24). IL-6 gene expression is inducible in different types of human cells (fibroblasts, monocytes, endothelial cells) by various stimuli, including cytokines such as TNF, IL-1, and platelet-derived growth factor; different viruses, and bacterial products such as endotoxin (3).

The IL-6 promoter region contains several potential transcriptional control elements, such as the glucocorticoid-responsive elements (GRE), an activator protein 1 (AP-1) binding site, a cyclic AMP–responsive element (CRE), a serum-responsive element (SRE) similar to that of the human c-*fos* gene, and NF-kB binding site (1,25). The similarity of transcriptional regulation between the IL-6 and the c-*fos* genes (26) is striking. Both are induced rapidly (within minutes of exposure to an inducer) without needing prior protein synthesis, and both are regulated by a broad range of stimuli in various tissues and cells. The two genes probably share some *cis*-acting 5′ regulatory elements. Ray et al. (26) showed that the 115-bp region from –225 to –111 in the IL-6 5′-flanking region, which shares nucleotide sequence similarity with the c-*fos* SRE and adjacent AP-1-like (the CGTCA motif) elements, confers responsiveness to several reagents, including serum, forskolin, and phorbol ester, upon the heterologous herpesvirus thymidine kinase (TK) promoter. They identified within the IL-6 enhancer region a 23-bp IL-6 MRE (–173 to –151) to which IL-1, TNF, and activators of the protein kinase A (forskolin) and protein kinase C (phorbol ester) signal transduction pathways converged. In a study by Isshiki et al. (27), the IL-1 responsive element in the IL-6 gene was mapped within the region of –180 to –111 bp. A gel shift assay and a methylation interference assay revealed an NF-IL-6 that specifically binds to a 14-bp palindrome (–158 to –145). NF-IL-6 is different from AP-1 and NF-κB, and direct cloning by the South-Western method showed close homology with C/EBP, a liver-specific nuclear factor (28). NF-IL-6 and C/EPB belong to the so-called basic leucine-zipper family, having a leucine-zipper–associated DNA binding domain. Recently, an additional member of the C/EBP gene family, termed NF-IL-6 β, has been cloned and characterized. This factor shows high sequence homology with NF-IL-6 in the basic and leucine zipper domains but differs in the N-terminal domain (29). The NF-IL-6 β gene is induced by LPS or inflammatory cytokines, similar to NF-IL-6. NF-IL-6 β forms a heterodimer with NF-IL-6, which synergistically enhances the transcriptional activity. This newly discovered member of the C/EBP family is potentially an important transcriptional activator in addition to NF-IL-6 in regulation of genes responsible for immune and inflammatory responses.

Shimizu et al. (30) reported that an IL-6 promoter element, whose sequence is homologous to the NF-κB motifs, is important for the IL-1/TNF-α responsiveness of the IL-6 gene. One of the nuclear factors interacting with this element, referred to as inflammatory lymphokine-responsive element (ILRE), is inducible by IL-1 and TNF-α and has sequence specificities, binding characteristics, and subcellular localization indistinguishable from those of NF-κB. NF-κB, originally identified as a nuclear factor binding to an enhancer element of the κ immunoglobulin light-chain gene, was subsequently found in other types of cells, binds to related sequence motifs in several viral and cellular enhancers, and plays a role in the transcription of several inducible genes (31,32). TNF-α and IL-1 activate NF-κB. Kashtan et al. (33) reported that induction of the IL-6 gene promoter in human mesangial cells in culture by serum, LPS, or IL-1β required an intact binding site for NF-κB. This was assessed by constructing a mutant promoter for IL-6 containing an altered binding site for the nuclear transcription factor NF-κB. Mesangial cells were transfected with wild-type or mutant promoter linked to the chloramphenicol acetyltransferase (CAT) reporter gene and then exposed to stimuli such as serum alone, LPS, or IL-1β. Induction of CAT activity was measured only in cells transfected with the wild-type promoter and was greater with LPS and IL-1β than with serum alone.

The IL-6 gene is strongly inhibited by glucocorticoids in different tissues. Ray et al. (34)

investigated the mechanism of repression of the IL-6 gene by dexamethasone in HeLa cells transiently transfected with plasmid constructs containing different IL-6 promoter elements linked to the herpesvirus thymidine kinase (tK) promoter and the bacterial CAT gene. The cells were cotransfected with cDNA vectors constitutively expressing either the active wild-type or inactive mutant human glucocorticoid receptor (GR). The induction by IL-1, TNF, phorbol ester, or forskolin of IL-6-tK-CAT chimeric constructs containing a single copy of the IL-6 DNA segment from −173 to −151 (MRE I) or from −158 to −145 (MRE II), which are derived from within the multiple cytokine- and second-messenger-responsive enhancer (MRE) region, was strongly repressed by dexamethasone in a wild-type GR-dependent fashion irrespective of the inducer used. Dexamethasone also repressed induction by a pseudorabies virus of an IL-6 construct containing the IL-6 TATA box and the RNA start site ("initiator" or Inr element) but not the MRE region (34). The purified DNA-binding domain fragment of GR generated footprints across both the MRE region and the basal promoter elements (TATA box and Inr element in the IL-6 promoter). These observations suggested that ligand-activated GR repressed IL-6 gene function by blocking of not only the IL-6 MRE enhancer region but also that of the basal promoter elements.

Protein Structure of IL-6

The open reading frame in the gene codes for a 211–amino acid protein in mouse and rat and 212 in humans. Depending on the site of cleavage of the signal peptide, this yields a mature protein of 183–185 amino acids. Human IL-6 contains two N-glycosylation sites and several O-glycosylation sites as well as phosphorylations on serine residues (35,36). The homology between human and mouse IL-6 is 42% at the protein level (37). There is very little homology in the N-terminal region, but the central portion is more conserved (57% for the region spanning residues 42 to 102). The four cysteine residues of the protein, which are located in this region, can be perfectly aligned and the intrachain disulfide bonds are identical (38,39). The N terminus of the molecule is not essential to functional integrity and in fact deletions of up to 28 residues of the mature protein do not affect its biological activity (40). However, the C terminus plays an important role in biological activity. Structure-function studies have recently identified an IL-6 receptor binding site in the C terminus of IL-6. When the sequence of IL-6 was compared with that of other known proteins, the same motif of four cysteines was found in human and mouse G-CSF (41,42) and in chicken myelomonocytic growth factor (43), suggesting an evolutionary relation.

IL-6 Receptors and Signal Transduction

In accordance with the multifunctional properties of IL-6, the specific receptor for IL-6 is expressed in various types of cells (1,44,45). The human IL-6 receptor (IL-6-R) is a glycoprotein with a molecular weight of 80 kDa, consisting of 449 amino acids with an intracytoplasmic portion of 82 amino acid residues. Molecular cloning showed that the IL-6-R has one Ig-like domain in the amino-terminal part of the extracellular portion (46). In this it differs from the IL-1 receptor, in which the entire extracellular portion consists of three Ig-like domains. The Ig-like domain in the IL-6-R is not involved in ligand-binding activity, but the remainder of the extracellular region is essential (47).

Other cytokine receptors—which include the IL-2 receptor β chain, IL-3, IL-4, IL-5, GM-CSF, and erythropoietin receptors—share striking structural similarities with the IL-6-R in their extracellular domains and represent a newly discovered "family" of cytokine receptors (48). The homologous region of this receptor family consists of about 200 amino acids with four conserved cysteine residues in the amino-terminal part and a Trp-Ser-X-Trp-Ser motif near the transmembrane portion.

Sequence similarity is less in the intracellular portion. Unlike other growth factor receptors, the intracytoplasmic portion of IL-6-R lacks a tyrosine kinase domain. Deletion of the intracytoplasmic domain of IL-6-R did not affect signal transduction, thus suggesting that transduction of the IL-6 signal could be mediated through another molecule associated with the receptor (47). Taga et al (49) reported that the IL-6 signal was mediated through a non-ligand-binding membrane glycoprotein, gp130, which associates with the 80-kDa IL-6-R. A cDNA encoding human gp130 has been cloned, revealing that it consists of 918 amino acids with a single transmembrane domain. The extracellular region comprises six units of a fibronectin type III module, and part of this region—about 200 amino acids—has features typical of a cytokine receptor family (50,51).

Bauer et al. (52) studied the regulation of expression of IL-6-R in vitro in human monocytes and found that LPS, IL-1, and IL-6 reduced it. We have recently observed that human glomerular mesangial cells in culture constitutively express the IL-6-R gene and the IL-6 signal transducer, gp 130 (53). Fukunaga et al. (54), investigating signal transduction mechanisms of IL-6 in cultured rat mesangial cells, found that IL-6 induced a transient increase of inositol 1,4,5-triphosphate followed by a transient but sustained rise in the intracellular calcium concentration, suggesting that IL-6 stimulates phosphoinositide turnover.

Renal Cellular Sources of IL-6 and Effects on the Kidney

Most nucleated cells express and synthesize IL-6 in vitro (3), especially LPS-stimulated monocyte-macrophages and cytokine-stimulated fibroblasts, and epithelial and endothelial cells. T and B cell lines, numerous tumor cell lines, and even polymorphonuclear leukocytes can also synthesize it. In the kidney, IL-6 is expressed by glomerular mesangial and epithelial cells and by tubular cells. Human mesangial cells in culture do not constitutively express the IL-6 gene, but they do so when stimulated with IL-1 or TNF (Figure 1). Upon such stimuli IL-6 protein is formed and released in the culture supernatant (8,9). This suggests that a complex network of cytokines modulates local immune-inflammatory responses. In diseases with cell proliferation and infiltrates into the glomeruli, stimuli for IL-6 synthesis, such as IL-1 and TNF, could originate from infiltrating monocyte/macrophages or from resident mesangial cells.

Earlier reports that IL-6 is also mitogenic for cultured rat mesangial cells (4,10) have not been confirmed: more recent experiments show that IL-6 fails to stimulate mesangial cell proliferation (9) and, if anything, inhibits mesangial cell growth (11). This conflicts, however, with the in vivo findings that IL-6 transgenic mice carrying a human IL-6 genomic gene fused with the human immunoglobulin heavy chain enhancer developed proteinuria and mesangioproliferative glomerulonephritis, with a high serum level of IL-6 (6). The causative role of IL-6 in mesangial proliferation was suggested by the fact that mice given antihuman IL-6 antibody were protected (7).

Because mesangial cell proliferation is the central feature of many forms of immune-mediated glomerulonephritis, van den Dobbelsteen et al. (55) recently investigated whether aggregated IgG or immune complexes were capable of modulating IL-6 production from rat mesangial cells in culture.

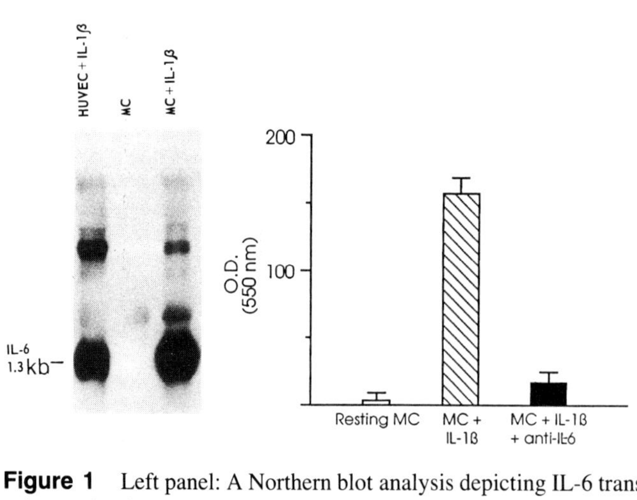

Figure 1 Left panel: A Northern blot analysis depicting IL-6 transcripts in human mesangial cells (MC) cultured for 6 hr with medium alone or IL-1β (10 ng/ml). RNA from human umbilical vein endothelial cells (HUVEC) stimulated with IL-1β (10 ng/ml) was used as positive control. Right panel: IL-6 production by resting or IL-1β-stimulated human mesangial cells (MC) and inhibitory effect of a specific anti-IL-6 antibody. IL-6 activity was measured as hybridoma growth factor using the 7TD1 cell line. (From Ref. 8.)

Aggregated IgG did bind to a specific Fc receptor on mesangial cells with a binding that was dose-dependent and served to enhance IL-6 synthesis. Similar results were obtained when mesangial cells were incubated with immune complexes of human albumin and rabbit antihuman albumin. These observations prompted the authors to suggest that binding of aggregated Ig or immune complexes to mesangial cells in vivo may favor IL-6 production and promote mesangial cell proliferation.

IL-6 can also play a direct role in renal disease progression, since it enhances the steady-state expression of messenger RNA coding for $\alpha 1$ collagen III, fibronectin, and laminin, at least in cultured mesangial cells (12).

Glomerular epithelial cells in culture also express the IL-6 gene and release the corresponding protein into the cell supernatant (56). LPS and IL-1β markedly increased IL-6 secretion. Incubating mesangial cells with increasing concentrations of recombinant IL-6 dose-dependently enhanced 3H-thymidine uptake, again suggesting an autocrine pattern of IL-6–dependent glomerular epithelial cell growth (57). These observations might cast some light on the pathogenesis of those inflammatory diseases involving epithelial cell proliferation, such as crescenteric glomerulonephritis.

The potential for expression of IL-6 is not confined to glomerular cells but applies to tubular epithelial cells as well (58,59). Thus a study explored the possibility that IL-6 participates in the process of tubulointerstitial damage often associated with proteinuric diseases. IL-6, which was not demonstrable in normal tubules, was expressed in tubular epithelial cells in various forms of renal diseases and was associated with tubular atrophy (58). Immunohistochemical studies provided evidence that IL-6 was localized in the cytoplasm around the nuclei of tubular cells with a diffuse or finely granular pattern (60). In tubules with advanced atrophy and thickened tubular basement membrane, IL-6 immunostaining had a diffuse, intense cytoplasmic pattern. It is difficult to establish the origin of IL-6 detected in the tubules because of the limitations of immunohistochemical methods. On the other hand, it is difficult to demonstrate IL-6 mRNA in isolated tubules because of contamination with vascular cells. The diffuse or fine granular distribution of IL-6 in the perinuclear cytoplasm, detected by confocal laser scanning microscopy, suggests that it is synthesized by the tubular cells (60). Its localization was more marked in tubular cells than in inflammatory cells infiltrating the interstitium. In tubules surrounded by inflammatory cells, IL-6 colocalized with HLA class II, suggesting a possible role in modulating antigen presentation by tubular cells, as recently documented.

IL-6 in Renal Disease

IL-6 appears to have some role in the pathogenesis of renal lesions (Table 1). IL-6 mRNA expression is increased in the glomeruli of mice with immune complex–mediated glomerulonephritis (61) and could originate from infiltrating inflammatory cells or from glomerular resident cells. In the MRL-lpr/lpr murine lupus nephritis model, plasma IL-6 levels are higher than normal (62) and glomerular IL-6 mRNA is also upregulated (61). Kiberd et al. (63) recently reported that treatment of MRL-lpr/lpr mice (15 weeks old) for 5 weeks with a neutralizing monoclonal antibody to the IL-6 receptor helped preserve glomerular function and structure. Thus IL-6 may play a role in lupus nephritis and its inhibition could be useful in the treatment of the disease.

Table 1 Renal Diseases Associated with Abnormal Production of IL-6

Mesangioproliferative glomerulonephritis	Urinary levels ↑ (19/38 pts)	Horii et al., 1989
IgA nephropathy	Urinary levels ↑ (10/32 pts)	Dohl et al., 1991
Active lupus nephritis	Urinary levels ↑ (24/29 pts)	Iwano et al., 1993
Chronic renal failure	Plasma levels ↑	Herbelin et al., 1991
Renal allograft rejection	Serum levels ↑	Van Oers et al., 1988
	urinary levels ↑	Ruggenenti et al., 1994
	mRNA in renal biopsies ↑	Vandenbroecke et al., 1991

Horii et al. (4) detected IL-6 by immunohistochemical staining of renal biopsies in mesangial cells of patients with mesangioproliferative glomerulonephritis, but not in cases of membranous nephropathy or minimal change. These authors also reported that urinary excretion of IL-6 was increased in patients with mesangioproliferative glomerulonephritis but not in healthy volunteers or in patients with other types of glomerular disease (4). In another study, urinary IL-6 was increased in IgA nephropathy and correlated with the degree of mesangial cell proliferation (64). In patients with lupus nephritis, a significant correlation has been found between urinary IL-6 and the histological indices of renal injury, suggesting that urinary IL-6 could be of value as a noninvasive marker of disease activity (5).

In uremia, levels of IL-6 in circulating blood were higher than normal and the hemodialysis procedure led to a further induction of IL-6 (65). Activated monocytes could be responsible at least in part for the increased cytokine levels. The presence of circulating endotoxin reported in uremic, not yet dialyzed patients could perhaps account for the activated state of monocytes (66). In uremic patients, activated T cells have also been observed, as reflected by increased expression of their membrane interleukin-2 receptors (IL-2-R) (67). Since IL-6 may induce IL-2 R expression by T cells (68), it is possible that activated monocytes producing IL-6 are involved in the mechanisms of T-cell activation in these patients. Moreover, activated T cells themselves may contribute to the increased plasma levels of IL-6. Chronic renal failure itself may directly raise IL-6 blood levels as a result of reduced renal clearance. In patients undergoing chronic hemodialysis, stimulation of monocytes to produce IL-6 and other cytokines, namely IL-1 and TNF, can occur due to complement activation by the dialyzer, the interaction of dialyzer polymer materials with monocytes, or microbial products diffusing into the blood from the dialysis bath (69).

Recently attempts have been made to define a role for urinary IL-6 as an early marker of renal transplant rejection. Urinary IL-6 increased in renal transplant patients coincident with acute rejection episodes (70,71), and elevated IL-6 mRNA was found by in situ hybridization in renal biopsies taken during such episodes (72). The most likely explanation is that IL-6 is generated in an increased amount in the kidney during the processes of allograft infiltration by inflammatory cells (71). This would be consistent with the findings of Raasveld et al. (73), who examined biopsies taken from seven patients during acute rejection by immunohistochemistry. They found an increased intensity for IL-6 in the tubules but not in infiltrating lymphocytes and endothelial cells, which correlated with the extent of the interstitial infiltrate. The staining was stronger in distal than in proximal tubules and was mainly located along the luminal side of the cells. However, whether increased tubular IL-6 synthesis is the consequence of lymphocyte-mediated tubular injury or is one of the triggers of interstitial accumulation of lymphocytes and monocyte/macrophages in acute allograft rejection still remains to be defined.

INTERLEUKIN-8

Gene Structure and Regulation

IL-8, also known as monocyte-derived neutrophil chemotactic factor (MDNCF) and neutrophil-activating peptide-1 (NAP-1), was originally described as a product secreted by LPS-stimulated human peripheral blood monocytes with neutrophil chemotactic and activating properties (13). IL-8 is a member of an emerging superfamily of cytokine polypeptides called the "intercrine" family, with a molecular mass of about 10 kDa (15,74). This superfamily is made up of proteins that share four conserved cysteine residues, which probably give rise to similar three-dimensional structures. The intercrine family can be divided into two subfamilies based on the spacing of the cysteine residues and chromosomal location. IL-8 belongs to the α subfamily that includes platelet factor 4 (PF4), β-thromboglobulin, the interferon-γ inducible gene IP-10, and growth regulatory gene/melanoma growth stimulatory activity (GRO/MGSA), among others. The two amino-terminal cysteines are separated by a single residue (CXC). The genes are mainly located closely together in the q12-21 region of human chromosome 4 (75). In the other subfamily (β-intercrines, like RANTES and the monocyte chemoattractant protein-1, MCP-1), the two cysteines are adjacent (CC) and the genes have been mapped to human chromosome 17 or mouse chromosome 11. IL-8 was molecularly cloned in 1988 by Matsushima et al. (76) and subsequently by Lindley et al. (77). The resulting cDNA sequence was identical to an enterotoxin-inducible gene in human leukocytes first reported in 1987

(78). The gene for IL-8 consists of four exons and three introns with a single "TATA"- and "CAT"-like structure (79). The 5′-flanking region of the IL-8 gene shows no overall sequence similarity with the flanking regions of other cytokines whose expression can be induced by IL-1 or TNF. The 5′-flanking region of the IL-8 contains several potential binding sites for known nuclear factors, including AP-1, AP-2, AP-3, NF-κB, hepatocyte nuclear factor-1, glucocorticoid receptor, and interferon regulatory factor-1 (15).

To delineate the sequences in the IL-8 gene involved in the regulation of gene expression in response to IL-1 or TNF, Mukaida et al. (80) constructed CAT expression plasmids into which serially deleted mutants of the 5′-flanking region of the IL-8 gene were inserted and transfected them into an IL-1/TNF-responsive human fibrosarcoma cell line. The authors found that the nucleotides between –94 and –71 bp from the start of the first exon are essential and sufficient for IL-8 induction by IL-1, TNF, and phorbol 12-myristate 13-acetate (PMA). This sequence is composed of two *cis*-elements; one is the potential binding site for an NF-κB-like factor and the other for a *cis*-regulatory enhancer binding protein-like factor. These two distinct but adjacent *cis*-elements must cooperate to induce IL-8 gene expression by the three stimuli. Mutation in either element abolished IL-1, TNF, and PMA responsiveness. The IL-8 gene can be induced by the protein X of the hepatitis B virus (HBV-X) as reflected by the enhanced IL-8 mRNA expression and IL-8 production observed in fibrosarcoma cells transfected with HBV-X (81). Mahé et al. (81) showed that both NF-κB and CCAAT/enhancer-binding protein-like *cis*-elements located at –94 to –71 bp of the IL-8 gene are necessary for the induction of the IL-8 gene by HBV-X and suggested the existence of a common pathway for HBV-X and the inflammatory cytokines IL-1 and TNF to activate the IL-8 gene. These observations might be relevant to the pathogenesis of inflammation in viral hepatitis, given the fact that during the acute phase of hepatitis an inflammatory neutrophil infiltration of the liver is commonly observed and that IL-8 can be induced in hepatocytes by IL-1 and TNF.

In a human gastric cancer cell line, it was observed that TNF and interferon γ synergistically induced IL-8 production through acting concurrently on AP-1 at –126 to –120 bp and NF-κB-like factor binding sites of the IL-8 gene (82). Thus, *cis*-regulatory enhancer elements required for the activation of the IL-8 gene by IL-1 or/and TNFα in these cells differ from those of human fibrosarcoma (81), whose minimal enhancer region in the activation of the IL-8 gene are at the region –94 to –71 bp. Different sets of nuclear factors may therefore be involved in the regulation of IL-8 gene transcription in a cell type-specific manner (82).

Recently Kunsch and Rosen (83) examined the ability of various NF-κB subunits to bind to, and activate transcription from, the IL-8 promoter. NF-κB is a heterodimeric complex consisting of a 50-kDA subunit (NF-κB1) and a 65-kDA subunit (Rel A) (32,84). The cloning of the genes for both NF-κB1 (85,86) and Rel A (87) revealed a high degree of homology to the protooncogene product c-Rel (88). All the members of the NF-κB/Rel gene family, which also includes NF-κB2 (89) and Rel B (90), share homology within a 300–amino acid region responsible for DNA binding and dimerization. Kunsch and Rosen (83), using purified kB/Rel subunits and nuclear extracts from PMA-treated Jurkat T cells, observed selective association of κB/Rel complexes with the κB element in the IL-8 promoter and demonstrated the direct involvement of Rel A in inducible nuclear factor binding, transcriptional activation, and regulation of endogenous IL-8 gene expression. Neither NF-κB1 nor heterodimeric NF-κB1-Rel A complexes could bind to the IL-8 κB element alone or in the context of the authentic IL-8 promoter. However, Rel A, NF-κB2, and c-Rel were capable of binding to this element. Although purified NF-κB2 and c-Rel were able to bind to the IL-8 promoter, antibody supershift experiments suggested that neither of these proteins represents a major component in the inducible nuclear protein-DNA binding complex in Jurkat T cells. Thus, there is a differential ability of members of the κB/Rel family to bind to, and activate transcription from, the IL-8 promoter.

Protein Structure of IL-8

Purification and sequencing of IL-8 from the culture supernatants of stimulated human blood monocytes showed that it has no significant homology with other cytokines produced by these cells, like IL-1, TNF, or colony-stimulating factors (13,77). IL-8 is generated as a 99–amino acid precursor with a characteristic leader sequence of 22 amino acids (76,78). Several mature forms have been identified; the main one consists of 72 amino acids and has been obtained by recombinant methodology using a synthetic gene expressed in *Escherichia coli* (77). It contains 14 basic amino acids (lysine and arginine), which contribute to the basic characteristics of the protein. The mature form of IL-8 contains four cysteine residues, which form disulfide bridges essential for activity (91). The three-dimensional structure of IL-8 has been investigated by x-ray crystallography and NMR spectrometry. It exists as a dimer of two identical subunits and may undergo a conformational change upon binding to the receptor (92–94).

IL-8 Receptors and Signal Transduction

Two distinct IL-8 receptors, designated type 1 and 2, with 77% amino acid identity, have been molecularly cloned from human neutrophils (95,96). The primary sequences show that these receptors contain a "seven-pass" motif consisting of seven hydrophobic membrane-spanning domains (97). This structural feature is characteristic of the superfamily of guanine nucleotide-binding protein (G-protein)-coupled receptors, indicating that IL-8 receptors may be a subfamily of this large supergene family. Although initial reports (96) indicated that type 2 was a low-affinity receptor for IL-8 and the structurally related cytokine GRO/MGSA (which also binds to and activates neutrophils), recent experiments with both receptor forms produced in COS cells showed little difference in their affinity for IL-8. Lee et al. (98) showed that both receptors bind IL-8 with high affinity in this system. The affinities differ for GRO/MGSA, however, with the type 1 IL-8 receptor showing low affinity and type 2 high affinity. Recently, using conserved restriction enzyme sites, a series of chimeric IL-8 receptor molecules were constructed between type 1 and type 2 receptors and transfected into human 293 kidney epithelial cells; it was thus established that the amino terminus of the IL-8 receptor is important for differential binding of GRO/MGSA and IL-8 (99). Peptides were then synthesized that identified the amino-terminal sequence of the receptor as the critical portion for interacting with IL-8.

Samanta et al. (100) studied the regulation of IL-8 receptor expression on human neutrophils by the IL-8 ligand itself and showed that IL-8 downregulates its own receptor expression and that this is accompanied by internalization of the ligand. IL-8 receptors reappeared on the cell surface within a few minutes. Since cycloheximide did not alter either the ligand internalization or the receptor reappearance, it was suggested that de novo protein synthesis of IL-8 receptors was not involved in their rapid turnover but that they were probably recycled. Rapid recycling would appear to be essential for the neutrophil chemotactic response to IL-8. The observation that *Bordetella pertussis* toxin inhibited some IL-8-induced cellular responses (such as the rapid rise in cytosolic free Ca^{+} concentration in human neutrophils) (15), similar to some other previously known G-protein-mediated responses, suggested that G proteins are involved in IL-8 signaling. In this context Sham et al. (101) recently demonstrated that IL-8–induced actin polymerization in human neutrophils was mediated through pertussis-toxin–sensitive G proteins. Moreover, that IL-8 acts through signal-transducing pathways involving specific G proteins has also been documented by Wu et al. (102). These authors investigated the pathways by which IL-8 activates inositide-specific phospholipase C (PLC) by coexpression of different components of the guanosine triphosphate binding protein (G protein) pathway in COS-7 cells.

Renal Cellular Sources of IL-8 and Effects on the Kidney

Like most of the intercrine superfamily members, IL-8 is produced by a large number of cell types—like fibroblasts, endothelial cells, monocytes, and macrophages—in response to a wide variety of endogenous and exogenous stimuli, inflammatory cytokines being the most common and potent (15).

Among renal cells, glomerular mesangial cells and tubular epithelial cells can produce IL-8. In 1991 four different groups found that human mesangial cells in culture activated by IL-1 or TNF expressed IL-8 mRNA and released the protein in the culture medium (8,9,16,17) (Figure 2). In situ hybridization experiments showed IL-8 mRNA in mesangial cells (17). Grain quantification indicated 13-fold and 8-fold increases in grains over IL-1-and TNF-stimulated mesangial cells compared to control cells.

Sedor et al. (103) cloned and sequenced the mesangial cell IL-8 using the polymerase chain reaction. The DNA sequence was identical to bases 1 to 293 of the protein coding segment reported by Matsushima et al. (76) for human monocyte cDNA for IL-8 and for bases 91 to 383 of a cDNA

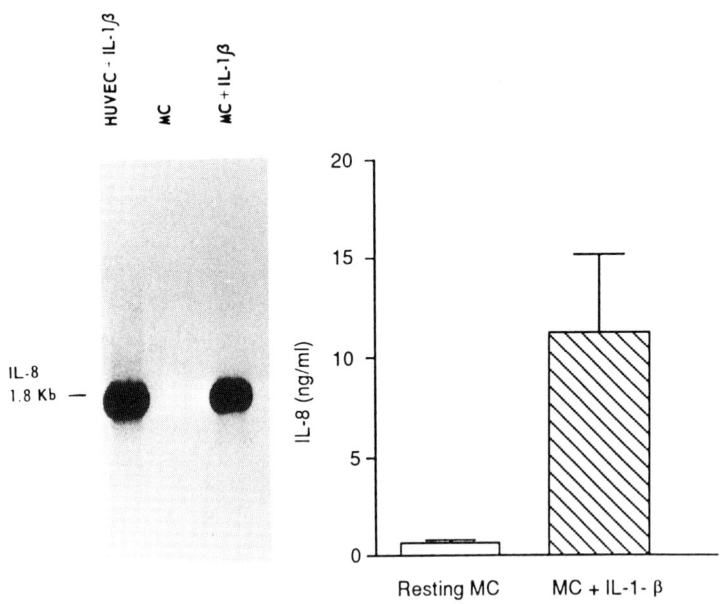

Figure 2 Left panel: Induction of IL-8 mRNA expression in human mesangial cells (MC) by 6-hr incubation with IL-1β (10 ng/ml). RNA from human umbilical vein endothelial cells (HUVEC) stimulated with IL-1β (10 ng/ml) was used as positive control. Right panel: Release of IL-8 measured by radioimmunoassay in supernatants of IL-1β-stimulated human MC. (From Ref. 8.)

coding for a "β-thromboglobulin-like" protein (later found to be IL-8) cloned from staphylococcal enterotoxin A–stimulated human peripheral blood leukocytes by Schmid and Weissman (78).

The amounts of IL-8 released into the medium of cytokine-stimulated mesangial cells are biologically important because they induce neutrophil migration, as evaluated by chemotaxis assay (17). Thus mesangial cell–derived IL-8 might play an important role in the recruitment of leukocytes during glomerular immune injury and may be involved in the progression of glomerular inflammation to scar and fibrosis. Tubular epithelia also produce IL-8. In vitro experiments by Shmouder et al. (104) showed that human renal cortical epithelial cells of tubular origin express and secrete IL-8. These cells respond to IL-1β, TNF, or LPS in both a time- and dose-dependent manner with the expression of IL-8 mRNA and the production of IL-8 antigen. The same authors also provided in vivo evidence that both proximal and distal tubular epithelial cells from three patients with acute allograft rejection produced IL-8 as established by immunohistochemical localization of the IL-8 antigen (104). Normal human renal tissue did not immunostain for IL-8. Thus IL-8 derived from tubular cells could help direct immune cell traffic into the renal interstitium. This would be particularly important in renal allograft rejection, where the recruitment of leukocytes could depend on activation of allograft tubular epithelial cells (104). However, other types of tubulointerstitial disease—including pyelonephritis, vasculitis, and allergic interstitial nephritis—could also be partly mediated by similar mechanisms.

IL-8 Involvement in Renal Disease

That IL-8 may modulate the glomerular inflammatory reaction in disease is suggested by the elevated urinary excretion of IL-8 in some patients with IgA nephropathy, acute glomerulonephritis, and lupus nephritis (105) (Table 2). In uremia and during hemodialysis, plasma IL-8 is higher than in healthy subjects (106,107), possibly because of monocyte activation. Moreover, reduced renal clearance could be directly responsible for the impaired clearance from the plasma of IL-8 and the other cytokines like TNF and IL-6 that are also elevated in uremia. In patients on continuous

Table 2 Renal Diseases Associated with Abnormal Production of IL-8

IgA nephropathy	Urinary levels ↑ (17/43 pts)	Hisada et al., 1993
Acute glomerulonephritis	Urinary levels ↑ (4/6 pts)	Hisada et al., 1993
Lupus nephritis	Urinary levels ↑ (11/15 pts)	Hisada et al., 1993
Uremia	Plasma levels ↑ PBMC mRNA ↑	Niwa et al., 1993
Hemolytic uremic syndrome	Serum levels ↑ (23/34 pts)	Fitzpatrick et al., 1992

ambulatory peritoneal dialysis, very high serum levels of IL-8 have been reported to coincide with peritonitis episodes and showed a rapid fall during clinical recovery (108).

Fitzpatrick et al. (109) recently reported high serum IL-8 levels in 20 of 25 children with diarrhea-associated hemolytic uremic syndrome (HUS) and in 3 of 9 children with non-diarrhea-associated HUS. IL-8 was undetectable by the same assay in control normal children. In diarrhea-associated HUS serum IL-8 correlated significantly with blood polymorphoneutrophil leukocyte count and also with circulating α1-antitrypsin-complexed elastase, a marker of neutrophil degradation. Whether IL-8 contributes to neutrophil recruitment and activation and plays a role in the microvascular lesions of diarrhea-associated HUS remains to be established.

REFERENCES

1. Kishimoto T. The biology of Interleukin-6. Blood 1989; 74:1–10.
2. Hirano T, Akira S, Taga T, Kishimoto T. Biological and clinical aspects of interleukin 6. Immunol Today 1990; 11:443–449.
3. Van Snick J. Interleukin-6: An overview. Annu Rev Immunol 1990; 8:253–278.
4. Horii Y, Muraguchi A, Iwano M, et al. Involvement of IL-6 in mesangial proliferative glomerulonephritis. J Immunol 1989; 143:3949–3955.
5. Iwano M, Dohi K, Hirata E, et al. Urinary levels of IL-6 in patients with active lupus nephritis. Clin Nephrol 1993; 40:16–21.
6. Suematsu S, Matsuda T, Aozasa K, et al. IgG1 plasmacytosis in interleukin 6 transgenic mice. Proc Natl Acad Sci USA 1989; 86:7547–7551.
7. Matsusaka T, Suematsu S, Horii Y, et al. Generation of mesangial proliferative glomerulonephritis in interleukin-6 transgenic mice. Proc XIth Intern Congr of Nephr, Tokyo, Japan 1990; July 15–20:374A.(Abstract)
8. Zoja C, Wang JM, Bettoni S, et al. Interleukin-1β and tumor necrosis factor $-\alpha$ induce gene expression and production of leukocyte chemotactic factors, Colony-stimulating factors, and interleukin-6 in human mesangial cells. Am J Pathol 1991; 138:991–1003.
9. Abbott F, Ryan JJ, Ceska M, et al. Interleukin-1β stimulates human mesangial cells to synthesize and release interleukins-6 and -8. Kidney Int 1991; 40:597–605.
10. Ruef C, Budde K, Lacy J, et al. Interleukin 6 is an autocrine growth factor for mesangial cells. Kidney Int 1990; 38:249–257.
11. Ikeda M, Ikeda U, Ohara T, et al. Recombinant Interleukin-6 inhibits the growth of rat mesangial cells in culture. Am J Pathol 1992; 141:327–334.
12. Zoja C, Benigni A, Piccinini G, et al. Interleukin-6 stimulates gene expression of extracellular matrix components in bovine mesangial cells in culture. Med Inflamm 1993; 2:429–433.
13. Yoshimura TK, Matsushima K, Oppenheim JJ, Leonard EJ. Neutrophil chemotactic factor produced by lipopolysaccharide (LPS)-stimulated human blood mononuclear leukocytes: Partial characterization and separation from interleukin 1(IL-1). J Immunol 1987; 139:788–793.
14. Baggiolini M, Walz A, Kunkel S. Neutrophil-activating peptide-1/interleukin 8, a novel cytokine that activates neutrophils. J Clin Invest 1989; 84:1045–1049.

15. Oppenheim JJ, Zachariae COC, Mukaida N, Matsushima K. Properties of the novel proinflammatory supergene "intercrine" cytokine family. Annu Rev Immunol 1991; 9:617–648.
16. Brown Z, Strieter RM, Chensue W, et al. Cytokine-activated human mesangial cells generate the neutrophil chemoattractant, interleukin 8. Kidney Int 1991; 40:86–90.
17. Kusner DJ, Luebbers EL, Nowinski RJ, et al. Cytokine- and LPS-induced synthesis of interleukin-8 from human mesangial cells. Kidney Int 1991; 39:1240–1248.
18. Larsen CG, Anderson AO, Appella E, et al. The neutrophil-activating protein (NAP-1) is also chemotactic for T lymphocytes. Science 1989; 243:1464–1466.
19. Tanabe O, Akira S, Kamiya T, et al. Genomic structure of the murine IL-6 gene: High degree conservation of potential regulatory sequences between mouse and human. J Immunol 1988; 141:3875–3881.
20. Northemann W, Braciak TA, Hattori M, et al. Structure of the rat interleukin 6 gene and its expression in macrophage-derived cells. J Biol Chem 1989; 264:16072–16082.
21. Yasukawa K, Hirano T, Watanabe Y, et al. Structure and expression of human B cell stimulating factor–2 (BSF-2/IL-6) gene. EMBO J 1987; 6:2939–2945.
22. Sehgal PB, Zilberstein A, Ruggieri RM, et al. Human chromosome 7 carries the β2 interferon gene. Proc Natl Acad Sci USA 1987; 84:3633–3637.
23. Bowcock AM, Kidd JR, Lathrop M, et al. The human "beta 2 interferon/hepatocyte stimulating factor/interleukin-6" gene: DNA polymorphism studies and localization to chromosome 7p21. Genomics 1988; 3:8–16.
24. Mock BA, Nordan RP, Justice MJ, et al. The murine IL-6 gene maps to the proximal region of chromosome 5. J Immunol 1989; 142:1372–1376.
25. Akira S, Hirano T, Taga T, Kishimoto T. Biology of multifunctional cytokines: IL-6 and related molecules (IL 1 and TNF). Faseb J 1990; 4:2860–2867.
26. Ray A, Sassone-Corsi P, Sehgal PB. A multiple cytokine- and second messenger-responsive element in the enhancer of the human interleukin-6 gene: Similarities with c-fos gene regulation. Mol Cell Biol 1989; 9:5537–5547.
27. Isshiki H, Akira S, Tanabe O, et al. Constitutive and IL-1 inducible factors interact with the IL-1 responsive element in the IL-6 gene. Mol Cell Biol 1990; 10:2757–2764.
28. Akira S, Isshiki H, Sugita T, et al. A nuclear factor for IL-6 expression (NF-IL-6) is a member of a C/EBP family. EMBO J 1990; 9:1897–1906.
29. Kinoshita S, Akira S, Kishimoto T. A member of the C/EBP family, NF-IL6β, forms a heterodimer and transcriptionally synergizes with NF-IL6. Proc Natl Acad Sci USA 1992; 89:1473–1476.
30. Shimizu H, Mitomo K, Watanabe T, et al. Involvement of a NF-κB-like transcription factor in the activation of the Interleukin-6 gene by inflammatory lymphokines. Mol Cell Biol 1990; 10:561–568.
31. Baeuerle PA. The inducible transcription activator NF-κB: regulation by distinct protein subunits. Biochim Biophys Acta 1991; 1072:63–80.
32. Lenard MJ, Baltimore D. NK-κB: A pleiotropic mediator of inducible and tissue-specific gene control. Cell 1988; 58:227–229.
33. Kashtan C, Libermann T, Kim Y, Van Ness B. Induction of the promoter of the interleukin-6 (IL-6) gene in human mesangial cells (HMC) requires an intact binding site for nuclear factor κB (NF- κB) (abstr). J Am Soc Nephrol 1993; 4:609.
34. Ray A, LaForge KS, Sehgal PB. On the mechanism for efficient repression of the interleukin-6 promoter by glucocorticoids: Enhancer, TATA box, and RNA start site (Inr motif) occlusion. Mol Cell Biol 1990; 10:5736–5746.
35. May LT, Grayeb J, Santhanam U, et al. Synthesis and secretion of multiple forms of β2-interferon/B-cell differentiation factor 2/hepatocyte-stimulating factor by human fibroblasts and monocytes. J Biol Chem 1988; 263:7760–7766.
36. May LT, Santhanam U, Tatter SB, et al. Phosphorylation of secreted forms of human β2-interferon/hepatocyte-stimulating factor/interlekin-6. Biochem Biophys Res Commun 1988; 152:1144–1150.
37. Tanabe O, Akira S, Kamiya T, et al. Genomic structure of the murine IL-6 gene: High degree of conservation of potential regulatory sequences between mouse and human. J Immunol 1988; 141:3875–3881.
38. Simpson RJ, Moritz RL, Van Roost E, Van Snick J. Characterization of a recombinant murine interleukin-6: Assignment of disulfide bonds. Biochem Biophys Res Commun 1988; 157:364–372.
39. Clogston CL, Boone TC, Crandall BC, et al. Disulfide structures of human interleukin-6 are similar to those of human granulocyte colony stimulating factor. Arch Biochem Biophys 1989; 272:144–151.
40. Brakenhoff JPJ, Hart M, Aarden LA. Analysis of human IL-6 mutants expressed in Escherichia coli—Biologic activities are not affected by deletion of amino acids 1-28. J Immunol 1989; 143:1115–1182.
41. Nagata S, Tsuchiya M, Asano S, et al. Molecular cloning and expression of cDNA for human granulocyte colony-stimulating factor. Nature 1986; 319:415–418.
42. Tsuchiya M, Asano S, Kaziro Y, Nagata S. Isolation and characterization of the cDNA for murine granulocyte colony-stimulating factor. Proc Natl Acad Sci USA 1986; 83:7633–7637.

43. Leutz A, Damm K, Sterneck E, et al. Molecular cloning of the chicken myelomonocytic growth factor (cMGF) reveals relationship to interleukin-6 and granulocyte colony stimulating factor. EMBO J 1989; 8:175–181.
44. Taga T, Kawanishi Y, Hardy R, et al. Receptors for B cell stimulatory factor 2: Quantitation, specificity, distribution and regulation of their expression. J Exp Med 1987; 166:967–981.
45. Coulie PG, Vanhecke A, Van Damme J, et al. High affinity binding sites for human 26-kDA protein (interleukin 6, B cell stimulatory factor-2, human hybridoma plasmacytoma growth factor, interferon-β2), different from those of type 1 interferon (alpha, β), on lymphoblastoid cells. Eur J Immunol 1987; 17:1435–1440.
46. Yamasaki K, Taga T, Hirata Y, et al. Cloning and expression of the human interleukin-6 (BSF-2/IFNβ2) receptor. Science 1988; 241:825–828.
47. Kishimoto T, Akira S, Taga T. Interleukin-6 and its receptor: A paradigm for cytokines. Science 1992; 258:593–597.
48. Bazan JF. A novel family of growth factor receptors: A common binding domain in the growth hormone, prolactin, erythropoietin and IL-6 receptors, and the p75 IL-2 receptor β-chain. Biochem Biophys Res Commun 1989; 164:788–795.
49. Taga T, Hibi M, Hirata Y, et al. Interleukin-6 triggers the association of its receptor with a possible signal transducer, gp130. Cell 1989; 58:573–581.
50. Hibi M, Murakami M, Saito M, et al. Molecular cloning and expression of an IL-6 signal transducer, gp130. Cell 1990; 63:1149–1157.
51. Murakami M, Narazaki M, Hibi M, et al. Critical cytoplasmic region of the interleukin 6 signal transducer gp130 is conserved in the cytokine receptor family. Proc Natl Acad Sci USA 1991; 88:11349–11353.
52. Bauer J, Bauer TM, Kalb T, et al. Regulation of interleukin 6 receptor expression in human monocytes and monocyte-derived macrophages. J Exp Med 1989; 170:1537–1549.
53. Rambaldi A, Bettoni S, Remuzzi G, Zoja C. Human mesangial cells in culture express interleukin-6 receptor and interleukin-6 signal tranducer, gp 130 (abstr). J Am Soc Nephrol 1992; 3:612.
54. Fukunaga M, Fujiwara Y, Fujibayashi M, et al. Signal transduction mechanism of interleukin 6 in cultured rat mesangial cells. FEBS Lett 1991; 285:265–267.
55. Van den Dobbelsteen MEA, Van der Woude FJ, Schroeijers WEM, et al. Soluble aggregates of IgG and immune complexes enhance IL-6 production by renal mesangial cells. Kidney Int 1993; 43:544–553.
56. Osawa H, Yamabe H, Ozawa K, et al. Production and gene expression of interleukin-6 (IL-6) by glomerular epithelial cells (GECs) (abstr). J Am Soc Nephrol 1992; 3:476.
57. Moutabarrik A, Namiki M, Ishibashi M, et al. Interleukin-6 (IL-6) and expression of its receptor on human glomerular epithelial cells (GEC) (abstr). J Am Soc Nephrol 1992; 3:606.
58. Fukatsu A, Matsuo S, Tamai H, et al. Distribution of interleukin-6 in normal and diseased human kidney. Lab Invest 1991; 65:61–66.
59. Frank J, Engler-Blum G, Rodemann HP, Muller GA. Human renal tubular cells as a cytokine source: PDGF-B, GM-CSF and IL-6 mRNA expression in vitro. Exp Nephrol 1993; 1:26–35.
60. Fukatsu A, Matsuo S, Yuzawa Y, et al. Expression of interleukin 6 and major histocompatibility complex molecules in tubular epithelial cells of diseased human kidneys. Lab Invest 1993; 69:58–67.
61. Iwano M, Dohi K, Hirata E, et al. Induction of interleukin 6 synthesis in mouse glomeruli and cultured mesangial cells. Nephron 1992; 62:58–65.
62. Kiberd BA. Interleukin 6 in murine lupus nephritis (abstr). J Am Soc Nephrol 1992; 3:598.
63. Kiberd BA. Interleukin-6 receptor blockage ameliorates murine lupus nephritis. J Am Soc Nephrol 1993; 4:58–61.
64. Dohi K, Iwano M, Muraguchi A, et al. The prognostic significance of urinary interleukin 6 in IgA nephropathy. Clin Nephrol 1991; 35:1–5.
65. Herbelin A, Urena P, Nguyen AT, et al. Elevated circulating levels of interleukin-6 in patients with chronic renal failure. Kidney Int 1991; 39:954–960.
66. Nisbeth U, Hallgren R, Eriksson O, Danielson BG. Endotoxemia in chronic renal failure. Nephron 1987; 45:93–97.
67. Beaurain G, Naret C, Marcon L, et al. In vivo T cell activation in chronic uremic hemodialyzed and non-hemodialyzed patients. Kidney Int 1989; 36:636–644.
68. Le JM, Fredrickson G, Pollack M, Vilcek J. Activation of thymocytes and T cells by interleukin-6. Ann NY Acad Sci 1989; 557:444–452.
69. Dinarello CA. Cytokines: Agents provocateurs in hemodialysis? Kidney Int 1992; 41:683–694.
70. Van Oers MHJ, Van der Heyden AAPAM, Aarden LA. Interleukin-6 (IL-6) in serum and urine of renal transplant recipients. Clin Exp Immunol 1988; 71:314–319.
71. Ruggenenti P, Noris M, Casizaghi F, et al. Urinary IL-6 but not serum IL-6 and urinary and serum soluble IL-2 receptor predicts acute rejection in renal transplant recipients (abstr). J Am Soc Nephrol 1994; 5:1035.

72. Vandenbroecke C, Caillat-Zucman S, Legendre C, et al. Differential in situ expression of cytokines in renal allograft rejection. Transplantation 1991; 51:602–609.
73. Raasveld MHM, Weening JJ, Kerst JM, et al. Local production of interleukin-6 during acute rejection in human renal allografts. Nephrol Dial Transplant 1993; 8:75–78.
74. Gomez-Chiarri M, Ortiz A, Seron D, et al. The intercrine superfamily and renal disease. Kidney Int 1993; 43(Suppl 39):S-81–S-85.
75. Modi WS, Dean M, Seuanez HN, et al. Monocyte-derived neutrophil chemotactic factor (MDNCF/IL 8) resides in a gene cluster along with several other members of the platelet factor gene family. Hum Genet 1990; 84:185–187.
76. Matsushima K, Morishita K, Yoshimura T, et al. Molecular cloning of a human monocyte-derived neutrophil chemotactic factor (MDNCF) and the induction of MDNCF mRNA by interleukin 1 and tumor necrosis factor. J Exp Med 1988; 167:1883–1893.
77. Lindley I, Aschauer H, Seifert JM. Synthesis and expression in Escherichia coli of the gene encoding monocyte-derived neutrophil-activating factor: Biological equivalence between natural and recombinant neutrophil-activating factor. Proc Natl Acad Sci USA 1988; 85:9199–9203.
78. Schmid J, Weissmann C. Induction of RNA for a serine protease and β-thromboglobulin-like protein in mitogen stimulated human leukocytes. J Immunol 1987; 139:250–256.
79. Mukaida N, Shiroo M, Matsushima K. Genomic structure of the human monocyte-derived neutrophil chemotactic factor (MDNCF), interleukin 8. J Immunol 1989; 143:1366–1371.
80. Mukaida N, Mahé Y, Matsushima K. Cooperative interaction of nuclear factor-κB- and cis-regulatory enhancer binding protein-like factor binding elements in activating the interleukin-8 gene by pro-inflammatory cytokines. J Biol Chem 1990; 265:21128–21133.
81. Mahé Y, Mukaida N, Kuno K, et al. Hepatitis B virus X protein transactivates human interleukin-8 gene through acting on nuclear factor kB and CCAAT/enhancer binding protein-like cis-elements. J Biol Chem 1991; 266:13759–13763.
82. Yasumoto K, Okamoto S, Mukaida N, et al. Tumor necrosis factor α and interferon γ synergistically induce interleukin 8 production in a human gastric cancer cell line through acting concurrently on AP-1 and NF-kb-like binding sites of the interleukin 8 gene. J Biol Chem 1992; 267:22506–22511.
83. Kunsch C, Rosen CA. NF-κB subunit-specific regulation of the interleukin-8 promoter. Mol Cell Biol 1993; 13:6137–6146.
84. Baeuerle PA. The inducible transcription activator NF-kB: Regulation by distinct protein subunits. Biochem Biophys Res Commun 1991; 1072:63–80.
85. Bours V, Villalobos J, Burd PR, et al. Cloning of a mitogen-inducible gene encoding a κB DNA-binding protein with homology to the rel oncogene and to cell-cycle motifs. Nature 1990; 348:76–79.
86. Kieran M, Blank V, Logeat F, et al. The DNA binding subunit of NF-κB is identical to factor KBF1 and homologous to the rel oncogene product. Cell 1990; 62:1007–1018.
87. Ruben SM, Dillon PJ, Schreck R, et al. Isolation of a rel-related human cDNA that potentially encodes the 65-kD subunit of NF-κB. Science 1991; 251:1490–1493.
88. Rice NR, Gilden RV. The rel oncogene. In: Reddy EP, Skalka AM, Curran T, eds. The Oncogene Handbook. New York, Elsevier, 1988.
89. Mercurio FJ, Didonato J, Rosette C, Karin M. Molecular cloning and characterization of a novel Rel/NF-κB family member displaying structural and functional homology to NF-κB p50-p150. DNA Cell Biol 1992; 11:523–537.
90. Ryseck RP, Bull P, Takamiya M, et al. RelB, a new Rel family transcription activator that can interact with DNA. Mol Cell Biol 1992; 12:674–684.
91. Peveri PA, Walz A, Dewald B, Baggiolini M. A novel neutrophil-activating factor produced by human mononuclear phagocytes. J Exp Med 1988; 167:1547–1559.
92. Clore CM, Appella E, Yamada M, et al. Determination of the secondary structure of interleukin 8 by nuclear magnetic resonance spectroscopy. J Biol Chem 1989; 264:18097–18911.
93. Clore MG, Appella E, Yamada M, et al. Three dimensional structure of interleukin 8 in solution. Biochemistry 1990; 29:1689–1696.
94. Baldwin ET, Franklin KA, Appella E, et al. Crystalization of human interleukin-8: A protein chemotactic for neutrophils and T lymphocytes. J Biol Chem 1990; 265:6851–6853.
95. Holmes WE, Lee J, Kuang WJ, et al. Structure and functional expression of a human interleukin-8 receptor. Science 1991; 253:1278–1280.
96. Murphy PM, Tiffany HL. Cloning of complementary DNA encoding a functional human interleukin-8 receptor. Science 1991; 253:1280–1283.
97. Taga T, Kishimoto T. Cytokine receptors and signal transduction. FASEB J 1992; 6:3387–3396.
98. Lee J, Horuk R, Rice G, et al. Characterization of two high affinity human interleukin-8 receptors. J Biol Chem 1992; 267:16283–16287.

99. Gayle RB, Sleath PR, Srinivason S, et al. Importance of the amino terminus of the interleukin-8 receptor in ligand interactions. J Biol Chem 1993; 268:7283–7289.
100. Samanta AK, Oppenheim JJ, Matsushima K. Interleukin 8 (MDNCF) dynamically regulates its own receptor expression on human neutrophils. J Biol Chem 1989; 265:183–189.
101. Sham RL, Phatak PD, Ihne TP, et al. Signal pathway regulation of interleukin-8-induced actin polymerization in neutrophils. Blood 1993; 82:2546–2551.
102. Wu D, LaRosa GJ, Simon MI. G protein-coupled signal transduction pathways for interleukin-8. Science 1993; 261:101–103.
103. Sedor JR, Konieczkowski M, Huang S, et al. Cytokines, mesangial cell activation and glomerular injury. Kidney Int 1993; 43(Suppl 39):S-65–S-70.
104. Schmouder RL, Strieter RM, Wiggins RC, et al. In vitro and in vivo interleukin-8 production in human renal cortical epithelia. Kidney Int 1992; 41:191–198.
105. Hisada Y, Wada T, Tomosugi N, et al. The elevated production of interleukin-8 in glomerular diseases (abstr). J Am Soc Nephrol 1993; 4:679.
106. Nakanishi I, Moutabarrik A, Okada N, et al. Interleukin-8 (IL-8) in chronic renal failure and dialysis patients (abstr). J Am Soc Nephrol 1993; 4:413.
107. Niwa T, Miyazaki T, Kambe F, et al. Effect of hemodialysis on plasma IL-8 and peripheral blood mononuclear cell (PBMC) IL-8 mRNA (abstr). J Am Soc Nephrol 1993; 4:373.
108. Brauner A, Hylander B, Wretlind B. Interleukin-6 and interleukin-8 in dialysate and serum from patients on continuous ambulatory peritoneal dialysis. Am J Kidney Dis 1993; 22:430–435.
109. Fitzpatrick MM, Shah V, Trompeter RS, et al. Interleukin-8 and polymorphoneutrophil leucocyte activation in hemolytic uremic syndrome of childhood. Kidney Int 1992; 42:951–956.

44

Interleukin-1: A Master Cytokine in the Renal Response to Injury

John R. Sedor
School of Medicine, Case Western Reserve University, and MetroHealth Medical Center, Cleveland, Ohio

INTRODUCTION

Mechanisms that initiate renal injury have been studied extensively. Recent interest has focused on the intermediary pathways, which are activated by these initial insults and that culminate in progressive nephron destruction (1,2). An increasing body of evidence demonstrates that cytokines, in part, mediate this process. The term "cytokine" refers to peptides that function as messengers between cells (cell-to-cell communication) to modify cellular growth, induce change in cellular differentiation, and alter cellular function.

In many ways, interleukin-1 (IL-1) is a master cytokine (Kunkel SL; personal communication). Synthesis and release of this proinflammatory peptide occurs rapidly after the induction of tissue injury and initiates production of a cascade of mediators that characterize the inflammatory milieu. IL-1 was described originally in the 1940s as an endogenous pyrogen. Systemic injection of nanogram quantities of IL-1 induces the "acute-phase response," which is characterized in part by fever, anorexia, neutrophilia, and hepatic synthesis of C-reactive protein (3,4). Higher concentrations of this cytokine induce hypotension and leukopenia (3), and IL-1 in concert with other cytokines has been implicated in the pathogenesis of septic shock syndrome (5). However, the synthesis and release of IL-1 within tissues after inflammatory injury was appreciated only after molecular probes and antibodies became available. In addition, IL-1 has been implicated in fibrosis, matrix remodeling, and endothelial cell activation, promoting intravascular coagulation and leukocyte adhesion. Both in vivo and in vitro studies have implicated intraglomerular synthesis and release of IL-1 in the pathogenesis of renal disease (1,2,6,7).

INTERLEUKIN-1 AND ITS RECEPTOR: GENOMIC STRUCTURE AND REGULATION OF SYNTHESIS

Interleukin-1α and Interleukin-1β

Several recent scholarly reviews have summarized much of the available data describing the genomic organization and the transcriptional and posttranscriptional regulation of IL-1 and IL-1 receptor (IL-1R) expression (3,4,8,9). This section emphasizes studies not previously reviewed by these investigators.

Dinarello and coworkers first demonstrated two forms of endogenous pyrogen with distinct isoelectric points (10). In 1984, cDNAs encoding two distinct IL-1 genes were identified. Interleukin-1β was cloned from human monocytes, and the IL-1α cDNA was isolated from a murine macrophage line cDNA library (see citations in Refs. 3 and 4). Subsequently, cDNAs for both proteins have been obtained from rat, mouse, rabbit, human, and bovine cells. Comparison of the IL-1α and IL-1β cDNA sequences reveals 40–45% nucleotide sequence homology and 20–25% deduced protein sequence homology. Both IL-1 forms are expressed in kidney and in cultured kidney cells (see below). The genes for IL-1α and IL-1β have been isolated. Despite the divergence in exon sequence, the IL-1α and IL-1β genes share an almost perfectly conserved intron-exon structure (11), which may have arisen by a reverse transcriptase–mediated duplication. Both the murine and the human IL-1 genes are located on chromosome 2. In this chapter, the term "IL-1" is used if the cited information applies to both isoforms or if the cited study did not distinguish between isoforms. Otherwise the specific isoform studied is indicated.

Transcription, translation, and release of IL-1 are distinct, independently regulated processes. Changes in IL-1 gene mRNA abundance can be induced by a variety of agents, but the kinetics and magnitude of the response can be quite varied (9). Neither IL-1 gene is expressed constitutively but is transcribed when competent cells are activated by an appropriate stimulus. Published studies suggest that transcriptional regulation of the IL-1 genes is complex, and upstream DNA elements that control basal and inducible expression have been described only recently for the IL-1β gene. The 5′-flanking region of the IL-1β gene contains both positive and negative regulatory elements (9), and the promoter is within 132 residues of the transcription start site (12). Maximal expression requires sequences within the first exon (12). Far upstream enhancer sequences are required for induction by either phorbol ester or lipopolysaccharide (12,13). Data conflict on the location of sequences conferring tissue specificity for IL-1β transcription. Two reports have identified sequences within the proIL-1β cap site–proximal (CSP) region (-131 bp upstream of the transcription start site to +12 bp downstream of the transcription start site) that are required for tissue specificity (13,14). However, other studies have failed to detect DNA sequences that controlled tissue-specific expression of IL-1β within 8 kb of the TATA motif (12) or within the CSP promoter (15). Functional binding sites for NF-IL-6, a member of the C/EBP family of transcription factors, NF-κB, and a novel protein or proteins termed NFIL-1βA have been demonstrated in the 5 ′-flanking region of the IL-1β gene (13,14,16,17). Novel proteins, which bind the cap site–proximal and NF-κB regions of the IL-1β gene, have been described (18); they can activate transcription from a heterologous promoter (15). Other DNA binding element motifs have been identified in both the IL-1β (AP-1 and CREB consensus sequences) and IL-1α (NF-κB and NF-IL6 consensus sequence) genes (13,17). However a functional role in IL-1 transcription of these *cis* elements has not been proven.

While several reports have demonstrated that both IL-1 mRNAs are posttranscriptionally regulated, the specific sequences mediating this effect have been identified only recently (9). Both the IL-1α and the IL-1β mRNAs contain AU-rich consensus sequences in the 3′-untranslated region, which decrease mRNA stability for other transcripts (19,20). Using a cell-free system, the instability determinant responsible for rapid turnover of the IL-1α transcript has been localized to a specific 3′-UTR sequence containing a cluster of four AU-rich motifs that lack nuclease activity but target this mRNA for degradation (21). Isolated AU sequences in the 3′-UTR have no appreciable effect on transcript abundance.

Both forms of IL-1 are synthesized as M_r 31-33K cytosolic precursor proteins, which are enzymatically processed to mature M_r 17K carboxyl peptides. The precise linkage between processing and secretion remains uncertain. The amount of IL-1 secreted depends on the cell type and the stimulus for secretion. Lipopolysaccharide-, but not IL-2- or IL-1α-, stimulated peripheral blood mononuclear cells efficiently secrete IL-1β, whereas IL-1α remains cell-associated, either within the cell or membrane-bound (3,4). In other cell types, considerable amounts of both isoforms remain cell-associated. The intracellular transport pathways for IL-1 appear to be novel. Both forms of IL-1 lack a typical N-terminal signal sequence; immunoelectron microscopy and subcellular fractionation studies have failed to demonstrate either IL-1α or IL-1β in secretory organelles but did identify these proteins in cytosol (see citations in Ref. 22). The functional significance of the retained intracellular amino and carboxyl IL-1 fragments is not clear. However, an exciting preliminary report has demonstrated that, in mesangial cells, the M_r 16K, N-terminal IL-1α segment is targeted to the nucleus following its cleavage from proIL-1α and may function as a transcription factor (23).

The proteases involved in the processing of both pro-IL-1 isoforms into mature carboxyl-fragment peptides have been characterized. Conversion of the IL-1α precursor to the mature peptide is mediated by a member of the calpain family of proteases (22). The IL-1β converting enzyme (ICE) has been purified and cloned (24,25). This protease is composed of two nonidentical subunits that are derived from a single proenzyme. ICE has been classified as a cysteine protease since it is inactivated by cysteine protease inhibitors, although the primary sequence shares no homology with other proteases or mammalian proteins (24,26). Modeling the primary structure of ICE using the three-dimensional structures for other proteases also fails to identify any structural similarities (26). However, a gene essential for cell death in the nematode *Caenorhabtidis elegans*, *ced-3*, has sequence similarity to ICE (27). Studies in fibroblasts and neurons have suggested that overexpressed ICE may regulate programmed cell death in vertebrates (27–29). This gene product may be intregral to the repair and restoration to normal function of inflamed tissues that often contain expanded populations of intrinsic and infiltrating cells.

The Interleukin-1 Receptor (IL-1R)

Two IL-1, cell-surface receptors have been cloned and characterized. Both receptors bind IL-1α and IL-1β and are members of the immunoglobulin superfamily. The high-resolution three-dimensional structure of IL-1β suggests the presence of three distinct binding sites that recognize the three immunoglobulin domains comprising the extracellular portion of the IL-1R (30). Both forms of the IL-1R are expressed constitutively in tissues of healthy patients (31) and appear to be unregulated in disease (32,33).

The M_r 80K, type I receptor (IL-1RtI) is present on many cell types. The 217–amino acid cytoplasmic domain contains sequences required for activation of cytosolic signaling pathways (34,35) but does not contain consensus sequences for either tyrosine or serine/threonine kinase activity or for protein tyrosine kinase phosphorylation acceptor sites. Serine/threonine phosphorylation of the IL-1RtI does occur early after IL-1 binding (36), but the functional importance of this observation remains unclear. The cytoplasmic region, in contrast to the extracellular domain of the protein, displays a striking degree of amino acid conservation in human, mouse, and chicken IL-1Rs and is related to cytoplasmic domain of the *Drosophila* morphogen Toll, suggesting that the cytosolic signals activated by these proteins control a cellular function conserved through phylogeny. After binding, the IL-1-IL-1RtI complex is internalized—a process that does not require the cytoplasmic domain of the receptor protein—but is not degraded. The ligand-receptor complex is translocated to the nucleus, where it binds DNA and may function as a transacting factor (37). In contrast to the amino terminus (23), the carboxyl IL-1 peptide must be receptor-associated to be localized to the nucleus (37).

The type II IL-1R (IL-1RtII) is a M_r 68K molecule with a relatively short cytoplasmic tail (29 amino acids). This receptor is predominantly expressed on B lymphocytes, monocytes, and neutrophils. The native IL-1RtII does not mediate gene activation. However, studies of a hybrid receptor composed of the extracellular and transmembrane domains of the IL-1RtII fused to the cytosolic domain of the IL-1RtI demonstrate that the IL-1RtII can transduce IL-1 binding into cytosolic and nuclear signals (38). Until recently, the biological function of the IL-1RtII was unknown. Several studies have now demonstrated that the IL-1RtII is an acceptor protein that functions as a molecular trap for IL-1 to inhibit IL-1 activity (39,40). The glucocorticoid dexamethasone and the cytokines IL-4 and IL-13 induce type II receptor expression and secretion, an effect which may contribute to the immunosuppressive and anti-inflammatory effects of these molecules (39–41).

The Interleukin-1 Receptor Antagonist (IL-1ra) and Other Naturally Occurring Interleukin-1 Inhibitors

Interleukin-1ra is a naturally occurring IL-1 inhibitor that was identified and subsequently cloned from monocytes adherent to immobilized IgG (42,43). Binding of IL-1ra to either IL-1 receptor does not initiate any biological response, but IL-1ra must be present in 100- to 1000-fold molar excess to effectively inhibit the actions of IL-1. The IL-1RtI binds IL-1ra, IL-1α, and IL-1β with equal affinity. Although all cells expressing the IL-1RtII can bind IL-1ra, certain cell types bind the antagonist with such low affinity that IL-1ra may not effectively block the actions of IL-1 (44,45). Interleukin-1ra is a member of the IL-1 gene family with a similar genomic organization (46); 1680 bp of the 5′-flanking region DNA from the IL-1ra gene have been isolated and contain consensus sequences for NF-κB, NFIL-1βA, AP-1, and CRE-binding sites (47). Although several studies have demonstrated clearly differential regulation of IL-1 and IL-1ra, the mechanisms for these observations have not been defined. This molecule has been used to reduce the severity of inflammation in several animal models of disease, including crescentic nephritis (see below).

Another inhibitory material, uromodulin, has been isolated from the urine of pregnant women and cloned (48–50). The primary structure of uromodulin is identical to the Tamm-Horsfall urinary glycoprotein, although uromodulin is more heavily glycosylated. Uromodulin inhibits IL-1 and TNFα activity by binding either cytokines via carbohydrate side chains (49,51). The biological significance of this observation has been questioned, since a subsequent study has shown that uromodulin binds only denatured but not native soluble cytokines (52).

Summary

Both IL-1α and IL-1β are regulated transcriptionally and posttranscriptionally. The precise contributions of transcription, transcript stability, and translational regulation to changes in cytokine message abundance have been defined in vitro but remain untested in vivo. Less is known about mechanisms controlling IL-1R and IL-1ra synthesis, but local levels of these two molecules could determine the effects of IL-1 in situ. Interleukin-1 is one of several important mediators of renal injury (see below). Further experimentation is needed to define regulatory mechanisms of IL-1, IL-1R, and IL-1ra expression in cell culture systems. Subsequently the pertinence of these pathways in mediating expression of these molecules in disease models must be determined for development of effective strategies to inhibit IL-1–induced inflammatory injury.

INTERLEUKIN-1 AND THE NORMAL KIDNEY: EXPRESSION AND EFFECTS ON STRUCTURE AND FUNCTION IN VIVO/IN SITU

Several studies have demonstrated that IL-1 infusion can alter both normal glomerular structure and tubular function. The results are discussed briefly, since effects on gene expression have not been examined. Rats, injected once with IL-1β (5 μg), develop within 4 hr a transient influx of neutrophils into the glomerulus that resolves within 24 hr (53). No damage to glomerular structure, assessed by light and electron microscopy, is apparent at 24 hr. Addition of IL-1 for 7 hr to an ex vivo recirculating kidney perfusion system causes a twofold increase in glomerular proteoglycan and free glycosaminoglycan synthesis (54). This IL-1–induced alteration in the relative abundance of the various matrix components could potentially disrupt the macromolecular structure of both matrix and basement membrane, resulting in altered cellular function and a disrupted filtration barrier. Both acute infusion or bolus administration of IL-1 stimulates a prostaglandin-dependent natriuresis and diuresis without altering glomerular filtration rate or systemic blood pressure, in part by inhibiting Na^+ reabsorption in both the cortical and inner medullary collecting duct (55). These findings may explain the diuresis and natriuresis characteristic of early endotoxemia.

Beyond the obvious physiological significance of these studies, the data suggest the presence of functional IL-1R in healthy kidney available to respond to IL-1 synthesized systemically or produced locally by either infiltrating or resident cells. Consistent with this supposition, we have demonstrated IL-1RtI mRNA in normal mouse kidney (32), and others have demonstrated high affinity, saturable, and reversible binding of radioiodinated IL-1 to crude kidney membranes (33). Receptor autoradiography shows a heterogeneous distribution of IL-1R in the kidney, with higher densities in the medulla compared to the cortex. In contrast, most investigators have not demonstrated IL-1 expression in normal kidney, although two groups did identify IL-1 mRNA in healthy murine and human kidney by in situ hybridization and Northern analysis, respectively (56,57).

INTERLEUKIN-1 AND INTERLEUKIN-1R IN EXPERIMENTAL AND HUMAN RENAL DISEASE

Molecular mechanisms of renal injury remain incompletely understood. The deposition of antibodies and complement and abnormalities in local physical forces clearly can initiate renal damage. Recent interest has focused on subsequent events, activated by these initial insults, that culminate in progressive nephron destruction and fibrosis. Cytokines—proteins that serve as messengers between cells to modify growth, differentiation, or function—have been implicated in these processes. Interleukin-1 was the first cytokine demonstrated in diseased renal tissue (58). Subsequently, enhanced IL-1 bioactivity, mRNA, and/or protein has been demonstrated in a number of animal models and, to a lesser degree, in human biopsies.

Interleukin-1 Expression and Actions in Experimental Models of Kidney Disease

Many studies have evaluated IL-1 expression in rodent models of primary glomerular injury (1,2). Interleukin-1 expression has been demonstrated in several models of immune complex glomerulonephritis (ICGN). By dot blot hybridization, we have demonstrated a two- to threefold increase of IL-1 transcripts in total RNA extracted from kidneys of rats with ICGN compared to that extracted from healthy rats (58). Akai and coworkers, using the reverse-transcription polymerase chain reaction, did not demonstrate IL-1α mRNA in glomeruli isolated from control mice (59). In contrast, IL-1α transcripts were expressed abundantly in glomeruli from mice with bovine serum albumin–induced ICGN, and transcript abundance correlated with the histological grade of renal damage. Rabbits with acute serum sickness develop a proliferative and exudative ICGN associated with a small increase in IL-1 synthesis (60). Further increasing local IL-1 levels, either indirectly by injecting phytohemagglutinin or directly by injecting of IL-1β itself, enhances the severity of the lesions, a finding which suggests that intraglomerular IL-1 can mediate glomerular injury. Urinary IL-1β excretion reflects the severity of the proliferative ICGN in rats with chronic serum sickness (61). A time-dependent increase in IL-1β but not IL-1α transcripts can be demonstrated, using solution hybridization, in rats with mesangiopathic glomerulonephritis (2). This model is induced by dextran immunization and is similar to human IgA nephropathy.

Interleukin-1 production has been evaluated in models of autoimmune glomerular disease induced by antibodies specific for glomerular basement membrane (GBM). Different protocols have been used to induce anti-GBM nephritis, and each has different effects on cytokine expression in this experimental disease. Space limitations preclude detailed discussion of each protocol for disease induction; the reader is encouraged to refer to the original papers for details. Both agonist-stimulated and unstimulated macrophage-infiltrated, isolated glomeruli produce IL-1 bioactivity (62–66), which is inhibitable by an anti-IL-1 antibody and has a molecular weight consistent with processed IL-1 (62). In contrast, IL-1 synthesis by glomeruli isolated from animals with macrophage-independent anti-GBM nephritis is similar to that of normal glomeruli (62), suggesting that in this model, IL-1 is synthesized by infiltrating macrophages rather than intrinsic glomerular cells (62–64). Wilson and coworkers have used a different protocol for anti-GBM nephritis induction. Despite a lack of macrophage infiltration in this model, they have demonstrated a concordant increase in glomerular IL-1 bioactivity and, using sensitive RNA solution hybridization assays, IL-1β mRNA transcripts that persists for 3 days after administration of anti-GBM antibody (67).

Rubin-Kelley and coworkers have carefully studied IL-1 expression in two strains of autoimmune mice that develop a kidney disease resembling lupus nephritis (68–70). Interleukin-1α was not detected in total RNA extracted from freshly isolated cortex, whereas IL-1β transcripts were expressed more abundantly in diseased animals than in control animals (69,70). In addition, more IL-1 bioactivity was released by nephritic glomeruli in culture. Interleukin-1β mRNA expression appears to correlate with the histopathological degree of renal injury and proteinuria (68). To localize the site of enhanced IL-1β expression anatomically in these animals, we have performed in situ hybridization. Glomerular grain counts increase with time in MRL-*lpr* but not the congenic MRL-+/+ mice. Expression was maximum when the animals were 36 weeks of age. Similar to effects of IL-1 in other experimental models of renal disease, administration of low doses of IL-1α can accelerate renal disease and increase mortality in these autoimmune mice. However, the dose given and the stage of disease activity at the time of administration determine if administered IL-1 has a pathogenic effect (70). Coffman and coworkers have shown that enhanced urinary thromboxane A_2 excretion and the development of renal dysfunction correlate temporally with the appearance of increased levels of IL-1β mRNA in the cortex (71). Treatment of autoimmune mice with a thromboxane receptor antagonist improves renal hemodynamic function, decreases proteinuria, and reduces the severity of renal inflammation (33). Interleukin-1β transcript abundance, however, is unchanged, suggesting that thromboxane does not induce IL-1β mRNA or acts through a receptor that does not bind the antagonist (33). In contrast to these results in overtly diseased mice, adherent peritoneal macrophages from multiple strains of autoimmune mice show defective expression of IL-1α and IL-1β mRNA and activity well before the onset of disease (72–74). This novel defect in autoimmune macrophage function may be integral to the immune dysregulation that characterizes autoimmunity. We have also demonstrated, by RNA-RNA solution hybridization, upregulation of IL-1R mRNA expression in kidneys of 24-week MRL-*lpr* mice when compared to MRL-+/+ animals (32) (Figure 1).

Interleukin-1 production has also been implicated in the pathogenesis of experimental glomerulosclerosis (GS). Administration of aminonucleoside of puromycin induces glomerular lesions in rats similar to human focal, segmental GS. Matsumoto and Atkins have demonstrated that glomeruli isolated from rats which had received repeated injections of puromycin synthesize IL-1 bioactivity early and persistently in the course of the disease and have suggested both mesangial cells and infiltrating monocytes as the cellular source of the cytokine (75). Subsequently, cells that express IL-1 have been detected by immunohistochemical techniques within the glomerular mesangium in kidneys of animals with this model of GS (76). Feeding nephrotic animals an essential fatty acid–deficient diet, which reduces circulating and glomerular macrophage numbers, significantly diminishes IL-1–positive glomerular cells (76). Enhanced IL-1 synthesis may also contribute to the development of diabetic GS. Glomerular basement membrane (GBM), isolated from rats with streptozotocin-induced diabetes, stimulates anti-IL-1 antibody-inhibitable IL-1 synthesis by peritoneal macrophages. Aminoguanidine treatment of the diabetic animals abrogates the effect of GBM on macrophage cytokine production, suggesting that accumulation of advanced glycation end products in the GBM mediates this process (77).

Lipopolysaccharide (LPS) injection or infusion in the rat, a model of endotoxemia, induces renal dysfunction and injury. Since LPS potently stimulates synthesis of a number of cytokines in vitro and in vivo, several studies have determined renal IL-1 production after infusion or injection of LPS. Although glomerular IL-1 activity could not be detected within 2 hr of LPS injection (78), other investigators have demonstrated by solution hybridization a transient increase in glomerular IL-1 mRNA 1 hr after a single LPS injection (67). The sensitivity of the bioassay used in the former study may have been insufficient to detect the cytokine, since LPS activates both IL-1 transcription as well as translation. Although a single injection of LPS fails to induce IL-1 in a sustained manner, infusion of LPS into the isolated erythrocyte-perfused kidney (IEPK) markedly increases cortical IL-1β mRNA expression (79). Since the IEPK lacks circulating leukocytes, these data have documented for the first time that cells within kidney parenchyma can express this cytokine without being placed into a cell culture system. In situ hybridization analysis localized IL-1β transcripts in the IEPK within peritubular capillary endothelial cells and less abundantly within glomerular mesangial and endothelial cells (79). Lipopolysaccharide also enhances the injury induced by anti-GBM antibodies, an effect associated with induction of glomerular IL-1β mRNA expression (53).

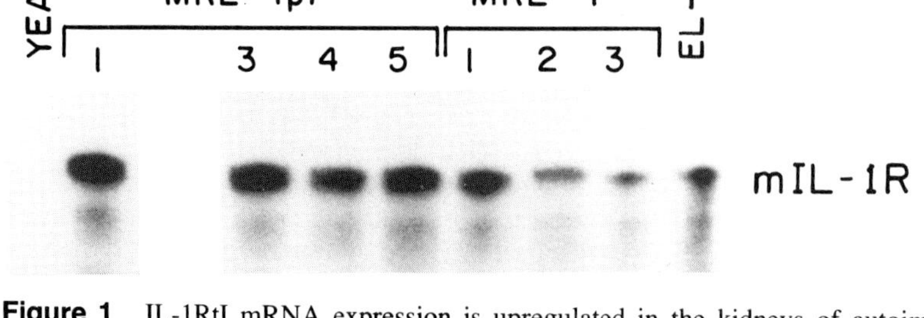

Figure 1 IL-1RtI mRNA expression is upregulated in the kidneys of autoimmune mice with lupus nephritis. IL-1RtI mRNA abundance has been assessed with RNA-RNA solution hybridization, using a [^{32}P]murine cRNA probe and digestion with S_1 nuclease. The MRL-*lpr* animals have an autoimmune syndrome that mimics systemic lupus erythematosus and develop lupus nephritis. The MRL-+ congenic mice, which develop disease mor indolently, serve as controls. The animals were sacrificed 24 weeks after birth. RNA from EL-4 cells served as a positive control.

Few investigators have evaluated, using molecular techniques, IL-1 expression in models of primary tubulointerstitial injury (1,2), although both in vitro and in vivo studies suggest that cytokines modulate tubular epithelial cell and interstitial fibroblast structure and function in both primary and secondary tubulointerstitial nephritis (80,81). Interleukin-1 mRNA transcripts have been identified, using the polymerase chain reaction, in the kidneys but not draining lymph nodes or spleens of mice with *Escherichia coli* pyelonephritis (82). Infected kidneys express mRNA for this cytokine at 12 hr and 1, 2, and 3 days after bacterial challenge. No transcripts were identified in kidneys of control animals. Interleukin-1 expression in other models of tubulointerstitial nephritis remains speculative, but the current understanding of mechanisms of damage to the interstitium would predict that infiltrating, activated T lymphocytes stimulate monocyte/macrophages to secrete cytokines, including IL-1 (81). Recent in vitro evidence supports this hypothesis (see below).

Interleukin-1 Expression and Actions In Human Renal Disease

Cytokine production during hemodialysis and continuous peritoneal dialysis has been assessed in a number of investigations but is not discussed in this chapter. The reader is referred to several excellent reviews which summarize this data (83–85). Studies of IL-1 expression in intrinsic human renal disease are considerably more limited. Several papers have focused on IL-1 production by peripheral blood mononuclear cells (PBMC). Monocytes, isolated from healthy donors and incubated with human GBM containing anti-GBM immune complexes, produce anti-IL-1 antibody–inhibitable IL-1 activity (86). Lipopolysaccharide-stimulated monocytes, isolated from patients with minimal change disease, synthesize less IL-1 activity than normal controls (87). In contrast, immune complex–stimulated monocytes isolated from patients with glomerulonephritides characterized by immune complex deposition and stimulated with heterologous soluble immune complexes produce more IL-1α and IL-1β activity than monocytes from healthy individuals (88). Interleukin-1β is overproduced by PBMC also during acute rejection of renal allografts (89).

Other studies have provided more compelling evidence that IL-1 mediates human renal injury. Interleukin-1 bioactivity is increased greatly in culture supernatants of glomeruli isolated from three patients with rapidly progressive crescentic nephritis (90). Interleukin-1β was detected by ELISA and bioassay in cyst fluids obtained from 13 patients with autosomal dominant polycystic kidney disease (91). The concentrations of IL-1β correlated with concentrations of other cytokines, stromelysin, and prostaglandin E_2 in cyst fluid and thymocyte mitogenesis in vitro—data suggesting that the IL-1 was biologically active in situ within the kidney. In situ production of IL-1β has been demonstrated by immunohistochemistry, the polymerase chain reaction and in situ hybridization in kidney biopsies from patients with ANCA-positive glomerulonephritis (92). Interleukin-1β mRNA transcript and protein abundance correlated with histological indices of disease activity and were expressed in both infiltrating mononuclear cells and resident renal cells. Transcription and translation of IL-1β has been demonstrated also in renal biopsies of acutely rejecting allografts but not in control kidneys (93). Consecutive analysis of serial sections by in situ hybridization and immunohistochemistry suggest a correlation between mRNA and protein expression. Cells expressing IL-1β were identified in periglomerular and perivascular interstitium and within glomeruli and arterial vessel wall, and the numbers of IL-1-positive cells correlated with clinical and histological evidence of acute cellular rejection.

Evidence That Interleukin-1 Mediates Renal Injury

Intrarenal IL-1 production suggests but does not prove that this cytokine has a pathogenic role in the induction and progression of glomerulonephritis. Several studies have now demonstrated the functional significance of IL-1 synthesis in kidney injury. Some data are correlative. Interleukin-6 can reduce both IL-1 and TNF-α synthesis by LPS-stimulated macrophages in vitro. Interleukin-6 pretreatment of animals with experimental nephritis ameliorates indices of glomerular inflammation induced by LPS and anti-GBM antibodies and concomitantly reduces glomerular IL-1 mRNA abundance (94). The effects of exogenous IL-1 on parameters of ongoing renal injury provide more convincing evidence. Pretreatment of rats with IL-1 prior to the administration of anti-GBM antibodies worsens renal injury by increasing the prevalence of glomerular capillary thrombosis, worsening albuminuria, markedly enhancing neutrophil influx, and increasing eicosanoid synthesis

(53,95). Indices of kidney injury also deteriorate in autoimmune mice and rats with ICGN given IL-1 (see above and Refs. 50 and 60).

However, improving renal injury by blocking the actions of IL-1 is necessary to establish that this cytokine is one mediator of kidney disease. Two groups of investigators have provided exciting, convincing data that demonstrate the pathogenetic significance of increased IL-1 in the diseased kidney. Administration of anti-IL-1β antibodies 1.5 hr before induction of anti-GBM nephritis in rats primed with small doses of LPS reduces albuminuria and diminishes the number of glomeruli with capillary thrombi by over 50% (96). The number of neutrophils within glomeruli also lessens, but creatinine clearances remain depressed. Interestingly, treatment of the animals with anti-IL-1α antibodies failed to improve proteinuria or glomerular histology. A preliminary report from this group of investigators further substantiates these findings. Animals with this model of glomerular injury excrete less protein if treated either with recombinant murine IL-1RtI to neutralize IL-1, with IL-1ra to block the IL-1R, or with IL-6 to reduce glomerular IL-1 synthesis (97). Atkins and coworkers also have used human recombinant IL-1ra to treat rats primed with heterologous IgG 5 days prior to injection of anti-GBM antibodies (98). Untreated animals develop marked proteinuria and renal dysfunction, but rats treated with IL-1ra for more than 1 day maintain normal renal function and excrete statistically less protein, although the treated animals continued to be profoundly nephrotic. Treatment with IL-1ra also improves indices of both glomerular and tubulointerstitial injury. Subsequent work from these investigators has shown one mechanism for the beneficial effects of IL-1ra in this model. Intercellular adhesion molecule-1 (ICAM-1) is upregulated and leukocyte infiltration is increased in the glomerulus and interstitium of saline-treated animals given nephrotoxic serum 14 days prior to analysis (99). In contrast, IL-1ra treatment moderately reduces glomerular ICAM-1 expression and white cell infiltration but dramatically inhibits interstitial ICAM expression, interstitial leukocyte influx, and tubulointerstitial damage (99). In contrast to these studies, another group of investigators has failed to show a beneficial effect of either IL-1 antibodies or IL-1ra on protein excretion, on the expression of leukocyte adhesion molecules, or on neutrophil accumulation in glomeruli of rats with anti-GBM nephritis (100). However, recombinant murine IL-1α was the immunogen for the anti-IL-1 serum, a reagent previously shown to be ineffective (96). In addition, the animals were sacrificed 24 hr after anti-GBM administration, a time in the disease process when other investigators have failed to identify a benefit of IL-1ra therapy (98).

INTERLEUKIN-1 EXPRESSION IN VITRO: RENAL CELL CULTURE MODEL SYSTEMS

These findings, taken together, suggest that in vitro studies to define mechanisms by which IL-1 alters glomerular cell structure and function are warranted and may provide insights into molecular mechanisms of glomerular disease. Interleukin-1 expression by cultured renal cells and the effects of IL-1 on renal cell gene expression in vitro are discussed specifically in this section. IL-1 does induce many other biochemical and functional responses in renal cells. The reader is referred to other reviews for further discussions of studies that describe actions of IL-1 and do not assess changes in gene expression (1,2,6,7).

Interleukin-1 Expression in Renal Cells

Interleukin-1 expression has been studied most extensively in glomerular mesangial cells. Lovett and coworkers first demonstrated that proliferating, cultured rat mesangial cells produced an IL-1–like cytokine, originally termed mesangial cell–derived thymocyte activating factor, which was an endogenous pyrogen (101,102). Both they and we demonstrated concurrently that cultured human and rat mesangial cells, respectively, contain IL-1α and IL-1β transcripts (58,103). The pI and molecular weights of the rat and human IL-1 proteins are indistinguishable from macrophage IL-1α and IL-1β (104–106). Serum, platelet-derived growth factor, and epidermal growth factor in combination, complement, and endotoxin increase mesangial cell IL-1 synthesis (103,106,107). Mesangial cell–derived as well as monocyte-derived IL-1α and IL-1β are myristylated after translation, which may target these proteins to the appropriate subcellular compartment (104).

Studies assessing IL-1 synthesis by other types of renal cells in vitro are limited. Human renal interstitial fibroblast cell lines, established from kidneys from patients with glomerulonephritis and interstitial fibrosis, express IL-1α and IL-1β mRNA and produce IL-1 as an autocrine growth factor (108). Recent studies have shown the endothelial cells play a critical role in the inflammatory response. Endothelial cells of blood vessels within renal cell carcinomas have been shown by immunohistochemistry to express IL-1 (109). Although few studies have described IL-1 synthesis by, or responses to, IL-1 by normal renal endothelium, data obtained using endothelial cells derived from other organs are undoubtedly pertinent to the kidney (110) and have been reviewed by Pober and Cotran (111).

Transcription control mechanisms of IL-1 expression have not been studied using in vitro renal cell systems. Experimental evidence to date provides no a priori reason to postulate that the kidney uses unique pathways to activate expression of the IL-1 gene.

Interleukin-1R expression on cultured renal cells has been assessed. We have measured binding of radioiodinated, recombinant human IL-1 to cultured human and mouse mesangial cells (112). Scatchard analysis of mesangial cell binding studies demonstrates a single class of high-affinity receptors with a K_d of 5.5×10^{-11} M and approximately 4000 receptors per cell on both human and rat mesangial cells (Figure 2). As with other cell types, steady-state binding of radioiodinated IL-1 to mesangial cells reaches equilibrium after 3 hr. RNA-RNA solution hybridization (Figure 2) and Northern analysis (113) has been used to demonstrate that mesangial cells maintained in serum constitutively express IL-1RtI mRNA. Several studies have used the specific IL-1ra to completely block effects of IL-1 on cultured mesangial cells (113–115). These data further documents that cultured mesangial cells express functional IL-1R.

We also analyzed radioiodinated IL-1 binding to rabbit tubular epithelial cells isolated by density gradient ultracentrifugation of cortical cellular homogenates (112,116). Proximal and distal tubular cells express 2000 to 4000 receptors per cell, with an approximate K_d of 10^{-10} M. Rabbit epithelia cultured from the thick ascending limb uniformly expressed Tamm-Horsfall (uromodulin) protein. Analysis of binding curves demonstrated a single class of high-affinity receptors ($K_d = 10^{-11}$ M to 10^{-10} M). Approximately 200 to 500 receptors were expressed per cell. Binding studies have demonstrated on cultured glomerular epithelial cells a single class of IL-1R with a dissociation constant of 0.3 n*M* and an apparent molecular weight of M_r 65K (117).

Genes Induced by Interleukin-1 in Renal Cells

Target Molecules

The binding of a cytokine or growth factor to its receptor initiates a progression of intracellular events that results in both short-term (e.g., prostaglandin synthesis) and long-term (e.g., a growth response) changes in cellular function. Changes in the profile of genes expressed often mediate this plasticity in the differentiated phenotype of a cell. Although many studies have demonstrated the profound effects of IL-1 on renal cell structure and function, few have specifically assessed whether alterations in the expression or abundance of a gene product are required for the measured changes in end point(s). Most studies of IL-1–regulated gene expression have used cultured mesangial cell model systems and have predominantly focused on four groups of target molecules: cytokines/ chemokines; leukocyte adhesion molecules; vasoactive, proinflammatory, nonpeptidic autacoids (eicosanoid and nitric oxide synthetic enzymes); and matrix and matrix-metabolizing enzymes.

Cytokines, Chemokines, and Growth Factors. Interleukin-1 is detectable early in the course of tissue injury, and the aggregate in vitro data suggest that IL-1 can function as a master cytokine, inducing the local synthesis of other cytokines integral to the generation of an inflammatory reaction. Exogenous IL-1 induces its own gene expression in both mesangial cells (113) and renal fibroblasts derived from normal and diseased human kidneys (118).

Dysregulated leukocyte infiltration and activation is an integral event in the pathogenesis of a number of experimental and human kidney diseases. Interleukin-1 is one of several critical, soluble signals, generated in injured kidney, that initiates production of leukocyte chemoattractants and growth factors. Interleukin-1β induces cultured human mesangial cells to express mRNAs for granulocyte-macrophage colony-stimulating factor (GM-CSF), macrophate colony-stimulating factor (M-CSF), and IL-6 (119,120). Both GM-CSF and IL-6 are secreted actively, but, as in other cell

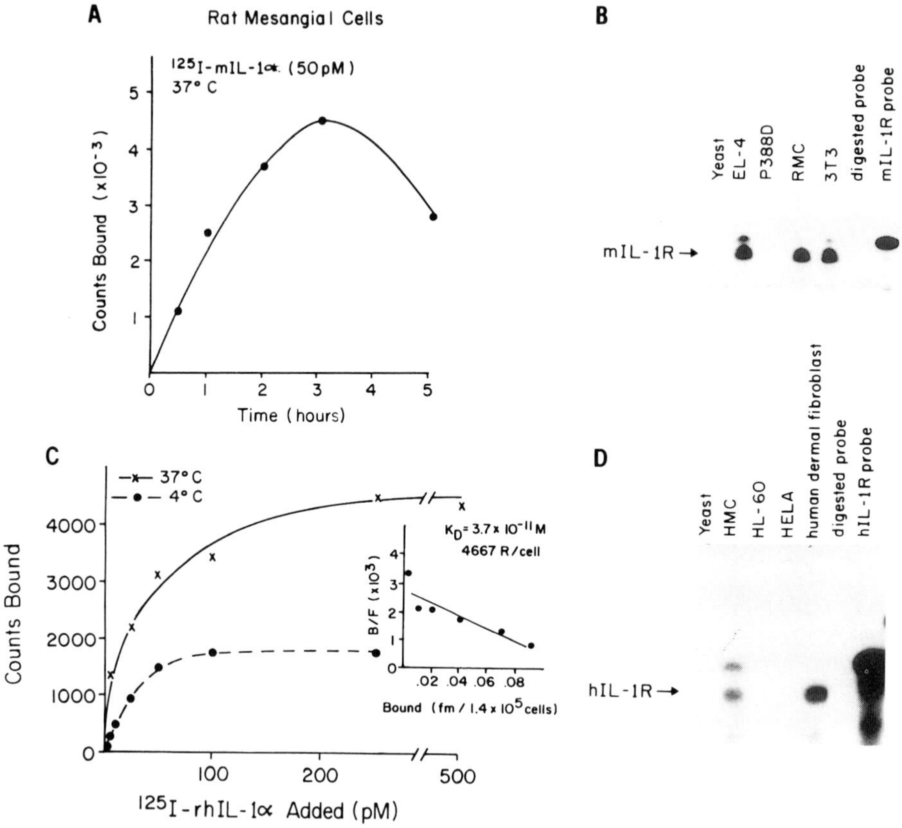

Figure 2 Rat and human mesangial cells bind radioiodinated IL-1α and express IL-1RtI mRNA. (A) Time course of [^{125}I] murine IL-1α binding to cultured rat mesangial cells. Counts bound has been corrected for nonspecific binding (counts bound in the presence of excess, unlabeled murine IL-1). (B) RNA-RNA solution hybridization, using a murine [^{32}P] cRNA probe and S_1 nuclease, demonstrates a specific IL-1tI transcript in EL-4 cells (positive control), rat mesangial cells (RMC), and 3T3 fibroblasts but not P388D macrophages. (C) Dose-response and Scatchard analysis (inset) of [^{125}I] human IL-1α binding to cultured human mesangial cells at 4°C and 37°C. (D) RNA-RNA solution hybridization, using a human [^{32}P] cRNA probe and digestion with RNase A and T_1, demonstrated IL-1RtI transcripts in human mesangial cells (HMC) and fibroblasts but not HL-60 or HeLa cells.

types, most M-CSF is retained intracellularly (119). Several intercrine chemokines, IL-8, monocyte chemoattractant protein (MCP-1), KC, *gro*, and Rantes are induced by IL-1 in both primary renal cell cultures and renal cell lines. Interleukin-1α- and IL-1β-stimulated human and rat mesangial cells produce the neutrophil chemokines IL-8 and the rat IL-8 homologue KC, respectively (119–123). Although the sequences of small molecular chemokines are related, solution hybridization has specifically identified IL-8 mRNA transcripts in cytokine-stimulated but not control human mesangial cells, a finding further confirmed by in situ hybridization (121). In rat mesangial cells, the induction of KC by IL-1 is inhibited at both a transcriptional and translational level by dexamethasone (123). The mononuclear leukocyte chemokines, Rantes and MCP-1, are also induced by IL-1 in mesangial cells and a cultured line of proximal tubular epithelial cells (114,119,124). Rantes is a chemoattractant for both CD4+ lymphocytes and monocyte/macrophages, while MCP-1 is a selective chemoattractant for monocyte/macrophages. An IL-1–stimulated kidney-derived epithelial cell line also expresses *gro* mRNA, a KC-related gene product (125,126). Taken together, these results suggest that IL-1–stimulated kidney cells produce a number of cytokines that may contribute through autocrine and paracrine mechanisms to structural and functional derangements characteristic of renal inflammatory injury. Interestingly, IL-1ra inhibits both IL-1–induced IL-8 and MCP-1 synthesis by mesangial cells in vitro, an action that may be a mechanism for its beneficial effect on renal inflammation in vivo (114,122).

Adhesion Molecules. Cell-cell interactions are critical events in both normal and pathological biological processes and are mediated by the interactions of adhesion molecule families. The importance of cell-cell interactions in kidney injury has been highlighted recently by Andres and coworkers, who have demonstrated that antibodies to the adhesion molecules, intercellular adhesion molecule-1 (ICAM-1) and lymphocyte function-associated antigen-1 (LFA-1), can prevent or retard kidney damage (127). Interleukin-1 increases the in vitro expression of adhesion molecules on glomerular endothelial cells, mesangial cells, and tubular epithelial cells and likely induces adhesion molecules during the evolution of human and experimental renal injury. An IL-1–mediated increase in cell adhesiveness results from de novo synthesis of integrins (CD11/CD18), immunoglobulin-like adhesion proteins (ICAM-1, vascular cell adhesion molecule-1), and/or selectins (L-selectin, E-selectin) and is transcriptionally regulated. These data have been included in several, excellent reviews (128–130) and are not discussed further here.

Vasoactive, Nonpeptidic, Proinflammatory Autacoids. Elevated eicosanoid synthesis is characteristic of many models of acute and chronic renal injury (6), and IL-1 stimulates eicosanoid formation in a variety of target renal cells (131–135). Several important studies, which have defined the role of IL-1 in the regulation of the enzymes that metabolize arachidonic acid to its active end products, have used renal cell systems (reviewed in Ref. 6). Interleukin-1 affects enzyme activity by both posttranslational mechanisms and de novo synthesis. Interleukin-1–induced changes in transcriptional regulation are emphasized in this chapter.

Phospholipase A_2 (PLA_2) activation provides the essential fatty acid precursor for eicosanoid formation, and PLA_2s are a growing, diverse class of enzymes with different structures, sites of action, and biochemical characteristics (reviewed in Ref. 136). Clearly PLA_2 isoforms function in cellular processes in addition to eicosanoid synthesis. Although the traditional group designations may better classify this diversity (136), the terms "secretory" ($sPLA_2$) and "cytosolic" PLA_2 ($cPLA_2$) are used for the M_r 14K (group II) and the M_r 97K PLA_2 (group IV) isoforms, respectively, to better correspond to pertinent published literature.

Pfeilschifter and coworkers and our laboratory concurrently have published a series of papers characterizing the PLA_2 isoforms required for IL-stimulated mesangial cell arachidonate release. After 6 to 10 hr, IL-1 stimulates the de novo synthesis of $sPLA_2$ (131,137,138). Although $sPLA_2$ mRNA and protein are not detectable under control conditions, they are induced markedly by the cytokine and coordinately increase with PLA_2 activity and PGE_2 synthesis (137,138). Interleukin-1–stimulated increases in steady-state $sPLA_2$ transcript abundance result from a moderate increase in PLA_2 transcription rate that is amplified by the prolonged persistence of the transcript (138). Conflicting results describing the effects of dexamethasone on mesangial cell $sPLA_2$ expression have been reported. Mühl and coworkers have demonstrated that dexamethasone minimally inhibits IL-1β-stimulated $sPLA_2$ mRNA expression, but completely prevents $sPLA_2$ synthesis and secretion (139). In contrast, we have reported that coincubation of mesangial cells with IL-1α and dexamethasone does not significantly change $sPLA_2$ transcript abundance or activity when compared to cells exposed to IL-1α alone (138). Interleukin-1–stimulated mesangial cell $sPLA_2$ gene expression is inhibited by TGFβ isoforms and PDGF-BB (50,138–140), suggesting that growth factor–dependent downregulation of $sPLA_2$ synthesis may limit tissue destruction and induce healing and tissue repair. The $sPLA_2$ secreted and purified from cytokine-activated mesangial cells hydrolyzes arachidonate from both glomerular epithelial and endothelial cells in culture (141) and may promote glomerular inflammation by this action.

Three observations suggested to us that a PLA_2 distinct from the $sPLA_2$ isoform must be activated in IL-1–stimulated mesangial cells. First, PGE_2 synthesis occurs prior to the induction of $sPLA_2$. Second, IL-1 potentiates or primes [^{3}H]arachidonate release or PGE_2 production by agonists proven to activate $cPLA_2$ (131,142). Third, IL-1–activated mesangial cell extracts contain an activity that hydrolyzes in vitro arachidonate from phosphatidylcholine, a poor substrate for $sPLA_2$. In contrast to $sPLA_2$ expression, both resting and serum-stimulated mesangial cells constitutively express $cPLA_2$ mRNA, protein, and activity (143). This study emphasizes the important effect of culture conditions on mesangial cell responses to IL-1. Interleukin-1 does not alter either $cPLA_2$ mRNA expression or mass in serum-stimulated mesangial cells but does activate $cPLA_2$ activity by a posttranslational phosphorylation (143,144). However, IL-1 treatment (24 hr) of serum-deprived mesangial cells doubles $cPLA_2$ mRNA, protein, and activity (143). We believe $cPLA_2$ activation to be a key step in the synthesis of proinflammatory, lipid mediators and an integral event in the phenotypic responses induced in target cells by this cytokine.

Two isoforms of prostaglandin endoperoxide synthase (PES), the enzyme required for further metabolism of arachidonate to prostaglandins and thromboxanes, are known. Morrison and coworkers originally reported that IL-1 stimulated de novo synthesis of a mesangial cell protein with a molecular weight and antigenic determinants similar to PES (145). Further work by this laboratory has demonstrated that the cytokine-stimulated increase in PES abundance was associated by a concordant induction of PES II mRNA (146). As with IL-1-stimulated $sPLA_2$ synthesis, control cells do not express PES II mRNA but constitutively express PES I (131,146). Interleukin-1 does not alter PES I mRNA abundance (131,146). Dexamethasone blocks translation but not transcription of IL-1–induced PES II, and cycloheximide superinduces PES II transcripts in both control and IL-1–treated mesangial cells (146). Unlike PES I mRNA, PES II mRNA contains AU-rich motifs in the 3′-untranslated region (UTR), and posttranslational mechanisms are quite important in regulating PES II transcript abundance (147,148).

Pfeilschifter and his group have also demonstrated that IL-1 increases mesangial cell cyclic GMP by inducing activity of the calcium- and calmodulin-independent isoform of nitric oxide synthase (iNOS) to generate nitric oxide (149,150). Indirect evidence, including the lag period required to increase cyclic GMP accumulation and the inhibitory effects of actinomycin D and cycloheximide on this process, suggest that increases in nitric oxide synthase activity require de novo synthesis of the enzyme. Recently this group of investigators has shown that IL-1β increases mesangial cell iNOS mRNA abundance (151). Although the mechanism for the increase in transcript number has not been assessed specifically in mesangial cells, transcriptional activation of the iNOS gene by IL-1 and other proinflammatory cytokines has been shown in a number of other cell types.

Matrix and Matrix-Metabolizing Enzymes. Significant glomerular injury leads to progressive accumulation of both normally and newly expressed extracellular matrix (ECM) proteins. Although the effects of IL-1 on transcription of ECM genes has been studied thoroughly using nonrenal cells, few published data have addressed this topic in renal cell culture systems. Interleukin-1-stimulated glomerular epithelial cells express more type IV collagen mRNA and synthesize more type IV collagen than control cells (117,152). The ECM turnover is controlled by several families of enzymes, including matrix metalloproteases (MMP). Lovett and coworkers have demonstrated synthesis of a specific M_r 72K type IV collagenase (MMP-2) in human and rat mesangial cells (see citations in Ref. 153). Although amino acid sequence analysis of this protein has suggested a high homology with a similarly sized type IV collagenase cloned from a transformed cell line, the regulation of the mesangial cell protein appears to be cell-specific. Interleukin-1 induces mesangial cell synthesis of the Mr 72K collagenase activity (52). In contrast, other cells constitutively express this protein. A homology-based PCR cloning strategy has identified a unique rat type IV collagenase transcript that is abundantly induced by IL-1, TNF, phorbol ester, and cyclic AMP agonists (153). Interleukin-1 and the other stimuli fail to induce expression of the mesangial cell M_r 92K collagenase (MMP-9), which typically is cytokine-inducible in other cell types.

Mechanisms of Interleukin-1–Induced Gene Expression

Binding of a ligand to its receptor initiates a cascade of intracellular events that activates a group of transcription factors to induce a specific gene set. The early signals generated by the IL-1-IL-1R interaction have been reviewed and are not discussed here in detail (6,7). The mechanisms linking these early events to changes in transcript abundance have been studied to a limited degree in renal cell systems and are poorly understood in other cell types.

We initially explored mechanisms of IL-1–stimulated gene expression by assessing whether activation of second messenger systems mimics or modulates $sPLA_2$ mRNA abundance. Our data showed that protein kinase C activation, cyclic AMP accumulation, or rapid changes in cytosolic Ca^{2+} or pH_i are not required for IL-1–directed gene expression and indicate that other signaling pathways are engaged directly by IL-1 to induce $sPLA_2$ mRNA expression (138). Interleukin-1-stimulated $sPLA_2$ gene expression is cycloheximide-insensitive, suggesting that cytosolic signals activate transcription factor(s) by posttranslational modifications. Based on these data, several model systems can be proposed to describe how IL-1-IL-1R interactions can directly alter gene activity in the nucleus. Traditional models of transmembrane signaling propose that a limited number of second messengers convey the information generated by a ligand-receptor interaction. Since published data have demonstrated that IL-1 either directly or indirectly activates protein kinases or inhibits phosphatase activity, we propose that this cytokine induces changes in mRNA transcript abundance by altering the phosphorylation state of a transcription factor or a transcription factor complex. An alternative model is suggested by recent work describing the pathways used by interferon α/β to induce gene expression (154). Extrapolation from these data, which suggest the existence of many ligand-specific, direct signaling pathways, would predict that binding of IL-1 to its receptor catalyzes a post-transcriptional modification of a specific, latent transcription factor(s). This latter model is consistent with our data demonstrating the inability of second-messenger mimics to induce $sPLA_2$ transcript expression (138). However, neither IL-1–specific transcriptional proteins nor specific IL-1–responsive DNA elements have been identified to date.

Additional work from this and other laboratories has focused on transcriptional mechanisms of IL-1–directed gene expression. Unpublished data from our laboratory suggest that tyrosine kinase activation is an important step in IL-1–mediated activation of the transcription factor NF-κB (Huang S, Konieczkowski M, and Sedor JR; unpublished data). We have also shown that arachidonic acid hydrolysis is necessary but not sufficient for IL-1–stimulated IL-6 mRNA expression in studies using IL-6 5′-flanking region deletion constructs ligated to a chloramphenicol acetyltransferase (CAT) reporter gene to identify arachidonate-responsive element(s) (155) (Figure 3). When a plasmid containing positions –742 to +11 has been transfected, IL-1 increases CAT activity three- to fivefold above control, an effect almost completely inhibited by the phospholipase inhibitor aristolochic acid. Exogenous arachidonate alone inconsistently induces CAT activity but completely restores IL-1–stimulated CAT activity in aristolochic acid–treated mesangial cells. In contrast, arachidonate does not restore IL-1–stimulated CAT activity in aristolochic acid–treated cells transfected with the –109 to +11 construct, which contains a κB binding element. These data suggest an arachidonate-responsive element resides between positions –742 to –109 of the IL-6 5′-flanking region, and we propose that a transcription factor, either directly or indirectly activated by arachidonate, is an integral signal in the cascade of cytosolic events required for IL-1-directed gene expression (Figure 4). Other data also are consistent with the premise that arachidonic acid hydrolysis is necessary for IL-1-directed gene expression. IL-1β-stimulated mesangial cell ecto-5′-nucleotidase activity is dependent, in part, on prostaglandin E_2 synthesis (156) and arachidonate activates heat shock factor 1 DNA-binding activity in HeLa S3 cells (157).

In both renal and nonrenal cell systems, IL-1 activates, as assayed by electrophoretic mobility shift assays, a number of ubiquitous transcription factors; but not all studies demonstrate that these factors are transcriptionally active. Several preliminary reports have provided evidence that the cytokine can activate NF-κB in mesangial cells (158,159). We have found that tyrosine kinase activity is necessary for κB binding to mesangial cell nuclear extracts (Huang S, Konieczkowski M, Sedor JR; unpublished data). NF-κB is a member of a family of rel-related transcription factors that derive their diversity by the pairing of different protein subunits to form a heterodimeric complex. In mesangial cells, IL-1β activates NF-κB (Figure 5), which consists of p50 and p65 subunits, since antibodies to these proteins eliminate binding of nuclear protein to probe in gel mobility shift assays (159). Interleukin-1–mediated activation of an IL-6 promoter-CAT reporter gene chimera in mesangial cells requires an intact κB element (160), suggesting that NFκB is transcriptionally active in these cells. Similar to other cell types, we have found that IL-1 induces c-*fos* and c-*jun* transcripts in mesangial cells (Huang S, Konieczkowski M, Sedor JR; unpublished data). In other cell types, IL-1-inducible nuclear factors bind to a unique 14-bp palindromic sequence (161) and a CCAAT/enhancer-binding protein element (162) and IL-1 induces c-*myc* (163).

Interleukin-1 can also change transcript number by posttranscriptional mechanisms (146,148, 164). It may increase PES II mRNA abundance by indirectly or directly activating a kinase that phosphorylates a cytosolic factor or factors binding to the 3′-UTR and consequently increases its half-life (147).

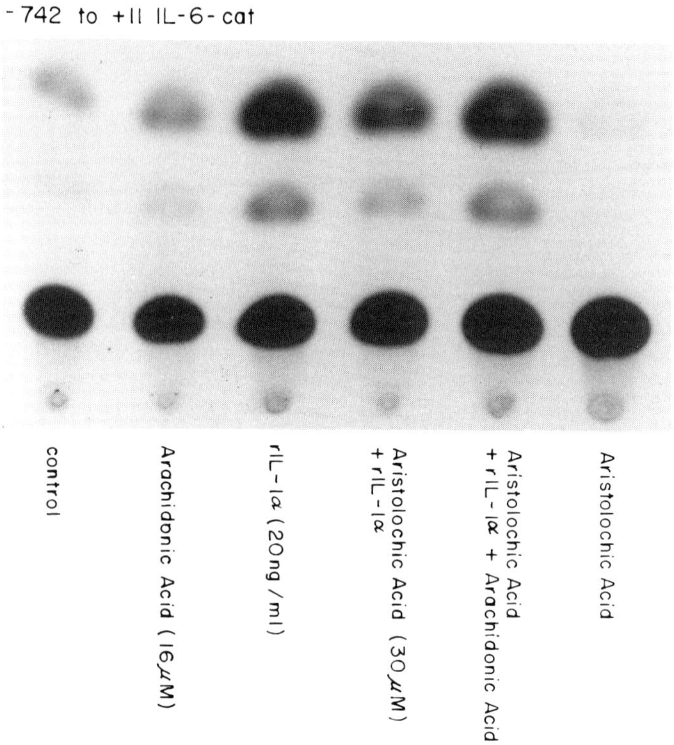

% conversion	3.7	7.9	30.5	17.4	23.9	1.2

Figure 3 The 5′ flanking region of the IL-6 gene contains an arachidonic acid–responsive element. Rat mesangial cells were transfected with the -742 to 11-bp region of the IL-6 5′-flanking region linked to a CAT reporter gene and CAT activity was assayed by standard techniques. The percent conversion of [^{14}C]chloramphenicol to acetylated forms is indicated below each lane. The PLA_2 inhibitor aristolochic acid inhibited IL-1–stimulated CAT activity. Exogenous arachidonate restored IL-1 induced CAT activity almost completely.

CONCLUSIONS AND PERSPECTIVES

As discussed by Johnson and Lovett (165), the in vitro and in vivo data reviewed here fulfill Koch's postulates in establishing IL-1 as a key mediator of renal injury. These studies have demonstrated that (a) IL-1 activates renal cells to express an inflammatory phenotype in vitro; (b) IL-1 is expressed within the kidney in experimental and human renal disease; (c) inhibition of IL-1 reduces indices of renal injury, and (d) infusion of IL-1 into animals with experimental kidney disease accelerates and worsens renal injury. The remaining criterion to be fulfilled is demonstrating that introduction of this cytokine in vivo into normal tissue by gene transfer results in structural and/or functional changes characteristic of inflammatory kidney injury. Ultimately data describing IL-1 in kidney disease must be integrated with information about the function of other cytokines/growth factors to generate models of cytokine interactions in the pathogenesis of renal injury and repair.

From a cell biological viewpoint, there are intriguing structural homologies between the intracellular domain of the IL-1R and *Drosophila* homeodomain protein Toll that are essential for IL-1–activated signal transduction (34). In addition, the sequence conservation between functionally equivalent signaling proteins in these two pathways is striking (166). Renal cells express distinct phenotypes in response to changes in their microenvironment. The conservation between pathways used by Toll to establish dorsoventral cell fate in the fruit fly and the pathways used by IL-1 to

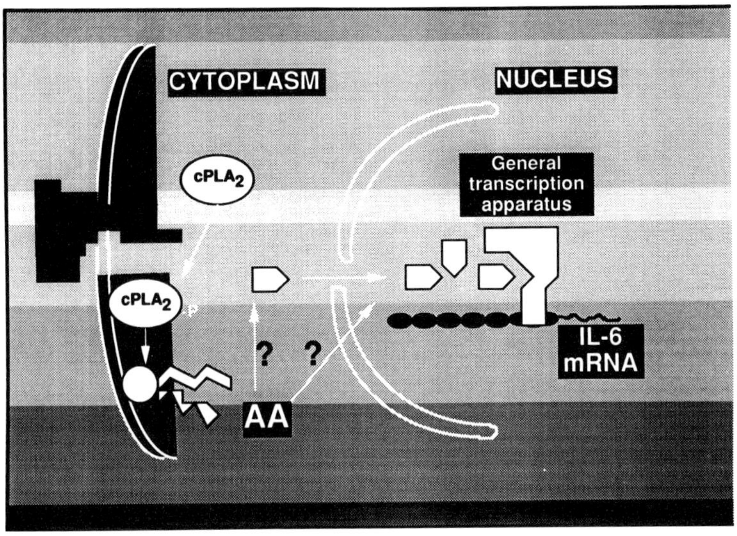

Figure 4 Arachidonic acid directly or indirectly activates a transcription factor to induce gene expression.

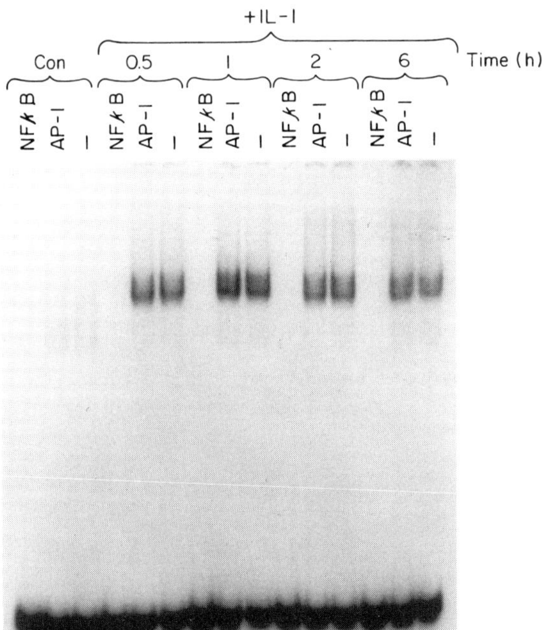

Figure 5 IL-1α activates NF-κB in a time-dependent manner in mesangial cells. Gel mobility shift assay demonstrating that mesangial cells express NF-κB. Lanes labeled NF-κB and AP-1 indicate reactions that contained 100-fold molar excess of unlabeled probe and demonstrate specificity of the binding reaction.

induce a specific gene set in mammalian cells suggests that IL-1 is an important activator of a conserved pathway for differentiation that is recapitulated during inflammatory injury. In fact, preliminary data demonstrate that inhibition of an IL-1–activated gene, using antisense expression vectors, causes cultured mesangial cells to revert from an inflammatory to a quiescent phenotype (167). Finally, the demonstration that the IL-1β converting enzyme may regulate the process of programmed cell death or apoptosis in the vertebrate suggests that this molecule may initiate renal repair by reducing expanded populations of cells that characterize many forms of kidney injury. Since apoptosis has been implicated in renal disease (168), this is particularly plausible. Further unraveling the molecular basis of renal injury may identify exciting possibilities for treatment of diseases that have few effective therapies.

ACKNOWLEDGMENTS

The work from Dr Sedor's laboratory cited in this chapter has been supported by DK-38558, DK-01404, DK-07470, the G. Harold and Leila Y. Mathers Charitable Trust, the Kidney Foundation of Ohio, the American Heart Association of Northeastern Ohio, the Community Dialysis Centers of Cleveland and Dean's Tax Funds (Case Western Reserve University/MetroHealth Medical Center). Dr. Sedor is an Established Investigator of the American Heart Association. The author thanks Drs. Konieczkowski, Ganz and Schelling for their careful reading of the manuscript and helpful discussions.

REFERENCES

1. Sedor JR. Cytokines and growth factors in renal injury. Semin Nephrol 1992; 12:428–440.
2. Emancipator SN, Sedor JR. Cytokines and renal disease. In: Kunkel SL, Remick DG, eds. Cytokines in Health and Disease. New York: Marcel Dekker, 1992:467–488.
3. Dinarello CA. Interleukin-1 and interleukin-1 antagonism. Blood 1991; 77:1627–1652.
4. Dinarello CA. Interleukin-1 and its biologically related cytokines. Adv Immunol 1989; 44:153–205.
5. Dinarello CA. The proinflammatory cytokines interleukin-1 and tumor necrosis factor and treatment of the septic shock syndrome. J Infect Dis 1991; 163:1177–1184.
6. Sedor JR, Konieczkowski M, Huang S, et al. Cytokines, mesangial cell activation and glomerular injury. Kidney Int Suppl 1993; 39:S65–S70.
7. Sedor JR, Nakazato Y, Konieczkowski M. Interleukin-1 and the mesangial cell. Kidney Int 1992; 41:595–599.
8. Dinarello CA. Modalities for reducing interleukin 1 activity in disease. Trends Pharmacol Sci 1993; 14:155–159.
9. Fenton MJ. Review: transcriptional and post-transcriptional regulation of interleukin 1 gene expression. Int J Immunopharmacol 1992; 14:401–411.
10. Dinarello CA, Goldin NP, Wolff SM. Demonstration and characterization of two distinct human leukocytic pyrogens. J Exp Med 1974; 139:1369–1381.
11. Clark BD, Collins KL, Gandy MS, et al. Genomic sequence for human prointerleukin 1 beta: Possible evolution from a reverse transcribed prointerleukin 1 alpha gene. Nucleic Acids Res 1986; 14:7897–7914.
12. Bensi G, Mora M, Raugei G, et al. An inducible enhancer controls the expression of the human interleukin 1 beta gene. Cell Growth Differ 1990; 1:491–497.
13. Shirakawa F, Saito K, Bonagura CA, et al. The human prointerleukin 1 beta gene requires DNA sequences both proximal and distal to the transcription start site for tissue-specific induction. Mol Cell Biol 1993; 13:1332–1344.
14. Hunninghake GW, Monks BG, Geist LJ, et al. The functional importance of a cap site-proximal region of the human prointerleukin 1 beta gene is defined by viral protein transactivation. Mol Cell Biol 1992; 12:3439–3448.
15. Buras JA, Monks BG, Fenton MJ. The NF-βA-binding element, not an overlapping NF-IL-6-binding element, is required for maximal IL-1bβ gene expression. J Immunol 1994; 152:4444–4454.
16. Hiscott J, Marois J, Garoufalis J, et al. Characterization of a functional NF-κB site in the human interleukin 1β promoter: Evidence for a positive autoregulatory loop. Mol Cell Biol 1993; 13:6231–6240.
17. Zhang Y, Rom WN. Regulation of the interleukin-1 beta (IL-1 beta) gene by myobacterial components and lipopolysaccharide is mediated by two nuclear factor–IL6 motifs. Mol Cell Biol 1993; 13:3831–3837.
18. Monks BG, Martell BA, Buras JA, Fenton MJ. An upstream protein interacts with a distinct protein that binds to the cap site of the human interleukin 1β gene. Mol Immunol 1994; 31:139–151.

19. Caput D, Beutler B, Hartog K, Thayer R, et al. Identification of a common nucleotide sequence in the 3′-untranslated region of mRNA molecules specifying inflammatory mediators. Proc Natl Acad Sci USA 1986; 83:1670–1674.
20. Shaw G, Kamen R. A conserved AU sequence from the 3′ untranslated region of GM-CSF mRNA mediates selective mRNA degradation. Cell 1986; 46:659–667.
21. Gorospe M, Kumar S, Baglioni C. Tumor necrosis factor increases stability of interleukin-1 mRNA by activating protein kinase C. J Biol Chem 1993; 268:6214–6220.
22. Garruth LM, Demezuk S, Mizel SB. Involvement of a caplain-like protease in the processing of the murine interleukin 1α precurser. J Biol Chem 1991; 266:12162–12167.
23. Stevenson FT, Turck J, Locksley RM, Lovett DH. Nuclear targeting of and intercellular form of interleukin-1a: A novel mechanism of IL-1 action (abstr). J Am Soc Nephrol 1993; 4:636.
24. Thornberry NA, Bull HG, Calaycay JR, et al. A novel heterodimeric cysteine protease is required for interleukin-1 beta processing in monocytes. Nature 1992; 356:768–774.
25. Cerretti DP, Kozlosky CJ, Mosley B, et al. Molecular cloning of the interleukin-1 beta converting enzyme. Science 1992; 256:97–100.
26. Ringe D. Enzymology. Proteases: To each his own. Nature 1992; 356:748–749.
27. Yuan J, Shaham S, Ledoux S, et al. The C. elegans cell death gene ced-3 encodes a protein similar to mammalian interleukin-1 beta-converting enzyme. Cell 1993; 75:641–652.
28. Gagliardini V, Fernandez PA, Lee RK, et al. Prevention of vertebrate neuronal death by the crmA gene. Science 1994; 263:826–828.
29. Miura M, Zhu H, Rotello R, et al. Induction of apoptosis in fibroblasts by IL-1 beta-converting enzyme, a mammalian homolog of the C. elegans cell death gene ced-3. Cell 1993; 75:653–660.
30. Clore GM, Wingfield PT, Gronenborn AM. High-resolution three-dimensional structure of interleukin 1 beta in solution by three- and four-dimensional nuclear magnetic resonance spectroscopy. Biochemistry 1991; 30:2315–2323.
31. Deyerle KL, Sims JE, Dower SK, Bothwell MA. Pattern of IL-1 receptor gene expression suggests role in noninflammatory processes. J Immunol 1992; 149:1657–1665.
32. Luebbers E, Nawaz A, Nowinski RJ, et al. MRL-1pr and MRL–+/+ mice differentially express IL-1β and IL-1R but not TNFα: Analysis by solution in situ hybridization (abstr). J Am Soc Nephrol 1994; 2:551.
33. Takao T, Mitchell WM, De Souza EB. Interleukin-1 receptors in mouse kidney: Identification, localization, and modulation by lipopolysaccharide treatment. Endocrinology 1991; 128:2618–2624.
34. Heguy A, Baldari CT, Macchia G, et al. Amino acids conserved in interleukin-1 receptors (IL-1Rs) and the Drosophila toll protein are essential for IL-1R signal transduction. J Biol Chem 1992; 267:2605–2609.
35. Kuno K, Okamoto S, Hirose K, et al. Structure and function of the intracellular portion of the mouse interleukin 1 receptor (type I): Determining the essential region for transducing signals to activate the interleukin 8 gene. J Biol Chem 1993; 268:13510–13518.
36. Gallis B, Prickett KS, Jackson J, et al. IL-1 induces rapid phosphorylation of the IL-1 receptor. J Immunol 1989; 143:3235–3240.
37. Weitzmann MN, Savage N. Nuclear internalisation and DNA binding activities of interleukin-1, interleukin-1 receptor and interleukin-1/receptor complexes. Biochem Biophy Res Commun 1992; 187:1166–1171.
38. Heguy A, Baldari CT, Censini S, et al. A chimeric type II/type I interleukin-1 receptor can mediate interleukin-1 induction of gene expression in T cells. J Biol Chem 1993; 268:10490–10494.
39. Colotta F, Re F, Muzio M, et al. Interleukin-1 type II receptor: A decoy target for IL-1 that is regulated by IL-4. Science 1993; 261:472–475.
40. Re F, Muzio M, De Rossi M, et al. The type II "receptor" as a decoy target for interleukin 1 in polymorphonuclear leukocytes: Characterization of induction by dexamethasone and ligand binding properties of the released decoy receptor. J Exp Med 1994; 179:739–743.
41. Colotta F, Re F, Muzio M, et al. Interleukin-13 induces expression and release of interleukin-1 decoy receptor in human polymorphonuclear cells. J Biol Chem 1994; 269:12403–12406.
42. Eisenberg SP, Evans RJ, Arend WP, et al. Primary structure and functional expression from complementary DNA of a human interleukin-1 receptor antagonist. Nature 1990; 343:341–346.
43. Hannum CH, Wilcox CJ, Arend WP, et al. Interleukin-1 receptor antagonist activity of a human interleukin-1 inhibitor. Nature 1990; 343:336–340.
44. Dripps DJ, Verderber E, Ng RK, et al. Interleukin-1 receptor antagonist binds to the type II interleukin-1 receptor on B cells and neutrophils. J Biol Chem 1991; 266:20311–20315.
45. Granowitz EV, Clark BD, Mancilla J, Dinarello CA. Interleukin-1 receptor antagonist competitively inhibits the binding of interleukin-1 to the type II interleukin-1 receptor. J Biol Chem 1991; 266:14147–14150.
46. Eisenberg SP, Brewer MT, Verderber E, et al. Interleukin 1 receptor antagonist is a member of the interleukin 1 gene family: Evolution of a cytokine control mechanism. Proc Natl Acad Sci USA 1991; 88:5232–5236.

47. Smith MF Jr, Eidlen D, Brewer MT, et al. Human IL-1 receptor antagonist promoter: Cell type–specific activity and identification of regulatory regions. J Immunol 1992; 149:2000–2007.
48. Muchmore AV, Decker JM. Uromodulin: An immunosuppressive 85-kilodalton glycoprotein isolated from human pregnancy urine is a high affinity ligand for recombinant interleukin 1 alpha. J Biol Chem 1986; 261:13404–13407.
49. Hession C, Decker JM, Sherblom AP, et al. Uromodulin (Tamm-Horsfall glycoprotein): A renal ligand for lymphokines. Science 1987; 237:1479–1484.
50. Mühl H, Geiger T, Pignat W, et al. PDGF suppresses the activation of group II phospholipase A_2 gene expression by interleukin 1 and forskolin in mesangial cells. FEBS Lett 1991; 291:249–252.
51. Sherblom AP, Decker JM, Muchmore AV. The lectin-like interaction between recombinant tumor necrosis factor and uromodulin. J Biol Chem 1988; 263:5418–5424.
52. Martin J, Lovett DH, Gemsa D, et al. Enhancement of glomerular mesangial cell neutral proteinase secretion by macrophages: role of interleukin 1. J Immunol 1986; 137:525–529.
53. Tomosugi NI, Cashman SJ, Hay H, et al. Modulation of antibody-mediated glomerular injury in vivo by bacterial lipopolysaccharide, tumor necrosis factor, and IL-1. J Immunol 1989; 142:3083–3090.
54. Kashihara N, Watanabe Y, Makino H, Kanwar YS. Interleukin-1-induced alterations in glomerular proteoglycans: Biochemical and tissue autoradiographic aspects. J Am Soc Nephrol 1992; 3:203–213.
55. Zeidel ML. Hormonal regulation of inner medullary collecting duct sodium transport. Am J Physiol 1993; 265:F159–F173.
56. Tovey MG, Content J, Gresser I, et al. Genes for IFN-beta-2 (IL-6), tumor necrosis factor, and IL-1 are expressed at high levels in the organs of normal individuals. J Immunol 1988; 141:3106–3110.
57. Takacs L, Kovacs EJ, Smith MR, et al. Detection of IL-1 alpha and IL-1 beta gene expression by in situ hybridization: Tissue localization of IL-1 mRNA in the normal C57BL/6 mouse. J Immunol 1988; 141:3081–3095.
58. Werber HI, Emancipator SN, Tykocinski ML, Sedor JR. The interleukin 1 gene is expressed by rat glomerular mesangial cells and is augmented in immune complex glomerulonephritis. J Immunol 1987; 138:3207–3212.
59. Akai Y, Iwano M, Kitamura Y, et al. Intraglomerular expressions of IL-1 alpha and platelet-derived growth factor (PDGF-B) mRNA in experimental immune complex-mediated glomerulonephritis. Clin Exp Immunol 1994; 95:29–34.
60. Camussi G, Tetta C, Bussolino F, et al. Effect of leukocyte stimulation on rabbit immune complex glomerulonephritis. Kidney Int 1990; 38:1047–1055.
61. Noble B, Ren K, Taverne J, et al. Mononuclear cells in glomeruli and cytokines in urine reflect the severity of experimental proliferative immune complex glomerulonephritis. Clin Exp Immunol 1990; 80:281–287.
62. Tipping PG, Lowe MG, Holdsworth SR. Glomerular interleukin 1 production is dependent on macrophage infiltration in anti-GBM glomerulonephritis. Kidney Int 1991; 39:103–110.
63. Matsumoto K. Interleukin-1 production by lipopolysaccharide-stimulated glomeruli from rats with nephrotoxic serum nephritis. Am J Nephrol 1989; 9:488–494.
64. Matsumoto K. Production of interleukin-1 by glomerular macrophages in nephrotoxic serum nephritis. Am J Nephrol 1990; 10:502–506.
65. Matsumoto K. Recombinant tumor necrosis factor stimulates interleukin-1 production in glomerular cultures from rats with nephrotoxic serum nephritis. Nephron 1990; 55:300–305.
66. Matsumoto K. Production of interleukin 1 in macrophage cultures from rats with nephrotoxic serum nephritis. Allergy Appl Immunol 1988; 87:435–438.
67. Feng L, Tang WW, Loskutoff DJ, Wilson CB. Dysfunction of glomerular fibrinolysis in experimental antiglomerular basement membrane antibody glomerulonephritis. J Am Soc Nephrol 1993; 3:1753–1764.
68. Boswell JM, Yui MA, Burt DW, Kelley VE. Increased tumor necrosis factor and IL-1 beta gene expression in the kidneys of mice with lupus nephritis. J Immunol 1988; 141:3050–3054.
69. Boswell JM, Yui MA, Endres S, et al. Novel and enhanced IL-1 gene expression in autoimmune mice with lupus. J Immunol 1988; 141:118–124.
70. Brennan DC, Yui MA, Wuthrich RP, Kelley VE. Tumor necrosis factor and IL-1 in New Zealand black/white mice: Enhanced gene expression and acceleration of renal injury. J Immunol 1989; 143:3470–3475.
71. Spurney RF, Bernstein RJ, Ruiz P, et al. Physiologic role for enhanced renal thromboxane production in murine lupus nephritis. Prostaglandins 1991; 42:15–28.
72. Levine J, Hartwell D, Beller DI. Imbalanced cytokine production by macrophages from autoimmune-prone mice. Immunol Lett 1991; 30:183–192.
73. Donnelly RP, Levine J, Hartwell DQ, et al. Aberrant regulation of IL-1 expression in macrophages from young autoimmune-prone mice. J Immunol 1990; 145:3231–3239.
74. Levine JS, Pugh BJ, Hartwell D, et al. Interleukin-1 dysregulation is an intrinsic defect in macrophages from MRL autoimmune-prone mice. Eur J Immunol 1993; 23:2951–2958.

75. Matsumoto K, Atkins RC. Glomerular cells and macrophages in the progression of experimental focal and segmental glomerulosclerosis. Am J Pathol 1989; 134:933–945.
76. Diamond JR, Pesek I. Glomerular tumor necrosis factor and interleukin 1 during acute aminonucleoside nephrosis: An immunohistochemical study. Lab Invest 1991; 64:21–28.
77. Hasegawa G, Nakano K, Sawada M, et al. Possible role of tumor necrosis factor and interleukin-1 in the development of diabetic nephropathy. Kidney Int 1991; 40:1007–1012.
78. Fouqueray B, Philippe C, Herbelin A, et al. Cytokine formation within rat glomeruli during experimental endotoxemia. J Am Soc Nephrol 1993; 3:1783–1791.
79. Xia Y, Feng L, Yoshimura T, Wilson CB. LPS-induced MCP-1, IL-1 beta, and TNF-alpha mRNA expression in isolated erythrocyte-perfused rat kidney. Am J Physiol 1993; 264:F774–F780.
80. Schreiner GF, Kohan DE. Regulation of renal transport processes and hemodynamics by macrophages and lymphocytes. Am J Physiol 1990; 258:F761–F767.
81. Strutz F, Neilson EG. The role of lymphocytes in the progression of interstitial disease. Kidney Int 1994; 45:S106–S110.
82. Rugo HS, O'Hanley P, Bishop AG, et al. Local cytokine production in a murine model of Escherichia coli pyelonephritis. J Clin Invest 1992; 89:1032–1039.
83. Haeffner Cavaillon N, Jahns G, et al. Induction of interleukin-1 during hemodialysis. Kidney Int Suppl 1993; 39:S139–S143.
84. Descamps Latscha B, Herbelin A. Long-term dialysis and cellular immunity: A critical survey. Kidney Int Suppl 1993; 41:S135–S142.
85. Chatenoud L, Jungers P, Descamps-Latscha B. Immunological considerations of the pyremic and dialyzed patient. Kidney Int 1994; 45:s92–s96.
86. Vissers MC, Fantone JC, Wiggins R, Kunkel SL. Glomerular basement membrane–containing immune complexes stimulate tumor necrosis factor and interleukin-1 production by human monocytes. Am J Pathol 1989; 134:1–6.
87. Matsumoto K. Decreased production of interleukin-1 by monocytes from patients with lipoid nephrosis. Clin Nephrol 1989; 31:292–296.
88. Matsumoto K. Interleukin-1 production by monocytes from patients with glomerulonephritis after stimulation in vitro with soluble immune complexes. Clin Nephrol 1991; 36:267–273.
89. Blancho G, Moreau JF, Chabannes D, et al. HILDA/LIF, G.CSF, IL-1 beta, IL-6, and TNF alpha production during acute rejection of human kidney allografts. Transplantation 1993; 56:597–602.
90. Matsumoto K, Dowling J, Atkins RC. Production of interleukin 1 in glomerular cell cultures from patients with rapidly progressive crescentic glomerulonephritis. Am J Nephrol 1988; 8:463–470.
91. Gardner KD Jr, Burnside JS, Elzinga LW, Locksley RM. Cytokines in fluids from polycystic kidneys. Kidney Int 1991; 39:718–724.
92. Noronha IL, Kruger C, Andrassy K, et al. In situ production of TNF-alpha, IL-1 beta and IL-2R in ANCA-positive glomerulonephritis. Kidney Int 1993; 43:682–692.
93. Noronha IL, Harley B, Cameron JS, Waldherr R. Detection of IL-1 beta and TNF-alpha message and protein in renal allograft biopsies. Transplantation 1993; 56:1026–1029.
94. Karkar AM, Tam FW, Proudfoot AE, et al. Modulation of antibody-mediated glomerular injury in vivo by interleukin-6. Kidney Int 1993; 44:967–973.
95. Ward PS, Fuller RW, Ritter JM, et al. Excretion of metabolites of prstacyclin and thromboxane by rats with nephrotoxic nephritis: Effects of interleukin-1. Br J Pharmacol 1991; 103:1663–1668.
96. Karkar AM, Koshino Y, Cashman SJ, et al. Passive immunization against tumour necrosis factor-alpha (TNF-alpha) and IL-1 beta protects from LPS enhancing glomerular injury in nephrotoxic nephritis in rats. Clin Exp Immunol 1992; 90:312–318.
97. Karkar AM, Tam FWK, Steinkasserer A, et al. Differential effects of inhibition of IL-1 and its glomerular expression (abstr). J Am Soc Nephrol 1994; 4:609.
98. Lan HY, Zarama M, Nikolic Paterson DJ, et al. Suppression of experimental crescentic glomerulonephritis by the interleukin-1 receptor antagonist. Kidney Int. 1993; 43:479–485.
99. Nikolic-Paterson DJ, Lan HY, Hill PA, et al. Suppression of experimental glomerulonephritis by the interleukin-1 receptor antagonist: Inhibition of intercellular adhesion molecule-1 expression. J Am Soc Nephrol 1994; 4:1695–1700.
100. Mulligan MS, Johnson KJ, Todd RF, et al. Requirements for leukocyte adhesion molecules in nephrotoxic nephritis. J Clin Invest 1993; 91:577–587.
101. Lovett DH, Ryan JL, Sterzel RB. A thymocyte-activating factor derived from glomerular mesangial cells. J Immunol 1983; 130:1796–1801.
102. Lovett DH, Sterzel RB, Ryan JL, Atkins E. Production of an endogenous pyrogen by glomerular mesangial cells. J Immunol 1985; 134:670–672.
103. Lovett DH, Larsen A. Cell cycle-dependent interleukin 1 gene expression by cultured glomerular mesangial cells. J Clin Invest 1988; 82:115–122.

104. Bursten SL, Locksley RM, Ryan JL, Lovett DH. Acylation of monocyte and glomerular mesangial cell proteins: Myristyl acylation of the interleukin 1 precursors. J Clin Invest 1988; 82:1479–1488.
105. Lovett DH, Szamel M, Ryan JL, et al. Interleukin 1 and the glomerular mesangium: I. Purification and characterization of a mesangial cell-derived autogrowth factor. J Immunol 1986; 136:3700–3705.
106. Lovett DH, Bursten SL, Gemsa D, et al. Activation of glomerular mesangial cells by gram-negative bacterial cell wall components. Am J Pathol 1988; 133:472–484.
107. Lovett DH, Haensch GM, Goppelt M, et al. Activation of glomerular mesangial cells by the terminal membrane attack complex of complement. Am J Pathol 1987; 133:472–484.
108. Lonnemann G, Shapiro L, Engler-Blum G, et al. Cytokines in human renal interstitial fibrosis: I. Interleukin-1 is an autocrine growth factor for cultured fibrosis-derived kidney fibroblasts. Kidney Int 1995; 47:837–844.
109. Kinjo T, Takashi M, Miyake K, Nagura H. In situ demonstration of immunological heterogeneity in vascular endothelial cells of renal cell carcinoma. J Surg Oncol 1990; 43:73–78.
110. Wardle EN. Cytokine growth factors and glomerulonephritis. Nephron 1991; 57:257–261.
111. Pober JS, Cotran RS. Cytokines and endothelial cell biology. Physiol Rev 1990; 70:427–451.
112. Sedor JR, Malone K, Njoku N, et al. Interleukin binds to both glomerular mesangial and tubular epithelial cells (abstr). Clin Res 1989; 37:501.
113. Zoja C, Rambaldi A, Remuzzi G. Interleukin-1 and glomerular mesangial cells. Renal Physiol Biochem 1993; 16:89–92.
114. Brown Z, Strieter RM, Neild GH, et al. IL-1 receptor antagonist inhibits monocyte chemotactic peptide 1 generation by human mesangial cells. Kidney Int 1992; 42:95–101.
115. Bursten SL, Harris WE, Bomsztyk K, Lovett D. Interleukin-1 rapidly stimulates lysophosphatidate acyltransferase and phosphatidate phosphohydrolase activities in human mesangial cells. J Biol Chem 1991; 266:20732–20743.
116. Sedor JR, Campbell L, Killian PL, et al. Interleukin-1 binds to culture thick ascending limb cells to stimulate diacyglycerol formation independent of polyphosphoinositide turnover. Kidney Int 1990; 37:431.
117. Hänsch GM, Braunger M, Mohring K, Wagner C. Identification of a receptor for interleukin 1 (IL-1) on human glomerular epithelial cells in culture. Cell Physiol Biochem 1993; 3:111–116.
118. Lonnemann G, Engler-Blum G, Müller GA, et al. Cytokines in human renal interstitial fibrosis: II. Autocrine interleukin (IL)-1 synthesis and IL-1–dependent production of IL-6 and IL-8 by cultured kidney fibroblasts. Kidney Int 1995; 47:845.
119. Zoja C, Wang JM, Bettoni S, et al. Interleukin-1 beta and tumor necrosis factor-alpha induce gene expression and production of leukocyte chemotactic factors, colony-stimulating factors, and interleukin-6 in human mesangial cells. Am J Pathol 1991; 138:991–1003.
120. Abbott F, Ryan JJ, Ceska M, et al. Interleukin-1 beta stimulates human mesangial cells to synthesize and release interleukins-6 and -8. Kidney Int 1991; 40:597–605.
121. Kusner DJ, Luebbers EL, Nowinski RJ, et al. Cytokine- and LPS-induced synthesis of interleukin-8 from human mesangial cells. Kidney Int 1991; 39:1240–1248.
122. Brown Z, Strieter RM, Chensue SW, et al. Cytokine-activated human mesangial cells generate the neutrophil chemoattractant, interleukin 8. Kidney Int 1991; 40:86–90.
123. Feng L, Xia Y, Kreisberg JI, Wilson CB. Interleukin-1α (IL-1) stimulates KC synthesis in rat mesangial cells: Glucocorticoids inhibit KC induction by IL-1. Am J Physiol 1994; 266:F713–F722.
124. Heeger P, Wolf G, Meyers C, et al. Isolation and characterization of cDNA from renal tubular epithelium encoding murine Rantes. Kidney Int 1992; 41:220–225.
125. Watanabe K, Konishi K, Fujioka M, et al. The neutrophil chemoattractant produced by the rat kidney epithelioid cell line NRK-52E is a protein related to the KC/gro protein. J Biol Chem 1989; 264:19559–19563.
126. Watanabe K, Nakagawa H. Cytokines enhance the production of a chemotactic factor for polymorphonuclear leukocytes by rat renal glomerular epithelioid cells. Nephron 1990; 54:169–175.
127. Nishikawa K, Guo YJ, Miyasaka M, et al. Antibodies to intercellular adhesion molecule 1/lymphocyte function-associated antigen 1 prevent crescent formation in rat autoimmune glomerulonephritis. J Exp Med 1993; 177:667–677.
128. Wuthrich RP. Intercellular adhesion molecules and vascular cell adhesion molecule-1 and the kidney. J Am Soc Nephrol 1992; 3:1201–1211.
129. Briscoe DM, Cotran RS. Role of leukocyte-endothelial cell adhesion molecules in renal inflammation: In vitro and in vivo studies. Kidney Int Suppl 1993; 42:S27–S34.
130. Brady HR. Leukocyte adhesion molecules and kidney diseases. Kidney Int 1994; 45:1285–1300.
131. Nakazato Y, Simonson MS, Herman W, et al. Interleukin-1α stimulates prostaglandin biosynthesis in serum-activated mesangial cells by induction of a non-pancreatic (type II) phospholipase A_2. J Biol Chem 1991; 266;14119–14127.
132. Topley N, Floege J, Wessel K, et al. Prostaglandin E_2 production is synergistically increased in cultured

human glomerular mesangial cells by combinations of IL-1 and tumor necrosis factor-alpha 1. J Immunol 1989; 143:1989–1995.
133. Floege J, Topley N, Wessel K, et al. Monokines and platelet-derived growth factor modulate prostanoid production in growth arrested human mesangial cells. Kidney Int 1990; 37:859–869.
134. Leighton JD, Pfeilschifter J. Interleukin 1- and tumor necrosis factor-stimulation of prostaglandin E_2 synthesis in MDCK cells, and potentiation of this effect by cycloheximide. FEBS Lett 1990; 259:289–292.
135. Lovett DH, Resch K, Gemsa D. Interleukin 1 and the glomerular mesangium. II. Monokine stimulation of mesangial cell prostanoid secretion. Am J Pathol 1987; 129:543–551.
136. Dennis EA. Diversity of group types, regulation, and function of phospholipase A_2. J Biol Chem 1994; 269:13057–13060.
137. Schalkwijk C, Pfeilschifter J, Marki F, Van den Bosch H. Interleukin-1 beta, tumor necrosis factor and forskolin stimulate the synthesis and secretion of group II phospholipase A_2 in rat mesangial cells. Biochem Biophys Res Commun 1991; 174:268–275.
138. Konieczkowski M, Sedor JR. Cell-specific regulation of type II phospholipase A_2 expression in rat mesangial cells. J Clin Invest 1993; 92:2524–2532.
139. Mühl H, Geiger T, Pignat W, et al. Transforming growth factors type-beta and dexamethasone attenuate group II phospholipase A_2 gene expression by interleukin-1 and forskolin in rat mesangial cells. FEBS Lett 1992; 301:190–194.
140. Schalkwijk C, Pfeilschifter J, Marki F, Van den Bosch H. Interleukin-1 beta- and forskolin-induced synthesis and secretion of group II phospholipase A_2 and prostaglandin E_2 in rat mesangial cells is prevented by transforming growth factor-beta 2. J Biol Chem 1992; 267:8846–8851.
141. Pfeilschifter J, Schalkwijk C, Briner VA, Van den Bosch H. Cytokine-stimulated secretion of group II phospholipase A_2 by rat mesangial cells: Its contribution to arachidonic acid release and prostaglandin synthesis by cultured rat glomerular cells. J Clin Invest 1993; 92:2516–2523.
142. Pfeilschifter J, Mühl H. Interleukin 1 and tumor necrosis factor potentiate angiotensin II- and calcium ionophore-stimulated prostaglandin E_2 synthesis in rat renal mesangial cells. Biochem Biophys Res Commun 1990; 169:585–595.
143. Gronich J, Konieczkowski M, Gelb MH, et al. Interleukin 1α causes rapid activation of cytosolic phospholipase A_2 by phosphorylation in rat mesangial cells. J Clin Invest 1994; 93:1224–1233.
144. Schalkwijk CG, de Vet E, Pfeilschifter J, Van den Bosch H. Interleukin-1 beta and transforming growth factor-beta 2 enhance cytosolic high-molecular-mass phospholipase A_2 activity and induce prostaglandin E_2 formation in rat mesangial cells. Eur J Biochem 1992; 210:169–176.
145. Coyne DW, Nickols M, Bertrand W, Morrison AR. Regulation of mesangial cell cyclooxygenase synthesis by cytokines and glucocorticoids. Am J Physiol 1992; 263:F97–F102.
146. Rzymkiewicz D, Leingang K, Baird N, Morrison AR. Regulation of prostaglandin endoperoxide synthase gene expression in rat mesangial cells by interleukin-1β. Am J Physiol (Renal Fluid Electrolyte Physiol) 1994; 266:F39–F45.
147. Srivastava SK, Tetsuka T, Daphna-Iken D, Morrison AR. IL-1β stabilizes COX II mRNA in renal mesangial cells: role of 3′ untranslated region. Am J Physiol (Renal Fluid Electrolyte) 1994; 267:F504–F508.
148. Ristimäki A, Garfinkel S, Wessendorf J, et al. Induction of cyclooxygenase-2 by interleukin-1α:: Evidence for post-transcriptional regulation. J Biol Chem 1994; 269:11769–11775.
149. Pfeilschifter J, Schwarzenbach H. Interleukin 1 and tumor necrosis factor stimulate cGMP formation in rat renal mesangial cells. FEBS Lett 1990; 273:185–187.
150. Pfeilschifter J, Rob P, Mulsch A, et al. Interleukin 1 beta and tumour necrosis factor alpha induce a macrophage-type of nitric oxide synthase in rat renal mesangial cells. Eur J Biochem 1992; 203:251–255.
151. Mühl H, Kunz D, Pfeilschifter J. Expression of nitric oxide synthase in rat glomerular mesangial cells mediated by cyclic AMP. Br J Pharmacol 1994; 112:1–8.
152. Torbohm I, Berger B, Schonermark M, et al. Modulation of collagen synthesis in human glomerular epithelial cells by interleukin 1. Clin Exp Immunol 1989; 75:427–431.
153. Marti HP, McNeil L, Davies M, et al. Homology cloning of rat 72 kDa type IV collagenase: Cytokine and second-messenger inducibility in glomerular mesangial cells. Biochem J 1993; 291:441–446.
154. Marx J. Taking a direct path to the genes. Science 1992; 257:744–745.
155. Huang S, Konieczkowski M, Sedor JR. Interleukin 1 induces IL-6 via arachidonate-stimulated activation of a transcription factor(s) (abstr). J Am Soc Nephrol 1994; 4:488.
156. Savic V, Stefanovic V, Ardaillou N, Ardaillou R. Induction of ecto-5′-nucleotidase of rat cultured mesangial cells by interleukin-1 beta and tumour necrosis factor-alpha. Immunology 1990; 70:321–326.
157. Jurivich DA, Sistonen L, Sarge KD, Morimoto RI, Arachidonate is a potent modulator of human heat shock gene transcription. Proc Natl Acad Sci USA 1994; 91:2280–2284.
158. Rovin B, Tan L. Intercellular regulation of interleukin-1-induced monocyte chemoattractant protein-1 in human mesangial cells (abstr). J Am Soc Nephrol 1994; 4:498.

159. Richardson CA, Bomsztyk K. IL-1β activates nuclear factor-κB in human mesangial cells (abstr). J Am Soc Nephrol 1994; 4:497.
160. Kashtan C, Libermann T, Kim Y, Van Ness B. Induction of the promoter of the interleukin-6 (IL-6) gene in human mesangial cells (HMC) requires an intact binding site for nuclear factor κB (NF-κB). J Am Soc Nephrol 1994; 4:609.
161. Isshiki H, Akira S, Tanabe O, et al. Constitutive and interleukin-1 (IL-1)–inducible factors interact with the IL-1-responsive element in the IL-6 gene. Mol Cell Biol 1990; 10:2757–2764.
162. Wilson DR, Juan TSC, Wilde M, et al. A 58-base-pair region of the human C3 gene confers synergistic inducibility by interleukin-1 and interleukin-6. Mol Cell Biol 1990; 10:6181–6191.
163. Kessler DJ, Duyao MP, Spicer DB, Sonenshein GE. NF-kappaB-like factors mediate interleukin 1 induction of c-myc gene transcription in fibroblasts. J Exp Med 1992; 176:787–792.
164. Stoeckle MY. Post-transcriptional regulation of gro alpha, beta, gamma, and IL-8 mRNAs by IL-1 beta. Nucleic Acids Res 1991; 19:917–920.
165. Johnson RJ, Lovett D. In vivo gene transfer, Koch's postulates, and renal disease. J Clin Invest 1993; 92:2568.
166. Shelton CA, Wasserman SA. pelle encodes a protein kinase required to establish dorsoventral polarity in the Drosophila embryo. Cell 1993; 72:515–525.
167. Turck J, Pollock AS, Lee LK, Lovett DH. Probing the biologic role of type IV collagenase: an anti-sense approach (abstr). J Am Soc Nephrol 1993; 4:668.
168. Savill J. Apoptosis: A mechanism for regulation of the cell complement of inflamed glomeruli. Kidney Int 1992; 41:607–612.

45

The Monocyte Chemoattractant Protein 1

Bruno Luckow and Detlef Schlöndorff
Ludwig-Maximilians-University Munich, Munich, Germany

Gunter Wolf
University of Hamburg, Hamburg, Germany

INTRODUCTION: MONOCYTES/MACROPHAGES AND RENAL INJURY

Monocytes/macrophages (M/M) play an important role in the initiation and progression of a variety of renal diseases. For example, glomerular M/M accumulation occurs in different types of immune-mediated glomerulonephritis (1–4), hyperlipidemia (5,6), diabetes mellitus (7), and unilateral nephrectomy (8). Similarly, recruitment of bone marrow–derived cells like M/M into the tubulointerstitial environment also occurs in a wide variety of diseases such as unilateral obstruction (9), two-kidney one-clip hypertension (10), infusion of angiotensin II into the kidney (11), tubulointerstitial nephritis (12), puromycin-induced proteinuria (13), allograft rejection (14), and several other pathophysiological situations (2).

The locally accumulated M/M can generate many different mediators, such as a variety of biologically active lipids, enzymes, cytokines, and growth factors, which all can alter the function and the structure of the surrounding renal tissue (15–19). For example, glomerular macrophages release vasoactive compounds like leukotriene D_4 and thromboxane A_2, which, in turn, reduce glomerular filtration rate and contribute to proteinuria (16,17). Other factors like proteolytic enzymes (collagenase, elastase) and active oxygen radicals can injure the glomerular basement membrane and disrupt the functional integrity of the filtration barrier, resulting in proteinuria (18,19). Furthermore, local release of factors such as transforming growth factor-β (TGF-β) by M/M may activate resident renal cells (like mesangial cells) to produce excess matrix components, such as collagens, resulting in glomerulosclerosis (20,21). A similar sequence of events has been proposed for tubulointerstitial injury involving influx of M/M, their activation, and various mediators of inflammation, leading to interstitial fibrosis with permanent loss of renal function (12,22).

Chemotaxis of "phagocytic" cells was already described by Metchnikoff in his classic treatise on inflammation around the turn of this century (23). The mechanisms responsible for the migration of M/M to specific anatomic target sites such as the glomerulus or interstitium in the kidney remain incompletely understood (2). In complement-dependent inflammatory processes (24), locally generated C5a or leukotrienes (25,26) can act as chemoattractants. However, accumulation of M/M in the kidney can also occur in some models independent of complement (2,27). Furthermore, many inflammatory mediators have some chemotactic activity but show little target cell selectivity and specificity.

CHEMOKINES

During the last decade, a new gene family of proinflammatory *chemo*tactic cyto*kines* has been established, the members of which have been termed *chemokines* (28). Alternatively, this family was called SIG (small inducible genes) family (29), platelet factor 4 (PF4) superfamily (30), or intercrine cytokine family (31). The different chemokines possess individual target cell specificity for subgroups of leukocytes. They are secreted proteins of 92–99 amino acids containing a cleaved leader sequence of 20–25 amino acids and are able to attract and activate specific types of leukocytes. The chemokine superfamily is subdivided and consists of the C-C and the C-X-C chemokine family, which both contain four conserved cysteine residues. In the C-X-C family, the first two conserved cysteines are separated by an additional amino acid; whereas in the C-C family, these two cysteines are located adjacent to each other. IL-8 is a prominent member of the C-X-C family, while the monocyte chemoattractant protein-1 (MCP-1) belongs to the C-C chemokine family (28,32,33). So far, seven different members of the human C-C chemokine family have been isolated (Table 1): MCP-1 (34), MCP-2 (35), MCP-3 (36,37), I-309 (38), RANTES (39), MIP-1α (40), and MIP-1β (41). It is noteworthy that several slightly different MIP-1β cDNAs have been isolated, which encode proteins that are at least 94% and at most 98% identical (32). These different cDNAs are derived from multiple nonallelic forms of the MIP-1β gene. The biological meaning of this family within the C-C chemokine family is at present unknown. An alignment of all human C-C chemokines is shown in Figure 1. The degree of sequence identity in comparison to human MCP-1 varies between 32.6% and 73.7%. Within the human C-C chemokine family, MCP-3 is most closely related to MCP-1 (73.7% identity and 77.8% similarity, respectively), whereas I-309 displays the weakest sequence conservation. For almost all human C-C chemokines, the corresponding mouse genes have been isolated as well (Table 1). Recently, a new mouse C-C chemokine has been isolated independently by two groups (42,43). This protein, designated either MARC or FIC, shows a degree of sequence homology to human MCP-1 (57.7% identity, 70.1% similarity), which exceeds even the homology to the mouse MCP-1 (JE) protein (53.5% identity, 69.7% similarity). Nevertheless, MARC seems to be the murine homologue to human MCP-3 and not MCP-1, because the homology between MARC and MCP-3 is even better (59.8% identity, 73.2% similarity). Table 1 shows all presently known human C-C chemokines and their corresponding murine homologues.

MONOCYTE CHEMOATTRACTANT PROTEIN 1

The monocyte chemoattractant protein 1 (MCP-1) belongs, as already mentioned, to the C-C chemokine subfamily. It is a small secreted protein with strong chemotactic activity for monocytes and to a lesser extent for basophil granulocytes. In the older literature, several alternative names for MCP-1 can be found: LDCF (lymphocyte-derived chemotactic factor) (44), TDCF (tumor-derived chemotactic factor) (45), JE (46), MCF (monocyte chemotactic factor) (47), MCAF (monocyte chemotactic and activating factor) (48), GDCF (glioma-derived chemotactic factor) (34), SMC-CF (smooth muscle cell–derived chemotactic factor) (49), HC11 (50), and TSG-8 (tumor necrosis factor stimulated gene 8) (51). To avoid confusion, we will use exclusively the term MCP-1 in this report. Several excellent reviews covering many aspects of the molecular biology of MCP-1 are available (52–57). In the meantime, however, considerable progress has been made, which is presented in this chapter. Furthermore, our current understanding of this cytokine in renal disease is summarized.

Table 1 Murine Homologues of Human C-C Chemokines

Human gene	Murine gene
MCP-1	JE
MCP-2 (=HC14)	Unknown
MCP-3	MARC (=FIC)?
I-309	TCA3
RANTES	RANTES
MIP-1α	MIP-1α
MIP-1β	MIP-1β
Unknown	C10

```
1  MKVSAALLCLLLIAATFIPQGLAQPDAINAPVTCCYNFTNRKISVQRLAS  MCP-1
1  ......................AQPDSVSIPITCCFNVINRKIPIQRLES  MCP-2
1  MKASAALLCLLLTAAAFSPQGLAQPVGINTSTTCCYRFINKKIPKQRLES  MCP-3
1  MQIITTALVCLLLAGMWPEDVDSKSMQVPFSR.CCFSFAEQEIPLRAILC  I-309
1  MKVSAARLAVILIATALCAPASASPYSSDT.TPCCFAYIARPLPRAHIKE  RANTES
1  MQVSTAALAVLLCTMALCN.QFSASLAADTPTACCFSYTSRQIPQNFIAD  MIP-1 alpha
1  MKLCVTVLSLLMLVAAFCSLALSAPMGSDPPTACCFSYTARKLPRNFVVD  MIP-1 beta

51 YRRITSSKCPKEAVIFKTIVAKEICADPKQKWVQDSMDHLDKQTQTPKT.  MCP-1
29 YTRITNIQCPKEAVIFKTKRGKEVCADPKERWVRDSMKHLDQIFQNLKP.  MCP-2
51 YRRTTSSHCPREAVIFKTKLDKEICADPTQKWVQDFMKHLDKKTQTPKL.  MCP-3
50 Y.RNTSSICSNEGLIFKLKRGKEACALDTVGWVQRHRKML.RHCPSKRK.  I-309
50 YF.YTSGKCSNPAVVFVTRKNRQVCANPEKKWVREYINSLEMS.......  RANTES
50 YF.ETSSQCSKPGVIFLTKRSRQVCADPSEEWVQKYVSDLELSA......  MIP-1 alpha
51 YY.ETSSLCSQPAVVFQTKRSKQVCADPSESWVQEYVYDLELN.......  MIP-1 beta
```

Figure 1 The protein sequences of all known human C-C chemokine precursors are shown. The signal peptide sequence for MCP-2 is not yet available. Amino acids identical in at least six different chemokines are boxed. (Protein sequences from Refs. 37–40, 50, 60, and 152.)

MOLECULAR CLONING AND CHARACTERIZATION OF THE MCP-1 GENE

Partial cDNA clones for mouse MCP-1 had been isolated fortuitously more than 10 years ago (58). When a cDNA library from BALB/c-3T3 cells was screened for PDGF-inducible genes by differential hybridization, one of the induced genes was designated JE. Nothing was known about its function, and only several years later did it become clear that the mouse homologue of the human MCP-1 gene had been isolated on that occasion. Since then, cDNA clones encoding MCP-1 have been isolated from seven different species (Table 2). Mouse MCP-1 was available first (46,58) followed by human (48,59,60), rat (61,62), rabbit (63), bovine (64), guinea pig (65), and sheep MCP-1 (65). Genomic clones have been isolated only from mouse (29,46), human (59,66), and rat (61). Southern blot analysis indicates that the human MCP-1 gene is a single-copy gene (59,60) consisting of 3 exons (59). These exons are 145, 118, and 478 bp long; the two introns represent 800 and 385 bp (66). The mouse and rat genes show a very similar structure. The exon-intron boundaries are precisely conserved between these three species. There is some controversy in the literature concerning the start site of transcription. If the transcription initiation site in the rat gene is taken as +1, then the start site of the mouse MCP-1 gene is either at position +3 (46) or –3 (29). Determinations of the start site of the human MCP-1 gene differ by a single nucleotide (59,66). In the mouse gene, two alternative polyadenylation sites have been identified in the third exon, which give rise to mRNAs of either 594 or 797 bases without poly(A) tail (46). In the rat and human genes, alternative polyadenylation site usage could not be detected and the mRNAs are 790 and 741 bases long. The MCP-1 mRNAs from all three species contain in the 3′ untranslated region one copy of the sequence AUUUA, characteristic of rapidly degraded mRNAs (67). This motif can be extended to TTATTTAA, which resembles the sequence TTATTTAT found in the 3′ untranslated region of several genes encoding inflammatory mediators (68). The time course of MCP-1 mRNA induction in human fibroblasts is rapid. A plateau is reached within the first 1 to 2 hr after stimulation and it is maintained for at least 16 hr. The induction is more than 100-fold (51). Similar results have been obtained in other cell types using different stimuli (Table 3). In the induced state, the MCP-1 mRNA can represent approximately 1% of the total cellular poly(A)$^+$ RNA (58). The human MCP-1 gene has been mapped to chromosome 17q11.2-12 (69). Other members of the human C-C chemokine family—like RANTES, MIP-1α, MIP-1β, and I-309—have been located at 17q11-21 (see Ref. 32 and references therein). The homologous mouse C-C chemokine genes including MCP-1 are clustered on the distal part of chromosome 11 (70), which is syntenic to human chromosome 17. The clustering of C-C chemokine genes on the same chromosome together with their sequence similarities strongly suggests a common origin of all C-C chemokines.

Table 2 Sequence Conservation of MCP-1 Proteins

Species	% Identity	% Similarity
Human	100.0	100.0
Cow	71.7	81.8
Sheep	67.7	78.8
Rabbit	73.7	80.8
Guinea pig	56.7	70.1
Mouse	53.5	69.7
Rat	55.1	68.4

The MCP-1 gene encodes in each species a small (8 to 10-kDa), secreted, basic (pI ≈ 10) glycoprotein. The size of the encoded protein varies between 99 amino acids (human, bovine, and sheep), 120 (guinea pig), 125 (rabbit), and 148 amino acids (mouse and rat). The reasons for these size differences are unclear. In terms of function, MCP-1 from different species behaves identically. An alignment of all seven MCP-1 protein sequences known at present is shown in Figure 2. The sequences include the signal peptide, which is cleaved to generate the secreted protein. The degree of sequence conservation between MCP-1 protein from humans and other species is given in Table 2. As already mentioned, the human MCP-1 gene consists of three exons. The first exon encodes amino acids 1 to 25, splitting the conserved aspartic acid residue at position 26. It includes the signal peptide, which encompasses amino acids 1 to 23. The second exon contains the information for the amino-terminal half of the mature protein from positions 26 to 65. The third exon encodes the remaining part of the protein from amino acids 65 to 99 and includes the 3′ untranslated region. The predicted molecular weight for the human MCP-1 protein precursor is 11025 Da. The mature secreted protein consists of only 76 amino acids and has a calculated molecular weight of 8685 Da. The amino terminus is blocked and starts with pyroglutamic acid (44). A consensus sequence for N-linked glycosylation (N-F-T) is present adjacent to the first two cysteines. Experiments with tunicamycin, an inhibitor of N-linked glycosylation, and glycopeptidase F, which removes N-linked carbohydrates, indicate, however, that this site is not utilized for glycosylation (71,72). Based on the MCP-1 protein sequence, several O-glycosylation sites have been predicted. Experiments by Jiang and coworkers demonstrate that the protein indeed contains O-linked carbohydrates, which are further modified by the addition of terminal sialic acid residues (72). The observed size heterogeneity of MCP-1 proteins produced by different cell types can therefore be explained by differences in O-linked carbohydrate processing. Further analyses of the carbohydrate structure revealed the presence of the disaccharide D-galactose β1-3D-N-acetyl galactoseamin (73). Although native human MCP-1 is a glycoprotein, glycosylation is not required for its chemotactic activity (55,73). Whether this type of posttranslational modification is required for other biological activities remains to be determined. Interestingly, the MCP-1 protein sequence contains several putative phosphorylation sites for PKA and PKC. To our knowledge, no experiments have been reported that address the question of whether MCP-1 is a phosphoprotein and whether phosphorylation influences the biological activity of this protein.

INDUCTION OF THE MCP-1 GENE IN DIFFERENT CELL TYPES

Many different agents are able to induce MCP-1 gene expression in a variety of cells (Table 3). As the gene was isolated originally because of its PDGF inducibility in mouse fibroblasts, PDGF was the first known MCP-1 inducer (58). Since then, an impressively long list of inducing agents has been established. It includes serum, bacterial endotoxin (LPS), IL-1, IL-4, TNF-α, TGF-β, EGF, LIF, retinoic acid, IFN-γ, PHA, ConA, infection with VSV, double-stranded RNA, phorbol esters like TPA or PMA, minimally modified low-density lipoprotein, IgG complexes, and others. Interestingly, some tumor cell lines secrete MCP-1 constitutively without the addition of any inducer. This fact facilitated the purification of the protein from cell culture supernatants considerably. Most

Table 3 Induction of MCP-1 in Different Cell Types by Various Inducers

Cell type	Species	Stimulus
Peripheral blood mononuclear leukocytes	Human	PHA, LPS, IL-1 (60)
Promyelocytic cell line	Human	PMA + RA + LPS + cycloheximide (48), PMA (59)
Monocytes	Human	(-) (59)
Peritoneal macrophages	Mouse	LPS, heat-killed *Listeria monocytogenes*, maleyl-BSA, fucoidan, PMA + A23187 (153), IFN-γ (85)
Macrophage cell lines	Mouse	LPS, PMA, IFN-γ (79)
B lymphocytes	Human	LPS (154)
Lymphocytes	Human	PHA (155)
Spleen cells	Rabbit	ConA, LPS (63)
Spleen cells	Rat	ConA (62)
Dermal fibroblasts	Human	IL-1α, TNF-α (156)
Pulmonary fibroblasts		
Fibroblast cell line	Mouse	PDGF, cycloheximide (58) double-stranded RNA, infection with VSV (157), PDGF, IL-1α (46), c-*sis* (PDGF B chain homodimer), bovine calf serum (59), TNF, cycloheximide, IFN-β, IFN-γ, IL-1α, EGF, PDGF, TGF-β, poly(I)-poly(C), TPA, A23187, dBcAMP, IBMX (51), cholera toxin (83)
Fibroblast cell lines derived from lung and skin	Human	PDGF (71)
Embryonic lung fibroblasts	Human	bovine calf serum
Foreskin fibroblasts	Human	IL-1β, TNF-α (158)
Endothelial cells from umbilical veins	Human	IL-1β, TNF-α, LPS (158,159), IL-1β, TNF, IFN-γ (160), IL-4 (161), TPA (66)
Aortic endothelial cells	Human	MM-LDL (162)
Smooth muscle cells	Human	MM-LDL (162)
Keratinocytes	Human	IFN-γ (163)
Retinal pigment epithelial cells	Human	IL-1β, TNF-α (164)
Pulmonary type II–like epithelial cells	Human	IL-1β, TNF-α (165)
Articular chondrocytes	Human	IL-1, TNF-α, LPS, PDGF, TGF-β, LIF, RA (78)
Synoviocytes	Human	IL-1, TNF-α, LPS, PDGF, TGF-β, RA (137)
Osteoblasts	Human	IL-1β (166)
Clonal osteoblastic cell line	Mouse	IL-1β, TNF-α, (167)
Astrocytes	Mouse	EAE (168)
Various tumors		
Glioma	Human	(-) (34, 49)
Fibrosarcoma	Human	(-) (49)
Osteosarcoma	Human	(-) (49)
Melanoma	Human	(-) (49)
Mesangial cells	Human	IL-1β, TNF-α (126, 169), LDL (170)
Mesangial cells	Mouse	IgG complexes (127), IFN-γ, TNF-α, IgG complexes (80), oxygen radicals (94)
Renal cortical epithelial cells	Human	IFN-γ, IL-1β, TNF-α, LPS (124)

```
  1  MKVSAALLCLLLIAATFIPQGLAQPDAINAPVTCCYNFTNRKISVQRLAS  Human
  1  MKVSAALLCLLLTVAAFSTEVLAQPDAINSQVACCYTFNSKKISMQRLMN  Cow
  1  MKFSAALLCLLLTVAAFSTEVLAQPDAINSQIACCYKFTNKKIPIQRLTN  Sheep
  1  MKVSATLLCLLLIAVAFSSHVLAQPDAVNSPVTCCYTFTNKTISVKRLMS  Rabbit
  1  MQRSSVLLCLLVIEATFCSLLMAQPDGVNTP.TCCYTF.NKQIPLKRVKG  Guinea pig
  1  MQVPVMLLGLLFTVAGWSIHVLAQPDAVNAPLTCCYSFTSKMIPMSRLES  Mouse
  1  MQVSVTLLGLLFTVAACSIHVLSQPDAVNAPLTCCYSFTGKMIPMSRLEN  Rat

 51  YRRITSSKCPKEAVIFKTIVAKEICADPKQKWVQDSMDHLDKQTQTPKT.  Human
 51  YRRVTSSKCPKEAVIFKTILGKELCADPKQKWVQDSINYLNKKNQTPKP.  Cow
 51  YRRVTTSKCPKEAVIFKTILGKEFCADPNLKWVQDAINHLNKKNQTPKP.  Sheep
 51  YRRINSTKCPKEAVIFMTKLAKGICADPKQKWVQDAIANLDKKMQTPKTL  Rabbit
 49  YERITSSRCPQEAVIFRTLKNKEVCADPTQKWVQDYIAKLDQRTQQKQNS  Guinea pig
 51  YKRITSSRCPKEAVVFVTKLKREVCADPKKEWVQTYIKNLDRNQMRSEPT  Mouse
 51  YKRITSSRCPKEAVVFVTKLKREICADPNKEWVQKYIRKLDQNQVRSETT  Rat

101  ..................................................  Human
101  ..................................................  Cow
101  ..................................................  Sheep
101  TSYSTT..................QEHTTNLSSTRTPSTTTSL.......  Rabbit
 99  T......APQTSKPLNIRFTTQDPKNRS......................  Guinea pig
101  TLFKTASALRSSAPLNVKLTRKSEANASTTFSTTTSSTSVGVTSVTVN.  Mouse
101  VFYKIASTLRTSAPLNVNLTHKSEANASTLFSTTTSSTSVEVTSMTEN.  Rat
```

Figure 2 An alignment of MCP-1 protein sequences from human, cow, sheep, rabbit, guinea pig, mouse, and rat is shown. The sequences of the signal peptides are included. The mature proteins start at the conserved glutamine residue at position 24. Amino acids identical in at least six different species are boxed. (Protein sequences from Refs. 46, 60, 61, and 63–65.)

cells must be stimulated with one of the agents listed above in order to detect MCP-1 expression. In several cases, so-called "constitutive" MCP-1 expression might have been induced by growth factors (like PDGF) present in the serum added to the cell-culture medium. As indicated, MCP-1 can be produced by many different cell types, including monocytes, macrophages, lymphocytes, fibroblasts, keratinocytes, endothelial cells, smooth muscle cells, osteoblasts, chondrocytes, many tumor cells, and mesangial cells. Table 3 summarizes the results with the induction of MCP-1 in different cell types using various inducers.

REPRESSION OF MCP-1 GENE EXPRESSION

In the human fibrosarcoma cell line 8387, induction of the MCP-1 gene by IL-1 or TNF-α is suppressed by the synthetic glucocorticoid dexamethasone (Dex) (74). Similar results have been obtained in murine Balb/c 3T3 fibroblasts. Induction of the mouse MCP-1 gene with either PDGF, serum, TPA or double-stranded synthetic RNA was inhibited by two different glucocorticoids, Dex, and methylprednisolone (75). Nonsteroidal anti-inflammatory agents like aspirin, ibuprofen, and phenylbutazone or other steroids like progesterone had no effect. In both cases, glucocorticoids reduced the transcription rate. In addition, the stability of MCP-1 mRNA was decreased in human cells but not in the murine cell line. In rat vascular smooth muscle cells, induction of the MCP-1 gene by serum or PDGF is also blocked by glucocorticoids (76). This effect appears mainly due to destabilization of MCP-1 mRNA. At present, it is not clear, whether these results represent real differences in the regulation of the mouse, rat, and human MCP-1 gene. Interestingly, the glucocorticoid effect became fully apparent only after a lag period of 1 to 2 hr and could be completely abolished by inhibitors of transcription (actinomycin D) or translation (cycloheximide, puromycin). These data suggest that the glucocorticoid effect is an indirect one and requires de novo transcription and protein synthesis. Therefore, it is most likely not mediated by direct binding of the glucocorticoid receptor to a DNA sequence in the vicinity of the MCP-1 gene. This conclusion was confirmed in a report by Brach et al. (77), who examined the effect of anti-inflammatory agents on the synthesis of MCP-1 in human monocytes. As expected, dexamethasone reduced the transcription rate and stability of the MCP-1 mRNA. In human articular chondrocytes, MCP-1 induction by serum, IL-1, cAMP, or the phorbol ester PMA could also be suppressed by the addition of Dex (78). Glucocorticoids are not the only substances that can inhibit MCP-1 induction. In murine macrophages, LPS induction of MCP-1 can be inhibited by the prostaglandin PGE_1, which elevates intracellular cAMP levels (79). Surprisingly, treatment of cells with dibutyryl cAMP gave a weaker inhibitory effect. Based on this indirect evidence, it was suggested that inhibition by PGE_1 may be partially independent of the cAMP signal transduction pathway. Experiments performed recently in our laboratory provide further evidence of a negative effect of cAMP on the induction of MCP-1 (80). In mouse mesangial cells, increased MCP-1 expression by IFN-γ, TNF-α, or IgG aggregates was attenuated by forskolin or PGE_2, both of which led to an increase in cAMP levels, as did 8-bromo-cAMP. The inhibitory effect was due to a decreased transcription rate. In human pulmonary fibroblasts, IL-1β–stimulated MCP-1 expression could also be suppressed by Dex as well as by PGE_2 (81). Steady-state mRNA levels as well as protein levels were significantly reduced in a dose-dependent manner. MCP-1 repression by glucocorticoids or cAMP was found not only in the established pulmonary fibroblast cell line 18Lu but also in primary pulmonary fibroblast cultures from five different patients. Interestingly, there are also reports describing a stimulatory effect of cAMP on MCP-1 expression. In human chondrocytes, for example, addition of cAMP led to induction of MCP-1 expression (78). Incubation of rabbit aortic endothelial cells with dibutyryl-cAMP increased MCP-1 mRNA levels 10-fold (82). The effect was even stronger if the cells were treated with cholera toxin, which can increase intracellular cAMP levels. However, in mouse cells, induction of MCP-1 by cholera toxin occurs via a cAMP-independent signaling pathway (83). These contradictory results may be explained by species- and cell-type–specific effects of cAMP. At present, most of the data are too indirect to permit firm conclusions about the different effects of cAMP.

SIGNAL TRANSDUCTION AND MCP-1 EXPRESSION

There are only a few reports covering signal transduction pathways involved in MCP-1 expression. In 1987, Hall and Stiles examined the response of the c-*myc*, c-*fos*, *KC*, and *JE* (mouse MCP-1) genes to PDGF and characterized the role of protein kinase C (PKC) in this process (84). Surprisingly, the four genes responded differentially. Transcription of the *MCP-1* gene could be induced by PDGF but not by PKC agonists. Depleting cells of PKC activity by prolonged TPA treatment did not prevent subsequent stimulation of MCP-1 transcription by PDGF. The authors concluded that PKC has no role in MCP-1 gene induction by PDGF. The response of murine macrophages to interferon-γ (IFN-γ) was analyzed by Prpic et al. (85). Binding of IFN-γ to its cell surface receptor ultimately leads to an enhanced expression of MCP-1. The first detectable effect, however, was a rapid (< 60 sec) increase in the intracellular pH by as much as 0.1 pH unit, paralleled by an influx of Na^+ ions. All IFN-γ–induced changes could be significantly inhibited by addition of amiloride, an inhibitor of the Na^+/H^+ antiporter. Therefore, it was postulated that alkalinization of the cytosol by the activated Na^+/H^+ antiporter may be the first step in this signal transduction pathway that can finally activate MCP-1. Furthermore, after a lag period of 5 to 10 min, an enhanced efflux of Ca^{2+} was observed. In several recent papers, it was shown that IFN-γ regulates gene expression by tyrosine phosphorylation of DNA-binding proteins (86–90). The protein tyrosine kinases involved in IFN-γ signal transduction are JAK1 and JAK2 (91,92). In mouse BALB/c 3T3 fibroblasts, MCP-1 can be induced by cholera toxin via a cAMP-independent pathway (83). Neither forskolin nor 8-bromo-cAMP could induce MCP-1. A recent report by Shyy et al. (93) proposes that induction of the MCP-1 gene in human endothelial cells involves at least three different pathways. Depending on the specific inducer, the signal is transmitted either by activation of PKC, by tyrosine phosphorylation or by an unknown third signal transduction pathway. Induction of the MCP-1 gene by TPA seems to involve PKC as well as tyrosine phosphorylation, because it is abolished only after addition of inhibitors for both pathways (staurosporine and genistein) (93). During LPS induction, a different third pathway might be active, because staurosporine and genistein could only partially repress the activation of the gene in TPA-desensitized cells. The third signal transduction pathway is probably not mediated by cAMP-dependent protein kinase (PKA), because treatment of cells with forskolin, an adenylate cyclase activator, had no effect. Recently, oxygen radicals have been implicated as second messengers for MCP-1 induction in mouse mesangial cells (94). Radical scavengers such as di- and tetra-methylthiourea attenuated the increase in MCP-1 mRNA levels after TNF-α and aggregated IgG stimulation. Generation of superoxide anions by xanthine oxidase and hypoxanthine led to an induction of the MCP-1 gene. Addition of NADPH to activate a membrane bound NADPH-oxidase generated superoxide, caused a dose-dependent increase in MCP-1 mRNA levels and further enhanced the stimulation by TNF-α and aggregated IgG. Free radicals can activate the transcription factor NF-κB, which might be directly involved in increased MCP-1 gene transcription.

Cis-ACTING ELEMENTS OF THE MCP-1 GENE

Little is known about regulatory elements and transcription factors involved in MCP-1 expression. First attempts to identify important regulatory sequences in the 5′ flanking region of the rat MCP-1 gene were performed by Timmers et al. (61). Their experiments demonstrated that the promoter region between -141 and -88 is required for TPA induction. The region between -70 and -38 is essential for basal activity and contains a sequence resembling an AP-1 binding site. However, in vitro binding assays indicated that the putative AP-1 site in the MCP-1 promoter bound common but also different proteins in comparison to a consensus AP-1 site. Sequences mediating induction of the mouse MCP-1 gene by PDGF have been identified by Freter et al. (95). Full inducibility required the presence of two widely separated regions located in the 5′ and the 3′-flanking region of the gene. Deletion of sequences between -2538 and -2298 resulted in complete loss of inducibility. The essential element in the proximal 3′-flanking region is a novel 7-bp motif, TTTTGTA, which does not resemble any known transcription factor binding sequence. This novel element appears to be position-dependent but orientation-independent. It is essential for MCP-1 induction not only by PDGF but also by serum, interleukin-1, and double-stranded RNA. Interestingly, this sequence motif is found in the 3′-flanking region of 25 immediate-early genes encoding either transcription factors or cytokines (95). Experiments suggesting a role for c-*fos* and c-*jun* in MCP-1 induction by TNF-α have recently been described (96). Using c-*fos* or c-*jun* antisense oligonucleotides, monocyte chemotactic activity could be partially inhibited. Furthermore, if mouse osteoblastic MC3T3-E1 cells were treated with curcumin, a specific inhibitor of c-*jun/AP-1*, the induction of MCP-1 by TNF-α was markedly inhibited. It is unclear, however, whether the observed effects on MCP-1 expression are direct or indirect ones. By sequence homology, a putative interferon response sequence has been identified in the promoter region of the mouse MCP-1 gene (46). This motif is not conserved in the human or rat MCP-1 gene. Its functional significance remains unclear. Experiments performed by Satriano et al. (94) provided circumstantial evidence for a possible role of NF-κB in MCP-1 induction. Activation and inhibition of the MCP-1 gene by various agents occurred in parallel with activation of nuclear NF-κB binding determined by gel shift experiments. By sequence comparison, a putative NF-κB binding site has been identified 148 bp upstream of the ATG codon in the human MCP-1 gene (66). It remains to be determined whether this potential NF-κB binding site plays a role in the regulation of the MCP-1 gene. This also applies for two sequences resembling TPA-responsive elements and an octamer binding site described by the same authors. As NF-κB can be activated by the same stimuli that increase mRNA levels for MCP-1 (phorbol esters, lipopolysaccharide, IL-1, TNF-α) (97,98), it is tempting to speculate about a role for NF-κB in the regulation of MCP-1 gene expression. The recent finding that NF-κB can form heterodimers with other transcription factors like AP-1 of Sp1 makes this possibility even more likely (99,100). By computer analysis, we have recently identified an additional binding site for NF-κB at position -398 and for Sp1 at -55 in the human MCP-1 gene (B.L., unpublished). Both, the NF-κB and the Sp1 consensus binding sites are present only in the 5′-flanking region of the human gene. They are missing in the mouse or rat gene, although the promoter sequences of the MCP-1 genes in these three species show a relatively high degree of sequence conservation. Thus, there could indeed exist species-specific differences in the regulation of the MCP-1 gene. Further experiments are required to answer this question.

MCP-1–SPECIFIC RECEPTORS ON TARGET CELLS

Evidence for MCP-1–specific receptors on human blood monocytes has been presented by Yoshimura and Leonard (101). Iodinated MCP-1 protein bound with high affinity only to monocytes but not to neutrophils or lymphocytes. The number of receptor molecules per cell was estimated to be at least 1700 ± 600 and a dissociation constant (K_d) of 1.9 n*M* ± 0.2 was determined. Similar results have been obtained by Valente et al. (102). They found approximately 1600 high-affinity binding sites per monocyte with a K_d of 1.1 n*M*. A synthetic peptide containing amino acids 13 to 35 from mature human MCP-1 was bound by the receptor and induced chemotaxis, whereas a peptide corresponding to amino acids 37 to 50 had no effect. A double mutation in human MCP-1 of tyrosine 28 and arginine 30 to leucine and valine, respectively, causes a loss of MCP-1 receptor recognition (103). Instead, the mutated MCP-1 protein bound to another specific chemokine receptor, which causes chemotaxis of neutrophils instead of monocytes. On human monocytic THP-1 cells, approximately 5000 high-affinity MCP-1–specific receptors/cell with a K_d of 0.44 n*M* have been found (104). In addition, MCP-1 was bound with low affinity by the RANTES specific receptor. Despite significant species-specific differences, human MCP-1 protein bound to mononuclear cells from rabbit, dog, and pig but failed to bind to rat cells. GTPγS sensitivity of MCP-1 binding to isolated THP-1 membranes provided direct evidence that the MCP-1 receptor belongs to the family of G protein–coupled receptors. Binding and competition studies involving MIP-1α, MIP-1β, and MCP-1 suggested the existence of three receptor subtypes in human monocytes (105): one specific receptor for MIP-1α and MIP-1β, another specific receptor for MCP-1, and a third promiscous receptor that bound all three chemokines. Recently, a promiscous chemokine receptor has also been identified on the surface of red blood cells (106). Its major role might be the one of a clearance receptor for chemotactic and inflammatory peptides in the blood. Erythrocytes contain a single class of high-affinity binding sites for different chemokines with K_d values of 9.5 n*M* ± 3.6 or 15.4 n*M* ± 5.0, depending on whether the receptor was membrane-bound or solubilized (107). Interestingly, the erythrocyte chemokine receptor functions as receptor for the malarial parasite *Plasmodium vivax* (108). Almost nothing is known about MCP-1–specific receptors on human basophils, although MCP-1 induces the release of histamine in this cell type (109–111). There is one report indicating that chemokines activate basophils via G protein–coupled receptors (112). Cross-desensitization experiments suggest the existence of different C-C chemokine receptors on basophils. The first C-C chemokine–specific receptor has been cloned recently by the group of Thomas Schall by screening a cDNA library prepared from phorbol ester–treated human HL60 cells (113). The isolated cDNA encodes a 41-kDa protein with seven transmembrane-spanning domains characteristic for G protein–coupled receptors. The C-C chemokines MIP-1α, MIP-1β, RANTES, and MCP-1 all bind to the receptor, although with different affinities. The binding affinity did not correlate with the strength of the intracellular signal generated. Only RANTES and human MIP-1α increased the level of intracellular free Ca^{2+} at physiological concentrations. The available data suggest that the isolated cDNA may encode the human MIP-1α receptor.

SIGNAL TRANSDUCTION IN MCP-1 TARGET CELLS

In human monocytes, MCP-1 causes chemotaxis, a rapid (< 5-sec) and transient (≈ 1.5-min) increase in intracellular Ca^{2+} by opening of plasma membrane channels and a respiratory burst (H_2O_2 production) (114,115). The increase in cytosolic free calcium as well as MCP-1–induced chemotaxis could be blocked by *Bordetella pertussis* toxin (115), consistent with coupling of the MCP-1 receptor to a pertussis-toxin–sensitive G protein (see previous paragraph). Experiments with various protein kinase inhibitors suggested that a serine/threonine kinase, possibly PKC, may be involved in MCP-1 signal transduction. A recent study by Sozzani and coworkers (116) provides further evidence that MCP-1 does not release Ca^{2+} from intracellular stores but causes Ca^{2+} or Mn^{2+} influx independent of changes in intracellular Ca^{2+} concentrations and voltage-dependent Ca^{2+} channels. The Ca^{2+} influx may involve a receptor-activated channel. As already mentioned, MCP-1 is not only a chemotactic factor for monocytes but also a potent histamine-releasing factor in basophils (109–111). MCP-1–mediated degranulation of basophils occurs at low concentrations (ED_{50} = 3 to 10 n*M*) and is also characterized by an increase in free intracellular Ca^{2+} (110). The effects of MCP-1 on basophils, similar to those on monocytes, can be inhibited by *B. pertussis* toxin. Therefore, the same receptor and signal transduction pathway might be activated in monocytes and basophils.

MCP-1–REGULATED GENES IN TARGET CELLS

Little is known about MCP-1–regulated gene expression in monocytes. A recent study by Jiang and coworkers (117) addresses the question of whether MCP-1 can influence the expression of adhesion molecules on the surface of human monocytes. Immunofluorescence flow cytometry experiments showed that MCP-1 induces the expression of the β-2 integrins CD11c (p150,95 α-subunit) and CD11b (Mac-1 α-subunit). The expression of CD11a, very late activation Ag-4, and leukocyte adhesion molecule-1 was not influenced. Antibodies against β-2 and β-4 integrins were able to block MCP-1 induced chemotaxis of monocytes. Furthermore, MCP-1 was able to induce IL-1 and IL-6 production in human monocytes but failed to increase TNF in those cells. It can be expected that these are not the only genes regulated by MCP-1. So far, nothing is known about MCP-1–induced changes in gene activity in basophils, the second type of MCP-1 target cell.

EXPRESSION OF MCP-1 IN THE KIDNEY AND IN RENAL DISEASE

In the kidney, MCP-1 is expressed in endothelium, glomerular epithelial cells, mesangial cells (MC), and the thick ascending limb (118–122). IL-1β and phorbol myristate acetate, an activator of protein kinase C, stimulated synthesis and release of MCP-1 from bovine glomerular endothelial cells (123). In human renal cortical epithelial cells, MCP-1 production and mRNA levels are stimulated by IL-1β, TNF-α, LPS, or IFN-γ (124). In cultured rat glomerular epithelial cells, IL-1 and TNF-α increased expression of MCP-1, while dexamethasone suppressed it (119). TNF-α, IFN-γ, IL-1, thrombin, and phorbol esters also induced expression of MCP-1 mRNA and protein product in cultured MC (80,120,125,126). Moreover, IgG complexes increased MCP-1 mRNA and protein product in cultured murine MC (127). This response is specific for IgG complexes, since monomeric IgG or $F(ab')_2$ fragments of IgG are without effect. Occupation of the mesangial Fc-receptor by IgG complexes is sufficient and phagocytosis is not necessary for the induction of MCP-1 mRNA (127). NADPH-dependent generation of reactive oxygen products may serve as a second messenger system for the induction of MCP-1 by TNF-α and IgG complexes in cultured MC (94). Oxygen radical scavengers suppressed the TNF-α and IgG-induced transcription for MCP-1, whereas exogenous superoxide anion enhanced MCP-1 expression. In contrast, agents increasing intracellular cAMP—like forskolin or prostaglandin E_2 (PGE_2)—are negative transcriptional regulators of MCP-1 (80).

Expression of MCP-1 has been described in a number of experimental animal models and human diseases. These include atherosclerosis (128–131), pulmonary fibrosis (132,133), and immune complex–induced lung disease (134), arthritis (135–137), allergic encephalomyelitis (138), cardiac allograft rejection (139), psoriasis (140), and various malignancies (45,49,141–143). In all of these, the local generation of MCP-1 is believed to contribute to the observed M/M infiltration. A similar in vivo role can be demonstrated for MCP-1 in the kidney.

Perfusion of the isolated rat kidney with 1 μg/ml LPS for 40 min increased expression of steady-state mRNA levels for MCP-1 (144). In situ hybridizations localized this expression mainly to endothelial cells, but MCs probably also contributed to enhanced MCP-1 expression in the LPS-perfused isolated kidney. Induction of MCP-1 was also detected in an animal model of unilateral ureteral obstruction (145). This model is characterized by an infiltration of M/M into the tubulointerstitial microenvironment, which parallels the MCP-1 expression (145).

To further test whether induction of MCP-1 occurs directly in renal inflammation in vivo, the expression of MCP-1 and CSF-1 has recently been studied in various models of glomerulonephritis. In the Thy-1.1 model of proliferative glomerulonephritis, expression of glomerular MCP-1 markedly increased in the early phase of mesangial immune complex formation 30 min after induction of nephritis but was reduced during the subsequent phase of mesangiolysis (24 hr after nephritis induction) (146). During proliferative glomerulonephritis (5 and 21 days postinduction), MCP-1 mRNA increased compared to nonnephritic controls. Immunofluorescence microscopy of kidney sections revealed primarily mesangial localization of the MCP-1 protein (146). Decomplementation of rats prevented this induction of MCP-1 and prevented the glomerular influx of M/M. In contrast to MCP-1 mRNA and protein expression, steady-state mRNA levels of CSF-1 did not significantly change in this model of proliferative glomerulonephritis (146). In the model of puromycin-induced proteinuria and interstitial nephritis, initial glomerular expression of MCP-1 was followed by interstitial location of MCP-1 and M/M. In spite of the expression of MCP-1, a neutralizing antibody for MCP-1 failed to reduce the M/M infiltration. It remains to be determined if the antibody levels obtained locally in the kidney were sufficient to neutralize the MCP-1 (147). In rats with nephrotoxic serum nephritis, glomerular MCP-1 mRNA was increased and correlated with M/M infiltration (148,149). Staining for MCP-1 antigen is positive in glomeruli from patients with lupus nephritis, proliferative glomerulonephritis, and Wegener's granulomatosis but not in minimal change disease or membranous glomerulonephritis (148). Increased renal levels of MCP-1 were also observed in patients with HIV nephropathy (150).

Enhanced expression of chemoattractive cytokines is not limited to inflammatory renal disease. MCP-1 mRNA and protein expression is enhanced after renal ischemia induced by a 50-min period of renal artery clamping (122). Levels for MCP-1 peaked 48 hr after release of the clamping and remained elevated for up to 96 hr. MCP-1 transcripts were also increased in the remaining kidney 2 weeks after 5/6 nephrectomy (151). This expression was partly reduced by feeding the animals a low (6%)-protein diet.

SUMMARY

During the last decade, enough data have accumulated supporting a role for chemokines, including MCP-1, in tissue injury and leukocyte recruitment to the site of injury. MCP-1 gene expression is enhanced in many different cell types (e.g., fibroblasts, endothelial cells, smooth muscle cells, keratinocytes, mesangial cells, chondrocytes, osteoblasts, macrophages, monocytes, etc.) after treatment with mediators involved in inflammation (e.g., PDGF, IFN-γ, lipopolysaccharide, IL-1, TNF-α, phorbol esters, aggregated IgG, etc.). Furthermore, locally generated oxygen radicals may serve as a signal for MCP-1 induction. Stimulated cells secrete MCP-1, which is bound by target cells (monocytes, basophils) via specific cell surface receptors. The activated receptors transduce the signal from the cell surface to the nucleus, where specific genes (β-2 integrins, IL-1, IL-6, etc.) are repressed or activated. These changes in the activity of specific genes lead finally to the observed biological effects of MCP-1 (i.e., chemotaxis, adhesion, and transmigration of monocytes; release of H_2O_2 and lysosomal enzymes; degranulation of basophils; etc.). Thus, chemokines like MCP-1 play an important role in the recruitment of specific types of leukocytes to sites of tissue injury. The multiple mediators—including oxygen radicals capable of inducing MCP-1 expression—may help to explain leukocyte infiltration into damaged tissue irrespective of the exact ethiology. A model for such interactions in the glomerulus is shown in Figure 3. Further understanding of the regulation of chemokine gene expression at the molecular level and its exact mode of action should considerably enhance our understanding of various inflammatory diseases, including glomerular and interstitial nephritis.

NOTE ADDED IN PROOF

Since submission of the manuscript several important papers have been published, which will be briefly summarized. The MCP-1 cDNA from pig has been isolated (171). Ueda and colleagues analyzed the transcriptional regulation of the human *MCP-1* gene and demonstrated the involvement of NF-κB and Sp1 (172). Bretz et al. showed that in lymphoblasts ectopic expression of C/EBP-related protein 2 is sufficient to confer inducibility by LPS (173). The group of Rollins published two papers dealing with structure/function relationship of human and murine MCP-1 protein (174,175). Carr et al. reported that MCP-1 acts also as a chemotactic factor for certain T lymphocytes (176). Rapid release of arachidonic acid from human monocytes was described as another new biological effect of MCP-1 (177). With respect to MCP-1 inducibility, it was shown that MCP-1 can be induced by IL-4 in mouse peritoneal macrophages (178) and by IFN-γ (179) as well as thrombin in human mesangial cells (180). There were also some new findings on the repression of the *MCP-1* gene. In mouse osteoblastic cells, the induction of MCP-1 by TNF-α can be suppressed by retinoic acid (181). In mouse peritoneal macrophages, MCP-1 induction by LPS is selectively inhibited by IFN-γ (182).

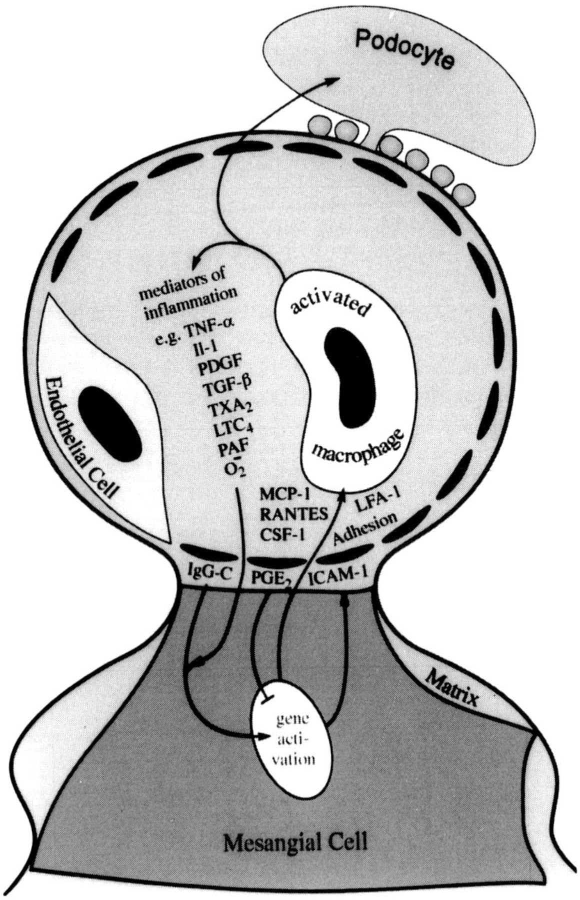

Figure 3 Model for the potential roles of inflammatory mediators, chemokines, and adhesion molecules in the interaction of circulating monocytes/macrophages with glomerular cells during glomerular injury. The scheme shows a glomerular capillary with the podocyte on the outside of the basement membrane and the fenestrated endothelium and the mesangial cell on the inside of the basement membrane. Activation of mesangial cells leads to release of chemokinetic cytokines such as MCP-1, RANTES, and CSF-1 and surface expression of ICAM-1. This, in turn, leads to chemoattraction, activation, and adhesion of macrophages. The release of mediators of inflammation causes further cell activation and influences the function of mesangial, endothelial, and epithelial cells. PGE_2 may act as a negative regulator in this scheme. A similar model can be envisioned for the interaction of circulating leukocytes in peritubular capillaries as well as epithelial, interstitial, and tubular cells during tubular and interstitial injury.

Concerning the MCP-1 receptor, cDNAs encoding the human receptor have been isolated (183). Finally, an extensive review on chemokines with more than 400 references was published (184).

REFERENCES

1. Couser WG. The pathogenesis of glomerulonephritis. Kidney Int 1993; 44(Suppl 42):S-19–S-26.
2. Schreiner GF. The role of the macrophage in glomerular injury. Semin Nephrol 1991; 11:268–275.
3. Schreiner GF, Contran RS, Pardo V, Unanue ER. A mononuclear cell component in experimental immunological glomerulonephritis. J Exp Med 1978; 1447:369–384.
4. Holdsworth SR, Neale TJ, Wilson CB. Abrogation of macrophage-dependent injury in experimental glomerulonephritis in the rabbit. J Clin Invest 1981; 68:686–698.

5. Diamond JR, Karnovsky MJ. A putative role of hypercholesterolemia in progressive glomerular injury. Annu Rev Med 1992; 43:83–92.
6. Schlondorff D. Cellular mechanisms of lipid injury in the glomerulus. Am J Kidney Dis 1993; 22:72–82.
7. Young B, Johnson R, Alpers C, et al. Mesangial cell proliferation precedes development of glomerulosclerosis in experimental diabetic nephropathy (abstr). J Am Soc Nephrol 1992; 3:770.
8. van Goor H, van der Horst M, Fidler V, Grond J. Glomerular macrophage modulation affects mesangial expansion in the rat after renal ablation. Lab Invest 1992; 66:564–571.
9. Schreiner GF, Harris KPG, Purkerson ML, Klahr S. Immunological aspects of acute ureteral obstruction: immune cell infiltrate in the kidney. Kidney Int 1988; 34:4487–4493.
10. Marcussen N. Atubular glomeruli in renal artery stenosis. Lab Invest 1991; 65:558–565.
11. Johnson RJ, Alpers CE, Yoshimura A, et al. Renal injury from angiotensin II-mediated hypertension. Hypertension 1992; 19:464–474.
12. Neilson EG. Pathogenesis and therapy of interstitial nephritis [clinical conference]. Kidney Int 1989; 35:1257–1270.
13. Diamond JR, Anderson S. Irreversible tubulointerstitial damage associated with chronic aminonucleoside nephrosis: Amelioration by angiotensin I converting enzyme inhibition. Am J Pathol 1990; 137:1323–1332.
14. Rao KV. Diagnosis of renal transplant rejection in the cyclosporine era. Curr Opin Nephrol Hypertens 1992; 1:280–1290.
15. Nathan CF. Secretory products of macrophages. J Clin Invest 1987; 79:319–326.
16. Lianos EA, Andres GA, Dunn MJ. Glomerular prostaglandin and thromboxane synthesis in rat nephrotoxic serum nephritis. J Clin Invest 1983; 72:14439–14488.
17. Storck JE, Dunn MJ. Hemodynamic roles of thromboxane A2 and prostaglandin E2 in glomerulonephritis. J Pharmacol Exp Ther 1985; 233:672–678.
18. Radeke HH, Resch K. The inflammatory function of renal glomerular mesangial cells and their interaction with the cellular immune system. Am J Kidney Dis 1992; 20:1–17.
19. Oberle GP, Niemeyer J, Thaiss F, et al. Increased oxygen radical and eicosanoid formation in immune-mediated mesangial cell injury. Kidney Int 1992; 42:69–74.
20. Coimbra T, Wiggins R, Noh JW, et al. Transforming growth factor-β production in anti-glomerular basement membrane disease in the rabbit. Am J Pathol 1991; 138:223–234.
21. Sharma K, Ziyadeh FN. The transforming growth factor-β system and the kidney. Semin Nephrol 1993; 13:116–128.
22. Nath KA. Tubulointerstitial changes as a major determinant in the progression of renal damage. Am J Kidney Dis 1992; 20:1–17.
23. Metchnikoff E. Lectures on the Comparative Pathology of Inflammation. London: Kegan, Paul, 1893:147.
24. Tipping PG, Boyce NW, Holdsworth SR. Relative contributions of chemoattractant and terminal components of complement to anti-glomerular basement membrane (GBM) glomerulonephritis. Clin Exp Immunol 1989; 78:444–448.
25. Baud L, Sraer J, Delarue F, et al. Lipoxygenase products mediate the attachment of rat macrophages to glomeruli in vitro. Kidney Int 1985; 27:855–863.
26. Gimbrone MA, Brock AF, Schafer AI. Leukotriene B4 stimulates polymorphonuclear leukocytes adhesion to cultured vascular epithelial cells. J Clin Invest 1984; 74:1552–1555.
27. Kennedy TL, Merrow M, Phillips SM, et al. Macrophage chemotaxis in anti-tubular basement membrane induced interstitial nephritis in guinea pigs. Clin Immunol Immunopathol 1985; 243–248.
28. Miller MD, Krangel MS. Biology and biochemistry of the chemokines: A family of chemotactic and inflammatory cytokines. Crit Rev Immunol 1992; 12:17–46.
29. Kawahara RS, Deuel TF. Platelet-derived growth factor-inducible gene JE is a member of a family of small inducible genes related to platelet factor 4. J Biol Chem 1989; 264:679–682.
30. Stoeckle MY, Barker KA. Two burgeoning families of platelet factor 4-related proteins: Mediators of the inflammatory response. New Biol 1990; 2:313–323.
31. Oppenheim JJ, Zachariae CO, Mukaida N, Matsushima K. Properties of the novel proinflammatory supergene "intercrine" cytokine family. Annu Rev Immunol 1991; 9:617–648.
32. Schall TJ. Biology of the RANTES/SIS cytokine family. Cytokine 1991; 3:165–183.
33. Baggiolini M, Dahinden CA. CC chemokines in allergic inflammation. Immunol Today 1994; 15:127–133.
34. Yoshimura T, Robinson EA, Tanaka S, et al. Purification and amino acid analysis of two human glioma-derived monocyte chemoattractants. J Exp Med 1989; 169:1449–1459.
35. Van Damme J, Proost P, Lenaerts JP, Opdenakker G. Structural and functional identification of two human, tumor-derived monocyte chemotactic proteins (MCP-2 and MCP-3) belonging to the chemokine family. J Exp Med 1992; 176:59–65.
36. Minty A, Chalon P, Guillemot JC, et al. Molecular cloning of the MCP-3 chemokine gene and regulation of its expression. Eur Cytokine Netw 1993; 4:99–110.
37. Opdenakker G, Froyen G, Fiten P, et al. Human monocyte chemotactic protein-3 (MCP-3): Molecular

cloning of the cDNA and comparison with other chemokines. Biochem Biophys Res Commun 1993; 191:535–542.
38. Miller MD, Wilson SD, Dorf ME, et al. Sequence and chromosomal location of the I-309 gene: Relationship to genes encoding a family of inflammatory cytokines. J Immunol 1990; 145:2737–2744.
39. Schall TJ, Jongstra J, Dyer BJ, et al. A human T cell-specific molecules is a member of a new gene family. J Immunol 1988; 141:1018–1025.
40. Obaru K, Fukuda M, Maeda S, Shimada K. A cDNA clone used to study mRNA inducible in human tonsillar lymphocytes by a tumor promoter. J Biochem Tokyo 1986; 99:885–894.
41. Lipes MA, Napolitano M, Jeang KT, et al. Identification, cloning, and characterization of an immune activation gene. Proc Natl Acad Sci USA 1988; 85:9704–9708.
42. Kulmburg PA, Huber NE, Scheer BJ, et al. Immunoglobulin E plus antigen challenge induces a novel intercrine/chemokine in mouse mast cells. J Exp Med 1992; 176:1773–1778.
43. Heinrich JN, Ryseck RP, Macdonald BH, Bravo R. The product of a novel growth factor-activated gene, fic, is a biologically active "C-C"-type cytokine. Mol Cell Biol 1993; 13:2020–2030.
44. Robinson EA, Yoshimura T, Leonard EJ, et al. Complete amino acid sequence of a human monocyte chemoattractant, a putative mediator of cellular immune reactions. Proc Natl Acad Sci USA 1989; 86:1850–1854.
45. Bottazzi B, Colotta F, Sica A, et al. A chemoattractant expressed in human sarcoma cells (tumor-derived chemotactic factor, TDCF) is identical to monocyte chemoattractant protein-1/monocyte chemotactic and activating factor (MCP-1/MCAF). Int J Cancer 1990; 45:795–797.
46. Rollins BJ, Morrison ED, Stiles CD. Cloning and expression of JE, a gene inducible by platelet-derived growth factor and whose product has cytokine-like properties. Proc Natl Acad Sci USA 1988; 85:3738–3742.
47. Matsushima K, Larsen CG, DuBois GC. Oppenheim JJ. Purification and characterization of a novel monocyte chemotactic and activating factor produced by a human myelomonocytic cell line. J Exp Med 1989; 169:1485–1490.
48. Furutani Y, Nomura H, Notake M, et al. Cloning and sequencing of the cDNA for human monocyte chemotactic and activating factor (MCAF). Biochem Biophys Res Commun 1989; 159:249–255.
49. Graves DT, Jiang YL, Williamson MJ, Valente AJ. Identification of monocyte chemotactic activity produced by malignant cells. Science 1989; 245:1490–1493.
50. Chang HC, Hsu F, Freeman GJ, et al. Cloning and expression of a γ-interferon-inducible gene in monocytes: A new member of a cytokine gene family. Int Immunol 1989; 1:388–399.
51. Lee TH, Lee GW, Ziff EB, Vilcek J. Isolation and characterization of eight tumor necrosis factor-induced gene sequences from human fibroblasts. Mol Cell Biol 1990; 10:1982–1988.
52. Matsushima K, Oppenheim JJ. Interleukin 8 and MCAF: Novel inflammatory cytokines inducible by IL-1 and TNF. Cytokine 1989; 1:2–13.
53. Leonard EJ, Yoshimura T. Human monocyte chemoattractant protein-1 (MCP-1). Immunol Today 1990; 11:97–101.
54. Rollins BJ. JE/MCP-1: An early-response gene encodes a monocyte-specific cytokine. Cancer Cells 1991; 3:517–524.
55. Yoshimura T, Leonard EJ. Human monocyte chemoattractant protein-1: Structure and function. Cytokines 1992; 4:131–152.
56. Mukaida N, Harada A, Yasumoto K, Matsushima K. Properties of proinflammatory cell type-specific leukocyte chemotactic cytokines, interleukin 8 (IL-8) and monocyte chemotactic and activating factor (MCAF). Microbiol Immunol 1992; 36:773–789.
57. Matsushima K, Baldwin ET, Mukaida N. Interleukin-8 and MCAF: Novel leukocyte recruitment and activating cytokines. Chem Immunol 1992; 51:236–265.
58. Cochran BH, Reffel AC, Stiles CD. Molecular cloning of gene sequences regulated by platelet-derived growth factor. Cell 1983; 33:939–947.
59. Rollins BJ, Stier P, Ernst T, Wong GG. The human homolog of the JE gene encodes a monocyte secretory protein. Mol Cell Biol 1989; 9:4687–4695.
60. Yoshimura T, Yuhki N, Moore SK, et al. Human monocyte chemoattractant protein-1 (MCP-1): Full-length cDNA cloning, expression in mitogen-stimulated blood mononuclear leukocytes, and sequence similarity to mouse competence gene JE. FEBS Lett 1989; 244:487–493.
61. Timmers HTM, Pronk GJ, Bos JL, van der Eb AJ. Analysis of the rat JE gene promoter identifies an AP-1 binding site essential for basal expression but not for TPA induction. Nucleic Acids Res 1990; 18:23–34.
62. Yoshimura T, Takeya M, Takahashi K. Molecular cloning of rat monocyte chemoattractant protein-1 (MCP-1) and its expression in rat spleen cells and tumor cell lines. Biochem Biophys Res Commun 1991; 174:504–509.
63. Yoshimura T, Yuhki N. Neutrophil attractant/activation protein-1 and monocyte chemoattractant protein-1 in rabbit. cDNA cloning and their expression in spleen cells. J Immunol 1991; 146:3483–3483.

64. Wempe F, Henschen A, Scheit KH. Gene expression and cDNA cloning identified a major basic protein constituent of bovine seminal plasma as bovine monocyte-chemoattractant protein-1 (MCP-1). DNA Cell Biol 1991; 10:671–679.
65. Yoshimura T. cDNA cloning of guinea pig monocyte chemoattractant protein-1 and expression of the recombinant protein. J Immunol 1993; 150:5025–5032.
66. Shyy YJ, Li YS, Kolattukudy PE. Structure of human monocyte chemotactic protein gene and its regulation by TPA. Biochem Biophys Res Commun 1990; 169:346–351.
67. Shaw G, Kamen R. A conserved AU sequence from the 3′ untranslated region of GM-CSF mRNA mediates selective mRNA degradation. Cell 1986; 46:659–667.
68. Caput D, Butler B, Hartog K, et al. Identification of a common nucleotide sequence in the 3′-untranslated region of mRNA molecules specifying inflammatory mediators. Proc Natl Acad Sci USA 1986; 83:1670–1674.
69. Rollins BJ, Morton CC, Ledbetter DH, et al. Assignment of the human small inducible cytokine A2 gene, SCYA2 (encoding JE or MCP-1), to 17q11.2-12: Evolutionary relatedness of cytokines clustered at the same locus. Genomics 1991; 10:489–492.
70. Wilson SD, Billings PR, D'Eustachio P, et al. Clustering of cytokine genes on mouse chromosome 11. J Exp Med 1990; 171:1301–1314.
71. Yoshimura T, Leonard EJ. Secretion by human fibroblasts of monocyte chemoattractant protein-1, the product of gene JE. J Immunol 1990; 144:2377–2383.
72. Jiang Y, Valente AJ, Williamson MJ, et al. Post-translational modification of a monocyte-specific chemoattractant synthesized by glioma, osteosarcoma, and vascular smooth muscle cells. J Biol Chem 1990; 265:18318–18321.
73. Jiang Y, Tabak LA, Valente AJ, Graves DT. Initial characterization of the carbohydrate structure of MCP-1. Biochem Biophys Res Commun 1991; 178:1400–1404.
74. Mukaida N, Hishinuma A, Zachariae CO, et al. Regulation of human interleukin 8 gene expression and binding of several other members of the intercrine family to receptors for interleukin-8. Adv Exp Med Biol 1991; 305:31–38.
75. Kawahara RS, Deng ZW, Deuel TF. Glucocorticoids inhibit the transcriptional induction of JE, a platelet-derived growth factor-inducible gene. J Biol Chem 1991; 266:13261–13266.
76. Poon M, Megyesi J, Green RS, et al. In vivo and in vitro inhibition of JE gene expression by glucocorticoids. J Biol Chem 1991; 266:22375–22379.
77. Brach MA, Gruss HJ, Riedel D, et al. Effect of antiinflammatory agents on synthesis of MCP-1/JE transcripts by human blood monocytes. Mol Pharmacol 1992; 42:63–68.
78. Villiger PM, Terkeltaub R, Lotz M. Monocyte chemoattractant protein-1 (MCP-1) expression in human articular cartilage: Induction by peptide regulatory factors and differential effects of dexamethasone and retinoic acid. J Clin Invest 1992; 90:488–496.
79. Martin CA, Dorf ME. Differential regulation of interleukin-6, macrophage inflammatory protein-1, and JE/MCP-1 cytokine expression in macrophage cell lines. Cell Immunol 1991; 135:245–258.
80. Satriano JA, Hora K, Shan Z, et al. Regulation of monocyte chemoattractant protein-1 and macrophage colony-stimulating factor-1 by IFN-γ, tumor necrosis factor-α, IgG aggregates, and cAMP in mouse mesangial cells. J Immunol 1993; 150:1971–1978.
81. Rolfe MW, Kunkel SL, Standiford TJ, et al. Expression and regulation of human pulmonary fibroblast-derived monocyte chemotactic peptide-1. Am J Physiol 1992; 263(5 Pt 1):pL536–545.
82. Parhami F, Fang ZT, Fogelman AM, et al. Minimally modified low density lipoprotein-induced inflammatory responses in endothelial cells are mediated by cyclic adenosine monophosphate. J Clin Invest 1993; 92:471–478.
83. Qureshi SA, Alexandropoulos K, Joseph CK, et al. Cholera toxin induces expression of the immediate-early response gene JE via a cyclic AMP-independent signaling pathway. Mol Cell Biol 1991; 11: 102–107.
84. Hall DJ, Stiles CD. Platelet-derived growth factor-inducible genes respond differentially to at least two distinct intracellular messengers. J Biol Chem 1987; 262:15302–15308.
85. Prpic V, Yu S-F, Figueiredo F, et al. Role of Na^+/H^+ exchange by interferon-γ in enhanced expression of JE and I-Aβ genes. Science 1989; 244:469–471.
86. Larner AC, David M, Feldman GM, Igarashi K, et al. Tyrosine phosphorylation of DNA binding proteins by multiple cytokines. Science 1993; 261:1730–1733.
87. Ruff JS, Chen K, Cohen S. Induction by EGF and interferon-γ of tyrosine phosphorylated DNA binding proteins in mouse liver nuclei. Science 1993; 261:1733–1736.
88. Sadowski HB, Shuai K, Darnell JJ, Gilman MZ. A common nuclear signal transduction pathway activated by growth factor and cytokine receptors. Science 1993; 261:1739–1744.
89. Shuai K, Stark GR, Kerr IM, Darnell JJ. A single phosphotyrosine residue of Stat91 required for gene activation by interferon-γ. Science 1993; 261:1744–1746.

90. Silvennoinen O, Schindler C, Schlessinger J, Levy DE. Ras-independent growth factor signaling by transcription factor tyrosine phosphorylation [see comments]. Science 1993; 261:1736–1739.
91. Müller M, Briscoe J, Laxton C, et al. The protein tyrosine kinase JAK1 complements defects in interferon-α/β and -γ signal transduction. Nature 1993; 366:129–135.
92. Watling D, Guschin D, Müller M, et al. Complementation by the protein tyrosine kinase JAK2 of a mutant cell line defective in the interferon-γ signal transduction pathway. Nature 1993; 366:166–170.
93. Shyy YJ, Li YS, Kolattukudy PE. Activation of MCP-1 gene expression is mediated through multiple signaling pathways. Biochem Biophys Res Commun 1993; 192:693–699.
94. Satriano JA, Shuldiner M, Hora K, et al. Oxygen radicals as second messengers for expression of the monocyte chemoattractant protein, JE/MCP-1, and the monocyte colony-stimulating factor, CSF-1, in response to tumor necrosis factor-α and immunoglobulin G: Evidence for involvement of reduced nicotinamide adenine dinucleotide phosphate (NADPH)-dependent oxidase. J Clin Invest 1993; 92:1564–1571.
95. Freter RR, Irminger JC, Porter JA, et al. A novel 7-nucleotide motif located in 3′ untranslated sequences of the immediate-early gene set mediates platelet-derived growth factor induction of the JE gene. Mol Cell Biol 1992; 12:5288–5300.
96. Hanazawa S, Takeshita A, Amano S, et al. Tumor necrosis factor-α induces expression of monocyte chemoattractant JE via fos and jun genes in clonal osteoblastic MC3T3-E1 cells. J Biol Chem 1993; 268:9526–9532.
97. Sen R, Baltimore D. Inducibility of kappa immunoglobulin enhancer-binding protein NF-κB by a posttranslational mechanism. Cell 1986; 47:921–928.
98. Osborn L, Kunkel S, Nabel GJ. Tumor necrosis factor α and interleukin 1 stimulate the human immunodeficiency virus enhancer by activation of the nuclear factor κ B. Proc Natl Acad Sci USA 1989; 86:2336–2340.
99. Perkins ND, Edwards NL, Duckett CS, et al. A cooperative interaction between NF-κB and Sp1 is required for HIV-1 enhancer activation. EMBO J 1993; 12:3551–3558.
100. Stein B, Baldwin AJ, Ballard DW, et al. Cross-coupling of the NF-κB p65 and Fos/Jun transcription factors produces potentiated biological function. EMBO J 1993; 12:3879–3891.
101. Yoshimura T, Leonard EJ. Identification of high affinity receptors for human monocyte chemoattractant protein-1 on human monocytes. J Immunol 1990; 145:292–297.
102. Valente AJ, Rozek MM, Schwartz CJ, Graves DT. Characterization of monocyte chemotactic protein-1 binding to human monocytes. Biochem Biophys Res Commun 1991; 176:309–314.
103. Beall CJ, Mahajan S, Kollatukudy PE. Conversion of monocyte chemoattractant protein-1 into a neutrophil attractant by substitution of two amino acids. J Biol Chem 1992; 267:3455–3459.
104. Van Riper G, Siciliano S, Fischer PA, et al. Characterization and species distribution of high affinity GTP-coupled receptors for human rantes and monocyte chemoattractant protein 1. J Exp Med 1993; 177:851–856.
105. Wang JM, Sherry B, Fivash MJ, et al. Human recombinant macrophage inflammatory protein-1α and -β and monocyte chemotactic and activating factor utilize common and unique receptors on human monocytes. J Immunol 1993; 150:3022–3029.
106. Neote K, Darbonne W, Ogez J, et al. Identification of a promiscuous inflammatory peptide receptor on the surface of red blood cells. J Biol Chem 1993; 268:12247–12249.
107. Horuk R, Colby TJ, Darbonne WC, et al. The human erythrocyte inflammatory peptide (chemokine) receptor: Biochemical characterization, solubilization, and development of a binding assay for the soluble receptor. Biochemistry 1993; 32:5733–5738.
108. Horuk R, Chitnis CE, Darbonne WC, et al. A receptor for the malarial parasite Plasmodium vivax: The erythrocyte chemokine receptor. Science 1993; 261:1182–1184.
109. Alam R, Forsythe PA, Lett BM, Grant JA. Interleukin-8 and RANTES inhibit basophil histamine release induced with monocyte chemotactic and activating factor/monocyte chemoattractant peptide-1 and histamine releasing factor. Am J Respir Cell Mol Biol 1992; 7:427–433.
110. Bischoff SC, Krieger M, Brunner T, Dahinden CA. Monocyte chemotactic protein 1 is a potent activator of human basophils. J Exp Med 1992; 175:1271–1275.
111. Kuna P, Reddigari SR, Schall TJ, et al. RANTES, a monocyte and T lymphocyte chemotactic cytokine releases histamine from human basophils. J Immunol 1992; 149:636–642.
112. Bischoff SC, Krieger M, Brunner T, et al. RANTES and related chemokines activate human basophil granulocytes through different G protein-coupled receptors. Eur J Immunol 1993; 23:761–767.
113. Neote K, DiGregorio D, Mak JY, et al. Molecular cloning, functional expression, and signaling characteristics of a C-C chemokine receptor. Cell 1993; 72:415–425.
114. Rollins BJ, Walz A, Baggiolini M. Recombinant human MCP-1/JE induces chemotaxis, calcium flux, and the respiratory burst in human monocytes. Blood 1991; 78:1112–1116.
115. Sozzani S, Luini W, Molino M, et al. The signal transduction pathway involved in the migration induced by a monocyte chemotactic cytokine. J Immunol 1991; 147:2215–2221.

116. Sozzani S, Molino M, Locati M, et al. Receptor-activated calcium influx in human monocytes exposed to monocyte chmotactic protein-1 and related cytokines. J Immunol 1993; 150:1544–1553.
117. Jiang Y, Beller DI, Frendl G, Graves DT. Monocyte chemoattractant protein-1 regulates adhesion molecule expression and cytokine production in human monocytes. J Immun 1992; 148:2423–2428.
118. Ohmori Y, Wyner L, Narumi S, et al. Tumor necrosis factor-α induces cell type and tissue-specific expression of chemoattractant cytokines in vivo. Am J Pathol 1993; 142:861–870.
119. Natori Y, Sekiguchi M, Natori Y, et al. Gene expression of monocyte chemoattractant protein-1 (MCP-1) by cytokine-treated glomerular epithelial cells (abstr). J Am Soc Nephrol 1993; 4:623.
120. Grandaliano G, Valente AJ, Abboud HE. A novel biologic activity of thrombin: Stimulation of monocyte chemotactic protein (MCP-1) production (abstr). J Am Soc Neprhol 1993; 4:604.
121. Taubman MB, Rollins BJ, Poon M, et al. JE mRNA accumulates rapidly in aortic injury and in platelet-derived growth factor-stimulated vascular smooth muscle cells. Circ Res 1992; 70:314–325.
122. Safirstein R, Megyesi J, Saggi SJ, et al. Expression of cytokine-like genes JE and KC is increased during renal ischemia. Am J Physiol 1991; 261(6 Pt 2):pF1095–1101.
123. Kakizaki Y, Sugimoto K, Waga S, Yokoyama M. Production of monocyte chemoattractant protein-1 (MCP-1) by bovine glomerular endothelial cells is enhanced by interleukin-1 (IL-1) and phorbol myristate acetate (PMA) (abstr). J Am Soc Nephrol 1993; 4:608.
124. Schmouder RL, Strieter RM, Kunkel SL. Interferon-γ regulation of human renal cortical epithelial cell-derived monocyte chemotactic peptide-1. Kidney Int 1993; 44:43–49.
125. Rovin B, Tan L. Intracellular regulation of interleukin-1 (IL-1)-induced monocyte chemoattractant protein-1 (MCP-1) in human mesangial cells (abstr). J Am Soc Nephrol 1993; 4:498.
126. Rovin BH, Yoshimura T, Tan L. Cytokine-induced production of monocyte chemoattractant protein-1 by cultured human mesangial cells. J Immunol 1992; 148:2148–2153.
127. Hora K, Satriano JA, Santiago A, et al. Receptors for IgG complexes activate synthesis of monocyte chemoattractant peptide 1 and colony-stimulating factor 1. Proc Natl Acad Sci USA 1992; 89:1745–1749.
128. Yla HS, Lipton BA, Rosenfeld ME, et al. Expression of monocyte chemoattractant protein 1 in macrophage-rich areas of human and rabbit atherosclerotic lesions. Proc Natl Acad Sci USA 1991; 88:5252–5256.
129. Yu X, Dluz S, Graves DT, et al. Elevated expression of monocyte chemoattractant protein 1 by vascular smooth muscle cells in hypercholesterolemic primates. Proc Natl Acad Sci USA 1992; 89:6953–6957.
130. Takeya M, Yoshimura T, Leonard EJ, Takahashi K. Detection of monocyte chemoattractant protein-1 in human atherosclerotic lesions by an anti-monocyte chemoattractant protein-1 monoclonal antibody. Hum Pathol 1993; 24:534–539.
131. Nelken NA, Coughlin SR, Gordon D, Wilcox JN. Monocyte chemoattractant protein-1 in human atheromatous plaques. J Clin Invest 1991; 88:1121–1127.
132. Antoniades HN, Neville GJ, Galanopoulos T, et al. Expression of monocyte chemoattractant protein 1 mRNA in human idiopathic pulmonary fibrosis. Proc Natl Acad Sci USA 1992; 89:5371–5375.
133. Standiford TJ, Rolfe MR, Kunkel SL, et al. Altered production and regulation of monocyte chemoattractant protein-1 from pulmonary fibroblasts isolated from patients with idiopathic pulmonary fibrosis. Chest 1993; 103(2 Suppl):133S.
134. Brieland JK, Jones ML, Clarke SJ, et al. Effect of acute inflammatory lung injury on the expression of monocyte chemoattractant protein-1 (MCP-1) in rat pulmonary alveolar macrophages. Am J Respir Cell Mol Biol 1992; 7:134–139.
135. Akahoshi T, Wada C, Endo H, et al. Expression of monocyte chemotactic and activating factor in rheumatoid arthritis: Regulation of its production in synovial cells by interleukin-1 and tumor necrosis factor. Arthritis Rheum 1993; 36:762–771.
136. Koch AE, Kunkel SL, Harlow LA, et al. Enhanced production of monocyte chemoattractant protein-1 in rheumatoid arthritis. J Clin Invest 1992; 90:772–779.
137. Villiger PM, Terkeltaub R, Lotz M. Production of monocyte chemoattractant protein-1 by inflamed synovial tissue and cultured synoviocytes. J Immunol 1992; 149:722–727.
138. Hulkower K, Brosnan CF, Aquino DA, et al. Expression of CSF-1, c-fms, and MCP-1 in the central nervous system of rats with experimental allergic encephalomyelitis. J Immunol 1993; 150:2525–2533.
139. Russell ME, Adams DH, Wyner LR, et al. Early and persistent induction of monocyte chemoattractant protein 1 in rat cardiac allografts. Proc Natl Acad Sci USA 1993; 90:6086–6090.
140. Gillitzer R, Wolff K, Tong D, et al. MCP-1 mRNA expression in basal keratinocytes of psoriatic lesions. J Invest Dermatol 1993; 101:127–131.
141. Graves DT, Valente AJ. Monocyte chemotactic proteins from human tumor cells. Biochem Pharmacol 1991; 41:333–337.
142. Graves DT, Barnhill R, Galanopoulos T, Antoniades HN. Expression of monocyte chemotactic protein-1 in human melanoma in vivo. Am J Pathol 1992; 140:9–14.

143. Rollins BJ, Sunday ME. Suppression of tumor formation in vivo by expression of the JE gene in malignant cells. Mol Cell Biol 1991; 11:3125–3131.
144. Xia Y, Feng L, Yoshimura T, Wilson CB. LPS-induced MCP-1, IL-1 β, and TNF-α mRNA expression in isolated erythrocyte-perfused rat kidney. Am J Physiol 1993; 264(5 Pt 2):pF774–780.
145. Restrepo N, Kees-Folts D, Ding G, et al. Tubulointerstitial macrophages, transforming growth factor β and monocyte chemoattractant peptide-1 after unilateral ureteral obstruction (abstr). J Am Soc Nephrol 1993; 4:781.
146. Stahl RA, Thaiss F, Disser M, et al. Increased expression of monocyte chemoattractant protein-1 in anti-thymocyte antibody-induced glomerulonephritis. Kidney Int 1993; 44:1036–1047.
147. Eddy AE, Warren JS. Expression and function of monocyte chemoattractant protein-1 (MCP-1) in puromycin aminonucleoside nephrosis (abstr). J Am Soc Nephrol 1993; 4:600.
148. Rumancik M, Rovin B. Glomerular expression of monocyte chemoattractant protein-1 (MCP-1) in experimental and human glomerulonephritis (abstr). J Am Soc Nephrol 1993; 4:630.
149. Tam FWK, Karkar Am, Largen PJ, et al. Glomerular expression of rat macrophage inflammatory protein-2 (MIP-2) in vitro and in vivo (abstr). J Am Soc Nephrol 1993; 4:637.
150. Kimmel PL, Bodi I, Abraham A, Phillips TM. Increased renal tissue cytokines in human HIV nephropathy (abstr). J Am Soc Nephrol 1993; 4:279.
151. Schiller-Moran B, DeLeo M, Warren E, et al. Modulation of monocyte chemoattractant protein (MCP-1) expression in the remnant kidney model by a low protein diet (abstr). J Am Soc Nephrol 1993; 4:632.
152. Zipfel PF, Balke J, Irving SG, et al. Mitogenic activation of human T cells induces two closely related genes which share structural similarities with a new family of secreted factors. J Immunol 1989; 142:1582–1590.
153. Introna M, Bast RCJ, Tannenbaum CS, et al. The effect of LPS on expression of the early competence genes JE and KC in murine peritoneal macrophages. J Immunol 1987; 138:3891–3896.
154. Strieter RM, Chensue SW, Standiford TJ, et al. Disparate gene expression of chemotactic cytokines by human mononuclear phagocytes. Biochem Biophys Res Commun 1990; 166:886–891.
155. Kaczmarek B, Calabretta B, Baserga R. Expression of cell cycle dependent genes in phytohemagglutinin-stimulated human lymphocytes. Proc Natl Acad Sci USA 1985; 82:5375–5379.
156. Larsen CG, Zachariae CO, Oppenheim JJ, Matsushima K. Production of monocyte chemotactic and activating factor (MCAF) by human dermal fibroblasts in response to interleukin 1 or tumor necrosis factor. Biochem Biophys Res Commun 1989; 160:1403–1408.
157. Zullo JN, Cochran BH, Huang AS, Stiles CD. Platelet-derived growth factor and double-stranded ribonucleic acids stimulate expression of the same genes in 3T3 cells. Cell 1985; 43:793–800.
158. Strieter RM, Wiggins R, Phan SH, et al. Monocyte chemotactic protein gene expression by cytokine-treated human fibroblasts and endothelial cells. Biochem Biophys Res Commun 1989; 162:694–700.
159. Sica A, Wang JM, Colotta F, et al. Monocyte chemotactic and activating factor gene expression induced in endothelial cells by IL-1 and tumor necrosis factor. J Immunol 1990; 144:3034–3038.
160. Rollins BJ, Yoshimura T, Leonard EJ, Pober JS. Cytokine-activated human endothelial cells synthesize and secrete a monocyte chemoattractant, MCP-1/JE. Am J Pathol 1990; 136:1229–1233.
161. Rollins BJ, Pober JS. Interleukin-4 induces the synthesis and secretion of MCP-1/JE by human endothelial cells. Am J Pathol 1991; 138:1315–1319.
162. Cushing SD, Berliner JA, Valente AJ, et al. Minimally modified low density lipoprotein induces monocyte chemotactic protein 1 in human endothelial cells and smooth muscle cells. Proc Natl Acad Sci USA 1990; 87:5134–5138.
163. Barker JNWN, Jones ML, Swenson CL, et al. Monocyte chemotaxis and activating factor production by keratinocytes in response to IFN-γ. J Immunol 1991; 146:1192–1197.
164. Elner SG, Strieter RM, Elner VM, et al. Monocyte chemotactic protein gene expression by cytokine-treated human retinal pigment epithelial cells. Lab Invest 1991; 64:819–825.
165. Standiford TJ, Kunkel SL, Phan SH, et al. Alveolar macrophage-derived cytokines induce monocyte chemoattractant protein-1 expression from human pulmonary type II-like epithelial cells. J Biol Chem 1991; 266:9912–9918.
166. Williams SR, Jiang Y, Cochran D, et al. Regulated expression of monocyte chemoattractant protein-1 in normal human osteoblastic cells. Am J Physiol 1992; 263:C194–C199.
167. Takeshita A, Hanazawa S, Amano S, et al. IL-1 induces expression of monocyte chemoattractant JE in clonal mouse osteoblastic cell line MC3T3-E1. J Immunol 1993; 150:1554–1562.
168. Ransohoff RM, Hamilton TA, Tani M, et al. Astrocyte expression of mRNA encoding cytokines IP-10 and JE/MCP-1 in experimental autoimmune encephalomyelitis. FASEB J 1993; 7:592–600.
169. Zoja C, Wang JM, Bettoni S, et al. Interleukin-1 β and tumor necrosis factor-α induce gene expression and production of leukocyte chemotactic factors, colony-stimulating factors, and interleukin-6 in human mesangial cells. Am J Pathol 1991; 138:991–1003.
170. Rovin BH, Tan LC. LDL stimulates mesangial fibronectin production and chemoattractant expression. Kidney Int 1993; 43:218–225.

171. Hosang K, Knoke I, Klaudiny J, et al. Porcine Luteal Cells Express Monocyte Chemoattractant Protein-1 (MCP-1)—Analysis by Polymerase Chain Reaction and cDNA Cloning. Biochem Biophys Res Commun 1994; 199:962–968.
172. Ueda A, Okuda K, Ohno S, et al. NF-kappa B and Sp1 regulate transcription of the human monocyte chemoattractant protein-1 gene. J Immunol 1994; 153:2052–2063.
173. Bretz JD, Williams SC, Baer M, et al. C/EBP-related protein 2 confers lipopolysaccharide-inducible expression of interleukin 6 and monocyte chemoattractant protein 1 to a lymphoblastic cell line. Proc Natl Acad Sci USA 1994; 91:7306–7310.
174. Zhang YJ, Rutledge BJ, Rollins BJ. Structure/activity analysis of human monocyte chemoattractant protein-1 (MCP-1) by mutagenesis—Identification of a mutated protein that inhibits MCP-1-mediated monocyte chemotaxis. J Biol Chem 1994; 269:15918–15924.
175. Ernst CA, Zhang YJ, Hancock PR, et al. Biochemical and Biologic Characterization of Murine Monocyte Chemoattractant Protein-1—Identification of Two Functional Domains. J Immunol 1994; 152:3541–3549.
176. Carr MW, Roth SJ, Luther E, et al. Monocyte Chemoattractant Protein 1 Acts as a T-Lymphocyte Chemoattractant. Proc Natl Acad Sci USA 1994; 91:3652–3656.
177. Baggiolini M. Novel aspects of inflammation: interleukin-8 and related chemotactic cytokines. Clin Investig 1993; 71:812–4.
178. Kikuchi H, Hanazawa S, Takeshita A, et al. Interleukin-4 acts as a potent stimulator for expression of monocyte chemoattractant JE/MCP-1 in mouse peritoneal macrophages. Biochem Biophys Res Commun 1994; 203:562–569.
179. Grandaliano G, Valente AJ, Rozek MM, Abboud HE. Gamma Interferon Stimulates Monocyte Chemotactic Protein (MCP-1) in Human Mesangial Cells. J Lab Clin Med 1994; 123:282–289.
180. Dahinden CA, Geiser T, Brunner T, et al. Monocyte chemotactic protein 3 is a most effective basophil- and eosinophil-activating chemokine. J Exp Med 1994; 179:751–6.
181. Hanazawa S, Takeshita A, Kitano S. Retinoic acid suppression of c-fos gene inhibits expression of tumor necrosis factor-alpha-induced monocyte chemoattractant JE/MCP-1 in clonal osteoblastic MC3T3-E1 cells. J Biol Chem 1994; 269:21379–21384.
182. Ohmori Y, Hamilton TA. IFN-gamma selectively inhibits lipopolysaccharide-inducible JE/monocyte chemoattractant protein-1 and KC/GRO/melanoma growth-stimulating activity gene expression in mouse peritoneal macrophages. J Immunol 1994; 153:2204–2212.
183. Charo IF, Myers SJ, Herman A, et al. Molecular Cloning and Functional Expression of Two Monocyte Chemoattractant Protein-1 Receptors Reveals Alternative Splicing of the Carboxyl-Terminal Tails. Proc Natl Acad Sci USA 1994; 91:2752–2756.
184. Baggiolini M, Dewald B, Moser B. Interleukin-8 and related chemotactic cytokines—CXC and CC chemokines. Adv Immunol 1994; 55:97–179.

46

Molecular Biology and Function of the Chemoattractant Cytokines RANTES and CSF-1

Gunter Wolf
University of Hamburg, Hamburg, Germany

Bruno Luckow and Detlef Schlöndorff
Ludwig-Maximilians-University, Munich, Munich, Germany

INTRODUCTION

RANTES is an acronym derived from several characteristics of the gene and its protein product: *R*egulated upon *A*ctivation, *N*ormal *T* cell *E*xpressed and *S*ecreted (1,2). *RANTES* is a member of the C-C chemokine subfamily with chemoattractant activity for monocytes/macrophages (M/M), eosinophil and basophil granulocytes, and T lymphocytes (see also previous chapter and Refs. 3 to 7). Below, we summarize the molecular biology and function of *RANTES*, emphasizing the kidney. Furthermore, the monocyte colony–stimulating factor CSF-1 is briefly reviewed, as the role of CSF-1 is not restricted to bone marrow hemopoesis but may also include an important local function during inflammatory renal disease.

RANTES GENE AND PROTEIN STRUCTURE

A systematic search for genes expressed specifically in T cells led several years ago to the fortuitous isolation of a cDNA clone encoding human *RANTES* (*huRANTES*). A (T minus B cell) cDNA library was screened with cDNA probes subtracted in the same manner and a previously known T cell–specific clone was isolated (1,2). Nothing was known about its biological function, and it took some time to realize that a novel chemokine had been isolated. The *huRANTES* mRNA is approximately 1200 bp long and encodes a protein of 91 amino acids with a typical signal peptide of 23 amino acids at the amino terminus. The open reading frame is followed by a 3′-untranslated region of more than 800 nucleotides, which contains three sets of Alu repeats. *The huRANTES* protein precursor has a molecular mass of 10 kDa, which is reduced to approximately 8 kDa by cleavage of the signal peptide (1,2). The first two of the four cysteines present in the secreted protein are located adjacent to each other, indicating that this protein is a member of the C-C chemokine subfamily (8). The 8-kDa *RANTES* protein is highly basic, with an isoelectric point of 9.5, and it does not seem to be glycosylated (1,2). By in situ hybridization and analysis of somatic cell hybrids, the human *RANTES* gene was mapped to the chromosome region 17q11.2-q12 (9).

Using the human cDNA as a probe, we and others have recently cloned the murine *RANTES* (*muRANTES*) cDNA (10,11). The *muRANTES* cDNA is approximately half as long as its human counterpart due to a relatively small 3′-untranslated region, but it encodes a protein of exactly the same length. An amino acid sequence comparison between secreted human and murine *RANTES* revealed the highest level of sequence conservation seen between species homologues within the chemokine family. Of 68 amino acids, 60 were identical in both species (10,11). Analysis of a 16-kb genomic clone containing the entire *muRANTES* gene revealed a three exon/two intron structure typical for all chemokine genes analyzed so far (14,15). Exon 1 encodes the 5′ untranslated region and the first 25 amino acids. Exon 2 encodes amino acids 26–63, whereas exon 3 encodes the remaining amino acids and the 3′ untranslated region. The *muRANTES* gene has been mapped to chromosome 11 in the vicinity of other members of the murine C-C chemokine subfamily (14,15).

In the original report, expression of *huRANTES* was described only for nontransformed antigen and interleukin 2–dependent $CD8^+$ T cells, and steady-state mRNA levels were dramatically reduced after stimulation with fresh antigen (1). In contrast, *RANTES* was not expressed in EBV-transformed B lymphoblasts, nonlymphoid hemopoietic, and established T cell tumor lines (1,2). Moreover, *muRANTES* mRNA was detected in antigen-specific T-cell clones ($CD8^+$, $CD4^+$), which recognize and react with a key antigen of tubulointerstitial nephritis (10,12). *RANTES* mRNA was also found in MCT cells, a murine proximal tubular cell line, and in a syngeneic mouse mesangial cell line (MMC) (10). Transcripts were induced in MCT cells by stimulation with IL-1 and TNF-α (10). In addition, treatment with TNF-α, IL-1, and LPS stimulated, in a dose-dependent manner, expression of *muRANTES* mRNA and protein in MMCs (13). Although the TNF-α–induced expression of *muRANTES* in MMCs could be abolished by coincubation with a neutralizing anti-TNF-α antibody, this antibody failed to block LPS-mediated induction of this chemokine. These findings suggest that LPS induction of *muRANTES* is not mediated by the generation of endogenous TNF-α (13). Studies performed in our laboratory showed that TNF-α induction of *muRANTES* in mesangial cells could be suppressed by radical scavengers. Furthermore, superoxide anion but not H_2O_2 also increased mRNA levels for *RANTES*. Thus, free radicals may be involved in *RANTES* gene activation (Satriano and Schlöndorff, unpublished). Regulatory sequences important for TNF-α induction of *muRANTES* seem to be located in the 5′-flanking region of the gene. A fusion gene consisting of 5′-flanking sequences of *muRANTES* and a luciferase reporter gene showed—after transfection into MCT cells and stimulation with TNF-α—an increase in luciferase activity (15). It remains to be determined whether a putative NF-κB site present in the *muRANTES* promoter at position –84 plays a role in this process.

RECEPTOR FOR *RANTES* AND FUNCTION OF THIS CHEMOKINE

Receptor binding studies with C-C chemokines revealed that MCP-1 and MIP-1α competeted for *RANTES* binding to M/M with a K_d of 6 and 1.6 n*M*, respectively (16). Both of these chemokines reduced Ca^{2+} mobilization induced by *RANTES* (17). In contrast, *RANTES* did not compete for MCP-1 or MIP-1α binding on M/M, suggesting the existence of promiscous receptors that recognize different C-C chemokines (16–18). The first C-C chemokine receptor has recently been isolated by Neote and colleagues (19). It belongs to the family of G protein–coupled receptors containing seven transmembrane-spanning domains. The isolated cDNA clone contained an open reading frame of 1065 bp, encoding a protein of 355 amino acids with a predicted molecular mass of approximately 41 kDa (19). Expression of this receptor cDNA (C-C CKR-1) in human kidney 293 cells demonstrated that several C-C chemokines (*RANTES*, MIP-1β, MCP-1) displaced ^{125}I-MIP-1α binding, but the C-X-C chemokine IL-8 did not, suggesting that the receptor was specific for the C-C chemokine subfamily (19). The available data suggest that the MIP-1α receptor has been isolated. Clones encoding a *RANTES*-specific receptor have not yet been published.

In a Boyden chamber assay, recombinant *huRANTES* attracts M/M and a subtype of T cells corresponding to the phenotype of memory T cells (20). In addition, recombinant *muRANTES* produced in the embryonic kidney cell line 293 has a chemotactic effect on human M/M in vitro (11). At least three different groups have independently shown that *huRANTES* is also a strong chemoattractant, but not an activator for human eosinophil granulocytes (21–23). Recent studies suggest that recombinant *huRANTES* is the most effective chemoattractant and activator for basophils (24).

RANTES EXPRESSION IN THE KIDNEY AND IN RENAL DISEASE

In general the expression of *RANTES* in leukocytes is more restricted than that of other chemokines. In the kidney, low levels of *RANTES* mRNA have been found in the cortex and in cultured renal tubular (MCT cells) and mesangial cells (MMCs) (10,13). Marked induction occurs after stimulation of MCT cells and MMCs with TNF-α and LPS (10,13). A preliminary report indicates that low density lipoprotein (LDL) may be able to induce *RANTES* mRNA and protein expression in cultured mesangial cells (25). IgG complexes are also capable of increasing mRNA levels for *RANTES* in murine MC. The increased expression of *RANTES* after TNF-α or IgG stimulation can be attenuated by free radical scavengers and by agents that increase cAMP, such as forskolin or PGE_2 (Satriano and Schlöndorff, unpublished). Furthermore, mRNA levels for *RANTES* were increased in glomeruli harvested from rats after in vivo perfusion with TNF-α (13). LPS injection into C3H/HeN mice also induced an increase in *RANTES* mRNA expression in glomeruli and renal cortices (26). This expression did not occur in the mouse strain C3H/HeJ known to be LPS resistent. Co-treatment of LPS-susceptible mice with prostaglandin E_1 (PGE_1) abolished the LPS-mediated increase in *muRANTES* mRNA (26). Preliminary experiments indicate that *muRANTES* mRNA is induced in glomeruli isolated from rats with a proliferative glomerulonephritis (Thy-1.1 model) (27). However, compared to MCP-1 expression in this model, *RANTES* expression occurs later, but remains elevated for a longer period. Since the glomerular accumulation of M/M is not preceded by *RANTES* expression in the Thy-1.1 model of glomerulonephritis, it is possible that the source of *RANTES* mRNA are infiltrating M/M rather than the intrinsic glomerular cells. PGE_1 treatment of nephritic animals reduced *RANTES* expression to control levels (27). It is intriguing to speculate that a PGE_1-mediated increase in intracellular cAMP may down-regulate *RANTES* transcription in this system as it does in cultured MC (Satriano and Schlöndorff, unpublished). *RANTES* transcripts were also induced in whole glomeruli from animals with autologous nephrotoxic serum nephritis (28). The glomerular source of this increased expression is currently unknown.

Recently, Pattison and coworkers studied *RANTES* expression in renal allograft biopsy specimens (29). During rejection periods, *RANTES* protein (immunofluorescence) and mRNA (in situ hybridization) were expressed by infiltrating M/M and by renal tubular epithelial cells. However, *RANTES* was not expressed in samples taken 1 hr after transplantation, or in native renal biopsies from patients with cyclosporin nephrotoxicity (29). These findings indicate that *RANTES* plays a role in allograft rejection and targeting of immune competent cells into the renal tubulo-interstitium. Thus, *RANTES* may be a prime target for immunomodulation in transplant rejection and other immune-mediated diseases (30).

STRUCTURE OF THE COLONY STIMULATING FACTOR 1 (CSF-1)

CSF-1, also called macrophage colony stimuating factor (M-CSF), is a specific growth factor for mononuclear phagocytic cells (31–34). Unlike the more pluripotent hemopoetic factor GM-CSF, CSF-1 specifically stimulates proliferation and differentiation of M/M and their committed bone marrow progenitors (32,33). CSF-1 is also required for the survival of peripheral resident monocytes. Furthermore, CSF-1 has some chemoattractive activity for M/M, as also indicated by transfection experiments with the receptor for CSF-1 (40). CSF-1 is a dimeric sialoglycoprotein that has been purified to homogeneity and cloned; it is the product of a single gene. The human CSF-1 gene consists of 10 exons spanning 21 kb encoding several alternatively spliced mRNAs (32,33,35). The human CSF-1 gene has been mapped to the long arm of chromosome 5 at band q 33.1 (33,35). Two CSF-1 transcripts of 4 kb and 1.6 kb can be detected in several cell types (33). The 4-kb mRNA encodes a precursor protein for CSF-1 consisting of 554 amino acids (36,37). The 554–amino acid precursor acquires both N- and O-linked oligosaccharides during intracellular trafficking (33,36,37). The membrane-associated homodimer is processed prior to secretion as a 86-kDa soluble protein. Biochemical analyses suggest that the protein product of the 4-kb mRNA accounts for almost all circulating CSF-1 (33,36,37). In contrast to the secreted form of CSF-1, the 256–amino acid precursor of the shorter 1.6-kb mRNA is not undergoing intracellular proteolysis, so that most of this form remains membrane-bound. These findings raise the possibility that membrane-associated CSF-1 may directly stimulate receptor-bearing cells through cell-to-cell interactions, independently from paracrine-secreted CSF-1 (33).

CSF-1 RECEPTOR AND SIGNAL TRANSDUCTION PATHWAYS

The CSF-1 receptor (CSF-1R) is encoded by the c-*fms* protooncogene and belongs to the family of receptor tyrosine kinases (38–40). The gene is approximately 60 kb long and composed of 22 exons.

It maps close to the gene encoding the B isoform of platelet-derived growth factor receptor (PDGF-R_B) on human chromosome 5, band q31-32, and is closely localized to the CSF-1 gene at band q33.1 (38–40). Human CSF-1R is an integral transmembrane glycoprotein of 972 amino acids (41). The extracellular ligand-binding domain of the CSF-1R is organized into five immunoglobulin-like domains (38). The intracellular portion contains two tyrosine kinase domains separated by a 72-amino acid spacer. Putative phosphorylation sites are the tyrosine residues at position 699, 708, 809, and 969. The protein contains a putative ATP binding site around lysine 616 (42). Binding of CSF-1 to its receptor activates an intrinsic protein kinase, which leads to autophosphorylation at tyrosine 809, followed by transphosphorylation of aggregated CSF-1R subunits (38,42). Activation of the tyrosine kinase activity leads to a further rapid phosphorylation of targets, probably including c-Raf, phospholipase C, phosphotidyl-inositol kinase, and the GTPase-activating protein (GAP), similar to the intrinsic kinase activities of other receptors (44). Furthermore, two novel cyclin-like (CYL) genes have recently been isolated which are also phosphorylated by CSF-1 during the G_1 phase of the M/M cell cycle (44). Such phosphorylation patterns play a pivotal role in the progression of quiescent M/M from the G_1 phase of the cell cycle toward mitosis.

CSF-1 EXPRESSION IN THE KIDNEY AND IN RENAL DISEASE

Although initially thought to be limited to hemopoetic cells, expression of CSF-1 occurs in many mesenchymal cells including MC (45). MC secrete CSF-1 and also display a cell surface form of CSF-1 (45–47). Mesangial induction of CSF-1 occurs in response to IFN-γ, TNF-α, and IgG complexes (47). These responses can be inhibited by cAMP (47) and partially by some thiol-containing scavengers for free radicals (48). Generation of superoxide anion also increases mRNA levels for CSF-1 in murine MC, indicating that free radicals may play a role in the expression of CSF-1 by MC (48).

The autoimmune renal injury of MRL-*lpr* mice shares many features with human lupus nephritis and is characterized by a prominent glomerular accumulation of M/M (50). Circulating CSF-1 is enhanced in the serum of MRL-*lpr* mice (51). CSF-1 transcripts were significantly elevated in the whole kidneys of these mice, suggesting a renal source of circulating CSF-1. In situ hybridization experiments demonstrated mesangial cells as the predominant source of renal CSF-1 (50). M/M isolated from glomeruli of MRL-*lpr* mice require CSF-1 to survive and proliferate (50). However, CSF-1 does not cause proliferation of MC (45,49). Whether the increase in renal CSF-1 expression—which is limited to MRL-*lpr* mice and does not occur in the NZB/W mice—is a primary or secondary event during development of nephritis remains unclear (51). A preliminary report indicates glomerular CSF-1 mRNA expression by in situ hybridization of biopsies from patients with IgA nephropathy (52). Future studies should help to define a potential role of CSF-1 in human renal disease.

SUMMARY AND PERSPECTIVES

Renal recruitment of M/M occurs in many inflammatory and noninflammatory kidney diseases and may present an initial step not only in acute renal injury but also in chronic glomerular and interstitial fibrosis (53,54). Recent evidence indicates that various chemotactic agents, including chemokines such as *RANTES* and MCP-1, can be locally released at sites of injury in the kidney and may play a pivotal role in the attraction of M/M and other inflammatory cells (Figure 1). Furthermore, locally generated CSF-1 may be important for the survival of resident and infiltrating M/M, and possibly for their local proliferation and their activation. In concert with the expression of the respective adhesion molecules on renal cells and inflammatory cells, this can result in further generation of cytokines, including PDGF and TGF-β, leading to cell proliferation and matrix expansion. Further studies will have to show that expression of chemokines and infiltration by inflammatory cells not only represents a correlation but also reflects a cause-effect relation. In vivo experiments with neutralizing antibodies against the specific cytokine and generation of knockout animals defective for these cytokines should help to further define the exact role of each chemokine in the attraction of M/M and the resulting pathophysiology. Identification of the exact sequence of events and the players involved should allow the development of new drugs that interfere with the pathophysiological

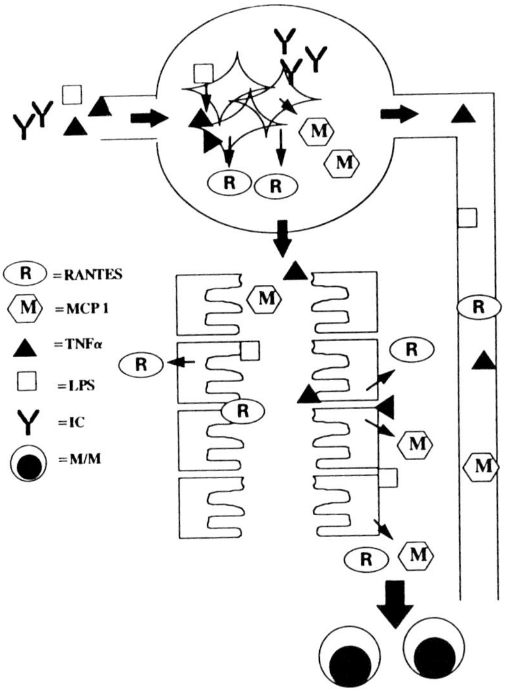

Figure 1 TNF-α, LPS, and immune complexes originating in the circulation or formed locally can bind to mesangial cells and release chemokines (MCP-1 and *RANTES*). Additionally, TNF-α and LPS may bind to either luminal or contraluminal receptors on proximal tubular cells and stimulate local synthesis and release of MCP-1 and *RANTES*. These chemoattractants may, in turn, stimulate the migration of M/M into glomerular tuft and tubulointerstitial microenvironment. Most likely, there exists a complex cytokine "bath" with interactions between systemically derived substances—cytokines generated in the glomerulus and at distinct tubular sites. Transport of cytokines to possible tubular target sites may be through glomerular ultrafiltration and/or postglomerular vessels. Such a scheme may help to explain the involvement of the tubulointerstitium in many forms of primary glomerular disease.

process and may enrich the therapeutic armentarium with more specific therapeutic agents for the treatment of renal diseases.

REFERENCES

1. Schall TJ, Jongstra J, Dyer BJ, et al. A human T cell-specific molecule is a member of a new gene family. J Immunol 1988; 141:1018–1025.
2. Jongstra J, Schall TJ, Dyer BJ, et al. The isolation and sequence of a novel gene from a human functional T cell line. J Exp Med 1987; 165:601–614.
3. Oppenheim JJ, Zachariae CO, Mukaida N, Matsushima K. Properties of the novel proinflammatory supergene "intercrine" cytokine family. Annu Rev Immunol 1991; 9:617–648.
4. Sherry B, Cerami A. Small cytokine superfamily. Curr Opin 1991; 3:56–60.
5. Clark SC, Kamen R. The human hematopoetic colony-stimulating factors. Science 1987; 236:1229–1237.
6. Hamilton JA. Colony stimulating factors, cytokines and monocyte-macrophages—Some controversies. Immunol Today 1993; 14:18–24.
7. Schall TJ. Biology of the *Rantes*/SIS cytokine family. Cytokine 1991; 3:165–183.
8. Rollins BJ, Stier P, Ernst T, Wong GG. The human homolog of the JE gene encodes a monocyte secretory protein. Mol Cell Biol 1989; 9:4687–4695.
9. Donlon TA, Krensky AM, Wallace MR, et al. Localization of a human T-cell-specific gene, *RANTES* (D17S136E), to chromosome 17q11.2-q12. Genomics 1990; 6:548–553.

10. Heeger P, Wolf G, Meyer C, et al. Isolation and characterization of cDNA from renal tubular epithelium encoding murine *Rantes*. Kidney Int 1992; 41:220–225.
11. Schall TJ, Simpson NJ, Mak JY. Molecular cloning and expression of the murine *RANTES* cytokine: Structural and functional conservation between mouse and man. Eur J Immunol 1992; 22:1477–1481.
12. Hines WH, Mann RA, Kelly CJ, Neilson EG. Biochemical and functional characterization of an antigen-specific helper T cell factor which induces the effector T cell repertoire in autoimmune interstitial nephritis. J Immunol 1990; 1444:75–83.
13. Wolf G, Aberle S, Thaiss F, et al. TNF-α induces expression of the chemoattractant cytokine *RANTES* in cultured mouse mesangial cells. Kidney Int 1993; 444:795–804.
14. Danoff TM, Heeger PS, Lalley PA, Neilson EG. Characterization of the murine *RANTES* (muR) gene (abstr). J Am Soc Nephrol 1992; 3:582.
15. Danoff TM, Chiang MY, Ortiz A, Neilson EG. Transcriptional regulation of murine *RANTES* (muR) in proximal tubular cells (abstr). J Am Soc Nephrol 1993; 4:599.
16. Wang JM, McVicar DW, Oppenheim JJ, Kelvin DJ. Identification of *RANTES* receptors on human monocytic cells: Competition for binding and desensitization by homologous chemotactic cytokines. J Exp Med 1993; 177:699–705.
17. Gao JL, Kuhns DB, Tiffany HL, et al. Structure and functional expression of the human macrophage inflammatory protein 1α/*RANTES* receptor. J Exp Med 1993; 177:1421–1427.
18. Van Riper G, Siciliano S, Fischer PA, et al. Characterization and species distribution of high affinity GTP-coupled receptors for human *RANTES* and monocyte chemoattractant protein 1. J Exp Med 1993; 177:851–856.
19. Neote K, DiGregorio D, Mak JY, et al. Molecular cloning, functional expression, and signaling characteristics of a C-C chemokine receptor. Cell 1993; 72:415–425.
20. Schall TJ, Bacon K, Toy KJ, Goeddel DV. Selective attraction of monocytes and T lymphocytes of the memory phenotype by cytokine *RANTES*. Nature 1990; 347:669–671.
21. Kameyoshi Y, Dörschner A, Mallet AI, et al. Cytokine *RANTES* released by thrombin-stimulated platelets is a potent attractant for human eosinophils. J Exp Med 1992; 176:587–592.
22. Alam R, Stafford S, Forsythe P, et al. *RANTES* is a chemotactic and activating factor for human eosinophils. J Immunol 1993; 150:3442–3447.
23. Rot A, Krieger M, Brunner T, et al. *RANTES* and macrophage inflammatory protein 1α induce the migration and activation of normal human eosinophil granulocytes. J Exp Med 1992; 176:1489–1495.
24. Kuna P, Reddigari SR, Schall TJ, et al. Characterization of the human basophil response to cytokines, growth factors, and histamine releasing factors of the intercrine/chemokine family. J Immunol 1993; 150:11932–1943.
25. Mondorf UF, Wolf G, März W, et al. Low density lipoprotein (LDL) stimulates the expression of mRNA for *RANTES* in mouse mesangial cells (abstr). J Am Soc Nephrol 1994; 4:494.
26. Thaiss F, Wolf G, Zahner G, et al. Lipopolysaccharide (LPS) induces mRNA expression of *muRANTES* in renal tissue (abstr). J Am Soc Nephrol 1993; 4:503.
27. Rau HP, Thaiss F, Wolf G, et al. Prostaglandin E_1 reduces the expression of the chemokine *RANTES* in glomeruli of rats with immune mediated mesangial cell injury (abstr). J Am Soc Nephrol 1993; 44:629.
28. Thaiss F, Helmchen U, Zahner G, et al. *muRANTES* mRNA expression in glomeruli isolated from rats with autologous nephrotoxic serum nephritis (abstr). J Am Soc Nephrol 1993; 4:638.
29. Pattison J, Nelson PJ, Huie P, et al. *RANTES* chemokine expression in cell-mediated transplant rejection of the kidney. Lancet 1994; 343:209–211.
30. McLean A. Regulation with *RANTES*. Lancet 1994; 343:189.
31. Metcalf D. The colony stimulating factor. Cancer 1990; 65:2185–2195.
32. Stanley ER, Chen DM, Lin HS. Induction of macrophage production and proliferation by a purified colony stimulating factor. Nature 1978; 274:168–170.
33. Sherr CJ, Rettenmier CW, Roussel MF. Macrophage colony-stimulating factor, CSF-1, and its proto-oncogene-encoded receptor. Cold Sping Harbor Symp Quant Biol 1988; 53:521–530.
34. Metcalf D. The molecular control of cell division, differentiation commitment and maturation in haemopoietic cell. Nature 1989; 339:27–30.
35. Kawasaki ES, Ladner MB, Wang AM, et al. Molecular cloning of a complementary DNA encoding human macrophage-specific colony-stimulating factor (CSF-1). Science 1985; 230:291–296.
36. Ladner MB, Martin GA, Noble JA, et al. cDNA cloning and expression of murine macrophage colony-stimulating factor from L929 cells. Proc Natl Acad Sci USA 1988; 85:6706–6710.
37. Rajavashisth TB, Eng R, Shadduck RK, et al. Cloning and tissue-specific expression of mouse macrophage colony-stimulating factor mRNA. Proc Natl Acad Sci USA 1987; 84:1157–1161.
38. Sherr CJ. Colony-stimulating factor-1 receptor. Blood 1990; 75:1–12.
39. Roussel MF, Dull TJ, Rettenmeier CW, et al. Transforming potential of the c-fms proto-oncogene (CSF-1 receptor). Nature 1987; 325:5449–5452.

40. Pierce JH, Di Marco E, Cox GW, et al. Macrophage-colony-stimulating factor (CSF-1) induces proliferation, chemotaxis, and reversible monocytic differentiation in myeloid progenitor cells transfected with the human c-fms/CSF-1 receptor cDNA. Proc Natl Acad Sci USA 1990; 87:5613–5617.
41. Fukunaga R, Ishizaka-Ikeda E, Nagata S. Growth and differentiation signals mediated by different regions in the cytoplasmic domain of granulocyte colony-stimulating factor receptor. Cell 1993; 74:1079–1087.
42. Vairo G, Hamilton JA. Signalling through CSF receptors. Immunol Today 1991; 12:362–369.
43. Bolen JB, Rowley RB, Spana C, Tsygankov AY. The Src family of tyrosine protein kinases in hemopoietic signal transduction. FASEB J 1992; 6:34403–3409.
44. Matsushime H, Roussel MF, Ashmun RA, Sherr CJ. Colony-stimulating factor 1 regulates novel cyclins during the G1 phase of cell cycle. Cell 1991; 65:701–713.
45. Mori T, Bartocci A, Satriano J, et al. Mouse mesangial cells produce colony-stimulating factor-1 (CSF-1) and express the CSF-1 receptor. J Immunol 1990; 144:4697–4702.
46. Brennan DC, Jevkinar AJ, Bloom RD, et al. Mesangial cells from autoimmune MRL/*lpr* mice have decreased secreted and surface M-CSF despite increased circulating and renal expression. Kidney Int 1992; 42:279–284.
47. Satriano JA, Hora K, Shan Z, et al. Regulation of monocyte chemoattractant protein-1 and macrophage colony-stimulating factor-1 by IFN-γ, tumor necrosis factor-α, IgG aggregates, and cAMP in mouse mesangial cells. J Immunol 1993; 150:1971–1978.
48. Satriano JA, Shuldiner M, Hora K, et al. Oxygen radicals as second messengers for expression of the monocyte chemoattractant protein, JE/MCP-1, and the colony-stimulating factor, CSF-1, in response to tumor necrosis factor-α and immunoglobulin G. J Clin Invest 1993; 92:1564–1571.
49. Bloom RD, Florquin S, Singer G, et al. Colony stimulating factor-1 in the induction of lupus nephritis. Kidney Int 1993; 43:1000–1009.
50. Rubin-Kelley V, Bloom RD, Yui MA, et al. Pivotal role of colony stimulating factor-1 in lupus nephritis. Kidney Int 1994; 45 (suppl 45):S83–S85.
51. Yui MA, Brissette WH, Brennan DC, et al. Increased macrophage colony-stimulating factor in neonatal and adult autoimmune MRL-*lpr* mice. Am J Pathol 1991; 139:255–261.
52. Niemir Z, Waldherr R, Noronha I, et al. In situ expression of cytokines in mesangial IgA-GN. (abstr). J Am Soc Nephrol 1993; 4:686.
53. Schreiner GF. The role of macrophage in glomerular injury. Semin Nephrol 1991; 11:268–275.
54. Nickolic-Paterson DJ, Lan HY, Hill PA, Atkins RC. Macrophages in renal injury. Kidney Int 1994; 45 (suppl 45):S79–S82.

47

Phospholipases A_2

Joseph V. Bonventre

Harvard Medical School, Massachusetts Institute of Technology, and Massachusetts General Hospital, Boston, Massachusetts

INTRODUCTION

Phospholipases are enzymes that hydrolyze phospholipids. The nomenclature for this class of enzymes is presented in Fig. 1. Phospholipases fall into two broad classes: acyl hydrolases (phospholipase A_1, PLA_1, which hydrolyzes the lipid at the sn-1-acyl ester bond; phospholipase A_2, PLA_2, which acts at the sn-2 position; and phospholipase B, PLB, which acts at both the sn-1 and sn-2 positions) and phosphodiesterases (phospholipase C, PLC, which cleaves the glycerol-phosphate bond, and phospholipase D, PLD, which removes the base from the phospholipid).

Phospholipases A_2 comprise a family of enzymes that act on phospholipids to generate a free fatty acid and lysophospholipid. Since the sn-2 position of phospholipids of mammalian cells is enriched with arachidonic acid, the precursor for eicosanoids, the regulation of PLA_2 activity has important implications for the control of eicosanoid production. Although arachidonic acid can be released from phospholipids by mechanisms not involving PLA_2 (1), it is likely that in many cells PLA_2 is the primary enzyme regulating arachidonic acid release. The free arachidonic acid and lysophospholipid, generated by PLA_2 activity, together with the metabolic products of arachidonic acid, generated by cyclooxygenases, lipoxygenases, and monooxygenases (Fig. 2), have many effects on cells, both as intercellular and intracellular messengers (2, 3). If the substrate lipid is a 1-O-alkyl, 2 acyl phospholipid, the lysophospholipid produced by PLA_2 can then be acetylated at the sn-2 position to form platelet activating factor. PLA_2 can be rate limiting for prostaglandin synthesis (4) and perhaps for platelet activating factor synthesis. Synthesis of noncyclooxygenase products requires both the release of arachidonic acid as well as activation of other enzymes (5).

PLA_2 and its products have been implicated in the control of a number of physiological processes, including activation of voltage-dependent channels (6,7), ligand-gated channels (8,9), smooth muscle contractility (10), mitogenesis (3,11), gene expression (12) modulation of neurotransmitter uptake (13,14) and release (15,16), and enhancement of the phosphorylation of important cellular proteins (17).

In addition to its role in physiological responses of the cell, PLA_2 activity is important for pathophysiological states in which activation is associated with membrane degradation and changes in plasma and mitochondrial membrane bioenergetics and permeability (18–20). Enzymes that metabolize arachidonic produce free radicals with destructive potential (21). Metabolites of arachidonic acid can modulate the production of inflammatory mediators (12,22) and hence are important modulators of inflammatory responses, including those associated with tubular interstitial diseases of the kidney (23).

CHARACTERISTICS OF PHOSPHOLIPASES A_2

The phospholipases A_2 (PLA_2s) comprise a family of ubiquitous enzymes that exist in both secretory and intracellular forms (Table 1). The secretory forms of the enzyme are prominent components of

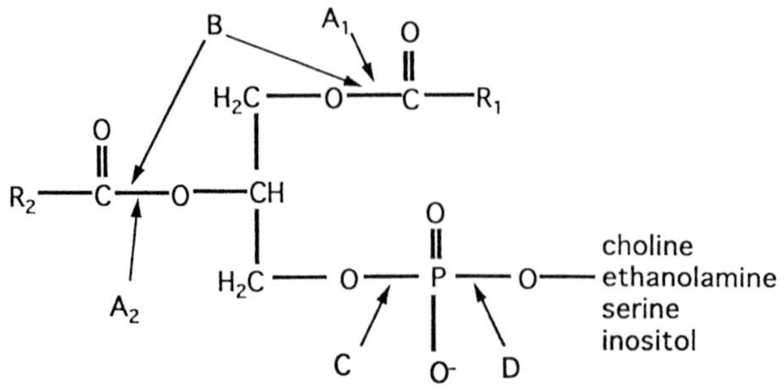

Figure 1 The site of hydrolysis of phospholipids by various phospholipases. Phospholipase A_1 hydrolyzes the 1-acyl ester; phospholipase A_2, the 2-acyl ester. Phospholipase B hydrolyzes both the 1 and 2 acyl ester bonds. Phospholipase C cleaves the glycerol-phosphate bond, whereas the base is removed by phospholipase D.

snake and insect venoms, inflammatory joint fluid, and pancreatic extracts, and it is from the study of these enzymes that most of our knowledge about PLA_2s derives. These enzymes are generally small proteins (mol mass ~12,000 to 18,000 Da), which depend upon millimolar concentrations of calcium for activity and have very high specific activities (>100 mmol/min/mg) (24). Many of these enzymes have been purified and their amino acid sequences determined (25). In general, much less is known about intracellular forms of PLA_2, some of which are involved in the hormonal regulation of arachidonic acid release. Both Ca^{2+}-dependent and independent forms of intracellular PLA_2s have been identified, and some intracellular forms have specific activities approaching those of the secretory forms of PLA_2 (26).

Phospholipases A_2 can be categorized into groups and subgroups based upon their amino acid structure and other characteristics. Groups I, II, and III PLA_2 have low molecular masses (13 to 18 kDa), are calcium-dependent for activity, and have many disulfide bonds. The secretory forms are subdivided into group I (elapid and hydrophid snakes) and group II (crotalid and viperid snakes) based upon positions of cysteine pairs in the protein sequence (27). The mammalian pancreatic enzyme is a group I enzyme (28). Group II PLA_2s can exist both as secretory forms or membrane-associated forms and are found in many tissues, where they are believed to play important roles in inflammation (28–36). Group III PLA_2, isolated from bee venom, has a slightly higher molecular mass (15 to 18 kDa) than group I and II forms (13 to 15 kDa) and different sequence

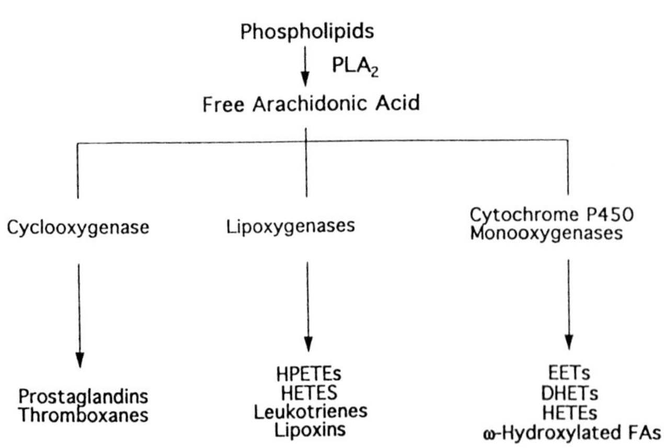

Figure 2 Metabolic pathways for arachidonic acid. After hydrolysis of the sn-2 position arachidonic acid from the phospholipid molecule, the released arachidonic acid can be metabolized by cyclooxygenase, lipoxygenases, or P450 monooxygenases. Some of the products of these metabolic pathways are listed.

Table 1 Characteristics of PLA_2s

Type	Size (kDa)	Origin	Ca^{2+} dependency	pH optimum	Acyl group selectivity	Other distinguishing characteristics
Ca^{2+}-dependent forms						
Group I	13–15	Snake venom Pancreas Gastric mucosa Spleen	Yes (mM)	8–9	None	Seven disulfide bonds including Cys^{11}-Cys^{77}
Group II	13–15	Snake venom Platelets Synovial fluid Mesangial cells Ascitic fluid Gastric mucosa Vascular smooth muscle cells	Yes (mM)	8–9	None	Cys^{50}-Cys^{32} replaces Cys^{11}-Cys^{77}
		Mitochondria of liver heart, kidney, brain	Yes (>1 μM)	8–9		
		Membrane-associated form in platelet, spleen, macrophage cell line ($P388D_1$)	Yes (mM)	8–9		
Group III	13–15	Bee venom Lizards	Yes (mM)	?	?	Not found in mammals (to date)
Group IV (cytosolic)	85–110	Kidney U937 cells Spleen Mesangial cells Platelets Macrophage cell lines (RAW 264.7 and J774)	Yes (>100 nM)	8–9	Arachidonic acid	Translocates to membrane in Ca^{2+}-dependent manner Ca^{2+} not required at the active site
	?180	Temporal cortex (human brain)	Yes	8.5	?	Membrane-associated

Table 1 *(Continued)*

Type	Size (kDa)	Origin	Ca^{2+} dependency	pH optimum	Acyl group selectivity	Other distinguishing characteristics
Ca^{2+}-independent forms						
	40	Heart, pancreas	No	6.4	None	Activity against 1-acylether-PC, 1,2-acyl PC and plasmalogen, with preference for plasmalogen; cytosolic
	97	Intestine	No	?	?	Lysophospholipase activity (PLB); membrane-associated
	80	$p388D_1$ cells	No	?	None	Activated by nucleotide triphosphates; active form is oligomer of 340 kDa
	110	Brain	No	7.4	Arachidonic acid	No activity against plasmalaogens
	40	Brain	No	8.0	Arachidonic acid	Activity against 1,2-acyl-PE and plasmenylethanolamine; inhibited by glycosaminoglycans
Lysosomal	?	Liver, heart	No	4.5	?	

? indicates not known.

homologies but is similar to the group I and II forms in catalytic function (37). Group IV PLA_2 is entirely different from those of groups I, II, and III. It is much larger in molecular mass (85 to 100 kDa), is activated by calcium concentrations in the high nanomolar range, is cytosolic in localization, and has a preference for arachidonic acid at the sn-2 position of its substrate phospholipid. In addition to these forms of the enzyme, there are other calcium-dependent and independent forms that are less well characterized. Thus the PLA_2 family represents a diverse family of heterogeneous proteins with varying characteristics. This chapter provides an overview of what is known about each of the different groups of this family. Space constraints prohibit coverage of all that is known in this rapidly expanding field.

GROUPS I, II, AND III AND CLOSELY RELATED PLA_2S

The PLA_2 forms in groups I, II, and III are evolutionarily related (37), with a great deal of sequence homology among the many group I and II forms that have been sequenced. Group I forms are found primarily in snake (elapid and hydrophid) venom and in pancreatic secretions. The pancreatic enzyme is synthesized in an inactive precursor form, whereas no such precursor form has been identified for the snake venom PLA_2s. Group I and II PLA_2s contain seven disulfide bonds. Six of these are conserved in all group I and II forms. Group I PLA_2s differ from group II forms by having Cys^{11} joined to Cys^{77}. In group II PLA_2, the seventh disulfide bond is between Cys^{50} and Cys^{132}. The first crystal structure of a PLA_2 to be characterized was that of the bovine pancreatic form (38). Approximately 50% of the group I and II PLA_2s consists of an α helix, and all contain an antiparallel β sheet. The active site resides in a hydrophobic pocket near His^{48} (39). Calcium also binds in this pocket. His^{48} is hydrogen-bonded to Asp^{99}. The catalytic mechanism of these forms of PLA_2 is similar to that of serine proteases in utilization of a His-Asp couple. Rather than a serine-OH group, a water molecule is polarized by the His-Asp couple, and this then attacks the carbonyl group of the substrate (39). The calcium ion that is required for catalysis acts to stabilize the transition state (40). These PLA_2s have much higher activity against aggregated substrates than on monomolecular ones. How the enzyme binds to the phospholipid substrate that is part of the lipid-water interface is not understood. Group I and II enzymes do not demonstrate any significant selectivity among fatty acids at the sn-2 position of phospholipids (41).

Group I PLA_2, although originally thought to be limited to pancreatic secretions and snake venoms, has been identified in a number of mammalian organs (42,43). When the pancreatic group I enzyme is added to cells, a number of responses have been described, including enhanced contractility, eicosanoid production, proliferation, and cell migration (44–46). The investigators that have carried out many of these studies have attributed these effects to receptor-mediated phenomena and have partially characterized a group I binding protein (44,47). By scatchard analysis, using ^{125}I-PLA_2, this group has described the presence of a binding protein on the rat mesangial cell with an equilibrium dissociation constant of 1.6 n*M* (46). Addition of group I PLA_2 to these cells results in marked increases in group II PLA_2 mRNA levels and PGE_2 synthesis.

Group II PLA_2s are produced and secreted by a number of cells, as indicated above. Large amounts of group II PLA_2 are found in inflammatory exudates (30). Administered group II PLA_2 is a potent inflammatory stimulus (48,49). Both group I and group II enzymes can exist in the same tissue (31,50). All group II forms are not secreted enzymes. Group II enzymes have been found in intracellular compartments, such as the mitochondria (51). Other 13- to 15-kDa forms of PLA_2 are associated with microsomal fractions of red cells, platelets, and a number of organs, including brain and kidney (32, 52–55). In some cases the forms have been characterized enough to confirm that they are group II forms, whereas in other cases they are insufficiently characterized. It is also apparent that intracellular group II enzymes represent distinct proteins. Antibodies raised against intracellular mitochondrial PLA_2, for example, fail to cross-react with a variety of secretory forms of PLA_2 (56) and fail to recognize other intracellular forms of the enzyme.

Cytokines enhance the production and secretion of PLA_2 by many cell types, including renal mesangial cells (57–59), and the presence of this enzymatic activity in the glomerulus may contribute in an important way to glomerular inflammatory processes. In the mesangial cell, Sedor, Pfeilschifter and colleagues have shown that IL-1α, and β, TNFα, forskolin, and lipopolysaccharide—but neither serum, EGF, PDGF, nor IL-2—enhance secretion of a group II PLA_2 (57–60). Nakazato et al. (57) found a sixfold increase in mRNA levels of group II PLA_2 after 24-hr of treatment of mesangial

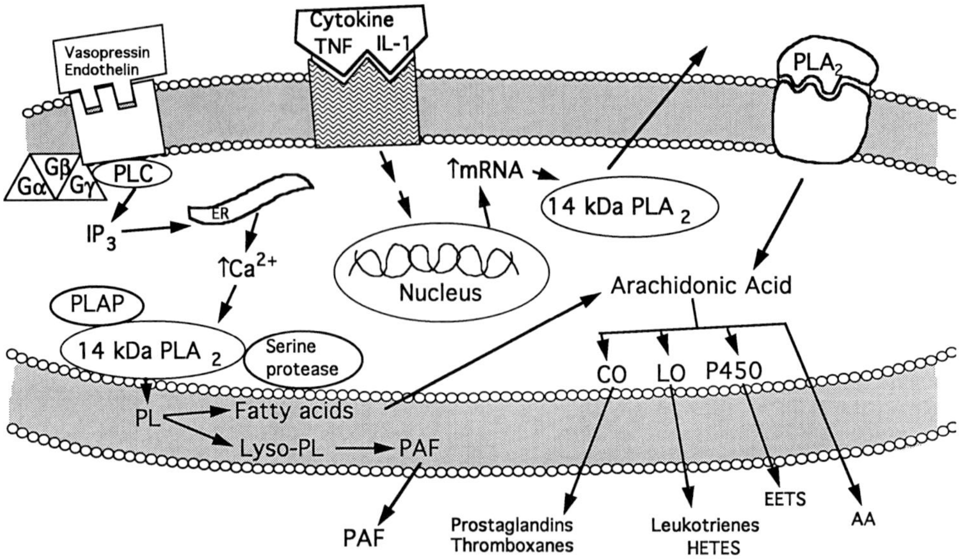

Figure 3 Signal transduction pathways involved in the activation of group II PLA_2. G protein–linked receptors, when occupied with ligands such as vasopressin or endothelin, increase phospholipase C (PLC) activity, and the resultant inositol trisphosphate (IP_3) formed releases calcium from intracellular storage sites, such as the endoplasmic reticulum (ER). The increased calcium, if raised to high enough levels locally, together with other proteins, such as serine proteases and PLA_2 activating protein (PLAP), activates PLA_2 resulting in the release of arachidonic acid from membrane stores. The released arachidonic acid can then be metabolized by cyclooxygenases (CO), lipoxygenases (LO), or P450 monooxygenases. Alternatively, cytokines such as interleukin-1 (IL-1) or tumor necrosis factor (TNF) can increase mRNA levels of PLA_2 and enhance its production and production and secretion. Extracellular group II PLA_2 can act on cells via a receptor.

cells with IL-1α. PDGF-BB inhibits the IL-1β and forskolin-induced increases in group II PLA_2 mRNA. This inhibition is blocked by genistein, a tyrosine kinase inhibitor, leading the authors to conclude that tyrosine phosphorylation is involved in the PDGF-induced effect on PLA_2 gene expression (57). Forskolin and tumor necrosis factor (TNF) increase mRNA levels of group II PLA_2 in cultured smooth muscle cells (61).

Endotoxin enhances the mRNA levels of group II PLA_2 in lung, spleen, stomach, and distal ileum of the rat (43,62). Serum PLA_2 levels increase markedly in patients with septic shock (63), and most of this activity is believed to be group II PLA_2. We have determined that large amounts of group II enzymes are present in the serum of patients receiving systemic heparin; this may account for the large changes seen in serum prostacyclin when patients are undergoing cardiac surgery and exposed to high doses of heparin (64).

Olivier et al. have characterized the promoter region of the group II PLA_2 gene using the cytokine IL-6 and chloramphenicol acetyl transferase (CAT) constructs of the 5′ flanking region of the human group II PLA_2 gene (65) transfected into HepG2 liver cells. The highest activity was obtained with the –210 to +20 promoter region, and the IL-6 responsive element was within this region. The 5′ (–1614 to –210) and 3′ flanking regions (+20 to +806) contain negative regulatory regions that act synergistically to repress expression of the group II gene and may account for the low baseline expression in the absence of IL-6. Three positive regulatory elements were identified within the region –210 to +20, one of which contained a TATA box and likely represented the binding site for TATA box–binding protein (TBP). One of these elements bound to members of the C/EBP family of transcription factors. This same element was necessary for the stimulatory effect of IL-6 to be observed. These observations suggest that C/EBP mediates the IL-6 stimulation of group II PLA_2 expression.

Dexamethasone inhibits the increase in Group II mRNA levels induced by IL-1, TNF, and endotoxin in a number of tissues, including the lung, distal ileum, spleen (43,59,62), cultured astrocyte (66), and renal mesangial cell (59). Dexamethasone also inhibits the increased group II mRNA levels observed in renal mesangial cells exposed to exogenous pancreatic group I PLA_2 (46). Whether dexamethasone works to inhibit group II PLA_2 production via inhibition of production of a cytokine, enhanced production of a PLA_2 inhibitory protein, or some other mechanism is not established. Identification of the mechanism of action of glucocorticoids on PLA_2 production may provide important insight into the anti-inflammatory mechanisms of action of these compounds.

Because of the requirement for millimolar concentrations of calcium, well out of the physiological range, and the nonselectivity for arachidonic acid, it has generally been considered that the group II PLA_2s were not important for regulation of intracellular arachidonic acid release and eicosanoid synthesis. This conclusion has been challenged recently, however, by investigators who have found that inhibition of group II PLA_2 expression impairs the production of eicosanoids (67). Treatment of P388D_1 cells with antisense oligonucleotides complementary to nucleotides encoding the calcium catalytic binding loop of group II PLA_2 resulted in a 63% reduction in homogenate PLA_2 activity directed against *Escherichia coli* membranes—an assay used by the authors for group II PLA_2. These antisense oligonucleotide-treated cells released significantly less prostaglandin E_2 (PGE_2) in response to lipopolysaccharide and platelet activating factor. Another group of cells were transfected to stably express an antisense group II PLA_2 RNA. These cells had a reduced level of basal PGE_2 production as well as a reduction in stimulated production to approximately one-third of activated control cells. The authors propose that group II PLA_2 may be secreted from the cell and then attached to the external cell membrane by interaction with proteoglycans to release arachidonic acid, which may then diffuse to the cyclooxygenase, where it can be converted to PGE_2. While the authors went to great lengths to associate the effects of reduction in PGE_2 production to reduced levels of group II PLA_2, the antisense oligonucleotides also decreased $cPLA_2$ and calcium-independent PLA_2 activities in the cells.

If the group II PLA_2 is functional inside the cell, then one must explain how it can function at physiological calcium concentrations. Marshall and colleagues (68,69) have reported that group II activity can be measured at lower than millimolar concentrations of calcium when EGTA is present in the assay. They speculated that the presence of the chelator may affect the interactions between enzyme and substrate phospholipid, reducing the EC_{50}. They propose that calcium binding proteins *in vivo* may serve a function similar to that of EGTA *in vitro*, resulting in enhanced calcium sensitivity of the group II enzyme.

The cloning and expression of a membrane receptor from rabbit skeletal muscle, which recognizes both group I and group II PLA_2 has recently been reported (70). The receptor has a molecular mass of 180 kDa and has 29% homology with the macrophage mannose receptor. By Northern blot analysis, the receptor is present in primary cultures of cells propagated from kidney, lung, brain, and heart in addition to skeletal muscle. Higher levels of transcripts were seen in cells derived from embryonic tissue. When expressed in 293 cells, the receptor-bound porcine pancreas group I PLA_2 with a Kd of 10.0 n*M* and group II human PLA_2 with a K_d of 0.8 n*M*. The receptor also recognizes glycosylated ligands that bind to the mannose receptor. The role that this receptor plays in secretory group I and II action is not clear at present. It is also not clear whether this receptor is the same as the binding protein partially characterized by Arita's group and described above. The binding selectivity of the expressed receptor is very different from that of the binding protein described by Koshino et al. (46), who found that group II PLA_2 did not compete with pancreatic group I for binding even at concentrations 60- to 70-fold higher than the K_d for Group I PLA_2.

A form of PLA_2 closely related to group I and II forms has been cloned from a human stomach cDNA library (71). The cDNA encodes a peptide with predicted molecular mass of 13,592. The predicted protein lacks one of the seven disulfide bonds that are characteristic of group I and II PLA_2s, identifying it as a member of a class of enzymes distinct from the group I and II forms. When the cDNA is expressed in human 293s cells, PLA_2 activity accumulated in the culture medium. Culture medium activity was greatest against phospholipids of ^{14}C-oleate-labeled *E. coli* in a calcium-dependent fashion with peak activity measured at a [Ca^{2+}] of 10 m*M*. PLA_2 activity remained high over a wide pH range (6.5 to 9.0). By Northern analysis, using the novel cDNA as a probe, it was found that there was an abundant 1.2-kb transcript present in heart and to a lesser extent in lung. A 1-kb transcript was abundant in placenta and less abundant in liver and skeletal muscle.

Group III PLA_2 has been identified in worker bee venom and in lizards. PLA_2 is a major component of bee venom and constitutes a principal allergen. To date, no group III PLA_2 has been found in mammals. This form of the enzyme has homology to the group I and II forms but contains only 10 cysteine residues implicated in the formation of 5 disulfide bonds (72).

GROUP IV PLA_2

We and others have purified a large-molecular-mass form of PLA_2 ($cPLA_2$) from cytosolic extracts of various organs and cell types (73–76). This enzyme also has lysophospholipase activity (77) and also a low CoA-independent transacylase activity, which results in the formation of phosphatidylcholine from lysophosphatidylcholine (78). This transacylase activity is likely not physiologically important because of the low levels of lysophospholipids usually present in the cell and the low activity of the enzyme.

A cDNA for this form of PLA_2 encoding a 85.2-kDa protein has been cloned from the mouse, human (75,79), chicken, and fish (80). Despite this predicted molecular mass, the protein migrates at 100 to 110 kDa by SDS-PAGE. $cPLA_2$ is likely the product of a single-copy gene. The human clone reacted with a single 3.4-kb transcript on Northern blot analysis (79). There has been a great deal of interest in this form of PLA_2 because of its preference for arachidonic acid at the sn-2 position of phospholipids and because of its activity at physiological calcium concentrations.

The promoter of the $cPLA_2$ has been partially characterized (81). The promoter does not have a canonical TATA or CCAAT box. A series of 18 CA repeats are present at approximately –240. Tay et al. (81) identified putative PEA-3 and modified AP-1 and NFκB recognition sites in the region from –844 to –276. Luciferase constructs, which included a region of the gene from –1003 to +40, provided the highest luciferase activity when transfected into rat mesangial cells. The human gene was localized to chromosome 1.

$cPLA_2$ expression can be regulated at the transcriptional level. In a human bronchial epithelial cell line Wu et al. (82) demonstrated that interferon-γ increases the amount of $cPLA_2$ protein by enhancing transcription as monitored by nuclear runoff assays. Transcription was enhanced within 15 min of addition of interferon-γ and remained elevated for at least 4 hr.

Much of what we know about $cPLA_2$ regulation deals with the influences of calcium and phosphorylation on the protein itself (Fig. 4). We demonstrated that activation can occur in submicromolar concentrations of calcium (73), an observation consistent with our previous finding that eicosanoid synthesis could be demonstrated in permeabilized mesangial cells when calcium concentrations were increased from resting levels of approximately 100 n*M* to levels measured when cells were activated by hormones or growth factors (83).

This large-molecular-mass PLA_2 is not dependent on calcium for its catalytic activity, as are the group I, II, and III forms; rather, calcium is required for this PLA_2 to associate with its substrate. We reported that Mn^{2+} could substitute for Ca^{2+} and Mg^{2+} could partially substitute for Ca^{2+} in the activation of rat mesangial cell $cPLA_2$ (84). Reynolds et al. subsequently added Sr^{2+} and Ba^{2+} to the list of divalent cations that could substitute for Ca^{2+} to give full enzymatic activity of the rat kidney (85) and human recombinant $cPLA_2$ (78). By contrast, heavy metals, Cd^{2+}, Cu^{+}, Cu^{2+}, Fe^{3+}, Hg^{2+}, and Zn^{2+} inhibited the enzyme. High concentrations of salt—either NaCl, Na_2SO_4, or $(NH_4)_2SO_4$—can substitute for Ca^{2+} or other divalent metals (78).

Calcium is necessary for group IV PLA_2 activity to translocate from the cytosolic to the membrane fraction of cells (84,86). When the recombinant (79) or purified (76) protein is incubated with membranes, it translocates when calcium concentration is increased within the physiological range. This does not mean, however, that there are not other proteins which may be important for this translocation, since they may be present in the membrane fractions. Clark and colleagues (79) reported that a 16-kDa NH_2-terminal fragment of $cPLA_2$ associated with membranes in a calcium-dependent manner. Furthermore, this part of the protein contains a 45–amino acid region, which they called the Ca^{2+}-dependent lipid-binding (CaLB) motif or C_2 domain, is homologous to similar regions in a number of enzymes including protein kinase C isoforms, which translocate to the membrane in a Ca^{2+}-dependent fashion; the synaptic vesicle protein p65, or synaptotagmin (87); the GTPase activating protein (GAP) (88); and phospholipase Cγ (89). It was suggested that this 45–amino acid region of these proteins determines Ca^{2+}-dependent phospholipid binding. Synaptotagmin I, an abundant synaptic vesicle membrane protein, is an important regulatory protein in neurotransmitter release and is known to associate with membranes in a calcium-dependent manner

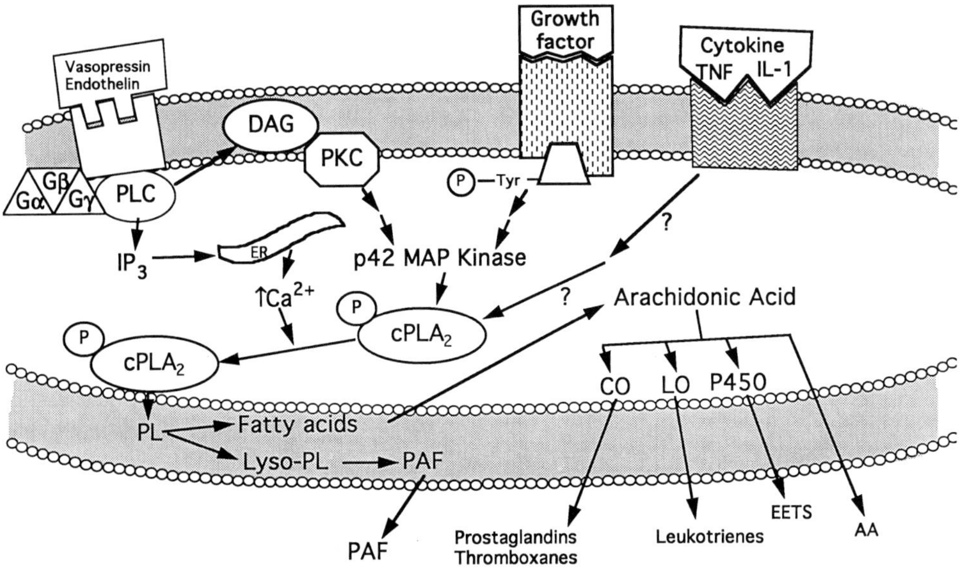

Figure 4 Cellular signaling pathways implicated in the regulation of group IV $cPLA_2$. G protein–linked receptors, when occupied with ligands such as vasopressin or endothelin, increase phospholipase C (PLC) activity, and the resultant inositol trisphosphate (IP_3) formed releases calcium from intracellular storage sites, such as the endoplasmic reticulum (ER). The increased calcium concentrations in the cellular cytosol are sufficient to mediate the translocation of the enzyme to the cell membrane. Another effect of PLC activation is the generation of diacylglycerol, which, in turn, together with calcium, will activate protein kinase C. This initiates the activation of a phosphorylation cascade, which results in the phosphorylation of $cPLA_2$. Phosphorylation and translocation result in enhanced PLA_2 activity. Once the enzyme has been translocated, calcium is no longer necessary for catalytic activity. Growth factors acting on receptors with tyrosine (tyr) kinase activity can initiate a phosphorylation cascade also leading to phosphorylation of $cPLA_2$. Alternatively, cytokines such as interleukin-1 (IL-1) or tumor necrosis factor (TNF) can, via unknown pathways, lead to phosphorylation of $cPLA_2$. Arachidonic acid, released from membrane stores, can then be metabolized by cyclooxygenases (CO), lipoxygenases (LO), or P450 monooxygenases.

(90). Another protein that has a C_2 domain is Rabphilin-3A. This protein is the putative target protein for *smg* p25A/*rab*3A p25A, a member of the rab subfamily of the ras p21-related small GTP-binding proteins implicated in intracellular vesicular traffic (91). Rabphilin-3A is particularly abundant in presynaptic vesicles and the synaptic plasma membrane, where it has been implicated in neurotransmission (92). Alignment of sequences demonstrating the homologies between $cPLA_2$, synaptotagmin, PKCα, and rabphillin-3A is presented in Fig. 5.

When the first 178 amino acids of $cPLA_2$ are fused to maltose-binding protein, the fusion protein translocates to membranes in a calcium-dependent way, thus demonstrating that this NH_2-terminal region of $cPLA_2$ can confer calcium-dependent membrane binding to a protein that normally does not associate with membranes (80). When a recombinant protein is made in which the Ca^{2+}-lipid-binding (CaLB) domain has been removed, there is no PLA_2 activity against micellar or liposomal substrates, but there is lysophospholipase activity toward monomeric lysophospholipids. It is difficult to present a monomeric diacylphospholipid to the enzyme because of the very low critical micellar concentration of the natural phospholipid substrate. This is consistent with the view that the CaLB domain is necessary for $cPLA_2$ to bind to aggregated substrates and that the region of $cPLA_2$ 3′ to the CaLB domain is sufficient for lysophospholipase catalytic activity against monomeric substrate, an activity which is calcium-independent. The CaLB domain is required for calcium-dependent lysophospholipase activity against micellar substrates.

When fusion proteins of glutathione-S-transferase and C_2 containing regions of synaptotagmin

cPLA2	37	D	M	L	D	T	P	D	P	Y	V	E	L	F	I	S	T	T	P	D	S	R	-	K	R	-
Synaptotagmin (A)	172	D	M	G	G	T	S	D	P	Y	V	K	V	F	L	L	P	E	K	K	-	-	K	K	F	E
PKCα	186	D	P	N	G	L	S	D	P	Y	V	K	L	K	L	I	P	D	P	K	N	E	S	K	Q	K
Rabphilin-3A	591	D	A	N	G	Y	S	D	P	F	V	K	L	W	L	K	P	D	M	G	K	K	A	K	H	K
consensus		D					P	D	P	Y	V	E	L		I		T							K		
							S			F		K	V		L		P									

cPLA2	T	R	H	F	N	N	D	I	N	P	V	W	N	E	T	F	E	F	I	L	D	P	N	Q	83
Synaptotagmin (A)	T	K	V	H	R	K	T	L	N	P	V	F	N	E	Q	F	T	F	K	V	P	Y	S	E	218
PKCα	T	K	T	I	R	S	T	L	N	P	R	W	D	E	S	F	T	F	K	L	K	P	S	D	235
Rabphilin-3A	T	Q	I	K	K	K	T	L	N	P	E	F	N	E	E	F	F	Y	D	I	K	H	S	D	639
consensus	T						D	I	N	P			N	E		F		F					N	Q	
							T	L					D					Y					S	E	
																								D	

Figure 5 Alignment of regions of cPLA2 and three other proteins that are homologous and likely mediate calcium dependent translocation to membranes. Synaptotagmin (87), bovine protein kinase Cα, and rabphilin-3A (123) have regions highly homologous to a region in cPLA2 (93). Each of these proteins translocates to membrane fractions in response to an increase in calcium concentration. Synaptotagmin has two regions that are homologous. The first (*A*) region is presented.

(93) or rabphillin-3A (94) are immobilized on glutathione columns and exposed to phospholipid liposomes and calcium, calcium-dependent phospholipid binding can be demonstrated. The binding is specific for negatively charged phospholipids, and half-maximal binding occurred at a calcium concentration of 4 to 6 μM (93).

Other factors besides calcium are important in the regulation of $cPLA_2$. The pH optimum of $cPLA_2$ from mesangial cells, whole kidney extracts, and brain is in the range of 8 to 9, although activity is present at physiological pH (54,55,73). Posttranslational modification of the enzyme, in particular phosphorylation, is believed to play an important role in its regulation. Agonists such as vasopressin (83,84) and endothelin (95) enhance PLA_2 activity in mesangial cells. These agonists not only increase $[Ca^{2+}]_i$ but also activate protein kinase C (14,96) and mitogen activated kinases via activation of the signal cascade intermediates, c-Raf and mitogen-activated protein kinase kinase (97). We evaluated whether protein kinase C might be involved in the activation of PLA_2 by examining whether the phorbol ester phorbol myristate acetate (PMA) modulates the $[Ca^{2+}]_i$-dependent activation of PLA_2 in the intact mesangial cell (83). PGE_2 production was determined in permeabilized cells where cytosolic Ca^{2+} was fixed at basal cellular levels of $[Ca^{2+}]_i$ (<200nM) or at levels of $[Ca^{2+}]_i$ (0.3 to 2.2 μM) that are measured in the presence of agonists such as vasopressin and endothelin. PMA had no effect on PGE_2 production when $[Ca^{2+}]_i$ was fixed at low basal levels. By contrast, at the higher (hormone-stimulated) levels of $[Ca^{2+}]_i$, there was a twofold increase in PGE_2 production when PMA was present. Thus protein kinase C enhances the Ca^{2+} sensitivity of PLA_2. In further support of this conclusion, we found that protein kinase C activation also potentiated Ca^{2+} ionophore (A23187)-stimulated PLA_2 activity in the intact mesangial cell (83). Activation of the kinase cascade, however, was insufficient to activate PLA_2 in the intact cell in the absence of an increase in intracellular $[Ca^{2+}]$. Permeabilized cells exposed to vasopressin and GTPγS, a maneuver that results in an increase in diacylglycerol levels due to activation of phospholipase C, did not increase PLA_2 activity when $[Ca^{2+}]_i$ was maintained at low basal cytosolic levels (83). Thus, in the mesangial cell, an increase in $[Ca^{2+}]_i$ was necessary in order for one or more members of the protein kinase cascade to enhance PLA_2 activity. We also directly examined $cPLA_2$ enzymatic activity in cytosolic fractions of mesangial cells previously stimulated with vasopressin or phorbol esters (84) and found that both stimuli enhanced the enzyme's activity further, suggesting that phosphorylation may be important for this activation process.

Sedor's group (98) has reported that interleukin 1 (IL-1) increases $cPLA_2$ enzymatic activity without increasing $cPLA_2$ mRNA or protein mass. This increase in activity is associated with enhanced ^{32}P incorporation into immunopreciptable $cPLA_2$ protein in mesangial cells. Consistent with our prior conclusion that phosphorylation alone does not enhance arachidonic acid release or eicosanoid production in mesangial cells, IL-1 added to cells did not result in stimulation of arachidonic acid release unless calcium ionophore was added with the IL-1.

Hormonal activation of $cPLA_2$ is associated with phosphorylation in a number of different cell types (99, 100). It has recently been demonstrated that p42 MAP kinase phosphorylates $cPLA_2$ on Ser^{505} and that phosphorylation of the enzyme results in an increase in activity when the assay is carried out in the presence of high calcium concentrations (100,101). Nemenoff et al. (101) reported that protein kinase C can directly phosphorylate and activate the enzyme but that the activation is much less than that seen with p42 MAP kinase. Lin et al. (100) reported phosphorylation by protein kinase C but concluded that this phosphorylation did not result in decreased mobility of $cPLA_2$ on SDS-polyacrylamide gels, and, in contrast to Nemenoff et al., found no significant increase in activity as a result of this phosphorylation. $cPLA_2$ containing a mutation at Ser^{505}, converting it to an alanine, is enzymatically active but no longer a substrate for MAP kinase. Furthermore, cells transfected with this mutated $cPLA_2$ release much less arachidonic acid in response to calcium ionophore, PMA + calcium ionophore, ATP and thrombin, as compared with cells transfected with the normal $cPLA_2$ (100). This further attests to the importance of Ser^{505} phosphorylation in activation of the enzyme. Thus, the paradigm that an increase in calcium concentration and phosphorylation are both necessary for optimal $cPLA_2$ activation continues to be supported by a large amount, but not all, of the published data.

$cPLA_2$ can be activated without an increase in cytosolic calcium concentration. We have found that platelet-derived growth factor (PDGF) increases arachidonic acid release prior to activating phospholipase C in mesangial cells (102). In addition, epidermal growth factor, which does not activate phospholipase C or increase cytosolic free calcium concentrations in mesangial cells under conditions we used for activation of the cells, results in a highly consistent increase in $cPLA_2$ enzymatic activity (103). Clark and Dunlop (104) subsequently found that EGF-stimulated PLA_2 activation could also be found in Chinese hamster ovarian (CHO) cells, transfected with the normal human EGF receptor, where phospholipase C is not activated. Goldberg et al. (105) reported that the EGF-induced activation of PLA_2 was dependent upon intact tyrosine kinase activity of the EGF receptor. Clark and Dunlop found that CHO cells did not respond to EGF with activation of PLA_2 if they were transfected with a mutant receptor that showed EGF-stimulated kinase activity but lacked the major autophosphorylation sites and was unable to undergo EGF-induced receptor internalization. This implicated a component of the growth factor–activated cell kinase cascade in the activation of $cPLA_2$. MAP kinase may play a role in this activation by EGF.

Winitz et al. have recently reported that a mutant $G\alpha_{i2}$, in which Gly^{203} is changed to Thr, when stably expressed in CHO cells results in inhibition of thrombin and ATP stimulation of arachidonic acid release, but did not affect calcium mobilization or MAP kinase activation (106). Phorbol ester was able to overcome this inhibition. We have found that transfection of the α_o subunit cDNA into a murine adrenal cell line results in a marked increase in expression of this protein and is associated with an increase in GTPγS-stimulatable release of arachidonic acid (107). Whether these results are explained by direct coupling of G proteins to $cPLA_2$ or by a G_i and G_o activated pathway that activates $cPLA_2$ is not known at this time.

ANOTHER Ca^{2+}-DEPENDENT FORM OF PLA_2

My laboratory has collaborated with that of Drs. Ross and Kish in Toronto in the initial characterization of a Ca^{2+}-dependent large-molecular-mass membrane-associated PLA_2 in human temporal cortex (108). While the enzyme is Ca^{2+}-dependent, 30% of the activity is maintained in the absence of added calcium. We cannot rule out at this time that this baseline activity in the presence of excess EGTA is not due to the presence of a Ca^{2+}-independent form together with a Ca^{2+}-dependent form in the human brain particulate fraction. The limited availability of human brain has made difficult the further purification and definitive characterization of the enzyme. This enzyme is activated *in vitro* with millimolar concentrations of calcium and has an alkaline pH optimum. It is weakly stimulated by DTT and inhibited by bromophenacylbromide, AACOCF3, γ-linolenoylamide, and *N*-methyl γ-linolenoylamide.

Ca^{2+}-INDEPENDENT PLA_2s

A Ca^{2+}-independent PLA_2 was purified from guinea pig intestinal brush-border membranes (109). By SDS-PAGE the molecular mass was estimated to be 97 kDa. The enzyme had roughly equal

PLA_2 and lysophospholipase activities. The purified enzyme had equivalent activities against PC and PE, with less activity when 1-O-alkyl phospholipids were used as substrates.

The best-studied Ca^{2+}-independent PLA_2 is a cytosolic form characterized in cardiac tissue by Gross and colleagues. The major isoform of canine (110), rabbit (111), and human (112) myocardial cytosolic PLA_2 is a 40-kDa protein that has a pH optimum of 7.0 and preferentially catalyzes the hydrolysis of plasmenylcholine substrate containing arachidonic acid at the sn-2 position. Since these lipids represent predominant constituents of the human myocardium (112) and the enzyme is rapidly activated with ischemia (111), it has been argued that this form of PLA_2 is of particular importance in the process of ischemia-induced phospholipid hydrolysis. It is important to note, however, that the enzyme does have activity against acyl and alkyl-ether phospholipids (110). This form of PLA_2 is also present in pancreatic islets from rats and humans. The enzyme is believed to participate in the D-glucose-stimulated phospholipid hydrolysis, which is necessary for glucose-induced insulin release (113).

This PLA_2 enzyme described by Hazen and Gross is activated and stabilized by ATP by mechanisms that are independent of phosphorylation (114). The ATP effects appear to be mediated by a cytosolic protein distinct from the purified PLA_2 (115). This calcium-independent form of PLA_2 has been reported to be modulated by a high-molecular-weight ATP-binding protein, which may be phosphofructokinase, a tetrameric protein composed of 85-kDa subunits (116). The 400-kDa phospholipase A_2 catalytic complex consists of one 40-kDa catalytic polypeptide and the tetrameric phosphofructokinase. Little is known about how this form of PLA_2 hydrolyzes phospholipids other than the fact that the enzyme can be inhibited by a mechanism-based suicide inhibitor, (*E*)-6-(bromomethylene)tetrahydro-3-(1-naphthalenyl)-2H-pyran-2-one (bromoenol lactone) (117).

Inhibition of the enzyme has been shown to decrease arachidonic acid release from a renal epithelial cell line (118), BSC-1, but further characterization of the inhibited activity was not carried out. An inhibitor has also been found to result in a reduction in the amount of hypoxia-induced arachidonic acid release and lactate dehydrogenase, a marker of cell injury, in isolated proximal tubules (119). These authors also found a considerable amount of Ca^{2+}-independent PLA_2 activity that was plasmalogen-selective, which increased with hypoxia in the isolated proximal tubules.

A different Ca^{2+}-independent form of PLA_2 has been purified from a macrophage-like cell line, $P388D_1$ (120). This enzyme did not show any preference for arachidonic acid at the sn-2 position or alkyl-ether linkage at the sn-1 position. The enzyme hydrolyzed dipalmitoyl-PC approximately fourfold faster than 1-palmitoyl-2-arachidonyl-PC and 15-fold faster than 1-O-hexadecyl-2-arachidonyl-PC. ATP and other nucleoside di- and triphosphates stimulated activity of the enzyme. SDS-PAGE of the purified enzyme revealed a single band at molecular mass of approximately 80 kDa. Radiation inactivation studies of cellular homogenates indicated a molecular mass of 337 kDa for the catalytically active form of the enzyme and Superose 6 chromatography and membrane filtration indicated a molecular mass of 300 to 400 kDa. One explanation for the apparent discrepancies in molecular size is that the active form of the enzyme exists as a tetramer of 80-kDa subunits. The pH optimum for this enzyme is 7.5.

Horrocks and colleagues have described two forms of calcium-independent PLA_2 in the cytosol of bovine brain, a 40-kDa and a 110-kDa form. The 40-kDa form of the enzyme has activity against 1,2-acyl-PE as well as plasmenylethanolamine (121). This enzyme is markedly inhibited by glycosaminoglycans with the following pattern of inhibition: heparin sulfate > hyaluronic acid > chondroitin sulfate > heparin (122). Whether this 40-kDa enzyme is related to the 40-kDa enzyme described by Hazen and Gross is not clear.

CONCLUSION

There are many forms of PLA_2. Although the small-molecular-mass forms of the enzyme have been well studied and a large number of this family cloned and sequenced, the intracellular forms of the enzyme are less well characterized. While information has been obtained about the structural domains and regulation of the large-molecular-mass $cPLA_2$ believed to be important for control of arachidonic acid release, a great deal more must be learned before the importance of this enzyme in physiological and pathophysiological function can be ascertained. Much less is known about the calcium-independent forms of the enzyme. None of these calcium-independent forms has been cloned, and potential relationships between the various forms described have not been clarified. We are at the earliest stages of the study of the molecular biology of PLA_2s; it is likely that as we learn more about these enzymes, we will find that they play critical roles not only in the regulation of arachidonic acid release and hence eicosanoid synthesis but also in other aspects of cellular signal transduction.

ACKNOWLEDGMENTS

The work presented in this chapter, derived from the author's laboratory, has been supported by NIH grants DK 39773, DK 38452, and NS 10828.

REFERENCES

1. Bonventre JV, Nemenoff R. Renal tubular arachidonic acid metabolism. Kidney Int 1991; 39:438–449.
2. Bonventre JV. Phospholipase A_2 and signal transduction. J Am Soc Nephrol 1992; 3:128–150.
3. Sellmayer A, Uedelhoven WM, Weber PC, Bonventre JV. Endogenous noncyclooxygenase metabolites of arachidonic acid modulate growth and mRNA levels of immediate-early response genes in rat mesangial cells. J Biol Chem 1991; 266:3800–3807.
4. Flower RG, Blackwell GJ. The importance of phospholipase A_2 in prostaglandin synthesis. Biochem Pharmacol 1976; 25:285–291.
5. Rouzer CA. Regulation and structure of human leukocyte 5-lipoxygenase. In: Crooke ST, Wong A, eds. Lipoxygenases and Their Products. San Diego, CA: Academic Press, 1991:51–65.
6. Haigler HT, Schlaepfer DD, Burgess WH. Characterization of lipocortin I and an immunologically unrelated 33-kDa protein as epidermal growth factor receptor kinase substrates and PLA_2 inhibitors. J Biol Chem 1987; 262:6921–6930.
6a. Schweitzer P, Madamba S, Siggins GR. Arachidonic acid metabolites as mediators of somatostatin-induced increase of neuronal M-current. Nature 1990; 346:464–467.
7. Ordway RW, Singer JJ, Walsh JV Jr. Direct regulation of ion channels by fatty acids. Trends Neurosci 1991; 14:96–100.
8. Massicotte G, Vanderklish P, Lynch G, Baudry M. Modulation of dl-alpha-amino-3-hydroxy-5-methyl-4-isoxazolepropionic acid/quisqualate receptors by phospholipase A_2: A necessary step in long-term potentiation? Proc Natl Acad Sci USA 1991; 88:1893–1897.
9. Miller B, Sarantis M, Traynelis SF, Attwell D. Potentiation of NMDA receptor currents by arachidonic acid. Nature 1992; 355:722–725.
10. Sohn UD, Kim DK, Bonventre JV, et al. Role of 100 kDa cytosolic PLA_2 in ACH-induced contraction of esophageal circular muscle. Am J Physiol (Gastro Liver Physiol) 1994; 267:G433–G441.
11. Beckman BS, Tou J-S, Mason-Garcia M. Phospholipase A_2 activation is an early event in erythropoietin stimulated murine fetal liver cell proliferation/differentiation. Adv Prost Thromb Leukotriene Res 1990; 21:831–834.
12. Horiguchi J, Spriggs D, Imamura K. Role of arachidonic acid metabolism in transcriptional induction of tumor necrosis factor gene expression by phorbol ester. Mol Cell Biol 1989; 9:252–258.
13. Barbour B, Szatkowski M, Ingledew N, Attwell D. Arachidonic acid induces a prolonged inhibition of glutamate uptake into glial cells. Nature 1989; 342:918–920.
14. Yu AC, Chan PH, Fishman RA. Effects of arachidonic acid on glutamate and gamma-aminobutyric acid uptake in primary cultures of rat cerebral cortical astrocytes and neurons. J Neurochem 1986; 47:1181–1189.
15. Lynch MA, Voss KL. Presynaptic changes in long-term potentiation: Elevated synaptosomal calcium concentration and basal phosphoinositide turnover in dentate gyrus. J Neurochem 1991; 56:113–118.
16. Moskowitz N, Shapiro L, Schnook W, Puszkin S. Biochem. Biophys Res Commun 1983; 115:94–99.
16a. Moskowitz N, Schook W, Puszkin S. Interaction of brain synaptic vesicles induced by endogenous Ca^{2+} dependent phospholipase A_2. Science 1982; 216:305–307.
17. Schaechter JD, Benowitz LI. Activation of protein kinase C by arachidonic acid selectively enhances the phosphorylation of GAP-43 in nerve terminal membranes. J Neurosci 1993; 13:4361–4371.
18. Malis CD, Bonventre JV. Mechanism of calcium potentiation of oxygen free radical injury to renal mitochondria: A model for post-ischemic and toxic mitochondrial damage. J Biol Chem 1986; 261:14201–14208.
19. Malis CD, Bonventre JV. Susceptibility of mitochondrial membranes to calcium and reactive oxygen species: Implications for ischemic and toxic tissue damage. Prog Clin Biol Res 1988; 282:235–259.
20. Malis CD, Weber PC, Leaf A, Bonventre JV. Incorporation of marine lipids into mitochondrial membranes increases susceptibility to damage by calcium and reactive oxygen species: Evidence for enhanced activation

of phospholipase A_2 in mitochondria enriched with n-3 fatty acids. Proc Natl Acad Sci USA 1990; 87:8845–8849.
21. Siesjo BK, Bengtsson F. Calcium fluxes, calcium antagonists and calcium related pathology in brain ischemia, hypoglycemia and spreading depression: A unifying hypothesis. J Cereb Blood Flow Metab 1989; 9:127–140.
22. Kunkel SL, Spengler M, May MA, et al. Prostaglandin E_2 regulates macrophage-derived tumor necrosis factor gene expression. J Biol Chem 1988; 263:5380–5384.
23. Kelly CJ, Zurier RB, Krakauer KA, et al. Prostaglandin E_1 inhibits effector T cell induction and tissue damage in experimental murine interstitial nephritis. J Clin Invest 1987; 79:782–789.
24. Waite M. Approaches to the study of mammalian cellular phospholipases. J Lipid Res 1985; 26:1379–1388.
25. Waite M. The phospholipases. In: Hanahan DJ, ed. Handbook of Lipid Research. New York: Plenum Press, 1987: 332 pp.
26. Pierik AJ, Nijssen JG, Aarsman AJ, Van den Bosch H. Calcium-independent phospholipase A_2 in rat tissue cytosols. Biochim Biophys Acta 1988; 962:345–353.
27. Hendrikson RL, Kreuger ET, Keim PS. Amino acid sequence of phospholipase A_2-α from the venom of Crotalus adamanteus. J Biol Chem 1977; 252:4913–4921.
28. deHaas GH, Postema NM, Nieuwenhuizen W, van Deenen LLM. Purification and properties of phospholipase A from porcine pancreas. Biochim Biophys Acta 1968; 159:103–117.
29. Verger R, Ferrato F, Mansbach CM, Pieroni G. Novel intestinal phospholipase A_2: Purification and some molecular characteristics. Biochemistry 1982; 21:6883–6889.
30. Frost S, Weiss J, Elsbach P, et al. Structural and functional properties of phospholipase A_2 purified from an inflammatory exudate. Biochemistry 1986; 25:8381–8385.
31. Ono T, Tojo H, Kuramitsu S, et al. Purification and characterization of a membrane-associated phospholipase A_2 from rat spleen: Its comparison with a cytosolic phospholipase A_2 S-1. J Biol Chem 1988; 263:5732–5738.
32. Hayakawa M, Kudo I, Tomita M, Inoue K. Purification and characterization of membrane-bound phospholipase A_2 from rat platelets. J Biochem 1988; 103:263–266.
33. Tojo H, Ono T, Kuramitsu S, et al. A phospholipase A_2 in the supernatant of rat spleen. J Biol Chem 1988; 263:5724–5731.
34. Olaison G, Sjodahl R, Tagesson C. Increased phospholipase A_2 activity in ileal mucosa in Crohn's disease. Digestion 1988; 41:136–141.
35. Stoner CR, Reik LM, Donohue M, et al. Human group II phospholipase A_2. Immunol Methods 1991; 145:127–136.
36. Mukherjee AB, Cordella-Miele E, Miele L. Regulation of extracellular phospholipase A_2 activity: Implications for inflammatory diseases. DNA Cell Biol 1992; 11:233–243.
37. Davidson FF, Dennis EA. Evolutionary relationships and implications for the regulation of phospholipase A_2: From snake venom to human secreted forms. J Mol Evol 1990; 31:228–238.
38. Dijkstra BW, Kalk KH, Hol WGJ, Drenth J. Structure of the bovine pancreatic phospholipase A_2 at 1.7Å resolution. J Mol Biol 1981; 147:97–123.
39. Verheij HM, Dijkstra BW. Phospholipase A2: Mechanism and structure. In: Woolley P, Petersen SB, eds. Lipases—their structure, biochemistry and application. Cambridge, England: Cambridge University Press, 1994:119–138.
40. Dennis EA. Diversity of group types, regulation, and function of phospholipase A_2. J Biol Chem 1994; 269:13057–13060.
41. Schalkwijk C, Marki F, Van den Bosch H. Studies on the acyl-chain selectivity of cellular phospholipases A_2. Biochim Biophys Acta 1990; 1044:139–146.
42. Sakata T, Nakamura E, Tsuruta Y, et al. Presence of pancreatic-type phospholipase A_2 mRNA in rat gastric mucosa and lung. Biochim Biophys Acta 1989; 1007:124–126.
43. Lilja I, Dimberg J, Sjodahl R, et al. Effects of endotoxin and dexamethasone on group I and II phospholipase A_2 in rat ileum and stomach. Gut 1994; 35:40–45.
44. Arita H, Hanasaki K, Nakano T, et al. Novel proliferative effect of phospholipase A_2 in Swiss 3T3 cells via specific binding site. J Biol Chem 1991; 266:19139–19141.
45. Tohkin M, Kishino J, Ishizaki J, Arita H. Pancreatic-type phospholipase A_2 stimulates prostaglandin synthesis in mouse osteoblastic cells (MC3T3-E1) via a specific binding site. J Biol Chem 1993; 268:2865–2871.
46. Kishino J, Ohara O, Nomura K, et al. Pancreatic-type phospholipase A_2 induces group II phospholipase A_2 expression and prostaglandin biosynthesis in rat mesangial cells. J Biol Chem 1994; 269:5092–5098.
47. Hanasaki K, Arita H. Characterization of a high affinity binding site for pancreatic-type phospholipase A_2 in the rat. J Biol Chem 1992; 267:6414–6420.
48. Vadas P, Pruzanski W, Kim J, Fornasier V. The proinflammatory effect of intra-articular injection of soluble human and venom phospholipase A_2. Am J Pathol 1989; 134:807–811.

49. Murakami M, Kudo I, Nakamura H, et al. Exacerbation of rat adjuvant arthritis by intradermal injection of purified mammalian 14-kDa group II phospholipase A_2. FEBS Lett 1990; 268:113–116.
50. Tojo H, Ono T, Kuramitsu S, et al. A phospholipase A_2 in the supernatant fraction of rat spleen: Its similarity to rat pancreatic phospholipase A_2. J Biol Chem 1988; 263:5724–5731.
51. Van den Bosch H, De Jong JGN, Aarsman AJ. Phospholipase A_2 from rat liver mitochondria. Meth Enzymol 1991; 197:365–373.
52. Aarsman AJ, de Jong JGN, Arnoldussen E, et al. Immunoaffinity purification, partial sequence, and subcellular localization of rat liver phospholipase A_2. J Biol Chem 1989; 264:10008–10014.
53. Kramer RM, Wuthrich C, Bollier C. Isolation of phospholipase A_2 from sheep erythrocyte membranes in the presence of detergents. Biochim Biophys Acta 1978; 507:381–394.
54. Nakamura H, Nemenoff RA, Gronich JH, Bonventre JV. Subcellular characteristics of phospholipase A_2 activity in rat kidney: Enhanced cytosolic, mitochondrial, and microsomal phospholipase A_2 enzymatic activity after renal ischemia and reperfusion. J Clin Invest 1991; 87:1810–1818.
55. Rordorf G, Uemura Y, Bonventre JV. Characterization of phospholipase A_2 (PLA_2) activity in gerbil brain: Enhanced activities of cytosolic, mitochondrial and microsomal forms after ischemia and reperfusion. J Neurosci 1991; 11:1829–1836.
56. de Jong JGN, Amesz H, Aarsman AJ, et al. Monoclonal antibodies against an intracellular phospholipase A_2 from rat liver and their cross-reactivity with other phospholipase A_2. Eur J Biochem 1987; 164:129–135.
57. Nakazato Y, Simonson MS, Herman WH, et al. Interleukin-1α stimulates prostaglandin biosynthesis in serum-activated mesangial cells by induction of a non-pancreatic (type II) phospholipase A_2. J Biol Chem 1991; 266:14119–14127.
58. Muhl H, Geiger T, Pignat W, et al. PDGF suppresses the activation of group II phospholipase A_2 gene expression by interleukin 1 and forskolin in mesangial cells. FEBS Lett 1991; 291:249–252.
59. Schalkwijk C, Vervoordeldonk M, Pfeilschifter J, et al. Cytokine- and forskolin-induced synthesis of group II phospholipase A_2 and prostaglandin E_2 in rat mesangial cells is prevented by dexamethasone. Biochem Biophys Res Commun 1991; 180:46–52.
60. Sedor JR, Sedlak TW, Hornbuckle K, et al. Inflammatory cytokines induce expression of a non-pancreatic (type II) mesangial cell phospholipase A_2 mRNA in a highly regulated manner. J Am Soc Nephrol 1990; 1:481.
61. Nakano T, Ohara O, Teraoka H, Arita H. Glucocorticoids suppress group II phospholipase A_2 production by blocking mRNA synthesis and post-transcriptional expression. J Biol Chem 1990; 265:12745–12748.
62. Nakano T, Arita H. Enhanced expression of group II phospholipase A_2 gene in the tissues of endotoxin shock rats and its suppression by glucocorticoid. FEBS Lett 1990; 273:23–26.
63. Pruzanski W, Vadas P. Phospholipase A_2—a mediator between proximal and distal effects of inflammation. Immunol Today 1991; 12:143–146.
64. Nakamura H, Kim DK, Philbin DM, et al. Heparin-enhanced plasma phospholipase A_2 activity and prostacyclin synthesis in patients undergoing cardiac surgery. J Clin Invest 1995; 95:1062–1070.
65. Olivier JL, Fan Q, Salvat C, et al. Positive and negative hepatic regulation of the human type II phospholipase A_2 gene. Biochemistry 1994; 33:7134–7145.
66. Oka S, Arita H. Inflammatory factors stimulate expression of group II phospholipase A_2 in rat cultured astrocytes: Two distinct pathways of gene expression. J Biol Chem 1991; 266:9956–9960.
67. Balbour SE, Dennis EA. Antisense inhibition of group II phospholipase A2 expression blocks the production of prostaglandin E2 by $P388D_1$ cells. J Biol Chem 1993; 268:21875–21882.
68. Andreoli SP, McAteer JA, Seifert SA, Kempson SA. Oxidant-induced alterations in glucose and phosphate transport in LLC-PK1 cells: mechanisms of injury. Am J Physiol 1993; 265:F377–F384.
69. Andreoli SP, McAteer JA. Reactive oxygen molecule-mediated injury in endothelial and renal tubular epithelial cells in vitro. Kidney Int 1990; 38:785–794.
70. Lambeau G, Ancian P, Barhanin J, Lazdunski M. Cloning and expression of a membrane receptor for secretory phospholipases A_2. J Biol Chem 1994; 269:1575–1578.
71. Chen J, Engle SJ, Seilhamer JJ, Tischfield JA. Cloning and recombinant expression of a novel human low molecular weight Ca^{2+}-dependent phospholipase A_2. J Biol Chem 1994; 269:2365–2368.
72. Kuchler K, Gmachl M, Sippl MJ, Kreil G. Analysis of the cDNA of phospholipase A_2 from honeybee venom glands: The deduced amino acid sequence reveals homology to the corresponding vertebrate enzymes. Eur J Biochem 1989; 184:249–254.
73. Gronich JH, Bonventre JV, Nemenoff RA. Purification of a high-molecular-mass phospholipase A_2 from rat kidney activated at physiological calcium concentrations. Biochem J 1990; 271:37–43.
74. Clark JD, Milona N, Knopf JL. Purification of a 110-kilodalton cytosolic phospholipase A_2 from the human monocytic cell line U937. Proc Natl Acad Sci USA 1990; 87:7708–7712.
75. Kramer RM, Roberts EF, Manetta J, Putnam JE. The Ca^{2+}-sensitive cytosolic phospholipase A_2 is a 100-kDa protein in human monoblast U937 cells. J Biol Chem 1991; 266:5268–5272.
76. Kim DK, Bonventre JV. Purification of a 100 kDa phospholipase A_2 from spleen, lung and kidney:

Antiserum raised to pig spleen phospholipase A_2 recognizes a similar form in bovine lung, kidney and platelets, and immunoprecipitates phospholipase A_2 activity. Biochem J 1993; 294:261–270.

77. Leslie CC. Kinetic properties of a high molecular mass arachidonoyl-hydrolyzing phospholipase A_2 that exhibits lysophospholipase activity. J Biol Chem 1991; 266:11366–11371.
78. Reynolds LJ, Hughes LL, Louis AI, et al. Metal ion and salt effects on the phospholipase A_2, lysophospholipase, and transacylase activities of human cytosolic phospholipase A_2. Biochim Biophys Acta 1993; 1167:272–280.
79. Clark JD, Lin L-L, Kriz RW, et al. A novel arachidonic acid-selective cytosolic PLA_2 contains a Ca^{2+}-dependent translocation domain with homology to PKC and GAP. Cell 1991; 65:1043–1051.
80. Nalefski EA, Sultzman LA, Martin DM, et al. Delineation of two functionally distinct domains of cytosolic phospholipase A_2, a regulatory Ca^{2+}-dependent lipid-binding domain and a Ca^{2+}-independent catalytic domain. J Biol Chem 1994; 269:18239–18249.
81. Tay A, Maxwell P, Li ZG, et al. Isolation of promoter for cytosolic phospholipase A_2 ($cPLA_2$). Biochim Biophys Acta 1994; 1217:345–347.
82. Beckman JK, Borowitz SM, Burr IM. The role of phospholipase A activity in rat liver microsomal lipid peroxidation. J Biol Chem 1987; 262:1479–1484.
83. Bonventre JV, Swidler M. Calcium dependency of prostaglandin E_2 production in rat glomerular mesangial cells: Evidence that protein kinase C modulates the Ca^{2+}-dependent activation of phospholipase A_2. J Clin Invest 1988; 82:168–176.
84. Gronich JH, Bonventre JV, Nemenoff RA. Identification and characterization of a hormonally regulated form of phospholipase A_2 in rat renal mesangial cells. J Biol Chem 1988; 263:16645–16651.
85. Ghomashchi F, Schuttel S, Jain MK, Gelb MH. Kinetic analysis of a high molecular weight phospholipase A_2 from rat kidney: divalent metal-dependent trapping of enzyme on product containing veicles. Biochemistry 1992; 31:3814–3824.
86. Channon JY, Leslie CC. A calcium-dependent mechanism for associating a soluble arachidonyl-hydrolyzing phospholipase A_2 with membrane in the macrophage cell line RAW 264.7. J Biol Chem 1990; 265:5409–5413.
87. Perin MS, Fried VA, Mignery GA, et al. Phospholipid binding by a synaptic vesicle protein homologous to the regulatory region of protein kinase C. Nature 1990; 345:260–263.
88. Vogel US, Dixon RAF, Schaber MD, et al. Cloning of bovine GAP and its interaction with oncogenic ras p21. Nature 1988; 335:90–93.
89. Stahl ML, Ferenz CR, Kelleher KL, et al. Sequence similarity of phospholipase C with non-catalytic region of src. Nature 1988; 332:269–272.
90. Bonventre JV. Phospholipase A2 and signal transduction. J Am Soc Nephrol 1992; 3:128–150.
91. Bonventre JV. Mechanisms of ischemic acute renal failure. Kidney Int 1993; 43:1160–1178.
92. Chakraborti S, Gurtner GH, Michael JR. Oxidant-mediated activation of phospholipase A_2 in pulmonary endothelium. Am J Physiol 1989; 257:L430–L437.
93. Clark JD, Lin L-L, Kriz RW, et al. A novel arachidonic acid-selective cytosolic PLA2 contains a Ca^{2+}-dependent translocation domain with homology to PKC and GAP. Cell 1991; 65:1043–1051.
94. Channon JY, Leslie CC. A calcium-dependent mechanism for associating a soluble arachidonoyl-hydrolyzing phospholipase A2 with membrane in the macrophage cell line RAW 264.7. J Biol Chem 1990; 265:5409–5413.
95. Schramek H, Wang Y, Konieczkowski M, et al. Endothelin-1 stimulates cytosolic phospholipase A_2 activity and gene expression in rat glomerular mesangial cells. Kidney Int 1994; 46:1644–1652.
96. Simonson MS, Wann S, Mené P, et al. Endothelin stimulates phospholipase C, Na^+/H^+ exchange, c-fos expression, and mitogenesis in rat mesangial cells. J Clin Invest 1989; 83:708–712.
97. Kyriakis JM, Force TL, Rapp UR, et al. Mitogen regulation of c-Raf-1 protein kinase activity toward mitogen-activated protein kinase-kinase. J Biol Chem 1993; 268:16009–16019.
98. Gronich J, Konieczkowski M, Gelb MH, et al. Interleukin 1-alpha causes rapid activation of cytosolic phospholipase A2 by phosphorylation in rat mesangial cells. J Clin Invest 1994; 93:1224–1233.
99. Lin L-L, Lin AY, Knopf JL. Cytosolic phospholipase A_2 is coupled to hormonally regulated release of arachidonic acid. Proc Natl Acad Sci 1992; 89:6147–6151.
100. Lin L-L, Wartmann M, Lin AY, et al. $cPLA_2$ is phosphorylated and activated by MAP kinase. Cell 1993; 72:269–278.
101. Nemenoff RA, Winitz S, Qian N-X, et al. Phosphorylation and activation of a high molecular weight form of phospholipase A_2 by p42 microtubule-associated protein 2 kinase and protein kinase C. J Biol Chem 1993; 268:1960–1964.
102. Bonventre JV, Weber PC, Gronich JH. PAF and PDGF increase cytosolic [Ca^{2+}] and phospholipase activity in mesangial cells. Am J Physiol (Renal Fluid Electrolyte Physiol. 23) 1988; 254:F87–F94.
103. Bonventre JV, Gronich JH, Nemenoff RA. Epidermal growth factor enhances glomerular mesangial cell soluble phospholipase A_2 activity. J Biol Chem 1990; 265:4934–4938.

104. Clark S, Dunlop M. Modulation of phospholipase A_2 activity by epidermal growth factor (EGF) in CHO cells transfected with human EGF receptor: Role of cytoplasmic subdomain. Biochem J 1991; 274:715–721.
105. Goldberg HJ, Viegas MM, Margolis BL, et al. The tyrosine kinase activity of the epidermal-growth-factor receptor is necessary for phospholipase A_2 activation. Biochem J 1990; 267:461–465.
106. Winitz S, Gupta SK, Qian N-X, et al. Expression of a mutant G_{i2} α subunit inhibits ATP and thrombin stimulation of cytoplasmic phospholipase A_2-mediated arachidonic acid release independent of Ca^{2+} and mitogen-activated protein kinase regulation. J Biol Chem 1994; 269:1889–1895.
107. Bloch DB, Bonventre JV, Neer EJ, Seidman JG. The G protein α_o subunit alters morphology, growth kinetics, and phospholipid metabolism of somatic cells. Mol Cell Biol 1989; 9:5434–5439.
108. Ross BM, Kim DK Bonventre JV, Kish SJ. Characterization of a novel phospholipase A_2 activity in human brain. J Neurochem. In press.
109. Gassama-Diagne A, Fauvel J, Chap H. Purification of a new, calcium-independent, high molecular weight phospholipase A_2/lysophospholipase (phospholipase B) from guinea pig intestinal brush-border membrane. J Biol Chem 1989; 264:9470–9475.
110. Hazen SL, Stuppy RJ, Gross RW. Purification and characterization of canine myocardial cytosolic phospholipase A_2. J Biol Chem 1990; 265:10622–10630.
111. Ford DA, Hazen SL, Saffitz JE, Gross RW. The rapid and reversible activation of a calcium-independent plasmalogen-selective phospholipase A_2 during myocardial ischemia. J Clin Invest 1991; 88:331–335.
112. Ford DA, Hazen SL, Saffitz JE, Gross RW. The rapid and reversible activation of a calcium-independent plasmalogen-selective phospholipase A_2 during myocardial ischemia. J Clin Invest 1991; 88:331–335.
113. Ramanadham S, Wolf MJ, Jett PA, et al. Characterization of an ATP-stimulatable Ca^{2+}-independent phospholipase A_2 from clonal insulin-secreting HIT cells and rat pancreatic islets: A possible molecular component of the β-cell fuel sensor. Biochemistry 1994; 33:7442–7452.
114. Goligorsky MS, Morgan MA, Lyubsky S, et al. Establishment of a hydrogen peroxide resistant variant of renal tubular epithelial cells: Role of calcium-independent phospholipase A_2 in cell damage. Arch Biochem Biophys 1993; 301:119–128.
115. Goldman R, Ferber E, Zort U. Reactive oxygen species are involved in the activation of cellular phospholipase A_2. FEBS Lett 1992; 309:190–192.
116. Hazen SL, Gross RW. The specific association of a phosphofructokinase isoform with myocardial calcium-independent phospholipase A_2. J Biol Chem 1993; 268:9892–9900.
117. Gronich J, Konieczkowski M, Gelb MH, et al. Interleukin 1-alpha causes rapid activation of cytosolic phospholipase A_2 by phosphorylation in rat mesangial cells. J Clin Invest 1994; 93:1224–1233.
118. Goligorsky MS, Morgan MA, Lyubsky S, et al. Establishment of a hydrogen peroxide resistant variant of renal tubular epithelial cells: Role of calcium-independent phospholipase A_2 in cell damage. Arch Biochem Biophys 1993; 301:119–128.
119. Portilla D, Shah SV, Lehman PA, Creer MH. Role of cytosolic calcium-independent plasmalogen-selective phospholipase A_2 in hypoxic injury to rabbit proximal tubules. J Clin Invest 1994; 93:1609–1615.
120. Ackermann EJ, Kempner ES, Dennis EA. Ca^{2+}-independent cytosolic phospholipase A_2 from macrophage-like $P388D_1$ cells: Isolation and characterization. J Biol Chem 1994; 269:9227–9233.
121. Hirashima Y, Farooqui AA, Mills JS, Horrocks LA. Identification and purification of calcium-independent phospholipase A_2 from bovine brain cytosol. J Neurochem 1992; 59:708–714.
122. Yang H-C, Farooqui AA, Horrocks LA. Effects of glycosaminoglycans and glycosphingolipids on cytosolic phospholipase A_2 from bovine brain. Biochem J 1994; 299:91–95.
123. Shirataki H, Kaibuchi K, Sakoda T, et al. Rabphilin-3A, a putative target protein for smg p25A/rab3A p25 small GTP-binding protein related to synaptotagmin. Mol Cell Biol 1993; 13:2061–2068.

48

The Renal Plasminogen Activating System

Eric Rondeau and Jean-Daniel Sraer
Hôpital Tenon, Paris, France

Wolf-Dieter Schleuning
Schering Research Laboratories, Berlin, Germany

BIOCHEMISTRY AND MOLECULAR BIOLOGY OF THE PLASMINOGEN ACTIVATING SYSTEM

Components of the Plasminogen Activating System

Plasmin is a trypsin-like serine protease that is formed by cleavage of plasminogen, an inactive circulating zymogen mainly synthesized in the liver (1,2). Plasmin is the main enzyme responsible for fibrinolysis (i.e., degradation of fibrin polymers to fibrin degradation products). Plasmin is also able to degrade several components—such as fibronectin, lamin, and thrombospondin—of extracellular matrices and basement membranes, to activate latent procollagenases and metalloproteases and to release latent growth factors bound to extracellular matrix proteins (3). (Table 1 and Figure 1.)

Activation of plasminogen into plasmin is mediated by two major activators, tissue-type plasminogen activator (t-PA) and urokinase-type plasminogen activator (u-PA), which cleave the Arg 560-Val 561 peptide bond in plasminogen. t-PA and u-PA are 40% identical at the amino acid level but are encoded by different genes. These have been cloned and sequenced (4–7) and are localized on different chromosomes (8,9). Both are serine proteases. t-PA has an affinity for fibrin and requires the presence of fibrin to be fully active, whereas u-PA activity is not much influenced by fibrin (10). t-PA and u-PA are secreted as single-chain proenzymes (sct-PA and scu-PA), which are converted to fully active enzymes by limited proteolysis in the presence of trace amounts of plasmin (10).

The activity of u-PA and t-PA is also tightly controlled by the specific plasminogen activator inhibitors, type 1 (PAI-1) (11) and type 2 (PAI-2) (12). These inhibitors are encoded by distinct genes, which have been cloned and sequenced (12–14). PAI-1 is produced by a wide variety of cell types, including endothelial cells, fibroblasts, vascular smooth muscle cells, hepatocytes, and platelets. It is secreted in an active form but converted after secretion into a latent inactive form which can be reactivated in vitro by protein denaturants. PAI-1 inhibits tct-PA, sct-PA, and tcu-PA but not scu-PA (15,16) by forming 1:1 molar complexes. PAI-1 secretion and gene expression are upregulated by interleukin 1 (17,18), thrombin (19), bacterial endotoxin, basic fibroblast growth factor, dexamethasone, tumor necrosis factor α, transforming growth factor β, and platelet-derived growth factor (18,20,21).

PAI-2 is produced by the placenta and monocytes-macrophages (22). A 47-kDa unglycosylated form is found intracellularly, whereas a 60-kDa glycosylated form is found extracellularly. Unlike PAI-1, extracellular PAI-2 remains functional over extended periods of time. It is primarily a rapid inhibitor of u-PA and to a much lesser degree of tct-PA. The secretion of PAI-2 by monocytes/macrophages is increased by colony stimulating factor 1, phorbol myristate acetate, cholera toxin, and bacterial lipopolysaccharide (13,23,24).

Table 1 Biochemistry and Molecular Biology of the Plasminogen Activating System

	Mr	Amino acid residues	Structural characteristics	Gene localization	mRNA	Properties
Plasminogen	92 kDa	790	Single chain 5 kringles 5 lysine binding sites		2.9 kb	Inactive zymogen Affinity for fibrin, for cellular receptors and matrix proteins
Plasmin	90 kDa	560	Two chains A and B Two disulfide bridges	20 kb		Trypsin-like serine protease
t-PA	70 kDa	527	Secreted as single chain Growth factor-like domain Two kringle structures One finger domain	Chromosome 8	2.7 kb	Affinity for fibrin serine Protease activity
u-PA	53 kDa	411	Secreted as single chain Growth factor-like domain One kringle structure	Chromosome 10	2.5 kb	Inactive scu-PA Serine protease activity of tcu-PA Affinity for cellular u-PA receptors
PAI-1	46–54 kDa	379	Single chain	12.2 kb on chromosome 7	2.3 and 3.2 kb	Inhibition of t-PA and tcu-PA Binding to vitronectin but not scu-PA
PAI-2	47 kDa 60kDa	415	Single chain Highly glycosylated	Chromosome 18	2.0 kb	Inhibition of u-PA
PAI-3	50 kDa			?	?	Inhibition of u-PA and thrombin, and tot-PA
Protease nexin 1	45–51 kDa	392		?	2.5 kb	Thrombin, plasmin, u-PA, trypsin
u-PA-R	55 kDa	313	Glycophosphatidyl inositol anchored protein	?	1.4 kb	High-affinity receptor for scu-PA and tcu-PA

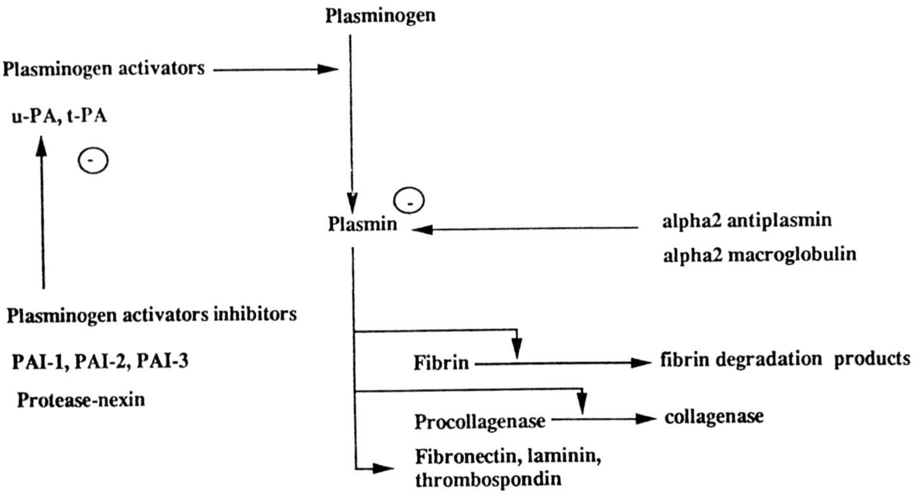

Figure 1 Schema of the plasminogen activating system.

Another plasminogen activator inhibitor, PAI-3, has been identified in human urine and in plasma (25). It is a single-chain 50-kDa glycoprotein forming 1:1 molar complexes with both u-PA and thrombin. It is immunologically identical to the heparin-dependent inhibitor of activated protein C. Protease nexin I is an inhibitor produced by a variety of cell types including fibroblasts, kidney epithelial cells, endothelial cells, and activated platelets (26,27). It inhibits thrombin, u-PA, plasmin, and trypsin.

Specific cell surface receptors of u-PA (u-PA-R) have been demonstrated (10,28,29). u-PA-R is a single-chain glycoprotein anchored to the plasma membrane by a glycosylphosphatidylinositol tail. It binds scu-PA and tcu-PA via the growth factor domain in the aminoterminal region of the molecule. u-PA-R cDNA has been cloned and sequenced (30).

Plasminogen/plasmin binding sites on various cell types have also been described. Their biochemical structure, however, remains unknown. The lysine-binding sites of plasminogen and plasmin are essential for this interaction. Plasmin attached to its binding site is protected from its circulating inhibitor, alpha2 antiplasmin (31).

Gene Structures and Promoters

The t-PA Gene

The human t-PA gene has been isolated and sequenced (32,33). The 2658-bases-long t-PA mRNA is encoded by a gene of approximately 33 kb overall length. The t-PA gene contains 14 coding regions interrupted by 13 introns. The gene and the 5′ flanking region contain 28 copies of Alu repetitive DNA and a single Kpn I repeat. The putative transcription start site is located 24 bp downstream a typical TATA consensus sequence. Two additional TATA motifs with unknown functions are found 93 and 226 bp upstream of the putative cap site. No sequences resembling the consensus for glucocorticoid receptor binding nor for cAMP or metal ion–mediated or interferon-stimulated induction were found in the 3530-bp 5′ region (33). In contrast, the 5′ region of the rat t-PA gene contains a cAMP-responsive element (CRE), the binding site for the transacting factor, termed CRE-binding protein (CREB) (34). Other potential recognition sequences for NF1 and SP1 and two sequence elements with homology to the consensus binding site for transcription factor AP2 have also been found in the 5′ flanking region of the rat t-PA gene (34). At the position −177 to −185 of the 5′ flanking region, where the CRE is located in the rat t-PA gene, both human and mouse genes have a 12-0 tetradecanoylphorbol-13-acctate-responsive element (TRE), a consensus recognition site for transcription factor AP1 coded for protooncogene *jun* (34,35). TRE has been shown to mediate induction by tumor-promoting phorbol esters. Furthermore, a DNA motif related to the CRE and an exon-located activator protein-2 binding site in the human tissue-type plasminogen activator gene promoter have been shown to cooperate in basal expression and to convey activation by phorbol esters and cAMP (36).

The u-PA Gene

The human u-PA gene is organized in 11 exons and is 6.4 kb long (37). The 5′ flanking region contains CAAT and TATA boxes, which are separated by a DNA fragment containing three sequences GGCGGG, previously found at similar regions in viral and eukaryotic promoters and shown to be essential for promoter activity. A fragment of 800 bp containing the entire 5′ flanking region shows promoter activity when introduced into human cells (37). A DNA fragment from −2350 to −1824 has enhancerless SV40 early promoter independently of orientation and distance (38). The removal of negative *cis*-acting sequences between −1824 and −1572 increases u-PA transcriptional activity if the more distal enhancer region is still retained. The pig (39) and mouse (40) u-PA genes have also been sequenced, including their 5′ flanking regions (41). A complex CRE between −3415 and −3340 is present in the pig promoter but is very poorly conserved in the mouse sequence. A combined PEA-3/AP1 site, implicated in phorbol ester/EGF induction of u-PA, is present in the human, mouse, and pig sequences about 2 kb from the transcription start site (41). u-PA promoters contain multiple AP1- and AP2-like DNA sequences. They also contain multiple binding sites for NF-κB. The conserved, transcribed 5′ noncoding sequences are also required for maximal gene expression, indicating the presence of multiple *cis* acting elements distributed over 7 kb 5′ to the translation start site of the u-PA gene.

The PAI-1 Gene

The human PAI-1 structural gene is approximately 12.2 kb pairs in length and consists of 9 exons (1206 bp coding for the 23 amino acids of the signal peptide and 379 amino acids of the mature PAI-1 protein), 8 introns (a total of 8978 bp), and a long 3′-untranslated region of about 1800 bp, which contains several polyadenylation sites (42,43). The length of the PAI-1 5′ untranslated region is 145 bp (43). The 5′ flanking DNA region (1520 bp) contains the essential eukaryotic *cis*-type proximal regulatory elements CCAAT and TATAA. The more distal 5′ flanking DNA region, as well as some introns, contains sequence elements that share identities with known eukaryotic enhances elements: SV40 enhancer, SV40 Sp1 protein binding site, a sequence element common to acute-phase reactant genes, and the possible human antithrombin III gene enhancer (43). Interestingly a large region (521 bp) of the 5′ flanking DNA of PAI-1 gene is 81% identical with the 5′ flanking DNA of the t-PA gene. These sequence identities are located on opposite DNA strands and their functional significance is not known. The rat PAI-1 gene structure resembles that of the human PAI-1 gene, including two regions in the 5′ flanking sequence (44). These two regions are involved in the glucocorticoid regulation of expression of the human PAI-1 gene (45), although they do not contain the hexamer consensus sequence for glucocorticoid-responsive elements (GRE). In the 5′ flanking region of the rat gene, five putative GRE and seven putative CRE have been identified, whereas there is only one CRE in the human gene (44).

The PAI-2 Gene

The cDNA of human PAI-2 have been cloned and sequenced from human placenta (46) and from the histiocytic lymphoma cell line U937 (13,47). To date, the structure of the PAI-2 gene is not known. A 2-kb region of the PAI-2 gene promoter has been sequenced and shown, by functional assays, to contain various *cis*-acting regions. In HT 1080 cells, constitutive expression of the gene requires more than 215 bp of the promoter sequence, whereas it is abolished by deletion to position −91 bp. This deletion also prevented any induction by phorbol esters. The promoter region between −215 and the transcription initiation site possesses numerous protected regions, including two AP1-like binding sites (AP1a and AP1b) and one CRE-like element, which seem necessary for constitutive expression and also for phorbol ester induction (48).

CELLULAR LOCALIZATION OF PLASMINOGEN ACTIVATORS AND THEIR INHIBITORS IN THE KIDNEY

Fibrinolytic activity in urine was recognized more than a hundred years ago (49). This PA was enriched and partially purified in 1951 (50). Epithelial cell lines derived from renal tissues of pigs, dogs, and monkeys have been shown to produce u-PA (51,52). By immunohistochemical studies, t-PA has been detected mainly in the glomerulus (53,54,55), whereas u-PA was found in the renal tubules (56). By sensitive enzymatic assays and zymography, supernatants of glomeruli isolated from rat and human renal cortex have been shown to contain a plasminogen activator activity (57,58), which was identified as free t-PA (Figure 2) accompanied by small amounts of t-PA-PAI-1 complexes and u-PA (53,55,59,60). Similar results were obtained recently with rabbit glomeruli (61).

By immunohistochemical methods, t-PA is localized in the glomerulus, in endothelial and/or mesangial cells of the normal adult human kidney, whereas PAI-1 and u-PA are not detectable (53). Similarly, using in situ zymography and in situ hybridization, Sappino et al. and Kristensen et al. demonstrated that in the adult mouse kidney, u-PA is synthesized by the epithelial cells lining the straight parts of both proximal and distal tubules (Figure 3), whereas t-PA is produced by glomerular cells and also by epithelial cells lining the distal part of the collecting ducts (62,63). The discrepancies between the results obtained by biochemical and immunohistochemical methods may be related to a difference in sensitivity and/or a tubular contamination during the isolation of the glomeruli. PAI-1 mRNA and protein expression in the mouse kidney is almost undetectable; however, it is increased after bacterial endotoxin injection and localized in glomerular and vascular endothelial cells (64). In the normal kidney, PAI-1 is not detectable, although a single study reported PAI-1 antigen expression in glomerular epithelial cells and to a lesser extent in mesangial and glomerular endothelial cells (65). The detection and localization of PAI-2 and u-PA-R in the kidney have as yet not been reported.

REGULATION OF PLASMINOGEN ACTIVATOR AND INHIBITOR BIOSYNTHESIS IN KIDNEY CELLS

Cultured kidney cells have been used to investigate PA gene regulation or to study the pathophysiology of glomerular fibrin deposition and glomerulosclerosis. However, due to changes in differentiation and culture conditions, cultured kidney cells may express PAs and PAIs with a different pattern from their normal counterparts in vivo. Therefore, results obtained with cultured cells have to be interpreted with caution.

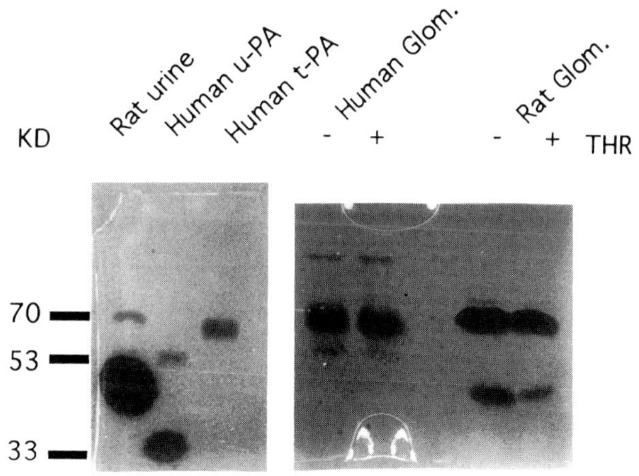

Figure 2 Zymographic analysis of human and rat glomerular plasminogen activators Glomeruli isolated from normal human or rat kidney cortex were incubated for 30 min at 37°C in the absence (–) or presence (+) of 10^{-8} M α thrombin. After centrifugation, the supernatants were analyzed by SDS-PAGE and zymography on a fibrin-agar underlay containing plasminogen. As controls of molecular weight and plasminogen activator activity, rat urine, human u-PA, and human t-PA were analyzed by the same method. t-PA (70 kDa) is the main plasminogen activator of rat and human glomeruli. Small amounts of u-PA are also detected.

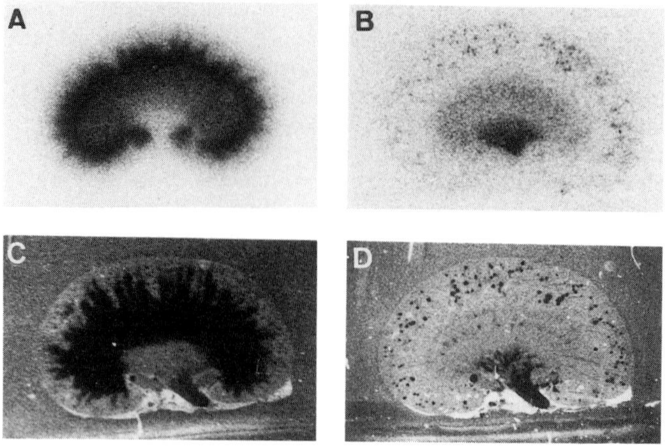

Figure 3 Regional localization of u-PA (A) and t-PA (B) mRNAs by in situ hybridizations of ^{32}P-labeled cRNA probes to cryostat tissue sections of adult kidneys. Photographs were taken after 24 hr (A) and 96 hr (B) exposure at room temperature (×3). Visualization of PA enzymatic activities by histological zymographies on cryostat tissue sections of adult kidneys. Incubations were performed in the absence (C) or in the presence of 1 mM amiloride (D) which selectively inhibits u-PA. Photographs were taken after 2 h (C) and 5 h (D) incubations at 37°C (×3). (Reproduced from Sappins et al., *J. Clin. Invest.*, 1991, with permission.)

Cultured Glomerular Cells

Glomerular Visceral Epithelial Cells

Human glomerular epithelial cells in culture, identified by morphological and immunocytochemical criteria as visceral epithelial cells or podocytes, synthesize mainly a 53-kDa form of sc-u-PA (66). Traces amounts of t-PA, complexed to PAI-1, are also released in the culture medium (Figure 4). GEC also express cell surface u-PA-R, partially autosaturated by endogenously secreted scu-PA. scu-PA and t-PA-PAI-1 complexes were identified by fibrin autography and by immunoblotting with specific antibodies (66). Free PAI-1, in a latent form, can also be demonstrated by reverse fibrin

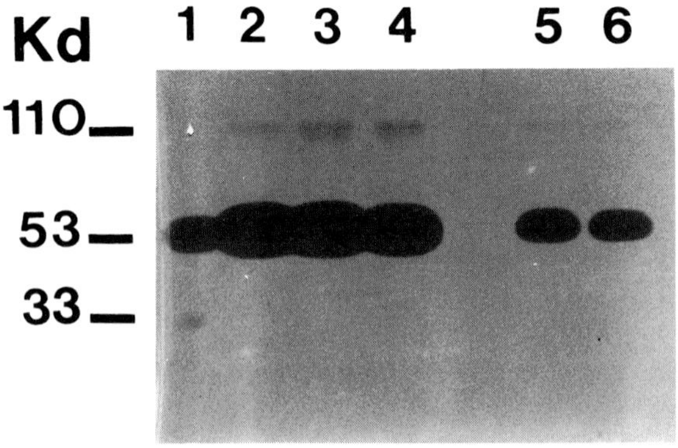

Figure 4 Zymography of culture medium conditioned by glomerular epithelial cells for 24 h. Lane 1 = 1 U/ml standard u-PA, lanes 2 to 5 = conditioned culture medium of GECs incubated in unstimulated conditions (lane 2), or in the presence of thrombin 10^{-9} M (lane 3), 5.10^{-9} M (lane 4), 10^{-8} M (lane 5), or 2.10^{-8} M (lane 6). As previously described (Rondeau et al, 1989), GECs release mainly 53 Kd u-PA and small amounts of PAI-1-t-PA and PAI-1-u-PA complexes. Thrombin decreased the activity of 53 Kd u-PA. (Reproduced from He' et al., *J. Cell Physiol.*, 1991, with permission.)

autography (67). Activation of protein kinase C with phorbol myristate acetate stimulates scu-PA, t-PA, and PAI-1 release by GEC in a time- and dose-dependent manner. This effect is associated with an increase in the steady-state level of u-PA mRNA and is inhibited by actinomycin D, suggesting that PMA induces an increase in u-PA gene transcription, as previously reported in other cell types (68). Activation of protein kinase A by 8-bromo cyclicAMP inhibits PMA-induced u-PA synthesis by GEC and PMA-induced u-PA mRNA increase. The exact mechanism of action of cAMP is not known. A cAMP-responsive element has been identified in the u-PA gene promoter, and cAMP has been shown to activate, not inhibit, u-PA gene transcription and u-PA biosynthesis in other cell types (69). Tissue or species specificity of u-PA regulation by protein kinase A activators may be the underlying cause for these discrepancies.

As fibrin deposition in the pericapillary space of the glomerulus requires local thrombin generation, the effects of thrombin on GEC in culture have been studied (70). Thrombin has a time- and dose-dependent proliferative effect on these cells. It also stimulates the synthesis of u-PA, t-PA, and PAI-1 via increased gene transcription. However, thrombin generates a double chain form of u-PA, which cannot be activated anymore. This results in decreased PA activity of thrombin-stimulated GEC-conditioned medium. Thrombin has also been shown to decrease the number of uPA-R at the GEC surface. Taken together, these results suggest that thrombin induces fibrin formation in Bowman's space of the glomeruli and possibly inhibits local fibrinolytic activity. IL-1 has been shown to stimulate t-PA and PAI-1 but not u-PA synthesis by GEC, whereas TNF-α increases u-PA and t-PA synthesis but has no effect on PAI-1. In the same study, γ interferon had no significant effect on the plasminogen activating system of GEC (71).

Human GEC produce endothelin 1 (ET-1) and express ET-1 receptors. These receptors are functional, since addition of ET-1 induced a rapid and transient increase in intracellular Ca^{2+} concentration (72). In an immortalized GEC line (E71 A1), ET-1 has been shown to have no effect on u-PA synthesis but to induce an increase in u-PA-R without change in receptor affinity (73). This effect is associated with an increase in u-PA-R mRNA steady-state level. The protein synthesis inhibitor cycloheximide blocks ET-1-induced u-PA-R increase at the cell surface but potentiates ET-1–induced u-PA-R mRNA augmentation. Human GEC also express low-affinity binding sites for plasminogen/plasmin. Activation of plasminogen to plasmin at the cell surface is promoted by u-PA bound to u-PA-R (74).

Mesangial Cells

Human mesangial cells in culture produce large amounts of PAI-1 and 100-fold less t-PA (75). They do not produce u-PA, although this remains controversial and may depend on cell passages, differentiation, and culture conditions (76). By zymography, only t-PA-PAI-1 complexes can be detected in the conditioned culture medium (Figure 5). Free PAI-1 is demonstrated by reverse fibrin autography. Activation of protein kinase C by phorbol myristate acetate induces a time- and

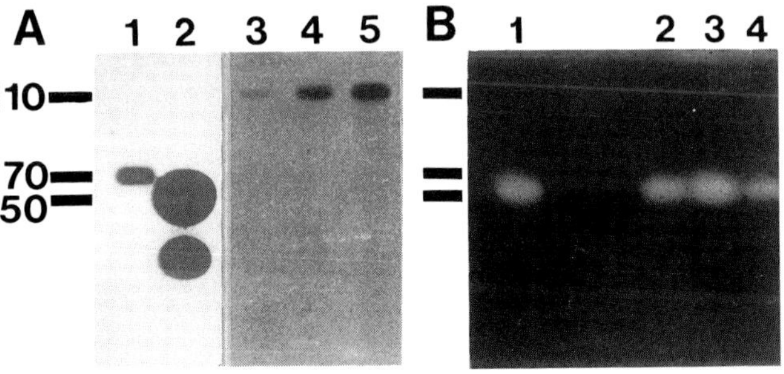

Figure 5 Effect of thrombin on t-PA and PAI-1 activities by zymography (A) and reverse fibrin autography (B). Zymography: lane 1: control human t-PA; lane 2: control human u-PA; lane 3: culture medium of unstimulated mesangial cells; lanes 4 and 5: culture medium of mesangial cells stimulated by 0.5 U/ml (lane 4) or 1 U/ml (lane 5) thrombin for 24 hr. (B) Reverse fibrin autography: lane 1: control human 50-kDa PAI-1; lane 2: culture medium of unstimulated mesangial cells; and lanes 3 and 4: culture medium of mesangial cells stimulated by 0.5 U/ml (lane 3) or 1 U/ml (lane 4) thrombin for 24 hr. Reproduced from Villamediana et al., *Kidney Int.*, 1990, with permission.)

dose-dependent increase in t-PA and PAI-1 release through an increase of gene transcription, as demonstrated by inhibition with alpha-amanitin and by Northern blot analysis. Activation of the protein kinase A pathway with 8-bromo cyclicAMP has no effect on basal production of t-PA and PAI-1 by HMC in culture (77). However 8 bromocyclic AMP was shown to decrease in a dose-dependent manner PMA-stimulated increase of t-PA and PAI-1 synthesis. At the mRNA level, cAMP inhibits PAI-1 mRNA accumulation induced by PMA but potentiates the t-PA mRNA accumulation, as also shown in other cell types. The inhibitory effect of cAMP on t-PA synthesis could therefore involve a posttranscriptional mechanism (77). Thrombin is also able to stimulate t-PA and PAI-1 synthesis by HMC, an effect that is mediated by protein kinase C activation, as suggested by the inhibition of the thrombin effect by H7 and by the downregulation of PKC. Thrombin induces an increase in t-PA and PAI-1 mRNA steady-state levels in HMC, and this effect is prevented by H7 (Figure 6) (78).

TNF α has been shown to selectively stimulate PAI-1 synthesis by HMC, whereas it has no effect on t-PA synthesis. It acts through an increase in PAI-1 gene transcription. The intracellular pathways stimulated by TNF α in HMC remain poorly understood but seem different from PKC activation (79).

PAI-1 has been shown to bind to the extracellular matrix of HMC in culture in a pericellular localization. As cell confluency increases, less matrix PAI-1 can be detected, suggesting that it can be removed by spreading cells. In vitro, addition of u-PA or t-PA to cultured HMC can remove matrix PAI-1, suggesting that cell surface–bound t-PA could complex matrix PAI-1. This process may play a role in mesangial matrix remodeling and mesangial cell migration (80).

In contrast to these results, some groups reported that rat and human MC produce u-PA, bound to a specific phospholipase C–sensitive u-PA-R alone or in a complex with PAI-1 (76,81). It has also been shown that antibodies to u-PA inhibit the loss of adhesion fragmentation of stress fiber and the shape changes induced by cAMP in rat mesangial cells. Similarly, thrombin was also able to inhibit u-PA activity of the conditioned medium and to prevent cAMP-induced shape changes by inactivating scu-PA released by rat mesangial cells (82). However, more recently, the same authors demonstrated that a synthetic peptide that is able to activate the thrombin receptor but has no enzymatic activity is also able to prevent cAMP-induced shape-changes in human mesangial cells (83). Taken together, these results indicate that the thrombin-induced inhibition of mesangial shape changes is not mediated by direct inactivation of scu-PA by thrombin.

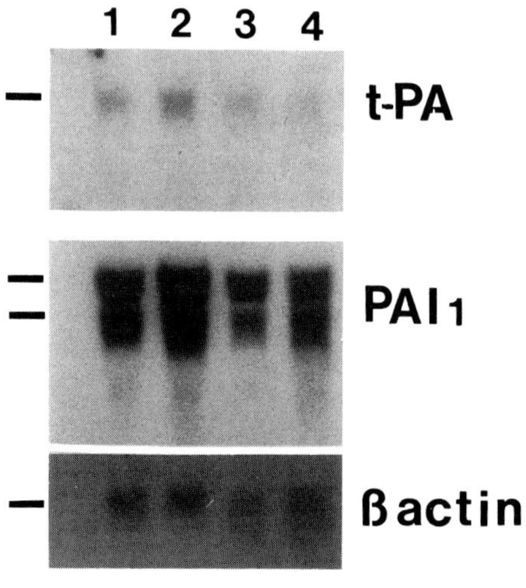

Figure 6 Northern blot analysis with a t-PA cDNA probe and PAI-1 cDNA probe. Ten μg of total RNA were used from mesangial cells incubated for 4 hr in control conditions (lane 1), in the presence of 1 U/ml thrombin (lane 2), in the presence of 12.5 μmol H7 (lane 3), and in the presence of 1 U/ml thrombin and 12.5 μmol H7 (lane 4). The control made with the β-actin cDNA probe shows that the same amount of total RNA was transferred in each lane. (Reproduced from Villamediana et al., *Kidney Int.*, 1991, with permission.)

Human Renal Microvascular Endothelial Cells

Wojta et al. have shown that renal microvascular endothelial cells isolated from human kidney cortex produce exclusively scu-PA but neither t-PA nor PAI-1. In contrast, omental microvascular endothelial cells and umbilical vein endothelial cells produce exclusively t-PA but not u-PA, indicating that the origin of the vascular bed influences the expression of plasminogen activators (84). Phorbol ester and thrombin were shown to increase u-PA mRNA and u-PA antigen in renal microvascular endothelial cells, whereas dexamethasone had no significant effect.

Tubular Epithelial Cells

Most studies of PA synthesis by tubular epithelial cells have been performed with LLC-PK1 and MDCK cells. These spontaneously transformed cell lines have been used as a model to study the molecular mechanisms of regulation of u-PA and PAI-1 synthesis (69). Some human renal carcinoma cell lines have also been shown to produce u-PA in vitro (85). No data are available concerning nontransformed tubular epithelial cells in primary culture. For this reason, the results obtained with transformed cell lines are of doubtful relevance for normal physiology or pathophysiology in vivo. To date, the exact role of u-PA in the kidney remains poorly understood.

Calcitonin and vasopressin have been shown to increase u-PA synthesis by LLC-PK1 cells (86). This effect is mediated by stimulation of adenylate cyclase, resulting in cAMP generation and protein kinase A activation. 8-bromo cAMP and other agents that increase intracellular cAMP concentrations, such as cholera toxin and the phosphodiesterase inhibitor isobutylmethylxanthine (IBMX), also increased u-PA synthesis.

The effects of cAMP-elevating agents on u-PA synthesis are inhibited by cycloheximide and actinomycin D, suggesting the requirement of transcription and translation. An early increase in u-PA mRNA level within 3 hr of stimulation by calcitonin has been demonstrated (87). Increased u-PA gene transcription in LLC-PK1, treated with calcitonin or with cAMP, was directly demonstrated by nuclear run-on transcription stimulation. Cycloheximide does not prevent mRNA accumulation for u-PA by calcitonin, indicating that gene induction by cAMP-mediated signal transduction is independent of de novo protein synthesis. Calcium potentiates cAMP-dependent expression of the u-PA gene through a calmodulin- and protein kinase C-independent mechanism (88).

Using a cell-free transcription system with various templates, deleted in the 5′-flanking region of the u-PA gene, it has been shown that sequences essential for cAMP induction and for basal expression of u-PA are located between 148 and 53 bp 5′ of the transcription initiation site. By DNAse I footprinting analysis, two protein-binding sites were identified within the u-PA promoter, with consensus sequences for the binding of transcription factors SP1 and AP1. The AP1-binding sequence, which mediates the phorbol myristate acetate action, could also mediate the cAMP induction of u-PA gene transcription, at least in the cell-free system. By transfecting a construct composed of u-PA gene promoter linked to a chloramphenicol acetyltransferase reporter gene in LLC-PK1 cells, it has been shown that other sequences further upstream were necessary for efficient transcription and cAMP induction (69).

Tumor promoters like phorbol myristate acetate and mezerein, which activate PKC, induce an accumulation of u-PA mRNA, but to a lesser extent than cAMP (68). PKC activation induces a rapid, transient increase of u-PA gene transcription. Within 2 hr, cells lose their response to PMA, while they retain responsiveness to cAMP-related agents (68). Furthermore, downregulation of PKC results in an enhanced induction of u-PA gene expression by cAMP-mediated signals without alterations in adenylate cyclase activity, suggesting a mechanism distal to adenylate cyclase (89). H7, an inhibitor of PKC, also inhibits the PMA-induced u-PA synthesis by LLC-PK1. Nordihydroguaiaretic acid (NDGA), an inhibitor of the lipoxygenase pathway, has a similar inhibitory effect. NDGA has been shown to inhibit PMA-stimulated PKC activity and to decrease u-PA mRNA level in PMA-stimulated LLC-PK1 cells (90). Other mechanisms leading to u-PA gene expression in LLC-PK1 are disruption of cytoskeletal structures by agents such as colchicine, nocodazole, or cytochalasin B (91) and inhibition of protein phosphatases 1 and 2A by okadaic acid (92). This effect occurs independently of cAMP-dependent protein kinase and protein kinase C and is sensitive to protein synthesis inhibition.

Dexamethasone has been shown to inhibit calcitonin induction of u-PA enzyme activity in

LLC-PK1 cells by at least two mechanisms: induction of an inhibitor of u-PA and reduction in u-PA mRNA levels. Dexamethasone reduces the transcription rate of the calcitonin-induced u-PA gene but does not affect the half life of u-PA mRNA (93).

POTENTIAL ROLES OF THE PLASMINOGEN ACTIVATING SYSTEM IN KIDNEY PHYSIOLOGY AND PATHOLOGY

Renal Ontogeny

As shown by Sappino et al., the kidney is the main site of synthesis of u-PA in the mouse embryo (Figure 7), whereas t-PA is produced in the brain and in the kidney cortex (62). Early expression of t-PA in the kidneys of human embryos has also been demonstrated, especially during glomerulogenesis. By immunohistochemical methods, t-PA has been localized in the developing glomerulus of human

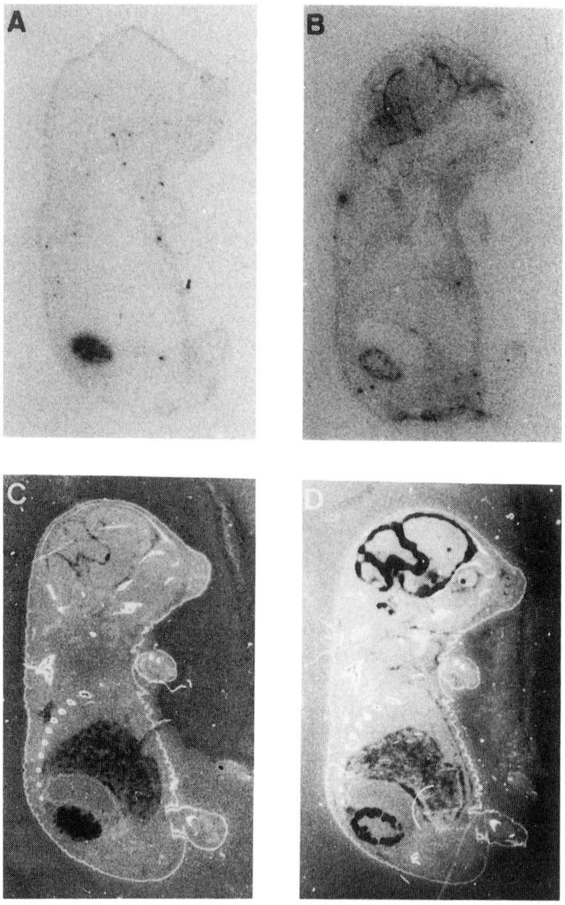

Figure 7 Regional localization of u-PA (A) and t-PA (B) mRNAs by in situ hybridizations of ^{32}P-labeled cRNA probes to cryostat tissue sections of 17.5-day-old mouse embryos. Photographs were taken after 72 hr (A) and 120 hr (B) exposure at room temperature (×2.5). Visualization of PA enzymatic activities by histological zymographies on cryostat tissues sections of 17.5-day-old mouse embryos. Incubations were performed in the absence (C) or in the presence of 1 m*M* amiloride (D), which selectively inhibits u-PA. In addition to the caseinolytic zones observed over the kidney, plasminogen-dependent proteolytic activity was observed over the liver and the brain. Photographs were taken after 2-hr (C) and 4-hr (D) incubations at 37°C (×2.5). Reproduced from Sappino et al., *J. Clin. Invest.*, 1991, with permission.).

embryonic kidneys. At the early stage formation of the S-shaped body, during glomerular differentiation, t-PA antigen is codistributed with a marker of invading endothelial cells, *Ulex europaeus* lectin. During further stages of glomerular maturation, t-PA is also found in developing and proliferating visceral epithelial cells or podocytes. By the same methods, u-PA has been localized in the proximal tubules but not in the glomerulus. These results suggest but do not prove that u-PA and t-PA could play a role in the formation of the tubules and the glomeruli, respectively. Interestingly, it has been shown that MDCK epithelial cells, grown in collagen or fibrin gels in the presence of fibroblasts or fibroblast-conditioned medium, form branching tubules instead of the spherical cysts, which develop under control conditions (94). The fibroblast-derived molecule responsible for epithelial tubulogenesis is hepatocyte growth factor (HGF) (95). In fibrin gels, the effect of HGF is inhibited by addition of exogenous serine protease inhibitors, suggesting a role for plasminogen activators in the matrix remodeling required for tubulogenesis. HGF has been shown to increase u-PA and u-PA receptor expression in MDCK cells and u-PA has been shown to activate the latent, secreted form of HGF (pro-HGF), which is mostly matrix-associated, into the active $\alpha\beta$ heterodimer of HGF (96). This effect of u-PA, however, has not been confirmed by all authors (97). These results suggest that HGF could regulate the cell surface proteolytic activity of epithelial cells required during tubule formation. It has to be noted that collagenases rather than u-PA are required for MDCK to form tubules in collagen gels. Whether u-PA and collagenases act in concert in vivo remains to be established.

Remodeling of Extracellular Matrix

TGFβ has been shown to play a pivotal role in the pathological accumulation of extracellular matrix in experimental glomerulonephritis induced by antithymocyte serum (ATS) in the rat. TGFβ increases the synthesis and deposition of extracellular matrix components by glomerular cells but also decreases matrix degradation. When added to isolated normal glomeruli, TGFβ decreases PA activity and increases PAI-1 synthesis (98). Diseased glomeruli from experimental animals injected with ATS also show decreased PA activity, increased PAI-1 synthesis, and increased PAI-1 deposition into matrix. These effects are prevented by administration of anti-TGFβ serum to glomerulonephritic rats. These results suggest that glomerular PA activity is required for glomerular matrix remodeling and the prevention of glomerulosclerosis. Cultured rat mesangial cells degrade extracellular matrix only in the presence of exogenously added plasminogen. Plasmin can directly degrade extracellular matrix but can also activate a latent 70-kDa gelatinase, which is released by mesangial cells (99).

Intrarenal Fibrinolysis

In an experimental model of intravascular coagulation induced by thrombin infusion in the rat, it has been shown that thrombi accumulate in glomerular capillaries. These thrombi progressively disappear after the end of thrombin infusion, indicating effective local fibrinolysis. Glomeruli isolated from rats injected with thrombin release more t-PA than glomeruli from control animals (57).

However, in human nephropathies, fibrin deposition is frequently observed in the absence of intravascular coagulation. A defective local fibrinolytic activity could explain the persistence of fibrin deposits either in the renal vasculature or in Bowman's capsule of glomeruli during extracapillary glomerulonephritis. Recombinant t-PA and streptokinase have been shown to decrease glomerular fibrin deposition in experimental models of glomerulonephritis (100,101). PAI-1 deposition has been demonstrated in human vascular and glomerular diseases associated with fibrin deposits (102), suggesting that hormones or cytokines such as TNF-α or IL-1, which induce PAI-1 synthesis (17,20,21), could promote fibrin accumulation in these cases. In the mouse, TNF-α, LPS, and TGFβ have been shown to increase the steady-state levels of mRNA for PAI-1 in the kidney within 3 hr (103). By in situ hybridization, PAI-1 mRNA was observed in glomerular and peritubular endothelial cells of LPS-injected mice but not in control mice (64). Thus intrarenal fibrinolysis, which seems mainly mediated by t-PA, can be inhibited by PAI-1 released by activated endothelial cells.

In an experimental model of anti-GBM glomerulonephritis in the rat, an increased PA release from isolated diseased glomeruli has been reported during the late phase of the disease (14 days) (104). This increased PA activity was correlated with the amount of glomerular fibrin deposition detected by immunofluorescence, suggesting that fibrin or factors leading to fibrin formation (cytokines, thrombin) stimulate PA release and that, as in human diseases, PAI could neutralize PA activity at the fibrin surface in vivo. Administration of anti-GBM antibody in the rat is associated with a rapid and transient increase in circulating plasma PAI-1 and an increased PAI-1 release from isolated glomeruli cultured for 4 and 24 hr in vitro. Concomitant administration of TNF-α induces a greater increase in PAI-1 release and in glomerular fibrin formation (105).

Mor recently Malliaros et al. showed that in anti-GBM glomerulonephritis in rabbits, glomerular fibrin deposition occurs only in the autologous phase of the disease and is dependent on macrophage infiltration and macrophage procoagulant activity. In this model, net glomerular fibrinolytic activity, measured 4 days after the induction of the disease, is significantly decreased compared to that in control animals or to animals with macrophage-independent anti-GBM induced glomerulonephritis (heterologous phase). The reduced glomerular fibrinolytic activity is associated with decreased expression of t-PA and increased expression of PAI-1 (61). Similarly, Feng et al. showed that glomerular PAI-1 mRNA level and PAI-1 bioactivity increase rapidly within 6 to 24 hr after the induction of an accelerated form of anti GBM glomerulonephritis in the rat. In contrast, there were no significant changes in u-PA and t-PA mRNA levels until day 6, where a slight increase in t-PA mRNA was observed. Interestingly these authors also showed an early increase in IL1 β mRNA expression within 6 hr and in TGFβ1 mRNA within 1 day, suggesting that these cytokines may play a role in the rapid and sustained increase in glomerular PAI-1 expression (106). By immunohistochemical methods, u-PA has been detected in the glomeruli of renal allograft during rejection episodes (107). However, by zymographic analysis of glomeruli obtained from rejected human kidney allografts, no u-PA was detected; rather, a decreased fibrinolytic activity was reported (108).

Tubular Permeability and Tubular Handling of Proteinases

Hypothetically, u-PA secreted by tubular epithelial cells could regulate intratubular protein degradation and prevent tubular obstruction. MDCK cells grown on polycarbonate filters do secrete u-PA predominantly at the apical site (109,110), but LLC-PK1 release u-PA at the basolateral site. PAI-1 was found in both compartments in equal amounts. Basolateral accumulation of u-PA, but not its apical targeting, requires functional intracellular acidic compartments and the integrity of the cytoskeleton (110). Thus u-PA released by tubular epithelial cells could also play a role in the pericellular proteolytic activity at the basolateral site of the cells. Whether urine acidification in vivo also modifies the basolateral release of u-PA is not known. Proximal tubular epithelial cells in the rat and human kidney express a 330-kDa glycoprotein called gp330, which is also expressed by rat but not human podocytes in vivo. gp 330 was originally identified as a target molecule in the kidney for autoimmune antibodies in rats with Heymann's nephritis. It is a calcium-binding receptor for endocytic uptake of proteins (111). Fragments of partial cDNA for gp330 have been cloned, and it has been shown that gp330 has homology with the LDL receptor and with the LDL receptor-related protein/alpha$_2$ macroglobulin receptor (LRP) involved in the binding and internalization of alpha$_2$ macroglobulin, alpha$_2$ macroglobulin-protease complexes, and of u-PA-or t-PA-PAI-1 complexes (112). More recently it has been shown that gp330 also binds several ligands of LRP, including t-PA-PAI-1 and u-PA-PAI-1 complexes (113). This binding is inhibited by a 39-kDa protein, known as alpha$_2$ macroglobulin receptor-associated protein or alpha$_2$-MRAP, which copurifies with LRP and gp330 and inhibits alpha$_2$ macroglobulin binding to LRP. The exact role of gp330 in the kidney is not clearly understood, but these results suggest that it could be involved in the internalization of u-PA-PAI-1 complexes and the regulation of intratubular proteolytic activity. Furthermore, Kanalas reported that plasminogen binds to gp330 in vitro and that it can be converted to active plasmin by urokinase. Plasmin bound to gp330 is protected from inactivation by its natural inhibitor, alpha$_2$ antiplasmin (114).

Renal Tumor Invasion and Dissemination

Using the in vivo chorioallantoic membrane, Ossowski et al. showed that tumor cells expressing both the surface u-PA-R and elevated levels of u-PA invade more efficiently than cells expressing either one of the components. Furthermore, to be effective in local invasion, a tumor cell has to be able to express at least u-PA, its receptor and interstitial collagenase, and possibly type IV gelatinase (115,116).

Although the plasminogen activating system may play a role in renal cancer invasion and metastasis, it has not been studied to date, in contrast to other carcinomas from the stomach, prostate, bladder, and colon.

Renal carcinoma cell lines (A 1251, Cur, and Caki-1) have been shown to produce u-PA, the production of which is increased by PMA (117,118). Interestingly, u-PA may also have a proliferative effect on various cell types, including malignant and normal renal cells (119,120). The proliferative effect of u-PA requires the binding to u-PA-R and in some cell types an intact proteolytic activity (119). The mechanism of this proliferative effect is still unknown but could be related to the activation of specific tyrosine kinases. It has recently been shown by immunoprecipitation that u-PAR is associated with a 38-kDa protein that is phosphorylated on tyrosine after u-PA treatment of cells (121).

CONCLUSIONS AND PERSPECTIVES

Plasminogen activators t-PA and u-PA are produced by kidney cells in specific parts of the nephron. While t-PA could be involved in glomerulogenesis and intravascular fibrinolysis, u-PA could be involved in tubular formation and intratubular proteolysis. PAI-1 does not seem to be expressed in normal conditions but is upregulated in endothelial and mesangial cells under pathological conditions. PAI-2 has not been detected within the kidney and no data are available concerning renal expression of u-PA-R.

Investigation of the plasminogen activating system in the kidney during aging and fibrosis could provide important clues for matrix degradation during these processes and provide potential leads to therapeutical intervention. Similarly, the role of the system in renal cell proliferation and tumor invasion is potentially important and remains to be studied.

REFERENCES

1. Collen D, Lijnen HR. The fibrinolytic system in man. Crit Rev Oncol Hematol 1986; 4:249–301.
2. Schleef RR, Loskutoff DJ, Fibrinolytic system of vascular endothelial cells: Role of plasminogen activator inhibitors. Haemostasis 1988; 18:328–341.
3. Mignatti P, Rifkin D. Biology and biochemistry of proteinases in tumor invasion. Physiol Rev 1993; 73:161–195.
4. Pennica D, Homes WE, Kohr WJ, et al. Cloning and expression of human tissue-type plasminogen activator cDNA in E. coli. Nature 1983; 301:214–221.
5. Verde P, Stoppelli MP, Galeffi P, et al. Identification and primary sequence of an unspliced human urokinase poly(A) + RNA. Proc Natl Acad Sci USA 1984; 81:4727–4731.
6. Fisher R, Waller EK, Grossi G, et al. Isolation and characterization of the human tissue-type plasminogen activator structural gene including its 5′ flanking region. J Biol Chem 1985; 260:11223–11230.
7. Riccio A, Grimaldi G, Verde P, et al. The human urokinase-plasminogen activator gene and its promoter. Nucleic Acids Res 1985; 13:2759–2771.
8. Tripputi P, Blasi F, Verde P, et al. Human urokinase gene is located on the long arm of chromosome 10. Proc Natl Acad Sci USA 1985; 82:4448–4452.
9. Tripputi P, Blasi F, Ny T, et al. Tissue-type plasminogen activator gene is on chromosome 8. Cytogenet Cell Genet 1986; 42:24–28.
10. Blasi F, Vassalli JD, Danø K. Urokinase-type plasminogen activator: Proenzyme, receptor, and inhibitors. J Cell Biol 1987; 104:801–804.
11. Loskutoff DS, Van Mourik SA, Erickson LA, Lawrence DA. Detection of an unusually stable fibrinolytic inhibitor produced by bovine endothelial cells. Proc Natl Acad Sci USA 1983; 80:2956–2960.
12. Antalis TM, Clark MA, Barnes T, et al. Cloning and expression of a cDNA coding for a human monocyte-derived plasminogen activator inhibitor. Proc Natl Acad Sci USA 1988; 85:985–989.
13. Schleuning WD, Medcalf RL, Hession C, et al. Plasminogen activator inhibitor2: Regulation of gene transcription during phorbol ester-mediated differentiation of U-937 human histiocytic lymphoma cells. Mol Cell Biol 1987; 7:4564–4567.
14. Ny T, Sawdey M, Lawrence D, et al. Cloning and sequence of a cDNA coding for the human β-migrating endothelial-cell-type plasminogen activator inhibitor. Proc Natl Acad Sci USA 1986; 83:6776–6780.
15. Erickson LA, Ginsberg MH, Loskutoff DJ. Detection and partial characterization of an inhibitor of plasminogen activator in human platelets. J Clin Invest 1984; 74:1465–1472.
16. Colucci M, Paramo JA, Collen D. Inhibition of one-chain and two-chain forms of human tissue-type

plasminogen activator by the fast-acting inhibitor of plasminogen activator in vitro and in vivo. J Lab Clin Med 1986; 108:53–59.
17. Bevilacqua MP, Schleef RR, Gimbrone MA Jr, Loskutoff DJ. Regulation of the fibrinolytic system of cultured human vascular endothelium by interleukin 1. J Clin Invest 1986; 78:587–591.
18. Schleef RR, Bevilacqua MP, Sawdey M, et al. Cytokine activation of vascular endothelium: Effects on tissue-type plasminogen activator and type 1 plasminogen activator inhibitor. J Biol Chem 1988; 263:5797–5803.
19. Gelehrter TD, Sznycer-Laszuk R. Thrombin induction of plasminogen activator-inhibitor in cultured human endothelial cells. J Clin Invest 1986; 77:165–169.
20. Medcalf RL, Kruithof EKO, Schleuning WD. Plasminogen activator inhibitor 1 and 2 are tumor necrosis factor/cachectin-responsive genes. J Exp Med 1988; 168:751–759.
21. Sawdey MS, Podor TJ, Loskutoff DJ. Regulation of type 1 plasminogen activator inhibitor gene expressed in cultured bovine aortic endothelial cells: Induction by TGFβ, LPS, and TNFa. J Biol Chem 1989; 264:10396–10401.
22. Vassalli JD, Dayer JM, Wohlwend A, Belin D. Concomitant secretion of prourokinase and of a plasminogen activator-specific inhibitor by cultured human monocytes-macrophages. J Exp Med 1984; 159:1653–1668.
23. Wohlwend A, Belin D, Vassalli JD. Plasminogen activator specific inhibitors in mouse macrophages: In vivo and in vitro modulation of their synthesis and secretion. J Immunol 1987; 139:1278–1284.
24. Genton C, Kruithof EKO, Schleuning WD. Phorbol ester induces the biosynthesis of glycosylated and non-glycosylated plasminogen activator inhibitor and urokinase-type plasminogen activator in U-937 cells. J Cell Biol 1987; 104:705–712.
25. Stump DC, Thienpont M, Collen D. Purification and characterization of a novel inhibitor of urokinase from human urine: Quantitation and preliminary characterization in plasma. J Biol Chem 1986; 261:12759–12766.
26. Baker JB, Low DA, Simmer RL, Cunningham DD. Protease-nexin: A cellular component that links thrombin and plasminogen activator and mediates their binding to cells. Cell 1980; 21:37–45.
27. Eaton DL, Baker JB. Evidence that a variety of cultured cells secrete protease nexin and produce a distinct cytoplasmic serine protease-binding factor. J Cell Physiol 1983; 117:175.
28. Vassalli JD, Baccino D, Belin D. A cellular binding site for the MR 55,000 form of the human plasminogen activator, urokinase. J Cell Biol 1985; 100:86–92.
29. Stoppelli MP, Corti A, Soffientini A, et al. Differentiation-enhanced binding of the amino-terminal fragment of human urokinase plasminogen activator to a specific receptor on U937 monocytes. Proc Natl Acad Sci USA 1985; 82:4939–4943.
30. Roldan A, Cubellis M, Masucci M, et al. Cloning and expression of the receptor for urokinase plasminogen activator, a central molecule in cell surface, plasmin dependent proteolysis. EMBO J 1990; 9:467–474.
31. Plow EF, Freaney DE, Plescia J, Miles LA. The plasminogen system and cell surfaces: Evidence for plasminogen and urokinase receptors on the same cell type. J Cell Biol 1986; 103:2411–2420.
32. Fisher R, Waller EK, Grossi G, et al. Isolation and characterization of the human tissue-type plasminogen activator structural gene including its 5′ flanking region. J Biol Chem 1985; 260:11223–11230.
33. Degen SJF, Tajput B, Reich E. The human tissue plasminogen activator gene. J Biol Chem 1986; 261:6972–6985.
34. Feng P, Ohlsson M, Ny T. The structure of the TATA-less rat tissue-type plasminogen activator gene. J Biol Chem 1990; 265:2022–20207.
35. Rickles RJ, Darrow AL, Strickland S. Differentiation response elements in the 5′ region of the mouse tissue plasminogen activator gene confer two-stage regulation by retinoic acid and cyclic AMP in teratocarcinoma cells. Mol Cell Biol 1989; 9:1691–1704.
36. Medcalf RL, Ruegg M, Schleuning WD. A DNA motif related to the cAMP responsive element and an exon-located activator protein-2 binding site in the human tissue-type plasminogen activator gene promoter cooperate in basal expression and convey activation by phorbol ester and cAMP. J Biol Chem 1990; 265:14618–14626.
37. Riccio A, Grimaldi G, Verde P, et al. The human urokinase plasminogen activator gene and its promoter. Nucleic Acids Res 1985; 13:2759–2771.
38. Verde P, Boast S, Franzè A, et al. An upstream enhancer and a negative element in the 5′ flanking region of the human urokinase plasminogen activator gene. Nucleic Acids Res 1988; 16:10699–10716.
39. Nagamine Y, Pearson D, Altus MS, Reich E. cDNA and gene nucleotide sequence of porcine plasminogen activator. Nucleic Acids Res 1984; 12:9525–9541.
40. Degen SJF, Heckel JL, Reich E, Degen JL. The murine urokinase-type plasminogen activator gene. Biochemistry 1987; 26:8270–8279.
41. Cassady AI, Stacey KJ, Nimmo KA, et al. Constitutive expression of the urokinase plasminogen activator gene in murine RAW264 macrophages involves distal and 5′ non-coding sequences that are conserved between mouse and pig. Nucleic Acids Res 1991; 19:6839–6847.

42. Loskutoff DJ, Linders M, Keijer J, et al. Structure of the human plasminogen activator inhibitor 1 gene: Nonrandom distribution of introns. Biochemistry 1987; 26:3763–3768.
43. Bosma PJ, van den Berg E, Kooistra T. Human plasminogen activator inhibitor-1 gene. J Biol Chem 1988; 263:9129–9141.
44. Bruzdzinski CJ, Riordan-Johnson M, Nordby EC, et al. Isolation and characterization of the rat plasminogen activator inhibitor-1 gene. J Biol Chem 1990; 265:2078–2085.
45. van Zonneveld AJ, Curriden SA, Loskutoff DJ. Type 1 plasminogen activator inhibitor gene: Functional analysis and glucocorticoid regulation of its promoter. Proc Natl Acad Sci USA 1988; 85:5525–5529.
46. Ye RD, Wun TC, Sadler JE. cDNA cloning and expression in Escherichia coli of a plasminogen activator inhibitor from human placenta. J Biol Chem 1987; 262:3718–3725.
47. Antalis TM, Clark MA, Barnes T, et al. Cloning and expression of a cDNA coding for a human monocyte-derived plasminogen activator inhibitor. Proc Natl Acad Sci USA 1988; 85:985–989.
48. Cousin E, Medcalf RL, Bergonzelli GE, Kruithof EKO. Regulatory elements involved in constitutive and phorbol ester-inducible expression of the plasminogen activator inhibitor type 2 gene promoter. Nucleic Acids Res 1991; 19:3881–3886.
49. Sahli W. Pflughs Arch Ges Physiol 1885; 36:209.
50. Sobel GW, Mohler SR, Jones NW, et al. Urokinase: An activator of plasma profibrinolysin extracted from urine. Am J Physiol 1952; 171:768–769.
51. Hull RN, Cherry WR, Weaver GW. The origin and characteristics of a pig kidney cell strain, LLC-PK1. In Vitro (Rockville) 1976; 12:670–677.
52. Rijken DC, Binnema DJ, Los P. Specific fibrinolytic properties of different molecular forms of pro-urokinase from a monkey kidney cell culture. Thromb Res 1986; 42:761–768.
53. Angles-Cano E, Rondeau E, Delarue F, et al. Identification and cellular localization of plasminogen activators from human glomeruli. Thromb Haemost 1985; 54:688–692.
54. Saksela O, Holthöfer H. Plasminogen activators during differentiation of the human kidney. Differentiation 1987; 34:131–148.
55. Bergstein JM, Riley M, Bang NU. Analysis of the plasminogen activator activity of the human glomerulus. Kidney Int 1988; 33:868–874.
56. Larsson LI, Skriver L, Nielsen LS, et al. Ditribution of urokinase-type plasminogen activator immunoreactivity in the mouse. J Cell Biol 1984; 98:894–903.
57. Sraer JD, Delarue F, Dard S, et al. Glomerular fibrinolytic activity after thrombin perfusion in the rat. Lab Invest 1975; 32:515–517.
58. Sraer JD, Blanc E, Delarue F, et al. Effect of calcium and hydrogen ion on the fibrinolytic activity of isolated renal glomeruli from rat. Kidney Int 1979; 15:238–245.
59. Rondeau E, Angles-Cano E, Delarue F, et al. Polyunsaturated fatty acids increase fibrinolytic activity of human isolated glomeruli. Kidney Int 1986; 30:701–705.
60. Rondeau E, Delarue F, Kanfer A, et al. Profibrinolytic and procoagulant activities of human glomeruli from normal kidneys and rejected renal allografts. Fibrinolysis 1988; 2:251–257.
61. Malliaros J, Holdsworth SR, Wojta J, et al. Glomerular fibrinolytic activity in anti-GBM glomerulonephritis in rabbits. Kidney Int 1993; 44:557–564.
62. Sappino AP, Huarte J, Vassalli JD, Belin D. Sites of synthesis of urokinase and tissue-type plasminogen activators in the murine kidney. J Clin Invest 1991; 87:962–970.
63. Kristensen P, Eriksen J, Danø K. Localization of urokinase-type plasminogen activator messenger RNA in the normal mouse by in situ hybridization. J Histochem Cytochem 1991; 39:341–349.
64. Keeton M, Eguchi Y, Sawdey M, et al. Cellular localization of type 1 plasminogen activator inhibitor messenger RNA and protein in murine renal tissue. Am J Pathol 1993; 142:59–70.
65. Aya N, Yoshioka K, Murakami K, et al. Tissue-type plasminogen activator and its inhibitor in human glomerulonephritis. J Pathol 1992; 166:289–295.
66. Rondeau E, Ochi S, Lacave R, et al. Urokinase synthesis and binding by glomerular epithelial cells in culture. Kidney Int 1989; 36:593–600.
67. Delarue F, Virone A, Hagège J, et al. Stable cell line of T-SV40 immortalized human glomerular visceral epithelial cells. Kidney Int 1991; 40:906–912.
68. Degen JL, Estensen RD, Nagamine Y, Reich E. Induction and desensitization of plasminogen activator gene expression by tumor promoters. J Biol Chem 1985; 260:12426–12433.
69. Nagamine Y, Altus MS, Nakagawa JI, et al. Urokinase-type plasminogen activator gene regulation as a model system for studying transcriptional activation by the cAMP-dependent protein kinase pathway. In: Cohen P, Foulkes JG, eds. The Hormonal Control Regulation of Gene Transcription. Amsterdam: Elsevier, 1991:197–222.
70. He CJ, Rondeau E, Medcalf RL, et al. Thrombin increases proliferation and decreases fibrinolytic activity of kidney glomerular epithelial cells. J Cell Physiol 1991; 146:131–140.
71. Iwamoto T, Nakashima Y, Sueishi K. Secretion of plasminogen activator and its inhibitor by glomerular epithelial cells. Kidney Int 1990; 37:1466–1476.

72. Rebibou JM, He CJ, Delarue F, et al. Functional endothelin 1 receptors on human glomerular podocytes and mesangial cells. Nephrol Dial Transplant 1992; 7:288–292.
73. He CJ, Nguyen G, Li XM, et al. Transcriptional activation of the urokinase receptor gene by endothelin-1. Biochem. Biophys Res Commun 1992; 186:1631–1638.
74. Becquemont L, Nguyen G, Peraldi MN, et al. Expression of plasminogen/plasmin receptors on human glomerular epithelial cells. Am J Physiol 1994; 257:F303–F310.
75. Lacave R, Rondeau E, Ochi S, et al. Characterization of a plasminogen activator and its inhibitor in human mesangial cells. Kidney Int 1989; 35:806–811.
76. Glass WF II, Radnik RA, Garoni JA, Kreisberg JI. Urokinase-dependent adhesion loss and shape change after cyclic adenosine monophosphate elevation in cultured rat mesangial cells. J Clin Invest 1988; 82:1992–2000.
77. Peraldi MN, Rondeau E, Medcalf RL, et al. Cell-specific regulation of plasminogen activator inhibitor 1 and tissue type plasminogen activator release by human kidney mesangial cells. Biochim Biophys Acta 1992; 1134:189–196.
78. Villamediana LM, Rondeau E, He CJ, et al. Thrombin regulates components of the fibrinolytic system in human mesangial cells. Kidney Int 1990; 38:956–961.
79. Meulders M, He CJ, Adida C, et al. Tumor necrosis factor α increases antifibrinolytic activity of cultured human mesangial cells. Kidney Int 1992; 42:327–334.
80. Hagège J, Peraldi MN, Rondeau E, et al. Plasminogen activator inhibitor 1 deposition in the extracellular matrix of cultured human mesangial cells. Am J Pathol 1992; 141:117–128.
81. Glass II WF, Kreisberg JI, Troyer DA. Two-chain urokinase, receptor, and type 1 inhibitor in cultured human mesangial cells. Am J Physiol 1993; 33:F532–F539.
82. Glass II WF, Rampt E, Garoni JA, et al. Regulation of mesangial cell adhesion and shape by thrombin. Am J Physiol 1991; 30:F336–F344.
83. Troyer D, Padilla R, Smith T, et al. Stimulation of the thrombin receptor of human glomerular mesangial cells by Ser-Phe-Leu-Arg-Asn-Pro-Asn-Asp-Lys-Tyr-Glu-Pro-Phe peptide. J Biol Chem 1992; 267:20126–20131.
84. Wojta J, Hoover RL, Daniel TO. Vascular origin determines plasminogen activator expression in human endothelial cells. J Biol Chem 1989; 264:2846–2852.
85. Stoppelli MP, Verde P, Grimaldi G, et al. Increase in urokinase plasminogen activator mRNA synthesis in human carcinoma cells is a primary effect of the potent tumor promoter, phorbol myristate acetate. J Cell Biol 1986; 102:1235–1241.
86. Dayer JM, Vassalli JD, Bobbitt JL, et al. Calcitonin stimulates plasminogen activator in porcine renal tubular cells: LLC-PK1. J Cell Biol 1981; 91:195–200.
87. Nagamine Y, Sudol M, Reich E. Hormonal regulation of plasminogen activator mRNA production in porcine kidney cells. Cell 1983; 32:1181–1190.
88. Ziegler A, Hagmann J, Kiefer B, Nagamine Y. Ca^{2+} potentiates cAMP-dependent expression of urokinase-type plasminogen activator gene through a calmodulin- and protein kinase C-independent mechanism. J Biol Chem 1990; 265:21194–21201.
89. Ziegler A, Knesel J, Fabbro D, Nagamine Y. Protein kinase C down-regulation enhances cAMP-mediated induction of urokinase-type plasminogen activator mRNA in LLC-PK1 cells. J Biol Chem 1991; 266:21067–21074.
90. Rondeau E, Guidet B, Lacave R, et al. Nordihydroguaiaretic acid inhibits urokinase synthesis by phorbol myristate acetate-stimulated LLC-PK1. Biochim. Biophys. Acta 1990; 1055:165–172.
91. Botteri FM, Ballmer-Hofer K, Rajput B, Nagamine Y. Disruption of cytoskeletal structures results in the induction of the urokinase-type plasminogen activator gene expression. J Biol Chem 1990; 265:13327–13334.
92. Nagamine Y, Ziegler A. Okadaic acid induction of the urokinase-type plasminogen activator gene occurs independently of cAMP-dependent protein kinase and protein kinase C and is sensitive to protein synthesis inhibition. EMBO J 1991; 10:117–122.
93. Pearson D, Altus MS, Horiuchi A, Nagamine Y. Dexamethasone coordinately inhibits plasminogen activator gene expression and enzyme activity in porcine kidney cells. Biochem Biophys Res Commun 1987; 143:329–336.
94. Montesano R, Schaller G, Orci L. Induction of epithelial tubular morphogenesis in vitro by fibroblast-derived soluble factors. Cell 1991a; 66:697–711.
95. Montesano R, Matsumoto K, Nakamura T, Orci L. Identification of a fibroblast-derived epithelial morphogen as hepatocyte growth factor. Cell 1991; 67:901–908.
96. Naldini L, Tamagnone L, Vigna E, et al. Extracellular proteolytic cleavage by urokinase is required for activation of hepatocyte growth factor/scatter factor. EMBO J 1992; 11:4825–4833.
97. Mizuno K, Takehara T, Nakamura T. Proteolytic activation of a single-chain precursor of hepatocyte growth factor by extracellular serine-protease. Biochem Biophys Res Commun 1992; 189:1631–1638.

98. Tomooka S, Border WA, Marshall BC, Noble NA. Glomerular matrix accumulation is linked to inhibition of the plasmin protease system. Kidney Int 1992; 42:1462–1469.
99. Wong AP, Cortez SL, Baricos WH. Role of plasmin and gelatinase in extracellular matrix degradation by cultured rat mesangial cells. Am J Physiol 1992; 263:F1112–F1118.
100. Tipping PG, Holdsworth SR. Fibrinolytic therapy with streptokinase for established experimental glomerulonephritis. Nephron 1986; 43:252–264.
101. Zoja C, Corna D, Macconi D, et al. Tissue plasminogen activator therapy of rabbit nephrotoxic nephritis. Lab Invest 1990; 62:34–40.
102. Rondeau E, Mougenot B, Lacave R, et al. Plasminogen activator inhibitor 1 in renal fibrin deposits of human nephropathies. Clin Nephrol 1990; 33:55–60.
103. Sawdey MS, Loskutoff DJ. Regulation of murine type 1 plasminogen activator inhibitor gene expression in vivo: Tissue specificity and induction by lipopolysaccharide, tumor necrosis factor-α, and transforming growth factor-beta. J Clin Invest 1991; 88:1346–1353.
104. Giroux L, Verroust P, Morel-Maroger L, et al. Glomerular fibrinolytic activity during nephrotoxic nephritis. Lab Invest 1979; 40:415–422.
105. Tomosugi N, Wada T, Naito T, et al. Role of plasminogen activator inhibitor on nephrotoxic nephritis and its modulation by tumor necrosis factor. Nephron 1992; 62:213–219.
106. Feng L, Tang WW, Loskutoff DJ, Wilson CB. Dysfunction of glomerular fibrinolysis in experimental antiglomerular basement membrane antibody glomerulonephritis. J Am Soc Nephrol 1993; 3:1753–1764.
107. Bukovsky A, Labarrere CA, Carter C, et al. Novel immunohistochemical markers of human renal allograft dysfunction—Antithrombin III, Thy-1, urokinase, and alpha-smooth muscle actin. Transplantation 1992; 54:1064–1071.
108. Rondeau E, Delarue F, Kanfer A, et al. Profibrinolytic and procoagulant activities of human glomeruli from normal kidneys and rejected renal allografts. Fibrinolysis 1988; 2:251–257.
109. Canipari R, Zurzolo C, Polistina C, et al. Polarized secretion of plasminogen activators by epithelial cell monolayers. Biochim Biophys Acta 1992; 1175:1–6.
110. Ragno P, Estreicher A, Gos A, et al. Polarized secretion of urokinase-type plasminogen activator by epithelial cells. Exp Cell Res 1992; 203:236–243.
111. Christensen EI, Gliemann J, Moestrup SK. Renal tubule gp330 is a calcium binding receptor for endocytic uptake of protein. J Histochem Cytochem 1992; 40:1481–1490.
112. Nykjaer A, Petersen CM, Møller B, et al. Purified alpha2-macroglobulin receptor/LDL receptor-related protein binds urokinase plasminogen activator inhibitor type-1 complex. J Biol Chem 1992; 267:14543–14546.
113. Willnow TE, Goldstein JL, Orth K, et al. Low density lipoprotein receptor-related protein and gp330 bind similar ligands, including plasminogen activator-inhibitor complexes and lactoferrin, an inhibitor of chylomicron remnant clearance. J Biol Chem 1992; 267:26172–26180.
114. Kanalas JJ. Analysis of plasmin binding and urokinase activation of plasminogen bound to the Heymann nephritis autoantigen, gp 330. Arch Biochem Biophys 1992; 299:255–260.
115. Ossowski L. Invasion of connective tissue by human carcinoma cell lines: Requirement for urokinase, urokinase receptor, and interstitial collagenase. Cancer Res 1992; 52:6754–6760.
116. Quax PHA, Pedersen N, Masucci MT, et al. Complementation between urokinase-producing and receptor-producing cells in extracellular matrix degradation. Cell Regul 1991; 2:793–803.
117. Ferraiuolo R, Stoppelli MP, Verde P, et al. Transcriptional induction of urokinase in cultured human kidney carcinoma cells by tetradecanoyl-phorbol-acetate. J Cell Physiol 1984; 121:368–374.
118. Nelson NF, Cieplak W, Dacus SC, Prager MD. Characterization of plasminogen activator from two human renal carcinoma cell lines. J Cell Physiol 1986; 126:435–443.
119. He CJ, Rebibou JM, Peraldi MN, et al. Growth factor-like effect of urokinase type plasminogen activator in human renal cells. Biochem Biophys Res Commun 1991; 176:1408–1416.
120. Kirchheimer JC, Wojta J, Christ G, et al. Mitogenic effect of u-PA on malignant and unaffected adjacent human renal cells. Carcinogenesis 1988; 9:2121–2123.
121. Dumler I, Petri T, Schleuning WD. Interaction of urokinase-type plasminogen activator (u-PA) with its cellular receptor (u-PAR) induces phosphorylation on tyrosine of a 38 kDa protein. FEBS Lett 1993; 322:37–40.

49
Leukocyte Adhesion Molecules

Hugh R. Brady
Brockton–West Roxbury Department of Veterans Affairs Medical Center and Brigham and Women's Hospital, Harvard Medical School, Boston, Massachusetts

LEUKOCYTE FUNCTION IN HOST DEFENSE AND INFLAMMATION

Overview of Leukocyte Trafficking During Inflammation

Circulating leukocytes play a central role in immune responses to invading microorganisms and in noninfectious tissue injury (e.g., trauma, radiation, thermal). Leukocytes also contribute to tissue injury in acute allograft rejection, ischemia-reperfusion, and many "autoimmune" diseases, including glomerulonephritis, vasculitis, and tubulointerstitial nephritis (1,2). The recruitment of circulating leukocytes from blood to extravascular tissue involves a coordinated series of cellular and molecular responses that include directed locomotion up gradients of chemoattractants (chemotaxis), rolling and immobilization on vascular endothelium (margination/adhesion), disruption of tight junctions and diapedesis between endothelial cells, and interactions with basement membrane and extracellular matrix components (Figure 1). The unacceptable immunologic and nonimmunologic toxicity of corticosteroids, cyclophosphamide, and cyclosporine has accelerated the search for molecular events in inflammation that are amenable to specific pharmacological manipulation. Given the array of chemoattractants generated within a local inflammatory milieu, it is probably not surprising that most agents that block the biosynthesis or bioactivity of individual mediators are only modestly successful in abrogating leukocyte-mediated tissue injury. Leukocyte adhesion, however, is a pivotal event in leukocyte trafficking that is provoked by many proinflammatory chemoattractants and cytokines and is an attractive target at which to direct therapy (reviewed in Refs. 3 to 13). Adhesion is supported by several classes of cell surface molecules that are members of larger superfamilies of receptors involved in immunosurveillance, inflammation, hemostasis, wound healing, morphogenesis, maintenance of tissue architecture, atherogenesis, and tumor metastasis. This chapter reviews (a) the discovery of leukocyte adhesion molecules; (b) their classification, structures, and cellular distribution; (c) the regulation of adhesion molecule biosynthesis and function by inflammatory mediators; (d) the evidence implicating leukocyte adhesion molecules in the pathogenesis of renal inflammation; (e) their potential as targets for anti-inflammatory agents, and (f) the possible involvement of related molecules in the pathophysiology of other renal diseases. In accordance with the aims of this book, special emphasis is placed on molecular aspects of adhesion molecule biology.

Leukocyte Adhesion Deficiency Syndromes I and II

The critical requirement of leukocyte adhesion molecules for normal host defense was initially recognised in studies of leukocyte adhesion deficiency (LAD) type 1, a rare inherited immunodeficiency disease of childhood (reviewed in Ref. 4). Afflicted children suffer recurrent and frequently fatal bacterial infections characterized by profound systemic neutrophilia and absence of pus formation at sites of infection; normal circulating immunoglobulin, complement, and

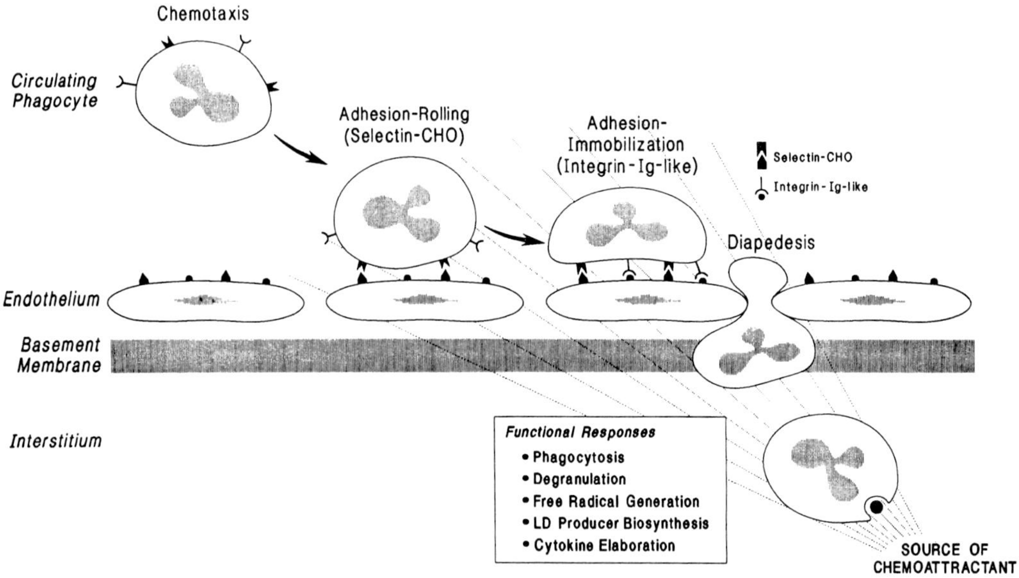

Figure 1 Model illustrating proposed involvement of adhesion molecules in the recruitment of leukocytes to sites of inflammation. Leukocytes migrate towards the endothelial wall overlying sites of inflammation in response to gradients of chemoattractants (chemotaxis), adhere to endothelial cells (margination), disrupt tight junctions, and migrate between endothelial cells to the extravascular space (diapedesis). The initial adhesion of circulating leukocytes and endothelial cells is supported by the interaction of selectins on leukocytes or endothelial cells with carbohydrate-containing ligands (e.g., mucins). Selectin-mediated adhesion causes leukocytes to roll on endothelium and facilitates their immobilization by interaction of leukocyte integrins with Ig-like molecules on endothelial cells. The molecular basis for diapedesis has not been established fully, but may involve the interaction of leukocytes with PECAM-1, an Ig-like molecule localized at intercellular junctions. (From Ref. 13.)

lymphocyte levels; and normal delayed-type skin hypersensitivity reactions and defense against fungal and viral infections. Phagocytic leukocytes from affected children display reduced adhesion to endothelium and other substrates in vitro and impairment of other adhesion-related functions such as transmigration, phagocytosis, and antibody dependent cellular toxicity. An elegant series of parallel immunological, biochemical, and molecular approaches determined that these individuals have heterogenous deletions or mutations in the gene encoding the common CD18 subunit of leukocyte CD11/CD18 $\beta 2$ integrins (see below). As a result there is impaired dimerization of CD18 and CD11 subunits of $\beta 2$ integrins, failure of normal trafficking of these molecules to the cell surface, and inability of neutrophils to diapedese from blood to extravascular tissue in response to chemoattractants and cytokines. Retrovirus-mediated gene transfer of a functional CD18 gene into lymphocytes of patients with LAD type 1 restores CD11/CD18 surface expression and adhesive function in vitro (14). These pioneering experiments heralded the discovery of four major classes of leukocyte adhesion molecules that act in concert to regulate leukocyte trafficking in health and disease: the selectins, which interact with the mucins and other carbohydrate-containing glycoproteins and glycolipids, and the integrins, which bind to immunoglobulin-like (Ig-like) ligands and other cellular and matrix components (3–13). A recent report indicates that deficiency of Sialyl-Lewis X, a carbohydrate ligand for several selectins, also predisposes to recurrent infections (LAD type II) and indicates that both categories of molecular interactions are essential for normal host defense (15).

STRUCTURE AND DISTRIBUTION OF MAJOR LEUKOCYTE ADHESION MOLECULES

The consensus model for leukocyte adhesion to vascular endothelium in health, host defense, and inflammation is summarized in Figure 1 and based largely on (a) in vitro studies of the influence of monoclonal antibodies (mAb) against specific adhesion molecules on leukocyte adhesion to cultured endothelial cells, (b) in vitro analyses of leukocyte adhesion to purified adhesion molecules adsorbed onto acellular substrates, (c) in vivo videomicroscopic analyses of the influence of adhesion-blocking mAb on leukocyte interactions with blood vessel walls in microvascular beds (e.g., hamster cheek pouch, mesentery, skin), and (d) assessment of the impact of "knockout" of adhesion molecules genes by targeted homologous recombination in embryonic stem cells on leukocyte binding to endothelium under physiological and disease conditions. The initial tethering of leukocytes to endothelium is achieved by interactions of leukocyte or endothelial cell selectins with carbohydrate-containing glycoproteins and possibly glycolipids (7,8,10). While the identity and structures of these selectin ligands are still being appreciated, some are members of a family O-glycosylated proteins known as mucins (16,17). Selectin-mediated adhesion is relatively resistant to shear stress but insufficient to immobilize circulating leukocytes on endothelium. Rather, selectin-mediated adhesion causes leukocytes to roll on endothelium, where they are subject to soluble and cell-associated signals from endothelial cells and extravascular tissue. These stimuli trigger binding of integrins with Ig-like molecules on endothelium, immobilization of leukocytes, dramatic changes in leukocyte morphology, and diapedesis (3–7,9,13). The molecular basis for diapedesis is not understood but may involve an Ig-like adhesion molecule, PECAM-1, that is expressed by leukocytes and at points of contact between endothelial cells (18,19).

Selectins

Three selectins have been characterized and named according to their cell of original discovery: P-selectin (platelet selectin; also expressed by endothelial cells), E-selectin (endothelial cell selectin), and L-selectin (leukocyte selectin) (Table 1) (7,8,10,20). Selectins share several structural features. Each contains a 120–amino acid NH_2 terminal lectin-binding domain that shares homology with C-type (calcium-dependent) carbohydrate recognition domains, a conserved epidermal growth factor–like domain of approximately 30 amino acids, a selectin-specific number of 60–amino acid repeat sequences that contain six cysteinyl residues and share homology with complement regulatory proteins, a single transmembrane domain, and a short intracellular COOH-terminal domain (Figure 2) (8,10). The genes encoding P-, E-, and L-selectin are localized in a tight cluster on the long arm of murine and human chromosome 1, in close proximity to the genes encoding complement-binding proteins (8,10). Accordingly, it has been suggested that these structurally related molecules may have evolved from a common ancestor by exon shuffling and gene duplication (10,11). Analyses of cDNAs for L-, P-, and E-selectin revealed striking preservation of structure among different species. In humans, the lectin domains of selectins share >60% homology (8,10). Selectins contain between 7 and 12 potential sites for N-linked glycosylation, and it is estimated that glycosylation accounts for >30% of their mass (10). The structures and functions of these carbohydrate residues have not been defined.

Selectins support adhesion of leukocytes and endothelial cells, and leukocytes and platelets (Table 1). L-selectin is constitutively expressed by most leukocytes, mediates adhesion of lymphocytes to endothelial cells of high endothelial venules (HEV) of lymph nodes and regulates physiological homing of lymphocytes to this vascular bed (8,10). Interestingly, adhesion of neutrophils, monocytes, and lymphocytes to cytokine-activated endothelium derived from other vascular beds, including glomerular capillaries, can be attenuated by mAb against this ligand, as can adhesion of a pre-B cell line transfected with L-selectin (21). These observations suggest that L-selectin may also support leukocyte adhesion to nonlymphoid endothelium during inflammation. P-selectin is expressed by endothelial cells and platelets where it is stored in intracellular granules (Weibel-Palade bodies and α-granules, respectively) and mobilized to the surface upon cell activation (8,10). P-Selectin supports adhesion of granulocytes, monocytes and some lymphocyte subsets. E-Selectin has only been detected on endothelial cells. This molecule is not expressed in most vascular beds under basal conditions, but is induced by cytokines and supports adhesion of

Table 1 Classification, Cellular Distribution, Ligands, and Target Cells for Major Leukocyte Adhesion Molecules

Major families	Individual members	Alternate nomenclature	Cellular distribution	Ligands on target cells	Target cells
Selectins	L-Selectin	LAM-1, LECCAM-1, MEL-14, Leu-8, TQ1 DREG.56	Leukocytes	MadCAM-1, CD34 ?GlyCAM-1, ?sLe^x, ?sLe^a, ?E- & P-selectin, other glycoproteins and/or glycolipids	Endothelial cells, ?other
	P-Selectin	CD62, GMP140, PADGEM, LECCAM-3	Platelets and endothelial	PSGL-1, ?others, mucins, glycoproteins and glycolipids (SLe^x Le^x, sLe^a, see text)	Granulocytes, monocytes, T-cell subsets, some cancer cells
	E-Selectin	ELAM-1, LECCAM-2	Endothelial	sLe^x, sLe^a, ?L-selectin other glycoproteins & glycolipids (see text)	Neutrophils, monocytes, lymphocyte subsets, some cancer cells
Carbohydrate ligands for selectins (including mucins)	GlyCAM-1	Sgp50, mucin	Endothelial	?L-selectin (see text)	Lymphocytes, ?other
	MadCAM-1	mucin	Endothelial	L-selectin, $\alpha4\beta7$ integrins	Leukocytes, lymphocytes
	CD34	mucin	Endothelial	L-selectin	Leukocytes
	PSGL-1	mucin	Leukocytes	P-selectin	Platelets, endothelial
	Sialyl Lewis^x	sLe^x	Leukocytes	E-selectin and P-selectin	Endothelium and platelets

Integrins	VLA-4 (beta-1)	LPAM-2, $\alpha_4\beta_1$	Monocytes, lymphocytes, eosinophils	VCAM-1, fibronectin	Endothelium, epithelial, mesangial, vascular smooth muscle
	CD11a/CD18 (beta-2)	LFA-1, TA-1	Leukocytes	ICAM-1, ICAM-2	Endothelial, epithelial, mesangial, vascular smooth muscle
	CD11b/CD18 (beta-2)	Mac-1, Mo1, OKM1, gp160	Granulocytes, monocytes	ICAM-1, C3bi, fibrinogen, factor x, other	Endothelial, epithelial, mesangial, vascular smooth muscle, other
	CD11c/CD18 (beta-2)	p150,95, LeuM5	Granulocytes, monocytes	Not characterized	Endothelial, mesangial
Ig-like	ICAM-1	CD54	Endothelial, epithelial, mesangial, smooth muscle, some cancer cells	CD11a/CD18, CD11b/CD18	Most leukocytes
	ICAM-2		Endothelial	CD11a/CD18	Most leukocytes
	VCAM-1	INCAM 110	Endothelial, epithelial, mesangial, smooth muscle	VLA-4	Monocytes, lymphocytes, eosinophils
	PECAM-1	EndoCAM,CD31	Endothelial, platelets, some leukocytes	PECAM-1	Some leukocytes, endothelial, platelets

Source: From Ref. 13.

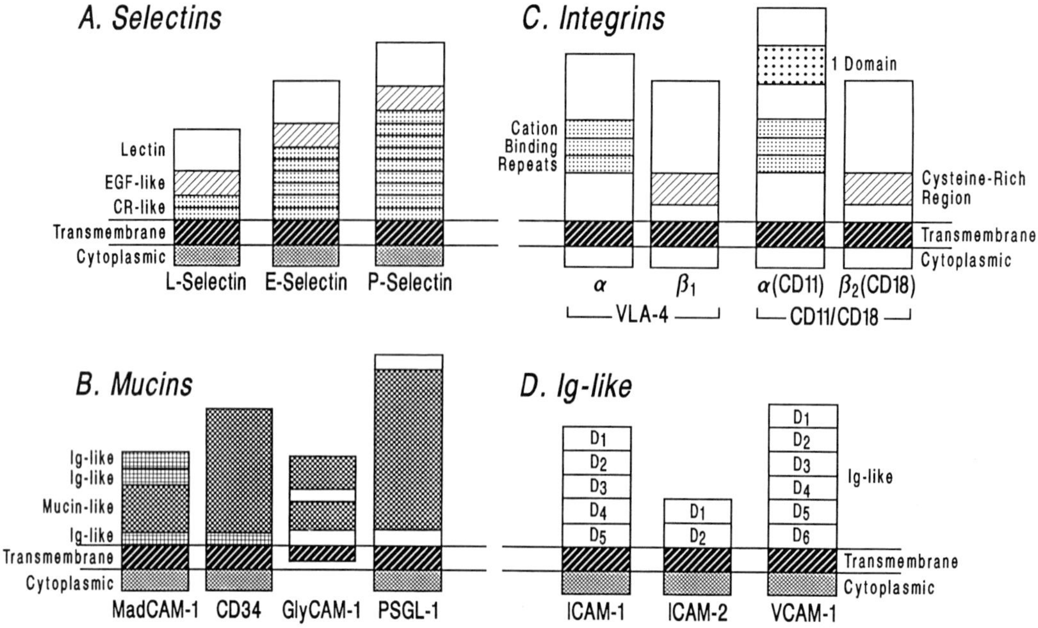

Figure 2 Structural characteristics of some members of the four major families of leukocyte adhesion molecules: selectins, mucins, integrins and Ig-like molecules. See text for explanation. EGF-like, epidermal growth factor-like domain; CR-like, complement regulatory protein-like domain; sLe^X, Sialyl Lewis^X; Ig-like, immunoglobulin-like; D, domain. (From Ref. 13.)

granulocytes, monocytes, some memory T-lymphocytes, natural killer cells and some carcinoma cells (Table 1).

Mucins and Other Selectin Ligands

The structures, cell distribution and functional characteristics of the carbohydrate-containing ligands for selectins are the focus of intensive investigation and have yet to be defined fully. Selectins bind at least three broad categories of natural or synthetic carbohydrates through their lectin binding domain: (a) glycoproteins bearing sulphated polysaccharides (e.g., mucins); (b) oligosaccharides such as sialyl Lewis^X (sLe^X); and (c) soluble phosphorylated mono- and polysaccharides (Table 1) (7,8,10,16). Three mucins have been cloned that are potential ligands for L-selectin: MadCAM-1, CD34 and GlyCAM-1 (Figure 2) (16). These structurally related proteins each contain a high local density of O-linked sugars on their extracellular domains that probably extend beyond the glycoprotein and polysaccharide glycocalyx that normally surrounds cells (16,17). The cDNA for MadCAM-1 contains a potential site for O-glycosylation and three potential N-glycosylation sites. MadCAM-1 is preferentially localized to mucosal lymphoid tissue (16,22,23). MadCAM-1 isolated from mesenteric lymph nodes bears a sialic acid-containing carbohydrate residue that supports adhesion of L-selectin transfected lymphoid cells and thus may regulate lymphocyte homing to this region (16,22,23). The tissue distribution of CD34 is still being appreciated (16). In contrast to GlyCAM-1 and MadCAM-1, CD34 is expressed by nonlymphoid endothelium, including glomerular endothelium, raising the possibility that this ligand may support leukocyte adhesion during inflammation. Cloning of the genes for CD34 and MadCAM-1 has demonstrated the presence of Ig-like domains similar to those found on the Ig-like ligands for leukocyte integrins (see below), suggesting that these L-selectin ligands possess molecular characteristics that facilitate both leukocyte rolling and immobilization (16). Indeed, MadCAM-1 is also a ligand for the $\alpha 4\beta 7$ integrin that supports lymphocyte adhesion to endothelium of Peyer's patches (22,23), further suggesting a role for MadCAM-1 in lymphocyte homing in mucosal tissue. This economy of adhesive function may have evolved to facilitate the physiological trafficking of lymphocytes within lymphoid tissue that is essential for normal immune function. GlyCAM-1 is a sulphated, fucosylated, and sialylated 50-kDa O-glycosylated mucin that has been postulated to support L-selectin-mediated lymphocyte adhesion to HEV of peripheral lymph nodes (24,25). However, GlyCAM-1 lacks a transmembrane spanning domain and is secreted and may alternatively serve to modulate L-selectin binding to HEV (24,25).

The structural characteristics of the leukocyte ligands for P- and E-selectin are less well defined. Sialyl Lewis^x (SLe^x), a sialylated, fucosylated cell surface tetrasaccharide that decorates many proteins, is a potential ligand for both E-selectin and P-selectin (7,8,10). In support of this contention, mAb against SLe^x and purified SLe^x presented in liposomes inhibit leukocyte adhesion mediated by E- and P-selectin in some assays. Furthermore, Chinese Hamster ovary cells (CHO) expressing SLe^x bind soluble forms of these selectins. Similar lines of evidence have implicated two related carbohydrates Lewis^x and Sialyl-Lewis^a as other ligands for P- and E-selectin (8,10). It has not been determined if these carbohydrate residues are presented by mucins or other molecules. In this regard, it is notable that a mucin, P-selectin glycoprotein ligand (PSGL-1), may be a ligand for P-selectin (Figure 2) (16,26,27). The extracellular domain of this glycoprotein is sialylated and contains three potential sites for N-linked glycosylation and a region of 15 decameric repeats with potential sites for O-linked glycosylation. Enzymatic disruption of O-linked, but not N-linked moieties results in loss of P-selectin binding. Immunoprecipitation of neutrophil proteins with chimeras of P- and E-selectin and the Fc portion of human IgG revealed two other potentially novel and distinct glycoprotein leukocyte receptors for P- and E-selectin of 160 and 130 Kda, respectively, that, unlike the sialomucins, require N-linked carbohydrates for adhesion (28). The functional significance of these ligands remains to be elucidated.

Integrins

Integrins are heterodimeric cell surface glycoproteins, composed of noncovalently associated α and β subunits (Figures 1 and 2), that mediate diverse cell-cell and cell-matrix interactions and are classified according to the structure of their β subunits (3–7,9,13). In general, members of each class share a common β subunit, of which there are at least nine, and are distinguished by their unique α subunits. The integrins that appear most important in leukocyte-endothelial adhesion are the very late activation antigen-4 $\beta 1$ integrin (VLA-4) and the CD11/CD18 $\beta 2$ integrins (Figure 2).

Very late activation antigen-4 (VLA-4) is an $\alpha 4\beta 1$ integrin (CD49d/CD29), named because it was identified on lymphocytes after prolonged activation by concanavalin A. VLA-4 is constitutively expressed by lymphocytes, monocytes, basophils, and eosinophils, but not neutrophils, and is a ligand for the inducible Ig-like vascular cell adhesion molecule-1 (VCAM-1), fibronectin, and possibly other matrix components (7). It is probable that lymphocyte and monocyte adhesion through VLA-4 and VCAM-1 accounts for the normal cellular immunity in children with LAD type 1. This contention is supported by in vitro and in vivo studies in which blockade of both VLA-4 and CD11/CD18-mediated adhesion is usually necessary to inhibit lymphocyte and monocyte trafficking (7). Three β-2 integrins have been characterized: CD11a/CD18, CD11b/CD18, and CD11c/CD18; CD11 and CD18 referring to their α and β subunits, respectively (Figure 2) (3,4,6). CD18 is a 678–amino acid protein, encoded by a single gene on chromosome 21, that has a short, highly conserved cytoplasmic tail of 46 amino acids, which contains several potential phosphorylation sites, a highly conserved transmembrane domain, and a longer extracellular region containing a conserved cysteine-rich region that is necessary for surface expression (Figure 2). Point mutations in the latter region can lead to the LAD type 1 immunodeficiency syndrome (4). CD11a, CD11b, and CD11c are made up of 1063, 1136, and 1144 amino acids, respectively, and are encoded by distinct genes in a cluster on chromosome 16 (4). Notable structural features on CD11 subunits include short nonhomologous cytoplasmic regions containing potential phosphorylation sites, highly conserved transmembrane regions, and a longer extracellular region that contains several cation-binding repeats and an "I" (interactive) domain that is relatively highly conserved across integrin subfamilies and may be an important adhesion domain (Figure 2) (3,4,6). CD11a shares 36% homology with CD11b and CD11c and is constitutively expressed by granulocytes, monocytes, and lymphocytes (Table 1). In contrast, CD11b and CD11c share 63% homology and are expressed by granulocytes and monocytes, but not lymphocytes (Table 1). Recent analyses indicate that CD11b, but not CD11c, is also expressed on subpopulations of B and T lymphocytes and natural killer (NK) cells (29). The major ligands for CD11a/CD18 are the Ig-like intercellular adhesion molecules (ICAM) 1 and 2. ICAM-1 is also a ligand for CD11b/CD18; however, the CD11b/CD18 also supports leukocyte adhesion to cellular and acellular substrates by mechanisms that are independent of ICAM-1 (Table 1). The biochemical structure of the cognate ligand(s) for CD11c/CD18 and precise role of this molecule in leukocyte migration have not been defined.

Immunoglobulin-like Molecules and Other Integrin Ligands

ICAM-1, ICAM-2, VCAM-1, and PECAM-1 are members of the immunoglobulin superfamily of cell surface receptors. Other members of this superfamily that are involved in immunoregulation include immunoglobulin itself, the T-cell receptor/CD3 complex, CD4, CD8, and class I and class I MHC molecules (6,7,9). Cloning and sequencing of the cDNAs for the Ig-like adhesion molecules revealed that each contains one or more regions of homology to Ig, each consisting of a disulfide-bridged loop containing antiparallel β-pleated strands arranged into two sheets, a transmembrane domain, and a short cytoplasmic tail (6). ICAM-1 is a glycoprotein of molecular weight 76 to 114 kDa that contains five tandem immunoglobulin domains (D1–D5) and, as discussed above, is a ligand for CD11a/CD18 and CD11b/CD18, but not CD11c/CD18. Single amino acid substitutions in the amino terminal D1 and, to a lesser extent, D2 domains reduce the avidity of ICAM-1 for CD11a/CD18, while deletions of the D3, D4, and D5 domains and the cytoplasmic tail have little effect on ICAM-1 adhesiveness for this ligand. ICAM-1 is constitutively expressed at low levels by endothelial cells, and its expression is markedly increased upon exposure to cytokines such as tumor necrosis factor (TNF) and interleukin-1 (see below). In addition, cytokines can induce de novo biosynthesis and expression of ICAM-1 by a variety of other cell types, including mesangial cells and renal epithelial cells. ICAM-1 is also expressed by lymphocytes and some other leukocytes, and homotypic and heterotypic lymphocyte adhesion mediated by interaction of ICAM-1 and CD11a/CD18 facilitates other important lymphocyte functions, including antigen recognition, lymphocyte co-stimulation, and cytotoxicity. ICAM-2 is a noninducible Ig-like adhesion molecule that is constitutively expressed at high levels by endothelial cells and is also a ligand for CD11a/CD18, but not other $\beta2$ integrins (Table 1) (6,7). In addition, low levels of ICAM-2 are detected on mononuclear cells, including lymphocytes and NK cells. ICAM-2 is a glycoprotein of molecular weight 60 kDa and contains two extracellular Ig-like domains that bear close homology to the amino terminal D1 and D2 domains of ICAM-1 (Figure 2). Because resting T lymphocytes express ICAM-2 but minimal levels of ICAM-1, it has been suggested that ICAM-2 may play a central role in the initial interaction of lymphocytes with antigen-presenting cells. Functional studies suggest that lymphocytes express a third Ig-like ligand for CD11a/CD18, designated ICAM-3, that supports homotypic lymphocyte adhesion and may be an important costimulatory signal during lymphocyte activation.

VCAM-1 is a 110-kDa glycoprotein that contains seven Ig-like domains, a 22–amino acid transmembrane domain, and a short 19–amino acid cytoplasmic tail (Figure 2) (6,7,9,30–32). A second form of VCAM-1, consisting of six Ig-like domains, is generated in some tissues by alternate splicing (30–32). The seven-domain species predominates in endothelial cells; the functional significance of the alternatively spliced form is unclear. VCAM-1 is absent or expressed at low levels on endothelial cells and can be induced by cytokines on endothelial cells and other cell-types, including mesangial cells, renal epithelial cells, and vascular smooth muscle cells (see below). VCAM-1 is constitutively expressed by parietal epithelial cells of Bowman's capsule; the functional significance of VCAM-1 in this location is unclear (9,11–13). Interestingly, mice that are rendered deficient in VCAM-1 by targeted homologous recombination in embryonic stem cells (VCAM-1 "knockout") usually die in utero, suggesting that VCAM-1 also plays a critical role in fetal development (33). VCAM-1 supports adhesion of eosinophils, basophils, monocytes, and lymphocytes but not neutrophils through interaction with VLA-4. Accordingly, it has been suggested that the interaction of VLA-4 and VCAM-1 may be important in the pathophysiology of allergic and delayed hypersensitivity reactions. PECAM-1 is a 130-kDa integral membrane glycoprotein expressed by platelets, some leukocytes, and endothelial cells. Recent studies suggest that PECAM-1 is constitutively expressed preferentially at tight junctions of endothelial cells and may regulate leukocyte diapedesis between endothelial cells during inflammation (18,19).

MOLECULAR REGULATION OF ADHESION MOLECULE EXPRESSION AND FUNCTION

The maintenance of leukocytes and endothelium in an antiadhesive phenotype is critical in preventing indiscriminate intravascular leukocyte adhesion, activation, and tissue injury in health. Inflammatory mediators provoke adhesion during host defense and inflammation by enhancing the avidity and/or expression of preformed molecules for cognate ligands and by stimulating de novo synthesis of adhesion molecules. It is probable that the initial recruitment of phagocytes is achieved by regulation of the surface expression and function of preformed molecules and that the induction of adhesion molecule biosynthesis by cytokines serves to sustain and amplify inflammatory responses.

Regulation of Expression and Avidity of Preformed Molecules

Mediators that rapidly increase leukocyte adhesiveness for endothelium include complement components (C5a), eicosanoids (leukotrienes B_4), and other lipid mediators (platelet activating factor), cytokines (monocyte chemotactic peptide-1, interleukin-8, granulocyte-macrophage colony-stimulating factor, tumor necrosis factor alpha), and some anti-neutrophil cytoplasmic antibodies (ANCA) (3–13,34,35). Most of these compounds activate leukocytes through specific cell surface receptors (36) and the ability of certain mediators to selectively recruit either granulocytes, monocytes, or lymphocytes (e.g., MCP-1 and monocytes; IL-8 and neutrophils) is probably determined by the differential expression of receptors on subpopulations of leukocytes. The engagement of receptors sets in motion an orchestrated cascade of signal transduction events that ultimately provoke mobilization of preformed molecules (e.g., CD11b/CD18, CD11c/CD18) from "specific" tertiary granules to the cell surface and/or an increase in the avidity of constitutively expressed molecules for their cognate ligands (e.g., CD11/CD18 integrins, L-selectin) (3–13). Qualitative changes in avidity appear to be relatively more important in determining leukocyte adhesion that quantitative changes in adhesion molecule expression. The mechanism(s) by which binding of inflammatory mediators to cell surface receptors is transduced to alterations in adhesion molecule function are still being elucidated. Signal transduction events that appear to play a role in leukocyte adhesion stimulated by bacterial wall peptides, C5a, leukotriene B_4 (LTB_4), and platelet-activating factor (PAF) include activation of phospholipase C (and possibly phospholipase D) through guanine nucleotide binding proteins/tyrosine kinase activity, hydrolysis of phosphatidyinositol bisphosphate and generation of inositol trisphosphate and diacylglycerol, elevation of intracellular calcium concentration, activation of protein kinases (reviewed in Ref. 36). These perturbations in cellular biochemistry occur within the same temporal framework as adhesion and chemoattractant-stimulated adhesion can be attenuated by pharmacological inhibitors of some of these events. Formal proof of their involvement will require the utilization of more specific molecular approaches to selectively delete individual components of signal transduction cascades. The distal signal transduction events that ultimately enhance the avidity of adhesion molecules probably involve phosphorylation of adhesion proteins and/or cytoskeletal elements (reviewed in Refs. 4 and 7). The cytoplasmic domain of the CD18 chain of $\beta 2$ integrins possesses multiple serine/threonine residues that are potential targets for phosphorylation and many compounds that provoke leukocyte adhesion (e.g., fMLP, PMA) also stimulate phosphorylation of these residues. Furthermore, deletion of the cytoplasmic domain of CD18 is associated with loss of adhesive function. These observation provide compelling evidence that the avidity of the CD11 ligand-binding chain of $\beta 2$ integrins is regulated by the phosphorylation state of the CD18 component. An intact cytoskeleton is an absolute requirement for most adhesive interactions assessed to date and leukocyte integrins, and possibly L-selectin, are intimately associated with cytoskeletal components (5,7). Indeed, in addition to receptor-mediated events inducing changes in integrin avidity through changes in the cytoskeleton ("inside-out signaling"), adhesion molecules themselves appear capable of transmitting information into cells ("outside-in signaling"), regulating cytoskeletal processes such as actin assembly, and other cellular events such as free radical generation and lipoxygenase product generation (see below) (5,7).

Endothelial cells are also subject to rapid changes in their adhesiveness for leukocytes. Thrombin, histamine, leukotrienes C_4 and D_4 (LTC_4, LTD_4), reactive oxygen species, and the membrane attack complex of complement (MAC) increase endothelial cell adhesiveness for granulocytes and monocytes by mobilizing preformed P-selectin from intracellular Weibel-Palade bodies to the surface of endothelial cells (7,8,10). How P-selectin is mobilized is unclear but appears to require an increase in intracellular calcium concentration and activation of protein kinase C. The time course of mobilization of P-selectin by histamine and thrombin (peak, 1 to 2 min) differs markedly from that of LTC_4 and LTD_4 (peak, 15 to 30 min), suggesting that endothelial cell P-selectin expression may be regulated by different signal transduction pathways. Interestingly, L-selectin and P-selectin are either shed rapidly or reinternalized following cell activation, a process that may limit adhesion and facilitate diapedesis in vivo (7,8,10).

Induction of Adhesion Molecule Gene Expression and Biosynthesis

Prolonged exposure (hours to days) of endothelial cells and other tissue cells to many cytokines augments their adhesiveness for leukocytes by stimulating de novo biosynthesis of adhesion molecules (3–13). Similarly, cytokines such as GM-CSF induce synthesis of CD11/CD18 integrins and L-selectin by leukocyte precursors. In addition, cytokines promote leukocyte recruitment by inducing the generation of soluble and cell-associated stimuli for leukocyte adhesion such as IL-8, MCP-1 and PAF by endothelial cells (reviewed in Refs. 3–13).

The profile of adhesion molecules expressed by cytokine-activated cells varies depending on the cell-type, time of exposure and cytokine. ICAM-1 and VCAM-1 can be induced on a variety of cell-types, including endothelial cells, epithelial cells, vascular smooth muscles cells, and mesangial cells (3–13). In contrast, E-selectin appears to be restricted to endothelial cells (3–13). Interestingly, cytokine-activated endothelial cells, including glomerular endothelial cells (20), also express a ligand(s) for leukocyte L-selectin that appears to be distinct from those expressed by high endothelial venules. In addition, cytokine-activated endothelial cells may display augmented levels of P-selectin, at least in some species (37). These findings support the contention that selectin-mediated adhesion may have evolved as a specialized function that facilitates the initial tethering of circulating leukocytes to endothelium under conditions of shear stress. Increased levels of ICAM-1 and VCAM-1 are usually sustained for at least 24 to 48 hr in the presence of a stimulatory cytokine in vitro (3–13). In contrast, E-selectin expression is usually transient, at least in vitro (peaks 4 hr, basal levels ~24 hr), although endothelial expression may be more sustained in some vascular beds (e.g., skin) during inflammation in vivo. Endothelial cell expression of E-selectin, VCAM-1 and ICAM-1 is markedly enhanced by TNFα and β, IL-1α and β, and lipopolysaccharide in contrast. Interferon-γ (IFNγ) induces relatively higher levels of ICAM-1 than VCAM-1, whereas IL-4 is relatively selective for VCAM-1. Endothelial expression of ICAM-1, VCAM-1 and E-selectin is either not enhanced or only slightly increased upon exposure to IFN α and β, IL-2, IL-3, IL-5, IL-6, IL-7, IL-8, or TGFβ. Intriguingly, IFNγ appears to be a more potent stimulus for adhesion molecule biosynthesis by epithelial cells, including renal tubular epithelial cells, than either TNF or IL-1.

The induction of ICAM-1, VCAM-1 and E-selectin by cytokines is associated with increased levels of mRNA for these molecules and can be attenuated by inhibitors of protein (cycloheximide) and mRNA (actinomycin D) synthesis. These observations provide compelling evidence that cytokines enhance adhesion molecule biosynthesis by stimulating gene transcription and have been confirmed in more direct fashion by nuclear run-off studies of RNA synthesis. The mechanism(s) by which cytokines promote transcription is currently the focus of intensive investigation. Several lines of evidence suggest that cytokines induce ICAM-1 expression, at least in part, through activation of members of the protein kinase C family and induction of binding of the transcription regulatory protein AP-1 to a binding site on the ICAM-1 promoter (3–13,38,39). Direct activation of protein kinase C by phorbol myristate acetate mimics the stimulatory effect of cytokines on ICAM-1 synthesis and pharmacologic inhibitors of protein kinase C afford partial inhibition of ICAM-1 expression, albeit at high concentrations (39). Activation of protein kinase C induces AP-1 activity in endothelial cells and cloning of the promotor on the 5′-flanking region of the ICAM-1 gene has revealed consensus sequences for promoter elements (TATA box, CAAT box, SP1 binding site) and enhancer elements, including several AP-1 and AP-2 binding sites (also IFN responsive and glucocorticoid responsive elements).

The mechanism of induction of VCAM-1 and E-selectin gene expression by cytokines appears to involve the pleiotropic transcription regulatory factor NFκB (40–43). The 5′-flanking region of both genes contain multiple consensus DNA binding sites for NFκB, and many cytokines (e.g., TNFα, IL-1β, LPS) that induce the expression of these adhesion molecules also induce NFκB binding activity. Purified p50 and p65 subunits of NFκB stimulate expression of reporter genes linked to the promoter for E-selectin or VCAM-1. Furthermore, site-directed mutagenesis studies of the NFκB binding sites on the VCAM-1 and E-selectin promoters have demonstrated that their NFκB binding sites are necessary, although not sufficient, for cytokine-induced adhesion molecule expression. Along these lines, it is noteworthy that the 5′-flanking regions of both genes contain multiple other elements that are required for induction of transcription by NFκB, namely an ATF-2 binding site, four positive regulatory domains (PRD I-IV), and an HMG-1 site that appears to enhance binding of ATF-2 and NFκB to the promoter. The mechanism by which engagement of cytokines with their receptors causes activation of NFκB has not been resolved but may involve the intracellular actions of free radicals or fatty acids and/or changes in the cellular redox state (44). In contrast to ICAM-1, the bulk of evidence suggests that PKC is not a potent stimulus for induction of VCAM-1 or E-selectin. Most cytokines do not activate PKC at concentrations that induce NFκB activity and VCAM-1 or E-selectin expression, and pharmacological inhibition of PKC does not block these processes. The molecular basis for the postinduction transcriptional repression that accounts for the transience of E-selectin expression, and for the restriction of E-selectin expression to endothelial cells has yet to be determined. Elucidation of the mechanisms by which cytokines regulate transcription may suggest strategies for inhibition of synthesis of adhesion molecules during inflammation.

Endogenous Inhibitors of Leukocyte Adhesion

Several compounds have been identified that are potent inhibitors of leukocyte-endothelial cell interactions in vitro and may potentially serve to maintain leukocytes and endothelium in an "antiadhesive" phenotype in health and limit or reverse adhesion during inflammation. Nitric oxide inhibits leukocyte adhesion to endothelial cells induced by exogenous PAF or cytokine activation of endothelium in vitro and neutrophil adhesion to resting endothelium in vivo (45,46). Given these observations, it is noteworthy that reduced nitric oxide synthesis and increased leukocyte–endothelial cell adhesion have been implicated as important events in the pathophysiology of ischemia-reperfusion injury in many organs, including the kidney. Prostacyclin (PGI_2), a potent vasodilator and inhibitor of platelet aggregation, also attenuates neutrophil adhesion in vitro (47). Thus, it is possible that nitric oxide and PGI_2, through their similar actions on smooth muscle cells, platelets, and leukocytes, act in concert to maintain tissue perfusion and prevent thrombosis and leukocyte activation in the microvasculature. The recent discovery of cytokine-inducible forms of nitric oxide synthetase and cyclooxygenase suggests that these compounds may also modulate leukocyte recruitment during inflammation. It would be premature, however, to label nitric oxide as an "anti-inflammatory" compound as nitric oxide itself is a chemoattractant and peroxynitrite, generated by interaction of nitric oxide with superoxide anion, appears to be an important cytotoxic species derived from monocytes-macrophages at sites of inflammation.

Leukotrienes derived from the 5-lipoxygenase pathway are potent stimuli for leukocyte chemotaxis and adhesion, as discussed above, and inhibitors of leukotriene biosynthesis inhibit leukocyte recruitment and tissue injury in several models of acute inflammation, including glomerulonephritis (48,49). There is an expanding body of evidence suggesting that the products of the 5- and 15-lipoxygenase pathways exert counterregulatory actions on leukocyte recruitment in a manner analogous to the opposing actions of thromboxane and PGI_2 on vascular tone and platelet aggregation. 15-HETE is an eicosanoid generated by numerous cell types through the actions of 15-lipoxygenase (also cyclooxygenases and epoxygenases) whose levels are elevated in inflamed tissues and exudates in several diseases. Intradermal and intrarticular administration of exogenous 15-HETE reduces inflammation in human psoriasis and experimental arthritis, respectively (reviewed in 50). 15(S)-HETE is rapidly esterified into neutrophil membrane phospholipids and blunts chemoattractant-induced neutrophil adhesion and migration across endothelium in vitro by inhibiting chemoattractant-stimulated signal transduction events with the cell membrane (51,52). Lipoxin A_4 (LXA_4) is generated by granulocytes and monocytes via the actions of 15- and 5-lipoxygenases on arachidonic acid (48). In addition, LXA_4 is formed during interactions of neutrophils and platelets via the sequential actions of leukocyte 5-lipoxygenase and platelet 12-lipoxygenases on arachidonic acid (53). LXA_4 is a potent inhibitor of several leukotriene-induced responses, including LTB_4- and LTC_4-induced neutrophil adhesion to endothelial cells supported by P-selectin or $\beta 2$ integrins,

LTD_4-induced phagocyte-mesangial cell adhesion, and LTB_4-induced chemotaxis (49,54–58). As with 15-HETE, elevated levels of LXA_4 have been recently reported in inflammatory diseases, including acute glomerulonephritis (59,60). Prolonged exposure of endothelial cells to certain cytokines may also reduce their adhesiveness for leukocytes (reviewed in Ref. 7). TGFβ diminishes basal endothelial adhesiveness and blunts the proadhesive effects of TNFα and IL-1β on endothelium, in part by inhibiting E-selectin expression. IL-4, a potent inducer of endothelial VCAM-1 expression, attenuates ICAM-1 and E-selectin expression by these cells. The relevance of these findings in vivo has yet to be established; however, it seems reasonable to conclude that the profile of adhesion molecules expressed by resident tissue cells during inflammation reflects the complex interplay of pro- and antiadhesive cytokines. Further characterization of such endogenous inhibitors of adhesion may prove fruitful in defining novel approaches to the treatment of inflammation.

ROLE OF ADHESION MOLECULES IN THE PATHOPHYSIOLOGY OF RENAL DISEASE

The pattern of expression of adhesion molecules in normal and diseased kidneys has been examined in humans and experimental animals using immunohistochemical and/or molecular biological approaches; the latter studies usually utilizing either northern analysis or in situ hybridization to assess gene expression.

Expression of Leukocyte Adhesion Molecules in Healthy and Diseased Kidneys

Normal Kidneys

ICAM-1 is normally expressed at low levels on the luminal surface of endothelial cells of large vessels, glomeruli, and peritubular capillaries, by some cells in the mesangium, on the luminal surface of some parietal epithelial cells of Bowman's capsule, on the brush border of proximal tubule cells, and by fibroblast-like interstitial cells (Table 2) (61–79). Constitutive expression of VCAM-1 is usually detected only on parietal epithelial cells of Bowman's capsule and occasional endothelial cells of large vessels or peritubular capillaries (76,80–84). E-selectin is not constitutively expressed in normal kidney (59,85–87).

Glomerulonephritis and Tubulointerstitial Disease

Increased glomerular expression of ICAM-1 is a common finding in patients with active crescentic glomerulonephritis, mesangioproliferative glomerulonephritis, IgA nephropathy, Henoch-Schönlein

Table 2 Expression of Leukocyte Adhesion Molecules in Healthy and Diseased Kidneys

Site of expression		ICAM-1 Normal	ICAM-1 Disease	VCAM-1 Normal	VCAM-1 Disease	E-Selectin Normal	E-Selectin Disease
Endothelium	Larger vessels	+	+/++	–/+	++	–	–/+
	Glomerular	+	+/++	–	+	–	–/+
	Peritubular	+	+/++	–/+	++	–	–/+
Epithelium	Bowman's capsule	+	++	+	++	–	–
	Tubule epithelium	–	++	–	++	–	–
	Mesangium	–/+	++	–	++	–	–
	Interstitium	–/+	++	–	+	–	–

Abbreviations: –, not detected; –/+, detected by some, but not all investigators; +, expression consistently reported; ++ marked increase in expression. # There are few published reports of expression of ICAM-2, P-selectin or ligands for L-selectin in renal disease. PECAM-1 is constitutively expressed by all renal vascular endothelium (not shown here). See text for details of expression in specific renal diseases.
Source: From Ref. 13.

purpura, proliferative grades of lupus nephritis, and in rats with experimental nephrotoxic serum nephritis (62–65). Marked upregulation of ICAM-1 expression on the luminal surface of proximal tubules, distal convoluted tubule, and collecting duct cells and on fibroblast-like interstitial cells are common additional findings in these diseases (62–65,69). In general, the level of expression correlates with disease activity and the intensity of the local leukocyte infiltrate. Glomerular ICAM-1 levels may revert toward normal or below baseline in patients with advanced sclerotic disease. Although upregulation of ICAM-1 expression has been reported in some patients with minimal change nephropathy, ICAM-1 levels are usually unchanged or reduced in this disease (62–65). Variable patterns of ICAM-1 expression have also been reported in patients with focal segmental glomerulosclerosis and membranous nephropathy; some investigators reporting increased mesangial and/or tubulointerstitial staining, and others reporting a focal and segmental decrease in glomerular expression (62–65). It is possible that these differences reflect sampling at different stages in the disease process. Soluble forms of ICAM-1 have been detected in normal blood and an intriguing preliminary report suggests that circulating levels of ICAM-1 may be elevated in acute glomerulonephritis (88–90). It will be of interest to define the source of ICAM-1 in this setting and to determine whether this increased concentration of circulating ICAM-1 represents either another level of regulation of leukocyte adhesion, proves useful as a serological marker of disease activity, or merely reflects accumulation of soluble ICAM-1 as a result of a fall in glomerular filtration rate.

Seron et al. assessed VCAM-1 expression 50 biopsy specimens from patients with a variety of glomerulonephritides or tubulointerstitial diseases (80). Induction of VCAM-1 expression was observed on proximal tubule cells of virtually all patients with vasculitis and crescentic nephritis, lupus nephritis (class II, III, IV, and V), IgA nephropathy, and acute interstitial nephritis induced by nonsteroidal anti-inflammatory drugs. As in studies of ICAM-1 expression, VCAM-1 levels were highest in patients with active inflammation (e.g., vasculitis), and there was a positive correlation, albeit weak, between the level of expression and the intensity of the surrounding leukocytic infiltrate. Interestingly, VCAM-1 expression was not observed on vascular endothelial cells in any of these diseases. Striking expression of VCAM-1 was also observed in proximal tubules of patients with diabetic nephropathy, amyloid, gouty nephropathy, minimal change disease, and membranous nephropathy, diseases that are not usually associated with leukocytic infiltration of the kidney (80). Rat and murine models have proved useful for further defining the expression of VCAM-1 and ICAM-1 in glomerulonephritis and tubulointerstitial inflammation. Wuthrich noted dramatic induction of VCAM-1 expression in cortical but not medullary tubule epithelial cells, on vascular endothelium, and in the glomerular mesangium of the MRL-lpr mouse model of lupus nephritis (81). Again, there was a positive correlation between VCAM-1 levels and disease activity as determined by proteinuria, histological assessment, and the intensity of the associated leukocytic infiltrate (81). Furthermore, kidney tissue sections from nephritic mice supported adhesion of T-cell and macrophage cell lines, a process that was inhibited by monoclonal antibodies against VCAM-1 and ICAM-1. These data suggest that VCAM-1 and ICAM-1 contribute to leukocyte recruitment in this disease and are not merely markers of cytokine release by infiltrating leukocytes. The stimulus for induction of ICAM-1 and VCAM-1 on tubular epithelium in patients with glomerulonephritis is unclear. Potential mechanisms include primary involvement of the tubulointerstitium and/or the "downstream" actions of glomerular cytokines that reach the tubulointerstitium via blood, urine, or diffusion through extravascular tissue. In support of the former hypothesis, T cells cloned from inflammatory renal infiltrates in experimental lupus nephritis demonstrate specific autoreactivity against renal tissue and induce ICAM-1 and MHC class II molecules on cultured tubule epithelial cells due, at least in part, to the actions of IFN-γ (69).

The pattern of expression of E-selectin in glomerulonephritis and tubulointerstitial inflammation is largely undefined. Cytokine-activated renal microvascular endothelial cells clearly express E-selectin in vitro (87–91) and a preliminary report suggests that E-selectin is also expressed by glomerular endothelial cells in some patients with acute glomerulonephritis, lupus nephritis, and IgA nephropathy but not in patients with focal segmental glomerulosclerosis or membranous nephropathy (90). Induction of E-selectin on endothelial cells of interstitial venules is a frequent additional finding in patients with lupus nephritis and prominent interstitial inflammation, and in patients with IgA nephropathy during acute exacerbations (90). E-Selectin has also been reported on glomerular endothelium in experimental models of septic shock (85,86) and acute glomerulonephritis (92). Interestingly, glomerular levels of E-selectin appear to be highest in patients with high circulating levels of TNFα (90), and glomerular expression of E-selectin, ICAM-1, and VCAM-1 can be induced in experimental animals by infusion of TNFα but not IL-1β, into the renal artery. Furthermore, upregulation of these molecules can be attenuated in rats with nephrotoxic serum nephritis by prior treatment of animals with either a monoclonal antibody against TNFα or soluble recombinant human TNF receptor-1 (92). Taken together, these data suggest that TNFα may be a major stimulus for induction of adhesion molecule expression in acute glomerulonephritis.

Allograft Rejection

The patterns of expression of ICAM-1, VCAM-1, and E-selectin in renal biopsy specimens from patients with allograft rejection differ markedly from those observed in acute glomerulonephritis (70–78). Glomerular levels of ICAM-1 and VCAM-1 are usually unchanged during acute rejection. In contrast, there is often a striking increase in ICAM-1 expression on the luminal surface of proximal tubule cells, on some distal tubule and collecting duct cells, and on infiltrating leukocytes. Most investigators have found it difficult to detect changes in ICAM-1 levels on vascular endothelium in rejection due to the constitutive expression of ICAM-1 at this site. De novo expression of VCAM-1 is usually observed in a focal distribution (30–50% of tubules) toward the basolateral surface of proximal tubule cells and on occasional distal tubules in renal allograft rejection in humans (76,77,82–85). In addition, striking induction of VCAM-1 is typically seen on the endothelium of peritubular capillaries, venules, and arterioles but not on glomerular cells. The distribution of E-selectin on endothelium in acute rejection tends to parallel that of ICAM-1 and VCAM-1 but is a less consistent finding (76,77), as has been observed in acute glomerulonephritis. It should be noted that the absence of staining in some patients does not preclude a role for this molecule in leukocyte recruitment and may reflect the transience of E-selectin expression or extensive endothelial injury. Indeed, focal absence of PECAM-1, which is constitutively expressed by healthy renal endothelium, has also been reported in acute allograft rejection, supporting the latter contention (77). As in the studies of acute glomerulonephritis discussed above, ICAM-1, VCAM-1 and E-selectin expression is usually greatest in areas of leukocyte infiltration, again suggesting that these molecules contribute to the recruitment process. Increased circulating levels of ICAM-1 have also been detected in acute rejection but not cyclosporine toxicity, and this parameter has been proposed as a means of differentiating these two diagnoses (93).

Other Adhesion Molecules

Albeit based on a limited number of reports, ICAM-2, PECAM-1, and the mucin CD34 appear to be constitutively expressed by microvascular endothelial cells in normal kidney, while P-selectin is not detected. There are few studies documenting the distribution of these ligands in renal disease. It is also worth noting that there are few reports on the expression of ICAM-1, VCAM-1, and E-selectin on the same pathology specimen or correlating the expression of these molecules with the relative numbers of different types of leukocytes in inflammatory infiltrates. Most resident renal cells, either in their basal state or following activation by cytokines, express ligands that may potentially support granulocyte, monocyte, or lymphocyte adhesion. Yet regional differences in the composition of leukocyte infiltrates are found in many inflammatory renal diseases and enhanced expression of adhesion molecules may be observed in the absence of leukocyte infiltration. These observations suggest that leukocyte recruitment is not regulated solely by the profile of adhesion molecules on invading and resident cells, but also by the complex interplay of chemoattractants and other soluble and cell-associated activation signals within a local inflammatory milieu.

Adhesion Promotes Bidirectional "Cross-Talk" Between Leukocytes and Renal Parenchymal Cells

In addition to regulating leukocyte recruitment, adhesion also facilitates a dynamic interplay between leukocytes and renal parenchymal cells that ultimately contributes to the impairment of function and destruction of tissue architecture. For example, leukocyte adhesion is an important event in T-cell activation and cytotoxicity during cellular immune responses (3–13,94–96). Activation of T-lymphocytes through interaction with antigen-bearing MHC molecules on antigen-presenting cells is markedly inhibited by mAb against CD11a/CD18 and ICAM-1 and other ligand pairs that support cell-cell adhesion (7,94,95). Similarly, mAb against CD11a/CD18 and ICAM-1 attenuates lysis of target cells, including renal tubule epithelial cells, by cytotoxic T-lymphocytes in vitro (96). Adhesion may also promote injury to renal cells and basement membrane mediated by phagocytic leukocytes by priming phagocyte respiratory bursts and degranulation to the actions of chemoattractants and cytokines (7,97–99). Phagocytes generate more superoxide anion when adherent to cytokine-activated mesangial cells in vitro than in suspension and mAb against CD18 attenuate adhesion, superoxide anion generation, and mesangial cell injury in this setting (98). Adhesion probably also contributes to tissue injury by promoting the release of reactive oxygen species and proteases in close proximity to glomerular cells and basement membrane, reducing the effectiveness of free radical scavengers and protease inhibitors in extracellular fluid (7).

Adhesion of phagocytic leukocytes to endothelial cells, other renal parenchymal cells, and platelets may serve to amplify the concentrations and array of lipid mediators at sites of inflammation by facilitating the generation of eicosanoids by transcellular routes (Figure 3) (100–102). For example, neutrophils and glomerular endothelial cells pool their enzymatic machinery during coincubations and generate markedly increased quantities of the vasoactive mediator LTC_4 than are formed in homogenous populations of either cell type. Monoclonal antibodies against CD11/CD18 integrins and L-selectin, which block leukocyte adhesion under these conditions, attenuate LTC_4 biosynthesis (100–102). These observations suggest that adhesion promotes transcellular routes LTC_4 generation either by approximating leukocyte and endothelial cell membranes and facilitating the transfer of the unstable lipophilic intermediate LTA_4 between cells (Figure 3) or by priming leukocyte 5-lipoxygenase pathways and LTA_4 generation and release, as with other functional responses (see above) (103).

Taken together, these in vitro observations suggest additional mechanisms by which adhesion may contribute to the pathophysiology of acute allograft rejection, glomerulonephritis, and other forms of renal inflammation. By extension, they suggest that agents that block adhesion may attenuate renal injury by mechanisms other than inhibition of leukocyte recruitment and mandate that these considerations be taken into account when interpreting the results of intervention studies (see below).

ADHESION MOLECULES AS TARGETS FOR THERAPY IN RENAL DISEASE

Glomerulonephritis

The influence of mAb directed against specific adhesion molecules on renal injury has been assessed in experimental models of glomerulonephritis, tubulointerstitial disease, allograft rejection, and renal ischemia-reperfusion injury (Table 3) (92,103–110). While the results of many studies have been encouraging and suggest that adhesion molecules are attractive targets for therapeutic intervention, it is clear that the ligands that support adhesion may differ markedly depending on the experimental model, species, and time of study. Mulligan et al. reported that mAb against CD18, CD11b, and ICAM-1 afford a marked reduction in proteinuria and glomerular neutrophil counts in Long-Evans rats with complement- and neutrophil-dependent nephrotoxic serum nephritis (92). In contrast, mAb against CD11a and E-selectin were not beneficial. Interestingly, mAb against VLA-4 also attenuated neutrophil recruitment and proteinuria in this model, even though this ligand does not play a direct role in neutrophil trafficking. These observations further suggest that some mAb may protect via mechanisms other than direct inhibition of neutrophil adhesion (see above). Along these lines, Wu et al. observed that infusion of anti-CD11b mAb 16 hr prior to induction of nephrotoxic serum nephritis in Lewis rats caused a striking decrease in proteinuria and neutrophil infiltration; however, administration of mAb 30 min before induction also afforded protection without affecting glomerular neutrophil counts (103). MAb against CD11a and ICAM-1 have also been shown to abrogate proteinuria and inhibit crescent formation in two studies of crescentic glomerulonephritis in Wistar-Kyoto rats (105–106), a model that is characterized by linear deposition of IgG in the glomerular basement membrane, upregulation of ICAM-1 on glomerular endothelium, early infiltration of glomeruli by T-lymphocytes and monocytes/macrophages, crescent formation, and glomerulosclerosis. Importantly, progression of disease was retarded significantly even when treatment was instituted after disease was established (106), an important consideration if such agents are to be therapeutically useful in humans. In contrast to these studies in rats, two groups did not

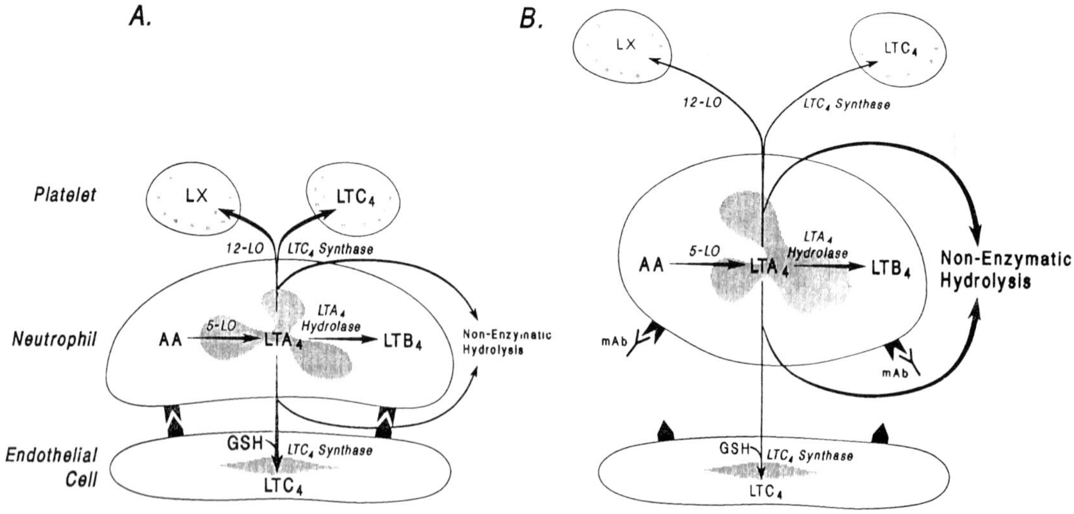

Figure 3 Proposed mechanism(s) by which leukocyte adhesion promotes the generation of lipoxygenase products by transcellular routes at sites of inflammation. Glomerular endothelial cells and platelets lack 5-lipoxygenase (5-LO) mRNA or catalytic activity, but transform leukocyte-derived LTA_4 to biologically active products. Glomerular endothelial cells conjugate LTA_4 with glutathione (GSH) to form LTC_4, a reaction catalysed by LTC_4 synthetase (glutathione-S-transferase). Platelets convert LTA_4 to both LTC_4 and lipoxins (LX) through the actions of LTC_4 synthetase and 12-lipoxygenase (12-LO), respectively. MAb which block leukocyte adhesion to glomerular endothelial cells, also block transcellular LTC_4 formation during coincubations of leukocytes and glomerular endothelial cells. These observations suggest that adhesion facilitates transfer of LTA_4, an unstable lipophilic and hydrophobic intermediate, from leukocytes to endothelial cells, thereby promoting the generation of LO products and minimizing nonenzymatic hydrolysis of LTA_4 to inactive products in extracellular fluid (100–102). Adhesion may also prime leukocyte lipoxygenase pathways and enhance LTA_4 biosynthesis (103). These observations highlight the dynamic interplay that occurs between leukocytes and renal parenchymal cells in the context of cell-cell adhesion and suggest that agents that block adhesion may have anti-inflammatory activity through mechanisms other than inhibition of leukocyte trafficking. (From Ref. 13.)

observe a protective effect of anti-CD18 mAb in nephrotoxic serum nephritis in rabbits using doses of mAb that saturate CD18 on circulating and glomerular neutrophils, inhibit neutrophil migration to other vascular beds, and have been shown previously to attenuate neutrophil-dependent tissue injury in other organs in this species (Table 3).

Tubulointerstitial Nephritis

Harning et al. assessed the influence of anti-ICAM-1 mAb on autoimmune tubulointerstitial nephritis in the kdkd variant of the CBA/Ca mice (107). These animals have normal kidneys at birth but develop progressive and ultimately lethal tubulointerstitial nephritis beginning after approximately 4 weeks. The disease process is associated with upregulation of ICAM-1 expression in the renal interstitium, on infiltrating leukocytes, and on the basolateral surface of renal tubule epithelium. The administration of anti-ICAM-1 mAb to mice with established disease caused a marked reduction in leukocyte infiltration, tubular injury, and proteinuria in this model; however, survival was unchanged.

Allograft Rejection

Cosimi et al. observed a marked delay in the onset of renal allograft rejection in cynomolgus monkeys and increased recipient survival when anti-ICAM-1 mAb was employed as the sole immunosuppres-

Table 3 Efficacy of Some Adhesion-Blocking Monoclonal Antibodies in Inflammatory Diseases and Ischemia-Reperfusion Injury of the Kidney

Renal disease	Species (strain)	Molecule	Antibody	Preparation	Dose	Timing[a]	Protection	Ref
Nephrotoxic serum nephritis	Rat (Long-Evans)	CD18	CL-26	$F(ab')_2$	33 μg IV	After	Yes	92
		CD11a	WT-1	Intact	200 μg IV	Simultaneous	No	
		CD11b	1B6c	Intact	300 μg IV	Not reported	Yes	
		VLA-4	TA-2	Intact	800 μg IV	Simult + after	Yes	
		ICAM-1	1A29	$F(ab')_2$	200 μg IV + IP	After	Yes	
		E-selectin	CL-3	$F(ab')_2$	45/133 μg IV	After	No	
Nephrotoxic serum nephritis	Rat (Lewis)	CD11b	OX42	Intact	0.15 mg/ 100g IV	Before	Yes	103
Nephrotoxic serum nephritis	Rat (Wistar)	ICAM-1	1A29	Intact	5 mg/kg IV	Before + after	Yes	104
Nephrotoxic serum nephritis	Rabbit (New Zealand White)	CD18	R15.7	Intact	2 mg/kg IV[b]	Before	No	[c]
		ICAM-1	R6.5	Intact	2 mg/kg IV	Before	No	
Nephrotoxic serum nephritis	Rabbit	CD18	60.3	Intact	saturating dose IV[b]	Before	No	[d]
Crescentic glomerulonephritis	Rat (Wistar-Kyoto)	CD11a	WT-1	Intact	1–5 mg/kg IP	Before + after	Yes	105
		ICAM-1	1A29	Intact	1–5 mg/kg IP	Before + after	Yes	
		CD11a + ICAM-1	WT-1 + 1A29	Intact	1 mg/kg of both IP	Before + after	Yes[e]	
Crescentic glomerulonephritis	Rat (Wistar-Kyoto)	CD11a + ICAM-1	WT-1 + 1A29	Intact	0.5 mg of both IV + IP	Before + after	Yes	106
Tubulointerstitial nephritis	Mouse (CBA/Ca, kdkd)	ICAM-1	YN1/1.7	Intact	10 mg/kg/ day IP	After	Yes	107
Acute allograft rejection	Monkey (Cynomolgus)	ICAM-1	R6.5	Intact	0.01–2 mg/kg/ day IV	Before + after	Yes	108
Acute allograft rejection	Human	ICAM-1	B1RR1	Intact	IV to achieve serum levels of ~10 μg/ml	Before + after	Yes	109

Table 3 (*Continued*)

Renal disease	Species (strain)	Molecule	Antibody	Preparation	Dose	Timing[a]	Protection	Ref
Ischemia-reperfusion	Rabbit (New Zealand White)	CD18	60.3	Intact	2 mg/kg IV	Before	No	112
Ischemia-reperfusion	Rabbit (New Zealand White)	CD18	R15.7	Intact	2 mg/kg IV	Before	No	[f]
		ICAM-1	R6.5	Intact	2 mg/kg IV	Before	No	
Ischemia-reperfusion	Rat	ICAM-1				Before or after	Yes	113

[a]Relative to induction of disease.
[b]Dose sufficient to saturate CD18 on circulating and glomerular leukocytes and cause demargination of leukocytes (leukocytosis) or inhibition of chemoattractant-stimulated leukocyte migration into skin. From Ref. 13.
[c]O'Meara YM, Salant DJ, Brady HR, and
[d]Tipping PG, Cornthwaite LJ, Holdsworth SR, XII International Congress of Nephrology, Jerusalem, Israel June 1993.
[e]Additive protection when compared with equivalent doses of individual mAb.
[f]Neuringer J, Brady HR, unpublished observations.

sive agent after transplantation (108). This protective effect of anti-ICAM-1 mAb was associated with partial inhibition of T lymphocyte (CD2, CD4, and CD8) and monocyte recruitment into the renal interstitium and arterial endothelium, respectively. Anti-ICAM-1 mAb also reversed established rejection in allograft recipients maintained on subtherapeutic doses of cyclosporine, on this occasion, without affecting the intensity of the leukocyte infiltrate. The preliminary results of a phase 1 clinical trial of anti-ICAM-1 in high risk allograft recipients suggests that this mAb may also prevent rejection in humans (109).

Ischemia-Reperfusion

There is compelling evidence that neutrophils contribute to ischemia-reperfusion injury in many vascular beds, including the pulmonary, coronary, cerebral, and splanchnic circulations (5), and that anti-CD18 mAb confer protection in many of these experimental models (reviewed in Ref. 7). The role of neutrophils in renal ischemic-reperfusion injury is less clear (111,112), and anti-CD18 and anti-ICAM-1 mAb did not confer functional or morphological protection in two studies of renal ischemia-reperfusion in rabbits (Table 3) (Ref. 112 and Neuringer J, Brady HR, unpublished observations). However, a recent report indicates that anti-ICAM-1 mAb can inhibit leukocyte recruitment, renal dysfunction, and morphological injury following renal ischemia in rats (113). As with glomerulonephritis and allograft rejection, it is encouraging that anti-ICAM-1 mAb afforded protection even when given hours after the renal insult. Which of these species bears closest resemblance to human disease remains to be determined, but this is clearly an important question given the high prevalence of renal ischemic-reperfusion injury in clinical practice.

INVOLVEMENT OF ADHESION MOLECULES IN OTHER BIOLOGICAL EVENTS

Leukocyte adhesion molecules are also potential targets for therapeutic intervention in several seemingly unrelated renal disorders: hemodialysis membrane incompatibility reactions, atherogenesis, tumor metastasis, and infections. Exposure of circulating blood to new cellulosic hemodialysis membranes frequently results in dramatic changes in CD11/CD18 and L-selectin surface expression on neutrophils and monocytes in association with increased leukocyte adhesiveness and may contribute to sequestration of leukocytes in the pulmonary vasculature and systemic granulocytopenia that characterizes the dialysis "first-use syndrome" (114–117). In keeping with this hypothesis, granulocytes from normal subjects undergo dramatic degranulation when exposed to cellulosic membranes in vitro, while degranulation is markedly attenuated with granulocytes from individuals with LAD type 1 disease (117). Increased expression of VCAM-1 and E-selectin on endothelium overlying intimal fatty streaks is an early event in the pathogenesis of experimental and human atherosclerosis (118–120). The mechanism of induction of adhesion molecule biosynthesis in this setting has not been elucidated fully but may involve direct stimulation of adhesion molecule gene transcription by oxidized LDL or the actions of cytokines released from resident tissue macrophages upon activation by oxidized LDL. Upregulation of endothelial cell VCAM-1 and E-selectin expression may subsequently play a role in monocyte recruitment into the vessel wall, a critical event in the formation of atheromatous plaques (118–120). Many adhesion molecules, in addition to supporting leukocyte adhesion, also support adhesion of tumor cells (121). These observations raise the intriguing possibility that tumor cells may usurp the function of endothelial cell adhesion molecules to extravasate from blood and establish metastatic lesions. These observations must be balanced, however, against the potential role of adhesion molecules in recruitment of lymphocytes to areas of tumor growth, frequently an indicator of a favorable prognosis (122). Similarly, rhinoviruses, some Coxsackie viruses, and *Plasmodium falciparum*-infected erythrocytes may usurp the function of ICAM-1 on airway epithelial cells and the cerebral vasculature, respectively, to infect their hosts (123,124). It remains to be determined whether it will be possible to develop orally active agents suitable for routine clinical use that selectively inhibit these diverse processes mediated by leukocyte adhesion molecules without compromising immunosurveillance and host defense mechanisms.

Although beyond the scope of this chapter, it should be noted that the leukocyte adhesion molecules are members of larger superfamilies of molecules that regulate renal development, maintenance of tissue architecture, and other important biological events and whose function may be perturbed in renal diseases. Beta-1 integrins, for example, are important anchors of renal parenchymal cells to their basement membranes. Several intriguing observations suggest that these interactions may be disrupted during glomerulonephritis (125–127), renal ischemia (128,129), and other forms of renal injury and contribute to the pathophysiology of these diseases. Further advances in our understanding of the molecular regulation of these events may herald the development of novel, potent, and relatively nontoxic therapies for common renal diseases.

ACKNOWLEDGMENTS

This work was supported by NIH grant DK44380 and an award from the W. F. Milton Fund, Harvard University.

REFERENCES

1. Eddy AA, Michael AF. Immunopathogenetic mechanisms of glomerular injury. In: Tisher CC, Brenner BM, eds. Renal Pathology. Philadelphia: Lippincott, 1989:111–155.
2. Couser WG. Mediation of glomerular immune injury. J Am Soc Nephrol 1990; 1:13–29.
3. Arnaout MA. Structure and function of leukocyte adhesion molecules CD11/CD18. Blood 1990; 75:1037–1050.
4. Arnaout MA. Leukocyte adhesion molecules deficiency: Its structural basis, pathophysiology and implications for modulating the inflammatory response. Immunol Rev 1990; 114:145–180.
5. Pober JS, Cotran RS. Cytokines and endothelial cell biology. Physiol Rev 1990; 70:427–451.
6. Springer TA. Traffic signals for lymphocyte recirculation and leukocyte emigration: The multistep paradigm. Cell 1995; 301–314.
7. Carlos TM, Harlan JM. Leukocyte-endothelial adhesion molecules. Blood 1994; 84:2068-2101.
8. Lasky LA. Selectins: interpreters of cell-specific carbohydrate information during inflammation. Science 1992; 258:964–969.
9. Wuthrich RP. Intercellular adhesion molecules and vascular cell adhesion molecule-1 and the kidney. J Am Soc Nephrol 1992; 3:1201–1211.
10. Bevilacqua MP, Nelson RM. Selectins. J Clin Invest 1993; 91:379–387.
11. Brady HR. Leukocyte adhesion molecules: Potential targets for therapeutic intervention in kidney diseases. Curr Opin Nephrol Hypertens 1993; 2:171–182.
12. Briscoe DM, Cotran RS. Role of leukocyte-endothelial cell adhesion molecules in renal inflammation: in vitro and in vivo studies. Kidney Int 1993; 44:S27–S36.
13. Brady HR. Leukocyte adhesion molecules and kidney diseases. Kidney Int 1994; 45:1285–1300.
14. Wilson JM, Ping AJ, Krauss JC, et al. Correction of CD18-deficient lymphocytes by retrovirus-mediated gene transfer. Science 1990; 248:1413–1416.
15. Etzioni A, Frydman M, Pollack S, et al. Recurrent severe infections caused by a novel leukocyte adhesion deficiency. N Engl J Med 1992; 327:1789–1792.
16. Shimizu Y, Shaw S. Mucins in the mainstream. Nature 1993; 366:630–631.
17. Carraway KL, Hull SR. Cell surface mucin-type glycoprotein and mucin-like domains. Glycobiology 1991; 1:131–138.
18. Muller WA, Weigl SA, Deng X, Phillips DM. PECAM-1 is required for transendothelial migration of leukocytes. J Exp Med 1993; 178:449–460.
19. Vaporciyan AA, DeLisser HM, Yan H-C, et al. Involvement of platelet-endothelial cell adhesion molecule-1 in neutrophil recruitment in vivo. Science 1993; 262:1580–1582.
20. Bevilacqua M, Butcher E, Furie B, et al. Selectins: A family of adhesion receptors. Cell 1991; 67:233.
21. Brady HR, Spertini O, Jimenez W, et al. Neutrophils, monocytes, and lymphocytes bind to cytokine-activated glomerular endothelial cells through L-selectin (LAM-1). J Immunol 1992; 149:2437–2444.
22. Briskin MJ, McEvoy LM, Butcher EC. MadCAM-1 has homology to immunoglobulin and mucin-like adhesion receptors and to IgA1. Nature 1993; 363:461–466.
23. Berg EL, McEvoy LM, Berlin C, Bargatze RF, Butcher EC. L-Selectin-mediated lymphocyte rolling on MadCAM-1. Nature 1993; 366:695–698.
24. Lasky LA, Singer MS, Dowbenko D, et al. An endothelial ligand for L-selectin is a novel mucin-like molecule. Cell 1992; 69:927–938.
25. Imai Y, Lasky LA, Rosen SD. Sulphation requirement for GlyCAM-1, an endothelial ligand for L-selectin. Nature 1993; 361:555–557.

26. Sako D, Chang XJ, Barone KM, et al. Expression cloning of a functional glycoprotein ligand for P-selectin. Cell 1993; 75:1179–1186.
27. Vorki A. Selectin ligands. Proc Natl Acad Sci USA 1994; 91:7390–7397.
28. Vestweber D, Levinovitz A, Lenter M. Monospecific and common glycoprotein ligands for E-selectin and P-selectin on myeloid cells (abstr). J Cell Biochem 1994; suppl 18A:263.
29. Andrew DP, Butcher EC. Subpopulations of B and T lymphocytes express CD11b/CD18 and are capable of CD11b/CD18 mediated adhesion (abstr). J Cell Biochem 1994; suppl 18A:294.
30. Osborn L, Hession C, Tizard R, et al. Direct expression cloning of vascular cell adhesion molecule-1, a cytokine-induced endothelial protein that binds to lymphocytes. Cell 1989; 59:1203–1211.
31. Cybulsky MI, Fries JW, William AJ, et al. Alternate splicing of human VCAM-1 in activated vascular endothelium. Am J Pathol 1991; 138:815–820.
32. Cybulsky MI, Fries JW, Williams AJ, et al. Gene structure, chromosomal location and basis for alternative splicing of the human VCAM-1 gene. Proc Natl Acad Sci USA 1991; 88:7859–7863.
33. Labow MA, Norton CR, Rumberger JM, et al. Characterization of E-selectin deficient mice: Demonstration of overlapping function of endothelial selectins. Immunity 1994; 1:709–720.
34. Falk RJ, Terrell RS, Charles LA, Jennette JC. Anti-neutrophil cytoplasmic antibodies induce neutrophils to degranulate and produce oxygen radicals in vitro. Proc Natl Acad Sci USA 1990; 87:4115–4119.
35. Ewert BW, Becker M, Jennette JC, Falk RJ. Anti-myeloperoxidase antibodies stimulate neutrophils to adhere to cultured human endothelial cells utilizing the beta-2 integrin CD11/CD18 (abstr). J Am Soc Nephrol 1992; 3:585.
36. Weissman G. The role of neutrophils in vascular injury: A summary of signal transduction mechanisms in cell/cell interactions. Springer Semin Immunopathol 1989; 11:235–258.
37. Weller A, Isenmann S, Vestweber D. Cloning of mouse endothelial selectins: expression of both E- and P-selectin is inducible by tumor necrosis factor alpha. J Biol Chem 1992; 267:15176–15183.
38. Stade BG, Messer G, Riethmuller G, Johnson JP. Structural characteristics of the 5′ region of the human ICAM-1 gene. Immunobiology 1990; 182:79–87.
39. Myers CL, Desai SN, Schembri-King J, et al. Discriminatory effects of protein kinase inhibitors and calcium ionophore on endothelial ICAM-1 induction. Am J Physiol 1992; 262:C365–C373.
40. Collins T, Williams A, Johnston GI, et al. Structure and chromosomal location of the gene foe ELAM-1. J Biol Chem 1991; 266:2466–2473.
41. Neish AS, Williams AJ, Palmer HJ. Functional analysis of the human vascular cell adhesion molecule-1 (VCAM-1) promoter. J Exp Med 1992; 176:1583–1593.
42. Shu HB, Agranoff AB, Nabel EG, et al. Differential regulation of VCAM-1 gene expression by specific NFκB subunits in endothelial and epithelial cells. Mol Cell Biol 1993; 13:6283–6289.
43. Read M, Whitley M, Williams A, Collins T. NFκB and IκB-α: An inducible regulatory system in endothelial activation. J Exp Med 1994; 179:503–512.
44. Marui N, Offerman MK, Swerlick R, et al. VCAM-1 gene transcription and expression are regulated through an anti-oxidant sensitive mechanism in human vascular endothelial cells. J Clin Invest 1993; 92:1866–1874.
45. Kubes P, Suzuki M, Granger DN. Nitric oxide: An endogenous modulator of leukocyte adhesion. Proc Natl Acad Sci USA 1991; 88:4651–4655.
46. Matsubara M, Takata S, Jimenez W, et al. Endothelial cell-derived nitric oxide limits neutrophil migration across TNF-activated endothelial cell monolayers (abstr). J Am Soc Nephrol 1992; 3:547.
47. Boxer LA, Allen JM, Schmidt M, et al. Inhibition of polymorphonuclear leukocyte adherence by prostacyclin. J Lab Clin Med 1980; 95:672–678.
48. Samuelsson B, Dahlen S-E, Lindgren JA, et al. Leukotrienes and lipoxins: Structures, biosynthesis, and biological effects. Science 1987; 237:1171–1176.
49. Badr KF. 15-Lipoxygenase products as leukotriene antagonists: Therapeutic potential in glomerulonephritis. Kidney Int 1992; 38:S101–S108.
50. Spector AA, Gordon JA, Moore SA. Hydroxyeicosatetraenoic acids. Prog Lipid Res 1988; 27:271–323.
51. Brezinski ME, Serhan CN. Selective incorporation of (15S)-hydroxyeicosatetraenoic acid in phosphatidylinositol of human neutrophils: Agonist-induced deacylation and transformation of stored hydroxyeicosanoids. Proc Natl Acad Sci USA 1990; 87:6248–6252.
52. Takata S, Matsubara M, Allen PG, et al. Remodeling of neutrophil phospholipids with 15(S)-hydroxyeicosatetraenoic acid inhibits leukotriene B_4-induced neutrophil migration across endothelium. J Clin Invest 1994; 93:499–508.
53. Fiore S, Serhan CN. Formation of lipoxins and leukotrienes during receptor-mediated interactions of human platelets and recombinant human granulocyte/macrophage colony stimulating factor-primed neutrophils. J Exp Med 1990; 172:1451–1457.
54. Brady HR, Persson U, Ballermann BJ, et al. Leukotrienes stimulate neutrophil adhesion to mesangial cells: Modulation with lipoxins. Am J Physiol 1990; 259:F809–F815.

55. Brady HR, Denton MD, Brenner BM, Serhan CN: Neutrophil adhesion to glomerular mesangial cells: Regulation by lipoxygenase-derived eicosanoids. In: Wong PK-Y, Serhan CN, eds. Cell-Cell Interaction in the Release of Inflammatory Mediators. New York: Plenum Press, 1992:347–359.
56. Lee TH, Horton CE, Kyan-Aung U, et al. Lipoxin A_4 and lipoxin B_4 inhibit chemotactic responses of human neutrophils stimulated by LTB_4 and N-formyl-L-methionyl-L-leucyl-L-phenylalanine. Clin Sci Lond 1989; 77:195–203.
57. Hedqvist P, Raud J, Palmertz J, et al. Lipoxin A_4 inhibits leukotriene B_4-induced inflammation in the hamster cheek pouch. Acta Physiol Scand 1989; 137:571–581.
58. Papayianni A, Takata S, Serhan CN, Brady HR. Counter-regulatory actions of leukotrienes and lipoxins on P-selectin expression on human endothelial cells and neutrophil-endothelial cell adhesion (abstr). J Am Soc Nephrol 1993; 4:627.
59. Lee TH, Crae AE, Gant V, et al. Identification of lipoxin A_4 and its relationship to the sulfidopeptide leukotrienes C_4, D_4 and E_4 in bronchoalveolar lavage fluids from patients with selected pulmonary diseases. Am Rev Respir Dis 1990; 141:1453–1458.
60. Papayianni A, Serhan CN, Phillips L, Rennke HG, Brady HR. P. selectin promotes transcellular generation of Lipoxin A_4 during platelet-neutrophil interactions in acute glomerulonephritis. Kidney Int 1995. In press.
61. Bishop GA, Hall BM: Expression of leukocyte and lymphocyte adhesion molecules in the human kidney. Kidney Int 1989; 36:1078–1085.
62. Muller GA, Markovic-Lipkovski J, Muller CA: Intercellular adhesion molecule-1 expression in human kidneys with glomerulonephritis. Clin Nephrol 1991; 36:203–208.
63. Lhotta K, Neumayer HP, Joannidis M, et al. Renal expression of intercellular adhesion molecule-1 in different forms of glomerulonephritis. Clin Sci 1991; 81:477–481.
64. Markovic-Lipkovski J, Muller CA, Risler T, et al. Mononuclear leukocytes, expression of HLA class II antigens and intercellular adhesion molecule-1 in focal segmental glomerulosclerosis. Nephron 1991; 58:286–293.
65. Dal Canton A, Fuiano G, Sepe V, et al. Mesangial expression of intercellular adhesion molecule-1 in primary glomerulosclerosis. Kidney Int 1992; 41:951–955.
66. Waldherr R, Eberlein-Gonska M, Noronha IL, et al. TNFα and ICAM-1 expression in renal disease (abstr). J Am Soc Nephrol 1990; 1:544.
67. Fuiano G, Sepe V, Ferrone S, et al. Expression of intercellular adhesion molecule-1 in necrotizing glomerulonephritis (abstr). J Am Soc Nephrol 1990; 1:560.
68. Wuthrich RP, Jevnikar AM, Takei F, et al. Intercellular adhesion molecule-1 expression is upregulated in autoimmune murine lupus nephritis. Am J Pathol 1990; 136:441–450.
69. Diaz Gallo C, Jevnikar AM, Brennan DC, et al. Autoreactive kidney-infiltrating T-cell clones in murine lupus nephritis. Kidney Int 1992; 42:851–859.
70. Faull RJ, Russ GR. Tubular expression of intercellular adhesion molecule-1 during renal allograft rejection. Transplantation 1989; 48:226–230.
71. Kanagawa K, Ishikura H, Takahashi C, et al. Identification of ICAM-1 positive cells in the nongrafted and transplanted rat kidney: An immunohistochemical and ultrastructural study. Transplantation 1991; 52:1057–1062.
72. Matsuno T, Sakagami K, Saito S, et al. Expression of intercellular adhesion molecule-1 and perforin on kidney allograft rejection. Transplant Proc 1992; 34:1306–1307.
73. Yoshizawa N, Oda T, Nakamura H: Expression of intercellular adhesion molecule-1 and HLA-DR by tubular cells and immune cell infiltration in human renal allografts. Transplant Proc 1992; 24:1308–1309.
74. Moolenaar W, Bruijn JA, Schrama E, et al. T-cell receptors and ICAM-1 expression in renal allografts during rejection. Transplant Int 1991; 4:140–145.
75. Andersen CB, Blaehr H, Ladenfoged S, Larsen S: Expression of intercellular adhesion molecule-1 in human renal allografts and cultured human tubular cells. Nephrol Dial Transplant 1992; 7:147–154.
76. Brockmeyer C, Ulbrecht M, Schendel DJ, et al. Distribution of cell adhesion molecules (ICAM-1, VCAM-1, ELAM-1) in renal tissue during allograft rejection. Transplantation 1993; 55:610–615.
77. Fuggle SV, Sanderson JB, Gray DWR, et al. Variation in expression of endothelial adhesion molecules in pretransplant and transplanted kidneys—Correlation with intragraft events. Transplantation 1993; 55:117–123.
78. von Willebrand E, Loginov R, Salmela K, et al. Relationship between intercellular adhesion molecule-1 and HLA class II expression in acute cellular rejection of human kidney allografts. Transplant Proc 1993; 25:870–871.
79. Hill PA, Lan HY, Nikolic-Paterson DJ, Atkins RC. ICAM-1 directs migration and localization of interstitial leukocytes in experimental glomerulonephritis. Kidney Int 1994; 45:32–42.
80. Seron D, Cameron JS, Haskard DO: Expression of VCAM-1 in the normal and diseased kidney. Nephrol Dial Transplant 1991; 6:917–922.
81. Wuthrich RP, Snyder TL: Vascular cell adhesion molecule-1 (VCAM-1) expression in murine lupus nephritis. Kidney Int 1992; 42:903–914.

82. Briscoe DM, Pober JS, Harmon HE, Cotran RS. Expression of vascular cell adhesion molecule-1 in human renal allografts. J Am Soc Nephrol 1992; 3:1180–1185.
83. Alpers CE, Hudkins KL, Davis CL, et al. Expression of vascular cell adhesion molecule-1 in human kidney allograft rejection. Kidney Int 1993; 44:805–816.
84. Lin Y, Kirby JA, Clark K, et al. Renal allograft rejection: Induction and function of adhesion molecules on cultured epithelial cells. Clin Exp Immunol 1992; 90:111–116.
85. Redl H, Dinges HP, Buurman WA, et al. Expression of endothelial leukocyte adhesion molecule-1 in septic but not traumatic/hypovolemic shock in the baboon. Am J Pathol 1991; 139:461–466.
86. Laszik Z, Nadasdy T, Johnson D, et al. Transient expression of ELAM-1 in endotoxin and E. coli-induced septic shock in rat kidney (abstr). J Am Soc Nephrol 1992; 3:601.
87. Nikolic-Paterson DJ, Yu Y, Atkins RC. Regulation of glomerular VCAM-1 and ELAM-1 gene expression by inflammatory stimuli (abstr). J Am Soc Nephrol 1992; 3:639–688.
88. Seth R, Raymond FD, Makgoba MW. Circulating ICAM-1 isoforms; Diagnostic prospects for inflammatory and immune disorders. Lancet 1991; 338:83–84.
89. Rothlein R, Mainolfi EA, Czajkowski M, Marlin SD. A form of circulating ICAM-1 in human serum. J Immunol 1991; 147:3788–3793.
90. Yokoyama H, Tomosugi N, Takaeda M, et al. Glomerular expression of cellular adhesion molecules and serum TNF alpha and soluble ICAM-1 levels in human glomerulonephritis (abstr). J Am Soc Nephrol 1992; 3:669.
91. Hancock WW, Cotran RS. Induction of activation antigens on human glomerular endothelium by interleukin-1, interferon-γ and endotoxin (abstr). Kidney Int 1987; 31:322.
92. Mulligan MS, Johnson KJ, Todd RF III, et al. Requirements for leukocyte adhesion molecules in nephrotoxic serum nephritis. J Clin Invest 1993; 91:577–587.
93. Stockenhuber F, Kramer G, Schenn G, et al. Circulating ICAM-1: Novel parameter of renal graft rejection. Transplant Proc 1993; 25:919–920.
94. Brennan DC, Jevnikar AM, Takei F, Reubin-Kelley V. Mesangial cell accessory functions: Mediation by intercellular adhesion molecule-1. Kidney Int 1990; 38:1039–1046.
95. Kelley VE, Jevnikar AM. Antigen presentation by renal tubular epithelial cells. J Am Soc Nephrol 1991; 2:13–26.
96. Suranyi MG, Bishop GA, Clayberger C, et al. Lymphocyte adhesion molecules in T-cell mediated lysis of human kidney cells. Kidney Int 1991; 39:312–319.
97. Nathan C, Srimal S, Farber C, et al. Cytokine-induced respiratory burst of human neutrophils: Dependence on extracellular matrix proteins and CD11/CD18 integrins. J Cell Biol 1989; 109:1341–1349.
98. Denton MD, Marsden PA, Luscinskas FW, et al. Cytokine-induced phagocyte adhesion to human mesangial cells: Role of CD11/CD18 integrins and ICAM-1. Am J Physiol 1991; 261:F1071–F1079.
99. Brady HR, Denton MD, Jimenez W, et al. Chemoattractants provoke monocyte adhesion to human mesangial cells and mesangial cell injury via CD11/CD18-ICAM-1 dependent and independent mechanisms. Kidney Int 1992; 42:480–487.
100. Brady HR, Serhan CN. Adhesion promotes transcellular leukotriene biosynthesis during neutrophil-glomerular endothelial cell interactions: Inhibition by anti-CD18 and L-selectin monoclonal antibodies. Biochem Biophys Res Commun 1992; 186:1307–1314.
101. Brady HR, Papayianni A, Serhan CN. Leukocyte adhesion promotes lipoxygenase product biosynthesis by transcellular routes. Kidney Int 1994; 45:590–597.
102. Brady HR, Lamas S, Papayianni A, Takata S, Matsubala M, Marsden PA. Lipoxygenase product formation and cell adhesion during neutrophil-glomerular endothelial cell interaction. Am J Physiol 1995; 268:F1–F12.
103. Wu X, Pippin J, Lefkowith JB: Attenuation of immune-mediated glomerulonephritis with an anti-CD11b monoclonal antibody. Am J Physiol 1993; 264:F715–F721.
104. Wada J, Makino H, Shikata K, Morioka S, Hirata K, Kashihara N, Ota Z: Role of intercellular adhesion molecule-1 in nephrotoxic serum nephritis (abstr). J Am Soc Nephrol 1992; 3:647.
105. Kawasaki K, Yaoita E, Yamamoto T, et al. Antibodies against intercellular adhesion molecule-1 and lymphocyte function-associated antigen-1 prevent glomerular injury in rat experiment crescentic glomerulonephritis. J Immunol 1993; 150:1074–1083.
106. Nishikawa K, Guo K-J, Miyasaki M, et al. Antibodies to ICAM-1/LFA-1 prevent crescent formation in rat autoimmune glomerulonephritis. J Exp Med 1993; 177:667–677.
107. Harning R, Pelletier J, Van G, et al. Monoclonal antibody to ICAM-1 reduces acute autoimmune nephritis in kdkd mice. Clin Immunol Immunopathol 1992; 64:129–134.
108. Cosimi AR, Conti D, Delmonico FL, et al. In vivo effects of monoclonal antibody to ICAM-1 (CD54) in nonhuman primates with renal allografts: J Immunol 1990; 144:4604–4612.
109. Haug CE, Colvin RB, Delmonico FL et al. A phase trial of immunosuppression with anti-ICAM-1 mAB in renal allograft recipients. Transplantation 1993; 55:766–773.

110. Linas SL, Shanley PF, Whittenburg D, et al. Neutrophils accentuate ischemia-reperfusion injury in isolated perfused rat kidneys. Am J Physiol 1988; 255:F728–F735.
111. Hellberg PO, Kallskog TO. Neutrophil-mediated post-ischemic tubular leakage in the rat kidney. Kidney Int 1989; 36:555–561.
112. Thornton MN, Winn R, Alpers CE: An evaluation of the neutrophil as a mediator of in vivo renal ischemic-reperfusion injury. Am J Pathol 1989; 135:509–515.
113. Kelly KI, Williams WW, Colvin RB, Bonventre JV. Antibody to intercellular adhesion molecule-1 protects the kidney against ischemic injury. Proc Natl Acad Sci USA 1994; 91:812–816.
114. Arnaout MA, Hakim RM, Todd RF III, et al. Increased expression of an adhesion-promoting surface glycoprotein in the granulocytopenia of hemodialysis. N Engl J Med 1985; 312:458–462.
115. Cheung AK, Hohnholt M, Gilson J. Adherence of neutrophils to hemodialysis membranes: Role of complement receptors. Kidney Int 1991; 40:1123–1133.
116. Himmelfarb J, Zaoui P, Hakim R. Modulation of granulocyte LAM-1 and Mac-1 during dialysis—A prospective randomized control trial. Kidney Int 1992; 41:388–395.
117. Cheung AK, Parker CJ, Hohnholt M. $\beta 2$ integrins are required for neutrophil degranulation induced by hemodialysis membranes. Kidney Int 1993; 43:649–660.
118. Ross R. The pathogenesis of atherosclerosis: A perspective for the 1990s. Nature 1993; 362:801–809.
119. Cybulsky MI, Gimbrone MA. Endothelial expression of a mononuclear leukocyte adhesion molecule during atherogenesis. Science 1991; 251:788–795.
120. Johnson-Tidey RR, Poston RN. Increase in P-selectin in the endothelium overlying human atherosclerotic plaques: Coexpression with ICAM-1 (abstr). J Cell Biochem 1994; suppl 18A:291.
121. Rice GE, Bevilacqua MP. An inducible endothelial surface glycoprotein mediates melanoma adhesion. Science 1989; 246:1303–1306.
122. Kelly CP, O'Keane JC, Orellano J, et al. Human colon cancer cells express ICAM-1 in vivo and support LFA-1 dependent lymphocyte adhesion in vitro. Am J Physiol 1992; 263:G864–G870.
123. Staunton DE, Dustin ML, Erickson HP, Springer TA: The arrangement of immunoglobulin-like domains of ICAM-1 and the binding sites for LFA-1 and rhinovirus. Cell 1990; 61:243–254.
124. Berendt AR, McDowall A, Craig AG, et al. The binding site on ICAM-1 for Plasmodium falciparum-infected erythrocytes overlaps, but is distinct from, the LFA-1 binding site. Cell 1992; 68:71–81.
125. Adler S. Integrin receptors in the glomerulus: potential role in glomerular injury (editorial). Am J Physiol 1992; 262:F697–F704.
126. Adler S, Chen X. Anti-FX1A antibody recognizes a beta-1 integrin on glomerular epithelial cells and inhibits adhesion and growth. Am J Physiol 1992; 262:F770–F776.
127. O'Meara YM, Natori Y, Minto AW, et al. Nephrotoxic anti-serum identifies a beta-1 integrin on glomerular epithelial cells. Am J Physiol 1992; 262:F1083–F1091.
128. Gailit J, Colflesh D, Rabiner I, et al. Redistribution and dysfunction of integrins in cultured renal epithelial cells exposed to oxidative stress. Am J Physiol 1993; 264:F149–F157.
129. Goligorsky MS, Lieberthal W, Racusen L, Simon EE. Integrin receptors in renal tubular epithelium: new insights into the pathophysiology of acute renal failure (editorial). Am J Physiol 1993; 264:F1–F8.

50

Molecular Biology of Renal Epithelial Antigens

Pierre J. Verroust and Pierre M. Ronco
INSERM U 064 Hôpital Tenon, Paris, France

Søren Nielsen and Erik Ilsø Christensen
University of Aarhus, Aarhus, Denmark

INTRODUCTION

The ability of the various components of the nephron to induce antibodies was first used to develop immunological models of renal diseases. This experimental approach using crude kidney preparations was first pioneered by Masugi (1) and more recently by Heymann et al. (2). Subsequently the refinement of biochemical purification techniques and the advent of monoclonal antibodies allowed the identification of the targets of at least some nephritogenic antibodies (3). At the same time, because of their exquisite specificity, antibodies have become a key tool in renal cell biology. To quote just a few examples, they have been used to dissect immunologically crude membrane preparations (4), to analyze the distribution of various nephron constituents, to determine their sites of expression at the subcellular level (5), and to identify critical molecular structures on enzymes or transporters (6–9). The development of molecular biology techniques provided a new level of sophistication, since it is now possible to prepare tailor-made peptide antigens from the predicted protein sequences.

In the context of recent molecular biology developments, this chapter is concerned with groups of proteins that have been selected either because they have been identified as the targets of immunological processes and or because their antigenic properties have played a central role in their identification, localization, or unraveling of their function. This probably applies to virtually all constituents of the kidney as illustrated in other chapters of this book; we therefore restrict this review to four groups of proteins, within our own research experience, most of which have not been covered.

Most of the proteins that will be considered are expressed by proximal tubule cells (Figures 1 and 2). The apical pole of these cells is separated by tight junctions from the basolateral domain and can be further subdivided into two microdomains: the microvilli supported by filaments of actin and the intermicrovillar domain characterized by a cytoplasmic coating of clathrin (10). Below, we successively review hydrolases that are a hallmark of the microvillar domain, gp330, and other proteins expressed by the intermicrovillar domain. The families of water channels and complement regulatory proteins are discussed separately. We then discuss Tamm-Horsfall protein (THP), a major protein of Henle's loop and the distal nephron. Finally, we list some "specific" glomerular epithelial proteins.

HYDROLASES

The typical localization of the hydrolases (reviewed in Refs. 11 and 12), listed with their basic properties in Table 1 is, as detected by immunohistological or histoenzymatic techniques, on the

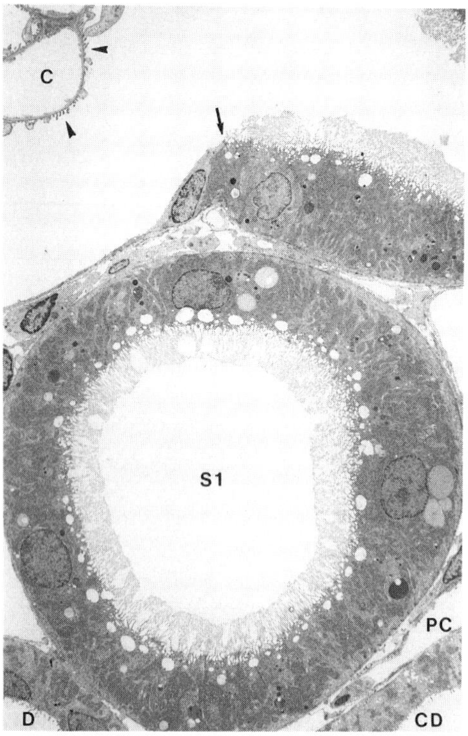

Figure 1 Electron micrograph of rat renal cortex, demonstrating a cross-sectioned proximal tubule, segment 1 (S1). In the upper part of the micrograph, the transition from the epithelium of Bowman's capsule and the initial part of the proximal tubule is seen (arrow). Upper left, glomerular capillaries (C) and foot processes of glomerular epithelial cells (arrowheads); lower left, distal tubule (D); and lower right, collecting duct (CD), peritubular capillaries (PC). ×2000.

apical pole of proximal tubule cells and more specifically in the microvillar domain. In the case of maltase (131) or gamma-glutamyl-transferase GGT (132), it has been further shown that the enzymes were excluded from the intermicrovillar domain. As also shown in Table 1, some brush border hydrolases can be localised in glomerular cells in intact glomeruli and often in glomerular cells in culture (13,96,97,62). As opposed to the tubular distribution, the glomerular expression is not or only partly polarized (133). It is likely that the development of new cell culture systems and the use of the more sensitive techniques based on in situ molecular amplification will modify this pattern established by immunohistology. For instance, the angiotensin converting enzyme (ACE) cannot be detected in vitro on glomerular endothelial cells and yet is probably expressed by these cells on the basis of its synthesis by a variety of endothelial cell types from which it has been cloned (85,86,88) and of in vivo antibody binding studies described below (134). Similarly, neutral endopeptidase (NEP) cannot be visualized on glomerular endothelial cells but can be amplified from endothelial cells in culture (135) and immunologically demonstrated in very small amounts on their membrane. NEP can also be demonstrated in cultures of vascular smooth muscle cells (136).

The exact role of brush border or glomerular hydrolases has not been defined, but the broad spectrum of potential substrates covered suggests that they hydrolyze a wide variety of bioactive peptides before they reach more distal sites of the nephron, including the macula densa. Regulation of their expression is difficult to study and requires in vitro cell culture systems and precise experimental conditions. Using primary cultures of proximal tubule cells (137), it was found that cells grown in the presence of serum or in serum free medium devoid of hormones (insulin and dexamethasone) expressed hydrolases in intracytoplasmic vesicles. Addition of dexamethasone did

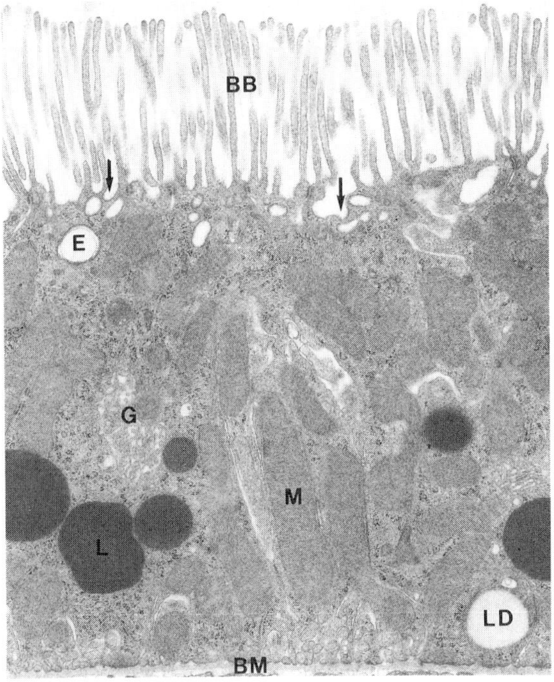

Figure 2 Electron micrograph of rat proximal tubule, segment 2, as shown by the dark electron-dense lysosomes (L) typical of this segment. Brush border (BB), coated pits (arrows), endosomes (E), mitochondria (M), Golgi apparatus (G), lipid droplet (LD), and basement membrane (BM). ×13,500.

not dramatically alter the amount of enzymes synthesized but allowed their targeting to the apical pole. In glomerular epithelial cells, dexamethasone, cAMP as well as agents which increase glomerular synthesis of cAMP, such as PGE2, and β adrenergic ligands, increased the expression of aminopeptidase A (Ap A) (13). This enzyme was unaffected by phorbolmyristylacetate, which, however, increased the mRNA levels of aminopeptidase N (Ap N) as well as the enzyme activity. A similar increase of (Ap N) could be induced by thrombin. Expression of di-peptidyl-peptidase IV (DPP IV) was not influenced by any of these agents but was increased by interferon gamma (31).

The availability of the full sequences for most of these enzymes has led to several important observations. It is first striking to note that a number of proteins identified by monoclonal antibodies on subpopulations of hematopoietic cells and found to be expressed on renal epithelial cells, such as the common lymphoblastic antigen (63), have subsequently been characterized as hydrolases. This was made possible through independent cloning of the lymphocyte proteins and renal enzymes and the availability of a relevant panel of monoclonal antibodies. As listed in Table 1, this applies to NEP (65,68), aminopeptidase N (16–20), aminopeptidase A (25,26) or DPP IV (37–39).

Systematic sequence comparisons have led to the identification of a "superfamily" of hydrolases characterized by the presence of a Zn-binding domain, which has been identified within a sequence HE--H. Most of these enzymes depend on Zn and there is abundant evidence (22) that mutations in this area dramatically alter the enzymatic activity, including that of aminopeptidase A (27), which requires calcium for full activity and is reportedly Zn-independent. It has thus been proposed that the Zn binding sequence not solely defines Zn dependent enzymes but reflects conserved evolutionary relationship within metalloproteases (27). In addition to the enzymes listed in Table 1 the family includes stromelysins, thermolysin, collagenases, and leukotriene A4 hydrolase (66,138). NEP has been particularly studied (70–77), and the role of at least one active-site arginine residue involved in substrate binding has been identified (71,74,75). But, as shown in Table 1, similar active site studies have been conducted or are in progress for most of the hydrolases.

Table 1 Brush Border Hydrolases

	Substrate and other ligands	MM (kDa)	Metal	Glomerulus	Tubule	Extrarenal	Anchor	cDNA	Gene	Site
Amino N[a] EC 3.4.11.2 CD 13	Neutral N-terminal amino acid, broad specificity	150	Zn (V--HE--H)	Podocytes (mouse, human) cult. hum. Mes/Epi (13)	+	Gut; myeloid progenitors, mature monocytes (14,15)	NH2	16–20	21	12,23
Amino A EC 3.4.11.7 gp 160 BP-1/6C3	Acidic N terminal ANG II	160	Ca (HE--H)	Podocytes (24) cult. Epi. (13)	+	Gut; early B progenitors (25)	NH2	26		27
DPP IV[b] EC 3.4.14.5 CD 26, gp 90	N terminal Gly/Ala-Pro, TNFα (28), collagen (29), fibronectin (30)	110		Podocytes, endothelium; cult. Hum. Epi (31–33)	+	Gut; activated T (34–36)	NH2	37–42		43–47
NEP EC 3.4.24.11 CD 10	Cys-Phe, ANF, BK, Il1, ET, Sub P, EK, bombesin, formyl pep, urodilatin, C-ANP, ANG, NT (48–61)	95–100	Zn (HE--H)	Podocytes (Rabbit, human); cult. epi. (32,62)	+ All PCT segments, S3 only in the rat	Gut, normal lymphoid progenitors, granulocytes (63,64)	NH2	65–68	69	70–77
EndopeptidaseII[c] Meprin EC 3.4.24.18	LHRH*, neuropeptide Y*, TGFα*, Sub P, BK, ANG	90–100	Zn (HE--H	–	+	Gut	COOH	78–82		
ACE[d] EC 3.4.15.1	ANG I, BK, Sub P, LHRH	140	Zn (HE--H)	? Endothelium	+	Endothelial cells	COOH	85–88	89–92	93–95
5'Nucleotidase[e] EC 3.1.3.5	5'AMP	67–73		Mes (96–101)	S1>S2>S3		GPI	102		
Gamma GT[f] EC 2.2.2.2	Glutathion	50/30	–	–	S3 only (103,104)		NH2	105	106–107	108
Maltase[g] EC 3.2.1.20	Maltose	300	–	–	+	Gut				

Alk Phos[h]	Monophosphate esters	57	–	–			GPI	116–117	118–120
EC 3.1.3.1								121–122	123
> "B/K/L"					S1, S2, S3	Bone, liver, gut			
> "I"					S3 only (115)	kidney			
Dipeptidase[i] EC 3.4.13.11	Glutathion, LTD4, β-lactam antibiotics	62	–	–	+		GPI	128–130	

Abbreviations: ANG = angiotensin; ANP = atrial natriuretic peptide; BK = bradikinin; ET = endothelin; EK = enkephalin; Epi = epithelial cells; GPI = glyco-phosphatidyl-inositol; Il-1 = interleukin 1; LHRH = luliberin; Mes = mesangial cells; MM = molecular mass in kilodaltons (kDa); PCT = proximal convoluted tubule; S1, 2, or 3 = first, second, or third segment of the PCT; Sub P = substance P; TGF = transforming growth factor.

Numbers in parentheses indicate references. The right-hand three columns concern structural data. cDNA lists references to full or partial sequence. "Gene" refers to studies reporting identification of at least some of the promoter elements and in some cases complete sequencing of the gene. "Site" provides references dealing specifically with identification of key structural elements of the binding site.

[a]Variable glycosylation has been demonstrated for Ap N, which in some cases may lead to masking of some structurally determined epitopes (23).

[b]Dipeptidyl-peptidase IV (DPP IV) has been cloned in rat (37,38); in human, where it is localized to chromosome 2 (39–41); and in the mouse (42). Enzymatic activity may be important for T-cell stimulation.

[c]Meprin A (EC 3.4.24.18) is the recommended name for the enzyme initially isolated from kidneys of mice with high meprin activity and for endopeptidase-2 isolated from kidneys of rats. Meprins have a broad substrate specificity which resembles that of NEP with some differences indicated by (*). At variance from NEP, meprins are not phosphoramidon sensitive. They are multimeric enzymes composed of homologous but distinct disulfide-linked α and β subunits. The 198 NH2 terminal amino acids of the meprin α chain constitute the astacin family protease domain (81), which includes a Zn binding site and terminates by an Ig/MHC complex protein signature. The carboxyl terminus EGF-like domain is followed by a transmembrane and a short intracytoplasmic domains. The meprin family is characterized by an extended Zn binding site (HE—H—GF-HE). Rat endopeptidase displays 87% identity with meprin A and 85% PABA peptide hydrolase of intestine (79). The β subunit, cloned in the rat (80), contains a potential membrane anchor and a Zn binding sequence. The α and β chains assemble by two to form a variety of tetramers, $\alpha 2\ \beta 2$, but also $\alpha 4$ or $\beta 4$, in some mouse strains (83,84). The mRNAs of NEP (EC 3.4.24.11) and meprin A (EC 3.4.24.18) colocalize in the proximal tubule (79). Together the two enzymes account for 10% of microvillar proteins in the rat.

[d]Official recommended denomination of angiotensin converting enzyme (ACE) is kininase II.

[e]mRNA of 5' nucleotidase colocalizes with erythropoietin mRNA in peritubular cells.

[f]Gamma-glutamyl-transferase (GGT) is a heterodimeric protein cleaved from a 75-kDa glycosylated prepropeptide to form (a) a 50-kDa subunit which is inserted in the membrane by an uncleaved amino-terminal signal and is N and O glycosylated, the latter sites being adjacent to the membrane anchor (109), and (b) a smaller 30-kDa noncovalently associated N-glycosylated subunit. A single gene, including 8 exons over 12 kb containing a sequence homologous to the SV40 enhancer, has been identified in the rat. It is driven by three separate promoters (104–107,111): two mRNAs with alternative 5' ends are expressed in the kidney pars recta and increase in level from birth to adult stage but are not transcribed in liver and seminal vesicles; a single 2.4-kb mRNA is detected in liver and seminal vesicles. At least four genes have been identified in humans (110,112,113) and localized on chromosome 22. Two mRNAs have been charaterized: type 1 is liver-specific whereas type II is expressed in the liver and kidney. In the mouse, six different mRNAs encoded by a single gene have been identified (114).

[g]The molecular mass of maltase, initially assessed by comparison with that of gp330, is likely to be substantially higher.

[h]B/K/L = bone, kidney, liver; I = intestine. The intestinal alkaline phosphatase (ALPI) shares 56% amino acid identity with the liver, bone, kidney (ALPL) and over 85% with the placental (ALPP1) and placental-like ALPP2 (located in testis and thymus) forms of the enzyme (124–127). In particular, catalytically important regions are conserved in this multigene family. The ALPL gene has been assigned to chromosome 1, whereas ALPI, ALPP1, and ALPP2 have been assigned to chromosome 2.

[i]Dipeptidase was long thought to be an endosomal enzyme. Recent data (130) show that it is expressed by the brush border.

Different transcription initiation sites under the influence of distinct promoters and different RNA species with, in some cases, a degree of organ specificity have been detected for a number of hydrolases, in particular for GGT (104–114) and alkaline phosphatase (119,120). In the case of NEP, the organization of the gene has been elucidated (69) and shown to consist of multiple miniexons and separate 5′ untranslated regions, an unusual structure, which suggested the possibility of alternative splicing events (139). In the case of ACE, the enzyme displays a high degree of internal homology between two large domains, which each bear a Zn-binding consensus sequence surrounded by nonhomologous regions. Both are catalytically active but have distinct reactivities (140–142). In contrast, the testicular enzyme encoded by the same gene displays only the carboxyl terminal domain of the endothelial enzyme and therefore a single Zn binding site preceded by a short, testicle-specific, heavily O-glycosylated sequence (143), which is not required for enzymatic activity. These results are best explained by a putative ancestral gene duplication (144; review in Ref. 91).

New Insights into the Sorting Mechanisms Provided by Hydrolases

The mechanisms of sorting of apical and basolateral proteins in epithelial cells remain imperfectly understood. Studies in MDCK cells (review in Ref. 145) suggest that sorting takes place in the trans-Golgi network, from which vesicles are directly targeted to the apical or basolateral pole. Pioneering work based on the polarized budding of viruses suggested that the primary sequence of the viral proteins was the prime determinant. There is also strong evidence in this system that glyco-phosphatidyl-inositol (GPI)–linked proteins are directly targeted to the apical pole, but the signals concerning non-GPI-linked hydrolases are not known. On the other hand, detailed studies in hepatocytes (review in Ref. 146) suggest that apical proteins such as Ap N or DPP IV are first delivered to the basolateral membrane and then transferred by endocytosis to the apical pole. Interestingly, a GPI linked enzyme, such as 5′ nucleotidase, is also transferred to the apical pole via an indirect route (147). A combination of the two processes is probably operating in Caco2 intestinal cells.

In order to determine whether these different pathways were related to distinct cell machineries or to distinct properties of the proteins themselves, it was important to compare the expression of the same proteins in several cell types. The availability for most of the hydrolases of the cDNA coding for their full sequences made this type of experiment possible. It has thus been shown that when constructs of Ap N (148), DPP IV (149,150), or NEP (151) were stably transfected in MDCK cells the corresponding proteins were directly targeted to the apical pole. In the case of Ap N, 20% of the enzyme was targeted to the basolateral domain but was not transcytosed to the apical pole. Extensive studies in which the transmembrane and intracytoplasmic domains of NEP were removed (151–153) showed that the enzyme was predominantly released in soluble form at the apical pole, indicating that the bulk of the required information was contained in its ectodomain. Mutations of the latter suggested that its integrity was probably necessary (154). Similar results were obtained with Ap N (155,156).

Interestingly, different results were observed when transfection studies were carried out in LLC/PK1 cells. Low et al. (157) reported that DPP IV was delivered to the apical pole both via a direct and a transcytotic route. Membrane-anchored GGT (158) and NEP were directly targeted to the apical pole, but the soluble form of NEP was found to be secreted equally on the basolateral and apical poles (154). In this context, further studies on DPPIV stably transfected in MDCK cells are particularly interesting. Weisz et al. (159) indeed showed that removal of the transmembrane and cytoplasmic domains leading to the production of a soluble form of DPPIV increased the efficiency of the apical targeting (>95%), suggesting the presence of competing basolateral targeting information in the cytoplasmic domain that could be demonstrated using chimeras composed of lysozyme fused with the cytoplasmic and intramembrane domain of DPP IV.

Taken together, these results strongly support the hypothesis that a given hydrolase may carry several sorting signals that are interpreted differently in various cell types. There are numerous ways in which the transfection models might contribute to our understanding of the regulating processes. Following studies demonstrating inhibition of apical secretion in MDCK cells by brefeldin A (160), it has been shown that this agent also induced mistargeting of DPP IV to the basolateral domain of the same cell type (161). The use of transfected cells may also permit new developments concerning the regulation of amount of enzyme synthesized (162). The combination of new culture and transfection studies should allow considerable progress in this area.

Hydrolases in Pathology

Little is known about the pathology potentially induced by dysregulation of the synthesis of hydrolases. It has been shown that the expression of NEP on murine-B-cell progenitors regulated stromal-dependent lymphopoiesis (64) and that cytokines increased NEP activity in the lung (163) suggesting that expression of hydrolases might regulate the actions of cytokines. This may be of significance in pathology since, as shown by Shipp et al. (54), NEP regulates the growth of small-cell carcinomas of the lung through its ability to hydrolyze bombesin-like peptides. A cDNA in which exon 16, which contains the sequence coding for the active site, was deleted has, for instance, been identified in the "normal lung" of a patient with small-cell carcinoma (164). It is conceivable that similar events could occur in cases of renal tumors. Nanus et al. (165) reported that, in some renal cell carcinomas in culture, the expression of aminopeptidase A was correlated with resistance to interferon.

At least three hydrolases expressed by glomerular cells can serve as targets of nephritogenic antibodies in experimental models. We have previously reported that antibodies to NEP or gp90/DPP IV induced transient glomerular deposits (33) but did not trigger proteinuria or nephritis. Subsequent studies by Mendrick et al. (166) indicated that, if the rats were preimmunized with Freund's adjuvant, proteinuria could be induced through some undetermined mechanisms. Further studies have shown that anti-DPP IV antibodies induced redistribution of the enzyme on the surface of the epithelial cells and were involved in graft versus host nephritis (167). Finally, Assmann et al. (24) reported that monoclonal anti-Ap A antibodies induced proteinuric glomerulonephritis via a non-complement-dependent route. The mode of action of the antibodies is most likely related to their inhibitory effect on the enzymatic activity, which includes degradation of angiotensin. This is strongly supported by recent experiments showing that proteinuria could be prevented by treating the rats with inhibitors of the angiotensin converting enzyme (ACE) (168).

A particularly interesting model has been described by Matsuo et al. (134), who have shown that antibodies specific for the angiotensin converting enzyme-induced subepithelial electron-dense deposits. This result may appear surprising, since ACE is not detectable by immunohistochemical techniques within rat glomeruli. The probable mechanism depends on the proteolytic membrane release of ACE, which has been elegantly demonstrated using cells transfected with ACE cDNA (169,170). It has thus been proposed that complexes initially formed on the membrane of endothelial cells were shed and forced by hydrodynamic forces to the subepithelial space.

GP330 AND OTHER INTERMICROVILLAR PROTEINS

Gp 330

Heymann nephritis (HN), an experimental glomerulonephritis, was originally induced in rats by autologous renal cortex (2) and subsequently by a crude renal cortical extract known as Fx1A (171) or by glycoproteins from isolated microvilli (172). The major antigen in Heymann nephritis, gp330 (173), was originally found in the glomerular epithelial cells and in proximal tubules (173) (Figure 3). In addition, gp330 is also expressed in coated pits of type II pneumocytes, epididymis, and epithelial cells of the visceral yolk sac (174,175), and recently the protein has been found in rat yolk sac carcinoma cell lines (176–179). In the renal glomerular epithelial cells, the protein is expressed in coated pits, also on the plasma membrane of the foot processes facing the glomerular basement membrane (180). In these cells, gp330 was also found in the granular endoplasmatic reticulum, Golgi elements, and multivesicular bodies (180). Initially, gp330 in renal proximal tubule cells was found to be restricted to the clathrin-coated pits at the base of the microvilli (Figures 1 and 2) and in apical endocytic vacuoles, at distinct variance with brush border proteins such as maltase (131). However, gp330 was later also detected in dense apical tubules (Figure 3) (181,182), an organelle known to be responsible for membrane recycling in these cells (183). Also, it appears that gp330 is not restricted to the apical endocytic apparatus of the proximal tubule cells, since several immunocytochemical studies using monoclonal and polyclonal antibodies subsequently have shown a certain degree of brush border labeling (Figure 3) (184–186), apparently with a certain segmental variation (185) between the three different segments of the proximal tubule, as described in rats (187). Kerjaschki et al. (188) identified in human kidney a 400-kDa protein that is similarly localized

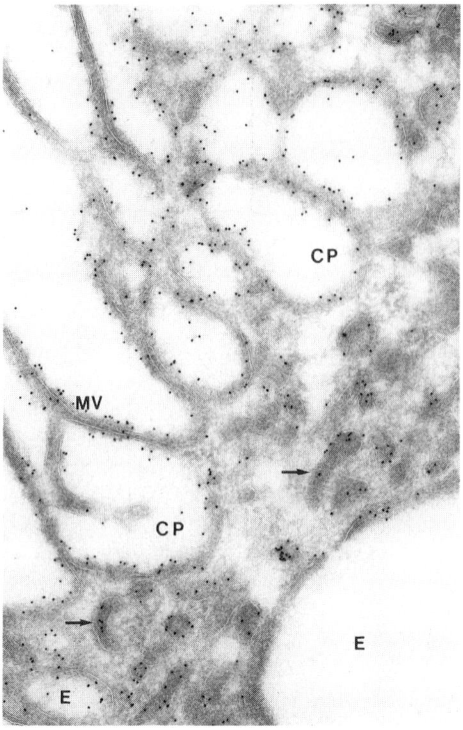

Figure 3 Immunocytochemical localization of gp330 in cryosections of rat proximal tubule, using a sheep anti-gp330 antibody and visualized by 10-nm protein-A gold particles. Gp330 is seen on microvilli (MV), in coated pits (CP), in endosomes (E), and in dense apical tubules (arrows). ×52,000.

in proximal tubules and immunologically cross-reacts with rat gp330. However, this protein is absent from podocytes of human glomeruli. During development of the kidney, gp330 is first detectable in the mesonephros and in the nephronic vesicle as well as in the ureteric bud (189). In the S-shaped body, gp330 is localized in areas that will give rise to the glomerulus, the proximal tubule, and the distal tubule; only later during development do the areas of expression narrow down to the glomerulus and the proximal tubule, being progressively concentrated in clathrin-coated pits simultaneously with the initiation of glomerular filtration (189). These results agree well with the observation that there is a close relationship between the ability of the proximal tubule to reabsorb peroxidase and the expression of gp330 in coated pits (181).

Under different experimental conditions, gp330 is redistributed in the proximal tubules. After treatment of rats with sodium maleate, which significantly reduces protein reabsorption and induces an extensive vacuolization apically in proximal tubule cells (190), gp330 was concentrated in newly formed apical vacuoles (132). In rats treated with colchicine, vesicles containing gp330 were found dispersed throughout the entire cell cytoplasm, indicating that microtubules are involved in the apical accumulation of gp330-containing vacuoles (191). In rats with Heymann nephritis, there is a loss of gp330 associated with the apical endocytic pathway together with a reduced uptake of dextran (192), which indicates a general perturbation in the endocytic process, since dextran is known to be taken up by fluid-phase endocytosis in these cells (193). Similarly, the endocytic uptake of horseradish peroxidase in proximal tubules is significantly reduced in rats with Heymann nephritis, not only in the early stages but also in later stages, when the brush border is in part regenerated (194).

Originally, the molecular weight of gp330 was estimated to be about 330 kDa. However, it is now generally accepted that the molecular weight is considerably higher, estimates varying from more than 440 kDa (195) up to about 600 kDa (196–198). Thus, its molecular weight appears to be similar to or slightly larger than that of the α2-macroglobulin receptor (α2MR)/low-density lipoprotein receptor–related protein (LRP), which is a 585-kDa protein. Recently, Raychowdhury et al. (195) in part elucidated the primary structure of gp330 by cDNA cloning and the protein was found to share considerable sequence identity with both the α2MR/LRP (199) and the low-density lipoprotein receptor (LDLR) (200,201), with which two receptors it shares clusters of 40–amino acid cysteine-rich repeats appearing as two distinct types, designated the epidermal growth factor repeats and the complement-type repeats. This latter type is responsible in the LDLR (202) and probably also in the α2MR/LRP (203) for the binding of Ca^{2+} and protein ligands. In addition, gp330 contains a transmembrane segment and a cytoplasmic tail containing a doublet of the NPXY sequence (195), which has been shown in the LDLR to be a signal for endocytosis (204). (See Note Added in Proof.)

The ultrastructure of the renal proximal tubule is characterized by a very well developed luminal endocytic apparatus (205) consisting of coated pits, small and large endocytic vacuoles, dense apical tubules, and an abundance of lysosomes (Figures 1 and 2). Proteins from the glomerular ultrafiltrate are removed highly efficiently in the proximal tubule by adsorptive endocytosis, and the specificity of the initial binding has been much debated, as recently reviewed (205–207). It was suggested, due to its location in coated pits, that gp330 is a receptor with (at that time) unknown ligands (131). In light of the structural homologies with α2MR/LRP and LDLR, it appeared very likely that gp330 would have similar functions. Several ligands for gp330 have now been identified, including the 40-kDa receptor–associated protein (RAP) (Figures 4 and 5) (182,197,198,207), plasminogen (209), extracellular matrix components (210), plasminogen activators in complex with their type-1 inhibitor (PAI-1) (196,197) (Figure 5), lipoprotein lipase (197,211), lactoferrin and apolipoprotein E–enriched lipoprotein particles (197), and aprotinin, a 6.5-kDa serine proteinase inhibitor (179). Endocytosis mediated by gp330 has been demonstrated for RAP in rat proximal tubules in vivo (182), for plasminogen activator complexed with PAI-1 in isolated perfused rabbit proximal tubules (196), and for aprotinin in cultured yolk sac carcinoma cells (179). Gp330 also binds Ca^{2+} (182), and the binding of the above-mentioned ligands is highly calcium-dependent (179,182,196). RAP was originally found as a 40-kDa (212) or 39-kDa (213) component of α2MR/LRP, but it is a gene product independent from the receptor (214,215). Instead, it is a ligand to this receptor, as also later found for gp330. It has been demonstrated immunocytochemically in the RER (195,208). This intracellular localization has led to the suggestion of a function as an intracellular regulator or a chaperone assisting correct folding of new synthesized receptors (216). In conclusion, gp330 appears to be a receptor mediating endocytosis of several ligands in certain epithelia (i.e., kidney, lung and yolk sac).

Gp330 in Pathology

The role of gp330 in the pathogenesis of HN was indicated by two distinct sets of experiments (180,217). First, antibodies eluted from the glomeruli of rats immunized with crude brush border

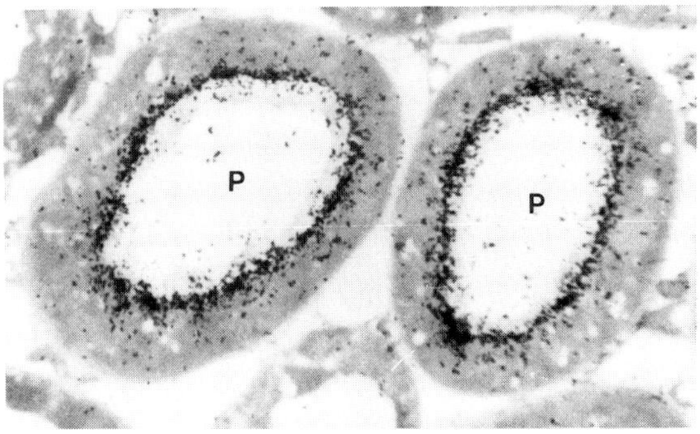

Figure 4 Light microscope autoradiograph of 0.8 μm cryosection of rat renal cortex incubated directly on the section with ^{125}I-RAP. The autoradiographic grains are located almost exclusively over proximal tubules (P) at the base of the microvilli. No labeling is seen over other nephron segments. $\times$1000.

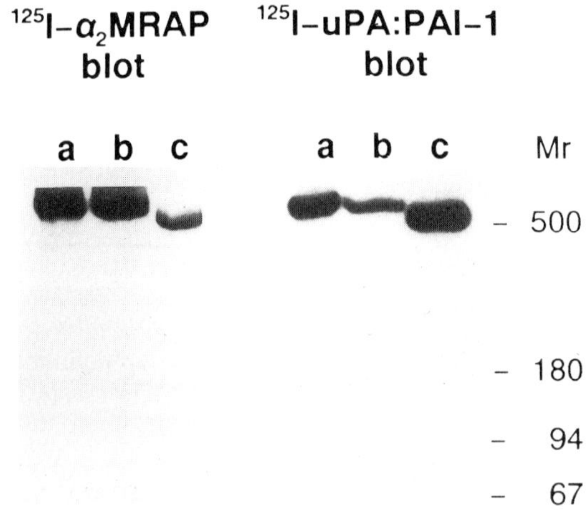

Figure 5 Ligand blot analysis of gp330 and α2MR/LRP using ^{125}I-labeled RAP and uPA.PAI-1. Ligand blotting with RAP and uPA.PAI-1 of approximately 150 μg of rabbit cortical membranes (lanes a), 0.5 μg of purified gp330 (lanes b), and 0.5 μg of α2MR/LRP (lanes c). (From Ref. 196.)

preparations react specifically with this molecule. Second, heterologous antibodies to gp330 can induce the typical subepithelial immune deposits in a matter of hours (218), as previously described in the passive form of HN classically induced with polyspecific antisera to renal brush border. In both the passive and active forms of HN, the specificity of the epitopes involved in the formation of the immune complexes is probably important (218,219). The identification of a target antigen led to studies concerning the mode of formation of the immune deposits. This requires the formation of large, highly reticulated immune complexes (218,220) on the surface of the podocytes, which are subsequently shed and become strongly adherent via undefined linkage to the basement membrane (218). The latter phenomenon probably accounts for the fact that the immune complexes formed in membrane areas usually destined to be internalized are in fact mainly released.

The debate on the significance of anti-gp330 in the pathogenesis of HN has been renewed by the cloning of a 40-kDa protein through screening of a renal cDNA expression library with Ig eluted from glomeruli of rats with HN (221). Subsequent observations described above indicated that this protein was the α2M receptor associated protein, RAP. It has now been established that gp330 can bind the 40-kDa RAP as well as most of the ligands of the α2M receptor. Membrane gp330 is associated with RAP and soluble complexes are released in the supernatant. The significance of RAP in HN is still uncertain, since antibodies to recombinant rat RAP could induce small-size immune deposits but did not reproduce the full spectrum of passive HN (208). Furthermore, study of the reactivity of glomerular eluates of rats with HN does not disclose reactivity with RAP but with gp330. When digested with CNBr, glomerular eluates react predominantly with fragments substantially larger than RAP, thus excluding the possibility that the reactivity with gp330 was due to complexed RAP. Finally, it appears that RAP is essentially an intracellular antigen. Active immunization experiments with RAP failed to induce HN (222). The effects of anti-gp330 are not limited to the glomerulus and the formation of electron-dense deposits. Antibodies are filtered by proteinuric animals and can bind to the brush border and induce, probably after internalization, a disturbed traffic of gp330 and dysfunction of the tubule cell as described above (192).

Gp280

This protein was initially identified during studies on gp330 (223) through the use of monoclonal antibodies raised against renal brush border. Initial survey indicated that it was expressed in the proximal tubule (Figure 6), particularly in the superficial cortex but not in glomeruli. When other

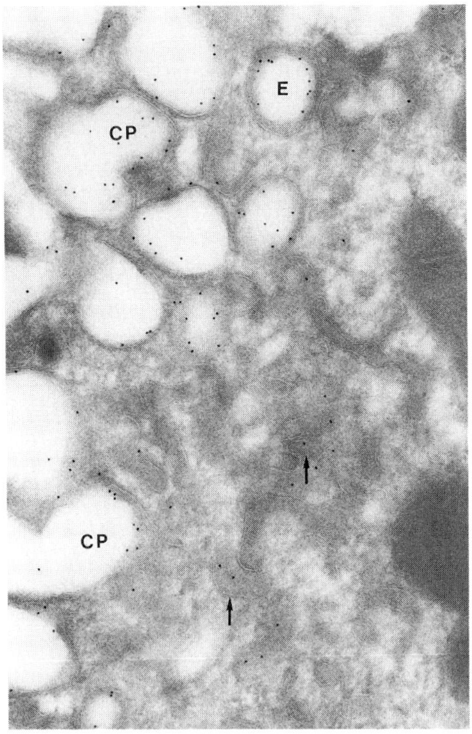

Figure 6 Immunocytochemical localization of gp280 on cryosection of rat proximal tubule, using a mouse monoclonal anti-gp280 antibody, visualized by 10-nm goat antimouse gold particles. Gold labeling is seen in coated pits (CP), endosomes (E), and dense apical tubules (arrows). ×58,000.

organs were studied, gp280 was detected only in the yolk sac (Figure 7) predominantly on the visceral layer but also on the parietal layer. At the ultrastructural level (Figures 6 and 7), gp280 was clearly concentrated in the intermicrovillar areas but also extended in the microvillar domain. Interestingly (224), during development, renal expression of gp280 resembles that of gp330. It is detectable on S-shaped bodies in the presumptive areas of the proximal tubule and glomerulus and initially assumes a diffuse pattern of membrane expression, which becomes restricted to the proximal tubule and concentrated in the intermicrovillar domain.

The molecular mass of gp280 was first estimated at 280 kDa by reference to gp330, which was initially ascribed a mass of 330 kDa. Since the latter is now estimated close to 585 kDa, it is likely that the molecular mass of gp280 is substantially higher than initially reported and close to 500 kDa. There is at present little information on the structure of gp280 although it is known that gp280 and gp330 share a number of CNBr peptides (224). Proteins similar to gp280 in terms of mass and tissue distribution have been detected in several species, including rabbit, mouse, and human (225). Comparative bidimensional maps of CNBr peptides derived from rat and human proteins suggest that its structure is conserved across species.

Potential ligands of gp280 have not yet been identified, but its expression in association with clathrin suggested that it could be involved in the endocytic process. In the rat, during the first days of pregnancy, the yolk sac is the only source of nutriment to the embryo through a process that relies on the internalization and degradation of maternal proteins. Since previous studies had shown that interference with the endocytic process induced fetal malformations, this provided a model to analyze the effects of anti-gp280 antibodies on endocytosis. It was thus found that anti-gp280 antibodies markedly inhibited embryonic development and induced fetal malformations. Alteration of endocytosis was confirmed by studies on embryos cultured in vitro showing that antibodies to gp280 disrupted the intracellular endocytic apparatus (226–228).

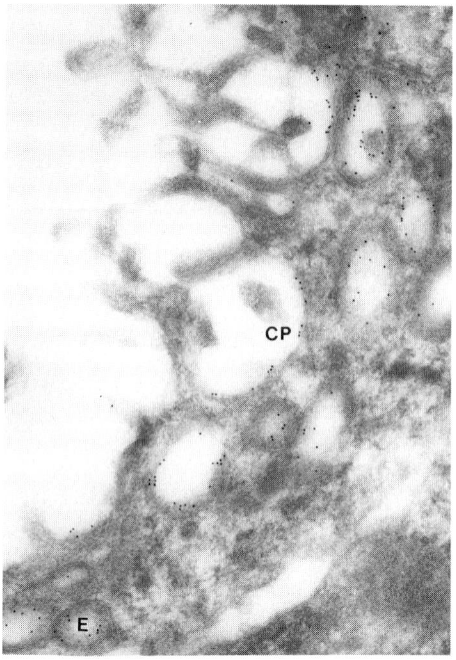

Figure 7 Immunocytochemical localization of gp280 on cryosection from rat yolk sac labeled as in Figure 6. The protein is localized in coated pits (CP) and in endosomes (E). ×47,000.

IGF-II/Man-6-P Receptors

We have recently localized the IGF-II/Man-6-P receptor in rat renal proximal tubules (229). The receptor is localized in apical coated pits, in endocytic vacuoles, and in dense apical tubule, as is gp330. In addition, we also found this receptor in cytoplasmic bodies, probably prelysosomes, which is not surprising, considering its function as Man-6-P receptor. However, the apical localization in the endocytic pathway probably to a large extent reflects its function as a receptor for IGF-II. Also due to this localization, it most probably functions in mediating endocytosis of IGF-II. As visualized by ligand binding on cryosections from renal cortex followed by autoradiography, the receptor bound IGF-II very strongly, IGF-I to a lesser extent, and did not bind insulin (229). Thus, contrary to gp330, which appears to have several ligands, this receptor seems to be rather specific in mediating endocytosis of IGF-II.

Folate-Binding Protein

Previous studies have localized folate binding protein (FBP) to the brush border membrane of renal proximal tubule cells (230–233) and have also indicated FBP to be responsible for the tubular reabsorption of folate (231,233). In addition to the brush border localization, we found, by immunocytochemistry, FBP to be located in the membranes of coated pits, endocytic vacuoles, and dense apical tubules and furthermore demonstrated by autoradiography that folate was taken up by endocytosis via the coated pits (234), a pathway different from that proposed by Rothberg et al. (235) in MA104 cells, in which folate apparently is internalized via noncoated pits (so-called caveolae). We further substantiated our findings in the proximal tubule, showing that antibodies against FBP were internalized via coated pits and recycled via dense apical tubules together with FBP (236).

AQUAPORINS—WATER CHANNELS

Aquaporins are integral membrane proteins that facilitate rapid and selective transmembrane water transport (reviewed in Ref. 237). Two types have been well characterized; in both cases, immunolocalization techniques based on affinity-purified antibodies played a key role in our understanding of their physiology. Aquaporin CHIP (AQP-CHIP), the first characterized molecular water channel, was originally isolated from red cells (238–240), and the corresponding cDNA was rapidly isolated (241). The function of AQP-CHIP as a selective water channel was established by expression cloning in *Xenopus* oocytes (237) and by reconstitution into liposomes (242) showing mercury-sensitive water permeability with low activation energy. AQP-CHIP excludes other small molecules including urea (242), H^+/OH^- or NH_3 (243), and the water conductance is independent of the membrane lipid composition (243). AQP-CHIP has six membrane-spanning domains and five connecting loops (240,241,243–245), the mercury-sensitive residue being localized to a single cysteine (246). It exists as homotetramers which can be visualized by freeze-fracture analysis, each monomer containing a separate pore (243,245,247). AQP-CHIP is abundant in proximal tubules and descending thin limbs (238,248) and accounts for approximately 4% of the apical plasma membrane protein content (248). The detailed localization in proximal tubules and thin limbs initially reported was later confirmed (249). It is localized on the apical pole over the entire length of the microvilli and in the invaginations between microvilli (Figure 8) but only in limited amounts in intracellular vesicles and vacuoles, probably reflecting a limited access to the endocytic pathway in contrast to, e.g., gp330 and gp280 (see above). The basolateral expression extends to both lateral and basal plasma membrane domains (Figure 8), with an almost equal distribution in apical and basolateral membranes. Heavy labeling is found in all segments 2 and 3 of the proximal tubules (248), whereas, for reasons still uncertain, this is not always the case in the initial part of segment 1 (248). The expression of AQP-CHIP (248) continues uninterrupted on the apical and basolateral membranes of the descending thin limbs (248) of both short and long loops. In contrast, the water-impermeable cells of the thin and thick segments of the ascending limb do not express AQP-CD, and the transition

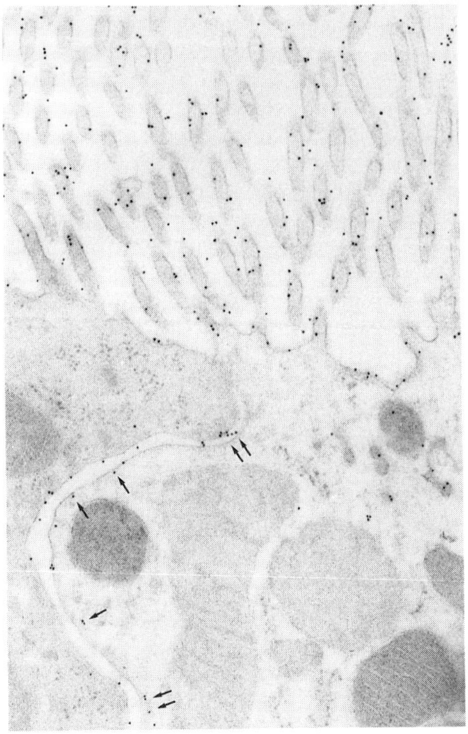

Figure 8 Immunolocalization of Aquaporin-CHIP water channels in proximal tubule cell. The labeling is localized to the apical plasma membrane corresponding to microvilli membrane and invaginations between microvilli. In addition, equally heavy labeling is observed of the basolateral plasma membrane (arrows), directly indicating the route of transcellular water reabsorption. ×60,000.

from labeled to unlabeled cells at the tip of the loops is abrupt (248). AQP-CHIP is not expressed in the rat collecting duct (248); thus, the vasopressin regulated pathway does not incorporate AQP-CHIP.

AQP-CHIP water channels are also localized in various other water-permeable epithelia, as revealed by Northern blot analysis (241,250,251), in situ hybridization (252), and immunocytochemistry (253,254). AQP-CHIP is detectable on the apical plasma membranes in choroid plexus of the brain (254) and in various structures of the eye, including the anterior parts of the ciliary body, the endothelium of the cornea, and the epithelium of the anterior lens (254); it may be involved in bile formation and modulation, since it is expressed in human biliary ducts and ductules (254) known to transport water (255), and is expressed in human gallbladder epithelium. Distinct expression is also detected in the nonfenestrated endothelium of capillaries and venules in muscle, lung, exocrine glands, and connective tissue (254). Thus, AQP-CHIP may be involved in the high water transport across capillary beds. In contrast, fenestrated endothelia in rat choroid plexus, intestine, liver (sinusoids), and kidney (glomerulus, capillaries) do not express AQP-CHIP (248,254), suggesting that other molecular structures are responsible for the water transport at these sites (254). CHIP is also present in the water reabsorptive epithelium of the rat male reproductive tract (253). The localization of AQP-CHIP at all the sites referred to (248,253,254) underscores the hypothesis that AQP-CHIP plays a major role in constitutive transcellular water transport throughout the body.

The gene expression of AQP-CHIP during development is complex. AQP-CHIP was transiently observed in periosteum, heart endothelium, large vessels, and cornea during fetal development but was permanently expressed in choroid plexus (252). A concurrent expression pattern was observed in red cells and kidney (252,256). AQP-CHIP was not detected in circulating prenatal red cells but was first identified on the third postnatal day and detectable on 100% of erythrocytes at day 14 (256). Correspondingly, a major induction of AQP-CHIP was observed in proximal tubules and thin descending limbs at birth, coincident with the development of renal concentrating mechanisms (256).

Aquaporin CD (AQP-CD) was subsequently cloned from a rat library using degenerate primers from the cDNA of AQP-CHIP and MIP26 (257) and is thought to be the vasopressin-sensitive water channel. Affinity-purified antibodies raised against a synthetic peptide deduced from the predicted amino acid sequence were used to establish its cellular and subcellular localization in order to analyze the mechanisms whereby vasopressin regulates water permeability of the apical plasma membrane of principal and inner medullary collecting duct cells (IMCD cells) and consequently water balance (for review, see Ref. 258). Vasopressin may regulate both activation and deactivation of the vasopressin response (259,260). The mechanisms may involve alterations in unit conductance of water channels or changes in the number of channels in the apical plasma membrane. Immunolabeling experiments revealed that AQP-CD is exclusively localized to the collecting duct, in principal cells (Figure 9) and in IMCD cells (261). It was not detected on intercalated cells, known to be engaged in acid-base transport. AQP-CD was localized in apical plasma membranes, and in addition, a substantial amount of AQP-CD was localized in subapical vesicles in the cytoplasm (261). Thus, there exists a large intracellular reservoir of water channels in subapical vesicles. The site and ultrastructure of the AQP-CD–bearing vesicles are in accordance with structures that incorporate endocytic markers (262). The localization pattern directly supports the "shuttle hypothesis" (263) which, based on indirect evidence, predicts that vasopressin stimulates exocytosis of water channels (for review, see Ref. 264). Of particular interest is also the observation that water restriction for 24 to 48 hr causes a marked enhancement in AQP-CD expression, as assessed by immunoblotting and immunolabeling (261). Thus, these data (261) strongly suggest two complementary modes of water-channel regulation in collecting duct cells. First, the data are compatible with control by vasopressin-stimulated exo- and endocytosis of water channel, corresponding to the shuttle hypothesis. Second, the absolute expression of water channel protein may be regulated by changes in hydration status.

COMPLEMENT REGULATORY PROTEINS

In vitro studies have shown that nucleated cells and in particular glomerular epithelial cells (GEC), are resistant to complement-induced lysis notably by homologous sources of complement (265). It is generally felt that this is mediated, at least in part (266–268), by membrane-bound regulators of complement activation listed in Table 2 (reviews in Refs. 269–271).

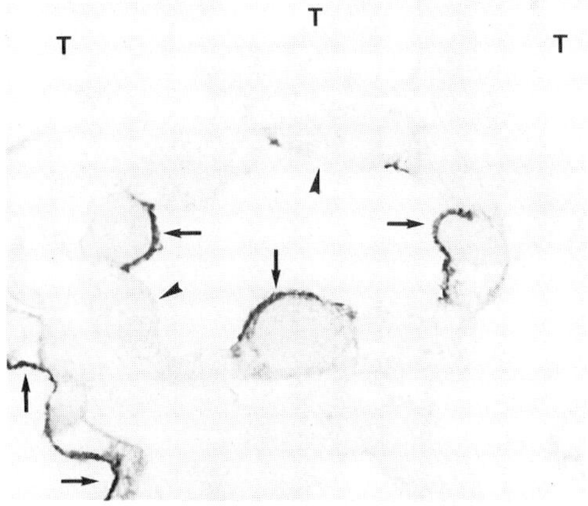

Figure 9 Immunolocalization of the vasopressin regulated water channel Aquaporin-CD in outer medullary collecting ducts. The labeling is confined to the apical domains of principal cells (arrows), whereas intercalated cells engaged in acid-base transport are unlabeled (arrowheads). Thick ascending limbs are also without labeling (T). ×1500.

The CR1 receptor for C3b is the best-known protein within this group. It was first identified on hematopoietic cells and rapidly shown to be expressed on podocytes, using erythrocyte-binding techniques and subsequently immunochemical staining. Although CR1 is synthesized by podocytes, the mRNA coding for the protein is only detectable in fetal kidneys (281).

Comparison of sequences has shown that CR1 (269,272,282,283) belongs to a family of proteins characterized by a series of 60 to 70 repeating amino acids, known as short consensus repeats (also found in gp330), which includes DAF (269,273) as well as CR2, MCP, and two serum complement inhibitors (factor H and C4 binding protein), which have all been mapped to band Iq32 of chromosome 1 (269). DAF is expressed by human glomerular epithelial cells and by tubular cells, whereas CR1 is detected only on podocytes.

In addition, recent studies show that there are yet other types of complement-inhibiting proteins (274–278) that act through binding C8 and have been shown to be expressed by glomerular podocytes. It is striking to note that three of these components are linked to the plasma membrane through a GPI bond. It has been proposed that this provides increased mobility and possibly efficiency to these proteins.

The formation of the attack complex of C is an important event in the pathogenesis of several immune-mediated glomerular diseases including Heymann nephritis (284), so that the mechanisms that control its biological activity are of importance. Antibodies to DAF increase lysis susceptibility of GEC (285), suggesting that it plays indeed a physiological role. In addition, the formation of immune complexes on the surface of human mesangial cells can induce the synthesis of DAF (286). Clinical studies implying a decreased expression of CR1 in lupus nephritis suggest that the regulation of these proteins may be important (287).

TAMM HORSFALL PROTEIN

Tamm Horsfall protein (reviewed in Refs. 288 and 289) was initially identified in human urine in 1950 by its ability to inhibit virus-induced hemagglutination. Found in all placental mammals, it is the most abundant protein in normal urine, from which it can be readily isolated by precipitation in the presence of NaCl. Its most striking property is indeed its ability to gel readily, particularly in the presence of various factors such as Ca, Na, low pH, albumin, and contrast media. The molecule exists mainly a polymer of high molecular weight (70,000 kDa), which can be dissociated in the presence of agents such as SDS or guanidine to monomers of 80 kDa. It is highly glycosylated, since carbohydrates account for 30% of its molecular weight. All chains are N-linked and several

Table 2 Complement Regulatory Proteins

Protein	Mol mass (kDa)	Cell distribution	Anchor	Glomerulus	Tubule	Mode of action	Ref.
CR1	190	Erythrocytes, PMN, monocytes, macrophages, B, some T, dendritic cells	COOH	Yes	No	Receptor, decay acceleration, cofactor activity[a,b]	272
DAF	70	Widespread	GPI	Yes	Yes	Decay acceleration	273
Protectin CD 59	18		GPI	Yes	Yes	C8 binding[c]	274–276
MIP	65	Widespread	GPI	Yes	Yes	C8 binding[c]	277, 278
CR2	145	B, some T, and dendritic cells, several epithelia	COOH	No	No		279
MCP (gp45–70)	58–63	Widespread	COOH	Likely[d]	Likely	Cofactor activity	280

Abbreviations: CR1 = complement receptor 1; CR2 = complement receptor 2; DAF = decay accelerating factor; MIP = membrane attack complex (MAC) inhibitory protein; MM = molecular mass in kilodaltons (kDa).

[a]Decay acceleration factor is the process of either preventing the association of or dissociating C3b or C4b from proteins of the complement cascade, such as Bb or C2a, which interact noncovalently with them as part of the convertase complexes.

[b]Cofactor activity refers to the ability of a molecule to promote the initial cleavage of C3b to the form iC3b, or the second cleavage of the reaction that generates C3c and C3dg.

[c]C8-binding proteins inhibit the activity of (MAC) via binding to C8.

[d]Tissue localization follows closely that of DAF, but to our knowledge, presence of MCP on renal tubule cells has not been directly reported.

contain unprocessed mannose-rich chains (290,291). As discussed below, carbohydrates play a key role in the ability of THP to aggregate and in its biological properties.

Using a variety of poly and monoclonal antibodies, THP was shown to be expressed by cells of the thick ascending limb of Henle's loop where it is localized both on the apical and basolateral domains and by most early distal tubule cells but not the macula densa cells. It was also detected in low amounts in the serum (292). During development, expression of THP coincides with the development of the TAL of Henle's loop.

THP has been cloned and found to be identical to uromodulin, a protein endowed with immunosuppressive properties independently identified in the urine of pregnant women by concanavalin A chromatography (293,294). THP/uromodulin has homologies with the cysteine rich domain of the epidermal growth factor precursor which has been described in several extracellular glycoproteins including the LDL receptor (see also above for gp330) and several clotting factors and expresses an RGD sequence found in matrix proteins. It does not have a classic transmembrane hydrophobic domain and has been shown to be anchored to the membrane via a GPI link (295).

Northern hybridization studies have confirmed that THP was synthesized by the kidney and in situ hybridization has shown the mRNA to be located in the TAL (296). Reactivity initially detected in various organs with polyclonal antibodies has not been confirmed using monoclonal antibodies, nor has mRNA for THP been detected in these tissues.

The physiological role of THP is unknown. Early studies suggesting that THP might be the Na-K-2Cl exchanger have not been supported by experimental data. There is good evidence that THP binds type 1 pili of *E. coli* in a mannose-dependent fashion and could thus play a role in the protection against urinary infection. The elucidation of the sequence of THP/uromodulin has not provided the key to this issue. Indeed, uromodulin is a high-affinity ligand for Il1, Il2, and TNF, but this occurs through the carbohydrate moiety of the molecule which differs from that of THP (297–299). Nevertheless, rIl1 and rTNF bind to tubular segments expressing THP which does have immunosuppressive properties 10 times less potent than uromodulin.

An interesting lead may be derived from the observation that THP/uromodulin shares, over a stretch of 450 amino acids encompassing the 28 cysteine residues, 85% similarity with gp2, the 78-kDa major zymogen granule protein of the exocrine pancreas, which is also GPI-anchored (300–301). Like THP, gp2 is released from the apical membrane and forms large aggregates in solution (302). It has been proposed that THP and gp2 may define a new gene family encoding for GPI-anchored proteins that utilize pH- and ion-dependent aggregation to establish membrane microdomains.

Tamm-Horsfall Protein in Pathology

THP can be involved in several pathogenic processes. It can experimentally be the target of antibodies which give rise to an inflammatory reaction around the TAL. In human and experimental pathology, THP is the main component of tubular casts. This has been related to its ability to form gels and has obvious implications in pathology. Recent studies using a panel of Bence Jones proteins point to a common peptidic binding site of these light chains to THP (303), the aggregation of which to form casts still depends on the carbohydrate chains. In cases of urinary obstruction and transplant rejection THP has been found in the tubular interstitium, possibly as a consequence of rupture of damaged tubules. THP has been found in renal stones, but it is not known whether it is an innocent bystander, a stone promoter, or, to the contrary, a component preventing the formation of stones. Finally, recent studies reveal that THP mRNA levels were decreased in the hyperprostaglandin E syndrome, a variant of Bartter's syndrome, (304), and in ureteral obstruction, which also decreases the preproepidermal growth factor (305).

PODOCYTE-SPECIFIC ANTIGENS

The role of protein components shared by the renal tubule and podocytes in glomerular pathology has been discussed above. Present evidence indicates that they probably are not relevant in human pathology. Substantial efforts have therefore been invested in the identification of components specific for glomerular epithelial cells. The technical approach used has essentially been the production of monoclonal antibodies against glomerular preparations or the isolation of proteins with specific biochemical properties such as podocalixin. Table 3 lists the components that have been

Table 3 Ultrastructural Distribution of Podocyte Membrane Antigens Identified with Monoclonal Antibodies[a]

Antigen Characteristics			Podocyte		Ultrastructural Localization: Glomerular endothelium		Bowman's cells		Peritubular capillaries			
Nature	MM (kDa)	Species	Bas.[b]	Ap.[c]	Bas	Ap	Bas	Ap	Bas	Ap	Tubule	Ref.
Podocalyxin	140	Human	–	+++	–	+	–	–	–	++	–	306, 307
		Rat										308
Podoendin	62	Rat	–	+++	–	++	–	+	–	++	–	309
?	120	Rat	+	–	–	–	–	–	–	–	Collecting (Bas)	310
Ganglioside	GD3	Rat	–	+++	–	–	–	–	–	–	–	310, 311
?	60	Human	+		?		?		+		–	312
?	70–80	Human	+		?		?		+		–	312
?	51	Rat	++	++	–	–	–	–	–	–	–	313
Integrin ?	115–150	Human	++	±	+	+	+	–	–	–	Mitochondria	314

[a]This table does not mention podocyte antigens coexpressed on the brush border of the proximal tubule (gp330 in the rat; DPP IV, neutral endopeptidase/CALLA, aminopeptidases A and N in most species).
[b]Bas = basal domain (facing the GBM; for podocytes, sole of the foot processes).
[c]Ap = apical domain (urinary domain for podocytes and Bowman's cells; luminal domain for endothelial cells).

identified at present. None has been cloned, but partial cDNA isolation has been reported for podocalyxin. These proteins clearly represent good candidates for future developments on their molecular biology and their potential role in glomerular pathology.

NOTE ADDED IN PROOF

Since this review was written, the full sequence of gp330 has been elucidated by Saito et al. (315), confirming and extending the partial structural data described.

REFERENCES

1. Masugi M. Über die experimentelle Glomerulonephritis durch das spezifische Antinierenserum: Ein Beitrag zur Pathogenese der diffusen Glomerulonephritis. Beitr Pathol Anat 1934; 92:429.
2. Heymann W, Hackel DB, Harwood S, et al. Production of nephrotic syndrome in rats by Freund's adjuvants and rat kidney suspensions. Proc Soc Exp Biol Med 1959; 100:660–664.
3. Verroust P, Ronco P, Chatelet F. Monoclonal antibodies and identification of glomerular antigens. Kidney Int 1986; 30:649–655.
4. Poujeol Ph, Ronco P, Tauc M, et al. Immunological segmentation of the rabbit distal, connecting and collecting tubules. Am J Physiol (Renal Fluid Electrolyte Physiol 21) 1987; 252:F412–F422.
5. Van Adelsberg JS, Edwards JC, Al-Awqati Q. The apical Cl/HCO3 exchanger of β intercalated cells. J Biol Chem 1993; 268:11283–11289.
6. Koepsell H, Korn K, Raszeja-Specht A, et al. Monoclonal antibodies against the renal Na+-D-glucose cotransporter: Identification of antigenic polypeptides and demonstration of functional coupling of different Na+-cotransport systems. J Biol Chem 1988; 263:18419–18429.
7. Barlet-Bas C, Arystarkhova E, Cheval L, et al. Are there several isoforms of Na, K-ATPase a subunit in the rabbit kidney? J Biol Chem 1993; 268:11512–11515.
8. Debiec H, Ronco PM. Identification and epitope analysis of the renal Na+/Pi cotransport protein using monoclonal antibodies. J Biol Chem 1993; 268:13356–13363.
9. Tse M, Levine S, Yun C, et al. The mammalian Na+/H+ exchanger gene family-Initial structure/function studies. J Am Soc Nephrol 1993; 4:969–975.
10. Rodman JS, Kerjaschki D, Merisko E, Farquhar MG. Presence of an extensive clathrin coat on the apical plasmalemma of the rat kidney proximal tubule cell. J Cell Biol 84; 98:1630–1636.
11. Semenza G. Anchoring and biosynthesis of stalked brush border membrane proteins: Glycosidases and peptidases of enterocytes and renal tubuli. Annu Rev Cell Biol 1986; 2:255–313.
12. Kenny AJ, Maroux S: Topology of microvillar membrane hydrolases of kidney and intestine. Physiol Rev 1982; 62:91–128.
13. Stefanovic V, Vlahovic P, Ardaillou N, et al. Characterization and regulation of cell surface aminopeptidase A and N activities in human glomerular epithelial cells. Kidney Int 1992; 41:1571–1580.
14. Gorvel JP, Vivier I, Naquet P, et al. Characterization of the neutral aminopeptidase activity associated to the mouse thymocyte-activating molecule. J Immunol 1990; 144:2899–2907.
15. Naquet P, Vivier I, Gorvel JP, et al. Activation of mouse T lymphocytes by a monoclonal antibody to a developmentally regulated surface aminopeptidase (THAM). Immunol Rev 1989; 111:177–193.
16. Look AT, Ashmun RA, Shapiro LH, Peiper SC. Human myeloid plasma membrane glycoprotein CD13 (gp150) is identical to aminopeptidase N. J Clin Invest 1989; 83:1299–1307.
17. Olsen J, Cowell GM, Konigshofer E, et al. Complete amino acid sequence of human intestinal aminopeptidase N as deduced from cloned cDNA. FEBS Lett 1988; 238:307–314.
18. Malfroy B, Kado-Fong H, Gros C, et al. Molecular cloning and amino acid sequence of rat kidney aminopeptidase M: A member of a super family of zinc-metallohydrolases. Biochem Biophys Res Commun 1989; 161:236–244.
19. Watt VM, Yip CC. Amino acid sequence deduced from a rat kidney cDNA suggests it encodes the Zn-peptidase aminopeptidase N. J Biol Chem 1989; 264:5480–5487.
20. Olsen J, Sjostrom H, Noren O. Cloning of the pig aminopeptidase N gene: Identification of possible regulatory elements and the exon distribution in relation to the membrane-spanning region. FEBS Lett 1989; 251:275–281.
21. Shapiro LH, Ashmun RA, Roberts WM, Look AT. Separate promoters control transcription of the human aminopeptidase N gene in myeloid and intestinal epithelial cells. J Biol Chem 1991; 266:11999–12007.
22. Ashmun RA, Shapiro LH, Look AT. Deletion of the zinc-binding motif of CD13/aminopeptidase N molecules results in loss of epitopes that mediate binding of inhibitory antibodies. Blood 1992; 79:3344–3349.

23. O'Connell PJ, Gerkis V, D'Apice AJ. Variable O-glycosylation of CD13 (aminopeptidase N). J Biol Chem 1991; 266:4593–4597.
24. Assmann KJM, van Son JPHF, Dijkman HBPM, Koene RAP. A nephritogenic rat monoclonal antibody to mouse aminopeptidase A: Induction of massive albuminuria after a single intravenous injection. J Exp Med 1992; 175:623–635.
25. Wu Q, Li L, Cooper MD, Pierres M, Gorvel JP. Aminopeptidase A activity of the murine B-lymphocyte differentiation antigen BP-1/6C3. Proc Natl Acad Sci USA 1991; 88:676–680.
26. Nanus DM, Engelstein D, Gastl GA, et al. Molecular cloning of the human kidney differentiation antigen gp160: Human aminopeptidase A. Proc Natl Acad Sci USA 1993; 90:7069–7073.
27. Wang J, Cooper MD. Histidine residue in the zinc-binding motif of aminopeptidase A is critical for enzymatic activity. Proc Natl Acad Sci USA 1993; 90:1222–1226.
28. Bauvois B, Sanceau J, Wietzerbin J. Human U937 cell surface peptidase activities: Characterization and degradative effect on tumor necrosis factor-α. Eur J Immunol 1992; 22:923–930.
29. Bauvois B. A collagen-binding glycoprotein on the surface of mouse fibroblasts is identified as dipeptidyl peptidase IV. Biochem J 1988; 252:723–731.
30. Piazza GA, Callanan HM, Mowery J, Hixson DC. Evidence for a role of dipeptidyl peptidase IV in fibronectin-mediated interactions of hepatocytes with extracellular matrix. Biochem J 1989; 262:327–334.
31. Ardaillou N, Stefanovic V, Placier S, et al. Interferon-γ (IFN-γ) induces dipeptidylpeptidase IV (DPP IV) expression in human glomerular epithelial cells (abstr). J Am Soc Nephrol 1992; 3:573.
32. Tauc M, Chatelet F, Verroust PJ, et al. Characterization of monoclonal antibodies specific for rabbit renal brush border hydrolases: Application to immunohistological localization. J Histochem Cytochem 1988; 36:523–532.
33. Ronco P, Allegri L, Melcion C, et al. A monoclonal antibody to brush border and passive Heymann nephritis. Clin Exp Immunol 84; 55:319–332.
34. van Leer EHG, Moullier Ph, Ronco P, Verroust P. Lymphocyte expression of a 90 kD brush border antigen. Clin Exp Immunol 1987; 67:572–580.
35. Vivier I, Marguet D, Naquet P, et al. Evidence that thymocyte-activating molecule is mouse CD26 (dipeptidyl peptidase IV). J Immunol 1991; 147:447–454.
36. Tanaka T, Kameoka J, Yaron A, et al. The costimulatory activity of the CD26 antigen requires dipeptidyl peptidase IV enzymatic activity. Proc Natl Acad Sci USA 1993; 90:4586–4590.
37. Ogata S, Misumi Y, Ikehara Y. Primary structure of rat liver dipeptidyl peptidase IV deduced from its cDNA and identification of the NH2-terminal signal sequence as the membrane-anchoring domain. J Biol Chem 1989; 264:3596–3601.
38. Hong WJ, Doyle D. Molecular dissection of the NH2-terminal signal/anchor sequence of rat dipeptidyl peptidase IV. J Cell Biol 1990; 111:323–328.
39. Darmoul D, Lacasa M, Chantret I, et al. Isolation of a cDNA probe for the human intestinal dipeptidylpeptidase IV and assignment of the gene locus DPP4 to chromosome 2. Ann Hum Genet 1990; 54:191–197.
40. Darmoul D, Lacasa M, Baricault L, et al. Dipeptidyl peptidase IV (CD 26) gene expression in enterocyte-like colon cancer cell lines HT-29 and Caco-2: Cloning of the complete human coding sequence and changes of dipeptidyl peptidase IV mRNA levels during cell differentiation. J Biol Chem 1992; 267:4824–4833.
41. Misumi Y, Hayashi Y, Arakawa F, Ikehara Y. Molecular cloning and sequence analysis of human dipeptidyl peptidase IV, a serine proteinase on the cell surface. Biochim Biophys Acta 1992; 1131:333–336.
42. Marguet D, Bernard AM, Vivier I, et al. cDNA cloning for mouse thymocyte-activating molecule: A multifunctional ectodipeptidyl peptidase IV (CD26) included in a subgroup of serine proteases. J Biol Chem 1992; 267:2200–2208.
43. Fujiwara T, Tsuji E, Misumi Y, et al. Selective cell-surface expression of dipeptidyl peptidase IV with mutations at the active site sequence. Biochem Biophys Res Commun 1992; 185:776–784.
44. Tsuji E, Misumi Y, Fujiwara T, et al. An active-site mutation (Gly633— : Arg) of dipeptidyl peptidase IV causes its retention and rapid degradation in the endoplasmic reticulum. Biochemistry 1992; 31:11921–11927.
45. David F, Bernard AM, Pierres M, Marguet D. Identification of serine 624, aspartic acid 702, and histidine 734 as the catalytic triad residues of mouse dipeptidyl-peptidase IV (CD26): A member of a novel family of nonclassical serine hydrolases. J Biol Chem 1993; 268:17247–17252.
46. Hong WJ, Piazza GA, Hixson DC, Doyle D. Expression of enzymatically active rat dipeptidyl peptidase IV in Chinese hamster ovary cells after transfection. Biochemistry 1989; 28:8474–8479.
47. Ogata S, Misumi Y, Tsuji E, et al. Identification of the active site residues in dipeptidyl peptidase IV by affinity labeling and site-directed mutagenesis. Biochemistry 1992; 31:2582–2587.
48. Erdos EG, Skidgel RA. Neutral endopeptidase 24.11 (enkephalinase) and related regulators of peptide hormones (review). FASEB J 1989; 3:145–151.

49. Vogt-Schaden M, Gagelmann M, Hock D, et al. Degradation of porcine brain natriuretic peptide (pBNP-26) by endoprotease-24.11 from kidney cortical membranes. Biochem Biophys Res Commun 1989; 161:1177–1183.
50. Skolovsky M, Galron R, Kloog Y, et al. Endothelins are more sensitive than sarafotoxins to neutral endopeptidase: Possible physiological significance. Proc Natl Acad Sci USA 1990; 87:4702–4706.
51. Vijayaraghavan J, Scicli AG, Carretero OA, et al. The hydrolysis of endothelins by neutral endopeptidase 24.11 (enkephalinase). J Biol Chem 1990; 265:14150–14155.
52. Okada K, Miyazaki Y, Takada J, et al. Conversion of big endothelin-1 by membrane-bound metalloendopeptidase in cultured bovine endothelial cells. Biochem Biophys Res Commun 1990; 171:1192–1198.
53. Skidgel RA, Jackman HL, Erdos EG. Metabolism of substance P and bradykinin by human neutrophils. Biochem Pharmacol 1991; 41:1335–1344.
54. Shipp MA, Tarr GE, Chen CY, et al. CD10/neutral endopeptidase 24.11 hydrolyzes bombesin-like peptides and regulates the growth of small cell carcinomas of the lung. Proc Natl Acad Sci USA 1991; 88:10662–10666.
55. Fagny C, Michel A, Leonard I, et al. In vitro degradation of endothelin-1 by endopeptidase 24.11 (enkephalinase). Peptides 1991; 12:773–778.
56. Yamaguchi T, Kido H, Fukase M, et al. A membrane-bound metallo-endopeptidase from rat kidney hydrolyzing parathyroid hormone: Purification and characterization. Eur J Biochem 1991; 200:563–571.
57. Indig FE, Pecht M, Trainin N, et al. Hydrolysis of thymic humoral factor gamma 2 by neutral endopeptidase (EC 3.4.24.11). Biochem J 1991; 278:891–894.
58. Soleilhac JM, Lucas E, Beaumont A, et al. A 94-kDa protein, identified as neutral endopeptidase-24.11, can inactivate atrial natriuretic peptide in the vascular endothelium. Mol Pharmacol 1992; 41:609–614.
59. Welches WR, Brosnihan KB, Ferrario CM. A comparison of the properties and enzymatic activities of three angiotensin processing enzymes: Angiotensin converting enzyme, prolyl endopeptidase and neutral endopeptidase 24.11 (review). Life Sci 1993; 52:1461–1480.
60. Kenny AJ, Bourne A, Ingram J. Hydrolysis of human and pig brain natriuretic peptides, urodilatin, C-type natriuretic peptide and some C-receptor ligands by endopeptidase-24.11. Biochem J 1993; 291:83–88.
61. Graf K, Grafe M, Bossaller C, et al. Degradation of bradykinin by neutral endopeptidase (EC 3.4.24.11) in cultured human endothelial cells. Eur J Clin Chem Clin Biochem 1993; 31:267–272.
62. Ardaillou N, Lelongt B, Turner N, et al. Characterization of a simian virus 40-transformed human podocyte cell line producing type IV collagen and exhibiting polarized response to atrial natriuretic peptide. J Cell Physiol 1992; 152:599–616.
63. Platt JL, Lebien TW, Michael AF. Stages of renal ontogenesis identified by monoclonal antibodies reactive with lymphohemopoeitic differentiation antigens. J Exp Med 1983: 157:155–172.
64. Salles G, Chen CY, Reinherz EL, Shipp MA. CD10/NEP is expressed on Thy 1 low B220+ murine B-cell progenitors and functions to regulate stromal cell-dependent lymphopoiesis. Blood 1992; 80:2021–2029.
65. Shipp MA, Richardson NE, Sayre PH, et al. Molecular cloning of the common acute lymphoblastic leukemia antigen (CALLA) identifies a type II integral membrane protein. Proc Natl Acad Sci USA 1988; 85:4819–4823.
66. Malfroy B, Kuang WJ, Seeburg PH, et al. Molecular cloning and amino acid sequence of human enkephalinase (neutral endopeptidase). FEBS Lett 1988; 229:206–210.
67. Jongeneel CV, Quackenbush EJ, Ronco P, et al. The common acute lymphoblastic leukemia antigen (Calla) expressed on leukemia and melanoma cell lines has neutral endopeptidase activity. J Clin Invest 1989; 83:713–717.
68. Letarte M, Vera S, Tran R, et al. Common acute lymphocytic leukemia antigen is identical to neutral endopeptidase. J Exp Med 1988; 168:1247–1253.
69. D'Adamio L, Shipp MA, Masteller EL, Reinherz EL. Organization of the gene encoding common acute lymphoblastic leukemia antigen (neutral endopeptidase 24.11): Multiple miniexons and separate 5′ untranslated regions. Proc Natl Acad Sci USA 1989; 86:7103–7107.
70. Helene A, Milhiet PE, Haouas H, et al. Effects of monoclonal antibodies raised against the common acute lymphoblastic leukemia antigen on endopeptidase-24.11 activity. Biochem Pharmacol 1992; 43:809–814.
71. Bateman RC Jr, Jackson D, Slaughter CA, et al. Identification of the active-site arginine in rat neutral endopeptidase 24.11 (enkephalinase) as arginine 102 and analysis of a glutamine 102 mutant. J Biol Chem 1989; 264:6151–6157.
72. Vijayaraghavan J, Kim YA, Jackson D, et al. Use of site-directed mutagenesis to identify valine-573 in the S′1 binding site of rat neutral endopeptidase 24.11 (enkephalinase). Biochemistry 1990; 29:8052–8056.
73. Le Moual H, Devault A, Roques BP, et al. Identification of glutamic acid 646 as a zinc-coordinating residue in endopeptidase-24.11. J Biol Chem 1991; 266:15670–15674.
74. Beaumont A, Le Moual H, Boileau G, et al. Evidence that both arginine 102 and arginine 747 are involved in substrate binding to neutral endopeptidase (EC 3.4.24.11). J Biol Chem 1991; 266:214–220.

75. Kim YA, Shriver B, Quay T, Hersh LB. Analysis of the importance of arginine 102 in neutral endopeptidase (enkephalinase) catalysis. J Biol Chem 1992; 267:12330–12335.
76. Dion N, Le Moual H, Crine P, Boileau G. Kinetic evidence that His-711 of neutral endopeptidase 24.11 is involved in stabilization of the transition state. FEBS Lett 1993; 318:301–304.
77. Le Moual H, Roques BP, Crine P, Boileau G. Substitution of potential metal-coordinating amino acid residues in the zinc-binding site of endopeptidase-24.11. FEBS Lett 1993; 324:196–200.
78. Jiang W, Gorbea CM, Flannery AV, et al. The alpha subunit of meprin A: Molecular cloning and sequencing, differential expression in inbred mouse strains, and evidence for divergent evolution of the alpha and beta subunits. J Biol Chem 1992; 267:9185–9193.
79. Corbeil D, Gaudoux F, Wainwright S, et al. Molecular cloning of the alpha-subunit of rat endopeptidase-24.18 (endopeptidase-2) and co-localization with endopeptidase-24.11 in rat kidney by in situ hybridization. FEBS Lett 1992; 309:203–208.
80. Johnson GD, Hersh LB. Cloning a rat meprin cDNA reveals the enzyme is a heterodimer J Biol Chem 1992; 267:13505–13512.
81. Dumermuth E, Sterchi EE, Jiang WP, et al. The astacin family of metalloendopeptidases. J Biol Chem 1991; 266:21381–21385.
82. Jiang W, Sadler PM, Jenkins NA, et al. Tissue-specific expression and chromosomal localization of the alpha subunit of mouse meprin A. J Biol Chem 1993; 268:10380–10385.
83. Gorbea CM, Flannery AV, Bond JS. Homotetrameric and heterotetrameric forms of the membrane-bound metalloendopeptidases meprin-A and meprin-B. Arch Biochem Biophys 1991; 290:549–553.
84. Flannery AV, Macadam GC, Beynon RJ. Report—Immunological characterisation of different meprin species in mice. Biochem Biophys Acta 1991; 1079:119–122.
85. Soubrier F, Alhenc-Gelas F, Hubert C, et al. Two putative active centers in human angiotensin I-converting enzyme revealed by molecular cloning. Proc Natl Acad Sci USA 1988; 85:9386–9390.
86. Bernstein KE, Martin BM, Bernstein EA, et al. The isolation of angiotensin-converting enzyme cDNA. J Biol Chem 1988; 263:11021–11024.
87. Ehlers MR, Fox EA, Strydom DJ, Riordan JF. Molecular cloning of human testicular angiotensin-converting enzyme: The testis isozyme is identical to the C-terminal half of endothelial angiotensin-converting enzyme. Proc Natl Acad Sci USA 1989; 86:7741–7745.
88. Bernstein KE, Martin BM, Edwards AS, Bernstein EA. Mouse angiotensin-converting enzyme is a protein composed to two homologous domains. J Biol Chem 1989; 264:11945–11951.
89. Hubert C, Houot AM, Corvol P, Soubrier F. Structure of the angiotensin I-converting enzyme gene: Two alternate promoters correspond to evolutionary steps of a duplicated gene. J Biol Chem 1991; 266:15377–15383.
90. Nadaud S, Houot AM, Hubert C, et al. Functional study of the germinal angiotensin I-converting enzyme promoter. Biochem Biophys Res Commun 1992; 189:134–140.
91. Costerousse O, Jaspard E, Wei L, Corvol P, Alhenc-Gelas F. The angiotensin I-converting enzyme (kininase II): Molecular organization and regulation of its expression in humans (review). J Cardiovasc Pharmacol 1992; 20 (suppl 9): S10–S15.
92. Testut P, Soubrier F, Corvol P, Hubert C. Functional analysis of the human somatic angiotensin I-converting enzyme gene promoter. Biochem J 1993; 293:843–848.
93. Chen YN, Riordan JF. Identification of essential tyrosine and lysine residues in angiotensin converting enzyme: Evidence for a single active site. Biochemistry 1990; 29:10493–10498.
94. Ehlers MR, Riordan JF. Angiotensin-converting enzyme: Zinc- and inhibitor-binding stoichiometries of the somatic and testis isozymes. Biochemistry 1991; 30:7118–7126.
95. Chen YN, Ehlers MR, Riordan JF. The functional role of tyrosine-200 in human testis angiotensin-converting enzyme. Biochem Biophys Res Commun 1992; 184:306–309.
96. Savic V, Sefanovic V, Ardaillou N, Ardaillou R. Induction of ecto-5′-nucleotidase of rat cultured mesangial cells by interleukin-1 beta and tumour necrosis factor-alpha. Immunology 1990; 70:321–326.
97. Savic V, Blanchard A, Vlahovic P, et al. Cyclic adenosine monophosphate-stimulating agents induce ecto-5′-nucleotidase activity and inhibit DNA synthesis in rat cultured mesangial cells. Arch Biochem Biophys 1991; 290:202–206.
98. Ardaillou R, Chansel D, Stefanovic V, Ardaillou N. Cell surface receptors and ectoenzymes in mesangial cells (review). J Am Soc Nephrol 1992; 2:S107–115.
99. Dawson TP, Gandhi R, Le Hir M, Kaissling B. Ecto-5′-nucleotidase: Localization in rat kidney by light microscopic histochemical and immunohistochemical methods. J Histochem Cytochem 1989; 37:39–47.
100. Bachmann S, Le Hir M, Eckardt KU. Co-localization of erythropoietin mRNA and ecto-5′-nucleotidase immunoreactivity in peritubular cells of rat renal cortex indicates that fibroblasts produce erythropoietin. J Histochem Cytochem 1993; 41:335–341.
101. Le Hir M, Kaissling B. Distribution and regulation of renal ecto-5′-nucleotidase: Implications for physiological functions of adenosine (editorial, review). Am J Physiol 1993; 264:F377–F387.
102. Misumi Y, Ogata S, Hirose S, Ikehara Y. Primary structure of rat liver 5′-nucleotidase deduced from the

cDNA: Presence of the COOH-terminal hydrophobic domain for possible post-translational modification by glycophospholipid. J Biol Chem 1990; 265:2178–2183.
103. Lebargy F, Bulle F, Siegrist S, et al. Localization by in situ hybridization of gamma-glutamyl transpeptidase mRNA in the rat kidney using 35S-labeled RNA probes. Lab Invest 1990; 62:731–735.
104. Darbouy M, Chobert MN, Lahuna O, et al. Tissue-specific expression of multiple gamma-glutamyl transpeptidase mRNAs in rat epithelia. Am J Physiol 1991; 261:C1130–C1137.
105. Laperche Y, Bulle F, Aissani T, et al. Molecular cloning and nucleotide sequence of rat kidney gamma-glutamyl transpeptidase cDNA. Proc Natl Acad Sci USA 1986; 83:937–941.
106. Rajagopalan S, Park JH, Patel PD, et al. Cloning and analysis of the rat gamma-glutamyltransferase gene. J Biol Chem 1990; 265:11721–11725.
107. Lahuna O, Brouillet A, Chobert MN, et al. Identification of a second promoter which drives the expression of gamma-glutamyl transpeptidase in rat kidney and epididymis. Biochemistry 1992; 31:9190–9196.
108. Ikeda Y, Fujii J, Taniguchi N. Significance of Arg-107 and Glu-108 in the catalytic mechanism of human gamma-glutamyl transpeptidase. Identification by site-directed mutagenesis. J Biol Chem 1993; 268:3980–3985.
109. Blochberger TC, Sabatine JM, Lee YC, Hughey RP. O-linked glycosylation of rat renal gamma-glutamyltranspeptidase adjacent to its membrane anchor domain. J Biol Chem 1989; 264:20718–20722.
110. Pawlak A, Lahuna O, Bulle F, et al. Gamma glutamyl transpeptidase: A single copy gene in the rat and a multigene family in the human genome. J Biol Chem 1988; 263:9913–9916.
111. Chobert MN, Lahuna O, Lebargy F, et al. Tissue-specific expression of two gamma-glutamyl transpeptidase mRNAs with alternative 5′ ends encoded by a single copy gene in the rat. J Biol Chem 1990; 265:2352–2357.
112. Pawlak A, Wu SJ, Bulle F, et al. Different gamma-glutamyl transpeptidase mRNAs are expressed in human liver and kidney. Biochem Biophys Res Commun 1989; 164:912–918.
113. Courtay C, Oster T, Michelet F, et al. Gamma-glutamyltransferase: Nucleotide sequence of the human pancreatic cDNA: Evidence for a ubiquitous gamma-glutamyltransferase polypeptide in human tissues. Biochem Pharmacol 1992; 43:2527–2533.
114. Rajagopalan S, Wan DF, Habib GM, et al. Six mRNAs with different 5′ ends are encoded by a single gamma-glutamyltransferase gene in mouse. Proc Natl Acad Sci USA 1993; 90:6179–6183.
115. Verpooten GF, Nouwen EJ, Hoylaerts MF, et al. Segment-specific localization of intestinal-type alkaline phosphatase in human kidney. Kidney Int 1989; 36:617–625.
116. Weiss MJ, Henthorn PS, Lafferty MA, et al. Isolation and characterization of a cDNA encoding a human liver/bone/kidney-type alkaline phosphatase. Proc Natl Acad Sci USA 1986; 83:7182–7186.
117. Terao M, Studer M, Gianni M, Garattini E. Isolation and characterization of the mouse liver/bone/kidney-type alkaline phosphatase gene. Biochem J 1990; 268:641–648.
118. Weiss MJ, Ray K, Henthorn PS, et al. Structure of the human liver/bone/kidney alkaline phosphatase gene. J Biol Chem 1988; 263:12002–12010.
119. Matsuura S, Kishi F, Kajii T. Characterization of a 5′-flanking region of the human liver/bone/kidney alkaline phosphatase gene: Two kinds of mRNA from a single gene. Biochem Biophys Res Commun 1990; 168:993–1000.
120. Toh Y, Yamamoto M, Endo H, et al. Isolation and characterization of a rat liver alkaline phosphatase gene: A single gene with two promoters. Eur J Biochem 1989; 182:231–237.
121. Berger J, Garattini E, Hua JC, Udenfriend S. Cloning and sequencing of human intestinal alkaline phosphatase cDNA. Proc Natl Acad Sci USA 1987; 84:695–698.
122. Henthorn PS, Raducha M, Edwards YH, et al. Nucleotide and amino acid sequences of human intestinal alkaline phosphatase: Close homology to placental alkaline phosphatase. Proc Natl Acad Sci USA 1987; 84:1234–1238.
123. Weissig H, Schildge A, Hoylaerts MF, et al. Cloning and expression of the bovine intestinal alkaline phosphatase gene: Biochemical characterization of the recombinant enzyme. Biochem J 1993; 290:503–508.
124. Kam W, Clauser E, Kim YS, et al. Cloning, sequencing, and chromosomal localization of human term placental alkaline phosphatase cDNA. Proc Natl Acad Sci USA 1985; 82:8715–8719.
125. Millan JL. Molecular cloning and sequence analysis of human placental alkaline phosphatase [published erratum appears in J Biol Chem 1991; 266:4023] J Biol Chem 1986; 261:3112–3115.
126. Watanabe S, Watanabe T, Li WB, et al. Expression of the germ cell alkaline phosphatase gene in human choriocarcinoma cells. J Biol Chem 1989; 264:12611–12619.
127. Millan JL, Manes T. Seminoma-derived Nagao isozyme is encoded by a germ-cell alkaline phosphatase gene. Proc Natl Acad Sci USA 1988; 85:3024–3028.
128. Satoh S, Keida Y, Konta Y, et al. Purification and molecular cloning of mouse renal dipeptidase. Biochim Biophys Acta 1993; 1163:234–242.
129. Satoh S, Kusunoki C, Konta Y, et al. Cloning and structural analysis of genomic DNA for human renal dipeptidase. Biochim Biophys Acta 1993; 1172:181–183.

130. Adachi H, Tawaragi Y, Inuzuka C, et al. Primary structure of human microsomal dipeptidase deduced from molecular cloning. J Biol Chem 1990; 265:3992–3995.
131. Kerjaschki D, Noronha-Blob L, Sacktor B, Farquhar MG. Microdomains of distinctive glycoprotein composition in the kidney proximal tubule brush border. J Cell Biol 1984; 98:1505–1513.
132. Rodman JS, Seidman L, Farquhar MG. The membrane composition of coated pits, microvilli, endosomes, and lysosomes is distinctive in the rat kidney proximal tubule cell. J Cell Biol 1986; 102:77–87.
133. Romco P, Ardaillou N, Verroust P, Lelongt B. Pathophysiology of the podocyte: A target and a major player in glomerulonephritis. Adv Nephrol. 1993.
134. Matsuo S, Fukatsu A, Taub ML, et al. Glomerulonephritis induced in the rabbit by anti-endothelial antibodies. J Clin Invest 1987; 79:1798–1811.
135. Llorens-Cortes C, Huang H, Vicart P, et al. Identification and characterization of neutral endopeptidase in endothelial cells from venous or arterial origins. J Biol Chem 1992; 267:14012–14018.
136. Dussaule JC, Stefanski A, Bea ML, et al. Characterization of neutral endopeptidase in vascular smooth muscle cells of rabbit renal cortex. Am J Physiol 1993; 264:F45–F52.
137. Ronco P, Antoine M, Baudouin B, et al. Polarized membrane expression of brush-border hydrolases in primary cultures of kidney proximal tubular cells depends on cell differentiation and is induced by dexamethasone. J Cell Physiol 1990; 145:222–237.
138. Minami M, Ohishi N, Mutoh H, et al. Leukotriene A4 hydrolase is a zinc-containing aminopeptidase. Biochem Biophys Res Commun 1990; 173:620–626.
139. Llorens-Cortes C, Giros B, Schwartz JC. A novel potential metallopeptidase derived from the enkephalinase gene by alternative splicing. J Neurochem 1990; 55:2146–2148.
140. Jaspard E, Wei L, Alhenc-Gelas F. Differences in the properties and enzymatic specificities of the two active sites of angiotensin I-converting enzyme (kininase II): Studies with bradykinin and other natural peptides. J Biol Chem 1993; 268:9496–9503.
141. Wei L, Alhenc-Gelas F, Corvol P, Clauser E. The two homologous domains of human angiotensin I-converting enzyme are both catalytically active. J Biol Chem 1991; 266:9002–9008.
142. Wei L, Clauser E, Alhenc-Gelas F, Corvol P. The two homologous domains of human angiotensin I-converting enzyme interact differently with competitive inhibitors. J Biol Chem 1992; 267:13398–13405.
143. Ehlers MR, Chen YN, Riordan JF. The unique N-terminal sequence of testis angiotensin-converting enzyme is heavily O-glycosylated and unessential for activity or stability. Biochem Biophys Res Commun 1992; 183:199–205.
144. Lattion AL, Soubrier F, Allegrini J, et al. The testicular transcript of the angiotensin I-converting enzyme encodes for the ancestral, non-duplicated form of the enzyme. FEBS Lett 1989; 252:99–104.
145. Rodriguez-Boulan E, Nelson WJ: Morphogenesis of the polarized epithelial cell phenotype. Science 1989; 245:718–725.
146. Mostov K, Apodaca G, Aroeti B, Okamoto C. Plasma membrane protein sorting in polarized epithelial cells. J Cell Biol 1992; 116:577–583.
147. Schell MJ, Maurice M, Stieger B, Hubbard AL. 5′nucleotidase is sorted to the apical domain of hepatocytes via an indirect route. J Cell Biol 1992; 119:1173–1182.
148. Wessels HP, Hansen GH, Fuhrer C, et al. Aminopeptidase N is directly sorted to the apical domain in MDCK cells. J Cell Biol 1990; 111:2923–2930.
149. Casanova JE, Mishumi Y, Ikehara Y, et al. Direct apical sorting of rat liver dipeptidylpeptidase IV expressed in Madin-Darby canine kidney cells. J Biol Chem 1991; 266:24428–24432.
150. Low SH, Wong SH, Tang BL, et al. Apical cell surface expression of rat dipeptidyl peptidase IV in transfected Madin-Darby canine kidney cells. J Biol Chem 1991; 266:13391–13396.
151. Corbeil D, Boileau G, Lemay G, Crine P. Expression and polarized apical secretion in Madin-Darby canine kidney cells of a recombinant soluble form of neutral endopeptidase lacking the cytosolic and transmembrane domains. J Biol Chem 1992; 267:2798–2801.
152. Lemay G, Waksman G, Roques BP, et al. Fusion of a cleavable signal peptide to the ectodomain of neutral endopeptidase (EC 3.4.24.11) results in the secretion of an active enzyme in COS-1 cells. J Biol Chem 1989; 264:15620–15623.
153. Roy P, Chatellard C, Lemay G, et al. Transformation of the signal peptide/membrane anchor domain of a type II transmembrane protein into a cleavable signal peptide. J Biol Chem 1993; 268:2699–2704.
154. Crine P, Jalal F, Lanctot C, et al. Targeting of neutral endopeptidase-24.11 in polarized cells. Biochem Soc Trans 1993; 21:668–672.
155. Vogel LK, Noren O, Sjostrom H. The apical sorting signal on human aminopeptidase N is not located in the stalk but in the catalytic head group. FEB S Lett 1992; 308:14–17.
156. Vogel LK, Spiess M, Sjostrom H, Noren O. Evidence for an apical sorting signal on the ectodomain of human aminopeptidase N. J Biol Chem 1992; 267:2794–2797.
157. Low SH, Wong SH, Tang BL, Hong WJ. Involvement of both vectorial and transcytotic pathways in the

preferential apical cell surface localization of rat dipeptidyl peptidase IV in transfected LLC-PK1 cells. J Biol Chem 1991; 266:19710–19716.
158. Altman RA, Orr AV, Lagenaur CF, et al. Expression of rat renal gamma-glutamyltranspeptidase in LLC-PK1 cells as a model for apical targeting. Biochemistry 1993; 32:3822–3828.
159. Weisz OA, Machamer CE, Hubbard AL. Rat liver dipeptidylpeptidase IV contains competing apical and basolateral targeting information. J Biol Chem 1992; 267:22282–22288.
160. Low SH, Wong SH, Tang BL, Tan P, et al. Inhibition by brefeldin A of protein secretion from the apical cell surface of Madin-Darby canine kidney cells. J Biol Chem 1991; 266:17729–17732.
161. Low SH, Tang BL, Wong SH, Hong W. Selective inhibition of protein targeting to the apical domain of MDCK cells by brefeldin A. J Cell Biol 1992; 118:51–62.
162. Oster T, Thioudellet C, Chevalot I, et al. Induction of recombinant human gamma-glutamyl transferase by sodium butyrate in transfected V79 and CHO Chinese hamster cells. Biochem Biophys Res Commun 1993; 193:406–412.
163. Kondepudi A, Johnson A. et al. Cytokines increase neutral endopeptidase activity in lung fibroblasts. Am J Respir Cell Mol Biol 1993; 8:43–49.
164. Iijima H, Gerard NP, Squassoni C, et al. Exon 16 del: A novel form of human neutral endopeptidase (CALLA). Am J Physiol 1992; 262:L725–729.
165. Nanus DM, Pfeffer LM, Bander NH, et al. Antiproliferative and antitumor effects of alpha-interferon in renal cell carcinomas: Correlation with the expression of a kidney-associated differentiation glycoprotein. Cancer Res 1990; 50:4190–4194.
166. Mendrick DL, Rennke HG: I. Induction of proteinuria in the rat by a monoclonal antibody against SGP-115/107. Kidney Int 1988; 33:818.
167. Bruijn JA, van Leer EHG, Baelde JJ, et al. Characterization and in-vivo transfer of nephritogenic autoantibodies directed against dipeptidyl peptidase IV and laminin in experimental lupus nephritis. Lab Invest 1990; 63:350–359.
168. Mentzel S, Assmann KJM, van Son JPHF, et al. Enalapril and losartan reduce considerably the acute albuminuria induced by injection of a monoclonal antibody against aminopeptidase A in mice. J Am Soc Nephrol 1993; 4:620.
169. Ehlers MR, Chen YN, Riordan JF. Spontaneous solubilization of membrane-bound human testis angiotensin- converting enzyme expressed in Chinese hamster overy cells. Proc Natl Acad Sci USA 1991; 88:1009–1013.
170. Wei L, Alhenc-Gelas F, Soubrier F, et al. Expression and characterization of recombinant human angiotensin I–converting enzyme: Evidence for a C-terminal transmembrane anchor and for a proteolytic processing of the secreted recombinant and plasma enzymes. J Biol Chem 1991; 266:5540–5546.
171. Edgington TS, Glassock RJ, Dixon FJ. Autologous immune complex nephritis induced with renal tubular antigen: I. Identification and isolation of the pathogenic antigen. J Exp Med 1968; 127:555–572.
172. Miettinen A, Tîrnroth T, Tikkanen I, et al. Heymann nephritis induced by kidney brush border glycoproteins. Lab Invest 1980; 43:547–555.
173. Kerjaschki D, Farquhar MG. The pathogenic antigen of Heymann nephritis is a membrane glycoprotein of the renal proximal tubule brush border. Proc Natl Acad Sci USA 1982; 79:5557–5561.
174. Chatelet F, Brianti E, Ronco P, et al. Ultrastructural localization by monoclonal antibodies of brush border antigens expressed by glomeruli: II. Extrarenal distribution. Am J Pathol 1986; 122:512–519.
175. Doxsey S, Kerjaschki D, Farquhar MG: A large glycoprotein (gp330) is a resident of coated pits of several absorbtive epithelia (abstr). J Cell Biol 1984; 98:178a.
176. Orlando RA, Farquhar MG. Identification of a cell line that expresses a cell surface and a soluble form of the gp330/receptor-associated protein (RAP) Heymann nephritis antigenic complex. Proc Natl Acad Sci USA 1993; 90:4082–4086.
177. Lundstrom M, Orlando RA, Saedi MS, et al. Immunocytochemical and biochemical characterization of the Heymann nephritis antigenic complex in rat L2 yolk sac cells. Am J Pathol 1993; 143:1423–1435.
178. Le Panse S, Galceran M, Lelongt B, et al. Expression by a yolk sac epithelial cell line of two proteins of the intermicrovillar areas of proximal tubule epithelial cells (abstr). J Am Soc Nephrol 1993; 4:903.
179. Moestrup SK, Christensen EL, Neilsen S, et al. Binding and endocytosis of proteins mediated by epithelial gp330. Ann NY Acad Sci. In press.
180. Kerjaschki D, Farquhar MG. Immunocytochemical localization of the Heymann nephritis antigen (GP330) in glomerular epithelial cells of normal Lewis rats. J Exp Med 1983; 157:667–686.
181. Biemesderfer D, Dekan G, Aronson PS, Farquhar MG. Assembly of distinctive coated pit and microvillar microdomains in the renal brush border. Am J Physiol (Renal Fluid Electrolyte Physiol 31) 1992; 262:F55–F67.
182. Christensen EI, Gliemann J, Moestrup SK. Renal tubule pg330 is a calcium-binding receptor for endocytic uptake of protein. J Histochem Cytochem 1992; 40:1481–1490.
183. Christensen EI. Rapid membrane recycling in renal proximal tubule cells. Eur J Cell Biol 1982; 29:43–49.

184. Chatelet F, Brianti E, Ronco P, et al. Ultrastructural localization by monoclonal antibodies of brush border antigens expressed by glomeruli: I. Renal distribution. Am J Pathol 1986; 122:500–511.
185. Abbate M, Bachinsky D, Zheng G, et al. Location of gp330/α2-m receptor-associated protein (α2- MRAP) and its binding sites in kidney: Distribution of endogenous α2-MRAP is modified by tissue processing. Eur J Cell Biol 1993; 61:139–149.
186. Bachinsky DR, Zheng G, Niles JL, et al. Detection of two forms of GP330: Their role in Heymann nephritis. Am J Pathol 1993; 143:598–611.
187. Maunsbach AB. Observations on the segmentation of the proximal tubule in the rat kidney. J Ultrastruct Res 1966; 16:239–258.
188. Kerjaschki D, Horvat R, Binder S, et al. Identification of a 400-kd protein in the brush border of human kidney tubules that is similar to gp330, the nephritogenic antigen of rat Heymann nephritis. Am J Pathol 1987; 129:183–191.
189. Sahali D, Mulliez N, Chatelet F, et al. Comparative immunochemistry and ontogeny of two closely related coated pit proteins. Am J Pathol 1993; 142:1654–1667.
190. Christensen EI, Maunsbach AB. Proteinuria induced by sodium maleate in rats: Effects on ultrastructure and protein handling in renal proximal tubule. Kidney Int 1980; 17:771–787.
191. Gutmann EJ, Niles JL, McCluskey RT, Brown D. Colchicine-induced redistribution of an apical membrane glycoprotein (gp330) in proximal tubules. Am J Physiol (Cell Physiol 26) 1989; 257:C397–C407.
192. Gutmann EJ, Niles JL, McCluskey RT, Brown D. Loss of antigens associated with the apical endocytotic pathway in proximal tubules from rats with Heymann nephritis. Am J Pathol 1991; 138:1243–1255.
193. Christensen EI, Maunsbach AB. Effects of dextran on lysosomal ultrastructure and protein digestion in renal proximal tubule. Kidney Int 1979; 16:301–311.
194. Kitazawa K, Gorfien S, Brentjens JR, et al. Reabsorption of horseradish peroxidase by proximal tubules in rats with Heymann nephritis. Am J Kidney Dis 1986; 7:58–68.
195. Raychowdhury R, Niles JL, McCluskey RT, Smith JA. Autoimmune target in Heymann nephritis is a glycoprotein with homology to the LDL receptor. Science 1989; 244:1163–1165.
196. Moestrup SK, Nielsen S, Andreasen P, et al. Epithelial glycoprotein-330 mediates endocytosis of plasminogen activator-plasminogen activator inhibitor type-1 complexes. J Biol Chem 1993; 268:16564–16570.
197. Willnow TE, Goldstein JL, Orth K, et al. Low density lipoprotein receptor-related protein and gp330 bind similar ligands, including plasminogen activator-inhibitor complexes and lactoferrin, an inhibitor of chylomicron remnant clearance. J Biol Chem 1992; 267:26172–26180.
198. Kounnas MZ, Argraves WS, Strickland DK. The 39-kDa receptor-associated protein interacts with two members of the low density lipoprotein receptor family, α2-macroglobulin receptor and glycoprotein 330. J Biol Chem 1992; 267:21162–21166.
199. Herz J, Hamann U, Rogne S, et al. Surface location and high affinity for calcium of a 500-kd liver membrane protein closely related to the LDL-receptor suggest a physiological role as lipoprotein receptor. EMBO J 1988; 7:4119–4127.
200. Yamamoto T, Davis CG, Brown MS, et al. The human LDL receptor: A cysteine-rich protein with multiple Alu sequences in its mRNA. Cell 1984; 39:27–38.
201. Goldstein JL, Brown MS, Anderson RGW, et al. Receptor-mediated endocytosis: Concepts emerging from the LDL receptor system. Annu Rev Cell Biol 1985; 1:1–39.
202. Russell DW, Brown MS, Goldstein JL. Different combinations of cysteine-rich repeats mediate binding of low density lipoprotein receptor to two different proteins. J Biol Chem 1989; 264:21682–21688.
203. Moestrup SK, Holtet TL, Etzerodt M, et al. α2-Macroglobulin-proteinase complexes, plasminogen activator inhibitor type-1-plasminogen activator complexes, and receptor- associated protein bind to a region of the α2-macroglobulin receptor containing a cluster of eight complement-type repeats. J Biol Chem 1993; 268:13691–13696.
204. Chen WJ, Goldstein JL, Brown MS. NPXY, a sequence often found in cytoplasmic tails, is required for coated pit-mediated internalization of the low density lipoprotein receptor. J Biol Chem 1990; 265:3116–3123.
205. Maunsbach AB, Christensen EI. Functional ultrastructure of the proximal tubule. In: Windhager EE, ed, Handbook of Physiology: Renal Physiology. Washington DC: New York: Oxford University Press, 1992:41–107.
206. Christensen EI, Neilsen S. Structural and functional features of protein handling in the kidney proximal tubule. Semin Nephrol 1991; 11:414–439.
207. Maack T, Park CH, Camargo MJF. Renal filtration, transport and metabolism of proteins, in Seldin DW, Giebisch G, eds. The Kidney: Physiology and Pathophysiology. New York: Raven Press, 1985:1773–1803.
208. Orlando RA, Kerjaschki D, Kurihara H, et al. GP330 associates with a 44-kDa protein in the rat kidney to form the Heymann nephritis antigenic complex. Proc Natl Acad Sci USA 1992; 89:6698–6702.
209. Kanalas JJ, Makker SP. Identification of the rat Heymann nephritis autoantigen (GP330) as a receptor site for plasminogen. J Biol Chem 1991; 266:10825–10829.

210. Mendrick DL, Chung DC, Rennke HG. Heymann antigen GP330 demonstrates affinity for fibronectin, laminin, and type I collagen and mediates rat proximal tubule epithelial cell adherence to such matrices in vitro. Exp Cell Res 1990; 188:23–35.
211. Kounnas MZ, Chappell DA, Strickland DK, Argraves WS. Glycoprotein 330, a member of the low density lipoprotein receptor family, binds lipoprotein lipase in vitro. J Biol Chem 1993; 268:14176–14181.
212. Jensen PH, Moestrup SK, Gliemann J. Purification of the human placental alpha2-macroglobulin receptor. FEBS Lett 1989; 255:275–280.
213. Ashcom JD, Tiller SE, Dickerson K, et al. The human alfa2-macroglobulin receptor: Identification of A420-kD cell surface glycoprotein specific for the activated conformation of alfa2-macroglobulin. J Cell Biol 1990; 110:1941–1048.
214. Kristensen T, Moestrup SK, Gliemann J, et al. Evidence that the newly cloned low-density-lipoprotein receptor related protein (LRP) is the α2-macroglobulin receptor. FEBS Lett 1990; 276:151–155.
215. Strickland DK, Ashcom JD, Williams S, et al. Sequence identity between the alpha 2-macroglobulin receptor and low density lipoprotein receptor-related protein suggests that this molecule is a multifunctional receptor. J Biol Chem 1990; 265:17401–17404.
216. Herz J. The LDL receptor related protein—Portrait of a multifunctional receptor. Curr Opin Lipid 1994; 4:107–113.
217. Ronco P, Neale TJ, Wilson CB, et al. An immunopathological study of a 330 kD protein defined by monoclonal antibodies and reactive with anti-RTEa5 antibodies and kidney eluates from active Heymann nephritis. J Immunol 1986; 136:125–130.
218. Kerjaschki D, Miettinen A, Farquhar MG. Initial events in the formation of immune deposits in passive Heymann nephritis. J Exp Med 1987; 166:109–128.
219. van Leer EHG, Ronco P, Verroust P, et al. Epitope-specificity of anti-gp330 autoantibodies determines the development of proteinuria in active Heymann nephritis (HN). Am J Pathol 1993; 142:821–829.
220. Allegri L, Brianti E, Chatelet F, et al. Polyvalent antigen-antibody interactions are required for the formation of electron-dense immune deposits in passive Heymann's nephritis. Am J Pathol 1986; 126:1–6.
221. Pietromonaco S, Kerjaschki D, Binder S, et al. Molecular cloning of a cDNA encoding a major pathogenic domain of the Heymann nephritis antigen gp330 Proc Natl Acad Sci USA 1990; 87:1811–1815.
222. Huang J, Makker SP. Role of 39-45 KD receptor associated protein (RAP) in active Heymann nephritis (HN). J Am Soc Nephrol 1993; 4:606.
223. Sahali D, Mulliez N, Chatelet F, et al. Characterization of a 280-kD protein restricted to the coated pits of the renal brush border and the epithelial cells of the yolk sac: Teratogenic effect of the specific monoclonal antibodies. J Exp Med 1988; 167:213–218.
224. Sahali D, Mulliez N, Chatelet F, et al. Comparative immunochemistry and ontogeny of two closely related coated pit proteins: The 280 kDa target of teratogenic antibodies and the 330 kDa target of neprhitogenic antibodies. Am J Pathol 1992; 142:1654–1667.
225. Sahali D, Mulliez N, Chatelet F, et al. Coexpression in man by kidney and fetal envelopes of a 280kDa coated pit restricted protein: Similarity with the murine target of teratogenic antibodies. Am J Pathol 1992; 140:33–44.
226. Sahali D, Mulliez N, Chatelet F, et al. Specific inhibition of endocytosis by monoclonal antibodies to a 280 kDa coated pit restricted brush border (BB) protein (abstr). J Am Soc Nephrol 1990; 1:730.
227. Le Panse S, Galceran M, Pontillon F, et al. Characterisation of a yolk sac epithelial cell line which expresses two proteins gp280 and gp330 of the intermicrovillar area of proximal tubule cells: Inhibition of endocytosis by the specific antibodies. Eur J Cell Biol 1995. In press.
228. Le Panse S, Galceran M, Roux Ch, et al. Antibodies to the 280 kDa coated pit protein target of teratogenic antibodies produce alterations in the traffic of internalised proteins. Am J Pathol 1994; 145:1526–1536.
229. Cui S, Flyvbjerg A, Nielsen S, et al. IGF-II/Man-6-P receptors in rat kidney: Apical localization in proximal tubule cells. Kidney Int 1993; 43:796–807.
230. Corrocher R, Abramson RG, King VF, et al. Differential binding of folates by rat renal cortex brush border and basolateral membrane preparations. Proc Soc Exp Biol Med 1985; 78:73–84.
231. Selhub J, Emmanouel D, Stavropoulos T, Arnold R. Renal folate absorption and the kidney folate binding protein: I. Urinary clearance studies. Am J Physiol (Renal Fluid Electrolyte Physiol 21) 1987; 252:F750–F756.
232. Selhub J, Franklin WA. The folate binding protein of rat kidney. Purification, properties and cellular distribution. J Biol Chem 1984; 259:6601–6606.
233. Selhub J, Nakamura S, Carone FA. Renal folate absorption and the kidney folate binding protein. II. Microinfusion studies. Am J Physiol (Renal Fluid Electrolyte Physiol 21) 1987; 252:F757–F760.
234. Hjelle JT, Christensen EI, Carone FA, Selhub J. Cell fractionation and electron microscope studies of kidney folate-binding protein. Am J Physiol (Cell Physiol 29) 1991; 260:C338–C346.
235. Rothberg KG, Ying Y, Kolhouse JF, et al. The glycophospholipid-linked folate receptor internalizes folate without entering the clathrin-coated pit endocytic pathway. J Cell Biol 1990; 110:637–649.

236. Birn H, Selhub J, Christensen EI. Internalization and intracellular transport of folate-binding protein in rat kidney proximal tubule. Am J Physiol Cell Physiol 1993; 264:C302–C310.
237. Agre P, Preston GM, Smith BL, et al. Aquaporin CHIP: The archetypal molecular water channel. Am J Physiol 1993; 265:F463–F476.
238. Denker BM, Smith BL, Kuhajda FP, Agre P. Identification, purification and partial characterization of a novel Mr 28,000 integral membrane protein from erythrocytes and renal tubules. J Biol Chem 1988; 263:15634–15642.
239. Agre P, Saboori AM, Asimos A, Smith BL. Purification and partial characterization of the Mr 30,000 integral membrane protein associated with the erythrocyte Rh(D)antigen. J Biol Chem 1987; 262:17497–17503.
240. Smith BL, Agre P. Erythrocyte Mr 28,000 transmembrane protein exists as a multisubunit oligomer similar to channel proteins. J Biol Chem 1991; 266:6407–6415.
241. Preston GM, Agre P. Isolation of the cDNA for erythrocyte integral membrane protein of 28 kilodaltons: Member of an ancient channel family. Proc Natl Acad Sci USA 1991; 88:11110–11114.
242. Zeidel ML, Ambudkar SV, Smith BL, Agre P. Reconstitution of functional water channels in liposomes containing purified red cell CHIP28 protein. Biochemistry 1992; 31:7436–7440.
243. Zeidel ML, Nielsen S, Smith BL, et al. Ultrastructure, pharmacological inhibition and transport selectivity of aquaporin CHIP in proteoliposomes. Biochemistry 1994; 33:1605–1615.
244. Preston GM, Jung JS, Guggino WB, Agre P. Membrane topology of aquaporin CHIP: Analysis of functional epitope-scanning mutants by vectorial proteolysis. J Biol Chem. In press.
245. Walz T, Smith BL, Zeidel ML, et al. Biologically active two-dimensional crystals of aquaporin CHIP. J Biol Chem 1994; 269:1583–1586.
246. Preston GM, Jung JS, Guggino WB, Agre P. The mercury-sensitive residue at cysteine 189 in the CHIP28 water channel. J Biol Chem 1993; 268:17–20.
247. Verbavatz JM, Brown D, Sabolic I, et al. Tetrameric assembly of CHIP28 water channels in liposomes and cell membranes: A freeze-fracture study. J Cell Biol 1993; 123:605–618.
248. Nielsen S, Smith B, Christensen EI, et al. CHIP 28 water channels are localized in constitutively water-permeable segments of the nephron. J Cell Biol 1993; 120:371–383.
249. Sabolic I, Valenti G, Verbavatz JM, et al. Localization of the CHIP28 water channel in rat kidney. Am J Physiol 1992; 263:C1225–C1233.
250. Deen PM, Dempster JA, Wieringa B, van Os CH. Isolation of a cDNA for rat CHIP28 water channel: High mRNA expression in kidney cortex and inner medulla. Biochem Biophys Res Commun 1992; 188:1267–1273.
251. Lanahan A, Williams JB, Sanders LK, Nathans D. Growth factor-induced delayed early response genes. Mol Cell Biol 1992; 12:3919–3929.
252. Bondy C, Chin E, Smith BL, et al. Developmental gene expression and tissue distribution of the CHIP28 water-channel protein. Proc Natl Acad Sci USA 1993; 90:4500–4504.
253. Brown D, Verbavatz JM, Valenti G, et al. Localization of the CHIP28 water channel in reabsorptive segments of the rat male reproductive tract. Eur J Cell Biol 1993; 61:264–273.
254. Nielsen S, Smith BL, Christensen EI, Agre P. Distribution of aquaporin CHIP in secretory and resorptive epithelia and capillary endothelia. Proc Natl Acad Sci USA 1993; 90:7275–7279.
255. Anwer MS. Anatomy and physiology of bile formation. In: Progress in Pharmacology and Clinical Pharmacology, Vol. 8/4. Stuttgart and New York: Gustav Fischer Verlag, 1991:3–23.
256. Smith BL, Baumgarten R, Neilsen S, et al. Concurrent expression of erythroid and renal aquaporin CHIP and appearance of water channel activity in perinatal rats [see comments]. J Clin Invest 1993; 92:2035–2041.
257. Fushimi K, Uchida S, Hara Y, et al. Cloning and expression of apical membrane water channel of rat kidney collecting tubule. Nature 1993; 361:549–552.
258. Knepper MA, Rector FC Jr. Urinary concentration and dilution. In: Brenner IBM, Rector FC, eds. The Kidney, Philadelphia and London: Saunders, 1991:445–482.
259. Nielsen S, Knepper MA. Vasopressin activates collecting duct urea transports and water channels by distinct physical processes. Am J Physiol 1993; 265:F204–F213.
260. Knepper MA, Nielsen S. Kinetic model of water and urea permeability regulation by vasopressin in collecting duct. Am J Physiol 1993; 265:F214–F224.
261. Nielsen S, Di Giovanni SR, Christensen EI, et al. Cellular and subcellular immunolocalization of vasopressin-regulated water channel in rat kidney. Proc Natl Acad Sci USA 1993; 90:11663–11667.
262. Nielsen S, Muller J, Knepper MA. Vasopressin- and cAMP-induced changes in the ultrastructure of isolated perfused inner medullary collecting ducts. Am J Physiol 1993; 265.
263. Wade JB, Stetson DL, Lewis SA, ADH action: evidence for a membrane shuttle mechanism. Ann NY Acad Sci 81; 372:106–117.
264. Brown D. Membrane recycling and epithelial cell function. Am J Physiol 1989; 256:F1–12.
265. Quigg RJ, Nicholson-Weller A, Cybulsky AV, et al. Decay accelerating factor regulates complement activation on glomerular epithelial cells. J Immunol 1989; 142:877–882.

266. Cosio FG, Sedmak DD, Mahan JD, Nahman NS Jr. Localization of decay accelerating factor in normal and diseased kidneys. Kidney Int 1989; 36:100–107.
267. White DJ, Oglesby T, Liszewski MK, et al. Expression of human decay accelerating factor or membrane cofactor protein genes on mouse cells inhibits lysis by human complement. Transplant Proc 1992; 24:474–476.
268. Molina H, Wong W, Kinoshita T, et al. Distinct receptor and regulatory properties of recombinant mouse complement receptor 1 (CR1) and Crry, the two genetic homologues of human CR1. J Exp Med 1992; 175:121–129.
269. Hourcade D, Holers VM, Atkinson JP. The regulators of complement activation (RCA) gene cluster (review). Adv Immunol 1989; 45:381–416.
270. Holers VM, Kinoshita T, Molina H. The evolution of mouse and human complement C3-binding proteins: Divergence of form but conservation of function (review). Immunol Today 1992; 13:231–236.
271. Krych M, Atkinson JP, Holers VM: Complement receptors (review). Curr Opin Immunol 1992; 4:8–13.
272. Klickstein LB, Wong WW, Smith JA, et al. Human C3b/C4b receptor (CR1): Demonstration of long homologous repeating domains that are composed of the short consensus repeats characteristics of C3/C4 binding proteins. J Exp Med 1987; 165:1095–1112.
273. Caras IW, Davitz MA, Rhee L, et al. Cloning of decay-accelerating factor suggests novel use of splicing to generate two proteins. Nature 1987; 325:545–549.
274. Davies A, Simmons DL, Hale G, et al. CD59, an LY-6-like protein expressed in human lymphoid cells, regulates the action of the complement membrane attack complex on homologous cells. J Exp Med 1989; 170:637.
275. Meri S, Morgan BP, Davies A, et al. Human protectin (CD59), an 18,000-20,000 MW complement lysis restricting factor, inhibits C5b-8-catalysed insertion of C9 into lipid bilayers. Immunology 1990; 71:1.
276. Rooney IA, Davies A, Griffiths D, et al. The complement-inhibiting protein, protectin (CD59 antigen), is present and functionally active on glomerular epithelial cells. Clin Exp Immunol 1991; 83:251–256.
277. Schonermark S, Rauterberg EW, Shin ML, et al. Homologous species restriction in lysis of human erythrocytes: A membrane derived protein with C8 binding capacity functions as an inhibitor. J Immunol 1986; 138:1772.
278. Watts MJ, Dankert JR, Morgan BP. Isolation and characterisation of a membrane attack complex inhibiting protein present in human serum and other biological fluids. Biochem J 1990; 265:471.
279. Moore MD, Cooper NR, Tack BF, Nemerow GR. Molecular cloning of the cDNA encoding the Epstein-Barr virus/C3d receptor (complement receptor type 2) of human B lymphocytes. Proc Natl Acad Sci USA 1987; 84:9194–9198.
280. Lublin DM, Liszewski MK, Post TW, et al. Molecular cloning and chromosomal localization of human membrane cofactor protein (MCP): Evidence for inclusion in the multigene family of complement-regulatory proteins. J Exp Med 1988; 168:181–194.
281. Appay MD, Kazatchkine MD, Levi-Strauss M, et al. Expression of CR1 (CD35) mRNA in podocytes from adult and fetal human kidneys. Kidney Int 1990; 38:289–293.
282. Hourcade D, Post TW, Holers VM, et al. Polymorphisms of the regulators of complement activation gene cluster (Review). Comp Inflamm 1990; 7:302–314.
283. Hourcade D, Miesner DR, Bee C, et al. Duplication and divergence of the amino-terminal coding region of the complement receptor 1 (CR1) gene: An example of concerted (horizontal) evolution within a gene. J Biol Chem 1990; 265:974–980.
284. Kerjaschki D, Schulze M, Binder S, et al. Transcellular transport and membrane insertion of the C5b-9 membrane attack complex of complement by glomerular epithelial cells in experimental membranous nephropathy. J Immunol 1989; 143:546–552.
285. Quigg RJ, Cybulsky AV, Salant DJ. Effect of nephritogenic antibody on complement regulation in cultured rat glomerular epithelial cells. J Immunol 1991; 147:838–845.
286. Shibata T, Cosio FG, Birmingham DJ. Complement activation induces the expression of decay-accelerating factor on human mesangial cells. J Immunol 1991; 147:3901–3908.
287. Kazatchkine MD, Fearon DT, Appay MD, et al. Immunohistochemical study of the human glomerular C3b receptor in normal kidney and in seventy-five cases of renal diseases: Loss of C3b receptor antigen in focal hyalinosis and in proliferative nephritis of systemic lupus erythematosus. J Clin Invest 82; 69:900–912.
288. Kumar S, Muchmore A. Tamm-Horsfall protein—uromodulin (1950–1990) (review). Kidney Int 1990; 37:1395–1401.
289. Ronco P, Brunisholz M, Geniteau-Legendre M, et al. Physiopathologic aspects of Tamm-Horsfall protein: A phylogenetically conserved marker of the thick ascending limb of Henle's loop. Adv Nephrol 1987; 16:231–250.
290. Serafini-Cessi F, Malagolini N, Hoops TC, Rindler MJ. Biosynthesis and oligosaccharide processing of human Tamm-Horsfall glycoprotein permanently expressed in HeLa cells. Biochem Biophys Res Commun 1993; 194:784–790.

291. Sathyamoorthy N, Decker JM, Sherblom AP, Muchmore A. Evidence that specific high mannose structures directly regulate multiple cellular activities. Mol Cell Biochem 1991; 102:139–147.
292. Brunisholz M, Geniteau-Legendre M, Ronco P, et al. Production and characterization of monoclonal antibodies specific for human Tamm Horsfall protein. Kidney Int 1986; 29:971–976.
293. Hession C, Decker JM, Sherblom AP, et al. Uromodulin (Tamm-Horsfall glycoprotein): A renal ligand for lymphokines. Science 1987; 237:1479–1484.
294. Pennica D, Kohr WJ, Kuang WJ, et al. Identification of human uromodulin as the Tamm-Horsfall urinary glycoprotein. Science 1987; 236:83–88.
295. Rindler MJ, Naik SS, Li N, et al. Uromodulin (Tamm-Horsfall glycoprotein/uromucoid) is a phosphatidylinositol-linked membrane protein. J Biol Chem 1990; 265:20784–20789.
296. Bachmann S, Metzger R, Bunnemann B. Tamm-Horsfall protein-mRNA synthesis is localized to the thick ascending limb of Henle's loop in rat kidney. Histochemistry 1990; 94:517–523.
297. Muchmore AV, Sathyamoorthy N, Decker J, Sherblom AP. Evidence that specific high-mannose oligosaccharides can directly inhibit antigen-driven T-cell responses. J Leuk Biol 1990; 48:457–464.
298. Winkelstein A, Muchmore AV, et al. Uromodulin: A specific inhibitor of IL-1-initiated human T cell colony formation. Immunopharmacology 1990; 20:201–205.
299. Sherblom AP, Sathyamoorthy N, Decker JM, Muchmore AV: Il-2, a lectin with specificity for high mannose glycopeptides. J Immunol 1989; 143:939–944.
300. Fukuoka S, Freedman SD, Yu H, et al. GP-2/THP gene family encodes self-binding glycosyl-phosphatidylinositol-anchored proteins in apical secretory compartments of pancreas and kidney. Proc Natl Acad Sci USA 1992; 89:1189–1193.
301. Hoops TC, Rindler MJ. Isolation of the cDNA encoding glycoprotein-2 (GP-2), the major zymogen granule membrane protein: Homology to uromodulin/Tamm-Horsfall protein. J Biol Chem 1991; 266:4257–4263.
302. Freedman SD, Sakamoto K, Venu RP. GP2, the homologue to the renal cast protein uromodulin, is a major component of intraductal plugs in chronic pancreatitis. J Clin Invest 1993; 92:83–90.
303. Huang ZQ, Kirk KA, Connelly KG, Sanders PW. Bence Jones proteins bind to a common peptide segment of Tamm-Horsfall glycoprotein to promote heterotypic aggregation. J Clin Invest 1993; 92:2975–2983.
304. Schroter J, Timmermans G, Seyberth HW, et al. Marked reduction of Tamm-Horsfall protein synthesis in hyperprostaglandin E-syndrome. Kidney Int 1993; 44:401–410.
305. Storch S, Saggi S, Megyesi J, et al. Ureteral obstruction decreases renal pre-pro-epidermal growth factor and Tamm-Horsfall expression. Kidney Int 1992; 42:89–94.
306. Kerjaschki D, Poczewski H, Dekan G, et al. Identification of a major sialoprotein in the glycocalyx of human visceral glomerular epithelial cells. J Clin Invest 1986; 78:1142–1149.
307. Kershaw D, Tomas P, Goyal M, et al. Isolation of glomerular epithelial cell podocalyxin cDNA (abstr). J Am Soc Nephrol 1993; 4:610.
308. Ronco P, Sahali D, Cittanova ML, et al. Monoclonal antibodies to glomerular antigens. Nephrol Dial Transplant 1992; suppl 1:9–15.
309. Huang TW, Langlois JC. Podoendin: A new cell surface protein of the podocyte and endothelium. J Exp Med 1985; 162:245–267.
310. Miettinen A, Dekan G, Farquhar MG. Monoclonal antibodies against membrane proteins of the rat glomerulus: Immunochemical specificity and immunofluorescence distribution of the antigens. Am J Pathol 1990; 137:929–944.
311. Reivinen J, Holthöfer H, Miettinen A. A cell-type specific ganglioside of glomerular podocytes in rat kidney: An O-acetylated GD3. Kidney Int 1992; 42:624–631.
312. Fukatsu A, Yuzawa Y, Olson E, et al. Interaction of antibodies with human glomerular epithelial cells. Lab Invest 1989; 61:389–403.
313. Orikasa M, Matsui K, Oite T, Shimizu F. Massive proteinuria induced in rats by a single intravenous injection of a monoclonal antibody. J Immunol 1988; 141:807–814.
314. Cittanova ML, Chatelet F, Ardaillou N, et al. Identification of a 135-kDa protein expressed at the sole of human podocyte foot processes and on the human podocyte clonal cell line HGVEC.SV1A4 (abstr). J Am Soc Nephrol 1992; 3:579.
315. Saito A, Pietromonaco S, Loo AK-C, Farquhar MG. Complete cloning and sequencing of rat gp330/"megalin," a distinctive member of the low-density-lipoprotein receptor gene family. Proc Natl Acad Sci USA 1994; 91:9725–9729.

51

Molecular Biology Approach to Human Kidney Biopsies

Liliane J. Striker, Emmanuel E. Peten, Chih-Wei Yang, and Gary E. Striker
National Institute of Diabetes, Digestive, and Kidney Diseases, National Institutes of Health, Bethesda, Maryland

INTRODUCTION

The aim of this chapter is to review the current knowledge on the application of molecular biology tools to renal biopsies and to propose a new strategy, based on our preliminary data, for the study of human diseases using renal biopsy material.

The general availability of molecular techniques has dramatically changed the face of the experimental pathology and cellular biology of the kidney, as reviewed in this book. However, there are very few data on renal biopsies, because many of these methods lack the sensitivity required for application to these small fragments of tissue.

This review may certainly have overlooked some publications, because many studies are still in abstract form. In addition, some studies contain very few cases, making their interpretation problematic.

Since the early 1960s, needle renal biopsies have contributed to a large body of descriptive information about a variety of renal diseases (1). However, the analysis of molecular events in renal biopsy tissue has been hampered by the difficulty of obtaining large enough samples. Large kidney tissue samples are not generally available, since most kidney diseases are not fatal and the incidental removal of renal tissue is not common. This contrasts with the situation encountered by cancer pathologists, for instance, who have large fragments of tumor tissue available for analysis, or by geneticists, who can obtain accurate information from blood samples. The amount of tissue that can be obtained from a renal biopsy is limited because the two or three cores of tissue provided to the renal pathologist are fully committed for clinical diagnostic purposes, light and immunofluorescence microscopy, and, in selected cases, electron microscopy and morphometry. Ethical considerations have sharply limited the amount of tissue that can be devoted to experimental techniques in the United States, as in many other countries, and this has certainly slowed progress in the understanding of the molecular events underlying human renal diseases (2). The potential availability of molecular analysis has raised expectations about their immediate application to human renal diseases. However, their use has been very limited because they often require the sacrifice of an additional core of renal biopsy, since the tissue requires different handling and preservation.

The scope of this chapter is limited to examination of the molecular analysis of responses that are thought to uniquely affect the diseased kidney. It does not consider genetic defects of a systemic nature, such as those occurring in Alport's syndrome or in Denys-Drasch syndrome, since the gene defect is present in all somatic cells and analysis can be performed with circulating cells (3–6). The detection of DNA or of mRNA in biopsy samples will be envisaged separately.

DETECTION OF DNA IN HUMAN BIOPSY SPECIMENS

Detection of Viral Genomic DNA

The detection of noneukaryotic DNA in a renal biopsy most often signals the presence of viruses, which have often been implicated in renal disease. Although new and interesting information has emerged from the use of molecular biology techniques, many questions remain about the link between virus infections and renal disease. Since the development of the polymerase chain reaction (PCR), the detection of viruses has been simplified (7). PCR provides an enormous advantage, since viruses can be found in a minute sample, but it has the drawback that the presence of an occasional infected blood-borne cell in a capillary or an arteriole could give a spuriously positive signal (8). This may lead to the incorrect conclusion that the viral material identified has relevance to a disease process.

Nevertheless, the analysis of viral sequences may solve some of the controversies concerning the role of hepatitis viruses, cytomegalovirus, and HIV in renal disease. These new data, and other information on the role of viruses in renal disease, must be interpreted with caution. The discovery of viral genome sequences in a renal biopsy constitutes only a presumption that a virus plays a causative role in a disease. The presence of viral sequences does not provide data on their expression or their significance in disease (9). However, the absence of viral sequences should serve to eliminate such a causative role.

Cytomegalovirus

Infection by cytomegalovirus (CMV) is a major cause of morbidity and of mortality in transplant recipients. Several studies, using PCR, report finding CMV DNA sequences in renal biopsies. Gnann et al. (8) found CMV gene sequences by in situ hybridization in infiltrating cells of renal biopsies obtained from infected transplant recipients. Chen et al. (10) examined paraffin-embedded material from 16 renal biopsies and from 21 nephrectomies fixed in Bouin's fixative or in formalin. After a sufficient number of sections were obtained for routine diagnosis, DNA was extracted from the biopsy tissue following deparaffinization. Using primers from the late antigen region of the CMV virus, they were able to detect amplified products by Southern blot analysis following electrophoresis and ethidium bromide staining in three biopsy and three nephrectomy specimens. All PCR-positive patients had a significant CMV infection, proven by a positive culture or by seroconversion. In addition, CMV-seropositive patients who did not have evidence of active infection were PCR-negative. The advantages of this method were its sensitivity, the absence of false-positive results, and the fact that it allowed a distinction between active and inactive infection. It may, therefore, have immediate clinical applications, particularly since the results can be obtained within a short time.

Another study (11) confirmed the fact that CMV DNA sequences were often present in transplant recipients and that PCR-based methods could yield positive results in samples negative by in situ hybridization.

Other diseases processes have recently been examined. Muller et al. (12) extracted DNA from cryostat sections of biopsies from patients with various glomerular diseases. They compared results in 10 patients with IgA nephropathy and 7 patients with focal sclerosis with 9 normal kidneys obtained from normal donors prior to transplantation. They found CMV DNA in all of the IgA nephropathies but in none of those with focal sclerosis. Three of the normal kidneys were also positive. In the recent study of Kadereit et al (9), PCR was utilized to detect CMV sequences in a series of 27 patients undergoing renal biopsy for a variety of renal diseases. No transplant recipients were included in the series. The detection of genomic DNA was performed on a core of renal tissue from which DNA was extracted by phenol following treatment with proteinase K. The incidence of a positive signal was quite high, since 37% of the specimens contained CMV DNA. Of the 20 patients with serologic evidence of CMV infection, 8 were PCR-positive. Interestingly, a dot-blot probe was positive in only 3 subjects from this group, confirming the higher sensitivity of the PCR-based method. Another group of samples came from seronegative patients and, surprisingly, 3 out of 10 samples contained CMV DNA. These data confirm the fact that PCR-based methods may detect CMV viral sequences in the absence of other signs of infection. It is interesting to note that patients from both groups had a wide variety of glomerular and other renal diseases. The significance of these findings is not yet fully understood and the role of CMV in renal disease unassociated with transplantation rejection is far from established. Finally, Liu recently found CMV DNA in several patients with IgA nephropathy and reached somewhat opposite conclusions than the previous article (13). She postulated that the virus may play a significant role in this disease.

HIV Virus

Epidemiological, immunochemical, and morphological data established a role for HIV in the development of glomerular disease (14). However, the demonstration of HIV in glomeruli awaited the study of Cohen et al. (15). They found viral DNA in renal biopsies or in kidneys of affected individuals by in situ hybridization, using paraffin slides from routinely fixed kidneys. Although the number of biopsy specimens was small, these investigators made several interesting observations. In patients with the glomerular lesion known as HIV-associated nephropathy, many positive cells were found both in the tubules and glomeruli. Parietal or visceral epithelial cells were the only positive glomerular cells. In contrast, in immune-complex–mediated glomerulonephritis in HIV patients, most of the viral sequences were found in tubular cells. There were apparently no false-positive findings, since samples from HIV-negative patients with other forms of renal disease contained no labeled cells. Finally, the tissues from patients with HIV infection but no renal disease contained only a few tubular cells positive for viral sequences. In summary, these observations suggest that HIV DNA is found only in glomerular cells of patients with glomerular disease but does not account for the differences in the types of glomerular disease.

Recently, Kimmel et al. examined DNA extracted from renal biopsy tissue for the presence of the *gag* region of the HIV proviral genome by PCR (16). They microdissected glomeruli, tubules, and even a few interstitial cells from paraffin sections routinely fixed for diagnostic purposes. They examined 28 biopsies from proteinuric patients with HIV infection and found that 95.5% were positive, irrespective of the type of glomerular lesion present. In contrast, no HIV DNA was found in 10 biopsies of patients who were HIV-negative and did not appear to carry any of the risk factor associated with HIV infection. However, they also found HIV DNA in HIV-infected patients without renal disease. This study confirmed the presence of HIV DNA in HIV-associated nephropathy but also suggested that it is only permissive and requires some other factors.

More recently, the same investigators (17) examined renal tissue from 4 HIV positive patients with immune-complex glomerular disease. They found HIV DNA in the circulating immune-complexes of 3 of 4 patients as well as in immune complexes eluted from 4 of 4 renal biopsies. This study illustrates the new possibilities offered by PCR-based techniques and is opening new avenues in the exploration of immune-complex–mediated disease.

Hepatitis C

There have been multiple attempts to define a role for hepatitis viruses in glomerular diseases, such as membranous and membranoproliferative glomerulonephritis (GN). Recently, Misiani and colleagues suggested that hepatitis C infection was a potential culprit in the development of type I membranoproliferative GN and mixed cryoglobulinemia (18). Johnson et al. (19) further confirmed these findings, and showed that the cryoprecipitate isolated from a group patients with mixed cryoglobulinemia and glomerular disease contained PCR-detectable hepatitis C nucleic acid material. Further demonstration will require the use of PCR-based methods directly applied to renal biopsy tissue. Since this would require only the detection of viral material, archival biopsies may provide the answer to this question.

In that respect, hepatitis C viral sequences were found by Davda et al. in two transplant recipients with membranous GN who had circulating antibodies against hepatitis C (20). RT-PCR was performed on formalin-fixed and paraffin-embedded biopsy tissue, revealing hepatitis C DNA in both samples. Interestingly, no positive signal was obtained by in situ hybridization using a digoxigenin-labeled probe. Furthermore, HCV antigens were not found by immunochemistry. These data were interpreted by the authors as consistent with the presence of only a small number of copies, which required the exquisite sensitivity of PCR methods for detection.

MRNA DETECTION AND MEASUREMENT

Introduction

The ultimate proof that a gene is expressed in human kidney and plays a role in a given disease requires the detection and/or measurement of the corresponding mRNA and ultimately of its product. If the mRNA is expressed in normal kidneys, quantitative methods are required to accurately measure the amplitude of the increase. This last point emphasizes the potential difficulty of obtaining valid control samples, since renal biopsies are never performed in subjects without renal disease. Several well-established methods provide accurate and quantitative measures of mRNA, such as Northern analysis and the S-nuclease protection assay. Unfortunately, since they require the use of large quantities of extracted RNA, they are not applicable to needle biopsy samples (21) and even less to isolated glomeruli. The use of in situ hybridization has yielded some interesting results, but this methodology can be applied only to high-signal molecules and is semiquantitative at best.

If we had at our disposal highly sensitive and quantitative methods capable of detecting mRNAs on paraffin sections, they could be easily applied to a large number of human biopsies without compromising the diagnosis and without submitting the patient to the extra risk involved in obtaining an additional sample for a "research biopsy" (2). The availability of nephrectomies performed for cancer has allowed preliminary analysis of human material, but these kidneys do not constitute perfect normal controls, nor do they adequately model the wide range of renal diseases (22). For these reasons, we developed a method that combines microdissection of human glomeruli and competitive PCR which is applicable to renal biopsies (23).

Several categories of genes have been examined in renal disease, depending on the nature of the questions to be addressed. These include several cytokines, a serine protease specific for cytotoxic T lymphocytes, and some components of the glomerular extracellular matrix (ECM) (22,24–29) type IV collagen α chains, and the tissue inhibitors of metalloproteinase (TIMPs). Because there are very few published data on renal biopsies, we will review data from our laboratory that have been generated from experimental animals and applied to nephrectomies and renal biopsies.

Cytokines

Experimental data suggest that multiple cytokines are implicated in glomerular and tubulointerstitial disease, even in the absence of signs of inflammation. Glomerular cells not only respond to multiple growth factors but also synthesize many growth factors in vitro (30–32). The exact contribution of the various cytokines to renal disease in humans is still largely unknown, and most of the current hypotheses are based on animal data (32–35).

Transplant Recipients

Several cytokines have been examined in biopsies from transplant recipients using in situ hybridization or PCR-based methods. The expression of IL-6, TNFα, and interferon gamma genes was investigated in a series of transplant recipients (25). Biopsies of five patients without signs of rejection and eight patients with acute rejection were compared with four biopsies and one nephrectomy specimen without morphological evidence of renal disease. The authors used in situ hybridization performed with RNA probes of high specific activity that could detect 1 to 5 copies per cell. They detected no transcript for any of these cytokines in the normal kidneys or in any of the transplants with stable renal function. Elevated levels of IL-6 were found in cells from all the compartments of the kidney in patients with acute rejection. TNF-α mRNA was found only in one patient with acute rejection, in clusters of cells surrounding some tubules.

Another study (24) of a large series of transplant biopsies, using a method based on PCR analysis, found somewhat opposite results. RNA was obtained by extraction from a core of renal biopsy, reverse-transcribed, and analyzed by PCR. The genes coding for IL-IB, TNF-α, IL-6, IL-2, IL-2RB, and serine protease were expressed in all the samples, but only serine protease was elevated in patients with acute rejection. The serine protease gene is specific for cytotoxic T lymphocytes. Since these determinations were done on fragments derived from whole kidney, any increase localized to certain compartments or a change of distribution in the gene activation would not be detected by this global approach. The discrepancy between the two series suggests that further investigation, based on PCR analysis and examination of specific renal compartments, will be required. Another problem complicating the interpretation of the data on cytokines is the poor correlation between mRNA levels and the active species.

Diseases of the Native Kidney

Several groups of investigators recently examined the role of cytokines in inflammatory renal disease. Yoshioka et al. (25) compared the distribution of TGF-β proteins by immunochemistry with that of the corresponding mRNA by in situ hybridization in a group of patients with IgA disease, Shönlein-Henoch purpura, and proliferative mesangial glomerulonephritis. They were able to detect mRNA coding for TGF-β, mostly in glomerular macrophages but also in occasional resident glomerular cells. Noronha et al. (26) examined the amount and distribution of TNF-α, IL-1 β, and IL-2-R in biopsies from 22 patients with vasculitis and ANCA-positive GN with a substantial inflammatory component. They compared the immunochemical analysis with PCR and with in situ hybridization, using normal kidneys from nephrectomies as control samples. There was an increase in mRNAs coding for all of these species except for IL2-R in infiltrating mononuclear cells, tubular cells, and Bowman's cells in biopsies with active lesions, and these data correlated with those obtained by immunostaining. In a comparable analysis of 40 biopsies from patients with IgA nephritis, Yoshioka et al. (28) examined both protein expression and mRNA for IL-1α, IL-6, and TNF-α. These cytokines were mainly expressed in macrophages infiltrating the glomeruli. A weak signal was noted in some resident cells. The relative insensitivity of the in situ hybridization technique utilized in this study does not allow clear conclusions on the potential role of cytokines on the nature and/or progression of the lesions.

The potential role of an upregulation of cytokines in certain forms of human diseases remain uncertain because the data published are at best semiquantitative.

Extracellular Matrix: Type IV Collagen

Introduction

Because the progression of glomerular disease is one of the most perplexing problems for the nephrologist, multiple attempts have been made to define predictors of progression based on renal biopsy material (1,31). A common feature of progressive glomerular diseases leading to end-stage renal disease (ESRD) is the accumulation of extracellular matrix (ECM) within the glomerulus. The determination of the nature of ECM as well as the rate of its accumulation in disease represent prerequisites for the understanding and possibly treating glomerulosclerosis. Prior to our studies, the molecular events involved in the synthesis and degradation of ECM had not been studied in humans. We initially undertook detailed studies addressing these issues in renal tissue obtained from nephrectomy specimens and then studied renal biopsies. We initially developed the methodology in animal models.

Type IV collagen is one of the major components of the glomerular extracellular matrix in normal individuals, and immunochemical studies of renal biopsies have shown that it accumulates in sclerosing diseases (38). The synthesis of extracellular matrix components in the glomerulus has been difficult to study, since type IV collagen mRNAs are at a low level in adult animals, precluding the use of in situ hybridization (39). Since glomeruli represent a small fraction of the renal cortex and changes in matrix synthesis are regulated independently of those of the other elements of the kidney, changes in whole kidney preparations do not accurately reflect those in glomeruli (37,40,41). For these reasons, we developed a method in mice consisting of microdissection of a single glomerulus followed by reverse transcription and PCR (23). This method has been successfully applied to renal biopsies.

Competitive PCR for Isolated Microdissected Mouse Glomeruli

Type IV collagen mRNA was found in glomeruli of young mice, up to 3 weeks of age, utilizing in situ hybridization (39). The levels of IV collagen mRNA decreased in adult mice, so that they were no longer detectable by in situ hybridization. These observations provided the rationale to develop a method to analyze mRNAs encoding subchains of type IV collagen, utilizing PCR, in adult glomeruli isolated by microdissection. The glomerular cells of the dissected glomeruli appeared preserved by electron microscopic examination, and we were able to culture cells from the glomeruli in vitro, providing evidence that they were not damaged by the isolation procedure. Furthermore, the Bowman's capsule was removed, allowing studies of the tuft itself. Following microdissection, in the presence of RNase inhibitors, the glomeruli were permeabilized and reverse transcribed in situ; the resulting cDNAs were examined by PCR. Since our aim was to analyze disease processes, we needed a method that would allow the reproducible quantitation of small changes in mRNA levels. We developed a PCR technique consisting of the synthesis of mutant cDNA templates, which were constructed to be identical to the test cDNA save for the introduction of a new restriction enzyme site or a short deletion (42). The mutant cDNA molecules competed with the test cDNA molecules on an equimolar basis and thus also served as internal standards. Thus, since the concentration of the added mutant cDNA was known, we could readily calculate the amount of test cDNA at the equivalence point (Figure 1). This method was previously called competitive PCR (42). We showed that the amount of mRNA coding for α1IV or α2IV collagen could be reproducibly determined in the attomolar range in one-tenth of a normal mouse glomerulus. Varying numbers of glomeruli were pooled because of the variation in size between glomeruli in mice. Multiple pools containing the same number of glomeruli gave similar results. We compared reverse transcription of extracted glomerular RNA with reverse transcription of intact permeabilized glomeruli and found that the yield of cDNA was greater in intact glomeruli than in extracted RNA. Glomerular α1IV and α2IV mRNA levels were measured in normal mice from 5 to 24 weeks of age. The levels were high at 5 weeks, a time at which there was still a nephrogenic zone; it decreased by 8 weeks; and it remained stable between 8 and 24 weeks in mice with normal glomeruli by light microscopy (Figure 2). In two of the three 24-week mice, which had mild glomerulosclerosis by light microscopy (a common finding in aging rodents) (23), there was a 1.8-fold increase in the levels of type IV collagen mRNAs. These data confirm the accuracy as well as the extreme sensitivity of the method. We also examined the amount of glomerular mRNA coding for α1 type IV collagen in a model of mouse glomerulosclerosis developed in the laboratory, which affects mice transgenic for bovine growth hormone (GH), and found that there was a marked upregulation in the expression of these genes (43) (Figure 3). The upregulation was detectable before the sclerosis was apparent by light microscopy and persisted at high levels throughout the disease. The fact that the gene upregulation occurred prior to the development of visible sclerotic lesions suggests that the level of gene activation is predictive of progression in this model.

Other variants of competitive PCR have been proposed. For instance, another technique utilizing a cRNA mutant, rather than a cDNA mutant, has recently been described (44). The potential advantage was that the tissue RNA is reverse-transcribed in presence of the mutant cRNA, providing an internal control for RT efficiency among different experiments. The main disadvantage of this technique is that it limits the number of mRNA species available for study to those for which mutants have been initially added to the reaction mixture. This difference will be critical for samples from human biopsies, since methods that allow storage of the cDNA without limiting the number or type of molecules to be analyzed may offer a substantial advantage.

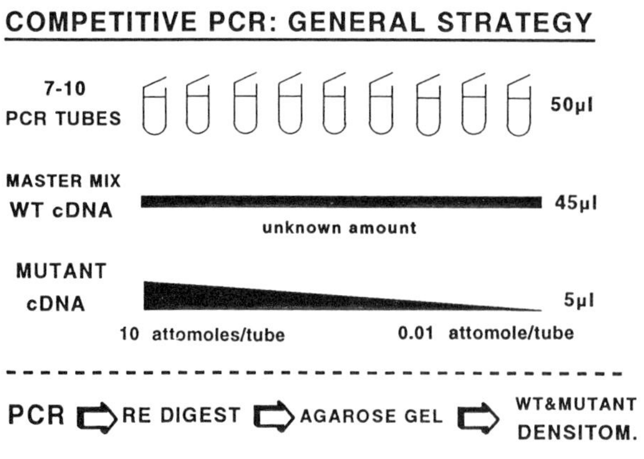

Figure 1 Schematic representation of the competitive PCR method.

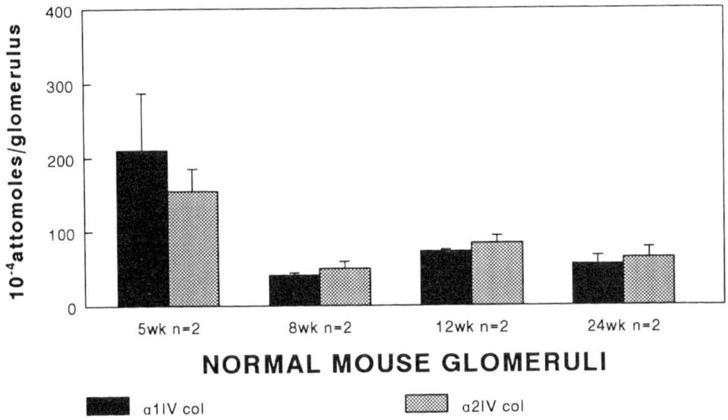

Figure 2 Quantitation of $\alpha1$ and $\alpha2$ type IV collagen in normal mouse glomeruli. As indicated in the text, the levels are high at 5 weeks in the presence of a persistent nephrogenic zone but decrease and remain stable for several months after. (From Ref. 23.)

Competitive PCR for Human Glomeruli: $\alpha2$ Type IV Collagen

The technique described above has recently been applied to human glomeruli in our laboratory. The use of microdissection yields a glomerular preparation free of tubular or vascular contaminants and may allow the isolation of essentially all the glomeruli available in a renal biopsy specimen. We took advantage of the availability of renal tissue from nephrectomies performed for renal carcinoma to measure the amount of $\alpha2$ type IV collagen subchain cDNA in individual glomeruli following

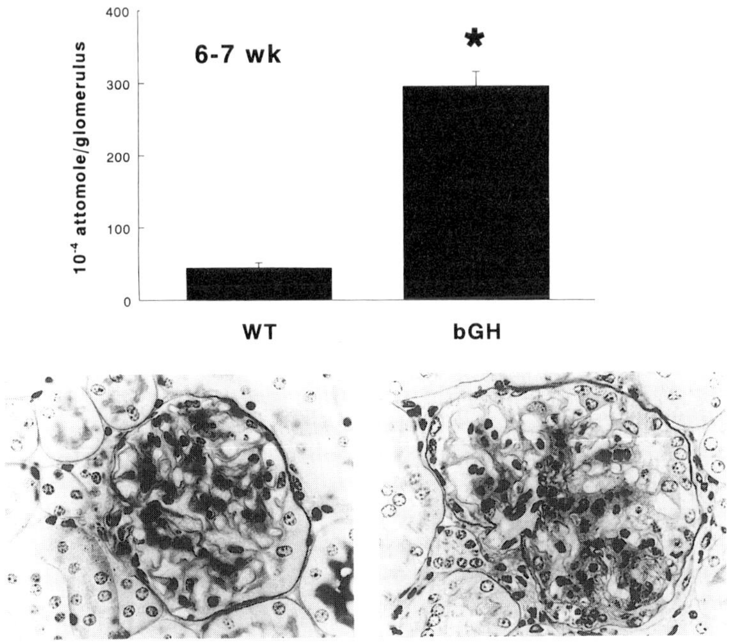

Figure 3 Comparison between a normal mouse (WT) and a mouse with glomerulosclerosis (GH), showing the upregulation of glomerular $\alpha1$ type IV mRNA in the latter.

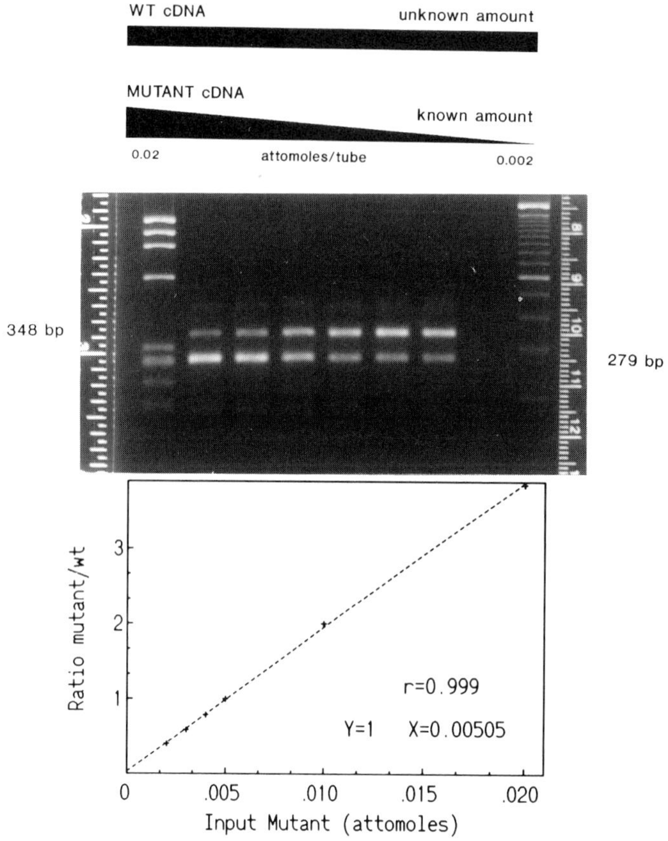

Figure 4 Competitive PCR for $\alpha 2$ type IV collagen using one-tenth of a human glomerulus as a template in each of the tubes. This represents an ethidium-bromide stained gel after PCR. Decreasing amounts of a mutant template were added in each tube. The mutant had a 69-bp deletion. The wild-type test CDNA and the mutant template were analyzed after 34 PCR cycles. The ratio of mutant/unknown cDNA was obtained by laser densitometry. The amount of cDNA was calculated from the point of equivalence ($Y = 1$). (From Ref. 22.)

reverse transcription. We were able to quantitate collagen type IV mRNA expression in the attomolar range, since we could measure cDNA expressed in a fraction of a glomerulus (Figure 4) by competitive PCR. Since a large proportion of patients with renal carcinoma have glomerulosclerosis, this material provided the means to assess the value of the technique for human specimens (1,22). We found that α2IV collagen cDNA was significantly elevated (3.8 times) in patients with glomerulosclerosis compared to those with normal glomeruli (Figure 5). We were unable to directly measure the minute amount of initial RNA present in the sample of isolated glomeruli that was reverse-transcribed, leaving open the important question as to whether the increment could be due to an increase in cell number associated with the glomerulosclerosis. Therefore, we used morphometric analysis to answer this question. We considered using a "house-keeping" gene in this study, but rejected the idea because of the possibility that this gene might be increased solely due to hypertrophy. The cDNA increase was not paralleled by cell number in the sclerotic glomeruli, since the average increase in cell number was 1.2 (Figure 6). This indicates that there was an upregulation in the level of ECM mRNA in each cell. Somewhat surprisingly, the glomerular α2IV collagen cDNA level was still high in one patient who had extensive glomerular scarring, suggesting that late sclerosis still remained as an active process in humans. These data confirm an earlier observation

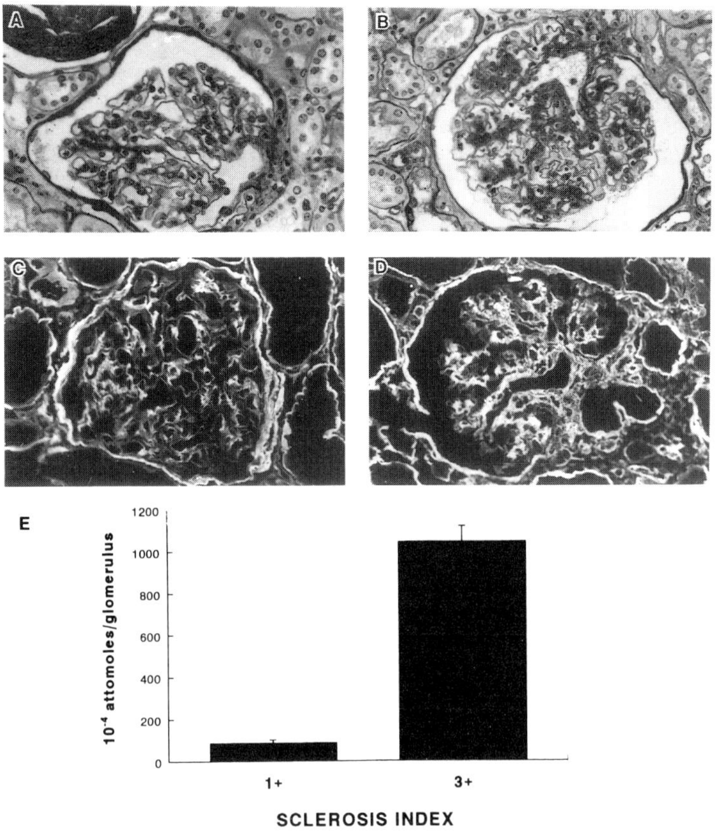

Figure 5 Comparison between two patients with normal glomeruli (left panel) and glomerulosclerosis (right panel). Glomeruli were stained by PAS for light microscopy and by an antibody to type IV collagen for immunofluorescence microscopy. The amount of $\alpha 2$ type IV collagen is ten times higher in the sclerotic glomeruli, as indicated in the lower panel. (From Ref. 22.)

that we made in GH transgenic mice (40,43). These observations raise the possibility that there may be a role for therapeutic intervention(s) at late stages of glomerular damage.

Degradation of ECM: Tissue Inhibitors of Metalloproteinase

The balance between ECM synthesis and degradation appears to be tightly regulated in the glomerulus in vivo. The enzymes that degrade the ECM (metalloproteinases including gelatinases) (45) and their inhibitors (tissue inhibitors of metalloproteinases, or TIMPs (29) play a role in determining the amount of ECM accumulation within the glomerulus. Very little is known about their regulation in human disease. For this reason, we examined the expression of TIMP-1 and TIMP-2 genes in normal and sclerotic human glomeruli and TIMP-2 protein in corresponding tissue sections. The kidney tissue was from the same patients as described above and the cDNA was an aliquot of the same glomerular isolates. TIMP cDNAs were quantitated by competitive PCR assays, using the above technique. TIMP-1 and TIMP-2 cDNA, detected in reverse-transcribed glomeruli from ten patients, were increased fourfold and threefold, respectively, in patients with glomerulosclerosis (29). These elevated levels could not be accounted for by an increased number of glomerular cells, based on a morphometric calculation. TIMP-2 protein was detected within both normal and sclerotic glomeruli. The fact that TIMP-1 and TIMP-2 genes were expressed in normal adult glomeruli and that their level of expression was increased in glomerulosclerosis suggests that they may play a role in disease.

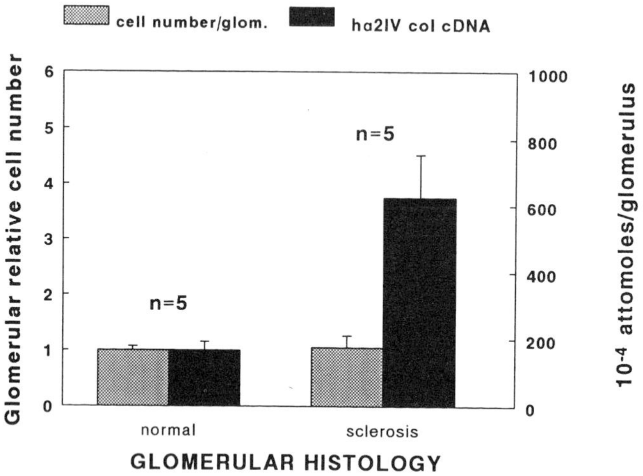

Figure 6 Comparison between the relative cell number per glomerulus and the amount of $\alpha2$ type IV cDNA in five patients without (left panel) and five patients with (right panel) sclerosis. The relative cell number did not differ between groups, in contrast to the cDNA levels. (From Ref. 22.)

INTERNATIONAL COLLABORATIVE STUDY

The application of these findings to progressive glomerular diseases in humans, principally IgA and the kidney disease of diabetes mellitus, is now being addressed. A group of nephrologists, the International Collaborative Group for Molecular Studies of Kidney Biopsies, from the United States and other countries (France, Belgium, Italy, China, Japan, Taiwan) was formed to examine whether competitive PCR of microdissected glomeruli from renal biopsies could be performed in multiple centers. The first phase was designed to teach the microdissection technique, to explore logistic problems, and to collect preliminary data from patients with progressive glomerular diseases. During this phase, glomeruli were isolated from tissue obtained from diagnostic renal biopsies after the clinician in charge was satisfied that there was no interference with the purpose for which the biopsy had been approved. The strategy adopted was the following: investigators were trained in our NIH laboratory over a period of 6 months to microdissect glomeruli from biopsies and to perform reverse transcription in situ. The glomeruli were microdissected in a solution containing RNase inhibitors at 4C°. In half the centers, they were reverse-transcribed on site, and in the other half they were frozen at –70°C, shipped in dry ice, and the reverse transcription was performed at the NIH laboratory. From the preliminary phase, we were able to analyze 75 samples originating from 15 centers. Investigators from all centers were trained and were able to isolate glomeruli, as evidenced by the presence of cDNA in all submitted samples. We measured the levels of α and $\alpha3$ type IV collagen mRNA. The results will be compared to normal glomeruli obtained either from nephrectomy specimens or those from biopsies without histological glomerular lesions. These data will become available in mid-1994.

CONCLUSIONS AND PERSPECTIVES

The quantitation of the mRNAs for ECM structural components, as proposed herein, may prove useful in the evaluation of initial responses or the potential to respond to injury. In addition, it may provide an opportunity to follow the course of glomerular disease and the response to therapy. The interpretation of current data requires validation, not so much of the findings but of their significance.

The availability of exquisitely sensitive methods, such as PCR, may create some confusion in the interpretation of studies of viral DNA or cytokines, since positive findings may be due to the presence of a small number of passenger blood-borne cells. This challenge is similar to the interpretation of a small number of interstitial mononuclear cell in transplanted kidneys. Most biopsies from renal transplants contain infiltrating lymphocytes, but renal pathologists have become accustomed to this baseline finding and interpret the renal biopsies accordingly (46). Similarly, we will have to recognize that a small number of viral copies or a modest amount of cytokines in a biopsy may only reveal that a patient has a viral infection or that there are a few activated inflammatory cells in a renal sample.

REFERENCES

1. Striker LJ. Modern renal biopsy interpretation: Can we predict glomerulosclerosis? Semin Nephrol 1993; 13:508–515.
2. Glassock RJ, Hirschman GH, Striker GE. Workshop on the use of renal biopsy in research on diabetic nephropathy: A summary report. Am J Kidney Dis 1991; 18:589–592.
3. Tryggvason K. Biochemistry and genetic diseases of glomerular basement membrane. Semin Nephrol 1993; 13:447–456.
4. Pelletier J, Bruening W, Kashtan CE, et al. Germline mutations in the Wilms' tumor suppressor gene are associated with abnormal urogenital development in Denys-Drash syndrome. Cell 1991; 67:437–447.
5. Knebelmann B, Deschenes G, Gros F, et al. Substitution of arginine for glycine 325 in the collagen alpha 5 (IV) chain associated with X-linked Alport syndrome: Characterization of the mutation by direct sequencing of PCR-amplified lymphoblast cDNA fragments. Am J Hum Genet 1992; 51:135–142.
6. Barker DF, Hostikka SL, Zhou J, et al. Identification of mutations in the COL4A5 collagen gene in Alport syndrome. Science 1990; 248:1224–1227.
7. Kiene P, Milde-Langosch K, Runkel M, et al. A simple and rapid technique to process formalin-fixed, paraffin-embedded tissues for the detection of viruses by the polymerase chain reaction. Virchows Arch A Pathol Anat Histopathol 1992; 420:269–273.
8. Gnann JW Jr, Ahlmën J, Svalander C, et al. Inflammatory cells in transplanted kidneys are infected by human cytomegalovirus. Am J Pathol 1988; 132:239–248.
9. Kadereit S, Michelson S, Mougenot B, et al. Polymerase chain reaction detection of cytomegalovirus genome in renal biopsies. Kidney Int 1992; 42:1012–1016.
10. Chen YT, Mercer GO, Cheigh JS, Mouradian JA. Cytomegalovirus infection of renal allografts: Detection by polymerase chain reaction. Transplantation 1992; 53:99–102.
11. Löning T, Stilo K, Rivière A, Helmchen U. Cytomegalovirus detection in kidney transplants: Results obtained from the polymerase chain reaction. Clin Nephrol 1992; 37:78–83.
12. Müller GA, Kühn W, Müller CA, et al. Detection of human cytomegalovirus-DNA in IgA nephropathy. Nephron 1991; 57:383–384.
13. Liu Z. Cytomegalovirus-DNA in serum and renal tissue of patients with IgA nephropathy. Chung Hua I Hsueh Tsa Chih 1992; 72:198–200.
14. Bourgoignie JJ. Renal complications of human immunodeficiency virus type 1. Kidney Int 1990; 37:1571–1584.
15. Cohen AH, Sun NC, Shapshak P, Imagawa DT. Demonstration of human immunodeficiency virus in renal epithelium in HIV-associated nephropathy. Mod Pathol 1989; 2:125–128.
16. Kimmel PL, Ferreira-Centeno A, Farkas-Szallasi T, et al. Viral DNA in microdissected renal biopsy tissue from HIV infected patients with nephrotic syndrome. Kidney Int 1993; 43:1347–1352.
17. Kimmel PL, Phillips TM, Ferreira-Centeno A, et al. HIV-associated immune-mediated renal disease. Kidney Int 1993; 44:1327–1340.
18. Misiani R, Bellavita P, Fenili D, et al. Hepatitis C virus infection in patients with essential mixed cryoglobulinemia. Ann Intern Med 1992; 117:573–577.
19. Johnson RJ, Gretch DR, Yamabe H, et al. Membranoproliferative glomerulonephritis associated with hepatitis C virus infection. N Engl J Med 1993; 328:465–470.
20. Davda R, Peterson J, Weiner R, et al. Membranous glomerulonephritis in association with hepatitis C virus infection. Am J Kidney Dis 1993; 22:452–455.
21. Miller DE, Noble NA, Yu X, Border WA. Molecular and cellular biological techniques in the study of glomerular diseases. Semin Nephrol 1992; 12:506–515.
22. Peten EP, Striker LJ, Carome MA, et al. The contribution of increased collagen synthesis to human glomerulosclerosis: A quantitative analysis of alpha 2IV collagen mRNA expression by competitive polymerase chain reaction. J Exp Med 1992; 176:1571–1576.
23. Peten EP, Garcia-Perez A, Terada Y, et al. Age-related changes in alpha 1- and alpha 2-chain type IV collagen mRNAs in adult mouse glomeruli: Competitive PCR. Am J Physiol 1992; 263:F951–F957.
24. Lipman ML, Stevens AC, Bleackley RC, et al. The strong correlation of cytotoxic T lymphocyte–specific serine protease gene transcripts with renal allograft rejection. Transplantation 1992; 53:73–79.

25. Vandenbroecke C, Caillat-Zucman S, Legendre C, et al. Differential in situ expression of cytokines in renal allograft rejection. Transplantation 1991; 51:602–609.
26. Noronha IL, Krüger C, Andrassy K, et al. In situ production of TNF-alpha, IL-1 beta and IL-2R in ANCA-positive glomerulonephritis. Kidney Int 1993; 43:682–692.
27. Yoshioka K, Takemura T, Murakami K, et al. Transforming growth factor–beta protein and mRNA in glomeruli in normal and diseased human kidneys. Lab Invest 1993; 68:154–163.
28. Yoshioka K, Takemura T, Murakami K, et al. In situ expression of cytokines in IgA nephritis. Kidney Int 1993; 44:825–833.
29. Carome MA, Striker LJ, Peten EP, et al. Human glomeruli express TIMP-1 mRNA and TIMP-2 protein and mRNA. Am J Physiol 1993; 264:F923–F929.
30. Striker LJ, Peten EP, Elliot SJ, et al. Mesangial cell turnover: effect of heparin and peptide growth factors. Lab Invest 1991; 64:446–456.
31. Striker LJ, Doi T, Elliot S, Striker GE. The contribution of glomerular mesangial cells to progressive glomerulosclerosis. Semin Nephrol 1989; 9:318–328.
32. Abboud HE. Growth factors in glomerulonephritis. Kidney Int 1993; 43:252–267.
33. Couser WG. Research opportunities and future directions in glomerular disease. Semin Nephrol 1993; 13:457–471.
34. Floege J, Eng E, Young BA, Johnson RJ. Factors involved in the regulation of mesangial cell proliferation in vitro and in vivo. Kidney Int 1993; 39:S47–S54.
35. Floege J, Burns MW, Alpers CE, et al. Glomerular cell proliferation and PDGF expression precede glomerulosclerosis in the remnant kidney model. Kidney Int 1992; 41:297–309.
36. Floege J, Eng E, Lindner V, et al. Rat glomerular mesangial cells synthesize basic fibroblast growth factor: Release, upregulated synthesis, and mitogenicity in mesangial proliferative glomerulonephritis. J Clin Invest 1992; 90:2362–2369.
37. Doi T, Striker LJ, Kimata K, et al. Glomerulosclerosis in mice transgenic for growth hormone: Increased mesangial extracellular matrix is correlated with kidney mRNA levels. J Exp Med 1991; 173:1287–1290.
38. Striker LJ, Killen PD, Chi E, Striker GE. The composition of glomerulosclerosis: I. Studies in focal sclerosis, crescentic glomerulonephritis, and membranoproliferative glomerulonephritis. Lab Invest 1984; 51:181–192.
39. Laurie GW, Horikoshi S, Killen PD, et al. In situ hybridization reveals temporal and spatial changes in cellular expression of mRNA for a laminin receptor, laminin, and basement membrane (type IV) collagen in the developing kidney. J Cell Biol 1989; 109:1351–1362.
40. Pesce CM, Striker LJ, Peten E, et al. Glomerulosclerosis at both early and late stages is associated with increased cell turnover in mice transgenic for growth hormone. Lab Invest 1991; 65:601–605.
41. Yang CW, Striker LJ, Kopchick JJ, et al. Glomerulosclerosis in mice transgenic for native or mutated bovine growth hormone gene. Kidney Int 1993; 39:S90–S94.
42. Gilliland G, Perrin S, Blanchard K, Bunn HF. Analysis of cytokine mRNA and DNA: Detection and quantitation by competitive polymerase chain reaction. Proc Natl Acad Sci USA 1990; 87:2725–2729.
43. Peten EP, Striker LJ, Garcia-Perez A, Striker GE. Studies by competitive PCR of glomerulosclerosis in growth hormone transgenic mice. Kidney Int 1993; 39:S55–S58.
44. Wang AM, Doyle MV, Mark DF. Quantitation of mRNA by the polymerase chain reaction. Proc Natl Acad Sci USA 1989; 86:9717–9721.
45. Woessner JF. Matrix metalloproteinases and their inhibitors in connective tissue remodeling. FASEB J 1991; 5:2145–2154.
46. Solez K, Axelsen RA, Benediktsson H, et al. International standardization of criteria for the histologic diagnosis of renal allograft rejection: The Banff working classification of kidney transplant pathology. Kidney Int 1993; 44:411–422.

52

Wilms' Tumor

Daniel A. Haber
Massachusetts General Hospital Cancer Center and Harvard Medical School, Charlestown, Massachusetts

INTRODUCTION: EPIDEMIOLOGY OF WILMS' TUMOR

Wilms' tumor is a pediatric kidney cancer, arising in 1 of 10,000 children, which is thought to originate in cells of the metanephric blastema (1). The characteristic "triphasic" histology of the tumor, consisting of blastemal, epithelial, and stromal elements, suggests an aberrant recapitulation of normal kidney differentiation within this embryonal cancer (see Figure 1). Features suggestive of further differentiation are also seen, primarily as skeletal muscle or neural elements. Rarely, Wilms' tumor can arise outside the kidney, particularly in the retroperitoneum or elsewhere in the genitourinary tract. These extrarenal Wilms' tumors are thought to arise in cells like the precursor cells of the genitourinary system. With modern therapeutic interventions, virtually 90% of children with Wilms' tumor are curable, usually by resection of the affected kidney, followed by radiation therapy or chemotherapy in cases with adverse prognostic features (2).

While most cases of Wilms' tumor appear to be sporadic, a subset of children appear to have an underlying genetic predisposition. True familial transmission of cancer susceptibility is rare (<1% of cases), but as many as 10% of children present with bilateral or multicentric tumors (3). The peak incidence for Wilms' tumor is 3 to 4 years of age, but children with bilateral tumors develop cancer 1 to 2 years earlier than those with sporadic tumors. These observations, presented by Knudson and Strong in their classic epidemiological analysis of Wilms' tumor incidence (4), established the genetic basis for cancer susceptibility. The Knudson model, as proposed for three pediatric cancers—retinoblastoma, Wilms' tumor, and neuroblastoma—predicted that two genetic "hits" are "rate-limiting" for tumor development (4–6) (Figure 2). In sporadic cases, these two hits represent two independent rare events that have occurred within the same somatic precursor cell. However, children with genetic susceptibility were predicted to harbor one hit in their germ line and to require only one additional hit in somatic tissues to initiate tumor formation, thus explaining both the early onset and mulifocal nature of these cancers. Subsequent studies identified the two hits as the inactivation of each allele of a tumor suppressor gene (7,8). The Kundson model was first confirmed with the isolation of *RB*, the tumor suppressor gene implicated in retinoblastoma (9). Mutational studies demonstrated that the first hit typically involves a point mutation within the gene, followed by loss of the remaining wild-type allele, along with a large fragment of neighboring DNA, constituting the second hit (10,11). Such large genetic lesions, detected by the loss of heterozygosity at polymorphic markers, have proved critical to the mapping of tumor suppressor genes. Together with the detection of germ-line abnormalities conferring predisposition to Wilms' tumor, these molecular studies have led to the identification of genetic loci involved in this cancer (reviewed in Ref. 12).

The genetic heterogeneity of Wilms' tumor is evidenced by the distinct congenital syndromes that have been associated with this cancer (Table 1). Although rare, these syndromes link the development of Wilms' tumor to other congenital abnormalities, resulting from the disruption of neighboring genes and comprising "contiguous gene syndromes." In some cases, these syndromes

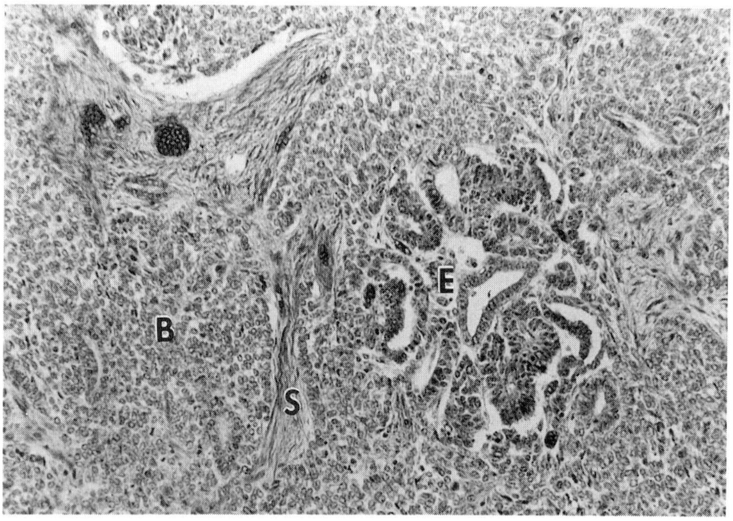

Figure 1 Wilms' tumor histology. Histologic section of Wilms' tumor, demonstrating the characteristic "triphasic" histology with blastemal (B), stromal (S), and epidermal (E) components. Hematoxylin and eosin stain, X100. (Photomicrograph provided by Drs. D. Hazen-Martin and A. J. Garvin, Medical University of South Carolina.)

are associated with germ-line cytogenetic abnormalities such as a chromosomal deletion at 11p13 (13) or a chromosomal duplication involving 11p15 (14,15). The tumor suppressor gene residing at the chromosome 11p13 locus has been identified and named *WT1* (16–18). The chromosome 11p15 locus appears to implicate genomic imprinting in its contribution to Wilms' tumorigenesis (19,20). Additional genetic loci that may lead to certain cases of familial Wilms' tumor are being sought (21–23).

THE WT1 TUMOR SUPPRESSOR GENE

Identification of WT1 at the Chromosome 11p13 Locus

In 1964, Miller and coworkers reported an association between two rare pediatric conditions: Wilms' tumor and aniridia, a malformation of the iris (24). While sporadic aniridia occurs in 1 in 70,000 children, this congenital abnormality is observed in 1 in 70 children with Wilms' tumor. Conversely, Wilms' tumor, which arises sporadically in 1 in 10,000 children, was found to develop in 1 in 3 children with aniridia. Wilms' tumors arising in the context of aniridia demonstrate an early age of onset and frequent bilaterality, consistent with the presence of underlying genetic susceptibility. The link between Wilms' tumor and aniridia results from a constitutional chromosomal deletion affecting two neighboring genes. This deletion, at chromosomal band 11p13, was first reported in children with the rare WAGR syndrome [an acronym for Wilms tumor, aniridia, genitourinary malformations, and (mental) retardation] (13). This constellation of symptoms is now understood to result from deletion of one allele of the *WT1* tumor suppressor gene, responsible for genitourinary malformations and the susceptibility to Wilms' tumor, and of the neighboring *Pax 6* gene, resulting in aniridia (25). The etiology of the mental retardation is unexplained.

The *WT1* gene was identified by positional cloning techniques, within the WAGR deletion at chromosome 11p13 (16,17). The gene encodes a transcription factor whose expression is developmentally regulated in the kidney. Normal expression of *WT1* is restricted to the condensed mesenchyme, renal vesicle, and glomerular epithelium of the fetal kidney (26). In the mouse, where serial studies are possible, *WT1* expression is detectable in the kidney at embryonic day 8, peaks at the time of birth, and drops precipitously by day 15 after birth (27). This transient pattern of

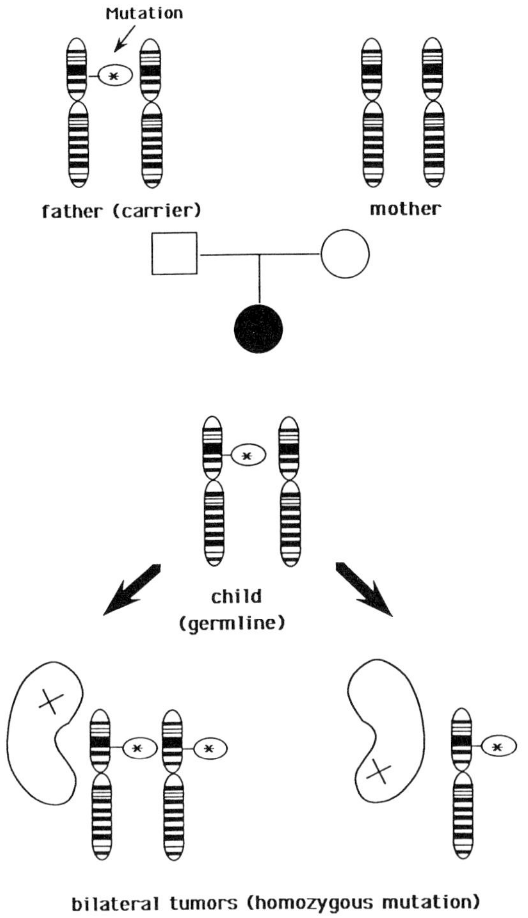

Figure 2 The Knudson model. Schematic representation of the "two-hit" model as it is now understood. A germ-line mutation in a tumor suppressor gene may be inherited from a parent, although in most cases of genetic susceptibility to Wilms' tumor, the *WT1* mutation appears as a de novo germ-line mutation in the child. Loss of the remaining wild-type allele in somatic target cells leads to homozygosity for the inactivated tumor suppressor gene, leading to the initiation of tumorigenesis. This reduction to homozygosity (also known as "loss of heterozygosity" or "LOH") at the tumor suppressor locus may occur by different mechanisms, typically involving gross chromosomal losses, such as chromosome nondisjunction or recombinational events, which are detectable using polymorphic markers.

expression, which contrasts dramatically with that of other tumor suppressor genes like *RB* and *p53*, suggests that *WT1* plays an important role during a critical period in kidney development. Loss of *WT1* function may thus result in aberrant developmental pathways within specific cells of the developing kidney, leading to the development of Wilms' tumor.

WT1: A Developmentally Regulated Transcription Factor

WT1 is encoded by 10 exons, spanning 50 kb of genomic DNA (28) (Figure 3). Two alternative splices are variably inserted into the *WT1* transcript, resulting in four distinct isoforms that are expressed in constant proportion in all *WT1*-expressing tissues. Alternative splice I results from the insertion of exon 5 and is present in 60% of *WT1* mRNA (28). Insertion of alternative splice II, detectable in 80% of *WT1* transcript, involves the use of an alternative splice donor site in exon 9,

Table 1 Characteristic Features of Wilms' Tumor–Associated Syndromes

Syndrome	Locus	Gene	Incidence of Wilms' tumor	Associated features
WAGR	11p13	*WT1*	>50%	Wilms' tumor Aniridia Genitourinary abn Mental retardation
Beckwith-Wiedemann	11p15	? *IGF2*? ?others?	<5%	Organomegaly (hemihypertrophy and umbilical hernia) Neonatal hypoglycemia Embryonal tumors (Wilms' tumor, adreno-cortical cancer, hepato-blastoma)

leading to the insertion of three amino acids (KTS) between exons 9 and 10. The carboxyl terminus of the *WT1* gene product (exons 7 to 10) contain four zinc-finger domains, loops of amino acids anchored by paired Cys-His residues, that mediate binding to a specific DNA sequence. Three of the four *WT1* zinc-finger domains have extensive amino acid homology with the zinc fingers of the early growth response 1 (EGR1) gene product (also known as NGFI-A, Krox 24, and Zif 268) (29–32). Expression of the *EGR1* gene is induced by mitogenic stimuli, and the gene product has been shown to bind to the DNA motif GCGGGGGCG, which is also recognized by recombinant WT1 protein (33). Insertion of alternative splice II (KTS) between zinc fingers 3 and 4 of *WT1* disrupts the critical spacing of these DNA binding domains and abolishes binding to the EGR1 consensus motif (33). The DNA-binding domain encoded by this alternatively spliced product, which constitutes the majority of cellular WT1 protein, appears to be capable of DNA binding, although the DNA target sequence remains unclear (34).

The amino terminus of *WT1* is rich in prolines and glutamines, a property shared by the transactivation domains of other transcription factors. This *WT1* domain appears to mediate

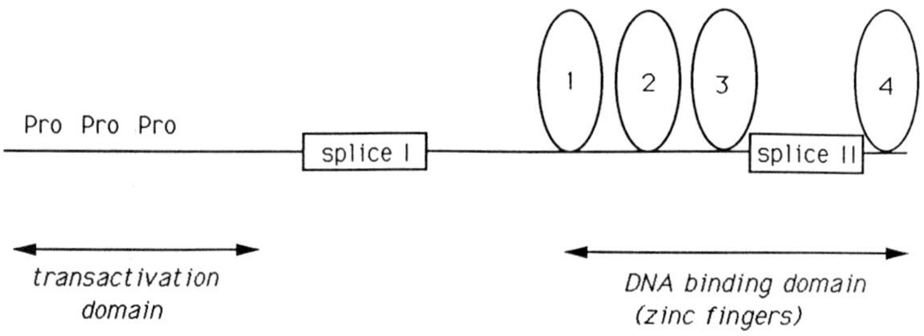

Figure 3 Schematic representation of WT1 protein. The protein encoded by the *WT1* tumor suppressor gene has functional domains characteristic of transcription factors. The carboxyl terminus encodes four zinc-binding domains, which mediate sequence-specific binding to DNA. The amino terminus of the protein is rich in prolines and glutamines and mediates the transactivational properties of the protein. Two alternative splices are variably inserted in the *WT1* transcript. Splice I encodes 17 amino acids that are inserted between the transactivation and DNA binding domains. Splice II encodes 3 amino acids that are inserted between zinc fingers three and four, altering DNA binding specificity. Four *WT1* isoforms, resulting from all combinations of alternative splices, are present in fixed proportion in tissues expressing *WT1*.

transcriptional repression, suppressing the expression of genes whose promoters may be a target of *WT1* (35). The apparent functional antagonism between the transactivator *EGR1* and the transcriptional repressor *WT1* has led to an attractive model involving a balance between growth-stimulating and growth-inhibitory signals during kidney development. Potential target genes of *WT1* have been identified in transient transfection assays, including *EGR1*, insulin-like growth factor II (IGF II), platelet-derived growth factor A (PDGF-A), *Pax 2*, GM-CSF among others (35–39). However, regulation of these genes by *WT1* in vivo remains to be demonstrated, as does the specificity and significance of these effects on kidney development and Wilms tumorigenesis. Transcriptional repression of target promoters by *WT1* appears to be linked to an interaction with p53 protein (40). This ubiquitously expressed tumor suppressor gene has been shown to form a physical complex with WT1 protein, both in immortalized baby rat kidney (BRK) cells and in Wilms' tumor specimens. In transient transfection experiments, *WT1* acts as a potent transcriptional activator of its target DNA sequence in the absence of *p53*, whereas it functions as a transcriptional repressor in the presence of *p53* (40).

Mutations of *WT1* in Wilms' Tumors

The majority of Wilms' tumor specimens demonstrate high levels of *WT1* expression, consistent with their postulated cells of origin (18,26). By RNA in situ hybridization, expression of *WT1* mRNA has been localized primarily to the epithelial and blastemal components, with low levels of expression in stromal cells (26). Consistent with the genetic heterogeneity of Wilms' tumor, inactivation of *WT1* in sporadic tumors occurs in a subset of cases. Gross DNA rearrangements are rare (approximately 1 in 50 cases), but PCR/sequencing analysis will reveal point mutations in approximately 1 of 10 cases (see Ref. 12). Point mutants within the DNA-binding domain of *WT1* result in abrogation of binding to the *EGR1* DNA consensus (41). Point mutants within the transactivation domain convert *WT1* from a transcriptional repressor to an activator (42,43), indicating that transcriptional repression may be important in the ability of *WT1* to function as a tumor suppressor gene.

Unlike retinoblastoma, in which homozygous mutations in *RB* appear to be required for tumorigenesis, not all *WT1* mutations in Wilms' tumors are homozygous (18,44). The presence of heterozygous mutations in tumor specimens suggests that a mutated gene product may act in a dominant manner to suppress the effect of the remaining wild-type gene product, thus providing the cell with a survival advantage. This "dominant negative" effect (45) appears to be a property of *WT1* mutants with a disrupted DNA binding domain, leading to the model that these altered proteins may mediate their effect by a nonproductive interaction with other cellular proteins. The dominant properties of a *WT1* mutant with a disrupted DNA binding domain have been demonstrated by its cooperation with the adenovirus gene *E1A* in the transformation of primary baby rat kidney cells (46).

In addition to point mutations in *WT1*, disruption of *WT1* function also appears to result from aberrant splicing of the *WT1* transcript (47). Wilms' tumor specimens contain variable amounts of a *WT1* mRNA species with an in-frame deletion of exon 2. This alternatively spliced exon, which is located within the *WT1* transactivation domain, is unlike other *WT1* alternative splices in that it is not found in normal *WT1*-expressing tissues. However, the majority of Wilms' tumors express low levels of this aberrant *WT1* transcript and ~10% express levels that are equal or higher than those of wild-type *WT1* mRNA. Like point mutants within the *WT1* transactivation domain, deletion of exon 2 from WT1 protein results in loss of transcriptional repressor activity, uncovering transcriptional activation. Thus, Wilms' tumors expressing the aberrant *WT1* mRNA species may contain two *WT1* proteins with antagonistic effects, one acting as a transcriptional activator and the other as a transcriptional repressor, resulting in the disruption of normal *WT1* function. The mechanism regulating this aberrant splicing of *WT1* mRNA is unknown, but appears to be in *trans*, implicating another gene in Wilms' tumorigenesis (47).

Germline Mutations in *WT1*

As predicted by the Knudson model, children with early-onset bilateral Wilms' tumor can be shown to harbor one mutated *WT1* allele in their germ line, with subsequent loss of the remaining wild-type allele in tumor cells (48,49). Conversely, children with WAGR syndrome, who have a large deletion of 11p13 in one germ-line chromosome, have a point mutation specifically inactivating the remaining *WT1* allele in their tumor (43,50,51). Not all children with bilateral Wilms' tumors harbor a *WT1* mutation. Although the incidence of germ-line *WT1* mutations among bilateral cases is unknown, children with genitourinary abnormalities (particularly males) appear to be more likely to have a *WT1* germ-line abnormality—evidence for the role of this Wilms' tumor gene in genitourinary development (49). While most cases reported to date have consisted of de novo germ-line mutations, at least one case has been reported in which a mutated *WT1* allele was transmitted from father to son, along with susceptibility to Wilms' tumor (49).

Just as dominant negative mutations have been implicated in Wilms' tumorigenesis, germ-line *WT1* mutations affecting the DNA-binding domain have a particularly dramatic effect. Children with Drash syndrome—a constellation of pseudohermaphrodism, early mesangial sclerosis, renal failure, and a predisposition to Wilms' tumor—have been shown to harbor a point mutation, typically within *WT1* zinc finger 3. The severity of the Drash phenotype, compared with that of children who have lost one *WT1* allele (i.e., WAGR syndrome) supports the concept of a dominant effect by dysfunctional WT1 proteins.

WT1 Expression in Gonadal and Mesothelial Cells

The developing kidney is not the sole organ expressing WT1 (Figure 4). High levels of expression have also been noted in the testis (Sertoli cells), ovary (granulosa cells), uterus, and placenta (26,52). In addition, high levels of *WT1* mRNA expression are found in the mesothelial lining and in the pericardial, pleural, and peritoneal, and stromal cells of the spleen and the capsule of the thymus (26,42). Expression of WT1 in these genitourinary and meothelial-derived structures differs from that of the kidney in that expression persists in adult tissues. The biological role of WT1 in these tissues may therefore differ from that in the developing kidney. The continued expression (and presumably continued role) of WT1 in these tissues may have implications for the timing of *WT1* mutations, as suggested by a mesothelioma in an adult patient, containing a mutation inactivating WT1 (42). *WT1* mutations have not been reported in tumors derived from other WT1-expressing tissues such as ovary, testis, or uterus.

Timing of *WT1* Inactivation and Reversal of Tumorigenicity

The presence of *WT1* mutations in the germ line of genetically predisposed individuals suggests that inactivation of *WT1* is an initiating event in Wilms' tumorigenesis. *WT1* inactivation is also an early

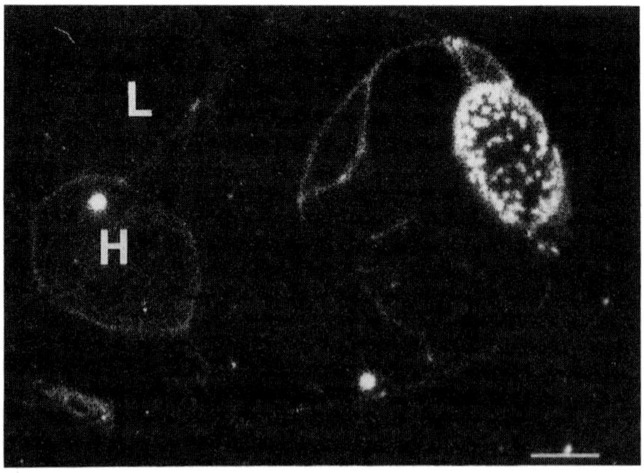

Figure 4 Tissue-specific expression of *WT1*. RNA in situ hybridization of antisense *WT1* probe to cross-section of mouse embryo (18 days). High levels of expression are detected in the developing kidney (primarily in glomerular precursors). *WT1* expression is also detected in a linear structure, the mesothelial lining of lung (L), heart (H), diaphragm, and abdominal viscera. *WT1* is also expressed in gonads and uterus (not seen in this picture). (From Ref. 42.)

event in sporadic Wilms' tumors. Nephrogenic rests, also known as nephroblastosis, are usually microscopic lesions that consist of primitive but not malignant blastemal cells (53). They are rarely seen in normal kidneys after 1 year of age but are present within the uninvolved kidney in virtually all cases of genetically predisposed Wilms' tumor. Approximately 30% of sporadic cases will also contain nephrogenic rests within the apparently normal kidney tissue. In two cases in which the Wilms' tumor had a somatic *WT1* mutation, the associated nephrogenic rest contained the same mutation. This observation indicates that nephrogenic rests may be clonal precursors to Wilms' tumor (54). Thus, inactivation of *WT1* appears to be an early genetic event in a renal stem cell, whose progeny can give rise to nephrogenic rests dispersed throughout the mature kidney. These nephrogenic rests may then provide an expanded population of preneoplastic cells, increasing the probability that additional genetic hits will lead to Wilms' tumor.

The observation that *WT1* inactivation is an early genetic event on the road to Wilms' tumorigenesis raises the question as to whether reintroduction of a functional *WT1* gene into Wilms' tumor cells will be sufficient to reverse the transformed phenotype. Early studies of Wilms' tumorigenesis demonstrated that the reintroduction of a normal chromosome 11 into G401 cells suppressed their tumorigenicity, a property associated with a chromosome fragment containing the 11p15, not the 11p13 locus (55,56). However, G401 cells have recently been shown to be derived from a rhabdoid tumor of the kidney rather than a Wilms' tumor (57). The cloning of *WT1* allowed direct testing of the gene's ability to suppress transformed growth. Indeed, transfection of constructs encoding all the alternatively spliced isoforms of *WT1* were capable of suppressing growth of a Wilms' tumor cell line, RM1, expressing an aberrantly spliced endogenous *WT1* transcript (47) (Figure 5). Wild-type *WT1*, like *RB* and *p53*, thus demonstrates the ability to suppress growth of tumor cells having a disrupted endogenous gene.

WT1 Inactivation in Mouse Models

Animal models of Wilms' tumor have been imperfect. In the rat, carcinogen-induced nephroblastoma shares some histological features with Wilms' tumor, although the proportion of blastemal cells appears to be far lower (58). Spontaneous nephroblastomas in the Japanese eel appear to most closely approximate the histological characteristics of human Wilms' tumor (59). The genetic etiology of these tumors is currently unknown.

In the mouse, an X-irradiation–induced mutant, Sey/Dey, has been shown to result from a hemizygous deletion on mouse chromosome 2, including a region syntenic to human chromosome

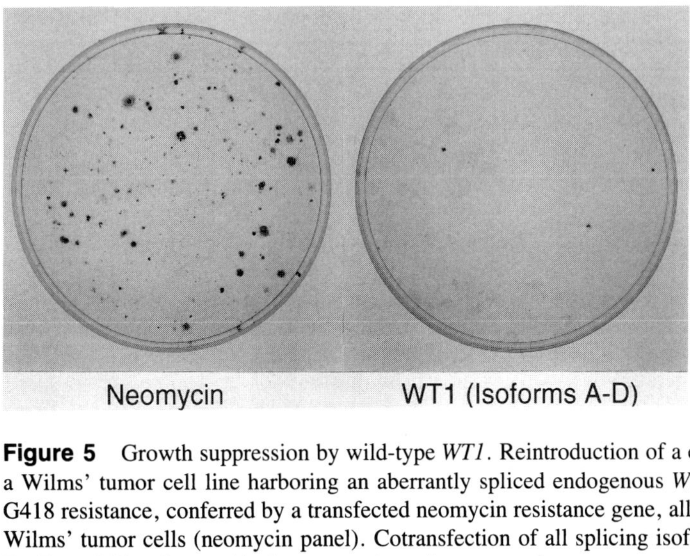

Figure 5 Growth suppression by wild-type *WT1*. Reintroduction of a cloned wild-type *WT1* allele into a Wilms' tumor cell line harboring an aberrantly spliced endogenous *WT1* transcript (47). Selection for G418 resistance, conferred by a transfected neomycin resistance gene, allows growth of stably transfected Wilms' tumor cells (neomycin panel). Cotransfection of all splicing isoforms of *WT1* (splice variants A, B, C, and D), along with the neomycin resistance marker, suppresses the emergence of drug-resistant colonies, demonstrating growth suppressive properties of this tumor suppressor gene [*WT1* (A to D) panel].

11p13 (60). Like the human WAGR deletion, the Sey/Dey deletion results in hemizygosity for the mouse *wt1* (27) and *pax 6* (25) genes. Sey/Dey mice have eye abnormalities that are comparable to the human aniridia lesions. However, they have no abnormalities of genitourinary development and no increased susceptibility to Wilms' tumor. Homozygosity for the Sey/Dey deletion is an early embryonal lethal (61,62).

The specific targeting of *WT1* in the mouse by homologous recombination has allowed the further study of the role of *WT1*. Mice bearing one inactivated *WT1* allele suffer no adverse effects, but homozygously deleted mice die within the second week of fetal development (63). These fetal mice show absence of both kidneys and gonads, implicating *WT1* as a critical gene in the normal development of these organs. The cause of death, however, has not been definitively determined and may involve cardiac malformations and diaphragmatic abnormalities. These defects may be related to aberrant inductive effects of mesothelial tissues in the pericardium and pleural/peritoneal spaces, a tissue with high levels of WT1 expression (42). The absence of kidney development in the homozygously *WT1*-deleted mouse prevents the possibility of Wilms' tumorigenesis in these animals. However, the absence of tumors in the *WT1*-hemizygous mice, like that in the Sey/Dey mutant, suggests that *WT1* may not be rate-limiting for kidney tumorigenesis in the mouse. Such species differences in tumor susceptibility have also been implicated in retinoblastoma, where *RB* inactivation in the mouse leads to pituitary tumors rather than retinoblastomas, as in humans (64). However, the absence of Wilms' tumors in the kidneys of *WT1*-hemizygous mice could also be explained by the infrequent loss of the remaining wild-type *WT1* allele in mouse somatic tissues. The generation of chimeric mice containing homozygously *WT1*-deleted cells within the kidney will be required to definitively exclude a role of *WT1* inactivation in mouse tumorigenesis.

THE 11p15 WILMS' TUMOR LOCUS

In addition to the *WT1* gene residing at the 11p13 locus, a second locus has been directly implicated in Wilms' tumorigenesis. Genetic susceptibility to Wilms' tumor is also present in children with Beckwith-Wiedemann syndrome (BWS), a congenital abnormality including visceromegaly, which may asymmetrical, so-called hemihypertrophy (65,66). Children with BWS may have a variable degree of abnormalities, including a large tongue and increased size of abdominal organs, resulting in umbilical hernia and neonatal hypoglycemia. The risk of developing cancer has been estimated at 7–8%, depending upon criteria for defining BWS, and is not restricted to Wilms' tumor but includes adrenocortical carcinoma and hepatoblastoma. Genetic lesions in patients with BWS are unusual for a tumor suppressor gene. They include duplication of the paternally derived 11p15 region, resulting in trisomy for that genetic locus (14,15), or paternal isodisomy (i.e., inheritance of both chromosomes 11 from the father and none from the mother) (67,68). These observations have suggested that genomic imprinting may play a critical role in BWS. For instance, expression of a gene whose expression is restricted to the paternal allele would be effectively doubled by these genetic mechanisms, and the extent of this epigenetic effect could be variable, thus resulting in the asymmetrical hypertophy. A potential candidate gene for BWS is *IGF II*, a growth-inducing gene residing at 11p15, which is imprinted in both humans and the mouse, with expression limited to the paternal allele. Loss or "relaxation" of *IGF II* imprinting, resulting in expression of *IGF II* from both alleles, has recently been demonstrated in the germ line of a child with BWS, directly implicating *IGF II* in the genesis of this pediatric syndrome (69,70).

However, the link between BWS and Wilms' tumorigenesis remains to be clarified. Loss of *IGF II* imprinting has also been reported in some Wilms' tumor specimens, suggesting that increased dosage of *IGF II* may contribute to Wilms' tumorigenesis (19,20). However, a subset of Wilms' tumors demonstrates classic allelic losses within 11p15 (71–73), implicating a more classic tumor suppressor gene mechanism at that locus. The identity of this putative second Wilms' tumor susceptibility gene (*WT2*) remains the subject of investigation.

MULTIPLE GENES INVOLVED IN WILMS' TUMORIGENESIS

The two Wilms' tumor loci on the short arm of chromosome 11, along with the unmapped familial Wilms' tumor locus, point to a genetic complexity that may reflect the diverse pathways involved in normal kidney development. Until the additional Wilms' tumor genes are isolated and characterized, it will be difficult to distinguish different genetic subtypes of Wilms' tumor and to appreciate the number of critical genetic abnormalities present within a single tumor. The existence of distinct genetic subsets of Wilms' tumor is supported by the characterization of preneoplastic nephrogenic rests. These precursor lesions (see above) have been divided into two classes based upon their topographical location within the kidney (74). Perilobar rests arise at the periphery of the kidney lobule and are seen primarily in the kidneys of children with BWS, as well as in sporadic cases. Intralobar rests, on the other hand, occur within the kidney lobule and are typical of the kidneys of patients with WAGR syndrome and aniridia (74). Thus, inactivation of the Wilms' tumor genes residing at different genetic loci may disrupt distinct steps in kidney development, resulting in the generation of Wilms' tumors that differ in their developmental origin.

However, molecular analyses in some cases of Wilms' tumor have suggested that more than one Wilms' tumor locus may contribute to the formation of a single tumor. For instance, such studies showed that a tumor arising in a child with WAGR syndrome, and hence a germ-line deletion within 11p13, contained somatic allelic losses restricted to 11p15 (72). Similarly, a Wilms' tumor developing in a child with familial Wilms' tumor (linked to neither of the chromosome 11 loci) showed loss of heterozygosity at 11p15 (21), and a sporadic Wilms' tumor demonstrated chromosome 11 loss and reduplication which had occurred prior to a mutation at the 11p13 gene (18). Thus, cumulative abnormalities in different Wilms' tumor genes may play a role in tumorigenesis. The isolation and characterization of these genes may lead to a better understanding of both Wilms' tumorigenesis and normal kidney development.

REFERENCES

1. Bennington J, Beckwith J. Tumors of the kidney, renal pelvis and ureter. In: Atlas of Tumor Pathology, series 2, fascile 12. Washington, DC: Armed Forces Institute of Pathology, 1975.
2. National Wilms' Tumor Study Committee. Wilms' tumor: status report, 1990. J Clin Oncol 1990; 9:877–887.
3. Matsunaga E. Genetics of Wilms' tumor. Hum Genet 1981; 57:231–246.
4. Knudson A, Strong L. Mutation and cancer: A model for Wilms' tumor of the kidney. JNCL 1972; 48:313–324.
5. Knudson A. Mutation and cancer: Statistical study of retinoblastoma. Proc Natl Acad Sci USA 1971; 68:820–823.
6. Knudson A, Strong L. Mutation and cancer: Neuroblastoma and pheochromocytoma. Am J Hum Genet 1972; 24:514–532.
7. Comings D. A general theory of carcinogenesis. Proc Natl Acad Sci USA 1973; 70:3324–3328.
8. Cavenee W, Dryja T, Phillips R, et al. Expression of recessive alleles by chromosomal mechanisms in retinoblastoma. Nature 1983; 305:779–784.
9. Friend S, Bernards R, Rogelj S, et al. A human DNA segment with properties of the gene that predisposes to retinoblastoma and osteosarcoma. Nature 1986; 323:643–646.
10. Dunn J, Philips R, Becker A, Gallie B. Identification of germline and somatic mutations affecting the retinoblastoma gene. Science 1988; 241:1797–1800.
11. Yandell D, Campbell T, Dayton S, et al. Oncogenic point mutations in the human retinoblastoma gene: Their application to genetic counselling. N Engl J Med 1989; 321:1689–1695.
12. Haber D, Housman D. The genetics of Wilms' tumor. Adv Cancer Res 1992; 59:41–68.
13. Riccardi V, Sujansky E, Smith A, Francke U. Chromosomal imbalance in the aniridia—Wilms' tumor association: 11p interstitial deletion. Pediatrics 1978; 61:604–610.
14. Waziri M, Patil S, Hanson J, Bartley S. Abnormality of chromosome 11 in patients with features of Beckwith-Wiedemann syndrome. J Pediatr 1983; 102:873–876.
15. Turleau C, Grouchy J, Nihoul-Fekete C, et al. Del 11p13/nephroblastoma without aniridia. Hum Genet 1984; 67:455–456.
16. Call K, Glaser T, Ito C, et al. Isolation and characterization of a zinc finger polypeptide gene at the human chromosome 11 Wilms' tumor locus. Cell 1990; 60:509–520.
17. Gessler M, Poustka A, Cavenee W, et al. Homozygous deletion in Wilms' tumours of a zinc-finger gene identified by chromosome jumping. Nature 1990; 343:774–778.
18. Haber D, Buckler A, Glaser T, et al. An internal deletion within an 11p13 zinc finger gene contributes to the development of Wilms' tumor. Cell 1990; 61:1257–1269.

19. Rainier S, Johnson L, Dobry C, et al. Relaxation of imprinted genes in human cancer. Nature 1993; 362:747–749.
20. Ogawa O, Eccles M, Szeto J, et al. Relaxation of insulin-like growth factor II gene imprinting implicated in Wilms' tumour. Nature 1993; 362:749–751.
21. Grundy P, Koufos A, Morgan K, et al. Familial predisposition to Wilms' tumour does not map to the short arm of chromosome 11. Nature 1988; 336:374–376.
22. Huff V, Compton D, Chao L, et al. Lack of linkage of familial Wilms' tumour to chromosomal band 11p13. Nature 1988; 336:377–378.
23. Schwartz C, Haber D, Stanton V, et al. Familial predisposition to Wilms' tumor does not segregate with the WT1 gene. Genomics 1991; 10:927–930.
24. Miller R, Fraumeni J, Manning M. Association of Wilms' tumor with aniridia, hemihypertrophy and other congenital malformations. N Engl J Med 1964; 270:922–927.
25. Ton C, Hirronen M, Miwa H, et al. Positional cloning and characterization of a paired box- and homeobox-containing gene from the aniridia region. Cell 1991; 67:1059–1074.
26. Pritchard-Jones K, Fleming S, Davidson D, et al. The candidate Wilms' tumour gene is involved in genitourinary development. Nature 1990; 346:194–197.
27. Buckler A, Pelletier J, Haber D, et al. Isolation, characterization, and expression of the murine Wilms' tumor gene (WT1) during kidney development. Mol Cell Biol 1991; 11:1707–1712.
28. Haber D, Sohn R, Buckler A, et al. Alternative splicing and genomic structure of the Wilms' tumor gene WT1. Proc Natl Acad Sci USA 1991; 88:9618–9622.
29. Sukhatme V, Cao X, Chang L, et al. A zinc finger encoding gene coregulated with c-fos during growth and differentiation and after cellular depolarization. Cell 1988; 53:37–43.
30. Milbrandt J. A nerve growth factor gene encodes a possible transcriptional regulatory factor. Science 1987; 238:797–799.
31. Christy B, Lau L, Nathans D. A gene activated in mouse 3T3 cells by growth factors encodes a protein with "zinc finger" sequences. Proc Natl Acad Sci USA 1988; 85:7857–7861.
32. Lemaire P, Revelant O, Bravo R, Charnay P. Two mouse genes encoding potential transcription factors with identical DNA-binding domains are activated by growth factors in cultured cells. Proc Natl Acad Sci USA 1988; 85:4691–4695.
33. Rauscher F III, Morris J, Tournay O, et al. Binding of the Wilms' tumor locus zinc finger protein to the EGR-1 consensus sequence. Science 1990; 250:1259–1262.
34. Bickmore W, Oghene K, Little M, et al. Modulation of DNA binding specificity by alternative splicing of the Wilms' tumor wt1 gene transcript. Science 1992; 257:235–237.
35. Madden S, Cook D, Morris J, et al. Transcriptional repression mediated by the WT1 Wilms' tumor gene product. Science 1991; 253:1550–1553.
36. Drummond I, Badden S, Rohwer-Nutter P, et al. Repression of the insulin-like growth factor II gene by the Wilms' tumor suppressor WT1. Science 1992; 257:674–678.
37. Wang Z, Madden S, Rauscher F III, Deuel T. The Wilms tumor gene product, WT1, represses transcription of the platelet-derived growth factor A-chain gene. J Biol Chem 1992; 267:21999.
38. Gashler A, Bonthron D, Madden S, et al. Human platelet-derived growth factor A chain is transcriptionally repressed by the Wilms' tumor suppressor WT1. Proc Natl Acad Sci USA 1992; 89:10984–10988.
39. Harrington M, Konicke B, Song A, et al. Inhibition of colony-stimulating factor-1 promoter activity by the product of the Wilms' tumor locus. J Biol Chem 1993; 268:21271–21275.
40. Maheswaran S, Park S, Bernard A, et al. Physical and functional interaction between WT1 and p53 proteins. Proc Natl Acad Sci USA 1993; 90:5100–5104.
41. Pelletier J, Bruening W, Kashtan C, et al. Germline mutations in the Wilms' tumor suppressor gene are associated with abnormal urogenital development in Denys-Drash syndrome. Cell 1991; 67:437–447.
42. Park S, Schalling M, Bernard A, et al. The Wilms' tumour gene WT1 is expressed in murine mesoderm-derived tissues and mutated in a human mesothelioma. Nature Genet 1993; 4:415–420.
43. Park S, Tomlinson G, Nisen P, Haber D. Altered trans-activational properties of a mutated WT1 gene product in a WAGR-associated Wilms' tumor. Cancer Res 1993; 53:4757–4760.
44. Little M, Prosser J, Condie A, et al. Zinc finger point mutations within the WT1 gene in Wilms' tumor patients. Proc Natl Acad Sci USA 1992; 89:4791–4795.
45. Herskowitz I. Functional inactivation of genes by dominant negative mutations. Nature 1987; 329:219–222.
46. Haber D, Timmers H, Pelletier J, et al. A dominant mutation in the Wilms' tumor gene WT1 cooperates with the viral oncogene E1A in transformation of primary kidney cells. Proc Natl Acad Sci USA 1992; 89:6010–6014.
47. Haber D, Park S, Maheswaran S, et al. WT1-mediated growth suppression of Wilms' tumor cells expressing a WT1 splicing variant. Science 1993; 262:2057–2059.
48. Huff V, Miwa H, Haber D, et al. Evidence for WT1 as a Wilms tumor (WT) gene: Intragenic germinal deletion in bilateral WT. Am J Hum Genet 1991; 48:997–1003.

49. Pelletier J, Bruening W, Li F, et al. WT1 mutations contribute to abnormal genital system development and hereditary Wilms' tumour. Nature 1991; 353:431–434.
50. Baird P, Groves N, Haber D, et al. Identification of mutations in the WT1 gene in tumours from patients with the WAGR syndrome. Oncogene 1992; 7:2141–2149.
51. Brown K, Watson J, Poirier V, et al. Inactivation of the remaining allele of the WT1 gene in a Wilms' tumour from a WAGR patient. Oncogene 1992; 7:763–768.
52. Pelletier J, Schalling M, Buckler A, et al. Expression of the Wilms' tumor gene WT1 in the murine urogenital system. Genes Dev 1991; 5:1345–1356.
53. Bove K, McAdams A. The nephroblastomatosis complex and its relationship to Wilms' tumor: A clinicopathologic treatise. Perspect Pediatr Pathol 1976; 3:185–223.
54. Weissman B, Saxon P, Pasquale S, et al. Introduction of a normal chromosome 11 into a Wilms' tumor cell line controls its tumorigenic expression. Science 1987; 236:175–180.
55. Park S, Bernard A, Bove K, et al. Inactivation of WT1 in nephrogenic rests, genetic precursors to Wilms' tumour. Nature Genet 1993; 5:363–367.
56. Dowdy S, Fasching C, Araujo D, et al. Suppression of tumorigenicity in Wilms tumor by the p15.5-p14 region of chromosome 11. Science 1991; 254:293–295.
57. Garvin A, Re G, Tarnowski B, et al. The G401 cell line, utilized for studies of chromosomal changes in Wilms' tumor, is derived from a rhabdoid tumor of the kidney. Am J Pathol 1993; 142:375–380.
58. Deshpande R, Hasgekar N, Chitale A, Lalitha V. Rat renal mesenchymal tumor as an experimental model for human congenital mesoblastic nephroma: II. Comparative pathology. Pediatr Pathol 1989; 9:141–151.
59. Masahito P, Ishikawa T, Okamoto N, Sugano H. Nephroblastoma in the Japanese eel, Anguilla japonica Teminck and Schlegel. Cancer Res 1992; 52:2575–2579.
60. Glaser T, Lane J, Housman D. A mouse model of the aniridia–Wilms' tumor deletion syndrome. Science 1990; 250:823–827.
61. Theiler K, Varnum D, Stevens L. Development of Dickie's small eye, a mutation in the house mouse. Anat Embryol 1978; 155:81–86.
62. Hogan B, Horsburgh G, Cohen J, et al. Small eyes (Sey): A homozygous lethal mutation on chromosome 2 which affects the differentiation of both lens and nasal placodes in the mouse. J Embryol Exp Morphol 1986; 97:95–110.
63. Kreidberg J, Sariola H, Loring J, et al. WT1 is required for early kidney development. Cell 1993; 74:679–691.
64. Jacks T, Fazeli A, Schmitt E, et al. Effects of an Rb mutation in the mouse. Nature 1992; 359:295–300.
65. Beckwith J. Macroglossia, omphalocele, adrenal cytomegaly, gigantism and hyperplastic visceromegaly. Birth Defects 1969; 5:188–196.
66. Wiedemann H. Complexe malformatif familial avec hernie ombilicale et macroglossie—Un syndrome nouveau? J Genet Hum 1964; 13:223–232.
67. Henry I, Bonaiti-Pellie C, Chehensse V, et al. Uniparental paternal disomy in a genetic cancer-predisposing syndrome. Nature 1991; 351:665–667.
68. Grundy P, Telzerow P, Haber D, et al. Chromosome 11 uniparental isodisomy in a child with hemihypertrophy and embryonal neoplasms. Lancet 1991; 338:1079–1080.
69. Ogawa O, Becroft D, Morison I, et al. Constitutional relaxation of insulin-like growth factor II gene imprinting associated with Wilms' tumour and gigantism. Nature Genet 1993; 5:408–412.
70. Weksberg R, Shen D, Fei Y, et al. Disruption of insulin-like growth factor 2 imprinting in Beckwith-Wiedemann syndrome. Nature Genet 1993; 5:143–149.
71. Mannens M, Slater R, Heyting C, et al. Molecular nature of genetic changes resulting in loss of heterozygosity for chromosome 11 in Wilms' tumor. Hum Genet 1988; 81:41–48.
72. Henry I, Grandjouan S, Couillin P, et al. Tumor-specific loss of 11p15.5 alleles in del 11p13 Wilms' tumor and in familial adrenocorical carcinoma. Proc Natl Acad Sci USA 1989; 86:3247–3251.
73. Reeve A, Sih S, Raizis A, Feinberg A. Loss of allelic heterozygosity at a second locus on chromosome 11 in sporadic Wilms' tumor cells. Mol Cell Biol 1989; 9:1799–1803.
74. Beckwith J, Kiviat N, Bonadio J. Nephrogenic rests, nephroblastomatosis and the pathogenesis of Wilms' tumor. Pediatr Pathol 1990; 10:1–36.

53
Alport Syndrome

Karl Tryggvason and Niina Heiskari
University of Oulu, Oulu, Finland

INTRODUCTION

Alport syndrome, also termed hereditary nephritis, was initially described in 1927 by A. L. Alport (1) as an inherited kidney disease characterized by hematuria and sensorineural deafness. Later, ocular lesions were also associated with the syndrome and, with the introduction of the electron microscope, irregularities and disruptions in the glomerular basement membrane (GBM) were shown to be typical for this disorder as well (2). During the last few years, mutations in the genes for the basement membrane–specific type IV collagen have been shown to underlie the disease (3,4).

Alport syndrome is primarily inherited as an X chromosome–linked dominant trait with an estimated gene frequency of 1:5000, but autosomal forms have also been reported (2,4). The defective gene in X-linked Alport syndrome was located in 1988 and 1989 by three groups to the middle of the long arm of the X chromosome (5–7). Based on the electron microscopic findings, it was suggested already in the early seventies that the defect was in a gene coding for type IV collagen (8). This triple-helical molecule, which is the major structural component of the basement membrane network, is composed of three α chains (4). The involvement of type IV collagen in the pathogenesis of Alport syndrome was indeed established in 1990, when mutations were found in the newly discovered α5(IV) collagen chain gene, which was localized to the q22 region on chromosome X (3,9–11). More recently, mutations have also been reported in the genes for the α3(IV) and α4(IV) collagen chains in the rarer autosomal forms of Alport syndrome (4). Presently over 60 different mutations are now identified in type IV collagen genes in Alport patients (11,12). These mutations can be considered responsible for abnormalities in the structural framework of the GBM, thus leading to the kidney manifestations observed in the disease.

CLINICAL FEATURES

The clinical picture of Alport syndrome is quite heterogeneous (2). Characteristically, Alport patients have recurrent microscopic or gross hematuria as early as in childhood, earlier in males than in females. The hearing loss is sensorineural and primarily affects high tones. Electron microscopy usually reveals thinning and thickening of the GBM with longitudinal splits into thin layers with a basket-weave pattern (Figure 1). Accumulation of electron-dense particles is also often seen. Anterior lenticonus, a peculiar change of lens shape in which the anterior lens pole shows a conical deformation, is also frequently observed in Alport patients. Absence of family history in Alport syndrome is present in about 15% of the cases. These may represent new mutations (2).

All the symptoms described above need not be present in all Alport patients, and their degree of severity may also vary greatly between individuals. Therefore, there has been some confusion among clinicians about the diagnostic criteria for and definition of Alport syndrome. Flinter et al. (13) proposed that Alport syndrome can be diagnosed if at least three of the four following criteria are fulfilled: (a) positive family history of hematuria/chronic renal failure; (b) electron microscopic

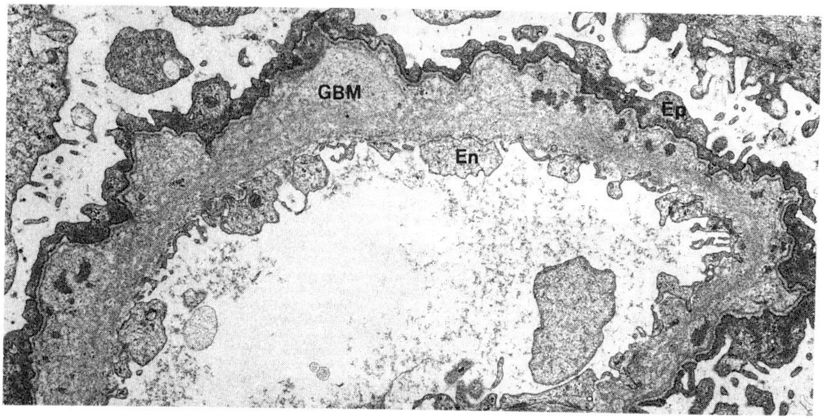

Figure 1 Electron micrograph of a glomerular capillary loop showing characteristic GBM lesions in Alport syndrome. The GBM shows irregular thickening and electron-dense particles. Abbreviations: En, endothelial cell; Ep, epithelial cell. ×10,000. (Courtesy Dr. Tom Törnoth, University of Helsinki.)

evidence on renal biopsy of Alport syndrome; (c) progressive high-tone sensorineural deafness, and (d) characteristic eye signs. While it is almost certain that patients who fulfil these criteria have mutations in some of the type IV collagen genes, many patients with renal failure who do not meet the criteria have been shown to have mutations in type IV collagen (11,12). Therefore, clinicians should consider Alport syndrome as a possible diagnosis for patients with hematuria and/or renal failure even though they lack symptoms such as hearing loss and ocular lesions or family history.

THE TYPE IV COLLAGEN PROTEIN FAMILY

Type IV collagen forms the structural network of basement membranes in all tissues, including the GBM (4). The type IV collagen molecules are 400-nm, flexible, triple-helical rods composed of three α chains (Figure 2). Each molecule has a large globule at the carboxyl terminal end. In recent years, it has become apparent that type IV collagen is a highly complex protein made of at least six different α chains, α1(IV), α2(IV), α3(IV), α4(IV), α5(IV), and α6(IV), which can form different trimer combinations, the molecular formula $(\alpha 1(IV))_2\alpha 2(IV)$ being the most common. At the present, it is not known whether the α3(IV), α4(IV), α5(IV), and α6(IV) chains are present in homo- or heterotrimer molecules. The α chains have molecular weights of 170 to 185 kDa and contain long collagenous Gly-X-Y-repeat sequences that are interrupted between 21 and 23 times by nocollagenous sequences. With regard to glycine mutations in type IV collagen in Alport syndrome (see below), it is important to appreciate that the location of a glycine residue in every third position of the collagenous domain of the α chain is essential for maintenance of the triple-helical conformation, as this amino acid is the only one small enough to fit into the center of the helix. The normally occurring interruptions in the collagenous sequence provide the molecules and meshwork structure with flexibility. Each α chain contains a carboxyl-terminal noncollagenous domain (NC1 domain), which contributes to the large globule. The NC1 domains that can be released separately from the otherwise insoluble GBM matrix by digestion with bacterial collagenase and then purified individually have molecular weights between 26 and 28 kDa, depending on the chain they are derived from. The α1(IV), α2(IV), and α5(IV) chains have been completely sequenced from humans (14–17) and partial sequence of the human α3(IV), α4(IV), and α6(IV) chains has also been obtained (18–20). Together, the amino acid sequence data have shown that all the chains are highly homologous, with some presumably functional sequences completely conserved, even between distant species such as *Drosophila* and humans (4). Furthermore, the sequence comparisons show that there are two homologous sets of chains, the α1(IV), α3(IV), and α5(IV) on the one hand and the α2(IV), α4(IV) and α6(IV) on the other. The conservation of amino acid sequences in all the chains is particularly

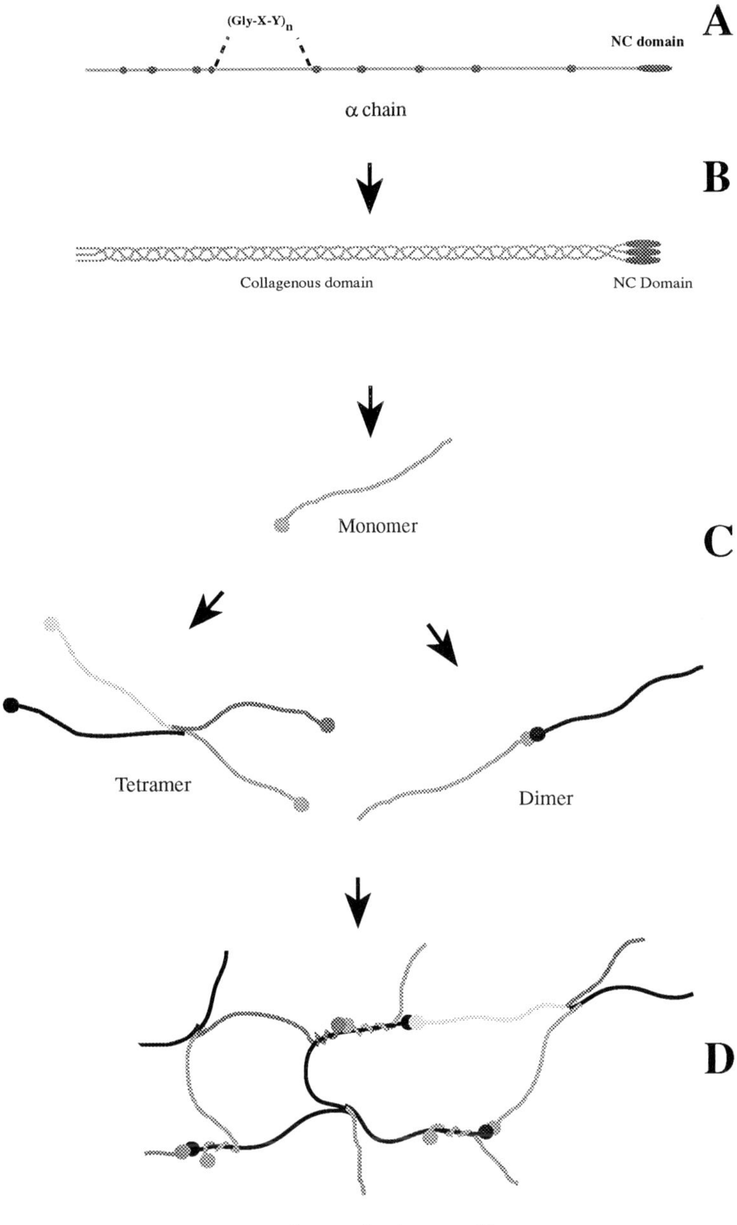

Figure 2 Schematic illustration of the structure and supramolecular assembly of type IV collagen. (A) Each α chain has a 400-mm-long collagenous domain characterized by a frequently interrupted Gly-X-Y-repeat sequence. A globular noncollagenous domain (NC1 domain) is located at the carboxyl-terminal end. (B) Three α chains, which can be of types $\alpha 1$, $\alpha 2$, $\alpha 3$, $\alpha 4$, $\alpha 5$, or $\alpha 6$, form the triple-helical molecule forming the building blocks (monomers) of the basement membrane meshwork. (C) Individual monomers associate into dimers via their disulfide bonds between NC1 domains or tetramers through disulfide bonds between the amino termini. (D) The supramolecular network is formed by assembly of dimers and tetramers strengthed by lateral association and partial winding of some molecules around each other. The other basement membrane components—such as laminin, proteoglycans and entactin (nidogen)—are bound into the type IV collagen meshwork in an as yet largely unclarified manner.

significant in the globular carboxyl-terminal NC1 domain, which is characterized by two homologous symmetrical halves and 12 completely conserved cysteine residues. These cysteine residues participate in intra- and intermolecular disulfide bonds. In general, over 60% of the amino acids of the NC1 domain are conserved in all type IV collagen α chains across species from *Drosophila* to human (4). This high conservation implies that the NC1 domains of any α chain has a certain function that requires almost identical structure, regardless of species. Several studies, particularly those carried out by Timpl et al. and Yurchenco et al. (see Refs. 21 and 22), have elucidated how the type IV molecules assemble to form the basement membrane network. Following secretion out of the cell, the triple-helical type IV collagen molecules (monomers) assemble into a complex network so that disulfide bonds are formed between the carboxyl-terminal NC1 domains of two molecules (dimers) or the amino termini of four molecules (tetramers). The dimers and tetramers then assemble further to form a complex network. Additionally, the type IV collagen molecules are believed to align laterally and/or twist around each other to form a stronger structure as illustrated in Figure 2.

The six type IV collagen α chains differ substantially with respect to tissue distribution (4). By antibody staining, the α1 (IV) and α2(IV) chains appear to be present in all basement membranes, while the minor chains have more limited distribution. Within the kidney, the α3(IV) and α4(IV) chains have similar distribution and are located in the GBM (23,24), as is the α5(IV) chain (9). In contrast, the α1(IV) and α2(IV) chains are located mainly in the mesangial matrix and vascular and tubular basement membranes in the kidney (23). The α1(IV) and α2(IV) chains are presumably also present in the GBM. In other tissues, the α5(IV) chain is also present, but detailed immunohistochemical studies have not been reported. The α6(IV) chain is expressed in kidney, but it is strongly expressed—e.g., in the esophagus—the expression pattern being different than that of the α5(IV) chain (20). The α3(IV) and α4(IV) chains are present in basement membranes of synaptic muscle fibrers but not in extrasynaptic muscle fibers, endoneurial and perineurial nerves, or arteries (4).

TYPE IV COLLAGEN GENES

The genes for type IV collagen in mammals have been shown to have an unusual arrangement in that they are located pairwise in a head-to-head manner on three different chromosomes (20,25,26), as depicted in Figure 3. This suggests that the genes have evolved by initial duplication and inversion of an ancestor gene followed by divergence to α1- and α2-like genes (4). This gene pair was then duplicated twice, resulting in the three gene pairs. The genes are seemingly all large and complex, the *COL4A1* and *COL4A5* genes encoding the α1(IV) and α5(IV) chains having sizes of more than

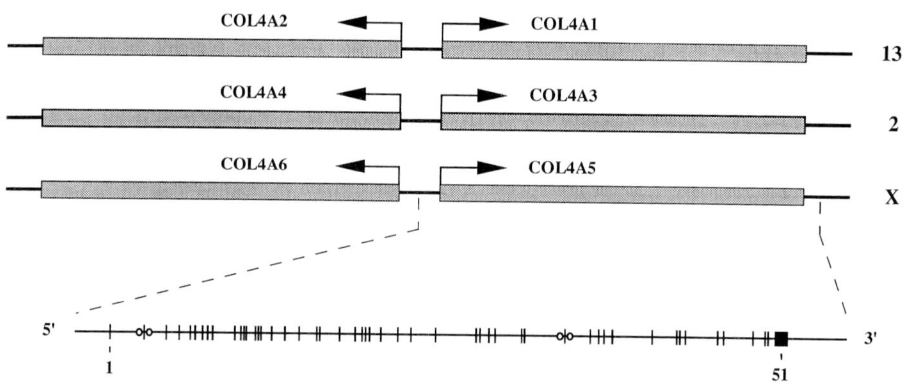

Figure 3 Schematic illustration of the organization and chromosome location of the human type IV collagen genes. The genes encoding the six type IV collagen chains are located pairwise in a head-to-head fashion on three different chromosomes. The genes are designated by boxes and flanking sequences by solid lines. The chromosomal number is shown on the right. For the *COL4A5* gene below, the location of exons is shown by vertical bars and that of introns by a horizontal line. The exons are numbered from the 5′ end of the gene. Intron sequences of unknown size are indicated by circles.

100 kb and 52 and 51 exons, respectively (27,28). Comparison of the *COL4A1* and *COL4A1* genes shows extensive homology in exon size pattern (27,28) and, similarly, the α2-like genes share high structural homology (20,29,30). The *COL4A1* and *COL4A2* genes, that code for the α1(IV) and α2(IV) chains share a common 127-bp common promoter region (25,31), which contains *cis*-acting elements with uni- and bidirectional activities (31,32). The properties of the promoters for the other two gene pairs have not yet been determined, but the distance between the first exons of *COL4A5* and *COL4A6* is known to be less than 452 bp (20).

IMMUNOHISTOPATHOLOGY OF TYPE IV COLLAGEN

Electron microscopic studies carried out in the late sixties already indicated molecular abnormalities in a structural component(s) of the GBM. In 1976, McCoy et al. (33) showed by immunohistochemical staining with autoantibodies from Goodpasture patients that some Alport patients lacked the Goodpasture antigen, a finding that was confirmed later in several studies. The Goodpasture antigen has been shown to be located in the NC1 domain of the α3(IV) chain (34). This NC1 domain, which can be purified from the GBM after digestion with bacterial collagenase, has a molecular weight of 28 kDa. This led researchers to believe that the α3(IV) chain gene was defective in Alport syndrome. However, as shown later and described above, this could not be the case in the X-linked disease, since the gene is on chromosome 2. Indications for the existence of another then unidentified component of type IV collagen that might be involved in Alport syndrome came from studies by McCoy et al. (35) and later by several other investigators showing that some Alport patients developed antibodies against renal allografts. Some of these antibodies have been shown to actually react with the 28-kDa NC1 domain of the α3(IV) chain, but some identify an NC1 domain–like protein of 26 kDa (36). This 26-kDa component is now believed to represent the NC1 domain of the α5(IV) chain, which is known to be mutated in a number of patients with X-linked Alport syndrome. The reason for the occasional absence of α3(IV) and α4(IV) chains from kidneys of Alport patients with X-linked disease remains a mystery but, as discussed below, they could be associated with α5(IV) chains in vivo.

MUTATIONS IN *COL4A5*

To date, numerous reports have described mutations in the *COL4A5* gene, the number already exceeding 60, of which 28 had been published when this was written (3,10,17,37–53). The published mutations are listed in Tables 1 and 2. These include large and small gene rearrangements such as deletions, insertions, inversions, and duplications as well as single-base changes. Furthermore, complete loss of the gene has been reported in one case. A striking finding is that the mutations identified so far in *COL4A5* are highly dispersed in this huge gene, which contains 51 exons and is ~250 kb in size (28). The same mutation has been found in two apparently unrelated kindreds in only a few cases. This sharply contrasts with findings in other diseases such as cystic fibrosis, where approximately 70% of the patients have the same mutation (54). The dispersion of mutations in *COL4A5* resembles the situation reported for osteogenesis imperfecta, a brittle-bone disease involving a variety of mutations in type I collagen genes (55).

The mutations present in the *COL4A5* gene in Alport syndrome can in most cases well explain the structural and pathophysiological changes in the GBM. The mutations can result in changes that affect (a) the synthesis of the primary transcript; (b) posttranscriptional modification of the transcript, such as splicing; (c) translation of the mRNA; (d) posttranslational modifications of nascent α chains; (e) assembly and folding of three α chains into a triple-helical molecule; (f) the stability of the helix structure; and (g) formation of cross-links between individual triple-helical molecules. Large gene rearrangements can result in total loss of expression of the gene, and small mutations in regulatory elements can have the same effects. Large and small mutations can also affect splicing of the primary transcript. Abnormal splicing and skipping of exons can cause two types of changes. First, if the exon skipping occurs in frame, the result is a shortened polypeptide, so that it lacks a segment; second, if the exon skipping occurs out of frame, the result is a protein partially containing a nonsense amino acid sequence. Duplications of the gene segments can lead to abnormally long α chains.

All the mutations leading to the absence of the α5(IV) chain or extensive alterations in protein

Table 1 Single Base Mutations in COL4A5 in Alport Syndrome

				Phenotype							
Mutation	Nucleotide change	Exon	RFLP	Juvenile	Adult	Hearing loss	Eye lesions	GBM splitting	Kidney transplant	Anti-GBM nephritis	Ref.
Missense											
Gly325→Arg	G→A at 1176[a]	17	–MspI		+	+	–	+	–		(39)
Gly325→Glu	G→A at 1177	17	–MspI	+		–	–	+			(42)
Gly521→Cys	G→T at 1764	23	+HindIII	+		+	–	n.d.	+	–	(17)
Gly1143→Ser	G→A at 3631	38	–MspI		+	+	+	+	–		(51)
Gly1143→Asp	G→A at 3632	38	–MspI	+		+	+	+	+		(44)
Pro1517→Thr	C→A at 3638	48		+		+	–	n.d.	–		(45)
Trp1538→Ser	G→C at 4702	48			+	–	–	+	+	–	(41)
Arg1563→Gln	G→A at 4777	48		+		+	+/–	+	+	–	(45,47)
Cys1564→Ser	G→C at 4780	49	+PstI		+	+	–	+	+		(3,10)
M1601→Ile	G→C at 4892	49		+		–	–	+			(49)
Nonsense											
Arg1563-Stop	C→T at 4776	48		+		+	–	n.d.			(47)
Splicing											
	G→C at 3657 + 1[b]	intron 38				+	–	+			(46)
	G→A at 3942 – 1	intron 41		+		+	–	+		–	(45)

[a]Numbering in cDNA sequence according to Ref 17.
[b]Numbering of intron mutations according to Ref. 58 refers to coding sequences in the first base of intron 38 following exon 38.

Table 2 Major Rearrangements in COL4A5 in Alport Syndrome

Mutation	Phenotype							
	Juvenile	Adult	Hearing loss	Eye lesions	GBM splitting	Kidney transplant	Anti-GBM nephritis	Ref.
Deletions								
Exons 42–47		+	+	–	nd	–		(3)
13 kb from 3' end of gene	+		+	–	+	+	–	(37)
Exon 1 extending upstream	+		+	+	+	–		(38)
Exon 1 extending upstream	+		–	+	+	+		(38)
Several 5' end exons and upstream	+		–	+	+	–		(38)
>38 kb in 5' end	+		+	–	nd			(43)
Large deletion in 3' end	+		+	–	+	+	+	(41)
34 kb, exons 38–51	+		+	+	nd			(40)
Entire gene			+	+	nd	+	+	(40)
Deletion GGGTGAA in exon 39								(50)
Deletion TGGA in exon 41								(50)
Deletion of A at 3142 in exon 34	+		+	+	+	+		(53)
Deletion of G at 3710 in exon 39	+		+	+	+			(52)
Deletion of C at 4016 in exon 42	+		+		+	+		(52)
Deletion of G at 5033 in exon 50								(50)
Insertion/duplication/deletion								
Part of 3' end of gene			+	+	+	+		(37)
Duplication/inversion								
Part of 3' end of gene	+		+	+	+	+	–	(37)
4767dupl10 exon 49		+	+	–	+			(45)

size would obviously lead to abnormal structure of any type IV collagen network where the α5(IV) chain is required as a normal component. Complete loss or presence of an abnormal α5(IV) chain may explain the clinical manifestations observed in Alport syndrome. In the kidney, the α5(IV) chain is normally present only in the GBM, as shown by immunostaining techniques (9). Very similar GBM staining is observed for the α3(IV) and α4(IV) chains (23,24). Although it is not known in what type of chain combinations the α5(IV) chain is in type IV collagen trimer molecules, its strict GBM location indicates a specific role for the structure and function of the GBM. Consequently, the absence of a normal α5(IV) chain may weaken the structural network of the GBM in one way or another, leading to leakage of large proteins or even large blood cells into the urinary space. It is important to note, however, that heterozygous females usually exhibit only mild phenotypes, and they seldom develop end-stage renal disease. This suggests that the synthesis of low amounts a normal α5(IV) chain is sufficient to maintain normal GBM function, even though the abnormal chain is present. This fact is particularly important in considering future possibilities for gene therapy which may be accomplished by supplementation of expression of a normal transgene in addition to that of the mutated gene.

Single-base mutations in exons leading to amino acid changes in the α5(IV) chain can be expected to render the protein malfunctional in most but not necessarily all cases, since such changes can affect proteins in a number of ways. This raises the question of how we can know if an amino acid substitution actually causes disease instead of being silent. This is important, especially from a clinical point of view, in making decisions about the termination of pregnancy after a mutation in the fetus has been identified. Actually, this is also a very difficult question to answer and, in fact, the only definite way of proving that a mutation is causative for the disease is to generate transgenic animals with the same mutation and observe whether this results in Alport syndrome–like phenotype. However, it is possible that a mutation causing disease in humans does not cause the same disease in mice. Clinicians will, therefore, have to rely on strong "circumstantial" evidence in predicting the potential pathogenic effect of mutations. Such evidence can be linkage or segregation of the mutations with the phenotype in an Alport kindred, knowledge about the role of certain amino acids for the function of the protein, or conservation of the amino acids during evolution. It is assumed that amino acids evolutionarily conserved in a protein between widely distant species have such functional importance that their substitution cannot be tolerated. This can be illustrated by several examples.

The amino acid sequence of about 230 residues at the C-terminal NC1 domain of the type IV collagen α chains contains two homologous halves (see Figure 2) with about 50% of the amino acids conserved in all six mammalian chains and also in type IV collagen α chains of *Drosophila*, *Caenovhabditis elegans*, and sea urchin (4). The conserved amino acids include 12 cysteines, 6 in each homologous half of the NC1 domain. It is apparent that the NC1 domain of all type IV collagen chains has the same biological function and that the highly conserved amino acids and three-dimensional structure of the NC1 domain are essential for correct alignment of three α chains prior to their folding and twisting into a triple helix, and subsequently for the formation of intermolecular cross links in the extracellular space (Figure 2). Therefore, substitution of conserved amino acids in this domain may affect these functions. To date, five single-base mutations leading to amino acid substitutions in the NC1 domain of the α5(IV) chain have been published in Alport syndrome (Figure 4 and Table 1). One mutation resulted in the change of cysteine 1564 to serine (10). The mutation would abolish one of the intrachain disulfide bonds, destroying bonds either between cysteines 1476 and 1564, or cysteines 1508 and 1564. The mutation that alters the conformation of the NC1 domain can have several effects. One possibility is that it interferes with the alignment of chains and formation of the triple helix, so that helix formation is slowed down, abolished completely, or the alignment of Gly-X-Y repeats is out of register. Alternatively, the triple-helical molecule may be formed and the protein secreted from the cell, but the loss of the cysteine can cause weak intermolecular cross links of the type IV collagen in the basement membrane meshwork.

The effects of amino acid changes in the NC1 domain other than those of cysteines are more difficult to predict, as the function of these amino acids is not known. Examples for such mutations are the mutations proline 1517→threonine, tryptophan 1538→serine and arginine 1563→glutamine (Table 1 and Figure 5) (41,45). In those cases one can, if possible, (a) study to see whether the mutation cosegregates in the families with the Alport phenotype, (b) see if the mutation is the result of a normal polymorphism and exists in normal individuals, or (c) examine whether the amino acids are conserved during evolution. As can be seen in Figure 5, all the amino acids listed above are

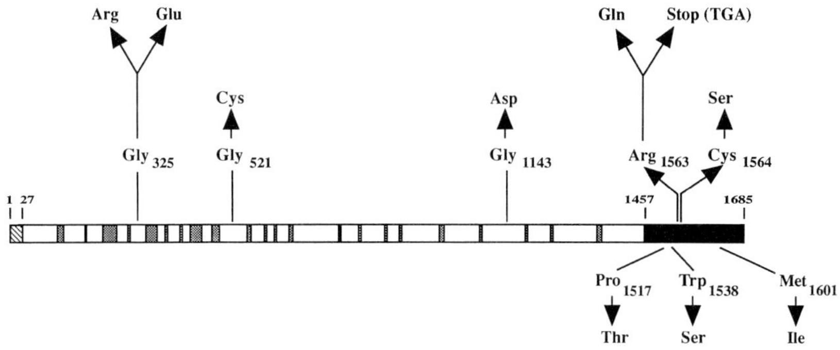

Figure 4 Illustration of amino acid substitutions in the α5(IV) collagen chain resulting from single-base mutations in the COL4A5 gene (see Table 1). The signal peptide (residues 1-26) is depicted by a cross-hatched pattern, the collagenous domain (residues 27-1456) by a white pattern interrupted by short noncollagenous sequences (shade); the NC domain (residues 1457-1685) is shown as a black box.

conserved in all known type IV collagen α chains even between distant species. Consequently, it can be assumed that these amino acids are essential for the normal function of the NC1 domain and that changes in them cannot be tolerated.

Several mutations converting a glycine residue in the Gly-X-Y-repeat–containing collagenous domain to another amino acid have been published (Figure 4 and Table 1). These mutations can, without doubt, affect the stability of the molecule's triple helix because, as mentioned above, glycine is the only amino acid small enough to fit into the center of the triple helix and an uninterrupted Gly-X-Y repeat sequence is essential for the maintenance of the triple-helical conformation. The result of glycine substitution is, therefore, that the helix is destabilized, creating kinks in the molecule that are not tolerated. Although this has not been demonstrated at the protein level for type IV collagen, a number of similar glycine mutations, either inhibiting helix formation or causing kinks in the molecule, have been described in type I collagen in osteogenesis imperfecta (55).

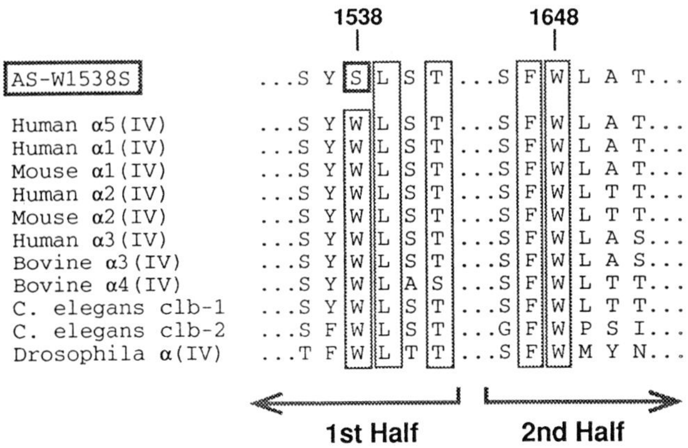

Figure 5 A mutation causing substitution of a conserved tryptophan 1538 to serine (W1538S) in an Alport patient (45). The actual effect of the mutation on the α5(IV) chain is difficult to predict. Sequence comparison shows, however, that the tryptophan residue in question is conserved in both symmetrical halves of the NC domain in all type IV collagen α chains characterized thus far from *Drosophila* to human. Since this amino acid residue has been completely conserved during evolution, it is extremely likely to be essential for the conformation and/or function of the NC domain, which is important both for the assembly of three α chains into a triple helix and the formation of intermolecular cross-links.

The dispersion of mutations in the *COL4A5* gene is a characteristic of Alport syndrome. Thus far, no "hot spots" particularly prone to mutagenic changes have been found. However, of the 12 single-base mutations published thus far in Alport syndrome, two codons (Gly325 and Arg1563) have been mutated in six apparently unrelated families (39,42,45,47). It remains to be seen whether or not these exons or these particular codons represent real "hot spots." Such regions, which are highly susceptible to mutations, would be of significant clinical value because they could greatly facilitate the search for mutations in Alport patients.

RELATIONSHIP OF *COL4A5* MUTATIONS WITH PHENOTYPES

Alport syndrome is a heterogeneous disease, with onset of end-stage renal disease at varying age and with or without other manifestations such as hearing loss and deafness, ocular lesions, thrombocytopenia, and so on (2). Since so many mutations have been identified in the *COL4A5* gene, it is of interest from a clinical point of view to correlate them with the phenotypes they produce. As can be seen from Tables 1 and 2 and references therein, this analysis is disappointing in the sense that it does not seem to be possible to predict the phenotype based on the type of mutation. For example, the point mutations generated by substitution of glycine residues in the collagenous domain or conserved amino acids in the NC1 domain result in quite wide spectra of phenotypes (Table 1). Most but not all patients have juvenile-onset end-stage renal disease; the presence of hearing loss and ocular lesions varies among individuals.

A similarly heterogeneous picture is seen for large changes in the gene (Table 2). Even entire loss of the gene does not necessarily produce more severe disease than a single glycine substitution in the collagenous domain of the $\alpha5$(IV) chain. Although this finding is disappointing, it does not come as a surprise, as the same phenomenon has been observed for defects in the genes for fibrillar collagens causing osteogenesis imperfecta, chondrodysplasia, Stickler syndrome, and Ehlers-Danlos syndrome (55). One particularly interesting Alport phenotype displays diffuse leiomyomatosis in addition to the classic symptoms (38). A clinically important group are the ~15% of posttransplantation Alport patients who develop anti-GBM antibodies. About one-third of those patients reject the transplant. Initial studies on Alport mutations and phenotypes gave hope that, based on the nature of the mutation, it might be possible to predict which patients develop anti-GBM nephritis and thus who should obtain a transplant and who not. It seemed reasonable that a mutation deleting the highly antigenic NC1 domain of the $\alpha5$(IV) chain would provoke recognition of the corresponding domain in the allograft as a foreign protein and that the patient should, therefore, not receive an allograft, as this would lead to anti-GBM nephritis. However, more recent data on transplanted patients with similar kinds of gene defects (Table 2) have shown that this explanation is not totally valid. In light of current and still limited knowledge, it is not possible to predict which patients are going to develop anti-GBM nephritis following kidney transplantation.

INVOLVEMENT OF *COL4A3*, *COL4A4*, AND *COL4A6* COLLAGEN GENES

Although Alport syndrome is primarily considered to be an X chromosome–linked disease, autosomal forms have also been postulated based on pedigree data. After defects were demonstrated in the $\alpha5$(IV) collagen gene in the X-linked disease, it was logical to search for mutations in the *COL4A3* and *COL4A4* genes for the $\alpha3$(IV) and $\alpha4$(IV) collagen chains in the autosomal form of the disease, respectively, as these chains are present in the GBM. Now Reeders' group has in fact identified mutations in both the *COL4A3* and *COL4A4* genes in two Alport kindreds (4,56). The mutation in *COL4A3* was found in a girl with juvenile Alport accompanied by sensorineural deafness (56). Her brother had similar disease, but the parents were unaffected. The girl was transplanted at the age of 10 but developed anti-GBM nephritis. The mutation is a 5-bp deletion in exon 47, leading to a premature stop codon 34 or 35 amino acids downstream. Details about the *COL4A4* mutation had not been reported when this was written.

At present there is no direct evidence showing that mutations in the $\alpha6$(IV) collagen chain *COL4A6* gene (20) alone can cause Alport syndrome. Deletions in the 5′ end of the *COL4A6* gene extending into the adjacent *COL4A5* gene have been reported to cause Alport syndrome and diffuse leiomyomatosis (38). In our preliminary work, we have sequenced five exons in the 5′ end of the *COL4A6* gene in over 200 patients without finding any mutation (57). Considering the random localization of mutations in the *COL4A5* gene in Alport syndrome, it was assumed that the same would hold for *COL4A6* if it were involved in the disease. These initial data indicate that (a) either the *COL4A6* gene is not mutated in Alport syndrome or (b) the mutations are not located randomly in the gene. Present data support the former hypothesis, as the *COL4A6* gene appears to differ from *COL4A5* with respect to spatial expression (10). However, at present the presence of mutations in *COL4A6* cannot be excluded with certainty in some Alport kindred.

SUMMARY

The recent work on Alport syndrome is one of the many beautiful examples of how the power of molecular biology has led to the elucidation of the pathogenesis of a genetic disease. As a result of this work we have reached two important milestones. First of all, we have gained new insight into the structure and properties of the specialized basement membrane that makes up the glomerular filtration barrier of the kidney. It has been shown to contain a highly specific type IV collagen component, whose actual role, however, remains unknown. Still, the $\alpha5$(IV) collagen chain must be essential for this structure, because its absence, which can result from deletion of the entire gene, leads to the Alport phenotype. The second and more important consequence of the work is that we are now reaching the stage where we are able to accurately diagnose the most frequent X-linked form of Alport syndrome and also the autosomal recessive forms. A routine diagnostic laboratory method has not yet been developed, but we are currently able to detect both large and point mutations. As is the case for other genetic diseases, the large mutations, which in Alport syndrome represent 5–10% of the mutations, can be detected by Southern hybridization using cDNA probes. Point mutations, most of which are probably going to be found in exons or in their immediate proximity, can be identified by other techniques, which are quite laborious. The mutation containing exons can be detected by analysis of polymerase chain reaction (PCR)-amplified exon regions—e.g., by denaturing gel electrophoresis (DGGE), single-stranded conformation polymorphism (SSCP), or the so-called chemical cleavage method, after which a region likely to contain a mutation can readily be sequenced. Also, sequencing of the patient's lymphocyte mRNA can be accomplished by RT-PCR. However, these techniques are very time-consuming and require extensive manual work. They are, therefore, not likely to reach routine automation-based hospital laboratories. A more rational approach, which may soon become a reality both for Alport syndrome and other genetic diseases, involves PCR amplification and direct sequencing of all exon regions of the gene. It is not unlikely that this technology—which will be based on the use of reaction robots, automated DNA sequencing, and data processing—will be routinely available in the near future. In fact, this approach is already being used successfully for the Alport gene.

A further important result of the recent research on Alport syndrome is the fact that mutations can be present in type IV collagen genes in nephritis patients, although the phenotype does not fulfil commonly used diagnostic criteria for Alport syndrome. It is particularly important to note that lack of hearing loss in nephritic patients by no means excludes the possibility of hereditary nephritis caused by a type IV collagen defect. Thus, the definition of Alport syndrome needs to be adjusted or one should refer to only hereditary nephritis.

In conclusion, it is evident that a giant leap forward has been taken concerning our understanding of Alport syndrome and its diagnosis. In the near future, we can expect revolutionary changes in possibilities for exact DNA-based diagnosis, and the time is ripe for the initiation of studies aimed at gene therapy.

ACKNOWLEDGMENTS

This work was funded in part by grants from the Sigrid Juselius Foundation, Finland's Cancer Institute, Finland's Cancer Societies, and the Academy of Finland.

REFERENCES

1. Alport AC. Hereditary familial congenital haemorrhagic nephritis. Br Med J 1927; 1:504–506.
2. Atkin CL, Gregory MC, Border WA. Alport syndrome. In: Schrier RW, Gottschalk CW, eds. Diseases of Kidney, Boston: Little, Brown, 1988:617–641.
3. Barker DF, Hostikka SL, Zhou J, et al. Identification of mutations in the COL4A5 collagen gene in Alport syndrome. Science 1990; 248:1224–1227.
4. Hudson BG, Reeders ST, Tryggvason K. Type IV collagen: Structure, gene organization, and role in human diseases: Molecular basis of Goodpasture and Alport syndromes and diffuse leiomyomatosis. J Biol Chem 1993; 15:26033–26036.
5. Atkin CL, Hasstedt SJ, Menlove L, et al. Mapping of Alport syndrome to the long arm of the X-chromosome. Am J Hum Genet 1988; 42:249–255.
6. Brunner H, Schroder C, van Bennekom C. Localization of the gene for X-linked Alport's syndrome. Kidney Int 1988; 34:507–510.
7. Flinter FA, Abbs S, Bobrow M. Localization of the gene for classic Alport syndrome. Genomics 1989; 4:335–338.
8. Spear GS. Alport's syndrome: A consideration of pathogenesis. Clin Nephrol 1973; 1:336–337.
9. Hostikka SL, Eddy RL, Byers MG, et al. Identification of a distinct type IV collagen α chain with restricted kidney distribution and assignment of its gene to the locus of X chromosome–linked Alport syndrome. Proc Natl Acad Sci USA 1990; 87:1606–1610.
10. Zhou J, Barker D, Hostikka SL, et al. Single base mutation in the α5(IV) collagen chain gene converting a conserved cysteine to serine in Alport syndrome. Genomics 1991; 9:10–18.
11. Tryggvason K, Zhou J, Hostikka SL, Shows T. Molecular genetics of Alport syndrome. Kidney Int 1993; 43:38–44.
12. Tryggvason K. Mutations in type IV collagen genes and Alport phenotypes. In: Tryggvason K. ed. Molecular Pathology and Genetics of Alport Syndrome Basel; Karger, 1995. In press.
13. Flinter FA, Bobrow M, Chantler C. Alport's syndrome or hereditary nephritis? Pediatr Nephrol 1987; 1:438–440.
14. Brazel D, Oberbäumer I, Dieringer H, et al. Completion of the amino acid sequence of the α1 chain of human basement membrane collagen (type IV) reveals 21 non-triplet interruptions located within the collagenous domain. Eur J Biochem 1987; 168:529–536.
15. Soininen R, Haka-Risku T, Prockop DJ, Tryggvason K. Complete primary structure of the α1 chain of human basement membrane (type IV) collagen. FEBS Lett 1987; 225:188–194.
16. Hostikka SL, Tryggvason K. The complete primary structure of the α2 chain of human type IV collagen and comparison with the α1(IV) chain. J Biol Chem 1988; 263:19488–19493.
17. Zhou J, Herz JM, Leinonen A, Tryggvason K. Complete amino acid sequence of the human α5 collagen chain and identification of a single base mutation in exon 29 from the 3′ end converting glycine-521 in the collagenous domain to cysteine in an Alport syndrome patient. J Biol Chem 1992; 267:12475–12481.
18. Morrison KE, Mariyama M, Yang-Feng TL, Reeders ST. Sequence and localization of a partial CDNA encoding the human α3 chain of type IV collagen. Am J Hum Genet 1991; 49:545–554.
19. Sugimoto M, Oohashi T, Yoshioka H, et al. cDNA isolation and partial gene structure of the human α4(IV) collagen chain. FEBS Lett 1993; 330:122–128.
20. Zhou J, Mochizuki T, Smeets H, et al. Deletion of the paired α5(IV) and α6(IV) collagen genes in inherited smooth muscle tumors. Science 1993; 261:1167–1169.
21. Timpl R. Structure and biological activity of basement membrane proteins. Eur J Biochem 1989; 180:487–502.
22. Yurchenco P, O'Rear J. Supramolecular organization of basement membranes. In: Rohrbach, DH, Timpl, R, eds. Basement Membranes: Cellular and Molecular Aspects. New York: Academic Press, 1993, pp. 19–47.
23. Butkowski RJ, Wieslander J, Kleppel M, et al. Basement membrane collagen in the kidney: Regional localization of novel chains related to collagen IV. Kidney Int 1989; 35:1195–1202.
24. Kleppel M, Santi PA, Cameron JD, et al. Human tissue distribution of novel basement membrane collagen. Am J Pathol 1989; 134:813–825.
25. Soininen R, Huotari M, Hostikka SL, et al. The structural genes for α1 and α2 chains of human type IV collagen are divergently encoded on opposite DNA strands and have an overlapping promoter region. J Biol Chem 1988; 263:17217–17220.
26. Mariyama M, Zheng K, Yang Feng TL, Reeders ST. Colocalization of the genes for the α3(IV) and α4(IV) chains of type IV collagen to chromosome 2 bands q35-q37. Genomics 1992; 13:809–813.
27. Soininen R, Huotari M, Ganguly A, et al. Structural organization of the gene for the α1(IV) chain of human type IV collagen. J Biol Chem 1989; 264:13565–13571.

28. Zhou J, Leinonen A, Tryggvason K. Structure of the human type IV collagen COL4A5 gene. J Biol Chem 1994; 269:6608–6614.
29. Hostikka SL, Tryggvason K. Extensive structural differences between genes for the $\alpha 1$ and $\alpha 2$ chains of type IV collagen despite conservation of coding sequences. FEBS Lett 1987; 224:297–305.
30. Kamagata T, Mattei MG, Ninomiya Y. Isolation and sequencing of cDNAs and genomic DNAs encoding the $\alpha 4$ chain of basement membrane collagen type IV and assignment of the gene to the distal long arm of human chromosome 2. J Biol Chem 1992; 267:24677–24682.
31. Pöschl E, Pollner R, Kühn K. The genes for the $\alpha 1$(IV) and $\alpha 2$(IV) chains of human basement membrane collagen type IV are arranged head-to-head and separated by a bidirectional promoter of unique structure. EMBO J 1988; 7:2687–2695.
32. Heikkilä P, Soininen R, Tryggvason K. Directional regulatory activity of *cis*-acting elements in the bidirectional $\alpha 1$(IV) and $\alpha 2$(IV) collagen gene promoter. J Biol Chem 1993; 268:24677–24682.
33. McCoy RC, Johnson HK, Stone WJ, Wilson CB. Variation in glomerular basement membrane antigen in hereditary nephritis (abstr). Lab Invest 1976; 34:325–326.
34. Butkowski RJ, Langeveld JPM, Wieslander J, et al. Localization of the Goodpasture epitope to a novel chain of basement membrane collagen. J Biol Chem 1987; 262:7874–7877.
35. McCoy RC, Johnson HK, Stone WJ, Wilson CB. Absence of nephritogenic GBM antigen(s) in some patients with hereditary nephritis. Kidney Int 1982; 21:642–652.
36. Kleppel M, Fan WW, Cheong HI, et al. Immunochemical studies of the Alport antigen. Kidney Int 1992; 41:1629–1637.
37. Boye E, Vetrie D, Flinter F, et al. Major rearrangements in the $\alpha 5$(IV) collagen gene in three patients with Alport syndrome. Genomics 1991; 11:1125–1132.
38. Antignac C, Zhou J, Sanak M, et al. Alport syndrome and diffuse leiomyomatosis—Deletions in the 5′ end of the COL4A5 collagen gene. Kidney Int 1992; 42:1178–1183.
39. Knebelmann B, Deschenes G, Gros F, et al. Substitution of arginine for glycine-325 in the collagen $\alpha 5$(IV) chain associated with X-linked Alport syndrome: Characterization of the mutation by direct sequencing of PCR-amplified lymphoblast cDNA fragments. Am J Hum Genet 1992; 51:135–142.
40. Netzer KO, Renders L, Zhou J, et al. Deletions of the COL4A5 gene in patients with Alport syndrome. Kidney Int 1992; 43:1336–1344.
41. Smeets HJM, Melenhorst JJ, Lemmink HH, et al. Different mutations in the COL4A5 collagen gene in two patients with different features of Alport Syndrome. Kidney Int 1992; 42:83–88.
42. Renieri A, Seri M, Myers JC, et al. De novo mutation in the COL4A5 gene converting glycine 325 to glutamic acid in Alport syndrome. Hum Mol Genet 1992; 1:127–129.
43. Renieri A, Seri M, Myers JC, et al. Alport syndrome caused by a 5′ deletion within the COL4A5 gene. Hum Genet 1992; 89:120–121.
44. Zhou J, Hertz JM, Tryggvason K. Mutation in the $\alpha 5$(IV) collagen chain in juvenile-onset Alport syndrome without hearing loss or ocular lesions: Detection by denaturing gradient gel electrophoresis of a PCR product. Am J Hum Genet 1992; 50:1291–1300.
45. Lemmink HH, Schröder CH, Brunner HG, et al. Systematic screening for mutations in 16 exons of the COL4A5 in Alport syndrome. Genomics 1993; 17:485–489.
46. Netzer KO, Pullig O, Zhou J, et al. COL4A5 splice site mutation and $\alpha 5$(IV) collagen mRNA in Alport syndrome. Kidney Int 1993; 43:486–492.
47. Zhou J, Gregory MC, Hertz JM, et al. Mutations in the codon for a conserved arginine-1563 in the COL4A5 collagen gene in Alport syndrome. Kidney Int 1993; 43:722–729.
48. Boye E, Flinter FA, Bobrow M, Harris A. An 8 bp deletion in exon 51 of the COL4A5 gene of an Alport syndrome patient. Hum Mol Genet 1993; 2:595–596.
49. Nomura S, Osawa G, Sai T, et al. A splicing mutation in the alpha 5(IV) collagen gene of a family with Alport's syndrome. Kidney Int 1993; 43:116–1124.
50. Renieri A, Seri M, Galli L, et al. Small frameshift deletions within the COL4A5 gene in juvenile-onset Alport syndrome. Hum Genet 1993; 92:417–420.
51. Renieri A, Meroni M, Sessa A, et al. Variability of clinical phenotype in a large Alport family with gly 1143 ser change of collagen $\alpha 5$(IV) chain. Nephron 1994; 67:444–449.
52. Renieri A, Galli L, De Marchi M, et al. Single base pair deletions in exons 39 and 42 of the COL4A5 gene in Alport syndrome. Hum Mol Genet 1994; 3:201–202.
53. Peissel B, Rossetti S, Renieri A, et al. A novel frameshift deletion in type IV collagene $\alpha 5$ gene in a juvenile-type Alport syndrome patient. Hum Mut 1994; 3(4):386–390.
54. Kerem BS, Rommens JM, Buchanan JA, et al. Identification of the cystic fibrosis gene: Genetic analysis. Science 1989; 245:1073–1080.
55. Kuivaniemi H, Tromp F, Prockop DJ. Mutations in collagen genes: Causes of rare and some common diseases in humans. FASEB J 1991; 5:2052–2060.
56. Mochizyki T, Mariyama M, Smeets HJM, et al. Identification of the first mutation in the $\alpha 3$ type IV

collagen gene in autosomal recessive Alport syndrome (abstr). Second International Workshop on Alport Syndrome. New Haven, CT, 1993.
57. Heiskari et al. Unpublished observations.
58. Beaudet AL, Tsui LC. A suggested nomenclature for designating mutations. Hum Mut 1993; 2:245–248.

54
Goodpasture Syndrome

Manfred Weber, Martin Marx, and Frank Merkel
Medizinische Klinik IV mit Poliklinik, University Erlangen-Nürnberg, Erlangen, Germany

INTRODUCTION AND DEFINITION

During the influenza epidemic of 1917 and 1918, Ernest Goodpasture described the autopsy of a patient with lung hemorrhage and proliferative glomerulonephritis (1). Nearly 40 years later, Stanton and Tange reported nine patients with similar findings and applied Goodpasture's name to it before the immunological heterogeneity of this syndrome was appreciated (2). The classic linear staining of the glomerular basement membrane (GBM) on direct immunofluorescence was first recognized by Scheer and Grossmann in 1964 (3). Subsequently, Lerner et al. demonstrated that antibodies to GBM were deposited in a linear pattern along the GBM, could be eluted from the kidneys, and were also found in the patients' serum. Classic transfer experiments convincingly established the pathogenic role of these antibodies. Anti-GBM antibodies either obtained by elution from affected kidneys or from the circulation could fix to the GBM of squirrel monkeys in vivo and caused pathological glomerular changes (4). Moreover, most convincing evidence for the pathogenic nature of the anti-GBM antibodies came from the observation of disease recurrence in renal allografts transplanted to patients with circulating anti-GBM antibodies (4–7). The transient nature of the autoantibodies, and the disease as well, further supports their pathogenic relevance.

Subsequently, Goodpasture syndrome was defined as a disorder consisting of the triad of (a) glomerulonephritis, commonly of the rapidly progressive, crescentic variety; (b) lung hemorrhage; and (c) anti-GBM antibody formation. It must be emphasized that the clinical feature of pulmonorenal syndrome consisting of lung hemorrhage with concomitant renal disease may coexist in various other conditions, including ANCA-associated vasculitis (like Wegener's granulomatosis) and microscopic polyarteritis, hypersensitivity angiitis (Churg-Strauss syndrome), systemic lupus erythematosus, Schönlein-Henoch purpura, mixed cryoglobulinemia, renal vein thrombosis with pulmonary embolism, congestive heart failure with uremia, and other disorders. Hence, several authors have defined the syndrome as anti-GBM antibody–mediated disease in order to emphasize the importance of circulating or kidney-bound antibodies in this autoimmune disorder. By using this definition, patients who clinically display only two features of the syndrome have to be included. Such oligosymptomatic variants of Goodpasture syndrome may occur in about one-third of the patients who present with anti-GBM antibodies and glomerulonephritis alone. Pulmonary hemorrhage may rarely also exist in conjunction with anti-GBM antibodies, minor glomerular abnormalities, and few, if any, findings on urinalysis. Consequently, Goodpasture syndrome is now recognized as an anti-GBM antibody–mediated disorder including a broad spectrum of clinical features, ranging from massive pulmonary hemorrhage with little overt evidence of renal disease and fulminant crescentic glomerulonephritis with no evidence of pulmonary bleeding to classic pulmonorenal syndrome.

EPIDEMIOLOGY

Goodpasture disease is rare, with an estimated incidence of about 0.5 per million or up to 5% of all glomerulonephritis (7,8). Early studies showed a preponderance of young men. Later series demonstrated a greater number of older patients and of women (9–11). Our data show a second peak of incidence in the sixth and seventh decades. The male-to-female ratio in 35 cases from Germany was 1.7, which is still in contrast to those of other autoimmune disorders, most of which show a preponderance of the female gender (12).

ETIOLOGY

The etiology of the disease is unknown. In general, human autoimmune disorders are believed to be initiated by environmental influences on a genetically susceptible background. Attention has therefore been drawn to the specific role of major histocompatibility antigens, especially class II molecules. By contrast, the role of environmental factors still remains to be defined.

Immunogenetics

Genetic backgrounds for susceptibility to the disease showed that HLA DR-2 is carried by 88% of patients (13–15). These initial data were based on serological investigations. Recent studies using restriction fragment length polymorphism of genomic DNA and sequence-specific oligonucleotide probes (SSO)—which precisely hybridize only to specific DNA sequences in the hypervariable regions of HLA genes—confirmed the strong association to DR-2 and showed that all DR-2 patients were restricted to DRB1-1501 and DQB1-0602 alleles. These studies also showed a highly significant association between disease and the alleles DRB1-0301 and DQB1-0201. DR-4 alleles as a group were not significantly more frequent among the patients, but the allele DRB1.0404 appeared to be associated with the disease (16). Associations to the IgGm allotype 1,2,21 (axg), and restriction of the IgG subclasses to IgG1 and IgG4 were also found (17–20). The occasional occurrence of the disease in identical twins supports the genetic background of Goodpasture syndrome (21–24).

Environmental Factors

A history of recent inhalation of volatile hydrocarbons has been obtained in several patients. However, exposure to organic solvents has also been reported in other forms of glomerulonephritis (25). It therefore seems difficult to judge whether organic solvents can cause or simply precipitate Goodpasture syndrome. Strong evidence that pulmonary hemorrhage may indeed be precipitated by nonspecific irritants or toxic effects on the lung comes from the observation of an association between cigarette smoking and hemoptysis. Such a mechanism is further supported by reports of remissions and relapses of pulmonary hemorrhages in association with exposure to a putative toxic agent as well as from animal experiments (21): In such experiments, exposure to pulmonary toxins not only led to the binding of antibodies to the alveolar basement membrane but also precipitated lung hemorrhage. Anecdotally, clustering of cases associated with upper respiratory tract infections has been reported. In summary, these data provide evidence for the importance of extrinsic factors, although their precise role still remains to be defined.

CLINICAL AND HISTOLOGICAL FEATURES

Fever, arthralgias, and other systemic symptoms are generally mild or absent at the time of presentation. A flu-like illness may antedate the disease in about 50% of the cases. Frequent initial symptoms are hematuria, moderate proteinuria, elevated serum creatinine, and hemoptysis. Weakness, fatigue, and reduced physical strength are also common. Renal function usually deteriorates within days or weeks. Only a few patients initially present with microscopic hematuria and normal renal function. Anemia is usual, even when there has been little or no hemoptysis. Hypertension is unusual, and kidney size is normal. Oliguria is a late feature and a bad prognostic sign. Pulmonary hemorrhage occurs in about 60% of patients and may be mild or severe and life-threatening. Some patients may present with cough or shortness of breath. Hilar pulmonary infiltrates may be seen on x-ray, and hypoxia is frequent. In contrast to renal disease, pulmonary hemorrhage shows a marked tendency to remit and relapse (9–12).

Renal biopsy in Goodpasture syndrome may show a wide range of histological features on light microscopy from nearly normal tissue or segmental hypercellularity of mesangial matrix to focal proliferative and necrotizing glomerulonephritis (26). Most often there is extensive cresent formation due to extracapillary proliferation. Interstitial inflammation is usually present and may be severe. It has been correlated with the extent of antibodies bound to the basement membranes of distal convoluted tubules. On direct immunofluorescence microscopy, smooth linear fixation of IgG along the GBM is the classical finding. IgG is accompanied by other immunoglobulins (IgA, IgM) in about one-third of the cases. Linear C3 deposition accompanies the immunoglobulins in about 70%. Occasional reports mention IgA, or IgM alone. On electron microscopy, breaks in the GBM are commonly found. In the lung, material obtained by transbronchial biopsy may show intraalveolar hemorrhage accompanied by hemosiderin-containing macrophages, fibrin deposition, and alveolar cell hyperplasia. Patchy linear fixation of IgG can be seen by immunofluorescence in most patients. Electron microscopy usually shows thickened alveolar basement membranes with defects. However, lung biopsies are not reliable for diagnostic purposes.

Fixation of anti-GBM antibodies to other basement membranes have rarely been demonstrated. In one report, IgG binding to Bruch's membrane and to the basement membranes of choroid vessels has been demonstrated. Similarly, fixation of antibodies to the choroid plexus has been reported (27–28).

IMMUNOPATHOGENESIS

The immunopathogenesis of Goodpasture syndrome was investigated by several groups during the recent years. Much progress has been made in the understanding and characterization of basement membrane architecture in general and in the identification of the "Goodpasture antigen," the target antigen of human anti-GBM antibodies.

Basement Membrane Architecture

Basement membranes are heterogeneous, highly specialized electron-dense structures built from extracellular matrix proteins. These 20- to 200-nm wide sheet-like membranes compartmentalize tissues, provide anchorage for adjacent cells, and contribute important signals for cell differentiation, cell migration, and cell phenotype (29–31). Vascular basement membranes are normally produced by adjacent endothelial cells. In contrast, the GBM is a fusion product formed from two cell lines, the glomerular endothelial and the visceral epithelial cells (podocytes). The latter cover the GBM along the urinary space of the glomerulus and the Bowman's capsule. This special construction is responsible for the typical laminated structure of the GBM, which posesses a rather thick duplicated lamina densa sandwiched between two laminae rarae. Structurally, the GBM therefore lacks the lamina reticularis, which usually anchors the vascular basement membranes into the interstitium. Functionally, the GBM has unique properties as a sieving barrier for the filtration of macromolecules. Furthermore, the endothelial cells form "fenestrae," which easily allow the GBM to become exposed to plasma proteins. The GBM is also in close contact with the mesangial matrix. The biochemical composition of vascular basement membranes has been studied extensively by using appropriate models such as the Englebreth-Holm-Swarm (EHS) mouse tumor. These and other studies elucidated that basement membranes are built up from a number of components, including type IV collagen, laminin, heparan sulfate proteoglycan, and nidogen/entactin (30,31). The bulk of these components is also common to the GBM; however, some molecules are found uniquely in this particular basement membrane. The mechanical stability and size-selective sieving properties are thought to be mainly due to the supramolecular network of collagen IV. This collagen is the major structural component of all basement membranes.

Goodpasture syndrome turned out to be a type IV collagen disease. It is therefore important to discuss the composition and molecular architecture of type IV collagen in the GBM (32,33). Individual collagen IV monomers consist of a triple helix composed of three α chains. Each α(IV) chain is characterized by a long collagenous domain of ~1400 amino acid residues, built from Gly-X-Y repeats, which is terminated at the C-terminal end by a globular noncollagenous (NC1) domain of ~230 residues. The ~15-residues-long N terminus is referred to as the 7S domain. The Gly-X-Y repeats are interrupted at several sites by short, noncollagenous sequences evenly distributed along the helices, which endow the molecule with a high degree of flexibility. Each chain is extensively glycosylated. Based on data from the EHS-tumor matrix, the collagen IV molecule was originally believed to be a heterodimer constructed from two genetically distinct α chains, [$\alpha1(IV)_2$ and $\alpha2(IV)$]. The existence of these two classic chains was subsequently confirmed by cloning and complete sequence analysis (34–36). However, more recent studies have led to the discovery of four new chains [$\alpha3(IV)$ to $\alpha6(IV)$] of type IV collagen (37–42). The complete sequence of the $\alpha5(IV)$ chain is also known, and until now about one-third of the human $\alpha3(IV)$, $\alpha4(IV)$, and $\alpha6(IV)$ chains have been sequenced (30, 42–45). A high degree of sequence similarity exists between the six different type IV collagen α chains, which makes it possible to divide them into two classes with even higher homology. One class includes $\alpha1(IV)$, $\alpha3(IV)$, and $\alpha5(IV)$ chains and the other one the $\alpha2(IV)$, $\alpha4(IV)$, and $\alpha6(IV)$ chains. Theoretically, many different isoforms of triple-helical monomers may exist. However, until now, evidence has been obtained only for $\alpha1(IV)_2$, $\alpha2(IV)$, $\alpha3(IV)_2$, and $\alpha4(IV)$ heterotrimers and homotrimers of $\alpha1(IV)_3$ and $\alpha3(IV)_3$ composition (33). The specificity to form triple-helical monomers from individual α chains seems to reside within the NC1 domain.

Type IV collagen triple-helical monomers self-associate by side-to-side and end-to-end associations, forming a supramolecular, network-like structure. Several modes of interactions are known. The N-terminal 7S domains associate with one another to form tetramers by lateral alignment over a 30-nm distance, alternatively in a parallel and an antiparallel fashion. The C-terminal globular NC1 domains generate dimers by end-to-end interactions between two monomers. Both sites of interaction become stabilized by covalent cross-linking with interchain disulfide bonds (46–48). An early structural proposal suggested that collagen IV molecules may associate into an unlimited network by the alternating use of 7S and NC1 cross-linking domains (49). However, further investigations showed that the collagen IV network is far more complex and includes lateral intertwining along the triple helix and additional binding of NC1 segments into triple-helical domains, thereby forming supercoiled structures (Figure 1) (33,50). The control of self-association of type IV collagen monomers also appears to reside within the NC1 domain. This domain is highly conserved among various species and provides two homologous subdomains, each having six cysteine residues in invariant positions. The 12 cysteines form six disulfide bonds, which force the region into two symmetrical leaves of trefoil-like structures (Figure 2) (33).

While the "classic" $\alpha1(IV)$ and $\alpha2(IV)$ chains are common to all basement membranes, the tissue distribution of the newly detected $\alpha3(IV)$ to $\alpha6(IV)$ chains differs considerably. Within the kidney, the $\alpha3(IV)$ and $\alpha4(IV)$ chains have a similar distribution and are localized to the GBM but not to the

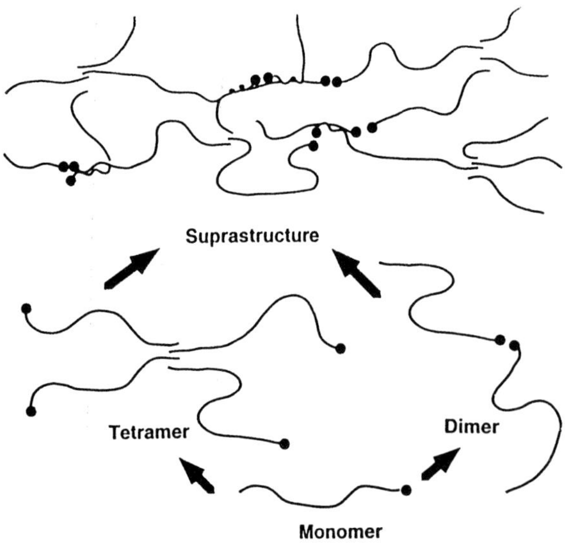

Figure 1 Model of type IV collagen self-association. Individual type IV collagen monomers self-associate side-to-side and end-to-end. By lateral intertwining along the triple helix, supercoiled network-like structures are formed which are assumed to cause the size-selective sieving properties of the GBM.

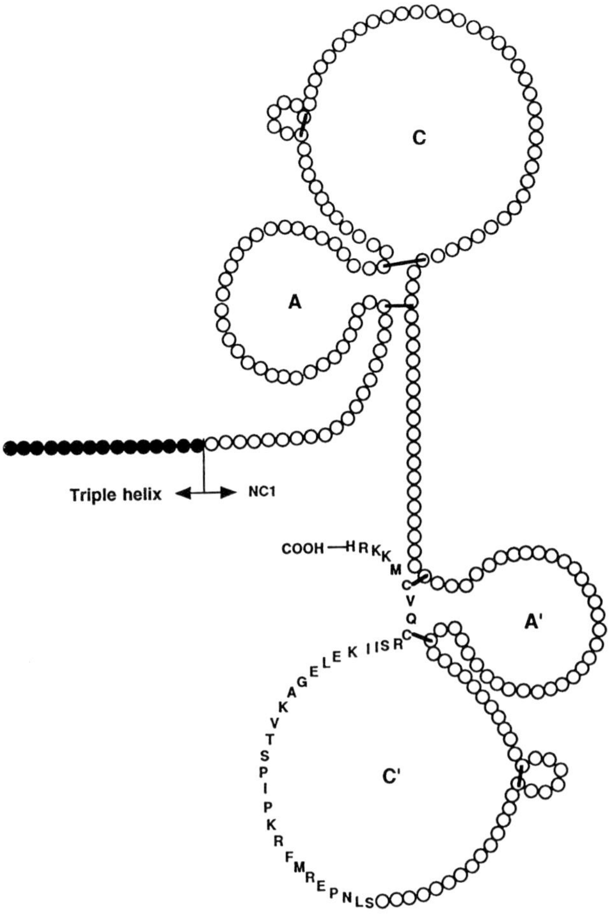

Figure 2 Presumed configuration of the C-terminal NC1 domain. Six S-S bridges force the domain into a symmetrical leaf of trefoil-like structure. The amino acid sequence of the putative C-terminal antibody binding site is given (63).

mesangial matrix or to the arteriolar basement membranes. In addition, monoclonal anti-α3(IV) antibodies bind to Bowman's capsule, distal tubules, alveolar capillaries, aorta, chorioid plexus, retina, lens capsule, synaptic muscle fibers, and cochlea (51,52). These immunohistological findings were confirmed by immunochemical studies based on NC1 globules isolated from GBM, tubular basement membrane, and lung (53). While these domains contained α3(IV), NC1 from placenta or small intestine did not. The α5(IV) chain was also found in GBM and some other tissues, but detailed immunohistological studies are lacking. The distribution of the α6(IV) chain has not been investigated at the protein level, but transcripts of the *COL4A6* gene can be detected in a variety of tissues. The highest mRNA levels have been observed in esophagus and lung (42). The heterogeneous distribution of the newer type IV collagen chains is assumed to determine the organ involvement in Goodpasture syndrome and other type IV collagen diseases as well.

The genes for the six different α-chains, *COL4A1* to *COL4A6*, have been localized on three different chromosomes. They are arranged pairwise on opposite strands in a unique head-to-head fashion. *COL4A1* and *COL4A2* were found on chromosome 13 (54). The genes for the α3(IV) and the α4(IV) chain were identified on chromosome 2 (30,44,55), while the *COL4A5* and *COL4A6* genes were localized on the X-chromosome (39,42,56). *COL4A1* and *COL4A2* share a 130-bp promoter region with uni- and bidirectional transcriptional activities; the intergenic region between

COL4A5 and *COL4A6* is 452 bp long. This region is not well defined, but it is larger between *COL4A3* and *COL4A4* (42,57).

Role of type IV Collagen in Goodpasture Syndrome

Extensive studies from several investigators identified the globular NC1 domain of type IV collagen α3(IV) chain as the target autoantigen for anti-GBM antibodies in Goodpasture syndrome (32,37,41, 58–61). The evidence was deduced from molecular and immunochemical studies performed with the soluble antigen obtained by collagenase digestion of alveolar, glomerular, and several other basement membranes. More recently, the identity of the C-terminal α3(IV) chain as target antigen for anti-GBM antibodies was further confirmed by studies using recombinant NC1 domains of the α1(IV) to α5(IV) chains (62). The epitope on the α3(IV) chain involves the last 36 residues of the NC1 domain as the primary interaction site (63). This could be confirmed by own investigations, however, microgram amounts of the oligopeptide were necessary to obtain sufficient antibody binding, which suggests that other parts of the domain may also participate in this event. The heterogeneity in the distribution of the α3(IV) chain explains the preferential clinical involvement of the lungs and the kidneys in this autoimmune disease. In vitro, the hexameric NC1 globule dissociates reversibly into monomers and dimers when exposed to denaturating agents or acid pH. Upon dissociation, the number of accessible epitopes increases 20 to 50-fold (60,64). Such disclosure of epitopes by infection or organic solvents is considered to play a role in the pathogenesis of the autoimmune disease.

Patients with Alport syndrome may develop anti-GBM antibodies and glomerulonephritis after renal transplantation. Alport syndrome is characterized by nonimmune thickening, thinning, and splitting of the GBM; progressive renal failure; sensorineural hearing loss; and ocular lesions (18,65). This mostly X-linked hereditary disease has recently been shown to result from mutations in the *COL4A5* gene encoding for the α5(IV) chain (66–68). More than 50 different mutations have now been identified in the *COL4A5* gene, including deletions, single-base mutations, inversions, insertions, and duplications. Moreover, evidence has been reported that the rare autosomal forms of the disease may be associated with mutations in the *COL4A3* or *COL4A4* gene (S.T. Reeders; unpublished). These molecular findings partially explain previous immunhistological and immunochemical observations that the Goodpasture antigen may be absent or altered in GBM from Alport patients (69,70). Our studies showed that the posttransplant Alport alloantibodies also target the α3(IV) chain even in a patient with a complete *COL4A5* deletion (human *COL4A5* knockout equivalent) (71,72). These observations suggest that α5(IV) mutations may additionally cause defective assembly of α3(IV) and some other type IV collagen chains. At present the mechanism linking a mutation in *COL4A5* with failure to incorporate the α3(IV) protein chain is unknown.

DIAGNOSIS

The diagnosis of Goodpasture syndrome is based on clinical features and on the demonstration of anti-GBM antibodies. The latter can be demonstrated as smooth, linear deposits of IgG along the GBM by direct immunofluorescence of renal biopsy material. In addition, demonstration of circulating anti-GBM antibodies may be used for diagnosis. While indirect immunofluorescence microscopy or assays based on crude GBM material often produced unreliable results, the identification of the Goodpasture antigen has greatly improved sensitivity and specificity of the anti-GBM antibody assays. Several groups now use radioimmunoassays or ELISA based on NC1 globules isolated from GBM. The ELISA performed in our laboratory is also based on purified NC1 antigen. For confirmation, positive samples subsequently become analyzed by immunoblotting (60). By using this appoach, anti-GBM antibodies were reliably uncovered in 45 of more than 4000 serum samples from patients with glomerulonephritis or pulmonary-renal syndrome. All positive cases were confirmed by biopsy.

In about one-third of Goodpasture patients, antineutrophil cytoplasmic antibodies (ANCA), most often with specificity for myeloperoxidase, may be detected (73,74). Clinically, there are some well-documented reports of the simultaneous occurrence of Goodpasture syndrome and microscopic polyarteritis or Wegener granulomatosis. In such rare overlapping cases, renal biopsy may show evidence of additional extraglomerular vasculitis. By contrast, the majority of "double-positive" patients do not have a distinctive clinical feature and most cases can be ascribed either to Goodpasture syndrome with low titers of additional ANCA or to the group of ANCA-associated vasculitis with secondary anti-GBM antibodies.

TREATMENT AND OUTCOME

In early studies, most untreated patients died shortly after diagnosis of pulmonary hemorrhage or renal failure (7,75–78). Subsequent uncontrolled studies suggested that administration of glucocorticoids improved pulmonary hemorrhage, while little effect on renal disease was documented. Similarly, cytotoxic agents have not generally been associated with beneficial effects on renal function. After the pathogenic relevance of anti-GBM antibodies had been recognized, a combination of plasma exchange with intensified immunosuppression was introduced in the mid 1970s in order to reduce antibody titers rapidly. Most centers now use protocols including corticosteroids, cyclophosphamide, and plasma exchange as basic therapy (i.e., prednisolone 1–2 mg/kg/day, cyclophosphamide 2–3 mg/kg/day, and plasma exchange until anti-GBM antibodies become undetectable). Although only one controlled study has been reported (79), prompt disappearance of pulmonary hemorrhage, stabilization of renal function in some patients, and a substantially improved survival have been observed compared to historical reports. Retrospective studies from Britain and subsequently from other countries showed that the severity of the disease at presentation is a powerful indicator of outcome, particularly whether or not any recovery of renal function can be expected (9,10,40). Poor results can be expected in oliguric patients or in those with advanced renal insufficiency (serum creatinine >600 μmol/L). In our retrospective study from Germany, patients with initial creatinine values greater than 600 μmol/L and more than 50% glomerular crescents on renal biopsy never recovered renal function. Among those who improved, most had an initial serum creatinine of less than 200 μmol/L (Figure 3). Only 11% died, which may reflect general improvements in intensive care therapy (12). Data from all reported studies confirm that the earlier immunosuppressive therapy starts, the better the results will be. These results underline that early diagnosis using reliable test systems seems to be the most promising approach to improve outcome.

Patients with Goodpasture syndrome have been shown to be suitable for transplantation (4–7). However, recurrence of the disease with subsequent loss of renal graft must be expected if circulating antibodies are still present at the time of transplantation. We and other centers postpone transplantation until anti-GBM antibodies are not detectable for at least 12 months. In patients with persisting antibodies, plasma exchange and immunosuppression may again be introduced prior to transplanta-

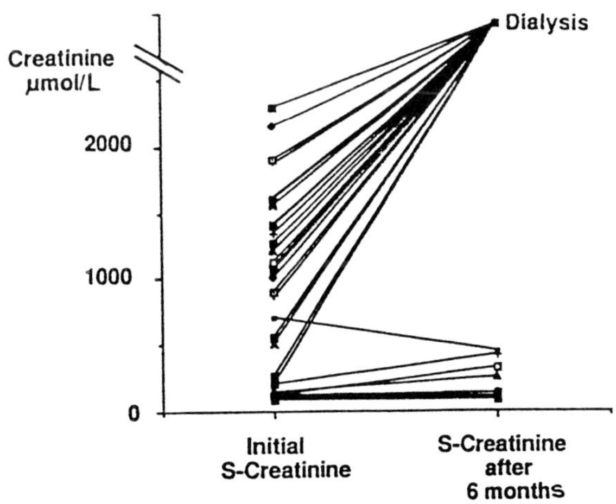

Figure 3 Initial serum-creatinine and outcome 6 months after diagnosis retrospectively analyzed in 35 patients with anti-GBM antibody-mediated disease (12).

tion. In any case, renal function, urinary sediment, and anti-GBM antibodies should be monitored after transplantation in Goodpasture patients.

REFERENCES

1. Goodpasture EW. The significance of certain pulmonary lesions in relation to the etiology of influenza. Am J Med Sci 1919; 158:863–870.
2. Stanton MC, Tange JD. Goodpasture's syndrome (pulmonary heamorrhage associated with glomerulonephritis). Aust NZ J Med 1958; 7:132–144.
3. Scheer RL, Grossman MA. Immune aspects of the glomerulonephritis associated with pulmonary haemorrhage. Ann Intern Med 1964; 60:1009–1021.
4. Lerner RA, Glassock RJ, Dixon FJ. The role of antiglomerular basement membrane antibody in the pathogenesis of human glomerulonephritis. J Exp Med 1967; 126:989–1004.
5. Beleil OM, Coburn JW, Shinaberger JH, Glassock RJ. Recurrent glomerulonephritis due to anti-glomerular basement membrane antibodies in two successive allografts. Clin Nephrol 1973; 1:377–380.
6. Briggs WA, Johnson JP, Teichman S, et al. Antiglomerular basement membrane antibody-mediated glomerulonephritis and Goodpasture's syndrome. Medicine (Baltimore) 1979; 58:348–361.
7. Wilson CB, Dixon FJ. Anti-glomerular basement membrane antibody-induced glomerulonephritis. Kidney Int 1973; 3:74–89.
8. Wilson CB, Dixon FJ. Diagnosis of immunopathologic renal disease. Kidney Int. 1974; 5:389–401.
9. Herody M, Bobrie G, Gouarin C, et al. Anti-GBM disease: Predictive value of clinical, histological and serological data. Clin Nephrol 1993; 40:249–255.
10. Savage COS, Pusey CD, Bowman C, et al. Antiglomerular basement membrane antibody mediated disease in the British Isles 1980-4. Br Med J 1986; 292:301–304.
11. Turner N, Rees AJ. Antiglomerular basement membrane disease. In: Cameron S, Davison AM, Grünfeld J-P, et al. (eds), Oxford Textbook of Clinical Nephrology. New York: Oxford University Press, 1992:438–456.
12. Merkel F, Pullig O, Marx M, et al. Course and prognosis of anti-basement membrane antibody (anti-BM-Ab)-mediated disease: Report of 35 cases. Nephrol Dial Transplant. Nephrol Dial Transplant 1994; 9:372–376.
13. Perl SI, Pussell BA, Charlesworth JA, et al. Goodpasture's (anti-GMB) disease and HLA-DRw2 (letter). N Engl J Med 1981; 305:463–464.
14. Rees AJ, Peters DK, Compston DA, Batchelor JR. Strong association between HLA-DRW2 and antibody-dedicated Goodpasture's syndrome. Lancet 1978; 1:966–968.
15. Rees AJ, Peters DK, Amos N, et al. The influence of HLA-linked genes on the severity of anti-GBM antibody-mediated nephritis. Kidney Int 1984; 26:445–450.
16. Huey B, McCormick K, Capper J, et al. Associations of HLA-DR and HLA-DQ types with anti-GBM nephritis by sequence-specific oligonucleotide probe hybridization. Kidney Int 1993; 44:307–312.
17. Bowman C, Ambrus K, Lockwood CM. Restriction of human IgG subclass expression in the population of auto-antibodies to glomerular basement membrane. Clin Exp Immunol 1987; 69:341–349.
18. Noel LH, Aucouturier P, Monteiro RC, et al. Glomerular and serum immunoglobulin G subclasses in membranous nephropathy and anti-glomerular basement membrane nephritis. Clin Immunol Immunopathol 1988; 46:186–194.
19. Rees AJ, Demaine AG, Welsh KI. Association of immunoglobulin Gm allotypes with antiglomerular basement membrane antibodies and their titer. Hum Immunol 1984; 10:213–220.
20. Weber M, Lohse AW, Manns M, et al. IgG subclass distribution of autoantibodies to glomerular basement membrane in Goodpasture's syndrome compared to other autoantibodies. Nephron 1988; 49:54–57.
21. Bernis P, Hamels J, Quoidbach A, et al. Remission of Goodpasture's syndrome after withdrawal of an unusual toxin. Clin Nephrol 1985; 23:312–317.
22. D'Apice AJ, Kincaid Smith P, Becker GH, et al. Goodpasture's syndrome in identical twins. Ann Intern Med 1978; 88:61–62.
23. Gossain VV, Gerstein AR, Janes AW. Goodpasture's syndrome: A familial occurrence. Am Rev Resp Dis 1972; 105:621–624.
24. Simonsen H, Brun C, Thomsen OF, et al. Goodpasture's syndrome in twins. Acta Med Scand 1982; 212:425–428.
25. Daniell WE, Couser WG, Rosenstock L. Occupational solvent exposure and glomerulonephritis: A case report and review of the literature. JAMA 1988; 259:2280–2283.
26. Heptinstall RH. Antiglomerular basement membrane antibody disease. In: Heptinstall RH, ed. Pathology of the Kidney. Boston: Little, Brown, 1992:677–712.
27. Jampol LM, Lahov M, Albert DM, Craft J. Ocular clinical findings and basement membrane changes in Goodpasture's syndrome. Am J Ophthalmol 1975; 79:452–463.

28. McIntosh RM, Copack P, Chernack WB, et al. The human choroid plexus and autoimmune nephritis. Arch Pathol 1975; 99:48–50.
29. Eble JA, Golbik R, Mann K, Kühn K. The $\alpha 1\beta 1$ integrin recognition site of the basement membrane collagen molecule $[\alpha 1(IV)]_2$ $\alpha 2(IV)$. EMBO J 1993; 12:4795–4802.
30. Timpl R. Structure and biological activity of basement proteins. Eur J Biochem 1989; 180:487–502.
31. Weber M. Basement membrane proteins. Kidney Int 1992; 41:620–628.
32. Hudson BG, Wieslander J, Wisdom BJ, Noelken ME. Goodpasture syndrome: Molecular architecture and function of basement membrane antigen. Lab Invest 1989; 61:256–269.
33. Hudson BG, Reeders, ST, Tryggvason K. Type IV collagen: Structure, gene organization, and role in human disease. J Biol Chem 1993; 268:26033–26036.
34. Brazel D, Oberbäumer I, Dieringer H, et al. Completion of the amino acid sequence of the $\alpha 1$ chain of human basement membrane collagen (type IV) reveals 21 non-triplet interruptions located within the collagenous domain. Eur J Biochem 1987; 168:529–536.
35. Hostikka SL, Tryggvason K. The complete primary structure of the $\alpha 2$ chain of human type IV collagen and comparison with the $\alpha 1(IV)$ chain. J Biol Chem 1988; 263:19488–19493.
36. Soinien R, Haka-Risku T, Prockop DJ, Tryggvason K. Complete primary structure of the $\alpha 1$ chain of human basement membrane (type IV) collagen. FEBS Lett 1987; 225:188–194.
37. Butkowski RJ, Langeveld JPM, Wieslander J, et al. Localization of the Goodpasture epitope to a novel chain of basement membrane collagen. J Biol Chem 1987; 262:7874–7877.
38. Gunwar S, Saus J, Noelken ME, Hudson BG. Glomerular basement membrane: Identification of a fourth chain, $\alpha 4$, of type IV collagen. J Biol Chem 1990; 265:5466–5469.
39. Myers JC, Jones TA, Pohjolainen E-R, et al. Molecular cloning of the $\alpha 5(IV)$ collagen and assignment of the gene to the region of the X chromosome containing the Alport syndrome locus. Am J Hum Genet 1990; 46:1024–1033.
40. Pihlajaniemi T, Pohjolainen E-R, Myers JC. Complete primary structure of the triple-helical region and the carboxyl-terminal domain of a new type IV collagen chain, $\alpha 5(IV)$. J Biol Chem 1990; 265:13758–13766.
41. Saus J, Wieslander J, Langeveld JPM, et al. Identification of the Goodpasture antigen as the $\alpha 3(IV)$ chain of collagen IV. J Biol Chem 1988; 263:13374–13380.
42. Zhou J, Mochizuki T, Smeets H, et al. Deletion of the paired $\alpha 5(IV)$ and $\alpha 6(IV)$ collagen genes in inherited smooth muscle tumors. Science 1993; 261:1167–1169.
43. Morisson KE, Germino GG, Reeders ST. Use of the polymerase chain reaction to clone and sequence a cDNA encoding the bovine $\alpha 3$ chain of type IV collagen. J Biol Chem 1991; 266:34–39.
44. Morrison KE, Mariyama M, Yang-Feng TL, Reeders ST. Sequence and localization of a partial cDNA encoding the human $\alpha 3$ chain of type IV collagen. Am J Hum Genet 1991; 49:545–554.
45. Zhou J, Herz JM, Leinonen A, Tryggvason K. Complete amino acid sequence of the human $\alpha 5$ collagen chain and identification of a single base mutation in exon 29 from the 3′end converting glycine-521 in the collagenous domain to cystein in an Alport syndrome patient. J Biol Chem 1992; 267:12475–12481.
46. Weber S, Engel J, Wiedemann H, et al. Subunit structure and assembly of the globular domain of basement membrane collagen type IV. Eur J Biochem 1984; 139:401–410.
47. Weber S, Dölz R, Timpl R, et al. Reductive cleavage and reformation of the interchain and intrachain disulfide bonds in the globular hexameric domain NC1 involved in network assembly of basement membrane collagen (type IV). Eur J Biochem 1988; 175:229–236.
48. Siebold B, Deutzmann R, Kühn K. The arrangement of intra- and intermolecular disulfide bonds in the carboxy terminal, noncollagenous aggregation and cross-linking domain of basement-membrane type IV collagen. Eur J Biochem 1988; 176:617–624.
49. Timpl R, Wiedemann H, Van Delden V, et al. A network model for the organization of type IV collagen molecules in basement membranes. Eur J Biochem 1981; 120:203–211.
50. Kleppel MM, Fan WW, Cheong HH, Michael AF. Evidence for separate networks of classical and novel basement membrane collagen: Characterization of $\alpha 3(IV)$-Alport antigen heterodimer. J Biol Chem 1992; 267:4137–4142.
51. Butkowski RJ, Wieslander J, Kleppel M, et al. Basement membrane collagen in the kidney: Regional localization of novel chains related to collagen IV. Kidney Int 1989; 35:1195–1202.
52. Kleppel MM, Santi PA, Cameron DJ, et al. Human tissue distribution of novel basement membrane collagen. Am J Pathol 1989; 134:813–825.
53. Weber M, Pullig O. Different immunologic properties of the globular NC1 domain of collagen type IV isolated from various human basement membranes. Eur J Clin Invest 1992; 22:138–146.
54. Griffin CA, Emanuel BS, Hansen JR, et al. Human collagen genes encoding basement membrane alpha1(IV) and alpha2(IV) chains map to the distal long arm of chromosome 13. Proc Natl Acad Sci USA 1987; 84:512–516.
55. Mariyama M, Kalluri R, Hudson BG, Reeders ST. The $\alpha 4(IV)$ chain of basement membrane collagen:

Isolation of cDNAs encoding bovine α4(IV) and comparison with other type IV collagens. J Biol Chem 1992; 267:1253–1258.
56. Hostikka SL, Eddy RL, Byers MG, et al. Identification of a distinct type IV collagen alpha chain with restricted kidney distribution and assignment of its gene to the locus of X-chromosome-linked Alport syndrome. Proc Natl Acad Sci USA 1990; 87:1606–1610.
57. Pöschl E, Pollner R, Kühn K. The genes for the α1(IV) and α2(IV) chains of human basement membrane collagen type IV are arranged head-to-head and separated by a bidirectional promoter of unique structure. EMBO J 1988; 7:2687–2695.
58. Butkowski RJ, Wieslander J, Wisdom BJ, et al. Properties of the globular domain of type IV collagen and its relationship to the Goodpasture antigen. J Biol Chem 1985; 260:3739–3747.
59. Kleppel MM, Michael AF, Fish AJ. Antibody specificity of human glomerular basement membrane type IV collagen NC1 subunits. J Biol Chem 1986; 261:16547–16552.
60. Weber M, Meyer zum Büschenfelde KH, Köhler H. Immunological properties of the human Goodpasture target antigen. Clin Exp Immunol 1988; 74:289–294.
61. Wieslander J, Barr JF, Butkowski RJ, et al. Goodpasture antigen of the glomerular basement membrane: Localization to noncollagenous regions of type IV collagen. Proc Natl Acad Sci USA 1984; 81:3838–3842.
62. Neilson EG, Kalluri R, Sun MJ, et al. Specificity of Goodpasture autoantibodies for the recombinant noncollagenous domains of human type IV collagen. J Biol Chem 1993; 268:8402–8405.
63. Kalluri R, Gunwar S, Reeders ST, et al. Goodpasture syndrome: Localization of the epitope for the autoantibodies to the carboxyl terminal region of the α3(IV) chain of basement membrane collagen. J Biol Chem 1991; 266:24018–24024.
64. Wieslander J, Langeveld J, Butkowski R, et al. Physical and immunochemical studies of the globular domain of type IV collagen. J Biol Chem 1985; 260:8564–8570.
65. Kashtan CE, Michael AF. Alport syndrome: From bedside to genome to bedside. Am J Kidney Dis 1993; 22:627–640.
66. Barker DF, Hostikka SL, Zhou J, et al. Identification of mutations in the COL4A5 collagen gene in Alport syndrome. Science 1990; 248:1224–1227.
67. Reeders ST. Molecular genetics of hereditary nephritis. Kidney Int 1992; 42:783–792.
68. Tryggvason K, Zhou J, Hostikka SL, Shows TB. Molecular aspects of Alport syndrome. Kidney Int 1993; 43:38–44.
69. Kleppel MM, Kashtan CE, Butkowski RJ, et al. Alport familial nephritis: Absence of the 28 kilodalton non-collagenous monomers of type IV collagen in glomerular basement membranes. J Clin Invest 1987; 80:263–266.
70. McCoy RC, Johnson HK, Stone WJ, Wilson CB. Absence of nephritogenic GBM antigen(s) in some patients with hereditary nephritis. Kidney Int 1982; 21:642–652.
71. Hudson BG, Kalluri R, Gunwar S, et al. The pathogenesis of Alport syndrome involves type IV collagen molecules containing the α3(IV) chain: Evidence from anti-GBM nephritis after renal transplantation. Kidney Int 1992; 42:179–187.
72. Kalluri R, Weber M, Netzer K-O, et al. COL4A5 gene deletion and production of posttransplant anti-α3(IV) collagen alloantibodies in Alport syndrome. Kidney Int 1994; 45:721–726.
73. Jayne DRW, Marshall PD, Jones SJ, Lockwood CM. Autoantibodies to GBM and neutrophil cytoplasm in rapidly progressive glomerulonephritis. Kidney Int 1990; 37:965–970.
74. Weber M, Andrassy K, Pullig O, et al. Antineutrophil-cytoplasmic antibodies and antiglomerular basement membrane antibodies in Goodpasture's syndrome and in Wegener's granulomatosis. J Am Soc Nephrol 1992; 2:1227–1234.
75. Beirne GJ, Wagnild JP, Zimmermann SW, et al. Idiopathic crescentic glomerulonephritis. Medicine (Baltimore) 1977; 56:349–381.
76. Benoit FL, Rulon DB, Theil GB, et al. Goodpasture syndrome: A clinicopathological entity. Am J Med 1964; 37:424–444.
77. Proskey AJ, Weatherbee L, Eaterling RE, et al. Goodpasture syndrome: A report of five cases and review of the literature. Am J Med 1970; 48:162–173.
78. Teague CA, Doak PB, Simpson IJ, et al. Goodpasture's syndrome: An analysis of 29 cases. Kidney Int 1978; 13:492–504.
79. Johnson JP, Moore J, Austin HA, et al. Therapy of antiglomerular basement membrane antibody disease: Analysis of prognostic significance of clinical, pathologic and treatment factors. Medicine 1985; 64:219–227.
80. Noel LH, Gubler MC, Bobrie G, et al. Inherited defects of renal basement membranes. Adv Nephrol 1989; 18:77–94.
81. Peters DK, Rees AJ, Lockwood CM, Pusey CD. Treatment and prognosis in antibasement membrane antibody–mediated nephritis. Transplant Proc 1982; 14:513–521.

82. Turner N, Mason PJ, Brown R, et al. Molecular cloning of the human Goodpasture antigen demonstrates it to be the $\alpha3$ chain of type IV collagen. J Clin Invest 1992; 89:592–601.
83. Walker RG, Scheinkestel C, Becker GJ, et al. Clinical and morphological aspects of the management of crescentic anti-glomerular basement membrane antibody (anti-GBM) nephritis/Goodpasture's syndrome. Q J Med 1985; 54:75–89.
84. Weber M, Köhler H, Manns M, et al. Identification of Goodpasture target antigens in basement membranes of human glomeruli, lung, and placenta. Clin Exp Immunol 1987; 67:262–269.

55

Molecular Genetics of Polycystic Kidney Disease

Stefan Somlo
Albert Einstein College of Medicine, Bronx, New York

Gregory G. Germino
Johns Hopkins University School of Medicine, Baltimore, Maryland

INTRODUCTION

Autosomal dominant polycystic kidney disease (ADPKD) refers to at least three genetically distinct disorders characterized by cystic enlargement of the kidneys. The incidence of ADPKD is between 1 in 600 and 1 in 1000 live births, making it one of the most common Mendelian disease traits in humans. The clinical spectrum of renal and extrarenal manifestations of this disorder has been the subject of several recent reviews (1–4) and is only briefly summarized here. The primary structural renal manifestation of ADPKD is progressive, bilateral, multiple cyst formation. It is uncertain from the available evidence whether this process involves recruitment of new nephrons to form cysts or progressive enlargement of existing cysts. Complications of the renal lesion include hypertension, which is very prevalent in the ADPKD population and the occurrence of which seems to correlate with cyst enlargement. Activation of the renin-angiotensin system is seen (5,6) and may be the result local intrarenal ischemia due to attenuation of blood vessels by the enlarging cysts. Of course, the most serious renal complication of ADPKD is end-stage renal disease (ESRD), which occurs in ~45% of affected individuals by the age of 60. Although the typical age of onset of ESRD is in middle life, the range is from infancy to 80 years. The renal disease is less aggressive in women than in men and is more aggressive in the setting of hypertension than in its absence.

Pain, both acute and chronic, is a common complication. Chronic pain can be the result of renal and/or cyst enlargement. Acute pain, with or without hematuria, is often the result of cyst infection, hemorrhage, or nephrolithiasis. The latter occurs in 20% of the ADPKD population (3). The extrarenal manifestations of ADPKD include cysts in the liver, which are common, as well as cysts in the ovary, pancreas, or spleen, which are rare. The appearance of liver cysts increases with age, affecting ~75% of patients over 60 years, and the number and size of liver cysts is influenced by female steroid hormones (7). Cardiac valvular abnormalities, most often mitral valve prolapse, are also associated with ADPKD (8). Intracranial saccular aneurysms occur in ADPKD patients, and their rupture is one of the catastrophic complications of the disease (4,9,10). Finally, ADPKD patients have an increased incidence of colonic diverticulosis relative to the non-ADPKD population.

The gene responsible for the majority of ADPKD resides on chromosome 16 and is referred to as *PKD1*. The second most common mutation occurs in a gene on chromosome 4, *PKD2* (see below). The PKD1 and PKD2 phenotypes are very similar both clinically and pathologically—so much so that there were no clinical grounds for suspecting genetic heterogeneity until it was demonstrated by linkage analysis (11,12). Once linkage heterogeneity was described, reports emerged showing that PKD2 may have a milder phenotype than PKD1 when assessed by age at renal death, at cyst appearance, and at onset of hypertension (13,14). Since there is marked intrafamilial—i.e., between individuals with identical disease genotypes—as well as interfamilial variation in the clinical expression of ADPKD, factors other than the disease genotype alone must act as significant determinants of disease progression in an individual.

Autosomal recessive polycystic kidney disease (ARPKD) is phenotypically and pathologically distinct from ADPKD (15–17). This is a rare disease with an incidence between 1 per 10,000 and 1 per 50,000. Parents of affected children are never affected and the pedigrees are small. ARPKD manifests two general clinical phenotypes—a presentation in infancy and a presentation in childhood. The infantile presentation includes oligohydramnios, difficult delivery due to markedly enlarged abdomen, and Potter facies. The major complications in this presentation are renal insufficiency and hypertension, often complicated by congestive heart failure and respiratory distress due to pulmonary hypoplasia, atelectasis, and pneumomediastinum (17). The proximate cause of death is most often pulmonary distress. Congenital hepatic fibrosis is present. The childhood presentation is characterized by progressive renal insufficiency and complications of portal hypertension due to congenital hepatic fibrosis. In ARPKD, there is much less intrafamilial variability than interfamilial variability. There is no evidence for locus heterogeneity in this disease.

Taken together, these disorders define the spectrum of "polycystic" diseases of the kidney, although a much longer list of conditions, both inherited and sporadic, manifest tubulocystic enlargement in the kidney (18). This chapter presents the available data on progress toward identification of these disease genes as well as some considerations regarding the pathogenesis of polycystic kidney disease that stem from molecular biological investigations.

MECHANISMS OF CYSTOGENESIS

In the absence of direct knowledge of the gene defect in any of the forms of polycystic kidney disease, investigations have centered on elucidating the mechanisms of cystogenesis. It is beyond the scope of the present discussion to review this topic, but a few hypotheses are highlighted, since they are useful adjuncts in the discussions of candidate genes to follow. Tubular epithelial cell proliferation is a central component of the polycystic phenotype, as evidenced by the presence of an increased number of cells in cyst walls (19) and the polypoid hyperplasia that has been described in cystic epithelium (20). Several in vitro cell culture models of cystogenesis (18) have been studied with respect to properties of cellular proliferation. Some studies have suggested that primary cyst-lining epithelial cell cultures show more rapid growth than normal tubular epithelium (21), but this finding has not been universal (22). Primary monolayer cultures of epithelial cells derived from human ADPKD cysts showed increased sensitivity to the mitogenic effects of epidermal growth factor (EGF), hydrocortisone, and insulin and a decreased sensitivity to the growth inhibitory activity of transforming growth factor β when compared to primary cultures of normal tubular epithelial cells (23,24).

In addition to cellular proliferation, fluid secretion is a prerequisite for cyst formation. In vitro studies of intact cysts from ADPKD patients demonstrated net fluid secretion into the cyst lumen (25). Native cyst fluid contained unidentified secretagogues and achieved a comparable secretory response to that obtained by stimulation with a nonspecific stimulator of adenylate cyclase (25). The authors suggest that interference with net fluid secretion into cysts may limit cyst growth and therefore may be a reasonable target for pharmacological intervention in ADPKD. The mislocalization of the Na^+, K^+-ATPase to the apical membrane of cyst lining epithelium in ADPKD (26) and in the *cpk/cpk* mouse model (27) is another potential explanation for the abnormal secretory function exhibited by cyst epithelium. This mislocalization of the Na^+, K^+-ATPase is not found in all models of polycystic disease and is therefore not likely to be an absolute requirement for cystogenesis. The finding that other membrane proteins are also mislocalized (e.g., Ref. 28) suggests that a general defect in intracellular protein trafficking may be a component of the polycystic phenotype. Primary defects in extracellular matrix and cellular differentiation have also been proposed as pathogenic in polycystic disease, and this topic has recently been reviewed (29).

Most recently, indirect evidence has suggested a role for the microtubule cytoskeleton in the pathogenesis of polycystic disease (30). Epithelial cells from human and murine polycystic kidneys in suspension culture spontaneously form cystic structures. This process is not blocked by inhibitors of DNA, RNA, or protein synthesis but is reversibly inhibited by blockade of Na^+, K^+-ATPase activity (ouabain, amiloride) and by treatment with the microtubule-specific inhibitors taxol, colchicine, and vinblastine (30). The effect of these agents was assessed in an in vivo murine model of recessive polycystic kidney disease—*cpk/cpk* (see below). Weekly intraperitoneal injections of taxol significantly extended the survival of *cpk/cpk* mice, which normally die a uremic death by day 28 postnatally (30). Pathological examination of the kidneys revealed only mild cystic changes compared to untreated controls, although there was more evidence of chronic fibrosis (30). Colchicine and vinblastine were lethal to the newborn mice. Methotrexate, an inhibitor of DNA synthesis and therefore of cellular proliferation, did not alter the course of the disease (30). The authors speculated that a defect in microtubular function related to intracellular trafficking may result in the polycystic phenotype (30). This is the first instance of a pharmacological intervention affecting the course of polycystic kidney disease in vivo.

ANIMAL MODELS OF POLYCYSTIC DISEASES

Animal models of human disease states often mimic selected aspects of the human disorder without entirely recapitulating the human phenotype. In addition, even for monogenic diseases in animal models, the phenotypic expression is greatly dependent on the genetic background onto which the mutation is bred. Interpretation of the relevance of an animal model to human disease based on the phenotypic spectrum observed in the former must be tempered by this variable factor.

There are a number of animal models for polycystic disease, some more intensively studied than others (Table 1). The large number of animal disease genes producing a cystic phenotype is not surprising given the number of human polycystic diseases (≥4) and the many syndromal disorders manifesting significant cystic changes in the kidney as part of their clinical spectrum. A possible interpretation of this variety is that the kidney responds to many injuries by the general phenomenon of cyst formation. This is further supported by the finding that nongenetic insults, such as prolonged exposure to dialysis in humans leading to acquired cystic disease (31) or diphenylthiazole induced kidney disease in mice (32), also result in cyst formation.

Autosomal Dominant Models of Polycystic Kidney

Three autosomal dominant animal models of polycystic disease have been reported—the Han:SPRD-*cy*/+ rat (33), the CFW_{wd} mouse (34), and the SR2-3 chimeric mouse (35). The Han:SPRD-*cy*/+ rat resembles human ADPKD in renal morphology and the delayed onset of renal failure in adult

Table 1 Animal Models of Polycystic Kidney Disease[a–c]

	Chromosome	Modifier loci	Human chromosome
Dominant models			
Han:SPRD-cy/+ (rat)	—	—	—
CFW_{wd}	—	—	—
SR2-3	—	—	—
Recessive models			
C57BL/6J-cpk/cpk	12		2p24-2p25
DBA/2FG-pcy/pcy	9	—	—
C57BL/6J-jpk/jpk	11	10(DBA)/1(BL/6)	—
Balb/c-bpk/bpk	—	—	—
nm1633/nm1633	8	19	—
TgN737Rpw/TgN737Rpw	14		13
bcl-2-/-	1	—	18q21

[a]Scc text for references and discussion.
[b]Organism is mouse unless otherwise noted.
[c]Mutations are spontaneously occurring except for SR2-3 (chimera), TgN737Rpw (insertional mutagenesis) and bcl-2-/- (targeted disruption).

rats. It differs by the absence of the associated extrarenal manifestations (e.g., liver cysts and berry aneurysms) and the fact that the disease is more severe in affected male rats than in female rats (36). As in human disease, cysts arise from all segments of the nephron but, unlike in human disease, cystic enlargement does not correlate well with azotemia. The renal cysts in CFW_{wd} mice (34) derive from all segments of the nephron and lead to slowly progressive renal failure. Interestingly, 20% of these mice also have liver cysts. Unlike human disease, kidney enlargement is not necessarily seen with cystic changes and cyst development in this model is environmentally controlled, since mice in germ-free colonies rarely develop disease while mice in ambient environment invariably do (34). The SR2-3 chimera, containing a single integrated copy of the v-*src* retroviral vector SR2, has renal cysts without extrarenal manifestations (35). No germ-line transmission has been reported to date. The genesis of the phenotype is due either to disruption of a mouse ADPKD gene or expression of the v-*src* oncogene carried by the retroviral vector used (35).

Naturally Occurring Autosomal Recessive Models of Polycystic Kidney Disease

There are a number of naturally occurring recessive mouse models for polycystic disease. The most extensively studied model is the C57BL/6J-*cpk*/*cpk* mouse. Heterozygous mice do not develop renal cysts, while homozygotes initially show proximal tubular dilatation in the fetus and newborn (37,38) but subsequently develop predominantly collecting duct cysts with concomitant renal enlargement and rapidly progressive azotemia leading to death by the third postnatal week (37,39). The *cpk* mutation has been localized to mouse chromosome 12 (40). The homologous region in the human genome is on chromosome 2p24-2p25 (41). Preliminary linkage studies in human disease with markers from the homologous region were not conclusive (L. Guay-Woodford, University of Alabama, Birmingham, AL; personal communication). The availability of refined genetic maps of the human genome should provide more conclusive data on the role of this syntenic region in human ARPKD.

The DBA/2FG-*pcy*/*pcy* homozygote animals show a slower rate of progression of disease—renal enlargement begins after the eighth week postnatally and uremia after the eighteenth week—with cysts arising from all segments of the nephron (42). The later stages of the disease are associated with cerebral artery aneurysms, but no liver abnormalities are seen (42). This mouse shows phenotypic features more associated with the dominant form of polycystic kidney disease in a recessively acting mutation. The *pcy* gene resides on mouse chromosome 9 (42). The C57BL/6J-*jpk*/*jpk* recessive mouse mutation gives rise to a phenotype intermediate between *cpk* and *pcy* with progressive cystic enlargement of the kidneys and no other organ involvement (42a). The *jpk* mutation has been mapped to mouse chromosome 11 and modifier loci have been identified on chromosome 10 from the DBA/2J strain and on chromosome 1 from the C57BL/6J strain (42b). Another recessively inherited model is the Balb/c-*bpk*/*bpk* mouse (43,44). This model is phenotypically similar to the *cpk* mouse, with rapid kidney enlargement and death from azotemia in the first month. It has the added features of liver involvement with intrahepatic biliary tract dysplasia and dilatation of the common bile duct (43,44). Chromosomal localization of the gene is unknown. Another spontaneous, recessively acting mouse mutation causing polycystic kidney disease has recently been identified (E. Birkenmeier, Jackson Laboratory, Bar Harbor, ME; Forefronts in Nephrology Symposium, May 1994). The *nm1633* mouse line shows progressive cystic enlargement of the kidneys and has the added phenotypic features of small body size, rounded facies, testicular hypoplasia, and severe progressive anemia. The mutation has been mapped to mouse chromosome 8 and, in what is becoming a recurrent theme in these studies, a modifier locus has been mapped to the distal tip of mouse chromosome 19 (E. Birkenmeier, Jackson Laboratory, Bar Harbor, ME; Forefronts in Nephrology Symposium, May 1994).

Autosomal Recessive Models of Polycystic Kidney Disease Created Through Genetic Engineering

Recently, a recessive polycystic mouse strain was produced by insertional mutagenesis (45). The mouse line *TgN(Imorpk)737Rpw* contains a single gene disruption at the *TgN737Rpw* locus on mouse chromosome 14 between the T cell receptor–α and retinoblastoma–1 genes (45). The homologous region of the human genome is on chromosome 13 (45). The normal *TgN737Rpw* gene encodes a widely expressed 3.2-kb messenger RNA that is present in fetal and adult life and encodes a putative 824–amino acid protein. This protein has no know homology with previously identified proteins but does contain 10 copies of the 34–amino acid tetratricopeptide repeat (TPR) motif (45). This motif has been described in nuclear proteins active in the cell cycle, and the authors speculate that this gene may have some cell cycle regulatory role in the epithelial component in the kidney. Homozygous disruption of this gene may lead to aberrant proliferation of epithelial cells and subsequent cyst formation (45). The renal lesions in the neonatal *TgN737Rpw/TgN737Rpw* animal show primarily proximal tubular dilation, and a progressive shift to a predominance of collecting duct cysts is noted with increasing age (45). Involvement of the intrahepatic biliary tract manifests primarily as hyperplasia, dysplasia, and portal fibrosis, which occur in homozygous mice (45). This phenotype closely resembles human ARPKD in some genetic backgrounds. A human homologue of the murine *TgN737Rpw* gene has been isolated and evaluated as a candidate gene for human ARPKD by direct sequencing (46, 46a). No mutations were identified in 34 affected individuals tested (L. F. Onunchic, Johns Hopkins University, Baltimore, MD; personal communication). This model represents the first renal cystic disease in which the primary, single gene defect has been identified. Although its direct relation to human polycystic disease is uncertain, the discovery of the function of the *TgN737Rpw* gene product will certainly contribute to the understanding of genetically determined cystogenesis in the kidney.

Targeted disruption of the *bcl-2* gene on chromosome 1 in mice recently produced another mouse line with polycystic kidneys (47). *Bcl-2* is an oncogene that acts by preventing or delaying the programmed cell death that normally results in response to apoptotic stimuli. It is normally widely expressed in virtually all developing tissues but shows tightly defined expression in mature organisms. The *bcl-2-/-* phenotype included massive cell death in lymphoid organs, coat hypopigmentation, and polycystic kidneys (47). The -/- mice develop enlarged, cystic kidneys between 10 days and 10 weeks of life. While cystic enlargement is not clearly age-dependent in this model, progressive azotemia is. The histological lesions are clearly proliferative. Proximal, distal, and convoluted tubules are involved and occasionally demonstrate tissue growing into the lumen, with multilayered epithelium and mitotic figures (47). Glomeruli with epithelial crescents are also seen (47). A transgenic mouse, SBM, that overexpresses c-*myc* (48) has some phenotypic similarities with the *bcl-2-/-* mouse, which is consistent with the reported cooperation between c-*myc* and *bcl-2* in promoting cell growth (49). The authors suggest that perhaps loss of functional *bcl-2* leads to unchecked endogenous c-*myc* activity leading to the excessive proliferation and the polycystic phenotype (47).

The region in the mouse genome homologous to the PKD1 locus on human chromosome 16 has been mapped to mouse chromosome 17 near the *t* complex and the globin pseudogene *Hbs-ps4* (50). It follows that any mouse model for the PKD1 human disease would have to involve a gene form this region. The syntenic region for PKD2 is not yet identified but is likely to lie on mouse chromosome 5 (or, less likely, 3), based on the present synteny map.

The significant advantage that the study of animal models possesses over the direct study of the human disease stems from the ability to manipulate the animal to better understand the pathobiology of the disease. For genetics-based approaches, the animal models afford the opportunity to breed the animals to optimally localize the disease gene interval and to identify modifier loci associated with disease progression. The disadvantages include the fact that positional cloning approaches in animal models are not more straightforward than in the human genome and, as is the case in the PKD models, the relationship of the mouse disease to the human disease is not always that certain.

MOLECULAR GENETICS OF HUMAN POLYCYSTIC KIDNEY DISEASES

Despite extensive and intensive studies directed at the mechanisms of cystogenesis, identification of the primary defects underlying the polycystic kidney diseases has not been forthcoming. The advent of molecular genetic techniques for directly analyzing the human genome have made possible approaches to disease gene identification that are not based on the study of complex phenotypes.

Rather, these approaches use the genetic basis of the disease as the means for directly identifying disease genes by an approach termed "positional cloning" (51–53). In the initial phase of this approach, the mutated gene is localized to a specific region of a chromosome by genetic linkage analysis and/or cytogenetic analysis. The genetic map is then refined to define closest flanking markers separated by less than 2 centiMorgan (cM, the unit of genetic distance), corresponding to ~2% recombination. A physical map is then generated in the region between the closest flanking genetic markers and the genomic interval is cloned in large-capacity vectors such as yeast artificial chromosomes, P1 bacteriophage, cosmids, etc. The cloned DNA obtained from the region thus defined is then screened for candidate expressed sequences. Such candidate sequences are then screened to detect alterations that are associated with the disease phenotype. These are not sequential processes; rather, they often proceed in parallel. Genomic cloning often begins with larger genetic intervals (>2 cM) since, such clones permit the isolation of additional polymorphic markers that may be useful in narrowing the interval. Conversely, even once the interval is <2 cM, one is always trying to refine it further because, in doing so, one can refine the physical interval and this is the easiest way in which to eliminate genes from further consideration.

The Chromosome 16-Linked Form of *ADPKD–ADPKD1*

Mutations in *PKD1* account for 79–91% of cases of ADPKD (54). This gene was first localized to chromosome 16p13.3 by the discovery of linkage to a hypervariable marker near the α-globin locus (55). The genetic distance between this marker and the disease locus is ~5 cM. A battery of genetic markers subsequently mapped to this region has been successfully used to define the genetic interval more precisely (56–58). Physical mapping has established that the closest flanking genetic markers are less than 500 kb apart (58,59). Two sets of overlapping genomic clones, separated by a gap of less than 20 kb, span virtually the entire interval (59). Southern blot hybridization studies comparing the genomic DNA restriction maps in this interval for individuals affected with ADPKD with that of unaffected individuals have so far failed to identify disease-producing mutations.

Identification of Candidate Genes

An intensive search for candidate genes within the PKD1 candidate interval has identified 20 independent sets of cDNA clones (60) (Figure 1). This likely represents an underestimate of the total number of genes in the region. A minimum of 60 kb of mRNA have been detected by hybridization of cDNA clones to Northern blots, including one very large transcript of ≥12 kb that is a member of a complex multigene family (G.G.G.; unpublished observations).* Most of the genes are expressed in multiple tissues, including normal and cystic kidney. Sequence analysis and comparison to the GenBank, Swissprot, and EMBL data bases using the BLASTX algorithm has identified a number of important homologies (Table 2). Hybridization studies using the cDNA clones on Southern blots of genomic DNA from affected individuals have, to date, failed to identify disease-specific variants. The candidate genes are presently being analyzed by single-strand conformational analysis (SSCA) (61) and direct genomic sequencing to identify oligo- or single-nucleotide sequence differences between the genomes of normal and affected individuals. It is this part of the positional cloning paradigm that has proved most refractory to the development of technological advances that have significantly expedited the other steps.

Refining the Genetic Interval: Recombination Mapping and Linkage Disequilibrium

Several genetic approaches have been attempted to reduce the number of candidate genes. One strategy has been to seek additional positional information by screening large number of meioses for recombinations between the closest flanking markers and the disease locus. Such recombination events can be further studied with internal polymorphic markers to identify new closest flanking markers. Unfortunately, such recombination events are rarely observed when the loci are as close as the markers flanking *PKD1* (*GGG1*, *NK92.6SH1.0*; Figure 1). Indeed, no recombinants between these markers have been found in the more than 1000 meioses segregating for ADPKD studied so far (58). Furthermore, one must be cautious in interpreting rare apparent recombinations between

*At the time of this writing, reports were emerging that this gene, identified by clones h,i,j,k,l in Figure 1, had been identified as the *PKD1* gene.

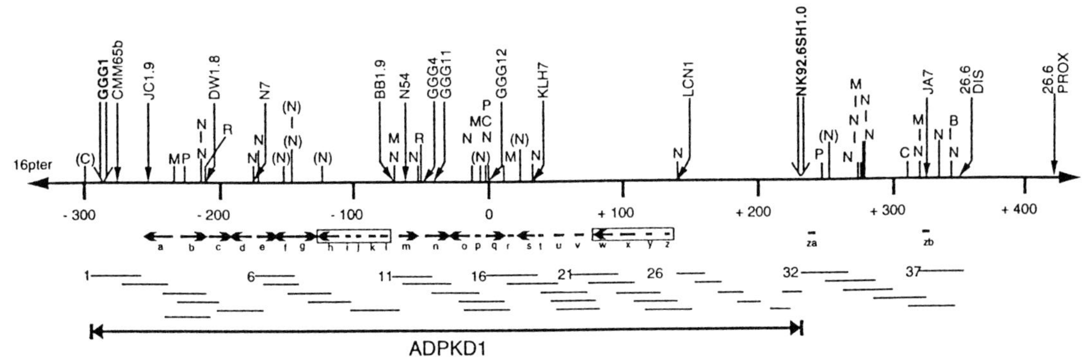

Figure 1 Map of the *PKD1* region on chromosome 16. Markers used in mapping are denoted by the vertical arrows above the line representing the linear array along the chromosome with 100-kb intervals indicated. The two polymorphic markers, *GGG1* and *NK92.6SH1.0*, are the closest flanking genetic markers for *PKD1* and define a ~500-kb physical segment. The single letter symbols above the line denote infrequent cutter restriction enzyme sites: *Cla*I (C), *Mlu*I (M), *Pvu*I (P), *Not*I (N), *Bss*HII (B). The numbered segments at the bottom (1-37) represent a set of cosmid and bacteriophage genomic clones that contain the entire region save ~20 kb in a gap between clones 29 and 30. Above the genomic clones, the cDNAs (a–z) corresponding to the genes in the region are shown. The arrowheads indicate the 5′ to 3′ orientation where such information is known and the boxes define a group of cDNAs from the same gene.

the disease phenotype and flanking markers, since the probability of an apparent recombination being a "pseudorecombinant" approaches that of it being a true recombinant. Apparent recombinations not due to true crossing-over events between homologous chromosomes can arise from gene conversion events, misdiagnoses, unusually late age of onset of disease, or laboratory error (e.g., mixup of DNA samples). In the case of *PKD1*, discordant genetic localization data provided by recombination mapping are likely due to one of the factors cited above (58). Genetic heterogeneity complicates the matter even further. In mapping recombinants, one presumes that the phenotype accurately reflects the genotype of the locus being studied rather than the genotype of an unlinked locus. An apparent recombination event detected in a small family with insufficient

Table 2 Clones from the ADPKD1 Region with Sequence Similarities to Members of Gene Families with Known Functions

Gene	Motif or homologous domain	Gene family "relatives"
AJ1	16kD H^+ATPase	16kD H^+ATPase
KG5	2 sets of C2H2 zinc-finger domains	ϕAP3, WT1, Kruppel
KG17	Cyclin family	Cyclin F
KG3	RING zinc-finger domain, β-transducin repeats	RAG-1, rpt-1, RAD18, PML, dTAFII 80 subunit of *Drosophila* TFIID, LIS-1
Nik9	Ankyrin repeats (six units), cytoplasmic tail of eph tyrosine kinase family	ankyrin, TAN-1, bcl-3, MAD3, NF-κBp105, eph, eck, elk, cek
Nik7	GTP-binding protein	Rab8, Rab4b, Rap2b
Nik1238	Two nucleotide-binding domains, two sets of six membrane-spanning domains	ABC family of transporters, MDR, CFTR
KM17	β-transducin repeats	As above
SAZD	β-transducin repeats	As above
SAZB	Unknown	ERV1 regulatory protein, yeast
SAZ20	GTP-ase activating protein	Tuberin

meioses to confirm chromosome 16 linkage may simply reflect a mutation at an unlinked disease locus (e.g., *PKD2*) in that family. In sum, recombination mapping has not been able to reduce the *PKD1* interval to less than 500 kb.

Searching for linkage disequilibrium is another means of refining the localization of disease genes. Linkage disequilibrium may occur when a disease mutation has spontaneously arisen or been imported through a founder effect into a population on a single or small number of ancestral chromosomes. Before discussing this concept further, a few terms need to be defined. The term "locus" refers to a unique position of a gene or marker along the linear array of a chromosome, and "allele" refers to one of several alternative forms of genetic information at a locus. Allelism is a direct consequence of the fact that there are a two copies (homologues) of every chromosome—one inherited from each parent. Thus, in an autosomal dominant trait like PKD1, an affected individual inherits one normal copy of the *PKD1* gene from the normal parent and one mutated copy of the gene from the affected parent. This affected individual is therefore heterozygous at the *PKD1* locus with one normal allele and one mutated allele of the *PKD1* gene. "Haplotype" refers to an associated group of alleles at two or more separate loci close together on a chromosome that tend to be inherited as a group due to their genetic proximity.

Linkage disequilibrium can be assessed by observing an association of the disease phenotype with a specific allele of a polymorphic locus among a group of unrelated individuals. This is in contrast to genetic linkage, where cosegregation of alleles at a locus and a disease phenotype is observed within families but not necessarily across families. Recombination events cause deviation from the ancestral haplotype, but the rate of this change depends on the genetic distance between loci, the time between introduction of the mutation and genetic testing, and the rate of new mutations developing at the disease locus. Generally, alleles of polymorphic loci very close to the disease locus maintain their association with the disease allele over long periods of time. Haplotype analysis, looking at multiple, closely spaced polymorphic loci near a disease gene, further increases the power of linkage disequilibrium analysis. The locus where a shared haplotype between unrelated individuals with the same disease phenotype becomes discordant likely represents one boundary of the genetic interval. Therefore, identifying a cluster of markers with alleles in linkage disequilibrium with a disease may direct the search for the mutant gene. This approach was extremely useful in the cloning of the Huntington disease gene (62,63), where discordant recombination mapping information had localized the disease locus to two unique, multimegabase intervals. Linkage disequilibrium was also instrumental in the identification of *CFTR* as the mutated gene in cystic fibrosis (64).

Testing for linkage disequilibrium in *PKD1* has not been definitive. The disease is associated with numerous haplotypes, even in relatively homogenous populations (65). This implies that *PKD1* is likely to have arisen spontaneously many times, consistent with the modest de novo mutation rate that has been reported (66). The latter may also help explain the high incidence of the disease. Evidence for linkage disequilibrium has been detected between *PKD1* and markers near the centromeric end of the genetic interval in several European populations (65,67–69, 69a). Haplotype analysis, while inconclusive, has suggested KG8 and 92.6SH1.0 as possible boundaries (65). Although this may reduce the number of candidates by one-third, a minimum of 12 genes, representing over 35 kb of coding sequence, remain as potential candidates (Figure 1).

Candidate Gene Functions and Their Possible Relationships to Kidney Disease

Probable functions for a number of the candidates have been determined by comparison of their partial sequences to data bases of known genes (Table 2). Perhaps the most striking observation is that many of the candidates encode proteins with functions consistent with current hypotheses of cystogenesis. For example, a defect in intracellular protein sorting mechanisms has been proposed as the primary cause of cyst formation in ADPKD (26) based on the discovery of altered polarity for several membrane proteins in cyst-lining epithelium–e.g., Na^+, K^+-ATPase (26,27), and epidermal growth factor receptor (EGF-R) (24,28). One of the PKD1 candidate genes is a novel member of the Rab family of proteins, a class of small GTP-binding proteins important in regulating intracellular membrane trafficking (70).

Alternative hypotheses suggest that cysts arise as a consequence of a primary abnormality of cellular proliferation (71) or cell fate determination (29). There are PKD1 candidates that may be important in these processes. The murine homologue of the zinc-finger gene *KG5* is a transcription factor found in its active, phosphorylated form in proliferating cells; it is thought to repress expression of genes that are important in inhibiting the cell cycle. The KG3 gene encodes a domain shared by a different class of transcription factors as well as a region of β-transducin repeats thought likely to mediate protein-protein interactions. Another candidate is a homologue of the cyclin F family. The ankyrin repeat motif, a feature of NIK9, is common to a number of transcription factors, cell-cycle proteins, and receptors important in cell fate determination. Last, the gene mutated in 30% of all cases of tuberous sclerosis (*TSC2*, tuberin) (72) was initially cloned as one of the PKD1 candidates (D. Weinstat-Saslow, Ph.D. thesis, Yale University, New Haven, CT, 1991). Tuberin encodes a GTPase that functions as a growth suppressor gene (73). Another prominent hypothesis for the molecular pathogenesis of ADPKD involves abnormalities of extracellular matrix components (29). To date, no genes mapping to the PKD1 interval have been discovered with homology to any of the known extracellular matrix proteins, although some of the genes for which no known homology exists may encode novel proteins that function in this capacity.

Tuberous Sclerosis (TSC2) and ADPKD1

A survey of the list of probable functions for the *PKD1* candidate genes (Table 2) suggests a clustering of genes with potentially complementary functions that may be important for normal renal morphogenesis and function. The discovery of altered levels of the gene products or mRNA in cystic kidney for several of the candidates (G.G.G.; unpublished observations) is consistent with this hypothesis. The colocalization of one form of tuberous sclerosis (TSC2) to the *PKD1* interval lends further support to this hypothesis. Renal manifestations are a common feature of this genetically heterogeneous, autosomal dominant disorder. Although benign tumors (angiomyolipomas) are the most common renal manifestation, renal cystic disease radiographically indistinguishable from that of ADPKD also is observed (74). Indeed, there have been instances of families initially diagnosed as having ADPKD who subsequently were reclassified as TSC after the discovery of a child with renal cystic disease and new-onset seizure disorder due to cortical tubers.

One possible explanation for the clinical overlap of ADPKD and TSC2 is that a subset of TSC2 patients have deletions (72) that include nearby genes (contiguous-gene syndrome). This could arise either at the germ-line level (all cells of the body inherit the same deletion) or as a consequence of a second mutation within somatic cells. The observation of loss of heterozygosity for PKD1 genetic markers in renal angiomyolipomas from tuberous sclerosis patients supports the hypothesis of a two-hit tumor or growth suppressor gene model for TSC (73). It should be noted that patients with the chromosome 9 form of tuberous sclerosis, TSC1, also develop renal cysts suggesting the possibility that defects in TSC2 alone may be sufficient to cause renal cysts.. Regardless the discovery of two diseases with common renal manifestations in a less than 500-kb segment of the human genome supports the hypothesis of a clustering of genes important in kidney structure and function.

The Second Major Gene for ADPKD–ADPKD2

Genetic and Physical Mapping to Define the Location of ADPKD2 as the Initial Step Toward Identifying the Gene

PKD2, the mutated gene in the second major form of ADPKD, has been localized to chromosome 4q in a region bounded by the polymorphic markers *D4S231* and *D4S423* (75,76). The genetic map around the *PKD2* gene locus, based on the integrated map produced by the Cooperative Human Linkage Center (CHLC) (77), is shown in Figure 2. The entire ~14 cM interval between the polymorphic loci *D4S400* and *D4S423* has been cloned in a minimal set of nine overlapping yeast artificial chromosome (YAC) clones with insert sizes ranging between 1.1 and 1.8 million bases. Such a panel of clones is called a “YAC contig” (78). Over 40 sequence tag sites (STS) have been mapped and unequivocally ordered on this contig. STS are short stretches of genomic DNA sequence for which primers exist that allow amplification of the segment by the polymerase chain reaction (PCR) (78). The cardinal feature of these STS are that they are unique loci and therefore represent a single “address” in the human genome. Their presence in a genomic clone such as a YAC identifies that clone as containing that portion of the genome for which the STS is the “address” or tag. If one assumes that, on a genomewide average, 1 cM of genetic distance corresponds to 1 million bases (based on 3×10^9 bases in the human genome $\div$ ~3000 cM in a sex-averaged genome), then the 14-cM *D4S400–D4S423* interval represents ~14 million bases and the average spacing of the STSs would be ~300,000 bases. There is no way to truly convert genetic distances to physical distances

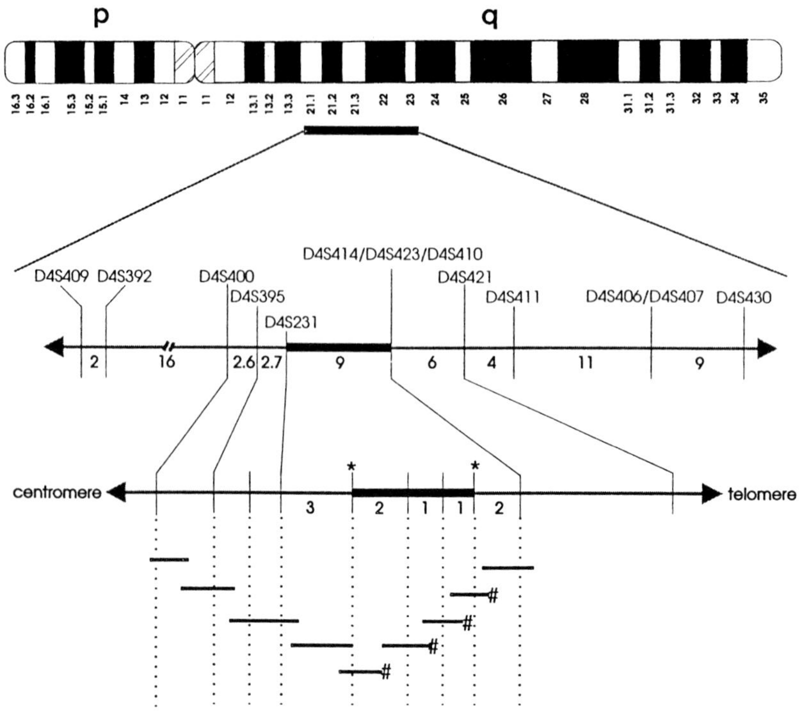

Figure 2 Schematic representation of the *PKD2* region on the long arm of chromosome 4. Below the chromosome ideogram showing the general Giemsa band localization for *ADPKD2* is the genetic map of that region with the 9-cM D4S231 to D4S423 interval of the initial linkage report in bold. The integers denote genetic distances in centiMorgans. These distances are approximate and are based on the integrated CHLC genetic map. The bottom panel shows a refined genetic map with additional, unpublished markers denoted by vertical bars not identified in the panel above. The pair of markers labeled with * are the new closest flanking markers which define a <4-cM interval for *PKD2*. Below this map is a schematic representation of the yeast artificial chromosome contig that spans the entire region. The four CEPH mega-YACs that now contain the interval between the closest flanking markers, are marked with #. It is important to note that the superposition of the genetic and physical maps in this figure is defined only by STS content—i.e., which YACs contain which markers—and that the relative genetic distance in the upper panels cannot be extrapolated to the actual physical distances covered by the YACs.

directly, so these figures are only valid as a genomewide average. These STS serve as physical landmarks on the YAC contig that ensure the fidelity of genomic clones obtained and provide a framework for ordering newly identified STS and genomic clones in the continued disease-gene cloning effort.

Since the nine cM *PKD2* genetic interval described in the original reports is too large for efficient positional cloning strategies (51), the recent effort has focused on identifying new polymorphic markers from the YACs spanning the *PKD2* genetic interval. The class of genetic markers sought are termed microsatellites and consist of simple sequence repeats, most commonly dinucleotide repeats of the $(CA)_n$ variety (79), which can be PCR amplified using primers designed to flanking unique sequence. These markers exhibit length polymorphism dependent on the number of repeat units present and alleles can be resolved on standard sequencing gels. The degree of polymorphism is related to the number of repeat units present, with stretches of more than 20 repeats being highly polymorphic and therefore very useful in genetic studies (a property called "informativeness") (80). Several such markers have been isolated in the PKD2 region (Figure 2) and have been useful in reducing the genetic interval to <4 cM. This reduced interval is wholly contained in a contig of four YACs, as illustrated in Figure 2. Low-stringency hybridization of cDNAs for *PKD1* candidate genes to these four YAC clones has not revealed any homologous sequences. The absence of *PKD1* homologs in the *PKD2* region in the setting of such similar phenotypes supports the hypothesis that the *PKD1* and *PKD2* genes may act at different steps along the same cellular pathway (e.g., control of proliferation, intracellular trafficking, etc.). A gene-by-gene search will be required to identify *PKD2* unless the discovery of *PKD1* sheds light on the functional and/or structural nature of *PKD* genes in general and thus facilitates the discovery of *PKD2*.

Future Directions in the Cloning of PKD2

As the PKD2 genetic interval is narrowed to <2 cM, the emphasis will shift to genomic clone-based strategies for isolating cDNAs. These strategies include various cDNA selection (81–83) and exon-trapping techniques (84–86). The goal will be the production of a transcription map of the region identifying all the candidate genes for *PKD2*. The strategies discussed previously with respect to identification of the *PKD1* gene will then be applied in the final step of disease gene identification.

Forms of ADPKD Unlinked to Either Chromosome 16 or Chromosome 4

One ADPKD family has been described that does not show genetic linkage to either chromosome 16 or chromosome 4 markers (87). The phenotype in this family was that of classical ADPKD with five affected children, two of whom had liver cysts as well. There was no clinical evidence that this family represented a "phenocopy" in the form of tuberous sclerosis or von Hippel-Lindau disease, two disorders that can mimic the radiographic findings of ADPKD in the kidney but not the liver. At least one additional unlinked family has since been identified (unpublished observation) making the existence of a third locus for ADPKD very likely. This finding has both clinical and scientific significance since further subclassification of families according to disease genotype may reveal additional differences in disease progression and response to therapy as well as hasten our understanding of the basic disease process and thereby improve our ability to develop rational therapeutic interventions.

Human Autosomal Recessive Polycystic Kidney Disease—ARPKD

Genetic studies of human ARPKD have been hampered by both a lack of large pedigrees and the infrequency of the disease (1 in 10,000 to 1 in 50,000). Genetic heterogeneity, if it exists, would serve to further dilute the power of linkage analysis in this group of families. Recently, however, genetic linkage to a single locus on 6p21-cen in 16 simplex ARPKD families was identified (87a), with a cumulative lod score of >7.0 (where a lod score >3.0 is considered proof of linkage). A marker that showed no recombination with disease was identified and there was no evidence for heterogeneity in these 16 families. However, this group of families did not include families with the neonatal form of ARPKD. Linkage in this latter subset of families has subsequently been confirmed (87b). In ARPKD, intrafamilial variability is much less than interfamilial variability. In the absence of linkage heterogeneity, this supports the notion that it is allelic heterogeneity (i.e., different mutant alleles at the same disease locus) that may produce the different phenotypes and phenotype/genotype correlation may prove instructive.

GENERAL CONSIDERATIONS

Variability in the expression of ADPKD is an important clinical phenomenon that is yet to be satisfactorily explained. Undoubtedly, allelic mutations account for at least some of the interfamilial variation, and mutation analyses are likely to yield important genotype/phenotype information for the ADPKD genes. These studies, however, may not explain the intrafamilial differences in disease severity nor do they explain the observation that only a small fraction of nephrons become cystic despite all cells inheriting an identical mutation.

One possible genetic explanation for these latter observations is that the mutation is not static within a family or an individual. A new class of mutations have been described which are notable for their molecular instability (88–90). GC-rich trinucleotide repeats, which frequently lengthen as a consequence of somatic and meiotic mutation, have been discovered within the 5′ or 3′ untranslated or coding regions of eleven disease genes (e.g., Refs. 91–93; reviewed in Ref. 93a). Clinical severity of these disorders within families directly correlates with the length of the repeats (94–96) and the diseases show the clinical phenomenon of anticipation—progressive increase in the severity of the phenotype with successive generations. These diseases are also characterized by a high apparent de novo mutation rate.

Unstable DNA elements have been proposed as a primary cause of the variation observed in ADPKD (90,97). In this model, children severely affected with ADPKD (98,99) are predicted to have greatly expanded repeats; apparent de novo mutations develop as a result of unstable repeat expansion on the background of a pre-mutation—a previous increase in repeat length that was insufficient to produce clinical disease (90,94,95); and renal cysts arise from nephron segments in which the repeats have undergone mitotic expansion (i.e., somatic mutation). An appealing aspect of this hypothesis is that it neatly explains many clinical features of ADPKD. Unfortunately, there are no molecular data currently available that support this hypothesis as applied to ADPKD. A search of the *PKD1* genomic clones for trinucleotide repeats that were unstable or greatly lengthened in severely affected children was negative (100). Such evidence does not exclude a role for unstable DNA elements in the molecular pathogenesis of ADPKD. Repetitive genomic sequences are frequently deleted by bacterial host cells, and our inability to identify expanded repeats may simply reflect their loss from our clones.

There is an alternative genetic explanation for the clinical variability. It is possible that loss of both *PKD1* alleles is required for cysts to form. According to this model, the *PKD1* gene would resemble many other tumor suppressor genes (e.g., retinoblastoma) in that it is inherited as an autosomal dominant trait but functions in a recessive manner at the molecular level. The germ-line mutation would be necessary but not sufficient for cyst formation. Sporadic mitotic mutations would inactivate the second (normal) allele and presumably result in the growth advantage, polarity differences, etc., observed in cyst epithelial cells. This explanation is appealing in its simplicity, but there is an important feature of this and the previous model that warrants further discussion.

Though only a small percentage of nephrons become cystic, the number of renal cysts is still very large. This suggests a much higher rate of somatic mutation involving the normal allele than has been observed for most other tumor suppressor genes. There are three possible explanations for this: (a) frequent nonmitotic mutations from carcinogens; (b) "conventional" mitotic mutations as seen involving other tumor suppressor genes that accumulate in a continuously proliferating organ like the colon; (c) unstable DNA elements that frequently mutate during the development of the kidney when there is a high mitotic rate—e.g., a trinucleotide repeat or a mutation "hot spot." The second option is unlikely given that the mature kidney is thought to have a low rate of mitosis. The first possibility is harder to exclude at this point, although there are no published examples of this mechanism for a "second hit." In the third model, mutations altering the previously normal allele arise spontaneously throughout the course of the development and growth of the kidney. One would predict that all tubular descendants of a progenitor cell that has undergone a second hit will inherit the same mutation at the previously normal allele. Cystic epithelium derived from another cell in the same kidney may have a different mutation in the previously normal allele. Of course, all cells in the kidney would have the same mutation in the allele of the *PKD1* gene carrying the germ-line mutation. A prediction of both the second and third explanations above is that epithelial cells lining renal cysts are likely to be clonal unless the second inactivating mutation results in the production of factors that act in an paracrine manner to recruit other tubular cells. This prediction of clonality in a molecular recessive model of cystogenesis of ADPKD can be assessed even before the gene is identified and studies are currently under way to determine if cyst lining epithelia in individual cysts from female kidneys are clonal in origin (G.G.G.; unpublished results).

Another prediction of the molecular "two hit" model is that homozygous individuals would be expected to have much more severe disease than heterozygous individuals, since they would have germ-line mutations involving both alleles. In the Han:SPRD-*cy*/+ autosomal dominant rat model, homozygous animals are more severely affected than heterozygotes (N. Gretz, Mannheim, Germany; personal communication), consistent with this hypothesis. The data available on human ADPKD do not provide a conclusive answer. In a report published only in abstract form (101), a single individual was inferred to have inherited a mutant *PKD1* gene from each of her affected parents. She was not more severely affected than her heterozygously affected siblings. Unfortunately, because of insufficient data, one cannot conclude with certainty that the individual truly is homozygously affected.

Another, more likely, cause for the variation in disease expression seen in ADPKD is the influence of genetic modifier loci. It is well recognized in animal models of cystic disease that breeding the mutant gene onto different genetic backgrounds significantly alters expression of the disease. As discussed above, this strategy has recently been used to localize genes important in modifying the expression of the cystic phenotype in *jpk/jpk* and *nm1633/nm1633* homozygous mice. Curiously, neither set of modifier loci mapped to other loci previously shown to harbor PKD genes. Obviously, breeding studies are not possible for identifying loci important in modifying the expression of human disease. However, large, carefully characterized clinical data bases such as that collected by the Polycystic Kidney Research Group at the University of Colorado may be very useful for comparing the phenotypic expression in affected siblings with genotype at candidate modifier loci such as the normal *PKD1* allele, *PKD2*, ARPKD, TSC1 and TSC2, the von Hippel-Lindau gene, hypertension genes, etc.

There is evidence to suggest that epigenetic and environmental influences also play an important role in affecting disease progression. In the Han:SPRD-*cy*/+ rat model, male rats are more severely affected than females. Human data are more ambiguous, but at least one study has implied a possible effect on the sex of the parent transmitting the disease mutation (99). Animal studies also imply a role for environmental influences. As discussed, CFW_{wd} mice raised in a pathogen-free animal facility do not develop cysts. There are two other observations that may suggest an important role for nongenetic factors. The first is the clinical course of the human disease. Cyst growth and possibly cyst number is not linear with time. The rapid expansion in cyst size over a relatively brief period of time in midlife may be the result of factors released by early cysts that act in a paracrine manner. In this scheme, cysts expand through a positive feedback mechanism, possibly recruiting previously unaffected segments. The second observation in support of this model is provided by the Han:SPRD-*cy*/+ rat model. Unilateral nephrectomy in these animals results in accelerated renal death (102). This effect may be mediated by the normal release of growth factors responsible for renal hypertrophy postnephrectomy. Finally, stochastic events have been reported to play an important role in the variable expression of other dominant diseases and may similarly be important in determining the fraction of nephroms that undergo cystic expansion in ADPKD (103).

It appears likely there are multiple steps in the pathway from an initial mutation to cyst formation and end-stage renal disease and that these factors may be at least as important as the primary mutation in the pathogenesis of cyst formation. Identifying and understanding the role of these factors may yield important insights into the pathophysiology of this disorder and thereby to the development of protective therapies. Given presently available technologies, targeting steps along the ADPKD pathway for therapeutic interventions may be more easily accomplished than treating this adult onset, autosomal dominant disease by gene therapy.

NOTE ADDED IN PROOF

The gene identified by clones h,i,j,k in Figure 1 has recently been identified as the *PKD1* gene through the discovery of a family with a balanced translocation and ADPKD (European Consortium. The polycystic kidney disease 1 gene encodes a 14kb transcript and lies within a duplicated region on chromosome 16. Cell 1994; 77:881–894). The initial study reported 40% of the cDNA sequence and did not identify any significant homologies with other known gene products. Analysis of the complete genomic sequence has revealed that the gene product is likely to be membrane glycoprotein with two leucine-rich repeats [American PKD1 Consortium, Analysis of the genomic sequence for the autosomal dominant polycystic kidney disease (PKD1) gene predicts the presence of a leucine rich repeat. Hum Mol Genet 1995; 4:575–582.]

ACKNOWLEDGMENT

This work was supported by Marion Merrell Dow PKD Research Merit Awards from the Polycystic Kidney Research Foundation (S.S. & G.G.G.) and NIH grants DK02015 (S.S.) and DK01423

(G.G.G.). The authors acknowledge the contributions of present and past members of the laboratories of Stefan Somlo, Gregory Germino, Stephen Reeders, and Anna-Maria Frischauf.

REFERENCES

1. Gabow PA. Autosomal dominant polycystic kidney disease. N Engl J Med 1993; 329:332–342.
2. Bennett WM, Elzinga LW. Clinical management of autosomal dominant polycystic kidney disease. Kidney Int Suppl 1993; 42:S74–S79.
3. Torres VE, Wilson DM, Hattery RR, Segura JW. Renal stone disease in autosomal dominant polycystic kidney disease. Am J Kidney Dis 1993; 22:513–519.
4. Chapman AB, Johnson AM, Gabow PA. Intracranial aneurysms in patients with autosomal dominant polycystic kidney disease: How to diagnose and who to screen. Am J Kidney Dis 1993; 22:526–531.
5. Chapman AB, Johnson A, Gabow PA, Schrier RW. The renin-angiotensin-aldosterone system and autosomal dominant polycystic kidney disease. N Engl J Med 1990; 323:1091–1096.
6. Chapman AB, Schrier RW. Pathogenesis of hypertension in autosomal dominant polycystic kidney disease. Semin Nephrol 1991; 11:653–660.
7. Everson GT. Hepatic cysts in autosomal dominant polycystic kidney disease. Am Kidney Dis 1993; 22:520–525.
8. Hossack KF, Leddy CL, Johnson AM, et al. Echocardiographic findings in autosomal dominant polycystic kidney disease. N Engl J Med 1988; 319:907–912.
9. Chapman AB, Rubinstein D, Hughes R, et al. Intracranial aneurysms in autosomal dominant polycystic kidney disease. N Engl J Med 1992; 327:916–920.
10. Huston J, Torres VE, Sulivan PP, et al. Value of magnetic resonance angiography for the detection of intracranial aneurysms in autosomal dominant polycystic kidney disease. J Am Soc Nephrol 1993; 3:1871–1877.
11. Kimberling WJ, Fain PR, Kenyon JB, et al. Linkage heterogeneity of autosomal dominant polycystic kidney disease. N Eng J Med 1988; 319:913–918.
12. Romeo G, Devoto M, Costa G, et al. A second genetic locus for autosomal dominant polycystic kidney disease. Lancet 1988; 2:8–11.
13. Parfrey PS, Bear JC, Morgan J, et al. The diagnosis and prognosis of autosomal dominant polycystic kidney disease. N Engl J Med 1990; 323:1085–1090.
14. Ravine D, Walker RG, Gibson RN, et al. Phenotype and genotype heterogeneity in autosomal dominant polycystic kidney disease. Lancet 1992; 340:1330–1333.
15. Zerres K. Autosomal recessive polycystic kidney disease. Clin Invest 1992; 70:794–801.
16. Shaikewitz ST, Chapman A. Autosomal recessive polycystic kidney disease: Issues regarding the variability of clinical presentation. J Am Soc Nephrol 1993; 3:1858–1862.
17. Cole BR. Autosomal recessive polycystic kidney disease, In: The Cystic Kidney. Dordrecht: Kluwer, 1990:327.
18. Wilson PD, Sherwood AC. Tubulocystic epithelium. Kidney Int 1991; 39:450–463.
19. Grantham JJ, Geiser JL, Evan AP. Cyst formation and growth in autosomal dominant polycystic kidney disease. Kidney Int 1987; 31:1145–1152.
20. Evan AP, Gardner KD JR, Bernstein J. Polypoid and papillary epithelial hyperplasia: A potential cause of ductal obstruction in adult polycystic disease. Kidney Int 1979; 16:743–750.
21. Wilson PD, Hreniuk D, Gabow PA. Abnormal extracellular matrix and excessive growth of human adult polycystic kidney disease epithelia. J Cell Physiol 1992; 150:360–369.
22. Carone FA, Nakamura S, Schumacher BS, et al. Cyst-derived cells do not exhibit accelerated growth or features of transformed cells in vitro. Kidney Int 1989; 35:1351–1357.
23. Wilson PD. Aberrant epithelial cell growth in autosomal dominant polycystic kidney disease. Am J Kidney Dis 1991; 17:634–637.
24. Wilson PD, Du J, Norman JT. Autocrine, endocrine and paracrine regulation of growth abnormalities in autosomal dominant polycystic kidney disease. Eur J Cell Biol 1993; 61:131–138.
25. Ye M, Grantham JJ: The secretion of fluid by renal cysts from patients with autosomal dominant polycystic kidney disease. N Engl J Med 1993; 329:310–313.
26. Wilson PD, Sherwood AC, Palla K, et al. Reversed polarity of Na(+) –K(+) –ATPase: mislocation to apical plasma membranes in polycystic kidney disease epithelia. Am J Physiol 1991; 260:F420–F430.
27. Avner ED, Sweeney WE JR, Nelson WJ. Abnormal sodium pump distribution during renal tubulogenesis in congenital murine polycystic kidney disease. Proc Natl Acad Sci USA 1992; 89:7447–7451.
28. Avner ED, Sweeney WE, Wilkinson JE, Woychik RP. Abnormal epidermal growth factor receptor (EGF-R) expression in congenital murine polycystic kidney disease (PKD) created through insertional mutagenesis. J Am Soc Nephrol 1993; 4:810.

29. Calvet JP. Polycystic kidney disease: Primary extracellular matrix abnormality or defective cellular differentiation? Kidney Int 1993; 43:101–108.
30. Woo DL, Miao SYP, Pelayo JC, Woolf AS. Taxol inhibits progression of congenital polycystic kidney disease. Nature 1994; 368:750–753.
31. Matson MA, Cohen EP. Acquired cystic kidney disease: occurrence, prevalence, and renal cancers. Medicine 1990; 69:217–226.
32. Kanwar YS, Carone FA. Reversible changes of tubular cell and basement membrane in drug-induced renal cystic disease. Kidney Int 1984; 26:35–43.
33. Kaspareit-Rittinghausen J, Deerberg F, Wcislo A. Hereditary polycystic kidney disease: Adult polycystic kidney disease associated with renal hypertension, renal osteodystrophy, and uremic enteritis in SPRD rats. Am J Pathol 1991; 139:693–696.
34. Werder AA, Amos MA, Nielsen AH, Wolfe GH. Comparative effects of germfree and ambient environments on the development of cystic kidney disease in CFWwd mice. J Lab Clin Med 1984; 103:399–407.
35. Boulter CA, Aguzzi A, Evans MJ, Affara N. A chimaeric mouse model for autosomal-dominant polycystic kidney disease. Contrib Nephrol 1992; 97:60–70.
36. Cowley BD JR, Gudapaty S, Kraybill AL, et al. Autosomal-dominant polycystic kidney disease in the rat. Kidney Int 1993; 43:522–534.
37. Gattone VH, Calvet JP, Cowley BD JR, et al. Autosomal recessive polycystic kidney disease in a murine model: A gross and microscopic description. Lab Invest 1988; 59:231–238.
38. Avner ED, Studnicki FE, Young MC, et al. Congenital murine polycystic kidney disease: I. The ontogeny of tubular cyst formation. Pediatr Nephrol 1987; 1:587–596.
39. Avner ED, Sweeney WE JR, Young MC, Ellis D. Congenital murine polycystic kidney disease: II. Pathogenesis of tubular cyst formation. Pediatr Nephrol 1988; 2:210–218.
40. Davisson MT, Guay-Woodford LM, et al. The mouse polycystic kidney disease mutation (cpk) is located on proximal chromosome 12. Genomics 1991; 9:778–781.
41. Simon EA, Cook S, Davisson MT, et al. The mouse congenital polycystic (cpk) locus maps within 1.3 cM of the chromosome 12 marker D12Nyu2. Genomics 1994; 21:415–418.
42. Takahashi H, Calvet JP, Dittemore-Hoover D, et al. A hereditary model of slowly progressive polycystic kidney disease in the mouse. J Am Soc Nephrol 1991; 1:980–989.
42a. Atala A, Freeman MR, Mandell J, Beier D. Juvenile cystic kidneys (jck): a new mouse mutation which causes polycystic kidneys. Kidney Int 1993; 43:1081–1085.
42b. Iakoubova OA, Dushkin H, Beier DR. Localization of a murine recessive polycystic kidney disease mutation and modifying loci that affect disease severity. Genomics 1995; 26:107–114.
43. Sweeney WE JR, Avner ED. Pathophysiology of renal tubular cyst formation in murine models of polycystic kidney disease. Contrib Nephrol 1992; 97:23–34.
44. Nauta J, Ozawa Y, Sweeney WE JR, et al. Renal and biliary abnormalities in a new murine model of autosomal recessive polycystic kidney disease. Pediatr Nephrol 1993; 7:163–172.
45. Moyer JH, Lee-Tischler MJ, Kwon HY, et al. Candidate gene associated with a mutation causing recessive polycystic kidney disease in mice. Science 1994; 264:1329–1333.
46. Onunchic LF, Schrick J, Guay-Woodford LM, et al. A human polymorphic site for the homolog of the gene mutated in the orpkd insertional mouse mutation identified by sequences analysis in ARPKD patients. J Am Soc Nephrol 1993; 4:820.
46a. Schrick JJ, Onuchic LF, Reeders ST, et al. Characterization of the human homologue of the mouse Tg737 candidate polycystic kidney disease gene. Hum Mol Genet 1995; 4:559–567.
47. Veis DJ, Sorenson CM, Shutter JR, Korsmeyer SJ. Bcl-2-deficient mice demonstrate fulminant lymphoid apoptosis, polycystic kidneys, and hypopigmented hair. Cell 1993; 75:229–240.
48. Trudel M, D'Agati V, Costantini F. C-myc as an inducer of polycystic kidney disease in transgenic mice. Kidney Int 1991; 39:665–671.
49. Vaux DL, Cory S, Adams JM: Bcl-2 gene promotes haemopoietic cell survival and cooperates with c-myc to immortalize pre-B cells. Nature 1988; 335:440–442.
50. Himmelbauer H, Pohlschmidt M, Snarey A, et al. Human-mouse homologies in the region of the polycystic kidney disease gene (PKD1). Genomics 1992; 13:35–38.
51. Collins FS. Positional cloning: Let's not call it reverse anymore. Nat Genet 1992; 1:3–6,
52. Germino GG, Somlo S, Weinstat-Saslow D, Reeders ST. Positional cloning approach to the dominant polycystic kidney disease gene, PKD1. Kidney Int Suppl 1993; 39:S20–S25.
53. Somlo S, Germino GG, Wirth B, et al. The molecular genetics of autosomal-dominant polycystic kidney disease of the PKD1 type. Contrib Nephrol 1992; 97:101–109.
54. Peters DJ, Sandkuijl LA. Genetic heterogeneity of polycystic kidney disease in Europe. Contrib Nephrol 1992; 97:128–139.
55. Reeders ST, Breuning MH, Davies KE, et al. A highly polymorphic DNA marker linked to adult polycystic kidney disease on chromosome 16. Nature 1985; 317:542–544.

56. Germino GG, Barton NJ, Lamb J, et al. Identification of a locus which shows no genetic recombination with the autosomal dominant polycystic kidney disease gene on chromosome 16. Am J Hum Genet 1990; 46:925–933.
57. Breuning MH, Snijdewint FG, Brunner H, et al. Map of 16 polymorphic loci on the short arm of chromosome 16 close to the polycystic kidney disease gene (PKD1). J Med Genet 1990; 27:603–613.
58. Somlo S, Wirth B, Germino GG, et al. Fine genetic localization of the gene for autosomal dominant polycystic kidney disease (PKD1) with respect to physically mapped markers. Genomics 1992; 13:152–158.
59. Germino GG, Weinstat-Saslow D, Himmelbauer H, et al. The gene for autosomal dominant polycystic kidney disease lies in a 750-kb CpG-rich region. Genomics 1992; 13:144–151.
60. Germino G, Weinstat-Saslow D, Somlo S, et al. The isolation and characterization of candidate genes for the chromosome 16-linked form of autosomal dominant polycystic kidney disease. J Am Soc Nephrol 1991; 2:253.
61. Orita M, Iwahana H, Kanazawa H, et al. Detection of polymorphisms of human DNA by gel electrophoresis as single-strand conformation polymorphisms. Proc Natl Acad Sci USA 1989; 86:2766–2770.
62. Snell RG, Thompson LM, Tagle DA, et al. A recombination event that redefines the Huntington disease region. Am J Hum Genet 1992; 51:357–362.
63. MacDonald ME, Lin C, Srinidhi L, et al. Complex patterns of linkage disequilibrium in the Huntington disease region. Am J Hum Genet 1991; 49:723–734.
64. Cutting GR, Antonarakis SE, Buetow KH, et al. Analysis of DNA polymorphism haplotypes linked to the cystic fibrosis locus in North American black and Caucasian families supports the existence of multiple mutations of the cystic fibrosis gene. Am J Hum Genet 1989; 44:307–318.
65. Peral B, Ward CJ, San Millan JL, et al. Evidence of linkage disequilibrium in the Spanish polycystic kidney disease 1 population. Am J Hum Genet 1994; 54:899–908.
66. Dalgaard OZ. Bilateral polycystic disease of the kidneys: A follow-up of 284 patients and their families. Acta Med Scand 1957; 158(suppl 328):1–255.
67. Pound SE, Carothers AD, Pignatelli PM, et al. Evidence for linkage disequilibrium between D16S94 and the adult onset polycystic kidney disease (PKD1) gene. J Med Genet 1992; 29:247–248.
68. Elles RG. Linkage disequilibrium between D16S94 and the locus for adult polycystic kidney disease (PKD1). J Med Genet 1992; 29:758.
69. Wright GD, Hughes AE, Larkin KA, et al. Linkage disequilibrium between the CA microsatellite D16S283 and PKD1. J Am Soc Nephrol 1993; 4:827.
69a. Snarey A, Thomas S, Schneider MC, et al. Linkage disequilibrium in the region of the autosomal dominant polycystic kidney disease gene (PKD1) Am J Hum Genet 1994; 55:365–371.
70. Simons K, Zerial M. Rab proteins and the road maps for intracellular transport. Neuron 1993; 11:789–799.
71. Grantham JJ. 1992 Homer Smith Award: Fluid secretion, cellular proliferation, and the pathogenesis of renal epithelial cysts. J Am Soc Nephrol 1993; 3:1841–1857.
72. The European Chromosome 16 Tuberous Sclerosis Consortium. Identification and characterization of the tuberous sclerosis gene on chromosome 16. Cell 1993; 75:1305–1315.
73. Green AJ, Smith M, Yates JR. Loss of heterozygosity on chromosome 16p13.3 in hamartomas from tuberous sclerosis patients. Nat Genet 1994; 6:193–196.
74. Bernstein J. Renal cystic disease in the tuberous sclerosis complex. Pediatr Nephrol 1993; 7:490–495.
75. Kimberling WJ, Kumar S, Gabow PA, et al. Autosomal dominant polycystic kidney disease: Localization of the second gene to chromosome 4q13-q23. Genomics 1993; 18:467–472.
76. Peters DJ, Spruit L, Saris JJ, et al. Chromosome 4 localization of a second gene for autosomal dominant polycystic kidney disease. Nat Genet 1993; 5:359–362.
77. Buetow KH, Weber JL, Ludwigsen S, et al. Integrated human genome-wide maps constructed using the CEPH reference panel. Nat Genet 1994; 6:391–393.
78. Green ED, Green P. Sequence-tagged site (STS) content mapping of human chromosomes: Theoretical considerations and early experiences. PCR Methods Appl 1991; 1:77–90.
79. Weber JL, May PE. Abundant class of human DNA polymorphisms which can be typed using the polymerase chain reaction. Am J Hum Genet 1989; 44:388–396.
80. Weber JL. Informativeness of human $(dC\text{-}dA)_n\text{-}(dG\text{-}dT)_n$ polymorphisms. Genomics 1990; 7:524–530.
81. Parimoo S, Patanjali SR, Shukla H, et al. cDNA selection: efficient PCR approach for the selection of cDNAs encoded in large chromosomal DNA fragments. Proc Natl Acad Sci USA 1991; 88:9623–9627.
82. Parimoo S, Kolluri R, Weissman SM. cDNA selection from total yeast DNA containing YACs. Nucleic Acids Res 1993; 21:4422–4423.
83. Tagle DA, Swaroop M, Lovett M, Collins FS. Magnetic bead capture of expressed sequences encoded within large genomic segments. Nature 1993; 361:751–753.
84. Duyk GM, Kim SW, Myers RM, Cox DR. Exon trapping: a genetic screen to identify candidate transcribed sequences in cloned mammalian genomic DNA. Proc Natl Acad Sci USA 1990; 87:8995–8999.

85. Buckler AJ, Chang DD, Graw SL, et al. Exon amplification: A strategy to isolate mammalian genes based on RNA splicing. Proc Natl Acad Sci USA 1991; 88:4005–4009.
86. Krizman DB, Berget SM. Efficient selection of 3′-terminal exons from vertebrate DNA. Nucleic Acids Res 1993; 21:5198–5202.
87. Daoust MC, Reynolds DM, Bichet DG, Somlo S. Evidence for a third genetic locus for autosomal dominant polycystic kidney disease. Genomics 1995; 25:733–736.
87a. Zerres K, Mucher G, Bachner L, et al. Mapping of the gene for autosomal recessive polycystic kidney disease (ARPKD) to chromosome 6p21-cen. Nature Genet 1994; 7:429–432.
87b. Guay-Woodford LM, Hopkins SD, Muecher G, Zerres K. The severe perinatal phenotype of ARPKD (autosomal recessive polycystic kidney disease) maps to chromosome 6p21-cen. J Am Soc Nephrol 1994; 5:624.
88. Kuhl DP, Caskey CT. Trinucleotide repeats and genome variation. Curr Opin Genet Dev 1993; 3:404–407.
89. Warren ST, Nelson DL. Trinucleotide repeat expansions in neurological disease. Curr Opin Neurobiol 1993; 3:752–759.
90. Caskey CT, Pizzuti A, Fu YH, et al. Triplet repeat mutations in human disease. Science 1992; 256:784–789.
91. Mahadevan M, Tsilfidis C, Sabourin L, et al. Myotonic dystrophy mutation: An unstable CTG repeat in the 3′ untranslated region of the gene. Science 1992; 255:1253–1255.
92. Kremer EJ, Pritchard M, Lynch M, et al. Mapping of DNA instability at the fragile X to a trinucleotide repeat sequence $p(CCG)_n$. Science 1991; 252:1711–1714.
93. The Huntington's Disease Collaborative Research Group. A novel gene containing a trinucleotide repeat that is expanded and unstable on Huntington's disease chromosomes. Cell 1993; 72:971–983.
93a. Willems PJ. Dynamic mutations hit double figures. Nature Genet 1994; 8:213–215.
94. Andrew SE, Goldberg YP, Kremer B, et al. The relationship between trinucleotide (CAG) repeat length and clinical features of Huntington's disease. Nature Genet 1993; 4:398–403.
95. Tsilfidis C, Mackenzie AE, Mettler G, et al. Correlation between CTG trinucleotide repeat length and frequency of severe congenital myotonic dystrophy. Nature Genet 1992; 1:192–195.
96. O'Hoy KL, Tsilfidis C, Mahadevan MS, et al. Reduction in size of the myotonic dystrophy trinucleotide repeat mutation during transmission. Science 1993; 259:809–812.
97. Reeders ST. Multilocus polycystic disease. Nature Genet 1992; 1:235–237.
98. Kaariainen H. Polycystic kidney disease in children: A genetic and epidemiological study of 82 Finnish patients. J Med Genet 1987; 24:474–481.
99. Fick GM, Johnson AM, Strain JD, et al. Characteristics of very early onset autosomal dominant polycystic kidney disease. J Am Soc Nephrol 1993; 3:1863–1870.
100. Somlo S, Schneider MC, Stevenson SA, et al. Is autosomal dominant polycystic kidney disease (ADPKD) the result of heritable unstable DNA sequences? J Am Soc Nephrol 1992; 3:302.
101. Bachner L, Armaignac C, Vinet M, et al. Possible homozygous subject for autosomal dominant polycystic kidney disease at PKD1 locus. Cytogenetics and Cell Genetics 1991; 58:2109.
102. Gretz N. Accelerated renal death after unilateral nephrectomy in a rat strain suffering from autosomal dominant polycystic kidney disease. J Am Soc Nephrol 1994; 4:1925–1926.
103. Prockop DJ, Colige A, Helminen H, Khillen JS, Pereira R, Vandenberg P. Mutations in type I procollagen that cause osteogenesis imperfecta: effects of the mutations on the assembly of collagen into fibrils, the basis of phenotypic variations, and potential antisense therapies. J Bone Miner Res 1993; 8(Suppl):S489–492.

56

Molecular Response to Ischemic and Nephrotoxic Acute Renal Failure

Robert L. Safirstein
University of Texas Medical Branch at Galveston, Galveston, Texas

Joseph V. Bonventre
Harvard Medical School, Massachusetts Institute of Technology, and Massachusetts General Hospital, Boston, Massachusetts

INTRODUCTION

The molecular response of the kidney to an ischemic or nephrotoxic insult is complex and incompletely understood. Complicating the interpretation of the array of genetic responses is the fact that while some genes may be expressed in a manner that is specific to the response of the kidney to the insult, other genes may be activated as nonspecific consequences of cell injury. For example, the injured cell is characterized by increases in cytosolic free calcium concentration and membrane depolarization (1,2)—changes that can activate a number of genes.

Gene induction may or may not have consequences for cell injury, survival or proliferation. Although most of the attention of investigators has been devoted to enhanced gene expression, resulting in increased levels of mRNA and protein, ischemia or nephrotoxic insults may also result in downregulation of genes, and this may be critically important for outcome. At present the integration of our phenomenological knowledge regarding gene induction and repression into a paradigm encompassing cell death, survival, and proliferation is rudimentary. Interpretation of the data is further complicated by the heterogeneous kidney architecture, which makes it important to identify spatial characteristics of gene expression within various kidney regions as well as among various tubular segments in that region.

This chapter provides an overview of the current state of knowledge of the molecular response to ischemic and nephrotoxic insults. It emphasizes the induced genetic programs that have been related to the regenerative process in the kidney after ischemia and reoxygenation. It also discusses, to a lesser degree, molecular responses that may play important roles in the injury itself as well as the process of cell death.

REGENERATION AND REPAIR

Recovery from ischemic and nephrotoxic acute renal failure requires replacement of damaged tubule cells with new ones that restore the morphological and functional integrity of the renal epithelium (2,3). During this process, normally quiescent renal cells increase their nucleic acid synthesis and undergo mitosis. This regenerative process has been documented to occur in the recovery phase of many forms of acute renal injury, including that caused by ischemia, gentamicin, folic acid, and cisplatin administration (4–8). Renal DNA synthesis often appears to peak at a time when renal function is at a nadir (9), suggesting, perhaps, some causal relationship between the two. Little is known, however, about the control and determinants of renal regeneration after injury. We will first discuss the effects of ischemia and nephrotoxic insults on genes that have been implicated in cell cycle control and then discuss genes that may be important for the regenerative response but are not directly associated with cell cycle control.

Genes Implicated in the Cell Cycle

The general characteristics of the renal DNA synthetic response to injury is shown in Figure 1, as measured by ^{3}H-thymidine incorporation in kidney cells (8). There is a sharp rise in ^{3}H-thymidine incorporation within 24 hr following release of a 50-min period of renal artery occlusion. This burst in renal DNA synthesis is seen with both ischemic and nephrotoxic insults, although the time course and extent vary with the severity of the damage to the kidneys. Increases in ^{3}H-thymidine incorporation (10) or 5-bromo-2′-deoxyuridine nuclear labeling (11,12) is also observed with systemic administration of growth factors, and growth factors have been proposed to be renotrophic agents accelerating the movement of cells through the cell cycle to replace damaged cells.

In order for mature, normally quiescent epithelial cells to divide, they must leave G_0 and enter the cell cycle. This likely entails the coordinated interplay of a number of cellular genes responding to stimuli transduced within the cell. Possible external stimuli may include growth factors such as platelet-derived growth factor (PDGF), epidermal growth factor (EGF), or insulin-like growth factor–1 (IGF-1). After the binding of a growth factor to its receptor, growth-promoting signals are generated which commit the cell to a new phase of the cell cycle, termed G_1. It is important to consider that a growth-promoting signal may also arise from within the cell. The transition to the G_1 phase has been well studied in tissue culture. While cells do not change their appearance in any obvious way, a number of genes are induced during this early transition from G_0 to G_1. Prominent among these are the so-called immediate early genes [13], whose expression is enhanced almost immediately after stimulation by many growth factors. This gene induction is transient and independent of new protein synthesis (14). Some of these immediate early genes encode DNA-binding transcription factors that likely initiate a genetic cascade ending in cell division. Others encode small secreted proinflammatory polypeptides and proteases whose role in cell division, if any, is less clear.

After a time delay that varies among different cell types, the cells move from G_0 into the next phase of the cycle, or G_1, where new protein and RNA synthesis occurs and the cells increase in size. The newly synthesized proteins and mRNAs are crucial for progression through the remainder of the G_1 phase as well as through the S phase, when DNA synthesis occurs. Additional protein and

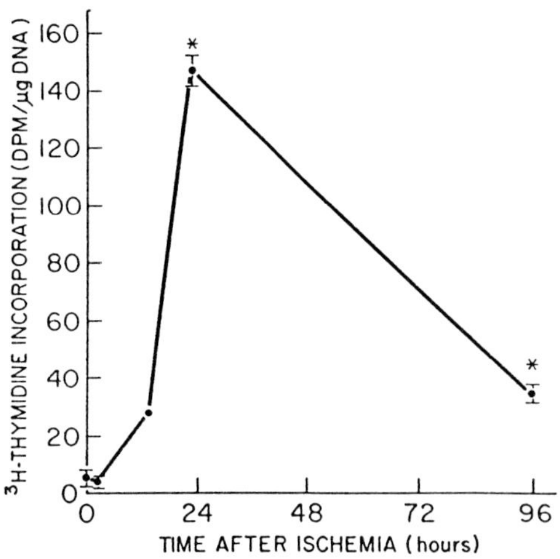

Figure 1 ^{3}H-Thymidine-specific activity (DPM/DNA) in whole kidney DNA in sham (n = 5), and animals 2 hr (n = 3), 16 hr (n = 1), 24 hr (n = 2), and 96 hr (n = 2) after ischemia. $^*p < 0.001$. (From Ref. 8.)

RNA synthesis is required for the cells to complete the cycle and undergo mitosis. Proliferating cell nuclear antigen (PCNA), a marker for the G_1-S transition in the cell cycle and hence mitogenesis, is a DNA polymerase–associated protein that can also be used as a marker for cell proliferation. Nuclei that stain positively for PCNA identify a population of cells in late G_1- and early S phases of the cell cycle (15). PCNA-positive nuclei are clearly detectable at 24 and 48 hr postischemia, with many more positive nuclei found in the S3 segment than in the S1 or S2 segments of the proximal tubule. The staining is particularly prominent in the S3 segment of the outer stripe (16) (Figure 2).

Table 1 lists the genes whose expression has been explored in various forms of nephrotoxic and ischemic damage. Renal injury—induced by ischemia, folic acid, glycerol, or cisplatin—and repair are associated with changes in expression of many genes with varied functions. The expression of transcription factors c-*fos* (6,8,17–20), c-*myc* (19–21), *Egr-1* (8,17,22), and NGF1-B (22) are all increased post-injury. Kid-1 expression is decreased after ischemia or folic acid (23); There are also increases in expression of small secreted cytokines (24), structural genes (6,18–20) as well as intracellular second-messenger proteins, including members of the Ras family [19] and c-*ros* (Safirstein; unpublished observation). There are also increases in expression of some growth factors (25–27) and decreased expression of others (6,8). In addition to changes in expression of these genes, which may be important for the regenerative process, there are also alterations in expression of genes that encode proteins—such as heat-shock proteins (28–30), clusterin (31–33), and superoxide dismutase (18)—which may play important roles in the injury process itself or in minimizing the injury. Finally, there is a change in expression of a number of other proteins, whose function, if any, in the injury or repair process is even less clear, including Tamm-Horsfall protein (24), renin (18), endothelin (34), parathyroid hormone–related protein (35), ADP-ATP translocase (20), histone H_4 (19), and histone H_{2b} (18).

For the immediate early genes examined, there is a striking parallel between the changes in gene expression induced by ischemic renal damage and those induced by growth factor stimulation of quiescent cells in culture. c-*fos* mRNA, the prototype of the nuclear binding members of the immediate early genes, increases almost immediately after release of renal hilar clamping (8,17,18). The expression of this gene is enhanced with many stimuli that potentiate cell division but also those that lead to cell activation or differentiation and are not linked to cell division. Pertinent in this regard is the observation that c-*fos* and *Egr-1* can be induced by cell depolarization (36), which occurs with cell energy depletion, and as such may be dissociated from the mitogenic response. c-*fos* gene induction with ischemia is short-lived and precedes the peak of renal DNA synthesis. The c-Fos protein localizes primarily to the nuclei of the medullary thick ascending limbs within the first few hours after ischemia (16). Some cells in the medullary collecting duct and the S3 segment of the proximal tubule also express the c-Fos protein.

An early postischemic increase in expression is also observed for the immediate early gene *Egr-1* (8,17). The c-Fos and Egr-1 proteins contain DNA binding motifs and regulate the transcription of other genes (37,38). While it is possible that these genes regulate the expression of downstream target genes that serve the renal regenerative response, the role, if any, that they play in the regenerative process is unknown. It is interesting that the c-Fos and Egr-1 proteins are induced to high levels in the thick ascending limbs, where there is minimal damage and regeneration during the postischemic period (16,39).

Another group of immediate early genes, the members of the small cytokine-like genes, are also expressed during renal ischemic injury. The expression of KC, which codes for a small secreted glycoprotein with potent chemotactic (40) and mitogenic (41) properties, increases to a maximum 1 hr after ischemia and returns to baseline levels by 4 hr postischemia in a pattern typical of the immediate early gene response. In contrast to c-Fos and Egr-1, the expression of JE, a potent monocyte chemoattractant (42), is increased at 48 hr after release of the hilar clamp. In contrast to its behavior in cells stimulated to grow in vitro, where the induction of the *JE* gene is brief, the expression of *JE* following ischemia is prolonged and persists for as long as 1 week (24). The significance of the expression of KC and JE is not known. Like c-Fos and Egr-1, the product of the *JE* gene is present primarily in the thick ascending limbs rather than the S3 segment of the proximal tubule, where most of the ischemic injury occurs. It is possible that KC and JE might be secreted by the thick ascending limb cells and act on the S_3 proximal tubule cells in a manner that enhances the regeneration of the damaged S_3 epithelium. A potentially detrimental effect of expression of

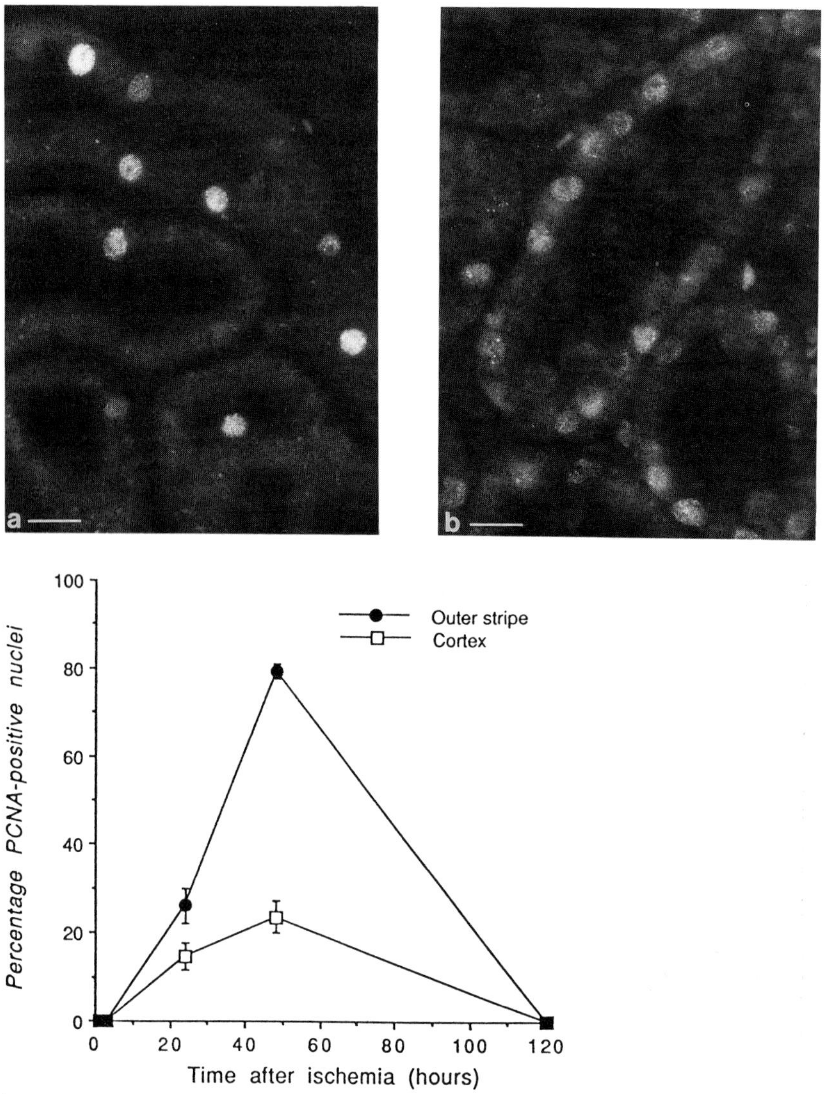

Figure 2 Expression of PCNA in cortex (a) and outer stripe of the outer medulla (b) of a postischemic kidney after 48 hr of reperfusion and time course of expression (c). (a and b) Sections of kidneys taken 48 hr after a 40-min. ischemic period were incubated with anti-PCNA antibodies. Nuclei stained in much greater numbers in the S3 segment of the proximal tubule in the outer stripe than in S1 and S2 segments located in the cortex. Bars = 20 μ. (c) A representative time course of PCNA staining of cortex and outer stripe taken from one set of animals studied at varying times of reperfusion after an ischemic period of 40 min. The peak of PCNA expression occurred at approximately 48 hr postischemia, although the percentage of positive nuclei in a given set of experiments varied somewhat at this peak time. At 120 hr, all cells were negative for PCNA. (From Ref. 16.)

Table 1 The Expression of Genes During Renal Regeneration

	Gene	Model	Direction	Ref.
Transcription factors				
	c-*fos*	Cisplatin	↑	(6)
		Ischemia	↑	(18)
				(17)
				(18)
		Folic acid	↑	(19)
				(20)
	c-*myc*	Folic acid	↑	(19)
				(20)
				(21)
	c-*jun*	Ischemia	↑	(56)
	Egr-1	Ischemia	↑	(17)
				(8)
		Folic acid	↑	(22)
	NGF1 B (glucocorticoid receptor-like)	Folic acid	↑	(22)
	Kid-1	Ischemia	↓	(23)
		Folic acid	↓	(23)
Small cytokine superfamily				
	KC	Ischemia	↑	(24)
	JE	Ischemia	↑	(24)
Structural genes				
	Actin	Ischemia	↑	(6)
				(18)
		Folic acid	↑	(19)
				(20)
	Vimentin	Folic acid	↑	(20)
Signaling				
	Ki-*ras* (G protein)	Folic acid	↑	(19)
	Ha-*ras*	Folic acid	↑	(19)
	c-*ros* (tyrosine kinase)	Ischemia	↑	Safirstein (unpublished observation)
Proteases				
	Tissue factor	Ischemia	↑	Safirstein (unpublished observation)
Growth factors				
	Hepatocyte growth factor	CCl_4	↑	(25)
		Ischemia	↑	(54)
	EGF	Cisplatin	↓	(6)
		Ischemia	↓	(8)
	IGF-I	Ischemia	↑	(26)

Table 1 (*Continued*)

	Gene	Model	Direction	Ref.
Genes associated with cell injury				
	Heat-shock protein	Ischemia	↑	(28)
				(29)
				(30)
	Clusterin	Ischemia	↑	(31)
		Glycerol	↑	(32)
				(33)
		Folic acid	↑	
	Superoxide dismutase	Ischemia	↓	(18)
Other				
	Tamm-Horsfall protein	Ischemia	↓	(24)
	Renin	Ischemia	↓	(18)
	Endothelin	Ischemia	↑	(34)
	Parathyroid hormone-related protein	Ischemia	↑	(35)
	ADP-ATP Translocase	Folic acid	↑	(20)
	Histone H_4	Folic acid	↑	(19)
	Histone H_{2b}	Ischemia	↑	(18)

these genes is the attraction of inflammatory cells, which may release reactive oxygen species and proteases, increase expression of leukocyte-endothelium adhesion molecules, and contribute to structural and functional deterioration of the kidney after ischemia (43,44).

In addition to these genes whose expression is upregulated in the postischemic period, the expression of other genes is downregulated. mRNA levels of a newly cloned putative kidney zinc-finger DNA-binding protein, Kid-1, is decreased following ischemic and folic acid–induced injury (23). This gene is downregulated under another condition where mitogenesis is induced: that is, early postnatal renal development. It is interesting that the non–zinc-finger region of the Kid-1 protein confers transcriptional repressor activity. Kid-1 may act, therefore, by inhibiting the expression of genes that encode proteins important for growth arrest or differentiation.

Not all cells participate equally in the genetic response to ischemic injury and regeneration. As indicated previously, it is the cells of the S3 segment of the proximal tubule that are most damaged by ischemia, and it is in this segment that much of the repair process occurs. The response of the cells of the thick ascending limb is interesting in this regard. While not featured prominently in the cellular necrosis provoked by either ischemic or nephrotoxic damage, these cells undergo both positive and negative regulation of gene transcription during renal injury, gaining the ability to express the nuclear-binding proteins Egr-1 (39) and c-Fos (16) while decreasing their synthesis of epidermal growth factor (EGF) and Tamm-Horsfall (TH) protein (see below), which they produce normally at high levels. Whether the thick ascending limb responds to a self-generated signal or to one arising from outside the cell membrane is unknown, but the close proximity of the thick ascending limb to the injured pars recta of the proximal tubule and activated interstitial cells (Figure 3) in the outer stripe of the outer medulla suggests that bidirectional communication is possible. Understanding of the renal regenerative response will require identification of the cells that initiate the growth-promoting signals and how these signals may affect events in the S3 segment cells.

Factors that Induce Renal DNA Synthesis

It is reasonable to consider that the regenerative processes occuring postischemia or after a nephrotoxic insult may be induced by growth factors. One growth factor that has been proposed to

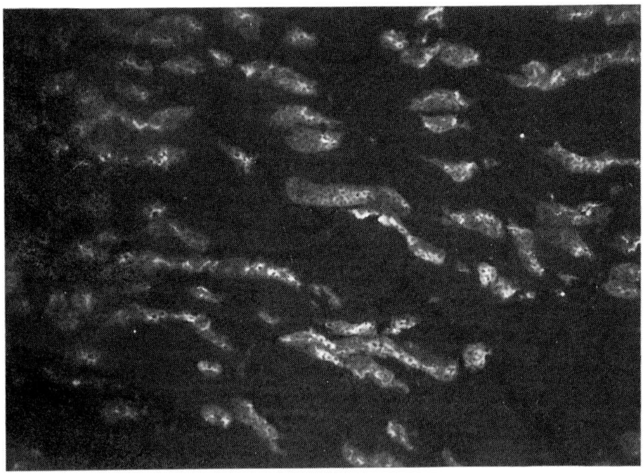

(a)

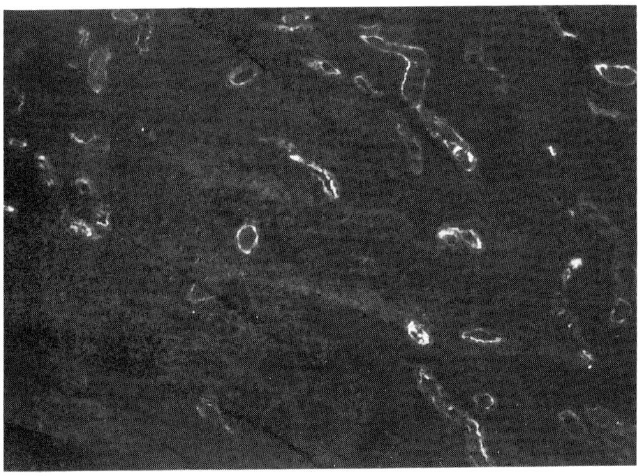

(b)

Figure 3 Thin sections (5 μm) of the outer stripe of the outer medulla from control rat kidney (a) and kidney removed 24 hr after 50 min-period of bilateral hilar clamping (b). Thick ascending limbs are labled using an FITC-labled anti–Tamm Horsfall (TH) antibody. TH staining is markedly reduced in the postischemic kidney, consistent with reduced TH mRNA levels at this time period (24). In the postischemic kidneys, thick ascending limbs are surrounded by islands of necrotic tubules.

potentiate the regenerative process is EGF, which, when administered to animals after ischemia, hastens recovery of renal function and enhances kidney tissue ^{3}H-thymidine incorporation (10,45). In a preliminary report (46), TGFα—which is related to EGF and binds the EGF receptor (47), and like EGF, is mitogenic for proximal tubule cells (48)—has been reported to accelerate renal recovery after acute renal failure. The EGF gene is highly expressed in the normal kidney (49) and EGF is mitogenic for the proximal tubule (50). The expression of preproEGF falls, however, and remains low for a prolonged period of time postischemia. Consistent with this finding, total renal content of EGF falls (51), as does the renal excretion of EGF (6,8) after an ischemic insult. As a counterbalancing factor, the number of renal EGF receptors increases (8). Furthermore, a small, soluble, and active species of EGF is retained by the kidney after ischemia (51), perhaps formed as a consequence of the posttranscriptional effects of ischemia on preproEGF processing (8). The significance of these alterations in EGF synthesis and receptor number is unknown at present. It is possible that the increase in the EGF receptor number is responsible for the beneficial effects of exogenously administered EGF and TGFα (10,45,46), but whether endogenous EGF can play a similar role postischemia is unknown. It has been suggested that EGF gene expression in the kidney is associated with differentiation of function rather than proliferation. The EGF gene is transcribed to a high degree by the mature kidney only and TGFα is believed to play a much more important role than EGF in fetal kidney (52), a developmental stage mimicked by the postischemic or nephrotoxin-exposed kidney. EGF, when administered to normal rats, does not provoke renal DNA synthesis (10), and the increase seen during acute renal failure may be dependent on the increase in EGF receptor number.

Increased renal expression of other growth factors known to be mitogenic to proximal tubules in vitro, such as insulin-like growth factor I (IGF-1) (26,53) or hepatocyte growth factor (HGF) (25,54), has been demonstrated after ischemic and nephrotoxic injury. The levels of these growth factors increase prior to regeneration of the proximal tubule epithelium. Exogenously administered IGF-1 to rats improved postischemic function and renal histology as well as mortality rates, although the mechanism of this protection is unclear (55). It is interesting that a protective effect is observed even when the IGF-1 is administered 24 hr after the ischemic renal insult in rats (12). EGF increases renal synthesis of IGF-1, and it is possible that the latter mediates EGF's effect on mitogenesis and recovery in the postischemic kidney.

The signal transduction pathways that mediate activation of *trans*-acting factors controlling kidney's genetic response to ischemia are unknown. Since c-*jun* is one of the immediate early response genes activated early in the postischemic period (56), Pombe et al. (57) recently evaluated whether the stress-activated protein kinases (SAPKs), which phosphorylate c-Jun within the N-terminal *trans*-activation domain, are activated in response to ischemia. SAPKs are a subfamily of the extracellular signal-regulated kinases (ERKs). SAPKs kinase activity was assayed using GST-c-Jun (1-135), containing the N-terminal *trans*-activation domain of c-Jun, as substrate. SAPKs were not activated by ischemia alone, but reperfusion for as little as 5 min was associated with a 4.6-fold increase in kinase activity. Kinase activity was increased 7.6-fold at 20 min following reperfusion and remained elevated at 90 min of reperfusion (4.9-fold). In contrast, activity of the related ERK-1 and -2 was increased only 1.4-fold and only at the 5-min reperfusion time point. SAPKs accounted for the majority of the N-terminal c-Jun kinase activity of kidney at 5 min following reperfusion. ATP repletion following ATP depletion in MDCK renal epithelial cells was associated with a 15- to 29-fold activation of SAPKs, with a similar time course of activation to that seen in the kidney after ischemia and reperfusion. This activation of SAPKs, possibly by *trans*-activating c-Jun, may function in the early stages of a complex genetic response to ischemia ultimately leading to mitogenesis and/or cytoprotection and repair (56).

Non–Cell Cycle Genes

The expression of a number of other genes not clearly related to the cell cycle also changes with induction of acute renal failure (Table 1). There is diminished expression of the Tamm-Horsfall (TH) protein (24) (Figure 4), which, like preproEGF, is produced by the thick ascending limb. Also, renin and superoxide dismutase mRNAs decrease in acute renal failure (18). Genes responsive to injury in other systems, such as HSP (heat-shock protein) (30) and clusterin (23,32,33), increase. If and how each of these changes in gene expression contributes to the regenerative response is not known. Because of the high evolutionary conservation and ubiquitous nature of the heat-shock response to a number of different types of insults to cells and tissues, it is tempting to propose that this response is protective. Heat shock protects against excitotoxicity in neurons (58). Heat shock has also been reported to protect porcine renal allografts from warm ischemic injury (59). At 15 min after reflow, Van Why et al. localized the expression of HSP-72 to the apical domain of proximal tubules at the site of loss and internalization of the brush border (30) at a time when there is loss of membrane polarity (60,61). Later the localization shifts to the cytoplasmic domain, where some of the HSP-72 protein is localized to lysosomes. Van Why and colleagues (30) propose that HSP-72 may be involved in apical membrane remodeling early in the postischemic period and proteolysis of irreversibly damaged proteins later.

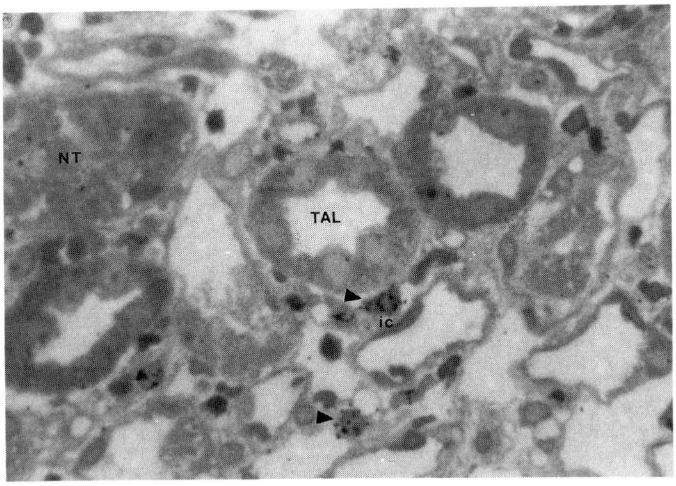

Figure 4 Photomicrograph of the outer stripe of the outer medulla of a kidney removed 24 hr after a 50-min period of ischemia and 1 hr after the rat was injected with ^{3}H-thymidine. Note the silver grains localized over the interstitial cell (ic) nuclei (arrows), some of which are adjacent to thick ascending limbs (TAL). Intact TALs are adjacent to necrotic tubules (NT). In other sections, silver grains could also been seen over nuclei of S3 segments of proximal tubule cells.

CELL DEATH

With ischemia, some cells die and have to be replaced; other cells survive but become depolarized (61); and other cells are not injured at all. Most of the attention devoted to ischemic cell death has focused on necrosis, as reflected by the term "acute tubular necrosis," which has been applied to the morphological consequences of ischemic injury to the kidney. Necrosis is the outcome of various metabolic processes that compromise the oxygen-deprived or toxin-exposed and ATP-depleted cell and ultimately lead to loss of cell viability. These metabolic processes include but are not limited to mitochondrial injury, phospholipase and protease activation, depolarization, reactive oxygen species, or calcium-induced dysfunction of vital cellular proteins or membranes [2]. In a sense, necrosis can be considered the passive consequence of various other processes.

Certain types of cell death, however, are finely controlled by active processes. This active process of cell death has been termed "apoptosis," from the Greek meaning "falling off," as apples from a tree (62). Apoptosis is characterized by compaction of chromatin to masses around the periphery of nuclei, cell blebbing, production of membrane-bound "apoptotic bodies," and rapid phagocytosis of these bodies by adjacent cells. In addition apoptosis is characterized by a DNA electrophoretic laddering pattern resulting from internucleosomal cleavage by endonucleases (62). During metamorphosis and development, "programmed cell death" represents an important cellular response to physiological stimuli that allow for the proper formation of the organism. Testosterone withdrawal results in involution of the prostate by a process involving programmed cell death (63). Abnormalities in the control mechanisms for programmed cell death may explain certain neurodegenerative diseases (64). Cell death genes have been identified in the nematode *Caenorhabditis elegans* (65). A mammalian homologue of the *C. elegans* cell death gene *ced-3* has recently been identified as IL1-β-converting enzyme (66). Another mammalian gene, *bcl-2*, is a protooncogene that inhibits most forms of apoptotic cell death. In a preliminary report, a 50–60% reduction in *bcl-2* mRNA levels was observed in the first 48 hr after folic acid–induced acute renal failure, at a time when clusterin expression was increased 10-fold (67). The extent to which apoptosis contributes to the cell death associated with ischemia or nephrotoxicity is unclear at present. Schumer and colleagues (31) found a small number of apoptotic bodies, with no associated necrosis, in kidneys 24 and 48 hr after reperfusion following 5 min of ischemia. In the kidney clamped for 30 or 45 min, apoptosis was found at 12, 24, and 48 hr of reperfusion. A ladder pattern of DNA fragmentation was also observed 24 hr after 30 min of ischemia. Apoptosis was seen often in clinical posttransplant acute tubular necrosis (68). In a preliminary study, another group failed to observe this DNA fragmentation pattern during equivalent degrees of ischemia (69).

To the extent that cell death secondary to ischemia or nephrotoxicity involves apoptosis, an identification of the precise genetic program responsible for such cell death may provide targets for intervention that may interfere with cell death and hence protect the organ. Our knowledge of the expression of "cell death" genes with ischemia is minimal. With ischemia and reperfusion, there is induction of the gene encoding clusterin, also called sulfated glycoprotein-2, or SGP-2, (16,31), a gene that has been implicated in apoptosis in the prostate (63). This gene has also been found to be expressed in normal cells, and its role in cell injury is not defined. When the same sections of outer medulla were stained with antibodies to proliferating cell nuclear antigen (PCNA), a marker of movement of cells through the cell cycle, vimentin, a marker of dedifferentiation, and clusterin, PCNA-positive cells did not stain with clusterin antibodies and clusterin-positive cells did not stain with PCNA antibodies (16). Furthermore, none of the cells that stained with clusterin antibodies were positively stained with vimentin antibodies. Likewise, none of the vimentin-positive cells expressed clusterin at detectable levels. Thus, the cells involved in the mitogenic response to replace damaged epithelial cells did not express clusterin (16). Dead cells exfoliated into the lumen of the tubule stained very strongly for clusterin.

Liver Regeneration

The liver, like the kidney, constitutes one of few normally quiescent organs that can undergo regeneration. It may be possible to understand the renal regenerative process better by examining a parallel process in the liver. Liver cells enter the cell cycle after either two-thirds hepatectomy or toxic injury (70). DNA synthesis is initiated 12 to 16 hr after partial hepatectomy and continues until liver mass is restored to its initial size. Nearly 95% of the remaining hepatocytes participate in this regenerative response. Many of the immediate early genes expressed by the kidney during the G_0/G_1 transition are also expressed by the regenerating liver, including *jun*, *Egr-1*, *actin*, *JE*, and *KC* (71). Not all of the immediate early genes respond to partial hepatectomy in the same way as that induced in insulin-activated H-35 liver cells in culture. For example there is a notable difference in the time course of expression of the *jun* and *fos* family of transcription factors when comparing liver regeneration and insulin treatment of H-35 cells (71). Multiple factors could contribute to these differences, including differences in cell response to a particular mitogen as well as differences in the mitogens present when comparing the complex organ response of regeneration with the relatively simple exposure of a cell in culture to insulin. Differences were also observed in the time course and intensity of the secreted immediate early protein response depending on which liver cell type was stimulated. This is similar to JE, whose expression is much more prolonged in the injured kidney after ischemia than in endothelial cell (42) or aortic vessel injury (72). Since the DNA-binding capacity of many transcription factors, including Fos and Jun proteins, depends upon dimerization, it is possible that differences in the mix of these dimers could shape the particular characteristics of the liver's regenerative response.

In the liver, it appears that multiple factors interact to initiate and support liver regeneration. These factors include circulating hormones, neural and liver-derived growth factors, α-adrenergic agonists, and hepatocyte growth factor (70). During CC14-induced liver injury, the Kupffer cell, a nonparenchymal cell, seems to be the source of the hepatocyte growth factor (73). This may have parallels in the regenerative process in the kidney, as there is a prominent nonparenchymal cell response to nephrotoxic injury as well (74).

In contrast to the increase in the number of EGF receptors during renal regeneration postischemia, there is a reduction in the number and activity of EGF receptors during hepatic regeneration (75). A portion of the EGF-receptor complex is localized to the nucleus in regenerating hepatocytes, suggesting a nuclear site of action of the activated receptor in regenerating cells (76).

Carbon tetrachloride–induced liver injury is followed by an even more impressive regenerative response than that provoked by partial hepatectomy (77). In contrast to partial hepatectomy, in which the differentiated function of the liver is well preserved, with carbon tetrachloride injury, there is a switch to a pattern of gene expression that is more characteristic of a dedifferentiated state. Albumin gene expression falls and α-fetoprotein gene expression increases, recapitulating the pattern of gene expression in the fetus. This dedifferentiation pattern is incomplete, however, since the expression of other liver-specific genes, such as ligandin and cytochrome P-450, remains unchanged. There is also evidence that stem cells may be involved in regeneration after massive hepatic necrosis (78), while no such involvement of a stem cell can be demonstrated after partial hepatectomy (70). These differences in the molecular response to partial hepatectomy and hepatotoxic injury reveal the diversity of the regenerative response of the liver. While a renal stem cell may exist in the adult kidney, it is clear that most, if not all, S3-segment proximal tubule cells have the capacity to be progenitor cells (16).

IMPLICATIONS OF THE OBSERVED CHANGES IN KIDNEY GENE EXPRESSION

Several themes emerge from study of the molecular response to renal injury. One paradigm is that the regeneration of a functional epithelium requires that subsets of the remaining viable cells undergo progression through the cell cycle. This has resulted in a search for potential growth factors that may be important for the entry of the cells into the cell cycle. While no one factor has been implicated as the important one, several investigators have attempted, with some success, to hasten the recovery process by administering growth factors to animals after the ischemic insult (10–12,45,55,79,80).

A second general paradigm that has evolved is the observation that regeneration postischemia or after a nephrotoxic insult recapitulates renal development (81,82). Thus the cells that enter the cell cycle after an ischemic (16) or toxic (83) insult express proteins, such as vimentin (16), that are expressed in those cell types only in early stages of renal development. In addition, the reduced expression of preproEGF, TH, and Kid-1 during acute renal failure, each of which is not expressed significantly in the developing kidney, is consistent with the hypothesis that the regenerating kidney assumes an earlier developmental stage. EGF excretion is also low in human renal diseases such as diabetic nephropathy, where it is an early indicator of deteriorating kidney function (84); polycystic kidney disease (85); and renal transplantation (86), where restoration of normal renal function is positively correlated with increasing EGF excretion. Thus, the reduced expression of each of these genes during renal injury may be a necessary component of the regenerative response.

A third paradigm is that inflammation may play an important role in the recovery process after an acute renal insult. This is supported by the fact that several of the changes in gene expression suggest the participation of the inflammatory cascade. The JE and KC proteins are chemotactic, and their expression may help to activate endothelial cells and recruit and activate leukocytes. Activated endothelial cells and leukocytes may release factors that alter vascular and epithelial cell function (87,88). Neutrophils accumulate in many tissues (89,90), including the kidney, after ischemia. Leukocyte depletion in the kidney limits postischemic damage in some studies (43,91) but not in others (92,93). Adding neutrophils to the perfusate of the isolated postischemic kidney adds to the functional damage (94). There is an increased adherence of leukocytes to endothelial cells in the postischemic tissue that is probably due, at least in part, to the upregulation of adhesion receptors, including ICAM-1 on the endothelium. This upregulation of ICAM-1 expression has been shown to occur in the heart postischemia and in cultured endothelial cells made hypoxic (95). Release of reactive oxygen species and proteases from the leukocytes will induce additional damage to the microvasculature. If this leukocyte-endothelial interaction occurs within the vasa recta, then it might enhance the tissue injury, resulting in S3 segment damage. If antibodies raised to ICAM-1 are administered to rats at the time of ischemia, or up to 2 hr after the ischemia, kidneys are markedly protected against acute renal failure (44). Thus, while possibly serving some regenerative role, the robust and early expression of these cytokine and adhesion genes may have deleterious effects on the kidney.

FUTURE RESEARCH DIRECTIONS

Acute renal failure continues to be a major cause of hospital morbidity. It is financially the most costly renal disease in hospitalized patients (96), and its high mortality has changed little in the postdialysis era (97). The goal of research in acute renal failure is to prevent or minimize injury and maximize the renal regenerative program. Prevention or reduction of injury depends upon better understanding of the factors that lead to cell death. In a complex organ like the kidney, this understanding depends not only on a more complete appreciation of the cellular factors but also on the vascular components that may contribute to the prolongation of local ischemia even when total renal blood flow is restored to near normal or normal levels. Understanding the inflammatory process and the role that adhesion molecules play in the reduction in blood flow to the outer medulla may provide important insight into vascular factors approachable with current and future therapies. At the level of the cell itself, a better understanding of how various biochemical factors contribute to necrotic cell death and a description of the role played by apoptotic cell death will be important for the development of therapeutic interventions. For example, if apoptosis contributes to cell death associated with ischemia and nephrotoxins, then it is reasonable to assume that therapies can be directed toward interference with this actively programmed cellular process.

Once damage to the kidney has occurred, approaches to therapy must be directed at hastening the regenerative process. This may take the form of administration of growth factors systemically. Results with this approach have been encouraging in that administered EGF (10,45), hepatocyte growth factor (11), or IGF-I (12,55) have been demonstrated to enhance rates of recovery in experimental animals; however, EGF and IGF have pleiotropic effects. For example, EGF is a potent renovascular constrictor (98) and induces bone resorption in vivo (99), while IGF-I causes hypoglycemia (100). Such effects may limit the clinical usefulness of these growth factors. An alternative strategy would involve a more kidney-specific approach. To achieve this goal, it will be necessary to identify what initiates renal dedifferentiation and mitogenesis, how the growth-promoting signal is transduced to the nucleus, and what the nuclear targets are that participate in regeneration. By studying the specific genes regulating the G_0/G_1 transition and the transactivating factors that bind to them, it may be possible to trace the growth-promoting signal back to its origin in the signal pathway. A similar approach may be used to trace the later downstream targets by studying a select group of genes not clearly related to the cell cycle but whose expression changes during the regenerative response. PreproEGF, TH, or Kid-1 would seem to be ideal for such studies because of their expression by the kidney, their uniform downregulation during renal injury, and their developmental pattern of expression. The goal for the future will be to manipulate the regenerative process, upregulating beneficial limbs of the pathway while downregulating potentially deleterious ones, so as to achieve full and rapid recovery of the kidney after injury.

Thus the investigators of acute renal failure must probe, together with developmental biologists and cancer/cell growth investigators, the fundamental issues of cell fate determination, cell cycle control, and growth factor signaling pathways; they must then apply this basic biology to this vital clinical problem. The implications of successful achievement of this search will likely extend beyond the kidney. By understanding the factors involved in cell death in the kidney, we likely will understand better the parallel processes that are likely to occur in brain and heart. Furthermore, by understanding the processes mediating repair in the kidney, we may understand why these processes do not occur in brain and heart. Possibly the kidney mechanisms can be copied to develop ways to regenerate heart and brain cells.

ACKNOWLEDGMENTS

The work from the authors' laboratories cited in this review was supported in part by NIH grants DK39773 and DK38452.

REFERENCES

1. Weinberg JM, Davis, JA, Roeser NF, Venkatachalam MA. Role of increased cytosolic free calcium in the pathogenesis of rabbit proximal tubule cell injury and protection by glycine or acidosis. J Clin Invest 1991; 87:581–590.
2. Bonventre JV. Mechanisms of ischemic acute renal failure. Kidney Int 1993; 43:1160–1178.
3. Toback FG. Regeneration after acute tubular necrosis. Kidney Int 1992; 41:226–246.
4. Cuppage FE, Neagry DR, Tate A. Repair of the nephron following temporary occlusion of the renal pedicle. Lab Invest 1967; 17:660–674.

5. Laurent G, Maldague P, Carlier MB, Tulkens PM. Increased renal DNA synthesis in vivo after administration of low doses of gentamicin to rats. Antimicrob Agents Chemother 1983; 24:586–593.
6. Safirstein R, Zelent A, Price P. Reduced preproEGF mRNA and diminished EGF excretion during acute renal failure. Kidney Int 1989; 36:810–815.
7. Threlfall G, Buck AT. The effect of folic acid on growth and deoxyribonucleic acid synthesis in the rat kidney. Lab Invest 1966; 15:1477–1485.
8. Safirstein R, Price PM, Saggi SJ, Harris RC. Changes in gene expression after temporary renal ischemia. Kidney Int 1990; 37:1515–1521.
9. Safirstein R, Winston J, Moel D, et al. Cisplatin nephrotoxicity: Insights into mechanism. Int J Androl 1987; 10:325–346.
10. Humes HD, Cieslinski DA, Coimbra TM, et al. Epidermal growth factor enhances renal tubule cell regeneration and repair and accelerates the recovery of renal function in postischemic acute renal failure. J Clin Invest 1989; 84:1757–1761.
11. Kawaida K, Matsumoto K, Shimazu H, Nakamura T. Hepatocyte growth factor prevents acute renal failure and accelerates renal regeneration in mice. Proc Natl Acad Sci USA 1994; 91:4357–4361.
12. Miller SB, Martin DR, Kissane J, Hammerman MR. Rat models for clinical use of insulin-like growth factor I in acute renal failure. Am J Physiol (Renal Fluid Electrolyte Physiol 35) 1994; 266:F949–F956.
13. Bravo R. Genes induced during the G0/G1 transition in mouse fibroblasts. Cancer Biol 1990; 1:37–46.
14. Greenberg ME, Ziff EB. Stimulation of 3T3 cells induces transcription of the c-fos proto-oncogene. Nature 1984; 311:433–438.
15. Connolly KM, Bogdanffy MS. Evaluation of proliferating cell nuclear antigen (PCNA) as an endogenous marker of cell proliferation in rat liver: A dual-stain comparison with 5-bromo-2′-deoxyuridine. J Histochem Cytochem 1983; 41:1–6.
16. Witzgall R, Brown D, Schwarz C, Bonventre JV. Localization of proliferating cell nuclear antigen, vimentin, c-fos, and clusterin in the postischemic kidney: Evidence for a heterogeneous genetic response among nephron segments, and a large pool of mitotically active and dedifferentiated cells. J Clin Invest 1994; 93:2175–2188.
17. Ouellette AJ, Malt RA, Sukhatme VP, Bonventre JV. Expression of two "immediate early" genes, Egr-1 and c-fos, in response to renal ischemia and during compensatory renal hypertrophy in mice. J Clin Invest 1990; 85:766–771.
18. Rosenberg ME, Paller MS. Differential gene expression in the recovery from ischemic renal injury. Kidney Int 1991; 39:1156–1161.
19. Cowley BD Jr, Chadwick LJ, Grantham JJ, Calvet JP. Sequential protooncogene expression in regenerating kidney following acute renal injury. J Biol Chem 1989; 264:8389–8393.
20. Norman JT, Bohman RE, Fischmann G, et al. Patterns of mRNA expression during early cell growth differ in kidney epithelial cells destined to undergo compensatory hypertrophy versus regenerative hyperplasia. Proc Natl Acad Sci USA 1988; 85:6768–6772.
21. Asselin C, Marcu KB. Mode of c-myc gene regulation in folic acid–induced kidney regeneration. Oncogene Res 1989; 5:67–72.
22. Kujubu DA, Norman JT, Hershman HR, Fine LG. Primary response gene expression in renal hypertrophy and hyperplasia: Evidence for different initiation processes. Am J Physiol 1991; 260:F823–827.
23. Witzgall R, O'Leary E, Gessner R, et al. Kid-1, a putative renal transcription factor: Regulation during ontogeny, and in response to ischemia and toxic injury. Mol Cell Biol 1993; 13:1933–1942.
24. Safirstein R, Megysesi J, Saggi SJ, et al. Expression of cytokine-like genes JE and KC is increased during renal ischemia. Am J Physiol 1991; 261:F1095–F1101.
25. Nagaike M, Hirao S, Tajima H, et al. Renotropic function of hepatocyte growth factor in renal regeneration after unilateral nephrectomy. J Biol Chem 1991; 266:22781–22784.
26. Matejka GL, Jennische E. IGF-I binding and IGF mRNA expression in the post-ischemic regenerating rat kidney. Kidney Int 1992; 42:1113–1123.
27. Igawa T, Matsumoto K, Kanda S, et al. Hepatocyte growth factor may function as a renotropic factor for regeneration in rats with acute renal injury. Am J Physiol (Renal Fluid Electrolyte Physiol 34) 1993; 265:F61–F69.
28. Polla BS, Mili N, Bonventre JV. Les proteines de stress: Quelles implications en nephrologie. Nephrologie 1991; 12:119–123.
29. Emami A, Schwartz JH, Borkan SC. Transient ischemia or heat stress induces a cytoprotectant protein in rat kidney. Am J Physiol (Renal Fluid Electrolyte Physiol 29) 1991; 260:F479–F485.
30. Van Why SK, Hildebrandt F, Ardito T, et al. Induction and intracellular localization of HSP-72 after renal ischemia. Am J Physiol 1992; 263:F769–F775.
31. Schumer M, Colombel MC, Sawczuk IS, et al. Morphologic, biochemical, and molecular evidence of apoptosis during the reperfusion phase after brief periods of renal ischemia. Am J Pathol 1992; 140:831–838.

32. Correa-Rotter R, Nath KA, Hostetter TH, Rosenberg ME. Clusterin expression in acute renal and chronic oxidative renal injury. J Am Soc Nephrol 1991; 2:660A.
33. Correa-Rotter R, Hostetter TH, Nath KA, Rosenberg ME. Interaction of complement and clusterin in renal injury. J Am Soc Nephrol 1991; 2:537A.
34. Terado Y, Tomito K, Nongudu H, Marumo F. Regulation of endothelin (ET) and two Type ET receptor mRNA in acute renal failure using competitive PCR (abstr). J Am Soc Nephrol 1992; 3:716A.
35. Soifer NE, Van Why SK, Dreyer BE, et al. Enhanced expression of parathyroid hormone-related protein in rat kidney after ischemic injury. J Am Soc Nephrol 1992; 3:715A.
36. Sukhatme VP, Cao X, Chang LC, et al. A zinc finger-encoding gene coregulated with c-fos during growth and differentiation, and after cellular depolarization. Cell 1988; 53:37–43.
37. Chiu R, Boyle WJ, Meek J, et al. The c-Fos protein interacts with c-Jun/AP-1 to stimulate transcription of AP-1 responsive genes. Cell 1988; 54:541–552.
38. Sukhatme VP. Early transcriptional events in cell growth: The Egr family. J Am Soc Nephrol 1990; 1:859–866.
39. Bonventre J, Sukhatme V, Bamberger M, et al. Localization of the protein product of the immediate early growth response gene, Egr-1, in the kidney after ischemia and reperfusion. Cell Reg 1991; 2:251–260.
40. Oquendo P, Alberta J, Duanzhi W. et al. The platelet-derived growth factor-inducible KC gene encodes a secretory protein related to platelet α-granule proteins. J Biol Chem 1989; 264:4133–4137.
41. Richmond A, Balentien E, Thomas HG, et al. Molecular characterization and chromosomal mapping of melanoma growth stimulatory factor structurally related to β-thromboglobulin. EMBO J 1988; 7:2025–2033.
42. Rollins BJ, Yoshimura T, Leonard EJ, Prober JS. Cytokine-activated human endothelial cells synthesize and secrete a monocyte chemotractant, MCP-1/JE. Am J Pathol 1990; 136:1229–1233.
43. Hellberg POA, Kallskog OK. Neutrophil-mediated post-ischemic tubular leakage in the rat kidney. Kidney Int 1988; 36:555–561.
44. Kelly KJ, Williams WW, Colvin RB, Bonventre JV. Antibody to intercellular adhesion molecule 1 protects the kidney against ischemic injury. Proc Natl Acad Sci USA 1994; 91:812–816.
45. Norman J, Tsau YK, Bacay A, Fine LG. Epidermal growth factor accelerates functional recovery from ischaemic acute tubular necrosis in the rat: Role of the epidermal growth factor receptor. Clin Sci 1990; 78:445–450.
46. Reiss R, Funke AJ, Cieslinski DA, Humes HD. Transforming growth factor-alpha (TGFα) accelerates renal repair and recovery following ischemic injury to the kidney (abstr). Kidney Int 1990; 37:493.
47. Massagué J. Transforming growth factor-α. J Biol Chem 1990; 265:21393–21396.
48. Humes HD, Beals TF, Cieslinski DA, et al. Effects of transforming growth factor-beta, transforming growth factor-alpha, and other growth factors on renal proximal tubule cells. Lab Invest 1991; 64:538–545.
49. Rall LB, Scott J, Bell GI. Mouse prepro-epidermal growth factor synthesis by the kidney and other tissues. Nature 313:228–231.
50. Norman J, Badie-Dezfooly B, Nord EP, et al. EGF-induced mitogenisis in proximal tubule cells: Potentiation by angiotensin II. Am J Physiol 253:F299–309.
51. Schaudies RP, Johnson JP. Multiple EGF containing proteins in rat kidney: Increase soluble EGF following ischemia is accompanied by a decrease in membrane associated immunoreactive EGF. Am J Physiol 1993; 264:F523–F531.
52. Popliker M, Shatz A, Avivi A, et al. Onset of endogenous synthesis of epidermal growth factor in neonatal mice. Dev Biol 119:38–44.
53. Rogers SA, Ryan G, Hammerman MR. Metanephric transforming growth factor-α is required for renal organogenesis in vitro. Am J Physiol 1992; 262:F533–F539.
54. Igawa T, Kanda S, Kanetake H, et al. Hepatocyte growth factor is a potent mitogen for cultured rabbit epithelial cells. BBRC 1991; 174:831–838.
55. Miller SB, Martin DR, Kissane J, Hammerman MR. Insulin-like growth factor I accelerates recovery from ischemic acute tubular necrosis in the rat. Proc Natl Acad Sci 1992; 89:11876–11880.
56. Megyesi J, DiMari J, Udvarhelyi N, et al. J Am Soc Nephrol. In press.
57. Pombe CM, Bonventre JV, Avruch J, et al. The stress-activated protein kinases (SAPKs) are major c-Jun amino-terminal kinases activated by ischemia and reperfusion. J Biol Chem. In press.
58. Rordorf G, Koroshetz WJ, Bonventre JV. Heat shock protects cultured neurons from glutamate toxicity. Neuron 1991; 7:1043–1051.
59. Perdrizet GA, Kaneko H, Buckley TM, et al. Heat shock and recovery protects renal allografts from warm ischemic injury and enhances HSP72 production. Transplant Proc 1993; 25:1670–1673.
60. Molitoris BA. Ischemia-induced loss of epithelial polarity: Potential role of the actin cytoskeleton. Am J Physiol 1991; 260:F769–F778.
61. Molitoris BA, Dahl R, Geerdes A. Cytoskeleton disruption and apical redistribution of proximal tubule Na^+-K^+-ATPase during ischemia. Am J Physiol 1992; 263:F488–F495.
62. Kerr JFR, Harmon BV. Definition and incidence of apoptosis: an historical perspective. In: Tomei LD,

Cope FO, eds. Apoptosis: the molecular basis of cell death. Cold Spring Harbor, NY: Cold Spring Harbor Laboratory Press, 1991:5–29.

63. Buttyan R. Genetic response of prostate cells to androgen deprivation: Insights into the cellular mechanism of apoptosis. In: Tomei LD, Cope FO, eds. Apoptosis: The Molecular Basis of Cell Death. Cold Spring Harbor, NY: Cold Spring Harbor Laboratory Press, 1991:157–173.
64. Ellis RE, Yuan J, Horvitz HR. Mechanisms and functions of cell death. Annu Rev Cell Biol 1991; 7:663–698.
65. Yuan J, Horvitz HR. The Caenorhabditis elegans genes ced-3 and ced-4 act cell-autonomously to cause programmed cell death. Dev Biol 1990; 138:33–41.
66. Miura M, Zhu H, Rotello R, et al. Induction of apoptosis in fibroblasts by IL-1b-converting enzyme, a mammalian homolog of the C. elegans cell death gene ced-3. Cell 1993; 75:653–660.
67. Ortiz A, Karp SL, Danoff TM, Neilson EG. Expression of survival promoting Bc12 oncogene by renal cells and whole kidney (abstr). J Am Soc Nephrol 1993; 4:742.
68. Olsen S, Burdick JF, Keown PA, et al. Primary acute renal failure ("acute tubular necrosis") in the transplanted kidney: Morphology and pathogenesis. Medicine 1989; 68:173–187.
69. Feurstenberg SM, Torok-Storb B, Zager RA. Evidence against apoptosis as a dominant mechanism for post-ischemic/post-hypoxic proximal tubular necrosis (abstr). J Am Soc Nephrol 4:753.
70. Michalopoulas G. Liver regeneration: Molecular mechanisms of growth control. FASEB J (1990); 4:176–187.
71. Mohn K, Laz T, Hsu J.-C, et al. The immediate-early growth response in regenerating liver and insulin-stimulated H-35 cells: Comparison with serum-stimulated 3T3 cells and identification of 41 novel immediate-early genes. Mol Cell Biol 1991; 11:381–390.
72. Poon M, Megyesi J, Green RS, et al. In vivo and in vitro inhibition of JE gene expression by glucocorticoids. J Biol Chem 1991; 266:22375–22379.
73. Noji S, Tashiro K, Koyama E, et al. Expression of hepatocyte growth factor gene in endothelial and Kupffler cells of damaged livers, as revealed by in situ hybridization. Biochem Biophys Res Comm 1990; 173:42–47.
74. Safirstein R, Megyesi J, Saggi SJ, et al. Molecular and cellular responses during renal ischemia (abstr). J Am Soc Nephrol 3:714.
75. Rubin RA, O'Keefe EJ, Earp HS. Alteration of epidermal growth factor–dependent phosphorylation during rat liver regeneration. Proc Natl Acad Sci USA 1982; 79:776–780.
76. Raper SE, Burwen SJ, Barker ME, Jones AL. Translocation of epidermal growth factor to the hepatocyte nucleus during rat liver regeneration. Gastroenterology 1987; 92:1243–1250.
77. Panduro A, Shalaby F, Weiner FR. Transcriptional switch from albumin to α-fetoprotein and changes in transcription of other genes during carbon tetrachloride induced liver regeneration. Biochemistry 1986; 25:1414–1420.
78. Gerber MA, Thung SN, Shen S, et al. Phenotypic characterization of hepatic proliferation. Am J Pathol 1983; 110:70–74.
79. Ding H, Kopple JD, Cohen AH, Hirshberg R. Recombinant human insulin-like growth factor-I improves recovery from acute renal failure in rats (abstr). J Am Soc Nephrol 1991; 3:705.
80. Lin J-J, Fine RN, Kaskal FJ. Effect of insulin-like growth factor-1 on recovery from postischemic acute renal failure in rats (abstr). J Am Soc Nephrol 3:709.
81. Toback FG. Control of renal regeneration after acute tubule necrosis. In: Robinson RR, ed. Nephrology. New York: Springer-Verlag, 1984:748–762.
82. Bacallao R, Fine LG. Molecular events in the organization of renal tubular epithelium: From nephrogenesis to regeneration. Am J Physiol 1989; F913–F924.
83. Wallin A, Zhang G, Jones TW, et al. Mechanism of nephrogenic repair response: Studies on proliferation and vimentin expression after ^{32}S-1,2-dichlorovinyl-L-cysteine nephrotoxicity in vivo and in cultured proximal tubule epithelial cells. Lab Invest 1992; 66:474–484.
84. Mathiesen ER, Nexo E, Hommel E, Parving H-H. Reduced urinary excretion of epidermal growth factor in incipient and overt diabetic nephropathy. Diabetic Med 1989; 6:121–126.
85. Gattone VH II, Andrews GK. Defective epidermal growth factor gene expression in mice with polycystic kidney disease. Dev Biol 1990; 138:225–230.
86. Kvist N, Nexo E. Epidermal growth factor in urine after kidney transplantation in humans. Urol Res 1989; 17:225–258.
87. Schreiner GF, Kohan DE. Regulation of renal transport and hemodynamics by macrophages and lymphocytes. Am J Physiol 1990; 258:F761–F767.
88. Springer T. Adhesion receptors of the immune system. Nature 1990; 346:425–434.
89. Hallenbeck JM, Dutka AJ, Tanishima T. Polymorphonuclear leukocyte accumulation in brain regions with low blood flow during the early postischemic period. Stroke 1986; 17:246–253.
90. Komatsu H, Koo A, Ghadishah E. Neutrophil accumulation in ischemic reperfused rat liver: Evidence for a role for superoxide free radicals. Am J Physiol 1992; 262:G669–G676.

91. Klausner JM, Paterson IS, Goldman G. Post-ischemic renal injury is mediated by neutrophils and leukotrienes. Am J Physiol 1989; 256:F794–F802.
92. Paller MS. Effect of neutrophil depletion on ischemic renal injury in the rat. J Lab Clin Med 1989; 113:379–386.
93. Thornton M, Winn R, Alpers C, Zager R. An evaluation of the neutrophil as a mediator of in vivo renal ischemia-reperfusion injury. Am J Pathol 1989; 135:509–515.
94. Linas SL, Shanley PF, Whittenburg D, et al. Neutrophils accentuate ischemia-reperfusion injury in isolated perfused rat kidneys. Am J Physiol 1988; 255:F728–F735.
95. Yoshida N, Granger DN, Anderson DC, et al. Anoxia/reoxygenation-induced neutrophil adherence to cultured endothelial cells. Am J Physiol 1992; 262:H1891–1898.
96. The National Kidney and Urological Diseases Advisory Board: 1990 Long-Range Plan, Window on the 21st Century.
97. Corwin HL, Bonventre JV. Factors influencing survival in acute renal failure. Semin Dial 1989; 2:220–225.
98. Harris RC, Hoover RL, Jacobson HR, Badr KF. Evidence for glomerular activity of epidermal growth factor in the rat. J Clin Invest 1988; 82:1028–1039.
99. Marie PJ, Hott M, Perheentupa J. Effects of EGF on bone formation and resorption in vivo. Am J Physiol 1990; 258:E275–E281.
100. Guler H-P, Zapf J, Froesch ER. Short term metabolic effects of recombinant human insulin-like growth factor I in healthy adults. N Engl J Med 1987; 317:137–140.

57

NF-κB Regulation of HIV-1 Gene Expression

Potential Role in the Pathogenesis of HIV-Associated Nephropathy

Leslie A. Bruggeman, Jeffrey B. Kopp, Jay Rappaport, and Paul E. Klotman

Mount Sinai School of Medicine, New York, New York

HIV-ASSOCIATED NEPHROPATHY

HIV-1-associated nephropathy (HIVAN) affects as many as 10% of patients infected with HIV-1. In these patients, renal disease is the cause of death or requires dialysis intervention (reviewed in Refs. 1 to 3). The syndrome has been observed sporadically in children infected perinatally, in women, and in asymptomatic HIV-1 carriers; however, over 90% of the cases in the United States are found in African-American males. HIVAN presents in the absence of hypertension and at any stage of HIV-1 infection. Approximately 50% of patients with HIVAN have no history of intravenous drug abuse. In addition to classic HIVAN, other renal complications have been described in HIV-infected patients, including acute tubular necrosis, immune complex glomerulonephritis, and IgA nephropathy. The pathogenesis of HIVAN remains largely unknown.

HIVAN is characterized clinically by heavy proteinuria and rapid progression to end-stage renal disease. Histologically, it is characterized by both glomerulosclerosis and tubulointerstitial disease (Figure 1A and B). There is extensive epithelial cell injury and microcystic tubular dilation. Reactive hyperplasia of both tubular (Figure 1A) and glomerular visceral epithelium (Figure 1B) can be observed. Renal biopsy material generally reveals coexistent segmental and global glomerulosclerosis (Figure 1A and B). Glomerular tuft collapse is often observed, but the mechanism for this phenomenon is unknown. Mesangial interposition, mesangial matrix deposition, and interstitial fibrosis are also common features, representing abnormalities in extracellular matrix metabolism and mesangial cell proliferation.

TRANSGENIC MOUSE MODEL OF HIVAN

To explore a direct role for viral gene products in the pathogenesis of HIVAN, we have studied a transgenic mouse model that expresses several genes from the infectious HIV-1 clone pNL4-3 (4). The pNL4-3 proviral DNA was modified for use as a transgene by deletion of the *gag/pol* genes. This deletion mutant is replication-incompetent but maintains the open reading frames for the regulatory proteins Tat, Rev, Nef, Vif, Vpr, and Vpu as well as Env. Three lines of transgenic mice develop renal disease and one of these lines, Tg26, has been studied in detail. Heterozygous mice are not immunodeficient and they have normal numbers of $CD20^+$ B cells, $CD3^+$ T cells, $CD4^+$ T cells, and $CD8^+$ T cells in the lymph node and spleen. They do not appear to be more susceptible to infections than normal mice housed in a conventional animal facility. The etiology of HIVAN has been obscured by potentially confounding variables such as drug abuse, hypertension, and socioeconomic factors. In the transgenic mouse model, however, expression of HIV-1 genes induces the development of renal disease with most of the clinical and histological features of HIVAN in

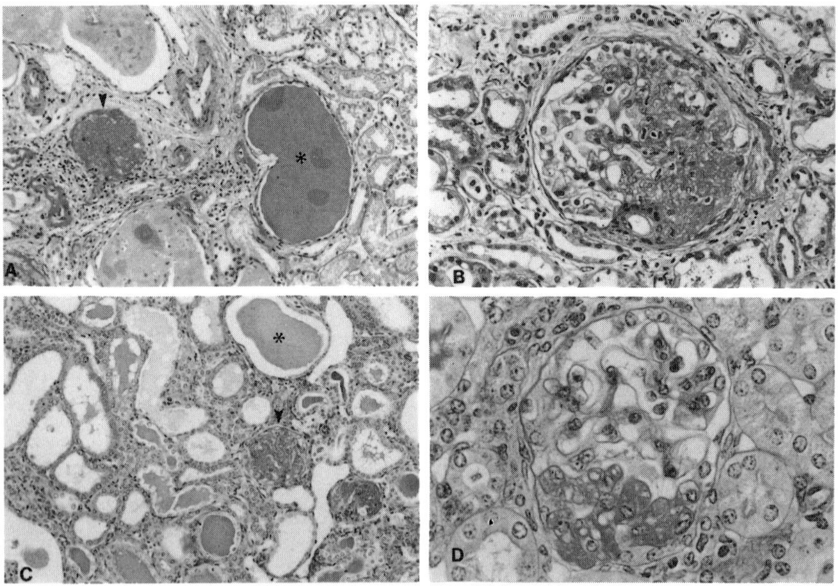

Figure 1 Kidney biopsies from an HIV-1-infected patient with HIV-associated nephropathy (A and B) and an HIV-1 transgenic mouse (C and D). In both the human and mouse models, segmental and global glomerulosclerosis are coexistent and tubulointerstitial disease is prominent. (From Ref. 1.)

humans, suggesting an essential role for the virus or viral proteins. Between 25 and 40 days of age, affected heterozygous mice develop proteinuria and, later, nephrotic syndrome with hypoalbuminemia and hypercholesterolemia. Late in the disease, they manifest ascites and peripheral edema as a preterminal event. Early renal involvement is characterized by focal segmental glomerulosclerosis, with tubular dilation and a mild mononuclear cell infiltrate (Figure 1C and D). Late in the disease, global sclerosis predominates, with extensive interstitial fibrosis, marked distortion of the renal architecture, and renal enlargement. Approximately 40% of the animals develop end stage renal disease within 300 days of age and renal disease is the cause of death in affected animals.

The level of expression of the transgene in heterozygous mice is tissue-dependent. In heterozygotes, muscle, skin, and gut are highly expressing tissues; lung, liver, and brain do not express the transgene; and lymphoid tissues and kidney are intermediate in the level of expression. In kidney, there is also a temporal pattern of expression. From 15 to 45 days of age, viral mRNAs are first detectable; then peak near weaning age (28 days). The expression declines to undetectable levels and does not appear to increase even in the setting of progressive renal disease. Thus, expression of the transgene in kidney appears to precipitate renal injury and initiate the events that lead to end-stage renal failure.

The presence of viral nucleic acids or infection of renal cells has not been clearly established in HIV-1 infected patients, but the expression of HIV-1 mRNA in the transgenic mice indicates that certain cell types in the kidney are able to support expression of the viral genome. This implies that tissue-specific factors are present in the kidney which are capable of supporting viral mRNA transcription. One of the inducible factors known to interact with the promoter of HIV-1, the LTR (long-terminal repeat), is the host protein nuclear factor kappa B (NF-κB). In addition to NF-κB, the viral LTR contains the consensus binding sites of several known eukaryotic transcription factors (Figure 2). Deletion mutant analysis has mapped a critical region of the LTR to the first 100 bp immediately upstream from the start site of transcription. This region contains the binding sites for NF-κB, Sp1, and TFIID, the transcription factor that binds to the TATA box (reviewed in Refs. 5 and 6). NF-κB has been implicated as one of the critical enhancer elements for high levels of viral mRNA expression.

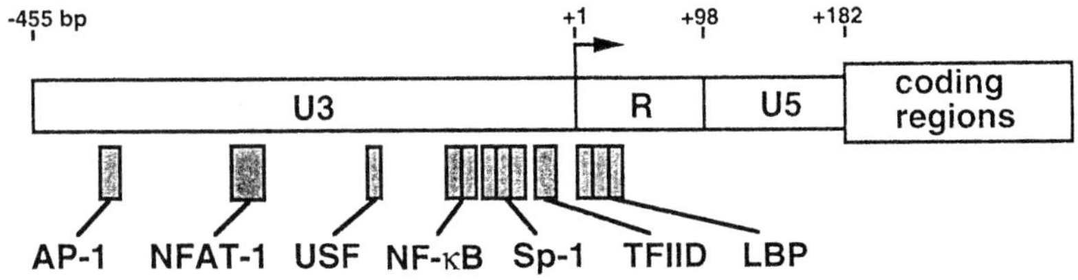

Figure 2 Transcriptional control region of the HIV-1 long terminal repeat (LTR). Consensus binding sites for known host transcriptional proteins present within the LTR are represented by boxes and their designations are shown below. There are two adjacent NF-κB sites from –105 to –84 numbered from the transcriptional start site (indicated by the arrow).

NF-κB AS A TRANSACTIVATOR OF TRANSCRIPTION

NF-κB was originally described as the nuclear protein bound to the B enhancer element of immunoglobulin kappa genes (reviewed in Refs. 7 to 9). Although it was originally thought to be a transcription factor specific to the B cell, it has been found in all cell types so far examined. NF-κB belongs to the *rel*-related family of transcriptional proteins, which are defined by the presence of ankyrin-like repeats. The Rel protein is the transforming element of the avian REV-T retrovirus and has a cellular homologue c-*rel* in mammals in addition to a similar protein Dorsal described in *Drosophila*. The transcription factor is a multiprotein complex made up of predominantly three proteins (see Figure 3A), including a subunit for transactivation p65, a subunit for DNA binding p50, and a subunit that functions to modulate these activities, IκB.

The transactivating subunit p65 represents a family of proteins, each a unique gene product. Presently, there are three known members: RelA, RelB, and c-*rel*; each molecule is approximately 65 kDa, but they have distinct primary structure. The DNA binding activity of the NF-κB complex is contained in the p50 subunit, which is similar to p65 in that it also represents a family of proteins, presently consisting of NFKB1 and NFKB2. The p50 subunit is translated as a larger protein of 100 to 105 kDa and is proteolytically cleaved in the cytoplasm to form the functional protein of approximately 50 kDa. The combination of one DNA-binding subunit (p50) with one transactivating subunit (p65) makes up the active transcription factor NF-κB. The activity of this heterodimer is controlled by a third protein IκB (inhibitor of NF-κB), which is also a family of proteins including IκBα, IκBβ, IκBγ, and the oncogene *bcl-3*. The IκBs are of variable molecular weight and are defined by their ability to bind the *rel*-related proteins. Their major function is to control the level of NF-κB activation.

NF-κB regulation is rapidly responsive; NF-κB is preformed and sequestered in the cytoplasm until it receives an activation stimulus through the signal transduction cascade (Figure 4). Since its activation does not require new protein synthesis, it is capable of inducing immediate changes in gene transcription. There are a variety of extracellular and intracellular signals that can activate NF-κB (Figure 4A). These signals include a diverse group of agents, including tumor necrosis factor-α, lymphotoxin, interleukin-1, interleukin-2, lipopolysaccharide, phorbol esters, viruses and viral proteins, reactive oxygen intermediates, and UV light (8). All of these agents stimulate second messengers of the signal transduction cascade primarily through receptor-mediated events (Figure 4B). These include seronine/threonine kinases (10), tyrosine kinases (11), phospholipase C–induced sphingomyelin breakdown (12,13), and reactive oxygen intermediates (14). There is also speculation that phosphatidyl inositol and prostaglandin metabolites will also be shown to play a role in NF-κB activation.

The various second messengers induce posttranslational modifications of the NF-κB complex including IκB; these include proteolytic cleavage, phosphorylation, and glycosylation events (Figure 4C). NF-κB is preformed in the cytoplasm. It is anchored by IκB which binds the p50/p65 heterodimer and sterically blocks the nuclear localization signal (NLS) found on p65. This steric hindrance prevents translocation of the active complex to the nucleus. The phosphorylation of IκB causes its release from NF-κB, revealing the NLS and allowing NF-κB to proceed to the nucleus, where it can initiate transcription.

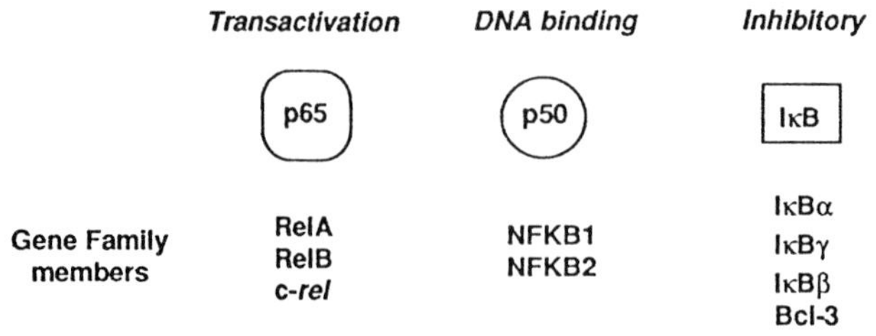

Figure 3 Protein subunits of the transcription factor NF-κB. There are three protein families which form the functional NF-κB complex, including a 65-kDa proteins ("p65") with primary transactivating function, 50-kDa proteins ("p50") with DNA binding activity, and a group of proteins regulating the function of the p50 and p65 proteins known as inhibitors of κB or "IκB."

In addition to the p50/p65 heterodimer universally known as "NF-κB," homodimers of p50 (15) and p65 (16,17) have now been shown to occur as well (Figure 4). The p50 homodimer, frequently detected in both the cytoplasm and nucleus, is able to bind a DNA target but contains no transactivation domain. These p50/p50 homodimers were believed to be a form of NF-κB that would suppress transcription because they block the NF-κB binding site from the active p50/p65 heterodimers. Recent studies have confirmed the suppressive effects of the p50 homodimers (15); interestingly, however, the combination of p50 homodimers in the nucleus with Bcl-3, a member of the IκB family, was found to have stimulatory properties on transcription (18,19). Whether Bcl-3 induces transactivation by removal of p50 homodimers from the target such that p50/p65 heterodimers can bind (15,20) or whether the p50/p50/Bcl-3 trimer can gain function is unclear at this time (19,21). Other members of the IκB family have specific interactions with NF-κB subunits that are analogous to those of Bcl-3 and p50. For example, IκBα binds NF-κB as long as the p65 subunit is not c-*rel*. IκBβ inhibits NF-κB binding to DNA but does not inhibit p50 homodimer binding. IκBγ inhibits both p50 homodimers and NF-κB binding to DNA (9). Thus, an understanding of the role and distribution of the family of IκB proteins may provide the greatest insight into the mechanisms of NF-κB activation and regulation.

A variety of genes contain binding sites for NF-κB and respond to activation of NF-κB by increasing transcription. These genes include (a) surface molecules involved in immune function, such as Ig light chains, interleukin-2 receptor, and MHC classes I and II; (b) soluble molecules involved in immune function, including interleukin-2, interleukin-6, tumor necrosis factor-α, lymphotoxin, and β-interferon; (c) acute-phase response genes such as NF-κB p50 itself, serum amyloid A, and complement C4; (d) selected oncogenes including c-*myc*; and (e) some viruses (8). Some of the genes that respond to NF-κB are also capable of stimulating NF-κB, thus establishing an autoregulatory positive feedback loop for sustaining high levels of gene expression. Included in this list are the genes for the p50/105 subunit and the IκBs; this provides a mechanism for replenishment of the pool of p50/105 and the IκBs following an activation event. The levels of p50/105 and the IκBs are maintained in excess in the cytoplasm to ensure that all of the p65 subunit containing the transactivating domain remains sequestered in the cytoplasm until needed.

Although, NF-κB is a ubiquitous transcription factor, stimulated by many agents and having broad effects on gene transcription, it retains specificity. Recently, Donnelly et al. investigated the stimulatory effects of interleukin-4 on interleukin-6 production by two cell lines (monocytes and fibroblasts). In monocytes, interleukin-4 induced the nuclear translocation of NF-κB and the stimulation of interleukin-6 gene expression; a similar phenomenon was not observed in fibroblasts (22). When ionizing radiation was used as the activation stimulus in fibroblasts, however, NF-κB was able to increase interleukin-6 gene expression (23). These studies indicate that specific signals are required for NF-κB translocation and that the events which follow are both cell-specific and stimulus-specific.

The specificity of the NF-κB signal transduction cascade is not surprising when viewed in the context of the large number of potential regulatory steps, subunit variations, and posttranslational modifications. For example, the HIV-1 promoter contains two NF-κB binding sites. Although TNFα, PMA, and bryostatin-1 each activate NF-κB in monocyte and T-cell lines, there are marked differences in the specific NF-κB subunits that appear in the nucleus, the kinetics of their appearance, and the

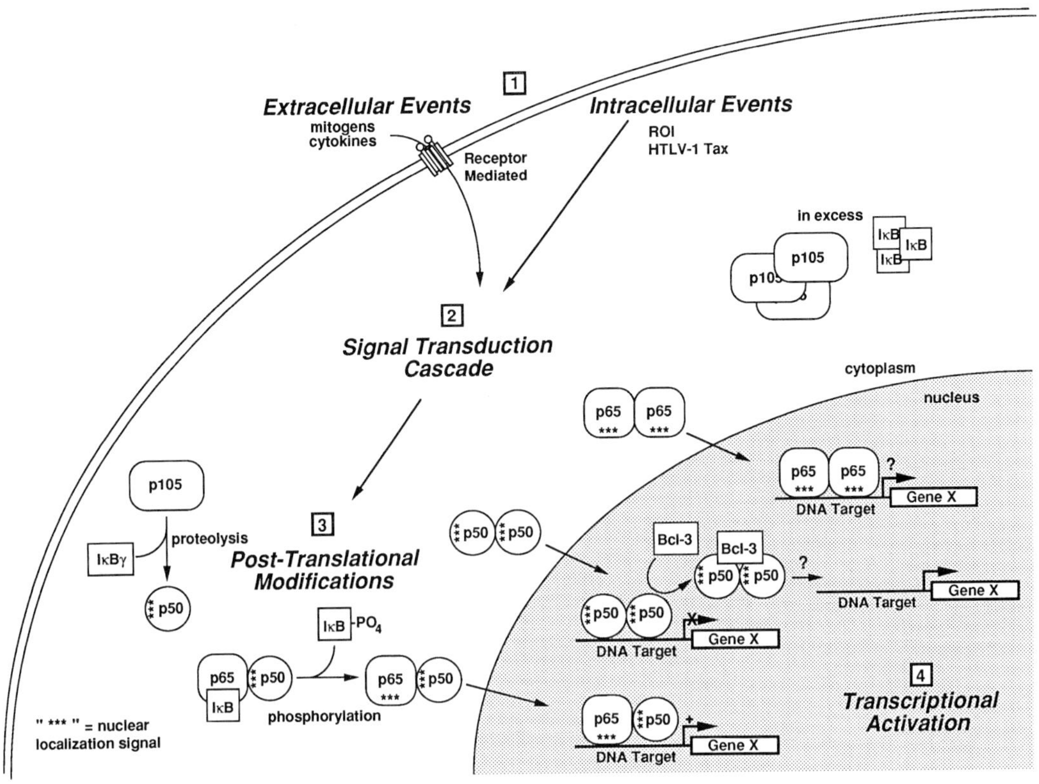

Figure 4 Mechanism of activation of NF-κB. Various extracellular and intracellular events associated with inflammatory and immune responses (1) induce the stimulation of the NF-κB signal transduction pathway (2). Posttranslational events (3) include phosphorylation and proteolytic cleavage of the protein components of the NF-κB complex. These changes allow for the formation of an NF-κB complex, which can translocate to the nucleus via a nuclear localization signal ("***"). Nuclear components of the NF-κB complex including p50 homodimers, p65 homodimers, or Bcl-3, may have additional effects on the NF-κB complex and gene expression. Once NF-κB is present in the nucleus, it can bind a DNA target and influence transcription (4).

effects of these stimuli on HIV-1 gene expression (24–26). The HIV-1 transgenic mouse model provides important in vivo correlation with the in vitro findings. For example, the expression of the transgene containing the HIV-1 promoter varies markedly in different tissues (Figure 5). Each tissue type produces mRNA for both p50 and p65 proteins and all tissue types possess an NF-κB complex that recognizes a consensus NF-κB target. The NF-κB complex in each tissue, however, is different in molecular weight, suggesting differences in the posttranslational modification of p50–p65 pairing. Thus, tissue-specific differences in the NF-κB complex result in different transactivational potential of the LTR. From both in vitro and in vivo studies, it appears that the response to a given stimulus is not generalized but is in fact very specific. Transcriptional activation depends not only on the tissue-specific expression of the NF-κB subunits but a cell-specific response as well. Although generally dismissed as an inappropriate therapeutic target, these findings suggest that it might be possible to design gene therapy strategies exploiting differences in the NF-κB signal transduction cascade.

ROLE FOR NF-κB IN VIRAL PATHOGENESIS

NF-κB plays a central role in viral pathogenesis by modulating gene expression of viruses, immediate response genes, and the genes encoding several inflammatory cytokines. In HIVAN, one of the major unresolved issues is whether HIV-1 infects primary renal cells. While several studies suggest

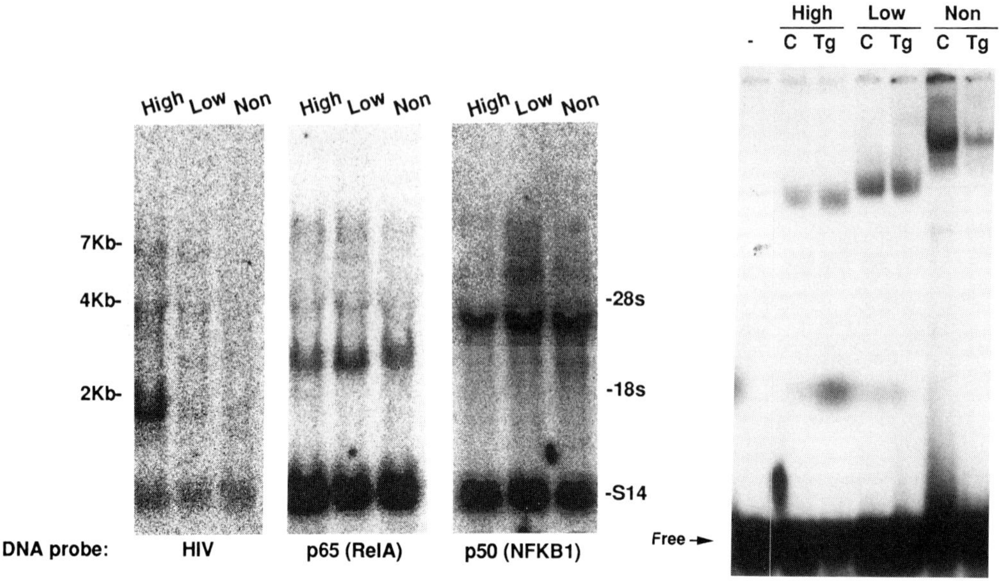

(A) (B)

Figure 5 Expression and Binding Activity of NF-κB in different tissues from HIV-1 transgenic mice. (A) Northern blot of total cellular RNA isolated from high expressing (intestine), low expressing (kidney), and non-expressing (lung) tissues. Blots were hybridized with the probes indicated: HIV-1, p50 (NFKB-1), and p65 (RelA). (B) Electrophoretic mobility shift assay (EMSA) of nuclear extracts isolated from the high, low, and non-expressing tissues with a radioactively labeled DNA frament containing a single NF-κB binding site. Unbound DNA is marked "free"; bands which migrate at a higher molecular weight indicate specific DNA/protein interactions.

this possibility (27–29), definitive studies have not yet been performed to substantiate this hypothesis (1,30). Data from the transgenic model indicate that should HIV-1 infect renal cells, the needed transcriptional machinery is available to allow for viral replication.

Renal injury may also occur through the activation of cytokines and growth factors either by the effects of viral replication in renal host cells or in response to circulating viral proteins or cytokines. Either circulating (31) or invading mononuclear cells (32) could provide a reservoir for toxic intermediates. In the transgenic model of HIVAN, the expression of HIV-1 in renal cells appears to induce renal injury manifested by dysregulated expression of extracellular matrix genes (collagen IV, laminin, and perlecan), at least two families of growth factors TGFβ and bFGF (22,33), and various cytokines. These processes contribute to renal pathogenesis, but a better understanding of the more proximate events in this model will be required for the development of effective therapy.

Activation of NF-κB and the stimulation of HIV-1 replication may be one of the early events in pathogenesis, and factors that affect this pathway may also predispose to disease. Previous attempts to explain the variable patient response to HIV-1 infection and the risks for the development of AIDS-related complications such as HIVAN have focused on putative cofactors for HIV-1 activation. Although a definitive environmental cofactor has not been identified for HIVAN (34,35), it is interesting to note the growing list of viruses that are known to respond to or can stimulate NF-κB (Table 1). Thus, NF-κB activation may represent one pathway in which simultaneous infections may compound the pathogenic role of HIV-1 in renal disease.

SUMMARY

A transgenic mouse model of HIVAN has provided perhaps the best evidence that expression of HIV-1 alone can induce renal pathogenesis independent of many confounding variables including

Table 1 Association of Viruses and NF-κB Activation

Stimulated by NF-κB activation	Ref.	Causes NF-κB activation	Ref.
JC virus	(36)	Sendai	(37)
CMV	(38)	CMV	(38)
Adenovirus	(39)	Adenovirus E1A	(40)
SV40	(41)	HTLV-1 Tax	(42–45)
HIV-1	(46)	Human herpesvirus VI	(47)
Herpes simplex II	(48)	Herpes simplex I	(49)
		Epstein-Barr LMP	(50)
		Hepatitis B virus HBx	(51)

immunodeficiency, drug abuse, and socioeconomic status. Mice expressing HIV-1 envelope and regulatory genes develop a fatal renal disease very similar to HIVAN in humans. Cytokine dysregulation appears to be a prominent component of renal pathogenesis. While the issue of direct HIV-1 infection in kidney remains unresolved, renal tissue appears to have the required transcriptional machinery, including NF-κB, to support viral replication. As a result, direct viral infection of renal epithelium appears likely. Tissue-specific differences in the level of transcription in the murine model appear to involve differences in the regulation of the transcription factor NF-κB.

Although NF-κB is a ubiquitous transcription factor, its activation can generate unique effects on gene expression. This flexibility results from NF-κB regulation at various levels including (1) the signal-transduction response and phosphorylation event, (2) the processing of cytoplasmic precursors, (3) the expression of tissue-specific isoforms, (4) developmental expression, (5) the combinatorial association subunits, and (6) the ultimate affinity of the complex for its DNA target. These various levels of NF-κB regulation can be viewed as primary and secondary responses to stimuli. The primary response is rapid, does not require new protein synthesis, and is associated with acute-phase responses to inflammatory and immune reactions. The secondary response involves new protein synthesis of various components of the NF-κB complex and constitutes an autoregulatory loop for NF-κB regulation. The mechanisms for gene activation by NF-κB are complex but very specific; thus, NF-κB may ultimately be found to be a reasonable therapeutic target.

REFERENCES

1. Rappaport J, Kopp JB, Klotman PE. Host-virus interactions and the molecular regulation of HIV-1: Role in the pathogenesis of HIV-associated nephropathy. Kidney Int 1994; 46:16–27.
2. Rao TK. Human immunodeficiency virus (HIV) associated nephropathy. Annu Rev Med 1991; 42:391–401.
3. Rao TK. A decade of human immunodeficiency virus-associated nephropathy (HIVAN). Transplant Proc 1993; 25:2439–2440.
4. Dickie P, Felser J, Eckhaus M, et al. HIV-associated nephropathy in transgenic mice expressing HIV-1 genes. Virology 1991; 185:109–119.
5. Cullen BR. Regulation of HIV-1 gene expression. FASEB J 1991; 5:2361–2368.
6. Zeichner SL, Kim JY, Alwine JC. Linker-scanning mutational analysis of the transcriptional activity of the human immunodeficiency virus type 1 long terminal repeat. J Virol 1991; 65:2436–2444.
7. Grilli M, Chiu JJ, Lenardo MJ. NF-kappa B and Rel: Participants in a multiform transcriptional regulatory system. Int Rev Cytol 1993; 143:1–62.
8. Grimm S, Baeuerle PA. The inducible transcription factor NF-kappa B: Structure-function relationship of its protein subunits. Biochem J 1993; 290:297–308.
9. Liou HC, Baltimore D. Regulation of the NF-kappa B/rel transcription factor and I kappa B inhibitor system. Curr Opin Cell Biol 1993; 5:477–487.
10. Finco TS, Baldwin AS Jr. Kappa B site-dependent induction of gene expression by diverse inducers of nuclear factor kappa B requires Raf-1. J Biol Chem 1993; 268:17676–17679.
11. Joshi Barve SS, Rangnekar VV, Sells SF, Rangnekar VM. Interleukin-1–inducible expression of gro-beta via NF-kappa B activation is dependent upon tyrosine kinase signaling. J Biol Chem 1993; 268:18018–18029.

12. Schutze S, Potthoff K, Machleidt T, et al. TNF activates NF-kappa B by phosphatidylcholine-specific phospholipase C-induced "acidic" sphingomyelin breakdown. Cell 1992; 71:765–776.
13. Dbaibo GS, Obeid LM, Hannun YA. Tumor necrosis factor-alpha (TNF-alpha) signal transduction through ceramide: Dissociation of growth-inhibitory effects of TNF-alpha from activation of nuclear factor-kappa B. J Biol Chem 1993; 268:17762–17766.
14. Schreck R, Albermann K, Baeuerle PA. Nuclear factor kappa B: An oxidative stress-responsive transcription factor of eukaryotic cells (review). Free Radic Res Commun 1992; 17:221–237.
15. Franzoso G, Bours V, Park S, et al. The candidate oncoprotein Bcl-3 is an antagonist of p50/NF-kappa B–mediated inhibition. Nature 1992; 359:339–342.
16. Fujita T, Nolan GP, Ghosh S, Baltimore D. Independent modes of transcriptional activation by the p50 and p65 subunits of NF-κB. Genes Dev 1992; 6:775–787.
17. Ganchi PA, Sun SC, Greene WC, Ballard DW. A novel NF-κB complex containing p65 homodimers: Implications for transcriptional control at the level of subunit dimerization. Mol Cell Biol 1993; 13:7826–7835.
18. Nolan GP, Fujita T, Bhatia K, et al. The bcl-3 proto-oncogene encodes a nuclear I kappa B-like molecule that preferentially interacts with NF-kappa B p50 and p52 in a phosphorylation-dependent manner. Mol Cell Biol 1993; 13:3557–3566.
19. Bours V, Franzoso G, Azarenko V, et al. The oncoprotein Bcl-3 directly transactivates through kappa B motifs via association with DNA-binding p50B homodimers. Cell 1993; 72:729–739.
20. Franzoso G, Bours V, Azarenko V, et al. The oncoprotein Bcl-3 can facilitate NF-κB–mediated transactivation by removing inhibiting p50 homodimers from select κB sites. EMBO J 1993; 12:3893–3901.
21. Fujita T, Nolan GP, Liou HC, et al. The candidate proto-oncogene bcl-3 encodes a transcriptional coactivator that activates through NF-kappa B p50 homodimers. Genes Dev 1993; 7:1354–1363.
22. Donnelly RP, Crofford LJ, Freeman SL, et al. Tissue-specific regulation of IL-6 production by IL-4. J Immunol 1993; 10:5603–5612.
23. Brach MA, Gruss HJ, Kaisho T, et al. Ionizing radiation induces expression of interleukin 6 by human fibroblasts involving activation of nuclear factor-kappa B. J Biol Chem 1993; 268:8466–8472.
24. Vlach J, Pitha PM. Activation of human immunodeficiency virus type 1 provirus in T-cells and macrophages is associated with induction of inducer-specific NF-kappa B binding proteins. Virology 1992; 187:63–72.
25. Roulston A, DAddario M, Boulerice F, et al. Induction of monocytic differentiation and NF-kappa B-like activities by human immunodeficiency virus 1 infection of myelomonoblastic cells. J Exp Med 1992; 175:751–763.
26. Kaufman PA, Weinberg JB, Greene WC. Nuclear expression of the 50- and 65-kD Rel-related subunits of nuclear factor-kappa B is differentially regulated in human monocytic cells. J Clin Invest 1992; 90:121–129.
27. Cohen AH, Sun NC, Shapshak P, Imagawa DT. Demonstration of human immunodeficiency virus in renal epithelium in HIV-associated nephropathy. Mod Pathol 1989; 2:125–128.
28. Alpers CE, McClure J, Bursten SL. Human mesangial cells are resistant to productive infection by multiple strains of human immunodeficiency virus types 1 and 2. Am J Kidney Dis 1992; 19:126–130.
29. Green DF, Resnick L, Bourgoignie JJ. HIV infects glomerular endothelial and mesangial but not epithelial cells in vitro. Kidney Int 1992; 41:956–960.
30. Kopp JB, Bruggeman LA, Klotman PE. Extracellular matrix gene expression in experimental glomerulonephritis. Curr Opin Nephrol Hypertens 1993; 2:609–617.
31. Rosenberg ZF, Fauci AS. Immunopathogenic mechanisms of HIV infection. FASEB J 1991; 5:2382–2390.
32. Weeks BS, Klotman ME, Dhawan S, et al. HIV-1 infection of human T lymphocytes results in enhanced alpha 5 beta 1 integrin expression. J Cell Biol 1991; 114:847–853.
33. Kopp JB, McCune BK, Notkins AL, et al. Increased expression of transforming growth factor β in HIV-transgenic mouse kidneys. J Am Soc Nephrol 1992; 3:318.
34. Bauer FA, Wear DJ, Angritt P, Lo SC. *Mycoplasma fermentans* (incognitus strain) infection in the kidneys of patients with acquired immunodeficiency syndrome and associated nephropathy: A light microscopic, immunohistochemical, and ultrastructural study. Hum Pathol 1991; 22:63–69.
35. di Belgiojoso GB, Genderini A, Vago L, et al. Absence of HIV antigens in renal tissue from patients with HIV-associated nephropathy. Nephrol Dial Transplant 1990; 5:489–492.
36. Ranganathan PN, Khalili K. The transcriptional enhancer element, kappa B, regulates promoter activity of the human neurotropic virus, JCV, in cells derived from the CNS. Nucleic Acids Res 1993; 21:1959–1964.
37. Lenardo MJ, Fan CM, Maniatis T, Baltimore D. The involvement of NF-kappa B in beta-interferon gene regulation reveals its role as widely inducible mediator of signal transduction. Cell 1989; 57:287–294.
38. Sambucetti LC, Cherrington JM, Wilkinson GW, Mocarski ES. NF-kappa B activation of the cytomegalovirus enhancer is mediated by a viral transactivator and by T cell stimulation. EMBO J 1989; 8:4251–4258.
39. Williams JL, Garcia J, Harrich D, et al. Lymphoid specific gene expression of the adenovirus early region 3 promoter is mediated by NF-kappa B binding motifs. EMBO J 1990; 9:4435–4442.

40. Shurman L, Sen R, Bergman Y. Adenovirus E1A products activate the Ig κ-chain enhancer in fibroblasts: A possible involvement of the NF-κB binding site. J Immunol 1989; 143:3806–3812.
41. Lattion AL, Espel E, Reichenbach P, et al. Characterization of a new tissue-specific transcription factor binding to the simian virus 40 enhancer TC-II (NF-kappa B) element. Mol Cell Biol 1992; 12:5217–5227.
42. Lacoste J, Cohen L, Hiscott J. NF-κB activity in T cells stably expressing the Tax protein of human T cell lymphotropic virus type I. Virology 1991; 184:553–562.
43. Crenon I, Beraud C, Simard P, et al. The transcriptionally active factors mediating the effect of the HTLV-I Tax transactivator on the IL-2R alpha kappa B enhancer include the product of the c-*rel* proto-oncogene. Oncogene 1993; 8:867–875.
44. Laherty CD, Perkins ND, Dixit VM. Human T cell leukemia virus type I Tax and phorbol 12-myristate 13-acetate induce expression of the A20 zinc finger protein by distinct mechanisms involving nuclear factor kappa B. J Biol Chem 1993; 268:5032–5039.
45. Arima N, Molitor JA, Smith MR, et al. Human T-cell leukemia virus type I Tax induces expression of the Rel-related family of kappa B enhancer-binding proteins: Evidence for a pretranslational component of regulation. J Virol 1991; 65:6892–6899.
46. Nabel G, Baltimore D. An inducible transcription factor activates expression of human immunodeficiency virus in T cells. Nature 1987; 326:711–713.
47. Horvat RT, Wood C, Josephs SF, Balachandran N. Transactivation of the human immunodeficiency virus promoter by human herpesvirus 6 (HHV-6) strains GS and Z-29 in primary human T lymphocytes and identification of transactivating HHV-6(GS) gene fragments. J Virol 1991; 65:2895–2902.
48. Feng CP, Kulka M, Aurelian L. NF-kappa B-binding proteins induced by HSV-1 infection of U937 cells are not involved in activation of human immunodeficiency virus. Virology 1993; 192:491–500.
49. Popik W, Pitha PM. Inhibition by interferon of herpes simplex virus type 1–activated transcription of *tat*-defective provirus. Proc Natl Acad Sci USA 1991; 88:9573–9577.
50. Hammarskjold ML, Simurda MC. Epstein-Barr virus latent membrane protein transactivates the human immunodeficiency virus type 1 long terminal repeat through induction of NF-kappa B activity. J Virol 1992; 66:6496–6501.
51. Kekulé AS, Lauer U, Weiss L, et al. Hepatitis B virus transactivator HBx uses a tumor promoter signaling pathway. Nature 1993; 361:742–745.

58

Molecular Features of Nephritogenic Antibodies, T-Cell Receptors, and MHC Molecules

Sharon L. Karp and Eric G. Neilson
University of Pennsylvania Medical Center, Philadelphia, Pennsylvania

INTRODUCTION

Many kidney diseases are immune-mediated, involving autoantibody production, the development of nephritogenic T cells, antigen presentation in the context of major histocompatibility complex (MHC) molecules and a myriad of cytokines associated with conventional immune responses. Antibodies directed toward both self and foreign antigens are observed in both glomerular and interstitial disorders, and T lymphocytes play a critical early role in aiming the specificity of the immune response in many renal diseases. T cells only recognize antigen in the context of MHC determinants, and this interaction is an essential event for the engagement of the immune system. In this chapter we examine some of the insights into the molecular biology of immune responses in various experimental renal diseases. Work in this area is limited, and there are only a few experimental systems that have been explored in any depth at the molecular level.

NEPHRITOGENIC B-CELL REPERTOIRES

Both B and T lymphocytes have cell surface multimeric receptors that recognize specific antigens complexed with accessory molecules which modulate cell function after antigen binding. On B cells, membrane-associated immunoglobulin molecules act as antigen receptors. Membrane-associated immunoglobulin differs from secreted immunoglobulin in that the heavy chain has transmembrane and cytoplasmic regions. Membrane-associated immunoglobulin is also complexed with another heterodimeric membrane-spanning protein needed for normal B cell function (1). Immunoglobulin molecules, both membrane-associated and secreted molecules, or antibodies, are composed of two identical heavy and two identical κ or λ light chains linked by disulfide bonds, each of which has a variable region and a constant region. The variable regions contain relatively conserved framework regions and hypervariable or complementarity-determining regions (CDR), which are important in antigen binding and may undergo somatic hypermutation during the maturation of immune responses. Immunoglobulin heavy and light chains are encoded by genes assembled from germ-line segments during lymphoid development. The heavy-chain variable region is encoded by V, D, and J genes and the light-chain variable regions are encoded by V and J genes. These germ-line gene segments are joined during lymphoid development by the process of V(D)J recombination, in which one of hundreds of V genes is ligated to one of several D genes and one of several J gene segments in a process that joins segments and allows deletion and addition of nucleotides at the joining sites (2–4). Usually the heavy chain rearranges first in pre-B cells with rearrangement of D to J_H preceding rearrangement of V_H to D-J_H. Subsequently there is rearrangement of the light-chain variable region

$V\kappa$ and $J\kappa$ genes (3). The mechanisms responsible for the process of gene recombination in immunoglobulin genes and TCR loci has not yet been completely elucidated. Two genes, RAG1 and RAG2, are both necessary for this process to occur, although their precise role is still under active investigation. Knockout mice lacking either RAG1 or RAG2 do not have mature B or T cells (5,6) indicating that both gene products are needed in the process of recombination. Transfection of both RAG1 and RAG2 genes into several types of nonlymphoid cells leads to V(D)J recombination (7).

During an immune response to protein-based antigens, antibody affinity increases. Most high-affinity antibodies directed against protein antigens have somatic mutations in their hypervariable regions which occur within germinal centers after the B cells bind antigen (8). Mature autoantibodies can be encoded either by pristine germ-line sequence (9) or by sequence modified by somatic mutation (10–12). In an autoantibody response, structural diversity depends on genes encoded by the germ line (13), on the combinatorial diversity arising from the rearrangements of V-D-J gene segments (2,14), and on somatic mutation (15).

The molecular structure of autoantibodies in an animal model of autoimmune interstitial nephritis, antitubular basement membrane (αTBM) disease is now known. Susceptible rodents develop αTBM antibodies 7 to 10 days after immunization with tubular antigen, and a mononuclear infiltrate appears in the interstitium of the kidney after several weeks. The target antigen of human and experimental αTBM disease is 3M-1, a glycoprotein synthesized by proximal tubular epithelium and expressed within their tubular basement membranes (16). The cDNA sequence encoding a nephritogenic domain (P1) has been deduced from peptide analysis (17). Serological studies of a library of rat monoclonal αTBM/α3M-1 antibodies revealed that they competitively inhibit one another as well as human and mouse α3M-1 antisera, indicating that they are directed against similar or identical epitopes of the 3M-1 antigen (18,19). Some of the α3M-1 antibodies as well as 3M-1 antigen reactive T cells express a cross-reactive idiotype by serological criteria that has been shown to alter the course of disease (18).

mRNA sequences of the immunoglobulin variable region heavy- and light-chain mRNA sequences of several of the monoclonal αTBM/α3M-1 antibodies as well as their germline V_H and $V\kappa$ genes were obtained in order to better understand the genetics of this autoimmune response (20). These antibodies have different affinities for the 3M-1 antigen. The seven heavy chains sequenced used only four different V_H genes, and the six κ light chains that were sequenced used six different $V\kappa$ genes. These data indicate that the specificity of αTBM/α3M-1 antibodies may therefore be favored by a selective use of V_H genes, but does not depend solely on a single pair of V_H and V_κ genes. Partial germ-line sequences of V_H and $V\kappa$ genes for some of the antibodies sequenced were compared to cDNA sequences to determine if somatic mutation plays a role in the generation of this autoimmune response. The three germ-line V_H genes used by six of the antibodies studied were identical to the cDNA sequences, indicating that no somatic mutations occurred in the region studied. Similarly, the two germ-line $V\kappa$ genes we studied were almost identical to the corresponding cDNA sequences of the light chains, with only one mutation in the first framework region of one of the $V\kappa$ regions. In the autoantibody response in αTBM disease, somatic mutation does not appear to be important in the generation of high-affinity antibodies (20).

Antibodies are also important in systemic lupus erythematosus, and the titer of dsDNA antibodies correlates with disease activity in patients. In the MRL-lpr/lpr mouse model of lupus, autoantibody gene usage in lupus has been investigated. MRL-lpr/lpr mice spontaneously develop autoimmune disease similar to human lupus, with nephritis, arthritis, antinuclear antibodies, and antibodies to ssDNA and dsDNA. They also develop lymphoproliferation of a T-cell subset. Studies by Weigert and colleagues have demonstrated that there are a limited number of V_H regions utilized by anti-DNA autoantibodies in these lupus mice. In their studies, anti-DNA antibodies were demonstrated to arise from clonal expansion of one or a few B cell clones in individual animals. Somatic mutation in the hypervariable CDR regions of these antibodies occurred during the autoimmune response. As a result of these mutations, arginine residues appear in the CDR regions and are thought to play an important role in determining antibody specificity (21).

Antibodies are found within glomerular immune deposits in lupus nephritis. Injection of anti-DNA antibodies derived from MRL-lpr/lpr mice into normal mice led to glomerular immune deposits, indicating that these antibodies recognized antigenic determinants within the glomerulus (22). Variable regions of glomerular immune deposit forming anti-DNA antibodies derived from

MRL-lpr/lpr lupus mice were characterized by sequence analysis. Their V regions appear to be encoded by an apparently unmutated germ-line sequence (23), indicating that germ-line sequence may encode variable regions of nephritogenic autoantibodies. Taken together, the data on the anti-DNA antibody variable region indicate that there are a limited number of variable-region gene families involved in the antibody response and that pathogenic antibodies can likely be encoded by both germ-line sequence (23,24) and sequences that have undergone somatic mutation (21).

The molecular structure of a cross-reactive idiotype present on several of the αTBM/α3M-1 antibodies has been investigated in experimental autoimmune interstitial nephritis. In other autoimmune diseases, some cross-reactive idiotypes have been demonstrated to be determined independently of V_H and V_κ genes (25) and others are associated with specific V_H or V_κ genes (26,27). The cross-reactive idiotype in αTBM disease was first localized to the antibody heavy chain by immunoblotting using anti-idiotype antisera. Comparison of the heavy-chain variable region sequences of antibodies positive and negative for the cross-reactive idiotype by radioimmunoassay was performed, and two αTBM/α3M-1 antibodies, cross-reactive idiotype positive α53R-4 and cross-reactive idiotype negative α53R-1, were found to differ only in the CDR3 regions. This observation allowed localization of the idiotype to the CDR3 region of the heavy chain (20).

Molecular modeling of the three-dimensional structure of this cross-reactive idiotype was done using sequence data from the antibodies positive and negative for the cross-reactive idiotype. The αTBM antibody V_H sequence data were compared to templates in the immunoglobulin crystallographic data base. A theoretical binding face for the antibodies was defined based on comparison of the topography of the hypervariable loops of structurally known antibodies. This model suggests that the residue in position four of the putative CDR3 turn along with residues in CDR1 and CDR2 make up the cross-reactive idiotype binding site (20).

Cross-reactive idiotypes are one mechanism by which immune responses can be modulated in an animal. The αTBM disease cross-reactive idiotype was found in T lymphocytes as well as in αTBM antibodies (28–30). Anti-idiotype antisera can attenuate αTBM disease in rats (18) and can lyse T cell in the presence of complement (E. Neilson; personal observation). Such findings demonstrate that highly focused responses to self antigen can be restrained specifically by anti-idiotype directed at different cell lineages and that approaches to prevention or amelioration of this autoimmune process through manipulation of the idiotypic network are feasible. This information may eventually lead to the development of idiotype or anti-idiotype vaccines.

NEPHRITOGENIC T-CELL REPERTOIRES

T lymphocytes are involved in the pathogenesis of many forms of glomerulonephritis (31) and interstitial nephritis (32). T lymphocytes play a major role in the immunopathogenesis of murine αTBM disease (29,32–35). T lymphocytes recognize antigenic peptide fragments bound to MHC molecules via antigen specific T-cell receptors (TCR). The T-cell antigen-recognition complex consists of several molecules, including TCR, CD3, and CD4, or CD8, which are necessary for antigen binding and signal transduction by the lymphocyte. The TCR is associated with the CD3 complex on the T-cell surface. The CD3 complex contains several membrane-spanning proteins, including γ, δ, ϵ, and ζ chains, which were initially characterized serologically by binding to the antibodies OKT3 and Leu 4. CD4 is a transmembrane protein that binds to MHC class II. CD8 consists of two chains, α and β, that form heterodimers or homodimers on the T-cell surface and bind to MHC class I. CD4 and CD8 molecules are members of the immunoglobulin supergene family (36).

T-cell activation requires costimulatory signals delivered by antigen-presenting cells in addition to ligation of the TCR with antigen, MHC and CD3 and either CD4 or CD8. One such costimulatory signal that may allow T cell activation is B7 on the antigen presenting cell, which interacts with CD28 or CTLA-4 on the T lymphocyte and leads to activation of tyrosine kinases (37). Lack of a costimulatory signal after T-cell antigen exposure with MHC and TCR engagement may lead to anergy instead of activation (37,38). Adhesion molecules involved in T-cell and antigen presenting cell interactions, including ICAM-1/LFA-1 and CD2/LFA-3, may also have a role in T-cell activation (39).

TCRs are heterodimers consisting of α and β chains (α/β) or γ and δ chains (γ/δ). Like antibody molecules, these chains have variable and constant regions, which are rearranged to form mature molecules. The α chain variable region is encoded by Vα and Jα gene segments. There are about 100 Vα and 50 Jα genes in the mouse. The β locus has two constant regions which are nearly identical, seven Jβ gene segments with one D gene 5′ to each, and about 24 Vβ genes in mice and about 70 in humans. The V gene encodes the CDR1 and CDR2 regions of the TCR and CDR3 is encoded by the V(D)J junction. The V(D)J segments are rearranged during T cell ontogeny and, after transcription, are joined to C region sequences by RNA splicing (40). The process of TCR recombination is thought to be similar to immunoglobulin recombination and also requires RAG1 and RAG2 (7). TCR diversity in an organism arises from recombination of different V(D)J genes, random α and β chain pairing, as well as imprecise joining of segments and the addition of nucleotides at junctions, a process analogous to immunoglobulin recombination. Mature T cells generally have either CD4 or CD8 on their cell surface as well as the TCR/CD3 complex.

The TCR recognizes processed antigenic peptide fragments bound to MHC molecules. MHC class I molecules, which are expressed by most cell types, normally present peptides derived from endogenous proteins. MHC class II molecules are usually expressed only on professional antigen presenting cells, B cells, macrophages, and dendritic cells; they generally present peptide antigens derived from exogenous molecules (40). Nonlymphoid somatic cells, including renal epithelial cells, can express MHC class II molecules on their cell surface under some circumstances (41). CD4+ helper T cells recognize antigen bound to self MHC class II molecules, and CD8+ cytotoxic T cells recognize antigen in the context of MHC class I. Protein antigens are processed into 14– to 18–amino acid peptide fragments, which bind to assembled MHC molecules. The MHC protein with bound peptide is transported to the cell surface, where it then may bind to antigen-specific TCRs. Peptide fragments that are immunogenic generally bind to MHC with high affinity (42). The variable region segments of the TCR bind to antigen and MHC, with the CDR3 segment of TCR probably contacting antigen, and the CDR1 and CDR2 loops of the TCR binding to residues of the MHC molecule adjacent to the peptide binding groove (43).

T cells are involved in the pathogenesis of many autoimmune diseases and have been studied in animal models of autoimmunity (44) as well as in human autoimmune diseases (45). For example, mice transgenic for a myelin basic protein–specific TCR develop spontaneous autoimmune encephalomyelitis (46). In the NOD mouse model of type I diabetes, thymectomy, or anti-T-cell therapy can prevent disease and the transfer of T cells from mice with disease leads to early onset of diabetes in young mice (47). When transgenic mice expressing α/β TCR from a diabetogenic CD4+ NOD T cell were constructed, transgenic mice bred back towards an NOD background developed more severe diabetes than nontransgenic controls indicating that self-reactive T cells expressing the transgene encoded TCR specificity are not tolerized in these animals (47). In some autoimmune diseases, preferential use of Vβ region genes during TCR recombination has been found (44). Some of this work has led to specific immunotherapy (44,48,49), but there is still controversy regarding the extent of restricted V gene usage in autoimmune T-cell repertoires.

The molecular basis of the T-lymphocyte response has been studied only in one model, autoimmune interstitial nephritis which produces αTBM disease. The selection of TCR variable region genes was investigated in mice after injection with tubular antigen. In this model, the development of disease depends on the emergence of CD4+ T-helper cells reactive to the 3M-1 antigen (17,35), which induce the development of 3M-1 antigen-specific CD8+ effector cells (34,35). CD4+ MHC class II–restricted T cells adoptively transfer interstitial nephritis 6 to 10 weeks after intravenous injection into naive syngeneic mice (35). CD8+ MHC class I–restricted T cells will induce disease 3 to 5 days after transfer under the renal capsule of syngeneic mice (29). Effector 3M-1 antigen-specific, TCR α/β CD8+ T cells have been cultured and cloned and have been shown to mediate antigen specific cytotoxicity in vitro as well as mediating an antigen-specific delayed type hypersensitivity response (50). A clone of MHC class I–restricted, CD8+ effector T cells harvested from SJL mice with αTBM disease transfer specific DTH response to the 3M-1 tubular antigen to naive syngeneic mice (50). This CD8+ T-cell clone also adoptively transfers αTBM disease and has also been demonstrated to be cytotoxic to tubular cells (MCT) which express both class I MHC and 3M-1 antigen (50). This cytotoxicity can be blocked by antibodies to class I MHC.

The peptide antigen specificity and TCR gene usage in CD4+ T-helper cell clones was evaluated in studies of the molecular basis of the helper T-cell repertoire in αTBM disease (51). T cells were isolated from the draining lymph nodes of several SJL mice with αTBM disease, cloned, and carried in long-term culture stimulated with antigen. The cells were confirmed to be CD4+ T-helper cells by flow cytometry. The antigen used was soluble renal tubular antigen (SRTA) or the synthetic peptides P1 or P2. The target antigen of αTBM disease, 3M-1, has been cloned and sequenced. Two potential antigenic peptides, P1 and P2, separated from each other by 22 amino acid residues, were identified by analysis of the deduced amino acid sequence (17). A third potentially antigenic peptide, P3, overlaps P1 and P2 (51). The antigen specificity of the T-helper cell clones was determined using a functional assay, the ability of each clone to induce an antigen-specific, delayed-type hypersensitivity (DTH) producing effector T-cell population. T-helper cells stimulated in culture with SRTA or P1 were able to induce an antigen specific DTH response with SRTA, P1, and P3 but not P2. Clones which were stimulated weekly with P2 induced an antigen-specific DTH response only to P2. Some of these results were confirmed by antigen-specific proliferation assays. A P1 reactive clone was also demonstrated to cause interstitial disease after subcapsular transfer into the kidneys of healthy syngeneic mice, while subcapsular injection of a P2-reactive clone did not cause interstitial infiltration and injury. These results suggest that the P1/P3 peptide is the sole antigenic epitope within the 3M-1 antigen in the SJL mouse (51). The overlap of P1 and P3 is eight amino acid residues in length. This region represents the core of the antigenic peptide, but the usual size of processed peptides eluted from MHC class II molecules have been 14 to 18 residues in length (52), which suggests that the antigenic region of 3M-1 probably is longer than these eight residues. A systemic evaluation using truncated and mutated peptides from this region of 3M-1 may identify optimal peptide size as well as residues that are essential in the recognition of this immunodominant peptide by T cells. The presence of this immunodominant epitope in αTBM disease may allow the development of specific immunotherapeutic interventions. In another animal model of autoimmunity, experimental allergic encephalomyelitis, immunization with an immunodominant peptide of myelin basic protein which had been mutated at one residue prevented or arrested the disease process (53).

TCR variable region sequences were determined for the eight P3-reactive T-helper cell clones and two P2-reactive clones. The eight P3-reactive clones used six different Vβ genes, only two different Dβ genes and five different Jβ genes with one gene, Jβ1.2, used by four clones. Three clones used Vβ14. These results suggest that this TCR repertoire may be biased toward use of Vβ14, but that several Vβ genes can be used in the response to 3M-1.

When the deduced amino acid sequences of the TCR variable regions were aligned, the eight nephritogenic P3-reactive T cell clones were similar across the VDJ junction which encodes the putative CDR3 region of the TCR (54). This region has been hypothesized to interact directly with the processed peptide, while other portions of the TCR variable region encode contact points between TCR and less polymorphic regions of the class II MHC molecule (43,54). The P2 reactive TCR clones share some homology in their CDR3 regions to the nephritogenic P3 reactive clones, except that the second to last residue is a charged amino acid, arginine or glutamine, in the P2 clones and a small nonpolar residue in the P3 reactive clones. The final residue of the CDR3 region of the two P2 reactive clones is also different from the asparagine residue present in most of the P3 reactive clones. Differences in these last two positions of CDR3 may explain the specific recognition of P3 versus P2 by these TCRs (51). The role of these two amino acids in the specific recognition of the P3 peptide bound to MHC class II will need to be confirmed through mutational analysis.

MHC GENES IN THE RECOGNITION OF RENAL STRUCTURES

The expression of MHC genes is another important step in the initiation and regulation of an immune response. Antigen-presenting cells express MHC determinants on their cell surface, which bind processed antigen fragments that can be recognized by antigen-specific T cells. As discussed above, MHC class I is expressed by most cells and presents antigen to CD8+ effector or regulatory T cells, whereas MHC class II expression is generally restricted to professional antigen-presenting cells (40). Some autoimmune diseases appear to be restricted to animals with specific MHC haplotypes. For example, in the kdkd mouse model of spontaneous autoimmune interstitial nephritis, adoptive transfer of disease is class I restricted and DTH-reactive cells are restricted specific class I haplotypes (55).

MHC molecules are heterodimers encoded by two different genes. The MHC class I gene product forms a heterodimer with a β2-microglobulin chain. MHC class II proteins are made up of α/β heterodimers. In the mouse, MHC class II molecules I-A and I-E are encoded by Aα, Aβ, Eα, and

Eβ genes on chromosome 17. In humans, analogous α and β genes are encoded on chromosome 6 at the DR, DQ, DP, DO, and DZ loci. In the endoplasmic reticulum, MHC class II α/β heterodimers associate with a protein called the invariant chain. This complex traverses the Golgi apparatus and then the invariant chain is cleaved from the class II heterodimer in endosomes, and the class II molecules are transported to the cell surface. The importance of the invariant chain has been demonstrated in studies of knockout mice lacking the invariant chain. These mice have abnormal trafficking of MHC class II to the cell surface, their class II molecules are reduced in number and have abnormal comformations (56).

MHC class I is expressed on most cells of the adult animal and can be upregulated by γ-interferon. The expression of MHC class I and β_2-microglobulin is mainly controlled at the transcriptional level (57). MHC class I gene expression is regulated by 5′ sequences including a TATA box, a CCAAT box, a class I regulatory element, enhancer A, and an interferon consensus sequence (58,59). Enhancer A is important in determining the level of constitutive class I expression. A second 5′ enhancer element B is also present in murine class I. The enhancer A element contains sequences responsible for the class I responsiveness to TNFα, phorbol esters, and cAMP. There is also a negative regulatory sequence in this region, which may be important in the embryo and in some neoplasms that do not express class I. The class I promoter region binds the transcription factor proteins NFκB, KBF1, the nuclear hormone receptor H-2RIIBP, and also has AP-1 and AP-2 binding sites. In mature animals, the level of β_2-microglobulin expression parallels class I expression. β_2-microglobulin contains a fragment of the class I regulatory element and a region similar to the interferon consensus sequence (58). Both class I and β_2-microglobulin promoters bind KBF1, and are upregulated by interferon-γ (57,58). In undifferentiated embryonic stem cells, treatment with interferon-γ leads to an increase in the mRNA levels of HAM-1 a peptide transporter important in class I cell surface expression (60).

MHC class II molecules present antigen to CD4+ T cells, most of which are helper T cells. Most antigen presentation to CD4+ T cells is done by professional antigen presenting cells such as B cells which constitutively express MHC class II on their cell surface, or macrophages and dendritic cells which express MHC class II in the presence of γ-interferon or tumor necrosis factor α (61). Other cell types normally express little or no MHC class II on their cell surface. Parenchymal cells may express MHC class II during an inflammatory response after exposure to cytokines, primarily γ-interferon (62,63). This upregulation of MHC class II expression has been noted in several diseases, including autoimmune interstitial nephritis (64), diabetes, and rheumatoid arthritis (63). In vivo, renal proximal tubule epithelial cells upregulate MHC class II expression during systemic infection (65). Under conditions of increased MHC class II expression, nonlymphoid cells (66,67), including renal epithelial cells (41,65,68,69), are capable of presenting antigen to CD4+ T cells. MHC class II protein expression correlates well with mRNA levels, which have been demonstrated to be regulated mainly by transcriptional control (63). Therefore, study of the transcriptional regulation of MHC class II genes should help elucidate mechanisms determining cell surface protein expression.

The regulation of MHC class II transcription of the murine Aβ gene is renal tubular cells has been another focus of study. The *cis*-acting promoter and enhancer elements involved in the positive regulation of MHC transcription and the transcription factor proteins which bind to these elements have been well characterized (63). MHC class II gene regulation elements include a 5′ promoter element, a 5′ enhancer, and an enhancer located in an intron within the gene (58). The 5′ promoter element contains sequences conserved among MHC class II genes in the region between 40 and 160 bp upstream of the transcription start site. These elements X1 and Y, are essential, but not sufficient, for both constitutive and inducible MHC class II expression (58,63). In between the X1 and Y boxes is a region, X2, which has homology to a cAMP response element or a TPA response element. Interferon-γ inducibility appears to require these elements as well as the S box located in the region about 30 base pairs 5′ to the X box. A negative element V, has been mapped to the region -193 through -179 in the human DRA gene (70). DNA transcription factor proteins (*trans*-acting factors) bind to the X and Y boxes and the S region and presumably modulate transcriptional activity of the MHC class II genes. Several proteins that bind to the X box and proteins that bind to the Y box have been identified and cloned (59,63). Interferon-γ is thought to increase MHC class II expression by altering the binding of transcription factors to these promoter elements (58). Fusions of MHC class II positive B cells and class II negative fibrosarcoma, plasmacytoma, or T-lymphoma cells lead to MHC class II negative hybrid cells, suggesting that class II negative cells contain a *trans*-acting suppressor factor that prevents class II expression (63).

In order to better understand the low MHC class II expression on parenchymal cells, studies were designed to characterize *cis*-acting elements essential to downregulate Aβ expression in murine renal tubular (MCT) cells. MCT cells normally express little or no I-A (Aα/Aβ^s) on their cell surface and express little Aβ mRNA (71). This low basal class II expression is not due to mutation in the Aβ coding sequence, as confirmed by the sequencing of MCT cell Aβ coding region cDNA (72). Interferon-γ has been demonstrated to increase cell surface MHC class II expression in MCT cells (64).

Plasmid constructs containing segments of the Aβ 5′ upstream region of DNA of various lengths linked to a chloramphenicol acetyl transferase (CAT) reporter gene were transfected into MCT cells in order to localize a presumptive *cis*-acting silencer element in the Aβ gene. CAT activity was assayed and found to be high in constructs containing short regions of 5′ sequence and decreased between -489 and -669, indicating the possible presence of a silencer region in this area of the gene. The silencing activity of the region between -669 and -489 was demonstrated to be position-independent by moving it downstream in the gene and ligating it directly to the homologous Aβ proximal promoter. When this construct was transfected into a class II expressing B cell line, no silencing of CAT activity occurred, suggesting the absence of a *trans*-acting protein needed for silencer activity in the B cells (71).

The core DNA binding site of the putative silencing protein was mapped by gel shift analysis utilizing an 88-bp probe from the 5′ upstream region -605 to -517 and nuclear protein extracts from MCT cells. Gel shift analysis using overlapping oligonucleotide probes and competitive binding with mutated probes allowed mapping of the core binding site to an 8- to 10-bp segment. The functional importance of this binding site was confirmed by introducing a mutation in this area of the 5′ upstream region of a CAT reporter construct. This mutation largely abrogated the silencing activity of the region as assayed by CAT activity (71). Our understanding of the mechanism of action of the nuclear factor recognizing this Aβ silencing element should be better elucidated after the protein has been isolated and characterized. Investigation of the mechanisms that normally maintain low MHC class II expression in epithelial cells may contribute to the understanding of organ-specific autoimmunity and peripheral tolerance.

CONCLUSIONS

Studies of immune processes in experimental autoimmune renal diseases have led to a better understanding of the genetics of antibody production, TCR gene usage, the antigenic focus of such autoimmune responses, and the mechanisms that normally prevent MHC class II expression on renal parenchymal cells and may protect against organ-specific autoimmune disease. Study of humoral and cell-mediated mechanisms of immunity in models of renal disease at the molecular level should lead to a better understanding of the pathogenesis of immune-mediated renal damage as well as normal mechanisms of protection from autoimmunity; it may then allow the development of specific interventions to treat these disease processes.

ACKNOWLEDGMENTS

This work was supported in part by grants DK-08592, AR-20553, DK-07006, DK-30280, DK-41110, and DK-45191 from the National Institutes of Health.

REFERENCES

1. Reth M, Hombach J, Wienands J, et al. The B-cell antigen receptor complex. Immunol Today 1991; 12:196–201.
2. Tonegawa S. Somatic generation of antibody diversity. Nature 1983; 302:575–581.
3. Blackwell TK, Alt FW. Immunoglobulin genes. In: Hames BD, Glover DM, eds. Molecular Immunology. Oxford: IRL Press.
4. Gellert M. V(D)J recombination gets a break. Trends Genet. 1992; 8:408–412.

5. Mombaerts P, Iacomini J, Johnson RS, et al. RAG-1-deficient mice have no mature B and T lymphocytes. Cell 1992; 68:869–877.
6. Shinkai Y, Rathbun G, Lam KP, et al. RAG-2-deficient mice lack mature lymphocytes owing to inability to initiate V(D)J rearrangement. Cell 1992; 68:855–867.
7. Oettinger MA. Activation of V(D)J recombination by RAG1 and RAG2. Trends Genet 1992; 8:413–416.
8. Jacob J, Kelsoe G, Rajewsky K, Weiss U. Intraclonal generation of antibody mutants in germinal centres. *Nature (Lond)* 1991; 354:389–392.
9. Trepicchio W, Maruya A, Barrett KJ. The heavy chain genes of a lupus anti-DNA antibody are encoded in the germline of a nonautoimmune strain of mouse and are conserved in strains of mice polymorphic for this gene locus. J Immunol 1987; 139:3139–3144.
10. Shlomchik MJ, Marshak-Rothstein A, Wolfowicz CB, et al. The role of clonal selection and somatic mutation in autoimmunity. *Nature* (*Lond*) 1987; 328:805–811.
11. van Es JH, Gmelig Meyling FHJ, van de Akker WRM, et al. Somatic mutations in the variable-regions of a human IgG anti double-stranded DNA antibody suggest a role for antigen in the induction of systemic lupus erythematosus. J Exp Med 1991; 173:461–470.
12. Marion TN, Tillman DM, Jou NT. Interclonal and intraclonal diversity among anti-DNA antibodies from an (NZB × NZW)F_1 mouse. J Immunol 1990; 145:2322–2332.
13. Kabat EA. Antibody diversity versus antibody complementarity. Pharmacol Rev 1982; 34:23–38.
14. Rolink A, Melchers F. Molecular and cellular origins of B lymphocyte diversity. Cell 1991; 66:1081–1094.
15. Manser T, Wysocki LJ, Gridley T, et al. The molecular evolution of the immune response. Immunol Today 1985; 6:94–101.
16. Clayman MD, Martinez-Hernandez A, Michaud L, et al. Isolation and characterization of the nephritogenic antigen producing anti-tubular basement membrane disease. J Exp Med 1985; 161:290–305.
17. Neilson EG, Sun MJ, Kelly CJ, et al. Molecular characterization of a major nephritogenic domain in the autoantigen of anti-tubular basement membrane disease. Proc Natl Acad Sci USA 1991; 88:2006–2010.
18. Clayman MD, Sun MJ, Michaud L, et al. Clonotypic heterogeneity in experimental interstitial nephritis. J Exp Med 1988; 167:1296–1312.
19. Clayman MD, Michaud L. Neilson EG. Murine interstitial nephritis: VI. Characterization of the B cell response in anti-tubular basement membrane disease. J Immunol 1987; 138:2242–2249.
20. Karp SL, Kieber-Emmons T, Sun MJ, et al. The molecular structure of a cross-reacting idiotype on autoantibodies recognizing parenchymal self. J Immunol 1993; 150:867–879.
21. Shlomchik M, Mascelli M, Shan H, et al. Anti-DNA antibodies from autoimmune mice arise by clonal expansion and somatic mutation. J Exp Med 1990; 171:265–297.
22. Madaio MP, Carlson J, Cataldo J, et al. Murine moloclonal anti-DNA antibodies bind directly to glomerular antigens and form immunee deposits. J Immunol 1987; 138:2883–2889.
23. Katz MS, Foster MH, Madaio MP. Independently derived murine glomerular immune deposit-forming anti-DNA antibodies are encoded by near-identical V_H gene sequences. J Clin Invest 1993; 91:402–408.
24. Foster MH, Madaio MP, Barrett KJ. Variable region sequence analysis of anti-DNA antibodies: Evidence for a family of closely related germ-line V_H genes encoding lupus autoantibodies. DNA Cell Biol 1992; 11:175–1832.
25. Bona CA. V genes encoding autoantibodies: Molecular and phenotypic characteristics. Annu Rev Immunol 1988; 6:327–358.
26. Carson DA, Chen PP, Fox RI, et al. Rheumatoid factors and immune networks. Annu Rev Immunol 1987; 5:109–126.
27. Pascual V, Victor K, Lelsz D, et al. Nucleotide sequence analysis of the V regions of two IgM cold agglutinins: Evidence that the V_H4-21 gene segment is responsible for the major cross-reactive idiotype. J Immunol 1991; 146:4385–4391.
28. Neilson EG, McCafferty E, Mann R, et al. Tubular antigen-derivatized cells induce a disease-protective, antigen-specific, and idiotype-specific suppressor T cell network restricted by I-J and Igh-V in mice with experimental interstitial nephritis. J Exp Med 1985; 162:215–230.
29. Neilson EG, McCafferty E, Mann R, et al. Murine interstitial nephritis: III. The selection of phenotypic (lyt and L3T4) and idiotypic (RE-Id) T cell preferences by genes in Igh-1 and H-2k characterizes the cell-mediated potential for disease expression: Susceptible mice provide a unique effector T cell repertoire in response to tubular antigen. J Immunol 1985; 134:2375–2382.
30. Neilson EG, Phillips SM. Suppression of interstitial nephritis by auto-anti-idiotypic immunity. J Exp Med 1982; 155:179–189.
31. Couser WG. Mechanisms of glomerular injury in immune-complex disease. Kidney Int 1985; 28:569–583.
32. Neilson EG. Pathogenesis and therapy of interstitial nephritis. Kidney Int 1989; 35:1257–1270.
33. Neilson EG, Phillips SM. Analysis of disease susceptibility and its relationship to pleiomorphic gene products defining both immune-response genes and a restrictive requirement for cytotoxic T cells at H-2K. J Exp Med 1982; 155:1078–1085.

34. Mann R, Kelly CJ, Hines WH, et al. Effector T cell differentiation in experimental interstitial nephritis: I. The development and modulation of effector lymphocyte maturation by I-J+ regulatory T cells. J Immunol 1987; 138:4200–4208.
35. Mann R, Zakheim B, Clayman M, et al. Murine interstitial nephritis: IV. Long-term cultured L3T4+ T cell lines transfer delayed expression of disease as I-A-restricted inducers of the effector T cell repertoire. J Immunol 1985; 135:286–293.
36. Hedrick SM. T lymphocyte receptors. In: Paul WE, ed. Fundamental Immunology. New York: Raven Press, 1989: 291–313.
37. Schwartz RH. Costimulation of T lymphocytes: The role of CD28, CTLA4, and B7/BB1 in interleukin-2 production and immunotherapy. Cell 1992; 71:1065–1068.
38. Neilson EG. Is immunologic tolerance of self modulated through antigen presentation by parenchymal epithelium? Kidney Int 1993; 44:927–931.
39. Springer TA. Adhesion receptors of the immune system. Nature (Lond) 1990; 346:425–434.
40. Theofilopoulos AN, Balderas RS, Baccala R, Kono DH. T-cell receptor genes in autoimmunity. Ann NY Acad Sci 1993; 681:33–46.
41. Haverty TP, Kelly CJ Hines WH, et al. Characterization of a renal tubular epithelial cell line which secretes the autologous target antigen of autoimmune experimental interstitial nephritis. J Cell Biol 1988; 107:1358–1368.
42. Sercarz EE, Lehmann PV, Ametani A, et al. Dominance and crypticity of T cell antigenic determinants. Annu Rev Immunol 1993; 11:729–766.
43. Jorgensen JI, Reay PA, Ehrich EW, Davis MM. Molecular components of T-cell recognition. Annu Rev Immunol 1992; 10:835–873.
44. Acha-Orbea H, Steinman L, McDevitt HO. T cell receptors in murine autoimmune diseases. Annu Rev Immunol 1989; 371–405.
45. Davies TF, Martin A, Concepcion ES, et al. Evidence of limited variability of antigen receptors on intrathyroidal T cells in autoimmune thyroid disease. N Engl J Med 1991; 325:238–244.
46. Goverman J, Woods A, Larson L, et al. Transgenic mice that express a myelin basic protein-specific T cell receptor develop spontaneous autoimmunity. Cell 1993; 72:551–560.
47. Katz JD, Wang B, Haskins K, et al. Following a diabetogenic T cell from genesis through pathogenesis. Cell 1993; 74:1089–1100.
48. Wraith DC, McDevitt HO, Steinman L, Acha-Orbea H. T cell recognition as the target for immune intervention in autoimmune disease. Cell 1989; 57:709–715.
49. Clayton JP, Gammon GM, Ando DG, et al. Peptide-specific prevention of experimental allergic encephalomyelitis. J Exp Med 1989; 169:1681–1691.
50. Meyers CE, Kelly CJ. Effector mechanisms in organ-specific autoimmunity. J Clin Invest 1991; 88:408–416.
51. Heeger PS, Smoyer WE, Saad T, et al. Molecular analysis of the helper T cell response in murine interstitial nephritis: T cells recognizing an immunodominant epitope use multiple TCR $V\beta$ genes with similarities across CDR3. J Clin Invest 1994; 94:2084–2092.
52. Rudensky AY, Preston-Hurlburt P, Al-Ramadi BK, et al. Truncation variants of peptides isolated from MHC class II molecules suggest sequence motifs. Nature (Lond) 1992; 359:429–431.
53. Smilek DE, Wraith DC, Hodgkinson S, et al. A single amino acid change in a myelin basic protein peptide confers the capacity to prevent rather than induce experimental autoimmune encephalitis. Proc Natl Acad Sci USA 1992; 88:9633–9637.
54. Chothia C, Boswell Dr, Lesk AM. The outline structure of the T-cell $\alpha\beta$ receptor. EMBO J 1988; 7:3745–3755.
55. Kelly CJ, Korngold R, Mann R, et al. Spontaneous interstitial nephritis in kdkd mice: II. Characterization of a tubular antigen-specific, H-2K-restricted lyt-2+ effector T cell that mediates destructive tubulointersitial injury. J Immunol 1986; 136:526–531.
56. Viville S, Neefjes J, Lotteau V, et al. Mice lacking the MHC class II-associated invariant chain. Cell 1993; 72:635–648.
57. Drezen JM, Babinet C, Morello D. Transcriptional control of MHC class I and β_2-microglobulin genes in vivo. J Immunol 1993; 150:2805–2813.
58. Halloran PF, Madrenas J. Regulation of MHC transcription. Transplantation 1990; 50:725–738.
59. Ting JPY, Baldwin AS. Regulation of MHC gene expression. Curr Opin Immunol 1993; 5:8–16.
60. Bikoff E, Jaffe L, Ribaudo R, et al. MHC class I surface expression in embryo-derived cell lines inducible with peptide or interferon. Nature (Lond) 1991; 354:235–238.
61. Chang RJ, Lee SH. Effects of interferon-γ and tumor necrosis factor-α on the expression of an la antigen on a murine macrophage cell line. J Immunol 1986; 137:2853–2856.
62. Bottazzo GF, Todd I, Mirakian R, et al. Organ-specific autoimmunity: A 1986 overview. Immunol Rev 1986; 94:137–169.

63. Glimcher, LH, Kara, CJ. Sequences and factors: A guide to MHC class-II transcription. Annu Rev Immunol 1992; 10:13–49.
64. Haverty TP, Watanabe M, Neilson EG, Kelly CJ. Protective modulation of class II MHC gene expression in tubular epithelium by target antigen-specific antibodies: Cell-surface directed down-regulation of transcription can influence susceptibility to murine tubulointerstitial nephritis. J Immunol 1989; 143:1133–1141.
65. Hagerty DT, Allen PM. Processing and presentation of self and foreign antigens by the renal proximal tubule. J Immunol 1992; 148:2324–2330.
66. Londei M, Lamb JR, Bottazzo GF, Feldmann M. Epithelial cells expressing aberrant MHC class II determinants can present antigen to cloned human T cells. Nature (Lond) 1984; 312:639–641.
67. Markman J, Lo D, Naji A, et al. Antigen presenting function of class II MHC expressing pancreatic beta cells. Nature (Lond) 1988; 336:476–479.
68. Hines W, Haverty T, Elias J, et al. T cell recognition of epithelial self. Autoimmunity 1989; 5:37–47.
69. Wuthrich RP, Glimcher LH, Yui MA, et al. MHC class II, antigen presentation and tumor necrosis factor in renal tubular epithelial cells. Kidney Int 1990; 37:783–792.
70. Cogswell JP, Basta PV, Ting JPY. X-box binding proteins positively and negatively regulate transcription of the HLA-DRA gene through interaction with discrete upstream W and V elements. Proc Natl Acad Sci USA 1990; 87:7703–7707.
71. Albert SE, Strutz F, Shelton K, et al. Characterization of a cis-acting regulatory element which silences expression of the class-II-A β gene in epithelium. J Exp Med 1994; 180:233–240.
72. Albert, SE, Shelton K, Sun MJ. Neilson EG. Analysis of the cDNA sequence encoding MHC Aβ in tubular epithelium from mouse kidney. Kidney Int 1991; 40:139–142.

59
Platelet-Derived Growth Factor and Renal Disease

Ashio Yoshimura, Hiroyuki Iida, Jürgen Floege, and Richard J. Johnson
University of Washington, Seattle, Washington

INTRODUCTION

Platelet-derived growth factor (PDGF) is a 28- to 32-kDa basic glycoprotein (pI 9.8-10) that contains two polypeptide chains, designated A (16 kDa) and B (14 kDa), that exists in disulfide linkage either as a cationic heterodimer or homodimer, resulting in three biologically active isoforms (PDGF-AA, PDGF-AB, and PDGF-BB) (1). Each of the PDGF chains is encoded by a separate gene (2,3). Although PDGF was initially isolated from the alpha granules of platelets, it is also synthesized and released by a variety of other cell types, including smooth muscle cells, activated macrophages, and activated endothelial cells (4). In the glomerulus, mesangial cells (5–7), glomerular endothelial cells (8–11), and visceral glomerular epithelial cells (12) also synthesize PDGF. Therefore, both infiltrating and endogenous glomerular cells in the injured glomerulus are capable of producing PDGF.

PDGF induces many biological responses in cells by binding to specific cell surface, high-affinity receptors (PDGF-R). At first it was believed that the biological actions of PDGF were induced via a single receptor. However, it has now been shown that the PDGF-R consists of two distinct subunits, termed α and β, that are encoded by two separate genes (13–15). The PDGF-R subunits are brought together upon PDGF binding to form one of three isoforms (PDGF-R$\alpha\alpha$, $\alpha\beta$, $\beta\beta$). Seifert et al. have demonstrated that the high-affinity binding of PDGF to the different PDGF-R isoforms involves binding specificity, in that the α-subunit can bind either the PDGF-A or B-chain, whereas the β subunit binds only the PDGF-B chain (14). Thus, PDGF-AA binds to the PDGF-R $\alpha\alpha$ receptor, PDGF-AB binds either to the PDGF-R $\alpha\alpha$ or to the $\alpha\beta$ receptor, and PDGF-BB binds to all three receptor subunit isoforms (PDGF-R $\alpha\alpha$, $\alpha\beta$, $\beta\beta$) (14). In a recent study, PDGF-AB was also shown to bind to the PDGF-R $\beta\beta$ subunit, but this binding occurs with low affinity and is probably biologically insignificant (16).

The PDGF-R contains a large ligand-binding domain in the extracellular region and a tyrosine kinase within the intracellular portion of the molecule (1–4). A rapid activation of the tyrosine kinase occurs following binding of PDGF to the PDGF-R, resulting in autophosphorylation of the PDGF-R as well as phosphorylation of cytoplasmic proteins such as phospholipase C, phosphatidylinositol kinase, and serine kinases. Activation of membrane phospholipases leads to prostaglandin formation; generation of inositol triphosphate (IP_3) which increases intracellular calcium; and diacylglyceride synthesis, which activates protein kinase C. Within minutes to hours, several "early response" proto-oncogenes, including c-*myc* and c-*fos*, are expressed, and a poorly defined sequence of intracellular signaling occurs that ultimately culminates in new DNA synthesis (4,17,18).

FUNCTIONS OF PDGF THAT MAY BE IMPORTANT IN GLOMERULAR DISEASE

Numerous biological functions of PDGF have been reported that may play an important role in glomerular disease. Most studies have focused on the role of PDGF in mesangial cell proliferation, as PDGF is a potent mitogen for mesangial cells in vitro (6,7,19). In addition to mesangial cell proliferation, other biological actions of PDGF have also been demonstrated that may contribute to the mechanisms of glomerular injury. For example, PDGF is a chemoattractant for mesangial cells in vitro (20) as well as for vascular smooth muscle cells (21) and therefore may be important for migration of mesangial cells within a damaged mesangium such as occurs with mesangiolysis. PDGF is also a powerful vasoconstrictor (22) and induces contraction of mesangial cells via a phospholipase C–dependent pathway (63); this may be important in the modulation of glomerular hemodynamics which occurs in glomerulonephritis. The interaction of PDGF with other growth factors or cytokines may also be important in glomerular injury. PDGF mediates the mitogenic effects of a variety of growth factors and cytokines on mesangial cells. For example, epidermal growth factor–mediated mesangial cell proliferation is partially inhibited by anti-PDGF antibodies (7). PDGF also stimulates the synthesis of various growth factors in mesangial cells, including interleukin-1 (IL-1) (23), transforming growth factor beta (TGF-β) (24), and PDGF itself (7). Regulation of matrix synthesis by mesangial cells may also involve PDGF directly or indirectly (24–26). Thus, the expression of type IV collagen mRNA in mouse mesangial cells that occurs in response to advanced glycosylation end products can be inhibited by anti-PDGF antibody (26). Prostaglandin generation by human mesangial cells is also increased by PDGF-BB or -AB when combined with IL-1 or interleukin 6 (IL-6) (27); this could be important in the regulation of glomerular hemodynamics in glomerular inflammatory processes. Furthermore, PDGF may function as a chemotactic factor for monocytes and neutrophils and, at higher concentrations, may induce release of lysosomal enzymes and proteases, thereby potentially influencing inflammatory cell accumulation and activation within the glomerulus (28–30).

APPLYING KOCH'S POSTULATES TOWARDS THE ESTABLISHMENT OF A ROLE FOR PDGF IN MESANGIAL CELL PROLIFERATION

Robert Koch (1843–1910) received the Nobel Prize in Medicine in 1905 for his discovery of the etiology of tuberculosis. In this landmark paper, he (a) identified the mycobacteria in disease tissue, (b) isolated these organisms from the diseased tissue and maintained them in culture, and (c) induced disease in susceptible animals by inoculating them with his purified bacterial cultures (31). The specific steps used by Koch in establishing the etiology and pathogenesis of disease have been adopted by many and have become known as Koch's postulates.

Abboud (32) and our group (33) have recently adopted Koch's postulates to the study of cytokines and growth factors in kidney disease. In order to prove that a cytokine mediates a particular effect in glomerular disease, we believe one must demonstrate that (a) the growth factor has a specific effect on the target cells in vitro; (b) the growth factor is expressed and/or localized in disease and correlates with the proposed effect; (c) exogenous administration of the growth factor in vivo (or overexpression as observed with transgenic animals or following in vivo gene transfer) reproduces the biological effect, and (d) blocking the growth factor prevents or inhibits the effect in disease. Important but less critical issues include whether or not the receptor expression is modulated, identification of the type of cell expressing the growth factor in disease, and determination of the factors that stimulate or turn off the expression of the growth factor(s) (33). These criteria have yet to be fulfilled for most cytokines and growth factors. However, all four major criteria mentioned above have been satisfied for the hypothesis that *PDGF is a significant mediator of mesangial cell proliferation in glomerulonephritis*.

MEDIATION OF MESANGIAL CELL PROLIFERATION IN VITRO BY PDGF

Mesangial cells in culture proliferate in response to numerous growth factors and cytokines, including PDGF (6,7,19,34–36). Several studies have suggested that PDGF is the most potent mitogen for cultured mesangial cells when compared to other peptide growth factors (6,7). However, whereas some studies have supported PDGF to be a "complete" growth factor for mesangial cells (19), in other studies PDGF acts as a "competence" factor and does not induce significant mesangial cell proliferation unless "progression" factors such as IL-1 or insulin-like growth factor 1 (IGF-1) are present (35,37). As mentioned above, PDGF may also mediate the effects of other growth factors and cytokines. Many growth factors, including PDGF itself, induce expression of PDGF and PDGF mRNA in mesangial cells (7). Furthermore, the mitogenic properties of EGF on mesangial cells (7) and of IL-1 on fibroblasts (38) can be inhibited by anti-PDGF antibody. This implies that PDGF may act as an autocrine growth factor for several types of cells, including mesangial cells.

In comparing the mitogenic effect of the three isoforms of PDGF on human mesangial cells, PDGF-AB and -BB have been shown to be potent mitogens, while PDGF-AA has little or no effect (19,39). This suggests that both α and β subunits are present on mesangial cells. Abboud has suggested that the relative lack of responsiveness to the PDGF-AA homodimer is due to downregulation of PDGF-R α-subunit in human mesangial cells (39). Indeed, both the PDGF-R α and β subunits have been demonstrated in cultured rat and human mesangial cells; however, the expression of the β subunit is predominant (19,39,40).

The PDGF-R may be modulated under several conditions. For example, TGF-β, which is usually considered an inhibitor of mesangial cell proliferation, may actually stimulate mesangial cell proliferation at low concentrations (34). This has recently been suggested to be a consequence of a TGF-β–mediated upregulation of the PDGF-R β subunit (41). A similar modulation of PDGF-R by TGF-β has been noted with other cell types [42].

Marx et al. have reported that rat mesangial cells grown in a three-dimensional type I collagen gel matrix are not responsive to PDGF due to *downregulation* of the PDGF-R β subunit on the cell surface (40). This has raised questions as to whether mesangial cells in vivo, which are surrounded by mesangial matrix, would be similarly unresponsive. However, recent studies have demonstrated that rats express PDGF-R β-subunit on mesangial cells in vivo (43). Similarly, both PDGF-R α- and β-subunit mRNA and protein have been localized by in situ hybridization and immunostaining to human mesangial cells in vivo (44–46).

EXPRESSION OF PDGF IN EXPERIMENTAL AND HUMAN GLOMERULAR DISEASES

PDGF in Proliferative Glomerulonephritis

The observation that PDGF may be a major growth factor for mesangial cells in vitro suggests that it may be involved in glomerular diseases associated with mesangial cell proliferation. The first report demonstrating the presence of PDGF in glomeruli was by Frampton et al., in which PDGF

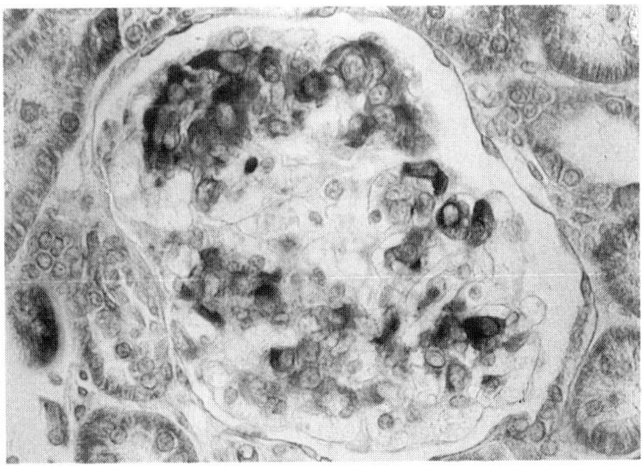

Figure 1 Immunostaining for the PDGF-B chain protein of a glomerulus from a rat with mesangial proliferative nephritis with anti-Thy 1 antibody (day 3 after disease induction). There is a marked increase in cells positive for PDGF-B-chain protein (×400).

was localized by immunostaining to the glomerular capillary wall of patients with diffuse proliferative lupus glomerulonephritis (47). Gesualdo et al. later reported increased expression of PDGF and PDGF-B-chain mRNA in whole kidneys in a murine model of IgA nephropathy (48). We have investigated whether PDGF is expressed in the anti-Thy 1 model of mesangial proliferative nephritis in the rat (43,49). The anti-Thy 1 model is induced by injection of complement-fixing antibody to the Thy 1.1 antigen that is present on the surface of mesangial cells (50). The initial phase is characterized by a decimation of the mesangial cell population ("mesangiolysis"), which peaks at 24 hr. A marked infiltration of platelets and monocyte/macrophages into the glomeruli occurs in association with the mesangiolysis (43,51). This is followed by a phase of mesangial cell proliferation and matrix expansion, resulting in a lesion resembling mesangial proliferative nephritis in humans (43). During this phase, mesangial cells undergo a phenotypic change with the de novo expression of α smooth muscle actin (52).

A marked increase (8- to 10-fold) in PDGF-A- and B-chain mRNA was demonstrated in isolated glomerular RNA by Northern analysis obtained 3 and 5 days after disease induction, which corresponded to the period of mesangial cell proliferation (43). Cells expressing PDGF-B-chain mRNA were also identified in mesangial locations by in situ hybridization using a nonradioactive digoxigenin-labeled cRNA probe (49) (Fig. 2). The use of digoxigenin-labeled cRNA probes had a number of advantages over classic radiolabeled probes, including (a) a short (< 72 hr) color reaction time, (b) no background signal, due to the fact that digoxigenin is not normally present in animal tissue; and (c) the avoidance of radioactive materials (49).

In addition to the demonstration of PDGF mRNA expression by Northern analysis and in situ hybridization, immunostaining with a monoclonal antibody to PDGF-B-chain protein documented the presence of numerous cells positive for PDGF-B-chain in mesangial regions of the rats with proliferative lesions (Fig. 1). In many cases the PDGF-B-chain positive cells could be shown to be in actual mitosis (43).

The PDGF expression correlated closely with the mesangial cell proliferation. First, the peak PDGF expression occurred at days 3 and 5 when PCNA expression was also maximal. Second, measures that reduced mesangial cell proliferation, such as complement or platelet depletion, also inhibited the expression of PDGF mRNA and PDGF-B-chain protein (43,49).

We have also studied the relationship of PDGF expression with glomerular cell proliferation in the remnant kidney model (53). This model is induced by right nephrectomy and infarction of two-thirds of the left kidney and results in a progressive and irreversible glomerulosclerosis within 10 to 12 weeks (53,54). In this model, mesangial cell proliferation can be documented prior to the development of glomerulosclerosis and correlates with an increased expression of PDGF-B-chain mRNA and protein in glomeruli (53).

PDGF expression is also upregulated in other experimental glomerular diseases models (Table 1)

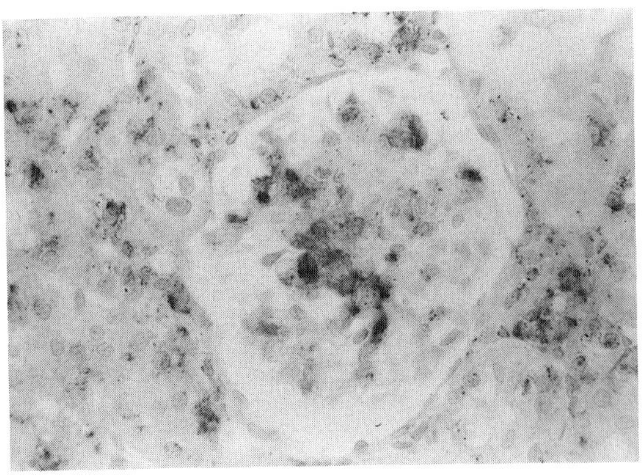

Figure 2 In situ hybridization for the PDGF-B-chain mRNA using a digoxigenin-labeled cRNA probe of a glomerulus from a rat with mesangial proliferative nephritis induced with anti-Thy 1 antibody (day 3 after disease induction). Cells positive for PDGF B-chain mRNA were identified in a mesangial distribution (×400).

Table 1 Expression of PDGF in Experimental and Human Glomerulonephritis

Disease	Ref.
Murine	
IgA nephropathy	(48,55)
Lupus nephritis	(55)
BSA nephritis	(59)
Rat	
Anti-Thy 1 nephritis	(43,49)
Remnant kidney model	(53)
Aminonucleoside nephrosis	(56)
Anti-GBM nephritis	(57)
Passive Heymann nephritis	(12)
Streptozotocin-induced diabetes	(61,62)
Habu snake venom-induced nephritis	(60)
DOCA-salt hypertension	(58)
Human	
Diffuse proliferative lupus nephritis	(47)
IgA nephropathy	(48,63,64,66)
Mesangial proliferative nephritis	(48,64,66)
ANCA-positive crescentic nephritis	(65)
Crescentic nephritis	(67)

(43,48–49,53,55–62). Examples include models of mesangial proliferative nephritis (e.g., Habu snake venom), focal sclerosis (e.g., aminonucleoside nephrosis), lupus (NZB/W F1 hybrid mice), diabetes (e.g. streptozotocin-induced diabetes), and hypertension (e.g., DOCA-salt) (55–62). In some of these models the expression of PDGF was correlated with glomerular cell proliferation (43,53,55,56,62). For example, Fukui et al. (56) demonstrated that PDGF mRNA expression correlates closely with PCNA mRNA expression in rats with aminonucleoside nephrosis. Furthermore, both the PDGF and PCNA expression are reduced by a low-protein diet (56). In streptozotocin-induced diabetes, a correlation of PDGF-B-chain and PCNA mRNA expression also can be shown (62).

Finally, studies have demonstrated that PDGF is expressed in human glomerular diseases (47,48,63–67) (Table 1). As mentioned above, PDGF was first localized to the glomerular capillary wall of some patients with diffuse lupus nephritis (47). In these cases, the PDGF was thought to originate from degranulating platelets, which then bound the capillary wall due to a charge interaction between the cationic PDGF and the anionic GBM. Subsequently, Gesualdo et al. demonstrated PDGF by immunocytochemistry in the mesangial regions of patients with IgA nephropathy (48). PDGF has also been localized by immunoelection microscopy to the mesangial deposits in this disease (63). Schena et al. have also reported an increase in PDGF mRNA by polymerase chain reaction from kidney biopsies of patients with IgA nephropathy (64). In these diseases, mesangial cells are proliferating, as evidenced by the presence of PCNA-positive, common leukocyte antigen-negative cells [68].

We (A. Yoshimura and colleagues) have also documented the upregulation of PDGF mRNA (Figure 3) and PDGF protein in mesangial regions of patients with IgA nephropathy (66). Mesangial cell proliferation was confirmed in these cases by staining with an antibody to Ki-67, a nuclear protein (69) expressed during the cell cycle.

PDGF-B-chain mRNA has also shown to be heavily expressed in crescents in patients with rapidly progressive glomerulonephritis (67). This is particularly interesting, as parietal epithelial cells expressed the PDGF-R β subunit (45). Expression was greatest in cellular as opposed to fibrotic crescents, and the origin of the PDGF was thought to be the macrophage (67). However, a contribution of the PDGF by parictal epithelial cells or fibroblasts cannot be excluded.

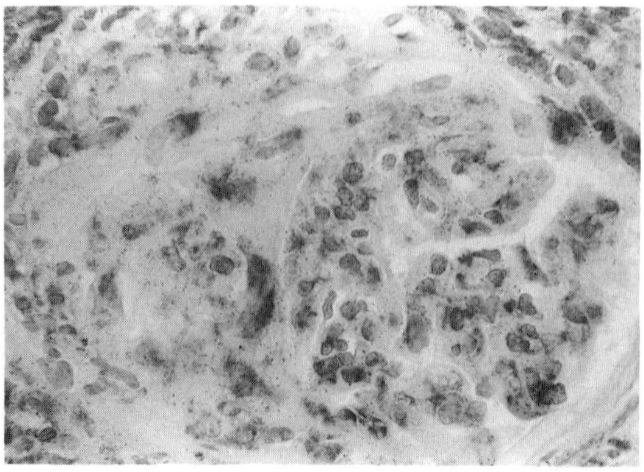

Figure 3 In situ hybridization for the PDGF-B-chain mRNA using a digoxigenin-labeled cRNA probe in a case of severe proliferative IgA nephropathy with crescent formation. A marked expression of PDGF-B-chain mRNA was shown in mesangial locations. Cells positive for PDGF B-chain mRNA were also present in crescents (×400).

Upregulation of PDGF-R in Proliferative Nephritis

Mesangial proliferative nephritis is also associated with an upregulation of the PDGF-R. We have studied the expression of the PDGF-R β subunit in both the anti-Thy 1 model and the remnant kidney model. In the anti-Thy 1 model, an 8- to 25-fold increase in PDGF-R β-subunit mRNA could be demonstrated by Northern analysis in isolated glomerular RNA from diseased rats compared to normal rats at 3 and 5 days after disease induction, respectively (43). The increased expression of PDGF-R β-subunit mRNA was associated with a corresponding increase in PDGF-R β-subunit protein by Western blot of isolated glomerular extracts (43). By immunostaining with a specific polyclonal antibody, the increased expression of PDGF-R β subunit was demonstrated in a mesangial cell pattern. The upregulation of the PDGF-R could be blocked if proliferation was inhibited by depleting rats of platelets or complement. In contrast to the PDGF-R β subunit, there was no PDGF-R α-subunit mRNA or protein expression in normal glomeruli or glomeruli in the anti-Thy 1 model (43). This suggests that in the rat, the PDGF-BB isoform is likely to be the main PDGF isoform mediating mesangial cell proliferation.

An increase in PDGF-R β-subunit mRNA and protein was also demonstrated in the remnant kidney model of progressive glomerulosclerosis (53). The increased PDGF-R protein staining was strictly observed in mesangial regions and occurred shortly after the onset of mesangial cell proliferation. A slight increase of PDGF-R β-subunit mRNA was also noted in rats with remnant kidneys when compared to sham-operated controls 2 weeks after renal ablation. As in the anti-Thy 1 model, expression of glomerular PDGF-R α-subunit mRNA could not be demonstrated (53). As in the rat, an increased mesangial expression of PDGF-R β mRNA and protein have also been observed in proliferative glomerular disease in humans and localizes to the mesangium by in situ hybridization and immunostaining, respectively (44,46).

The Source of the Cells Expressing PDGF in Glomeruli with Proliferative Nephritis

The source of PDGF in proliferative glomerular diseases could potentially derive from either exogenous (e.g., platelets and monocyte/macrophages) and/or endogenous (mesangial, endothelial, or visceral epithelial) cells, as all of these cell types have been shown to express or release PDGF.

Platelets

Platelets are likely to be a major source of PDGF. Platelets contain large quantities of PDGF in their α granules, which they can release upon activation (4). Platelets and platelet antigens can also be demonstrated in glomeruli in numerous types of human and experimental glomerulonephritis

(51,70–74, and reviewed in Ref. 75). An influx of platelets into glomeruli can be shown within minutes to hours after disease induction in several experimental glomerular models (51,53,70,71). Following the influx of platelets, glomerular cell proliferation can often be demonstrated (51,71). Furthermore, PDGF has been localized by immunoelectron microscopy in both platelets within capillary loops and in mesangial deposits in IgA nephropathy (63). In the anti-Thy 1 model, rats that have been depleted of platelets by an antiplatelet antibody have significantly reduced mesangial cell proliferation (76). Platelet depletion also reduces mesangial cell proliferation in the Habu snake venom model (77).

Monocyte/Macrophages

Activated macrophages may also be an important source of PDGF. It has been reported that macrophages are the principal source of PDGF in atherosclerotic blood vessels (78). In the Habu snake venom induced-injury model, glomerular PDGF-B-chain expression is closely associated with the early influx of monocytes/macrophages and platelets (60). Nakamura et al. have also reported that peripheral blood monocytes express increased amounts of PDGF B-chain mRNA in IgA nephropathy (79).

Mesangial Cells

Mesangial cells can also produce PDGF-A- and B-chain mRNA and protein (6,7). As mentioned above, most of the PDGF-B-chain mRNA and protein-positive cells are in mesangial locations in the anti-Thy 1 model (43,49). Although some of this PDGF probably originates from macrophages, >85% of the PDGF-B-chain positive cells were positive for α smooth muscle actin by double immunolabeling (43). α Smooth muscle actin is expressed by activated, proliferating mesangial cells in this model, whereas macrophages and glomerular epithelial cells are negative for this actin isoform (52). Therefore, the mesangial cell is likely to be the major source for the increased PDGF expression in this model of nephritis. Mesangial cells are also likely to be the major source of the PDGF-B-chain expression in the remnant kidney model, as the PDGF localizes to the mesangium and its expression can be shown to precede the influx of monocytes (53). This suggests that PDGF may in part act as an autocrine growth factor, and confirms in vitro observations made by Abboud's group (7).

Glomerular Endothelial Cells

Glomerular endothelial cells also synthesize PDGF in vitro (8,11). However, there are no reports to date demonstrating the expression of PDGF by glomerular endothelial cells in vivo.

Visceral Glomerular Epithelial Cells

In passive Heymann nephritis, an experimental model of membranous nephropathy, transient cell proliferation and expression of the PDGF B-chain mRNA and protein by visceral glomerular epithelial cells have been demonstrated (12). Although the proliferation of visceral glomerular epithelial cells correlated with PDGF expression in this model, it is unlikely that the PDGF is mediating the cell proliferation, as these cells do not express PDGF-R (12,43,45).

Parietal Epithelial Cells

As discussed above, PDGF-B-chain mRNA and protein have also been localized to cellular crescents in human glomerular disease (67). Although the source of PDGF is likely to be the macrophage, the possibility that the parietal epithelial cell can produce PDGF has not been excluded. Furthermore, human parietal epithelial cells express the PDGF-R β subunit (45), so it is likely to be responsive to PDGF in either a paracrine or autocrine fashion.

Factors that Stimulate PDGF Expression in Glomerular Diseases

The precise mechanism by which PDGF expression is stimulated in disease has not been identified. However, several factors are known to stimulate PDGF expression in vitro. Many different growth factors and cytokines, such as epidermal growth factor (EGF), basic fibroblast growth factor (bFGF), endothelin, and PDGF itself will upregulate PDGF expression in cultured mesangial cells (7,80). Thrombin is also a potent stimulus for mesangial production of PDGF (81). Shear stress has been shown to stimulate glomerular endothelial cell PDGF mRNA expression in vitro (10). Many of these factors are likely to be involved in glomerular disease. For example, in the anti-Thy 1 model, a variety of cytokines are released from platelets, macrophages, and lysed mesangial cells, including bFGF (82) and PDGF itself, and shear stress may also occur as a consequence of the initial mesangiolysis. Thrombin will be released during the formation of fibrin (83). Endothelin-1 expression is also upregulated during the cell proliferation (84). The reduction of PDGF expression in this model by platelet depletion (43,49), administration of anti-PDGF antibody (85), and administration of heparin (83) also supports a role for some of these factors in mediating the PDGF expression.

INDUCTION OF MESANGIAL CELL PROLIFERATION BY ADMINISTRATION OF PDGF OR OVEREXPRESSION OF PDGF IN VIVO

If PDGF were an important mediator of mesangial cell proliferation in vivo, then one would expect that overexpression of PDGF or administration of PDGF in normal animals should reproduce a proliferative lesion. Indeed, we have recently administered PDGF-B-chain protein intravenously to normal rats and rats that had received subnephritogenic doses of anti-Thy 1 antibody (86). The administration of PDGF to normal rats resulted in a proliferative lesion with active mitoses, an increase in glomerular PCNA expression, and an increase in glomerular cellularity. This was even more marked in rats that had received a subnephritogenic dose of anti-Thy 1 antibody, in which an increase in type IV collagen and laminin mRNA and protein was also documented. It was not clear how the subnephritogenic dose of anti-Thy 1 antibody made the mesangial cells more responsive to PDGF. A mild increase in PDGF-R β-subunit mRNA was noted in these rats, but it was of a magnitude thought to be unlikely to explain the increased mesangial cell proliferation. Alternative possibilities include a postreceptor modulation or perhaps alteration of the mesangial cell-matrix interaction such that greater access of the PDGF to the mesangial cell could result.

Recently, Isaka et al. have reported an exciting study in which the human PDGF-B-chain gene was transfected into the rat kidney (87). The method involved renal artery perfusion of a liposomal preparation in which hemagglutinating virus was incorporated into the liposome to facilitate fusion to cell membranes, and high-mobility group 1 nuclear protein was mixed with the plasmid DNA to facilitate entry into the nucleus. About 35% of glomeruli were transfected; the result was a markedly proliferative lesion with mild matrix expansion (87). Aside from confirming a role for PDGF in mesangial cell proliferation, the introduction of this method represents a major advance and should have great utility in studying the pathogenesis of other cytokines and growth factors. Indeed, these authors also reported in the same paper that transfection of glomeruli with the human TGF-β gene resulted in a lesion characterized principally by matrix expansion (87).

INHIBITION OF PDGF EXPRESSION IN PROLIFERATIVE NEPHRITIS RESULTS IN REDUCED MESANGIAL CELL PROLIFERATION

If PDGF is an important mediator of mesangial cell proliferation, then inhibition of PDGF-BB should reduce mesangial cell proliferation. We have tested this hypothesis using a neutralizing antibody to PDGF in the anti-Thy 1 model. Although the inhibition of PDGF by administration of its antibody did not reduce the initial mesangial cell proliferation at day 2 after the disease induction, a 60% reduction of mesangial cell proliferation, with a lesser inhibition of the mesangial matrix expansion, was observed at day 4 (85). Importantly, no effect of anti-PDGF treatment was seen on the initial mesangiolysis, serum complement levels, circulating platelet counts, or the number of macrophages infiltrating into glomeruli (85).

These results suggested that the initial mesangial cell proliferation is mediated by other factors, of which bFGF appears to be a prime candidate (82). After the initial cell proliferation, a secondary phase occurs that is PDGF-dependent and that would appear to be autocrine-driven. In this phase, upregulation of PDGF-R may increase the responsiveness of the mesangial cell to PDGF. It is possible that this upregulation depends on TGF-β, as TGF-β is upregulated in this model (88), and can increase PDGF-Rβ expression in mesangial cells in vitro [41]. TGF-β also appears to regulate much of the extracellular matrix expansion in this model (89,90).

Finally, it has been reported that trapidil, which is an antiplatelet agent, may also block the binding of PDGF to its receptor (91). Trapidil inhibits mesangial cell proliferation in vitro to either PDGF or to fetal bovine serum (91,92). Administration of trapidil to the anti-Thy 1 model also reduced total glomerular hypercellularity and PCNA expression (92).

CONCLUSION

There is now accumulating evidence that PDGF has a central role in proliferative glomerular disease. The fact that PDGF is also expressed in glomerular development (93) suggests that PDGF expression in diseases may be participating in the cell growth/proliferation and differentiation that occurs with the tissue remodeling and repair of an injured glomerulus. The balance between a healthy physiological response of PDGF and an altered PDGF synthesis leading to excess proliferation and matrix accumulation in disease must be clearly identified. However, glomerular cell proliferation is also intricately linked to an expansion of the mesangial matrix and development of glomerulosclerosis (94,95). The goal of future therapies in glomerular diseases should be to prevent excess mesangial cell proliferation and matrix expansion but to allow normal healing processes, so that glomerular architecture can be restored.

REFERENCES

1. Bowen-Pope DF, Hart CE, Seifert RA. Sera and conditioned media contain different isoforms of platelet-derived growth factor (PDGF) which bind two different classes of PDGF receptors. J Biol Chem 1989; 264:2502–2508.
2. Ross R, Raines EW, Bowen-Pope DF. The biology of platelet-derived growth factor. Cell 1986; 46:155–169.
3. Heldin CH, Westermark B. Platelet-derived growth factor: Mechanism of action and possible in vivo function. Cell Reg 1990; 1:555–566.
4. Ross R. Platelet-derived growth factor. Lancet 1989; 1:1179–1182.
5. Abboud HE, Poptic E, DiCorleto P. Production of platelet-derived growth factorlike protein by rat mesangial cells in culture. J Clin Invest 1987; 80:675–683.
6. Shultz PJ, DiCorleto PE, Silver BJ, Abboud HE. Mesangial cells express PDGF mRNA and proliferate in response to PDGF. Am J Physiol 1988; 255:F674–F684.
7. Silver BJ, Jaffer FE, Abboud HE. Platelet-derived growth factor synthesis in mesangial cells: Induction by multiple peptide mitogens. Proc Natl Acad Sci USA 1989; 86:1056–1060.
8. Daniel TO, Gibbs VC, Milfay DF, et al. Thrombin stimulates c-sis gene expression in microvascular endothelial cells. J Biol Chem 1986; 261:9579–9582.
9. Daniel TO, Gibbs VC, Milfay DF, Williams LT. Agents that increase cAMP accumulation block endothelial c-*sis* induction by thrombin and transforming growth factor-β. J Biol Chem 1987; 262:11893–11896.
10. Ott M, Ballermann BJ. Shear stress augments glomerular endothelial cell (GEN) PDGF mRNA expression and mitogen production (abstr). J Am Soc Nephrol 1992; 3:476.
11. Grandaliano G, Barnes JL, Woodruff K, et al. Thrombin stimulates platelet-derived growth factor (PDGF) production in cultured bovine glomerular endothelial cells (BG-ENDOS) (abstr). J Am Soc Nephrol 1992; 3:468.
12. Floege J, Johnson RJ, Alpers CE, et al. Visceral glomerular epithelial cells can proliferate in vivo and synthesize platelet-derived growth factor B-chain. Am J Pathol 1993; 142:637–650.
13. Hart CE, Forstrom JW, Kelly JD, et al. Bowen-Pope DF: Two classes of PDGF receptor recognize different isoforms of PDGF. Science 1988; 240:1529–1531.
14. Seifert RA, Hart CE, Phillips PE, et al. Two distinct subunits associate to create isoform-specific platelet-derived growth factor receptors. J Biol Chem 1989; 264:8771–8778.
15. Matsui T, Heidaran M, Miki T, et al. Isolation of a novel receptor cDNA establishes the existence of two PDGF receptor genes. Science 1989; 243:800–804.
16. Seifert RA, van Koppen A, Bowen-Pope DF. PDGF-AB requires PDGF receptor α-subunits for high-affinity, but not for low-affinity, binding and signal transduction. J Biol Chem 1993; 268:4473–4480.
17. Mene P, Abboud HE, Dubyak GR, et al. Effect of PDGF on inositol phosphates, Ca^{2+}, and contraction of mesangial cells. Am J Physiol 1987; 253:F458–F463.
18. Bonventre JV, Weber PC, Gronich JH. PAF and PDGF increase cytosolic [Ca^{2+}] and phospholipase activity in mesangial cells. Am J Physiol 1988; 254:F87–F94.
19. Floege J, Topley N, Hoppe J, et al. Mitogenic effect of platelet-derived growth factor in human glomerular

mesangial cells: Modulation and/or suppression by inflammatory cytokines. Clin Exp Immunol 1991; 86:334–341.
20. Barnes JL, Hevey KA. Glomerular mesangial cell migration in response to platelet-derived growth factor. Lab Invest 1990; 62:379–382.
21. Grotendorst GR, Chang T, Seppa HEJ, et al. Platelet-derived growth factor is a chemoattractant for vascular smooth muscle cells. J Cell Physiol 1982; 113:261–266.
22. Berk BC, Alexander RW, Brock TA, et al. Vasoconstriction: A new activity for platelet-derived growth factor. Science 1986; 232:87–90.
23. Lovett DH, Larsen A. Cell cycle-dependent interleukin 1 gene expression by cultured glomerular mesangial cells. J Clin Invest 1988; 82:115–122.
24. Abboud HE, Woodruff KA, Snyder SP, Bonewald LF. Polypeptide growth factors regulate the production of latent transforming growth factor β-1 in human mesangial cells (abstr). J Am Soc Nephrol 1991; 2:434.
25. Border WA, Okuda S, Languino LR, Ruoslahti E. Transforming growth factor-β regulates production of proteoglycans by mesangial cell. Kidney Int 1990; 37:689–695.
26. Doi T, Vlassara H, Kirstein M, et al. Receptor-specific increase in extracellular matrix production in mouse mesangial cells by advanced glycosylation end products is mediated via platelet-derived growth factor. Proc Natl Acad Sci USA 1992; 89:2873–2877.
27. Floege J, Topley N, Wessel K, et al. Monokines and platelet-derived growth factor modulate prostanoid production in growth arrested, human mesangial cells. Kidney Int 1990; 37:859–869.
28. Deuel TF, Senior RM, Huang JS, Griffin GL. Chemotaxis of monocytes and neutrophils to platelet-derived growth factor. J Clin Invest 1982; 69:1046–1049.
29. Tzeng DY, Deuel TF, Huang JS, et al. Platelet-derived growth factor promotes polymorphonuclear leukocyte activation. Blood 1984; 64:1123–1128.
30. Pierce GF, Mustoe TA, Lingelbach J, et al. Platelet-derived growth factor and transforming growth factor-beta enhance tissue repair activities by unique mechanisms. J Cell Biol 1989; 109:429–440.
31. Koch R. Die Aetiologie der Tuberkulose. Berl Klin Woschr 1882; 19:221.
32. Abboud HE. Growth factors in glomerulonephritis. Kidney Int 1993; 43:252–267.
33. Johnson RJ, Floege J, Couser WG, Alpers CE. Role of platelet-derived growth factor in glomerular disease. J Am Soc Nephrol 1993; 4:119–128.
34. Jaffer F, Saunders C, Shultz P, et al. Regulation of mesangial cell growth by polypeptide mitogens. Am J Pathol 1989; 235:261–269.
35. Lovett DH, Ryan JL, Sterzel RB. Stimulation of rat mesangial cell proliferation by macrophage interleukin 1. J Immunol 1983; 131:2830–2836.
36. Horii Y, Muraguchi A, Iwano M, et al. Involvement of IL-6 in mesangial proliferative glomerulonephritis. J Immunol 1989; 143:3949–3955.
37. Doi T, Striker LJ, Elliot SJ, et al. Insulinlike growth factor-1 is a progression factor for human mesangial cells. Am J Pathol 1989; 134:395–404.
38. Raines EW, Dower SK, Ross R: Interleukin-1 mitogenic activity for fibroblasts and smooth muscle cells is due to PDGF-AA. Science 1989; 393–396.
39. Abboud HE: Platelet-derived growth factor and mesangial cell. Kidney Int 1992; 41:581–583.
40. Marx M, Daniel TO, Kashgarian M, Madri JA. Spatial organization of the extracellular matrix modulates the expression of PDGF-receptor subunits in mesangial cells. Kidney Int 1993; 43:1027–1041.
41. Haberstroh U, Zahner G, Disser M, et al. TGF-beta stimulates rat mesangial cell proliferation in culture: Role of PDGF beta-receptor expression. Am J Physiol 1993; 264:F199–205.
42. Gronwald RGK, Seifert RA, Bowen-Pope DF. Differential regulation of expression of two platelet-derived growth factor receptor subunits by transforming growth factor-β. J Biol Chem 1989; 264:8120–8125.
43. Iida H, Seifert R, Alpers CE, et al. Platelet-derived growth factor (PDGF) and PDGF receptor are induced in mesangial proliferative nephritis in the rat. Proc Natl Acad Sci USA 1991; 88:6560–6564.
44. Fjellström B, Klareskog L, Heldin CH, et al. Platelet-derived growth factor receptors in the kidney-upregulated expression in inflammation. Kidney Int 1989; 36:1099–1102.
45. Alpers CE, Seifert RA, Hudkins KL, et al. PDGF-receptor localizes to mesangial, parietal epithelial, and interstitial cells in human and primate kidneys. Kidney Int 1993; 43:286–294.
46. Gesualdo L, Milani S, Di Paolo S, et al. Platelet derived growth factor (PDGF) receptor expression in normal and glomerulonephritic human kidney: An immunohistochemistry (IMH) and in situ hybridization (ISH) study. J Am Soc Nephrol 1993; 4:678.
47. Frampton G, Hildreth G, Hartley B, et al. Could platelet-derived growth factor have a role in the pathogenesis of lupus nephritis? Lancet 1988; 2:343.
48. Gesualdo L, Pinzani M, Floriano JJ, et al. Platelet-derived growth factor expression in mesangial proliferative glomerulonephritis. Lab Invest 1991; 65:160–167.
49. Yoshimura A, Gordon K, Alpers CE, et al. Demonstration of PDGF B-chain mRNA in glomeruli in mesangial proliferative nephritis by in situ hybridization. Kidney Int 1991; 40:470–476.

50. Yamamoto T, Wilson CB. Complement dependence of antibody-induced mesangial cell injury in the rat. J Immunol 1987; 138:3758–3765.
51. Johnson RJ, Pritzl P, Iida H, Alpers CE. Platelet-complement interactions in mesangial proliferative nephritis in the rat. Am J Pathol 1990; 138:313–321.
52. Johnson RJ, Iida H, Alpers CE, et al. Expression of smooth muscle cell phenotype by rat mesangial cells in immune complex nephritis. J Clin Invest 1991; 87:847–858.
53. Floege J, Burns MW, Alpers CE, et al. Glomerular cell proliferation and PDGF expression precedes glomerular sclerosis in the remnant kidney model. Kidney Int 1992; 41:297–309.
54. Floege J, Alpers CE, Burns MW, et al. Glomerular cells, extracellular matrix accumulation, and the development of glomerulosclerosis in the remnant kidney model. Lab Invest 1992; 66:485–497.
55. Nakamura T, Ebihara I, Nagaoka I, et al. Renal platelet-derived growth factor gene expression in NZB/W F1 mice with lupus and ddY mice with IgA nephropathy. Clin Immunol Immunopathol 1992; 63:173–181.
56. Fukui M, Nakamura T, Ebihara I, et al. Low-protein diet attenuates increased gene expression of platelet-derived growth factor and transforming growth factor-β in experimental glomerular sclerosis. J Lab Clin Med 1993; 121:224–234.
57. Feng L, Tang WW, Xia Y, Wilson CB. Growth factor (GF), extracellular matrix (ECM) and protease inhibitor (PI) mRNA expression in anti-GBM antibody (Ab) associated glomerulonephritis (GN) (abstr). J Am Soc Nephrol 1992; 3:468.
58. Nishimura M, Okamura M, Konishi Y, et al. Platelet-derived growth factor gene expression in the kidney of DOCA-salt spontaneously hypertensive rats (abstr). J Am Soc Nephrol 1992; 3:475.
59. Akai Y, Iwano M, Dohi Y, et al. Quantitative analysis for intraglomerular expression of platelet-derived growth factor (PDGF) mRNA in mice with BSA nephritis (abstr). J Am Soc Nephrol 1992; 3:572.
60. Barnes JL, Abboud HE. Temporal expression of autocrine growth factors corresponds to morphologic features of mesangial proliferation in habu snake venom (HSV) induced glomerulonephritis (abstr). J Am Soc Nephrol 1992; 3:574.
61. Young B, Johnson R, Alpers C, et al. Mesangial cell (MC) proliferation precedes development of glomerulosclerosis (GS) in experimental diabetic nephropathy (DN) (abstr). J Am Soc Nephrol 1992; 3:770.
62. Nakamura T, Fukui M, Ebihara I, et al. mRNA expression of growth factors in glomeruli from diabetic rats. Diabetes 1993; 42:450–456.
63. Nakajima M, Newitson TD, Mathews DC, Kincaid-Smith P. Platelet-derived growth factor mesangial deposits in mesangial IgA glomerulonephritis. Nephrol Dial Transp 1991; 6:11–16.
64. Schena FP, Ranieri E, Montinaro V, et al. Quantification of cytokine mRNA expression in human renal biopsies by reverse transcriptase-polymerase chain reaction (RT-PCR) (abstr). J Am Soc Nephrol 1992; 3:664.
65. Waldherr R, Noronha IL, Brecht H, et al. In situ expression of cytokines and cytokine receptors in ANCA-positive vasculitis (abstr). J Am Soc Nephrol 1992; 3:667.
66. Nabeshima K, Yoshimura A, Inui K, et al. Relationship of PDGF B-chain mRNA expression identified by in situ hybridization (ISH) and disease severity in various human glomerular diseases (abstr). J Am Soc Nephrol 1993; 4:777.
67. Yoshimura A, Inui K, Suzuki T, et al. Demonstration of PDGF B-chain mRNA expression in the cellular crescent in human glomerular diseases (abstr). J Am Soc Nephrol 1993; 4:692.
68. Alpers CE, Hudkins KL, Gown AM, Johnson RJ. Enhanced expression of "muscle-specific" actin in glomerulonephritis. Kidney Int 1992; 41:1134–1142.
69. Schwarting R. Little missed markers and Ki-67. Lab Invest 1993; 68:597–599.
70. Johnson RJ, Guggenheim SJ, Klebanoff SJ, et al. Morphologic correlates of glomerular oxidant injury induced by the myeloperoxidase-hydrogen peroxide-halide system of the neutrophil. Lab Invest 1988; 58:294–301.
71. Johnson RJ, Alpers CE, Pruchno C, et al. Mechanisms and kinetics for platelet and neutrophil localization in immune complex nephritis. Kidney Int 1989; 36:780–789.
72. Duffus P, Parbtani A, Frampton G, Cameron JS. Intraglomerular localization of platelet related antigens, platelet factor 4 and β-thromboglobulin in glomerulonephritis. Clin Nephrol 1982; 17:288–297.
73. Miller K, Dresner IG, Michael AF. Localization of platelet antigens in human kidney disease. Kidney Int 1980; 18:472–479.
74. Mezzano S, Burgos ME, Ardiles L, et al. Glomerular localization of platelet factor 4 in streptococcal nephritis. Nephron 1992; 61:58–63.
75. Johnson RJ. Platelets in inflammatory glomerular injury. Semin Nephrol 1991; 11:276–284.
76. Johnson RJ, Garcia RL, Pritzl P, Alpers CE. Platelets mediate glomerular cell proliferation in immune complex nephritis induced by anti-mesangial cell antibodies in the rat. Am J Pathol 1990; 136:369–374.
77. Cattell V. Focal mesangial proliferative glomerulonephritis in the rat caused by habu snake venom: The role of platelets. Br J Exp Pathol 1979; 60:201–208.
78. Ross R, Masuda J, Raines EW, et al. Localization of PDGF-B protein in macrophages in all phases of atherogenesis. Science 1990; 248:1009–1012.

79. Nakamura T, Ebihara I, Nagaoka I, et al. Activated peripheral blood mononuclear cells in IgA nephropathy express platelet-derived growth factor B-chain messenger RNA. J Lab Clin Med 1992; 120:212–221.
80. Jaffer FE, Knauss TC, Poptic E, Abboud HE. Endothelin stimulates PDGF secretion in cultured human mesangial cells. Kidney Int 1990; 38:1193–1198.
81. Shultz PJ, Knauss TC, Mene P, Abboud HE. Mitogenic signals for thrombin in mesangial cells: Regulation of phospholipase C and PDGF genes. Am J Physiol 1989; 257:F366–F374.
82. Floege J, Eng E, Linder V, et al. Rat glomerular mesangial cells synthesize basic fibroblast growth factor: Release, upregulated synthesis, and mitogenicity in mesangial proliferative glomerulonephritis. J Clin Invest 1992; 90:2362–2369.
83. Floege J, Eng E, Young BA, et al. Heparin suppresses mesangial cell proliferation and matrix expansion in experimental mesangioproliferative glomerulonephritis. Kidney Int 1993; 43:369–380.
84. Yoshimura A, Inui K, Iwasaki S, et al. Upregulated expression of endothelin-1 (ET-1) protein, ET-1 mRNA and endothelin B type receptor (ET_BR) are introduced in mesangial proliferative nephritis in the rat (abstr). J Am Soc Nephrol 1992; 3:624.
85. Johnson RJ, Raines EW, Floege J, et al. Inhibition of mesangial cell proliferation and matrix expansion in glomerulonephritis in the rat by antibody to platelet-derived growth factor. J Exp Med 1992; 175:1413–1416.
86. Floege J, Eng E, Young BA, et al. Infusion of platelet-derived growth factor or basic fibroblast growth factor induces selective glomerular mesangial cell proliferation and matrix accumulation in rats. J Clin Invest 1993; 92:2952–2962.
87. Isaka Y, Fujiwara Y, Ueda N, et al. Glomerulosclerosis induced by in vivo transfection of TGF-β or PDGF gene into the rat kidney. J Clin Invest 1993; 92:2697–2701.
88. Okuda S, Langiuno LR, Ruoslahti E, Border WA. Elevated expression of transforming growth factor-β and proteoglycan production in experimental glomerulonephritis. J Clin Invest 1990; 86:453–462.
89. Border WA, Okuda S, Languino LR, et al. Suppression of experimental glomerulonephritis by antisera against transforming growth factor β1. Nature 1990; 346:371–374.
90. Border WA, Noble NA, Yamamoto T, et al. Natural inhibitor of transforming growth factor-β protects against scarring in experimental kidney disease. Nature 1992; 360:361–364.
91. Gesualdo L, Di Paolo S, Di Cillo M, et al. Trapidil A PDGF-receptor antagonist, inhibits human mesangial cell (HMC) proliferation (abstr). J Am Soc Nephrol 1992; 3:453.
92. Futamura A, Iida H, Izumino K, et al. Effect of the platelet-derived growth factor (PDGF) antagonist trapidil on rat mesangial cell proliferation (abstr). J Am Soc Nephrol 1992; 3:588.
93. Alpers CE, Seifert RA, Hudkins KL, et al. Developmental pattern of PDGF B-chain, PDGF-receptor, and α-actin expression in human glomerulogenesis. Kidney Int 1992; 42:390–399.
94. Striker LJ, Doi T, Elliot S, Striker GE. The contribution of glomerular mesangial cells to progressive glomerulosclerosis. Semin Nephrol 1989; 9:318–328.
95. Eng E, Floege J, Young BA, et al. Does extracellular matrix expansion in glomerular disease require mesangial cell proliferation? Kidney Int 1994; 45:545–548.

60

The Molecular Biology of Congenital Nephrogenic Diabetes Insipidus

Eliezer J. Holtzman, Lee F. Kolakowski, Jr., and Dennis A. Ausiello
Massachusetts General Hospital and Harvard Medical School, Charlestown, Massachusetts

INTRODUCTION

The conservation or excretion of water by the human kidney is the function of the renal tubules, which are arranged in a complex architecture with blood vessels and contain selective cells responsive to the neurohypohyseal antidiuretic hormone arginine vasopressin (AVP). The major action of AVP is to facilitate urinary concentration (1,2).

The urinary concentrating mechanism requires sequential and interactive activity among the renal tubules. The reabsorbtion of NaCl but not water from both the thin and thick ascending limbs of Henle initiate countercurrent multiplication within the renal medulla. This process builds an osmotic gradient in the medullary interstitium that extends from the cortex to the papilla. Plasma AVP increases the water permeability of the renal collecting ducts, allowing for water to be transported passively down an osmotic gradient between the tubular fluid and the surrounding interstitium.

AVP is the major hormone involved in the regulation of water balance in mammals. Its mechanism of action has been studied in the key target epithelium, the renal collecting duct. In general, AVP-sensitive epithelia are remarkably impermeable to water in the resting state, in contrast to the usual high permeability of luminal membranes of epithelial cells in general. When stimulated by AVP, the permeability of the renal collecting duct increases to a level comparable to that of most other biological membranes (2). AVP induces this transformation in water permeability in its target cells by first binding to its V_2 receptor on the basolateral surface of the epithelial cell, stimulating adenylyl cyclase and increasing the cytoplasmic concentration of the second messenger, cyclic AMP (cAMP) (2). The increase in cAMP levels activates cAMP-dependent protein kinase (PKA) (Figure 1). While the substrates for PKA are obscure, the resulting morphological and functional events have been defined in the kidney collecting duct. It has been shown that, within minutes after stimulation by AVP, aggregates of small intramembranous particles that most probably contain water channels appear in the luminal membrane of the collecting duct of the mammalian kidney as a result of the insertion of intracellular vesicles containing water channels (3–5). When vasopressin is removed, functional water channels are retrieved from the apical membrane by an endocytic process involving clathrin-coated pits and are returned to an intracellular compartment, from which they may return to the apical membrane upon rechallenge with vasopressin (3,6,7).

Nephrogenic diabetes insipidus (NDI) is defined as the inability to maximally concentrate urine in the presence of adequate plasma concentration of AVP in conditions when the renal concentrating mechanism has been maximally stimulated. NDI can be divided to two categories: congenital and acquired (8). NDI may result from either a failure to create or maintain the renal corticopapillary interstitial osmotic gradient or the failure of AVP to increase water permeability in the presence of an adequate osmotic gradient (Table 1).

In this chapter we review the molecular basis for congenital disorders resulting from

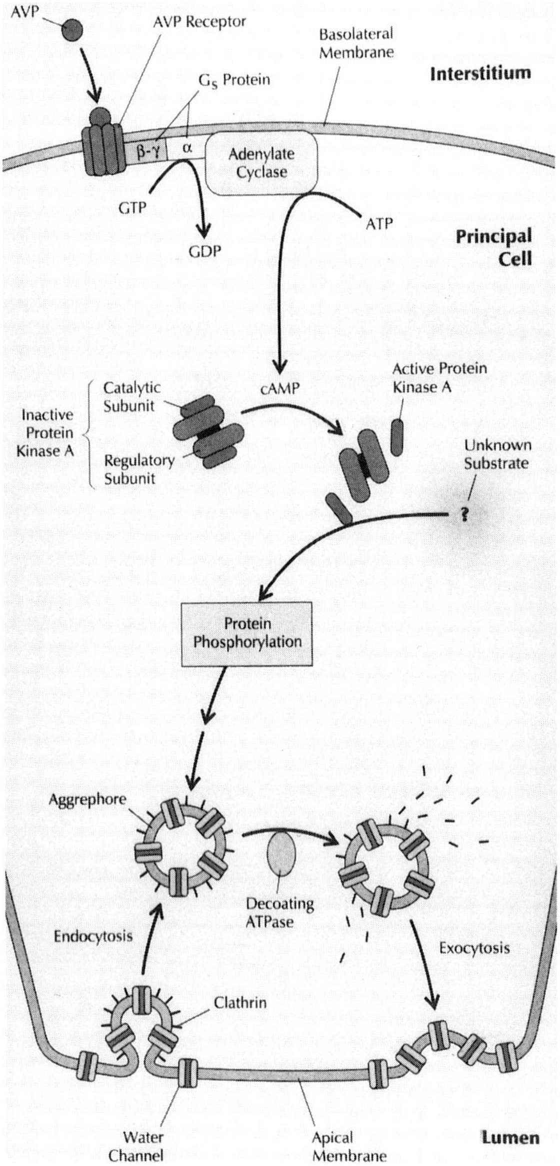

Figure 1 AVP-dependent signal transduction in collecting duct principal cell. AVP induces water permeability in principal cells of the renal collecting duct by binding to the AVP2R receptor and imitating a second messenger cascade. AVP binds to the receptors on the basolateral membrane. AVP regulated water channels (Aquaporin-2) are shuttled to the apical membrane after stimulation. (From Ref. 1.)

abnormalities in the AVP signaling pathways that occur in the presence of an adequate osmotic gradient. The molecular basis and mechanisms of two genetically distinct types of congenital diabetes insipidus (CNDI) are described:

1. Type I CNDI, the more frequent X-linked form, is caused by mutations in the V2-vasopressin receptor (AVPR2). These patients have been shown to have no enhancement of urine cAMP levels in response to the administration of AVP (9).

Table 1 Etiology of Nephrogenic Diabetes Insipidus According to Probable Mechanisms

I. Compromised ADH-induced cAMP rise or effect
  A. Congenital nephrogenic diabetes insipidus
  B. Elecrolyte abnormalities
    Hypercalcemia
    Hypokalemia
  C. Drugs
    Lithium
    Demeclocycline

II. Failure to create and/or maintain cortical-papillary osmotic gradient
  A. Renal medullary pathology
    Infiltration (amyloid, light chain nephropathy)
    Infections (pyelonephritis)
    Drug-induced
    Hypoxic damage (sickle cell anemia)
    Obstructive uropathy
    Polycystic kidney disease
  B. Compromised medullary hypertonicity
    Loop diuretics
    Osmotic diuresis: glucose, mannitol, urea
  C. Electrolyte abnormalities
    Hypokalemia
    Hypercalcemia

2. Type II CNDI is an autosomal recessive disease due to mutations in the collecting duct AVP-regulated water channel (aquaporin 2) and as yet undefined additional genes. Patients with this disorder have been reported to have increased urinary cAMP excretion in response to AVP administration (10). A single pedigree has been described as having an autosomal dominant form of CNDI and is also a member of this category.

THE MOLECULAR BIOLOGY OF X-LINKED CONGENITAL NEPHROGENIC DIABETES INSIPIDUS (TYPE I)

Clinical Background

X-linked CNDI is a rare hereditary disorder in which the production of AVP is normal but the AVP-responsive cells in the collecting duct of the kidney lack the expected response to the hormone and therefore are unable to reabsorb water in response to AVP stimulation. CNDI was first described 102 years ago by McIlraith (11). Recently, Brownstein and Lolait have reinterpreted McIlraith's findings in light of the current understanding of the molecular basis of the disease (12).

In the 1940s the clinical presentation of a number of families whose members presented with polyuria, polydipsia and the inability to form a concentrated urine due to end-organ resistance to AVP were detailed (13–15). These patients excreted large volumes of urine that was consistently hypotonic when compared to plasma, even under conditions where the plasma osmolarity and plasma AVP concentrations were increased significantly. Generally, half the males in affected families are symptomatic and usually do not give an antidiuretic response to the administration of either AVP or the strong antidiuretic V2 agonist 1-desamino (8-D-arginine) vasopressin (dDAVP), consistent with an abnormal renal V2 receptor response. Affected males become symptomatic early in infancy. There are varying degrees of genetic penetrance in female carriers, who are presumably heterozygous and show clinical manifestations ranging from no symptoms to marked polyuria. If unrecognized, CNDI can result in repeated episodes of severe hypertonic dehydration, causing growth and mental retardation and early death (Table 2). Laboratory evaluation of patients usually reveals extremely high levels of serum sodium and chloride, prerenal azotemia, metabolic acidosis, and dilute urine, despite very high serum sodium. Nocturia, enuresis, megaureter, and hydronephrosis are frequent in late childhood. The mental and physical development of patients who receive sufficient water at birth are found to be the same as their healthy counterparts, stressing the importance of early genetic based prenatal diagnosis (16).

Extrarenal Manifestations

The therapeutic use of the AVP analogue dDAVP led to the conclusion that vasopressin V2-like receptors exist outside of the collecting duct. The extrarenal actions of dDAVP include the release of coagulation factors, VIIIc and Von Willebrand factor, and hemodynamic changes such as a decrease in blood pressure and peripheral resistance with a concomitant increase in plasma renin activity. All of these effects are impaired in CNDI patients (17–20). These data support the existence of extrarenal vasopressin V2 receptors that appear to share the defect in patients with CNDI. Molecular biology studies however, have not yet confirmed the presence of AVPR2 in extrarenal tissues.

Prevalence and Historical Interest in CNDI

CNDI is an rare disease for which statistical frequencies have not been reported. The disease has been the focus of historical interest because of its prevalence among the descendants of the clan

Table 2 Clinical Manifestations of CNDI

History
Onset—in the first few months of life, sometimes noticed shortly after birth
Unexplained fevers—sometimes prompting misdirected workup
Vomiting—particularly over the first 3 months
Constipation—persistent; stools described as small, hard like pebbles
Irritability—whining and crying nearly constant, but improves when patient is given water
Polydipsa—many diapers soaked daily—literally dripping; nocturia frequent in older children
Growth failure—falling off of growth chart percentiles
Development delay
Physical Examination
Signs of dehydration—poor skin turgor, possibly doughiness to skin, mottled color, sunken anterior fontanel, tongue dry or parched, decreased tears, sunken eyes, weak pulses, hypotensive
Multiple abdominal massess—small mobile fecaliths
May soak several diapers with dilute urine during office visit
Marked irritability even in mother's arms
Often febrile or feels warm without obvious source of infection
Laboratory Evaluation
Hypernatremia, hyperchloremia, hyperosmolality
Usually mild metabolic acidosis—may be severe if dehydrated enough
Normokalemic
Hyperuricemic
Azotemic (prerenal—corrects when rehydrated)
Urine maximally dilute; no response to AVP

Source: From Ref. 95.

known as the Ulster Scots, who settled in Nova Scotia during the eighteenth century. In 1969, Bode and Crawford provided an analysis of published data and five new pedigrees with CNDI (21). They were able to link all the CNDI pedigrees to a common group of Ulster Scot immigrants who arrived in Halifax in 1761 aboard the ship *Hopewell*. A link between this family and a large Utah kindred (Cannon) was also suggested. They proposed the "Hopewell hypothesis," suggesting that most of North American patients suffering from this disorder are descendants of a common ancestor with a single genetic defect. Recent molecular data, discussed below, demonstrate that this conclusion is incorrect. Past reports of the occurrence of the disease in French Canadian (19,22), African American (23), Samoan (24), and Australian aboriginal (25) families also suggest a more heterogeneous distribution of the disease.

Mode of Inheritance and Gene-Linkage Analyses

The clinical occurrence of the disease, which is normally found in males, and the description of a subclinical as well as a rarer clinical form in carrier females, has suggested an X-linked recessive trait with variable penetrance in the female due to nonrandom X-chromosome inactivation.

Pedigrees of four New England families are shown in Figure 2. Family A is a large pedigree of Ulster Scot descent and family B is a member of the large Ulster Scot Hopewell kindred. Families C and D are of Spanish and European ancestry, respectively.

Linkage studies have demonstrated that the gene responsible for CNDI is located in the subtelomeric region of the long arm of the X chromosome in the region 28 (Xq28), close to DXS52 anonymous polymorphic DNA marker. Since the cDNA for the *AVPR2* gene has been cloned, several groups have utilized more detailed DNA mapping studies to determine the precise location of the *AVPR2* gene in the Xq28 region (26–28). The position of the *AVPR2* gene in the context of these markers is shown in Figure 3.

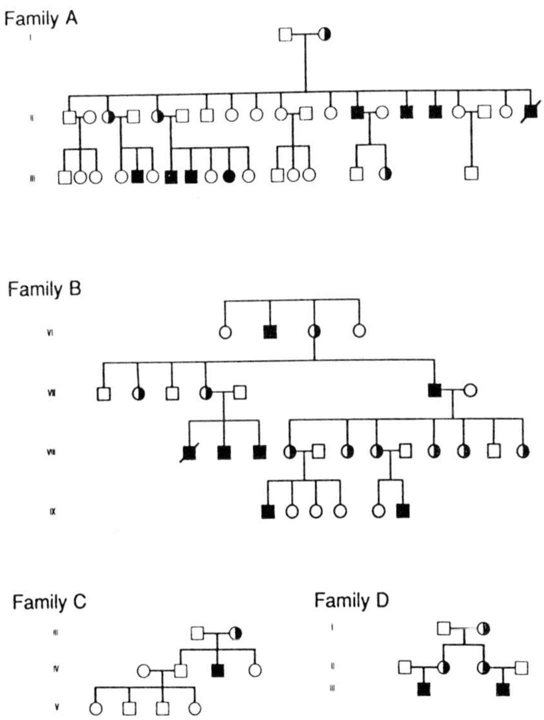

Figure 2 Pedigrees of four New England families with X-linked CNDI. Family A is a large pedigree of Ulster Scot descent and family B is a member of the large Ulster Scot *Hopewell* kindred. Families C and D are of Spanish and European ancestry, respectively. The phenotype of affected males ■, females ●, and obligate heterozygotes ◑ is indicated. (From Refs. 44, 48, and 49.)

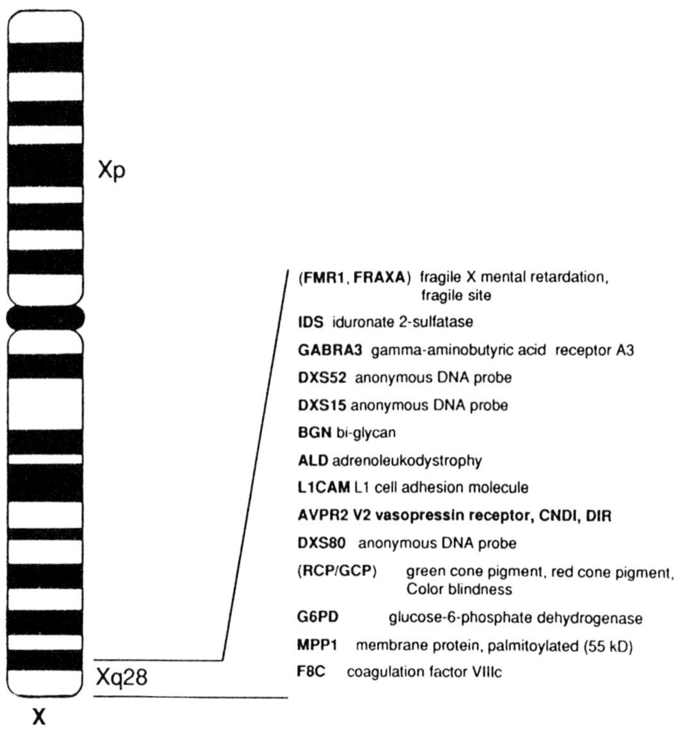

Figure 3 Chromosomal localization of CNDI and *AVPR2*. The gene for AVPR2 was found at the same locus on the long arm of the X-chromosome occupied by the gene for CNDI, suggesting that mutations of the *AVPR2* are responsible for the disease. Mapping positions of each of the listed markers is derived from the Fourth International Workshop in Chromosome X. (From Ref. 105.)

Markers in the region of Xq28 have been useful for testing hypotheses about the genetic origins of CNDI and assessing the historical accuracy of pedigrees. Bichet and colleagues have tested the Hopewell hypothesis by their analysis of a four-locus haplotype of RFLPs and St14 VNTR in the Xq28 region and have shown a different CNDI haplotype in several North American CNDI families, suggesting that no apparent familial relationship exists (29). These markers have been found to be useful for pedigree analysis and carrier detection in CNDI families (30).

AVPR2 Gene Expression

The physiological action of AVP in the human nephron requires binding of the nonapeptide hormone to the renal-type vasopressin receptor (AVPR2) on the basolateral membrane of collecting duct principal cells. This results in the activation of adenylyl cyclase and the generation of cAMP. Recently, a cDNA clone for the human AVPR2 has been described, and its mRNA has been found by Northern blot analyses and in situ hybridization to be expressed only in the kidney, specifically in the inner and outer renal medulla (31).

AVPR2 Structure and Homology

AVPR2 is a member of the family of seven transmembrane-spanning domain receptors which couple to heterotrimeric guanine nucleotide-regulatory (G) proteins (32,33). Despite the extraordinary diversity of ligands and signaling, all of the G protein–coupled receptors related to rhodopsin and the $\beta 2$-adrenergic receptor share a highly conserved structure, topology, and sequence similarity (34). Unlike many receptors in this gene family, the AVPR2 receptor gene is interrupted by two introns within the coding region (28) (Figure 4).

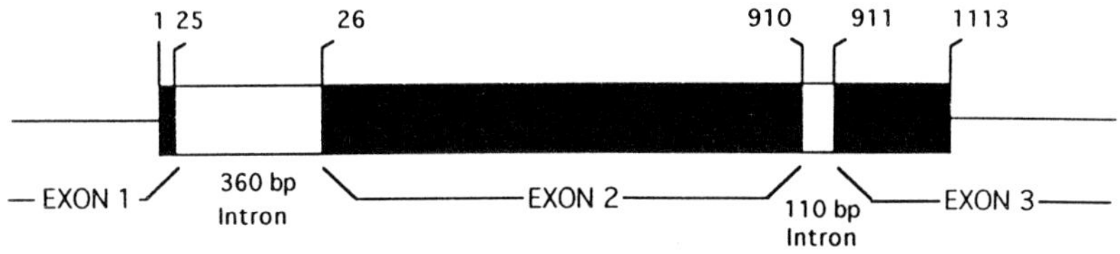

Figure 4 Intron/exon structure of the AVP2R gene. The coding region of the *AVP2R* gene is interrupted by two small introns. The first exon encodes only the amino-terminal nine amino acids of the receptor. The second exon encodes most of the receptor through transmembrane segment six. The final exon encodes transmembrane segment seven and the carboxyl-terminal tail. There is no evidence of additional 5′ or 3′ untranslated exons. (From Ref. 28.)

The AVPR2 protein is ~45% identical in sequence to the vasopressin V1a receptor (AVP1R) and the oxytocin receptor (OXTR). These receptors bind the related ligands AVP and oxytocin. The next most closely related G protein–coupled receptors to these are the vasotocin receptors and gonadotropin-hormone releasing hormone receptor (GnRHR). The amino acid sequences of each of the human receptors are shown in Figure 5 (32,35–37). To date, the homologue of the AVPR2 receptor has been cloned from human, rat and pig (32,33,38). These three receptor sequences are more than 90% identical (Figure 6).

Figure 7 depicts a topological model of the human AVPR2 receptor based on analyses of its hydrophobicity and by analogy with rhodopsin (39). AVPR2 shares all the characteristics of the G protein–coupled receptor family: (a) seven predicted transmembrane segments, each of which contain about twenty hydrophobic amino acids; (b) sequence similarity between members of the family in the transmembrane segments; (c) sequence divergence in the connecting hydrophilic loops (extracellular and intracellular); (d) extracellular N terminus with consensus sites for N-linked glycosylation; (e) a cytoplasmic carboxyl tail and large intracellular loop, which may contain several sites for phosphorylation by various kinases (serine and threonine) known to be involved in receptor desensitization or sequestration; (f) conserved site(s) for fatty acylation with palmitate, which may serve as a membrane anchor (situated at cysteines in the carboxyl-terminal tail); and (g) two highly conserved cysteine residues in the second and third extracellular loops, which are thought to form a disulfide bridge that stabilizes folding of the molecule and the binding pocket. The seven transmembrane segments are probably configured as amphipathic alpha helices with charged residues facing inward forming an AVP binding site. Recently, a photoaffinity labeling study of the bovine AVPR2 receptor has identified a portion of the second transmembrane segment and the first extracellular loop as being involved in AVP binding (40).

The intracellular portions of the transmembrane segments and the intracellular loops have been shown to interact selectively with the specific G proteins determining the signal transduction pathway and the ultimate biological response. Signal transduction by receptors in this family requires a ligand-receptor complex capable of binding to and activating the exchange of bound-nucleotide by the transducing G protein (Gs in the case of activation of adenylyl cyclase) in order to generate the physiological response.

Mutational Analysis—*AVPR2*

While several groups had suspected a tight link between CNDI and the AVPR2 gene, the finding by Lolait and colleagues that the human AVPR2 cDNA mapped to the Xq28 region prompted several groups to investigate the molecular basis of CNDI (33). Since the initial confirmation of this hypothesis (41), the search for AVPR2 mutations in CNDI families has resulted in a flurry of reports of different mutations (Figures 8 and 9; Tables 3, 4, and 5). Of the 53 different mutations described to date, half (27) are amino acid substitutions (missense mutations), seven of which involve an amino acid transition to cysteine. Of the remaining half, eight are substitutions of an amino acid to a termination codon (nonsense mutations), causing premature termination of translation; fourteen are deletions of codons in the open reading frame, causing a frame shift to nonreceptor codons followed by premature termination; and four families have insertions that cause the same physiological

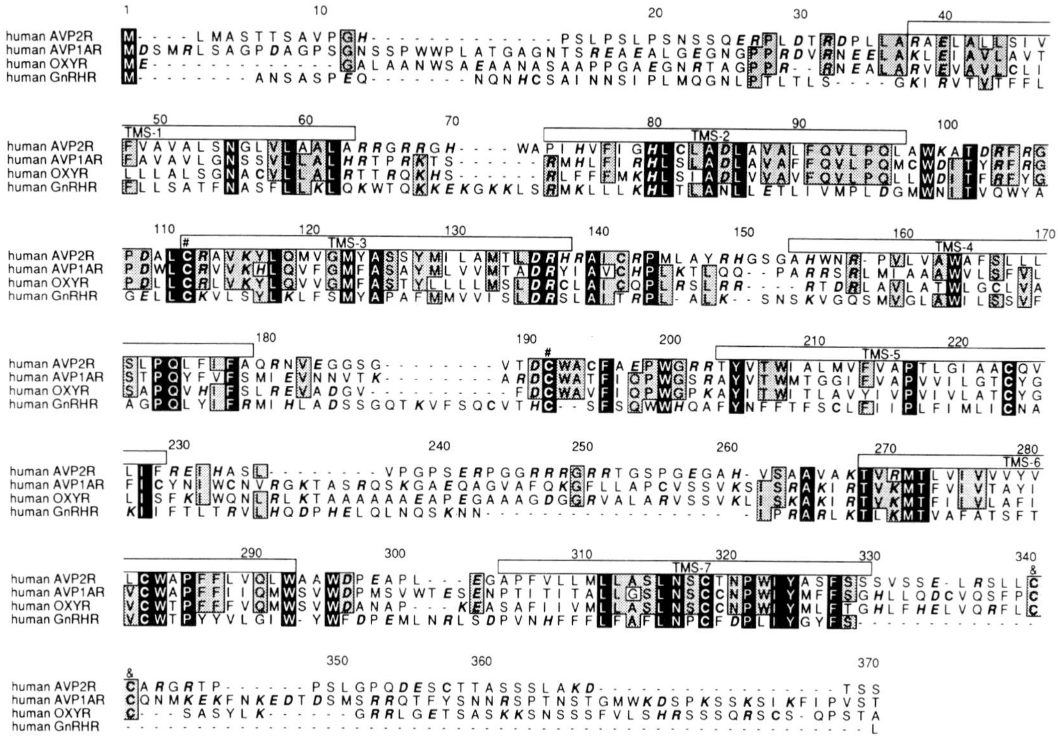

Figure 5 Sequence comparison of human receptors related to AVP2R. The sequences of the three human G protein–coupled receptors most closely related to AVP2R were aligned with the human AVP2R protein sequence. The amino acid positions which are identical in all four sequences are shown as white letters on a black background. Amino acids which are identical in three of four sequences are shaded with gray. The sequences shown are AVP2R: human V2 vasopressin receptor, AVP1R: human V1a vasopressin receptor (35), OXYR: human oxytocin receptor (36), and the GnRHR: gonadotropin releasing hormone receptor (37).

consequences (see Frame Shift Mutations, below). At least four apparently X-linked CNDI pedigrees have been characterized and no mutations were found in the coding region of the AVPR2 gene (42,43), suggesting that CNDI in these families results from a defect in regulatory areas, introns, or untranslated regions of the AVPR2 gene. Alternatively, some other gene product important to the physiological pathway for AVP action may also be located on the X-chromosome. We have tabulated all the known mutations in CNDI and discuss the functional characteristics of each mutation by their mutation class.

Missense Mutations

As shown in Table 3, missense mutations have been found in all transmembrane segments (TM) except TM7. Mutations were also reported in the first and second extracellular loops (EXL) as well as the second intracellular loop (INL) (see Figure 8).

Naturally occurring missense mutations are a very important tool for studying structure function-relationships of molecules in general and especially receptors. The Arg113 → Trp mutation is perhaps a hot-spot for mutations, as we and others have shown that five families with this mutation are likely of independent origin in Europe and North America (44). Two different St14 VNTRs were found in families with this mutation. Family A (Figure 2) and a Canadian family (29,45) have 1690- and 700-bp alleles, suggesting an independent origin for these mutations (unpublished observation). These observations have been extended by Bichet and colleagues (46). In family A, the affected individuals analyzed demonstrated a C → T transition at codon 113 of the AVPR2 gene which

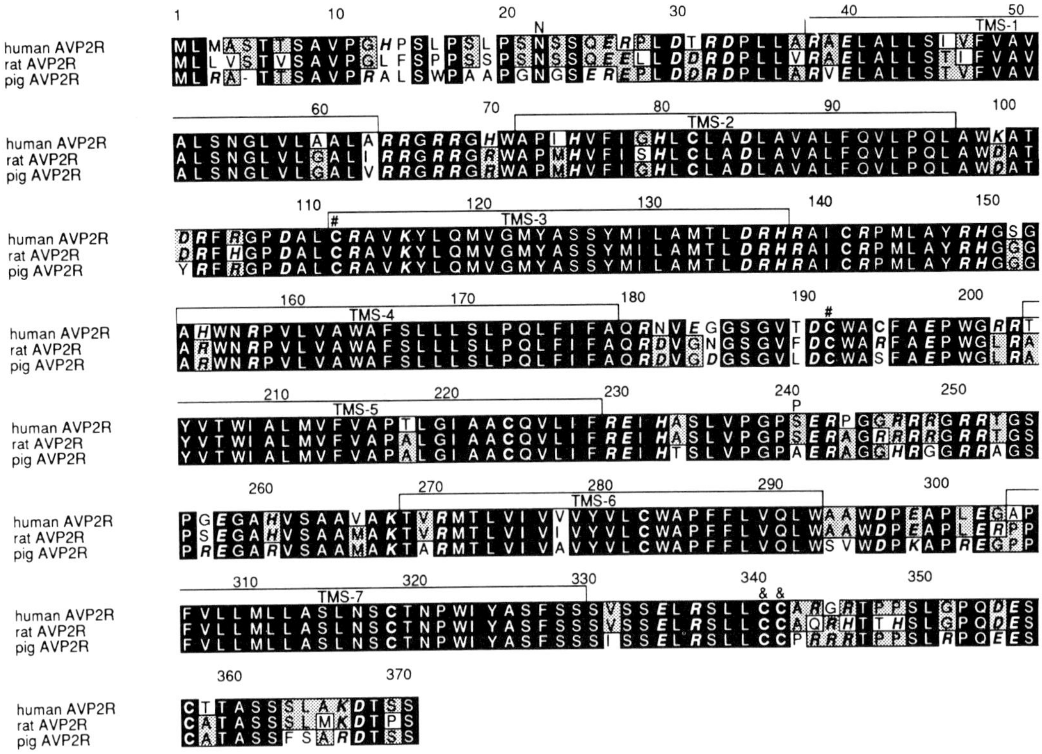

Figure 6 Sequence comparison of cloned AVP2R receptors. The sequences of the human, rat, and pig AVP2R receptors were aligned and identical amino acids highlighted as in Figure 5.

resulted in a missense mutation causing an arginine (codon CGG) to change to a tryptophan (codon TGG) (44). C → T transitions are the most common single-base mutations found in genes. Obligate heterozygotes were shown to be genotypically heterozygous (both a C and T) at this base pair. The female who manifested clinical symptoms of CNDI, was demonstrated by DNA sequencing to be heterozygous at this position, and presumably manifests nonrandom X-chromosome inactivation. The mutation in family A members (R113W) is one amino acid toward the carboxy terminus from a critical extracellular cysteine residue (cysteine 112) and is an arginine in the normal sequence. This cysteine residue, which is highly conserved among receptors in this class, is proposed to be involved in a critical extracellular disulfide bond. This mutation may impair function of AVPR2 by compromising a normal disulfide bridge between the first and second extracellular loops of the receptor. Of particular relevance to this CNDI mutation is the observation that similar mutations in the opsin gene cause it to be abnormally retained in the endoplasmic reticulum. A survey of all G protein–coupled receptors shows that disulfide bond formation between the first and second extracellular loops is a repeated theme in these receptors. Tryptophan, as demonstrated in the AVPR2 of family A, is not found adjacent to the cysteines responsible for disulfide bond formation in any G protein–coupled receptor (more than 400 characterized to date). The fact that a quarter of the identified amino acid substitutions of CNDI were to cysteine could also suggest that extra cysteines will interfere with the formation of the disulfide bridge, which may have an effect on receptor folding or hormonal binding. A new mutation in Cys112 → Arg has been found which is likely to cause CNDI by a similar mechanism. Recent biochemical data from analogous mutations in rhodopsin (Cys110 → Ala, Cys187 → Ala) suggest that this disulfide bond is not absolutely critical (47).

Nonsense Mutations

In this category, the two most famous kindred groups, the Nova Scotia/New England Hopewell and the Mormon Utah Cannon pedigrees, each have demonstrated different nonsense mutations. In family

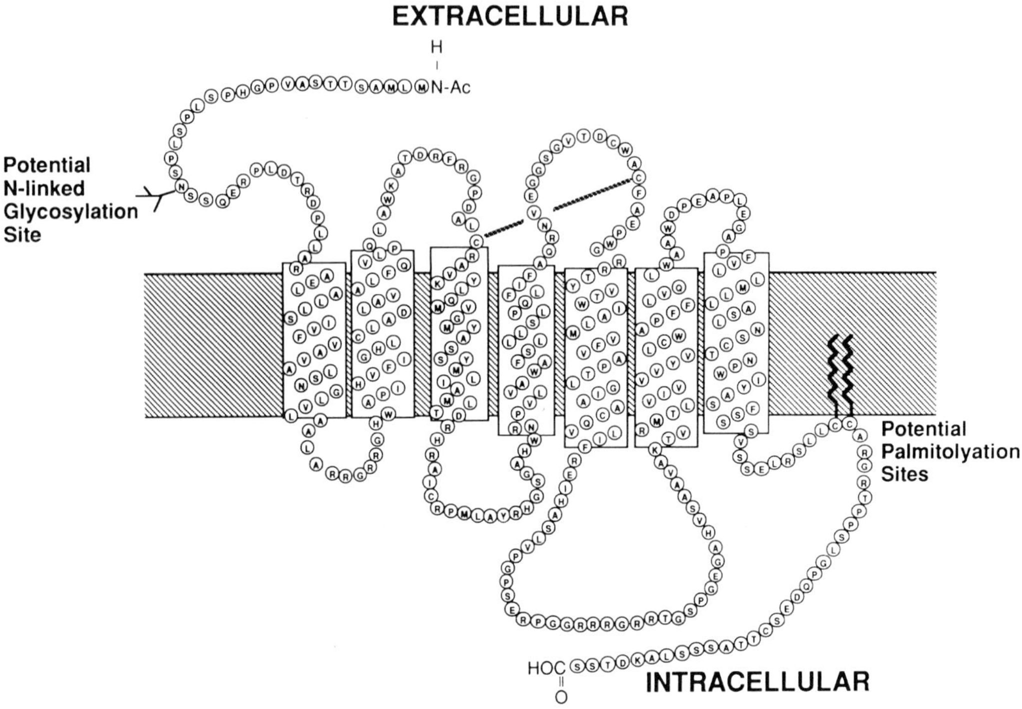

Figure 7 Topological model of the AVPR2 protein. The V2 vasopressin receptor encodes a 371–amino acid protein which is presumed to span the membrane seven times by homology to other members in the G protein–coupled receptor family. Shown are the potential sites for asparagine-linked glycosylation, acylation with palmitoyl derivatives, and an intrachain disulfide bond. Transmembrane boundaries were taken from the rhodopsin structural model developed by Baldwin (39). The extracellular regions and the transmembrane domains are implicated in ligand binding. The intracellular loops are thought to interact with intracellular G proteins. A postulated disulfide bridge is shown between amino acids Cys-112 and Cys-195.

B (Hopewell), the affected individuals analyzed demonstrated a G → A transition in codon 71 (Figure 10) (48). This mutation results in a tryptophan (codon TGG) becoming a termination codon (codon TGA), causing premature truncation of the encoded receptor protein after just one transmembrane domain. Obligate heterozygotes were shown to be genotypically heterozygous (both a G and A) at this base pair. The mutation resulted in a very short protein and is a clear null mutation. In this category is also the mutation Arg337 → Stop (#35, Table 4) which is located in the carboxyl-terminal tail in the proximity of the potential palmitoylation sites.

Frameshift Mutations

Several mutations have been found which disrupt the normal AVPR2 gene sequence by the insertion or deletion of nucleotides causing a frameshift (Table 5). Many of these mutations lead to a short region of nonsense codons followed by a stop codon in the new reading frame. Others however, proceed in the new, nonsense frame for many codons leading to the expression of a large protein, which is part AVPR2 and part nonsensical protein.

In one case we have described, there is an insertion of 28 basepairs in the pedigree shown in Figure 2 (49). The two affected individuals in family D show a 28-bp insertion at the very beginning of exon 2 downstream of the splice acceptor site. These inserted nucleotides duplicate a 28-bp sequence adjacent to the site of insertion. The context of this mutation provides some clues to a potential mechanism for this type of defect. Three identical 9-bp repeats (CTGCCCAGC) and an inverted repeat (palindrome) sequence (GCCTGGGCA) were found in the coding region of the normal gene in the area of the insertion.

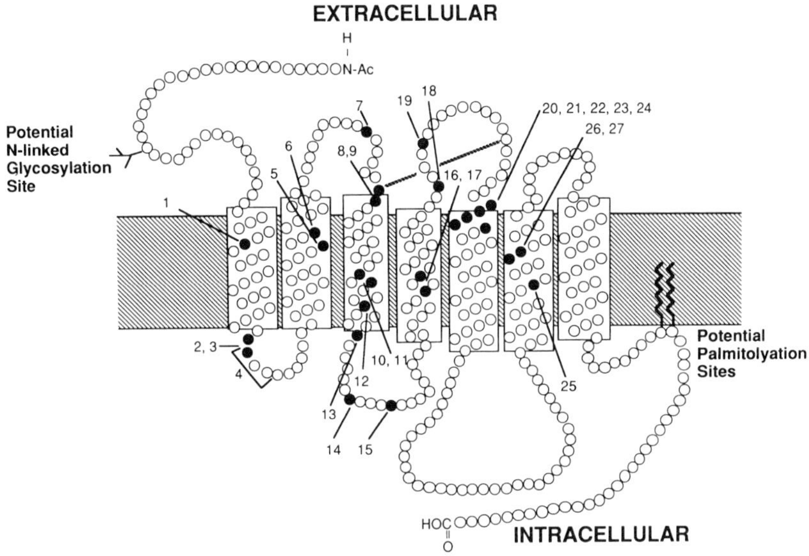

Figure 8 Missense mutations reported in AVP2R. Transmembrane model of AVP2R showing locations and identities of 27 CNDI missense mutations described. Numbers correspond to mutations listed in Table 3.

A small but growing proportion of gene mutations involve insertion of specific DNA sequences into a gene coding region (50) including p53 mutations (51). In a subset of these, the inserted nucleotide(s) duplicate the sequence preceding its insertion. These insertions are thought to arise from two potential mechanisms: (a) slipped mispairing at the replication fork mediated by direct

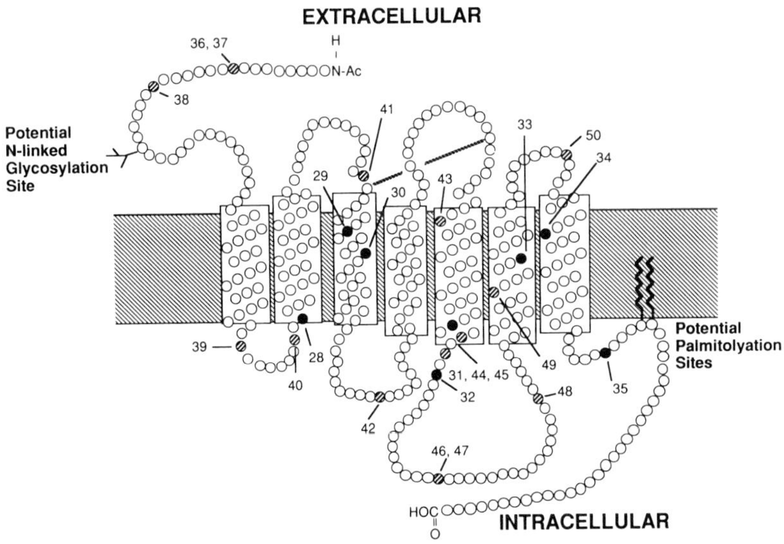

Figure 9 Nonsense and frameshift mutations reported in AVP2R. Transmembrane model of AVP2R showing locations and identities of 27 CNDI nonsense mutations described. Numbers correspond to mutations listed in Tables 4 and 5. The symbols ● and ⊘ indicate the sites of nonsense and frameshift mutations in Tables 4 and 5, respectively.

Table 3 Missense Mutations in AVPR2

No.	Codon changes	Domain	Comments	Ref.
1	Leu44 → Phe	TM1		(96)
2	Ala61 → Val	TM1	Normal ligand binding, normal cAMP production	(97)[a]
3	Leu62 → Pro	TM1		(96)
4	Leu62-Arg64 → Deletion	TM1	Deletion of 9 bp in frame	(46)
5	Asp85 → Asn	TM2		(96)
6	Val88 → Met	TM2		(96)
7	Arg106 → Cys	EXL-1		(46)
8	Cys112 → Arg	TM3		(46)
9	Arg113 → Trp	TM3	Reduced affinity, accumulation in the endoplasmic reticulum	(29, 44, 96, 98)[b]
10	Ser126 → Phe	TM3		(46)
11	Tyr128 → Ser	TM3	No ligand binding, no cAMP production	(43)[a]
12	Ala132 → Asp	TM3		(41)
13	Arg137 → His	TM3	Normal ligand binding, no G protein coupling	(99)
14	Arg143 → Pro	INL-2		(100)
15	ALa147 → Val	INL-2		(46)
16	Trp164 → Ser	TM4		(46)
17	Ser167 → Leu	TM4		(96)
18	Arg181 → Cys	EXL-2	Very reduced affinity for ligand, ⅓ level of cAMP production	(43)
19	Gly185 → Cys	EXL-2		(101)
20	Arg202 → Cys	EXL-2		(98)
21	Arg203 → Cys	TM5		(101)
22	Thr204 → Asn	TM5		(96)
23	Tyr205 → Cys	TM5		(101)
24	Val206 → Asp	TM5		(96)
25	Tyr280 → Cys	TM6		(52)
26	Ala285 → Pro	TM6		(46)
27	Pro286 → Arg	TM6	No ligand binding, no cAMP production	(43)[a]

[a]Y. Pan, personal communication.
[b]E. J. Holtzman, unpublished data.

repeats of runs of identical bases and/or, (b) the templated misincorporation of bases by secondary-structure intermediates whose formation is facilitated by palindromic (inverted repeat) sequences.

We have proposed that both mechanisms are involved in creating the germinal mutation found in family D, and this mechanism is shown schematically in Figure 11. The duplicating insertion in this family and a 28-bp deletion of the same region found in an unrelated family with CNDI (Ref. 52 and R. S. Wildin, personal communication) together with the demonstration of three adjacent repeats of nine identical base pairs with an inverted repeat between the first two, strongly suggests that the duplicating insertion as well as the deletion are a result of a non-random mutagenic event that is largely dependent upon the context of the DNA sequence in the AVPR2 gene. We have

Table 4 Nonsense Mutations in AVPR2

No.	Codon changes	Domain	Comments	Ref.
28	Trp71 → Stop	INL-1	(Hopewell), no ligand binding	(45, 48)[a]
29	Gln119 → Stop	TM3	No ligand binding	(43)[b]
30	Tyr124 → Stop	TM3		(46)
31	Gln225 → Stop	TM5		(96)
32	Glu232 → Stop	INL-3	no ligand binding	(49)[a]
33	Trp284 → Stop	TM6		(46)
34	Leu312 → Stop	TM7	(Cannon)	(45)
35	Arg337 → Stop	C-Tail		(96)

[a]E. J. Holtzman, unpublished data.
[b]Y. Pan, personal communication.

pointed out the potential relationships between this insertion mechanism and the similar insertion/deletion mutants in two hemoglobinopathies. Hb Gun Hill and Hb Koriyama (53,54) are caused by the deletion or insertion of five amino acid residues, respectively.

Bichet and colleagues have also characterized several mutations which, they suggest, have also been caused by slipped-mispairing as well as larger rearrangements of the AVPR2 locus which cause CNDI (46).

Table 5 Frame Shift Mutations in AVPR2

No.	Bp of insertion or deletion	Comments	Ref.
36	26 insertion of 28bp	Ala9 insertion	(49, 52)[a]
37	26 deletion of 28bp	Ala9 deletion	(52)[a]
38	42 deletion of 2 bp	Leu16 deletion	(46)
39	182 deletion of 35 bp	Leu62 deletion	(46)
40	203 insertion of 1 bp	Gly69 insertion	(46)
41	331 deletion of 2 bp	Leu111 deletion	(46)
42	457 deletion of 7 bp	Gly153 deletion	(96)
43	613 deletion of 2 bp	Tyr205 deletion	(46)
44	680 insertion of 1 bp	Ile228 insertion	(102)
45	692 deletion of 1 bp	Arg230 deletion	(43)
46	738 deletion of 1 bp	Gly246 deletion	(41)
47	738 insertion of 1 bp	Gly246 insertion	(46)
48	784 deletion of 1 bp	Val262 deletion	(97)
49	836 deletion of 1 bp	Val279 deletion	(100)
50	906 deletion of 1 bp	Leu302 deletion	(96)
51	deletion 3' at bp 110 large (>1KB) deletion		(46)
52	deletion 3' at bp 649 large (>1KB) deletion		(46)
53	deletion 3' at bp 850 Large (>1KB) deletion		(46)

[a]R. S. Wildin, personal communication.

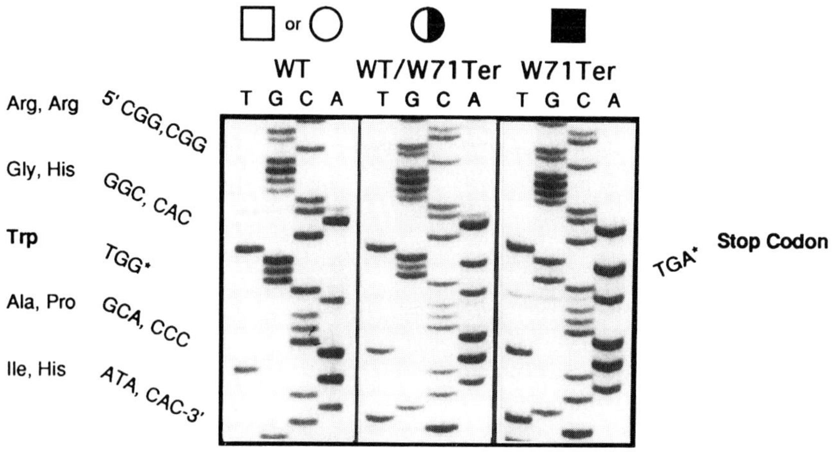

Figure 10 DNA sequencing of the Trp71 missense mutation. DNA sequences from cloned PCR fragments amplified from genomic DNA as described in the methods. Sequences from an unrelated normal male, a carrier female, and an affected male are shown. The nucleotide sequence and the translated amino acid sequences are shown. (From Ref. 48.)

Methods of Mutation Detection

In addition to direct DNA sequencing of the AVPR2 gene, developments in the polymerase chain reaction (PCR) and restriction fragment length polymorphism (RFLP) analyses have provided complementary diagnostic tools. One recently developed approach for the identification of mutations by PCR is ARMS (amplification refractory mutation system) (55,56). ARMS is a general method for the analysis of point mutations or deletions, the basis of which is a mismatch at the 3′ OH residue in the PCR primer, which does not function properly in PCR reactions under the appropriate conditions. We designed two oligonucleotide pairs which amplified either the wild-type DNA sequence (WT) or the mutant (M) and applied this technique to the analysis of the large pedigree (Family A); we characterized 23 patients and found 100% accuracy as compared with DNA sequencing. Typical results from this experiment are shown in Figure 12. Recently, ARMS-based approaches have been developed that incorporate multiplex PCR and RFLP or oligonucleotide ligation analyses, allowing for the rapid simultaneous characterization of the mutational spectrum in disease genes with heterogeneous haplotypes (57,58).

Many mutations that alter the nucleotide sequence of the gene also result in the creation or abolition of restriction enzyme sites. Judicious selection of such enzymes allows a difference in the restriction digest patterns of the wild-type and mutant alleles to be diagnostic in the rapid screening of large pedigrees. An example is the creation of BsiHKA1 site in Hopewell family members who are carriers or affected patients (Figure 12).

Functional Characterization of AVPR2 Mutations

In general, the expected phenotypes of the genetic mutations in AVPR2 causing CNDI will probably be characterized as (a) *binding mutations*: lack of ligand binding capacity but normal plasma membrane localization of the receptor; (b) *signaling mutations*: lack of G protein coupling but normal plasma membrane localization and binding; (c) *processing mutations*: unstable, truncated, and/or misfolded receptors that are retained partially or completely in the endoplasmic reticulum and/or rapidly degraded, and (d) *desensitization mutations*: change in receptor phosphorylation and desensitization processes. A final form of defects are ones which show completely wild-type characteristics in all in vitro assays yet are still the only explanation for the disease phenotype (59).

The common approach used to evaluate the biochemical defects associated with each mutation is to express the mutant and wild-type proteins in a tissue culture system and to characterize the expressed AVPR2 receptor proteins for their ability to bind AVP, to stimulate the accumulation of

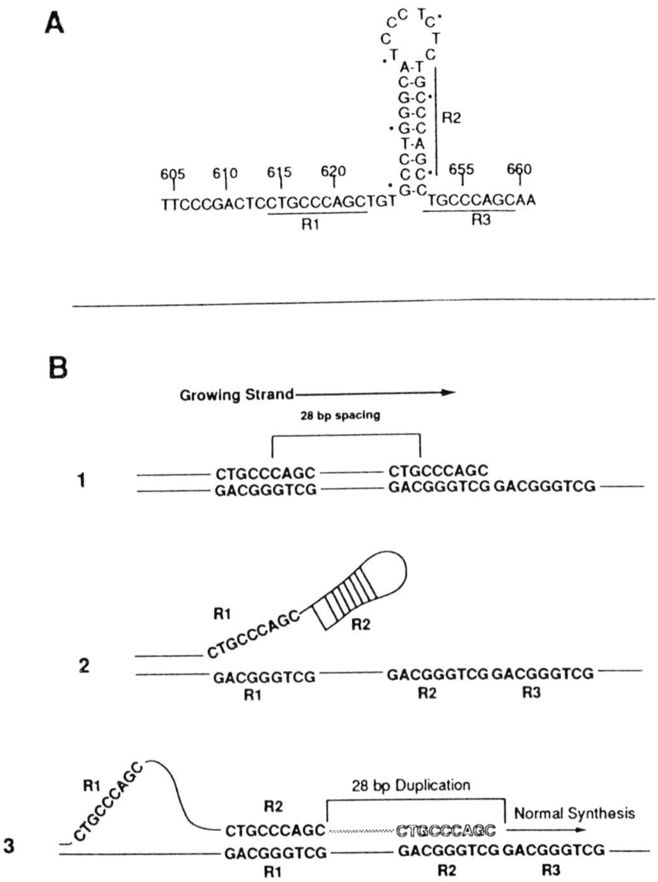

Figure 11 Proposed mechanism of the 28-bp insertional mutagenesis in family D. (A) Structure of the inverted repeat-hairpin loop. The hairpin loop contains the repeat 2 (R2) and the self complementary inverted repeat and is flanked by the direct repeats, R1 and R3. (B) Mechanism of insertion. Line 1: normal AVPR2 gene replication. The distance between repeats R1 and R2 is 28 bp. Line 2: Inverted repeat-mediated hairpin loop formation on the nascent strand behind the advancing DNA replication fork. Line 3: Continued DNA synthesis would be templated now by the bottom strand with a parallel slipped mispairing when the repeat R2 in the replicating (upper) DNA strand will base-pair with the complementary R1 repeat in the templated (lower) strand, resulting in a duplication in the 28-bp sequence which contains the R2 repeat and the inverted repeat. (From Ref. 48.)

cAMP, and their cellular (or subcellular) localization. It has been generally difficult to raise antibodies against other members of the G protein–coupled receptor family. In order to bypass this difficulty, many workers have introduced peptide epitopes within the genes in order to facilitate protein surveillance (60). Several different epitope tags have been used in studies of these receptors (FLAG, HA, and myc tags, notably). A limited set of functional results are listed in Tables 3 to 5.

Alterations in G Protein–Coupled Receptors Causing Human Diseases

To date, a number of G protein–coupled receptors have been implicated in causing human disease (61,62). Specific degenerative diseases of the retina (autosomal dominant retinitis pigmentosa, autosomal recessive retinitis pigmentosa, color blindness, and stationary night blindness) have been

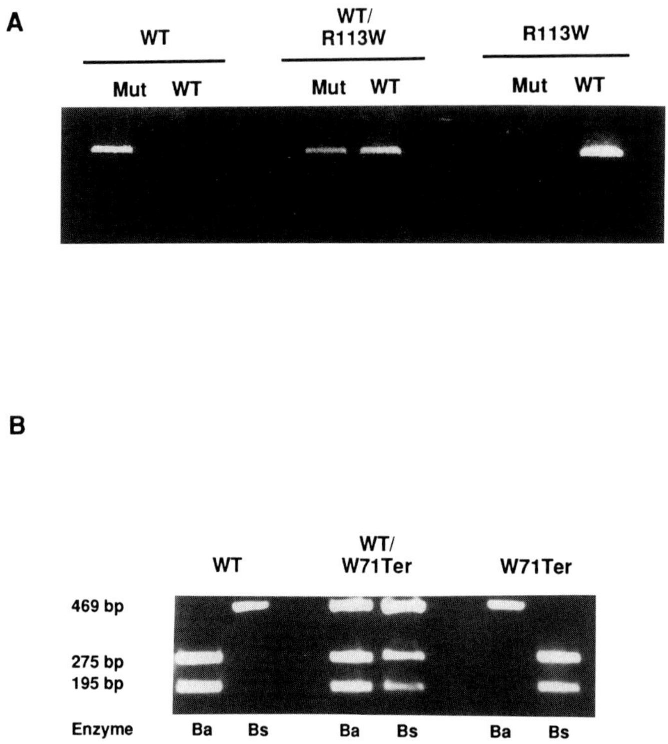

Figure 12 ARMS and RFLP analysis of mutations in AVP2R. (A) Using a pair of PCR primers designed to selectively amplify the wild-type (WT) or mutant allele (M), genomic DNA from patients in the pedigree was analyzed. This PCR based method provides a convenient tool for analyzing the prevalence of this allele. (B) Restriction digest patterns of a 469-bp PCR product containing the mutation. A PCR product from an unrelated normal male, a carrier female, and an affected male are shown digested with *BanI* (Ba) and *Bsi*HKAI (Bs). The mutation destroys the *BanI* site and creates the *Bsi*HKAI site. (From Refs. 44 and 48.)

shown to result from mutations in the genes for opsins (63–65). The hallmarks of retinitis pigmentosa are early loss of rod function followed by progressive degeneration of the retina. Mutations within the rhodopsin gene are found in approximately 25–30% of patients with autosomal dominant disease. Forty three mutations, 39 of which lead to amino acid substitutions, have been reported in the heterozygous state among patients with autosomal dominant retinitis pigmentosa (AD-RP) (Figure 13). The distribution of AD-RP mutations within the opsin protein is similar to that seen in the AVPR2 protein (Figures 8 and 9). Abnormally folded rhodopsin, due to a missense mutation, which has been retained in the endoplasmic reticulum inexorably kills the rod cells and causes the disease. Very recently, this cell death has been attributed to apoptotic processes in a mouse model (66). Autosomal recessive retinitis pigmentosa was described in a patient homozygous for a nonsense mutation. Both alleles must be affected to cause clinically apparent disease (67), suggesting that null alleles, in single dose, are relatively innocuous. Red/green color vision is usually associated with gross rearrangements in the X-linked red/green opsin gene array (64,68,69). Occasionally, point mutations of critical amino acids in the red and green visual pigments also account for defective color vision (70).

ACTH receptor mutations have been found to cause congenital isolated glucocorticoid deficiency (71–73), which is an autosomal recessive syndrome of failure of adrenal cortisol responsiveness to ACTH. Tsigos et al. demonstrated that a young patient with the disease had inherited two different mutations in the gene for the ACTH receptor (71). Weber found additional mutations in several families; in one of them the point mutation S74I shifts the dose response curve to the right to an extent that would be compatible with the biochemical finding in vivo (72,73).

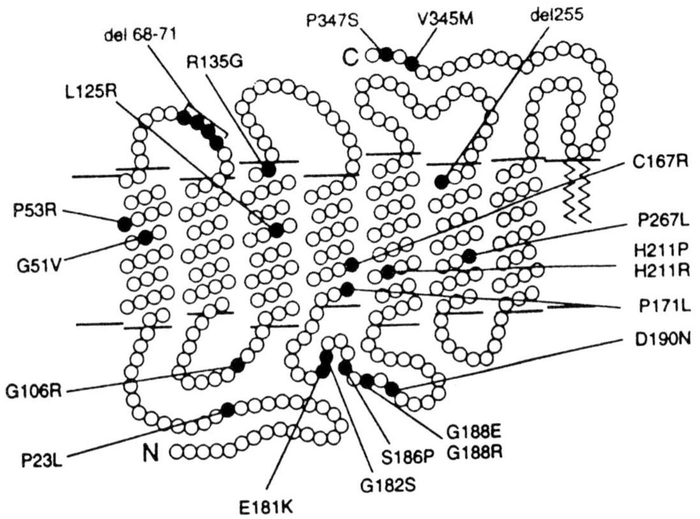

Figure 13 Retinitis pigmentosa mutations in rhodopsin. Transmembrane model of rhodopsin showing locations and identities of 21 AD-RP mutations studied. N and C represent amino and carboxyl termini, respectively. The amino terminus faces the extracellular space. Each shaded amino acid corresponds to an AD-RP mutation. (From Ref. 59.)

Parma et al. and Shenker et al. described the identification of defects responsible for an uncommon form of hyperthyroidism and for familial precocious puberty, respectively, in which the receptors remain constitutively active due to conformational changes influencing the activation of downstream effector molecules (74,75). Somatic mutations were found in the carboxyl-terminal portion of the third cytoplasmic loop of the thyrotropin receptor in three of eleven hyperfunctioning thyroid adenomas. This mutant receptor confers constitutive activation of adenylyl cyclase when tested by transfection in COS-7 cells. Familial male precocious puberty is a gonadotropin-independent disorder that is inherited in an autosomal dominant, male-limited pattern. Affected males generally exhibit signs of puberty by the age of 4. The disease was found to be caused by a mutant receptor that is activated in the presence of no agonist. A single-base substitution of glycine to aspartate in position 578 in the sixth transmembrane domain of the LH receptor was found in affected individuals from eight different families. COS-7 cells expressing the mutant LH receptor exhibit markedly increased cAMP production in the absence of agonist.

Mutations in the recently cloned calcium-sensing receptor, which senses the level of free calcium in the blood (76), appear to cause familial hypocalciuric hypercalcemia and neonatal severe hyperparathroidism (77). The two inherited conditions are characterized by altered calcium homeostasis and show abnormal parathyroid and renal responsiveness to changes in extracellular levels of calcium. Three nonconservative missense mutations were reported in affected families; two occurred in the extracellular N-terminal domain and one in the third intracellular loop of the receptor. These data suggest that G protein–coupled receptors are susceptible to many different mutations, which often result in the loss of function of the receptor, causing a similar clinical phenotype and, in the minority of cases, hyperfunction of the receptor.

MOLECULAR MECHANISMS IN AUTOSOMAL RECESSIVE (TYPE II) CONGENITAL NEPHROGENIC DIABETES INSIPIDUS

Clinical Background

Autosomal recessive nephrogenic diabetes insipidus is very rare compared to the more prevalent X-linked form. Only a handful of families have been described. Three autosomal recessive families and one clearly autosomal dominant family have been reported and probably belong to type II CNDI.

Langley reported two intellectually normal sisters with severe AVP-resistant diabetes insipidus born to healthy consanguineous Pakistani parents (78) (Figure 14, family E). Both patients presented in early infancy with dehydration associated with polyuria, hypernatremia, and hyposthenuria, which were unresponsive to treatment with AVP. A kidney biopsy performed on one patient was normal. The sex of the patients, the history of parental consanguinity, and the fact that both parents formed normally concentrated urine suggested that the CNDI in the two sisters was the result of inheritance of an autosomal recessive mutation affecting renal tubular water reabsorption. The results of DNA analysis of DXS52 locus with the use of St14 VNTR (30), which has been shown to be tightly linked to the CNDI locus, showed that each girl inherited different Xq28 regions of the maternal X-chromosome, ruling out a diagnosis of classic X-linked disease. However, the absence of increased levels of cAMP excretion in the urine in response to AVP stimulation is inconsistent with type II CNDI and needs further study.

Ohzeki et al. reported an extensive Japanese kindred in which cAMP excretion increased in response to AVP and inheritance was clearly autosomal dominant (Figure 14, family F). In four generations, nine persons were affected with three instances of male-to-male transmission (79). A Dutch family has been described in which mutations in aquaporin-2 account for the functional defects

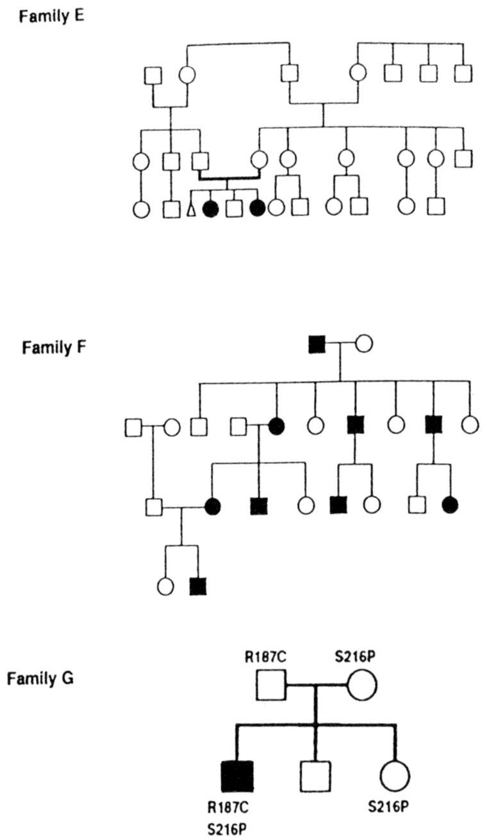

Figure 14 Autosomal CNDI pedigrees. Pedigrees E, F, and G show clear autosomal recessive or dominant genetics. Pedigrees E and F have not been characterized at the molecular level for mutations in either AVP2R or aquaporin-2. Pedigree E: A Pakistani family has been described in which there are two affected females (78). Pedigree F: A Japanese family with numerous affected individuals which show a potential autosomal dominant mode of inheritance (79). Pedigree G: Inheritance of the R187C and S216P mutations in the family of the patient with a variant of NDI. The shaded square is the patient studied (80). (From Refs. 78, 79, and 80.)

(see mutation analysis section) (80) (Figure 14, family G). In a final family, there was a 3-year-old female with severe NDI but a negative family history. She responded to AVP administration with an 89% increase in urinary cAMP concentration but no change in urinary osmolarity (10).

Collecting Duct Water Channel(s): The Candidate Gene(s) for Mutations in Autosomal Recessive Nephrogenic Diabetes Insipidus

The high water permeability of the plasma membrane of several cell types is accounted for by the presence of channel-forming proteins that act as hydrophilic pores in the lipid bilayer. An integral membrane protein, CHIP28, responsible for high constitutive water permeability in erythrocytes and in the kidney, has been identified (81). CHIP28 was found to be homologous to a major intrinsic protein of lens fibers (MIP26) as well as to certain channel-forming proteins in bacteria and plants (82). The water channel properties of CHIP28 were determined by functional expression in *Xenopus* oocytes (81) and by reconstitution into proteoliposomes (83,84). CHIP28 was found to be abundant in the basolateral and apical membranes of proximal tubules and highly expressed also in the thin descending limb of Henle (85,86). This protein is expressed in all the tubular regions that have constitutively high permeability to water, and it is probable that this CHIP28 is responsible for this function.

CHIP28, however, is not expressed in the renal collecting duct. The cDNA of a homologous protein located in the apical membrane of the rat kidney collecting tubule has been cloned (87). This channel, called aquaporin-2, is a strong candidate to be the AVP-regulated water channel, has 42% identical amino acid sequence to CHIP28, and is expressed only in the collecting tubule of the kidney (87). Sasaki et al. cloned a cDNA for the human homologue, which was found to have 91% amino acid identity to the rat protein (88). Figure 15 shows the immunohistochemical localization of aquaporin-2 in the collecting duct of a human kidney. In situ hybridization revealed that the gene was assigned to 12q13, very close to the site of MIP26 gene, whose cDNA shows 59% homology to aquaporin-2.

Functional studies have shown that the basolateral plasma membrane of kidney collecting duct

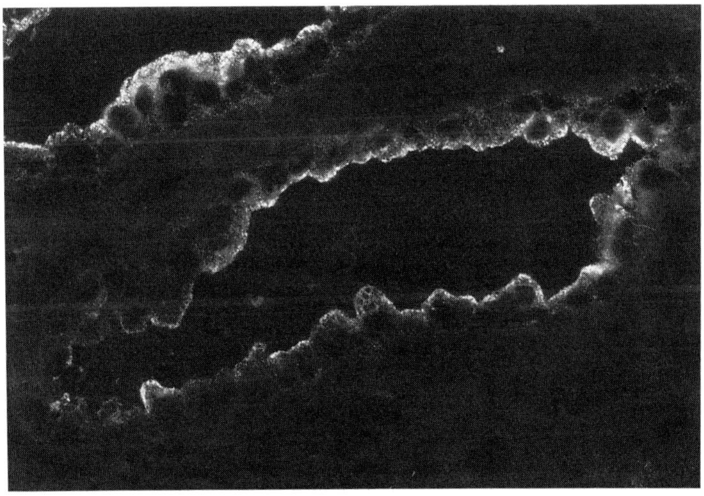

Figure 15 Aquaporin-2 localization in the kidney. Collecting duct from a frozen section of a human kidney papilla stained by indirect immunofluorescence to localize the AVP-sensitive water channel protein WCH-CD (aquaporin-2). Collecting duct principal cells are heavily labeled, the staining is concentrated at the apical pole of these cells. This staining pattern probably indicates staining of the apical plasma membrane as well as subapical vesicles in the cytoplasm. The kidney used was a nephrectomy specimen from a patient with a renal tumor. The antibody was a rabbit polyclonal raised against the 15 amino acids carboxyl-terminal sequence of aquaporin-2 (87). Goat antirabbit FITC was used as the secondary antibody. Bar = 10 μm. (Figure kindly provided by D. Brown, D. Bachinsky and G. Zheng.)

principal cells is constitutively permeable to water (7,89,90). The basolateral membrane of granular cells in another AVP-sensitive epithelium, the amphibian urinary bladder, also has a high AVP-independent water permeability (91). In kidney, the high constitutive water permeability of the basolatateral membrane of collecting duct principal cells is not accounted for by the presence of either CHIP28 or aquaporin-2 based on immunocytochemistry (85–87). In addition in situ hybridization confirmed that CHIP28 mRNA is not detectable in the kidney collecting duct (92). Valenti et al. provided evidence that the basolateral membrane of collecting duct principal cells contains a protein that is related to but distinct from the previously described members of the aquaporin/MIP26 protein family (93). In the absence of functional studies, the authors could not determine whether this novel protein is a transmembrane water channel. Recent work from Ishibashi et al. has also identified a basolateral protein (aquaporin-3) with water channel function in principal cells (94). The relationship between these two proteins is at present unknown.

From the point of view of pathophysiology, mutations in each of the principal cell water channels (aquaporin-2 or -3) could account for an autosomal recessive form of nephrogenic diabetes insipidus.

Mutational Analysis of Water Channels

The search for mutations in the aquaporin-2 gene has been conducted in one family to date. Deen et al. described a male patient with nephrogenic diabetes insipidus with an abnormal dDAVP response that was restricted only to the kidney and in which the coding region of the AVPR2 was found to be normal (80). The patient was found to be a compound heterozygote for two mutations in the gene encoding aquaporin-2. The first mutation was a substitution of cysteine for arginine in position 187 (R187C) in a strongly conserved region in the MIP family (Figure 16). The arginine itself is conserved

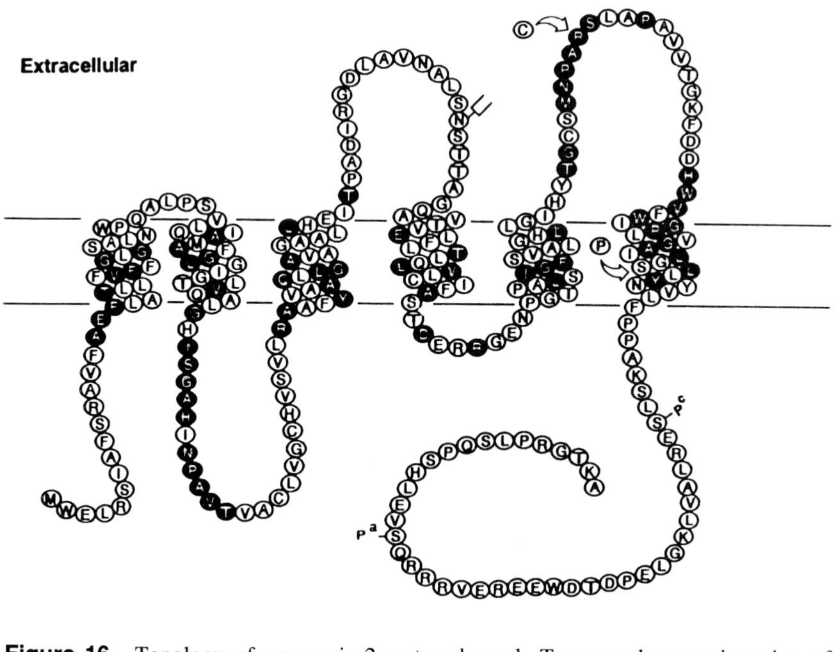

Figure 16 Topology of aquaporin-2 water channel. Transmembrane orientation of the aquaporin-2 protein, based on the proposed topology of the rat homologue (87) and the human CH1P28 protein (81). The two point mutations are indicated by arrows. The amino acid residues that are represented in the consensus sequence of the MIP family, which is conserved in at least 9 of 17 analyzed members from bacteria, yeast and plants and animals (82), are indicated by filled symbols. Consensus sequences for potential N-linked glycosylation sites (two-pronged symbol) and phosphorylation sites for protein kinase A (P^a) and protein kinase C (P^c) are indicated. (From Ref. 80.)

Table 6 Diseases in Humans Linked to G Protein–Coupled Receptors

Disease	Receptor	Mode of inheritance	Type and function of mutation	Ref.
Retinitis pigmentosa	Rhodopsin	AD	(–) Apoptosis of rod cells	(59, 64, 66)
Retinitis pigmentosa	Rhodopsin	AR	(–) Null mutations	(67)
Color blindness	Color opsins	X-linked	(–) X chromosome rearrangements	(103, 104)
Nephrogenic DI	V2-receptor	X-linked	(–)	(41)
Isolated glucocorticoid deficiency	ACTH-receptor	AR	(–)	(71–73)
Hyperfunctioning thyroid adenomas	TSH-receptor	Somatic mutation	(+) missense	(75)
Familial precocious puberty	LH-receptor	AD male limited	(+) Missense	(74)
Familial hypocalciuric hypercalcemia	Ca^{+2} sensing receptor	AD	(–) Missense	(77)
Neonatal severe hyperparathroidism	Ca^{+2} sensing receptor	AR	(–) Missense	(77)

in 15 out of 17 members of the MIP family. The second mutation was a substitution of proline for serine in position 216 (S216P). This residue is less conserved and, in the other members of the MIP family, is either serine or an aliphatic amino acid. The authors speculate that the introduction of proline residue might distort the alpha-helical structure of the molecule in this part of the transmembrane region. Sequence analysis revealed that the R187C mutation was inherited from the father and the S216P mutation from the mother (Figure 14, family F).

Functional Expression Studies of Water Channels

Deen et al. performed functional studies in *Xenopus* oocytes with cRNAs and revealed that the mutations described above failed to increase the osmotic water permeability, P_f, above that of the water control when the wild type cRNA increased the P_f 10-fold (80). Coinjection of either of the mutant cRNA with the wild-type cRNA had no effect on the activity of the wild-type aquaporin-2, which is in agreement with the autosomal recessive inheritance observed in the family (Table 7).

Table 7 Functional Properties of Human AVP-Sensitive Water Channel Mutations

cRNA injected into oocyte	P_f (μm/s)
5 ng of aquaporin-2	196 ± 26 (22)
Water control	20 ± 13 (16)
10 ng of R187C aquaporin-2	17 ± 11 (10)
10 ng of S216P aquaporin-2	18 ± 7 (11)
5 ng of aquaporin-2 + 5 ng of R187C aquaporin-2	187 ± 38 (19)
5 ng of aquaporin-2 + 5 ng of S216P aquaporin-2	192 ± 41 (18)

Source: From Ref. 80.

SUMMARY

In summary, there have been dramatic advances in the understanding of the molecular biological aspects of the etiology of X-linked congenital nephrogenic diabetes insipidus. The chromosome localization, cDNA sequence, gene structure, and specific mutations are all now known. Over fifty different mutations of the vasopressin V2 receptor gene (*AVPR2*) have been determined and are strongly associated with the disease. As the functional characterization of these mutants progresses, it is clear these mutations are the cause of CNDI in these families. This X-linked form of the disease is providing important structural and functional information concerning the specific interaction of the AVPR2 receptor with its circulating hormone ligand, AVP, and the components in the intracellular signal transduction cascade. We can expect additional insights into the AVP receptor's activities that will facilitate the understanding of its signal transduction mechanisms as well as further the development of therapeutic agents that might modify the function of this renal-specific receptor.

Non-X-linked causes of CNDI are beginning to be described at the molecular and genetic level. The work of Deen and colleagues described above has provided confirmation that other proteins which are specific to the AVP-stimulated pathway in the kidney can also be the direct cause of CNDI. The further characterization of mutations in aquaporin-2 and probably other genes will be important in elucidating the complete biochemical and cell biological process that is initiated by AVP on the basolateral membrane of the collecting duct and propagated to the apical side, ending with the flow of water through the principal cells in the collecting duct.

ACKNOWLEDGMENTS

We are grateful to Drs. Daniel Bichet, Jane Gitschier, Nine Knoers, and Robert Wildin for providing data before publication on CNDI pedigrees and functional data of CNDI mutations. This work has been supported in part by NIH grant DK19406 to D.A.A.

REFERENCES

1. Holtzman EJ, Ausiello DA. Nephrogenic diabetes insipidus causes revealed. Hosp Pract 1994; 29:89–104.
2. Skorecki KL, Brown D, Ercolani L, Ausiello DA. Molecular mechanisms of vasopressin action in the kidney. In: Windhager EE, ed. Handbook of Physiology: Section 8: Renal Physiology. New York: Oxford University Press, 1992:1185–1218.
3. Brown D, Orci L. Vasopressin stimulates formation of coated pits in rat kidney collecting ducts. Nature 1983; 302:253–255.
4. Muller J, Kachadorian WA, DiScala VA. Evidence that ADH-stimulated intramembrane particle aggregates are transferred from cytoplasmic to luminal membranes in toad bladder epithelial cells. J Cell Biol 1980; 85:83–95.
5. Wade JB. Membrane structural specialization of the toad urinary bladder revealed by the freeze-fracture technique: III. Location, structure and vasopressin dependence of intramembrane particle arrays. J Membr Biol 1978; 281–296.
6. Brown D, Weyer P, Orci L. Vasopressin stimulates endocytosis in kidney collecting duct epithelial cells. Eur J Cell Biol 1988; 46:336–340.
7. Strange K, Spring KR. Cell membrane water permeability of rabbit cortical collecting duct. J Membr Biol 1987; 96:27–43.
8. Moses AM, Scheinman SJ. Hereditary vasopressin resistance in man and mouse. Ann NY Acad Sci 1993; 689:233–249.
9. Bell NH, Clark CMJ, Avery S, et al. Demonstration of a defect in the formation of adenosine 3′,5′-monophosphate in vasopressin-resistant diabetes insipidus. Pediatr Res 1974; 8:223–230.
10. Zimmerman D, Green OC. Nephrogenic diabetes insipidus-typeII: Defect distal to the adenylate cyclase step. Pediatr Res 1975; 9:381.
11. McIlraith CH. Notes on some cases of diabetes insipidus with marked family and heridatary tendencies. Lancet 1892; 2:767–768.
12. Brownstein MJ, Lolait SJ. Hereditary nephrogeneic diabetes insipidus. In: Gross P, Richter D, Robertson GL, eds. Vasopressin. Paris: John Libbey, 1993:33–43.
13. Williams RH, Henry C. Nephrogenic diabetes insipidus transmitted by females and appearing during infancy in males. Ann Intern Med 1947; 27:84–95.
14. Waring AG, Kajdi L, Tappan V. Congenital defect of water metabolism. Am J Dis Child 1945; 69:323.

15. Forssmann H. On hereditary diabetes insipidus. Acta Med Scand 1945; 121 (suppl 159):9–46.
16. Uttley WS, Paxton J, Thistlethwaite D. Urinary concentrating ability and growth failure in urinary tract disorders. Arch Dis Child 1972; 47:436–441.
17. Moses AM, Miller LJ, Levine MA. Two distinct pathophysiological mechanisms in congenital diabetes insipidus. J Clin Endocrinol Metab 1988; 66:1259–1264.
18. Knoers N, Brommer EJ, Willems H, et al. Fibrinolytic responses to 1-desamino-8-D-arginine-vasopressin in patients with congenital nephrogenic diabetes insipidus. Nephron 1990; 54:322–326.
19. Bichet DG, Razi M, Lonergan M, et al. Hemodynamic and coagulation responses to 1-desamino[8-D-arginine] vasopressin in patients with congenital nephrogenic diabetes insipidus. N Engl J Med 1988; 318:881–887.
20. Kobrinsky NL, Doyle JJ, Israels ED, et al. Absent factor VIII response to synthetic vasopressin analogue (DDAVP) in nephrogenic diabetes insipidus. Lancet 1985; 1:1293–1294.
21. Bode HH, Crawford JD. Nephrogenic diabetes insipidus in North America–The Hopewell hypothesis. N Engl J Med 1969; 280:750–754.
22. Bichet DG, Razi M, Arthus MF, et al. Epinephrine and dDAVP administration in patients with congenital nephrogenic diabetes insipidus: Evidence for a pre-cyclic AMP V2 receptor defective mechanism. Kidney Int 1989; 36:859–866.
23. Feigin RD, Rimoin DL, Kaufman RL. Nephrogenic diabetes insipidus in a Negro kindred. Am J Dis Child 1970; 120:64–68.
24. Nakano KK. Familial nephrogenic diabetes insipidus. Hawaii Med J 1969; 28:205–208.
25. Schultz P, Lines DR. Nephrogenic diabetes insipidus in an Australian aboriginal kindred. Humangenetik 1975; 26:79–85.
26. Faust CJ, Gonzales JC, Seibold A, et al. Comparative mapping on the mouse and human X chromosomes of a human cDNA clone encoding the vasopressin renal-type receptor (AVP2R). Genomics. 1993; 15:439–441.
27. Frattini A, Zucchi I, Villa A, et al. Type 2 vasopressin receptor gene, the gene responsible nephrogenic diabetes insipidus, maps Xq28 close to the LICAM gene. Biochem Biophys Res Commun 1993; 193:864–871.
28. Seibold A, Brabet P, Rosenthal W, Birnbaumer M. Structure and chromosomal localization of the human antidiuretic hormone receptor gene. Am J Hum Genet 1992; 51:1078–1083.
29. Bichet DG, Hendy GN, Lonergan M, et al. X-linked nephrogenic diabetes insipidus: from the ship Hopewell to RFLP studies. Am J Hum Genet 1992; 51:1089–1102.
30. Richards B, Heilig R, Oberle I, et al. Rapid PCR analysis of the St14 (DXS52) VNTR. Nucleic Acids Res 1991; 19:1944.
31. Ostrowski NL, Lolait SJ, Bradley DJ, et al. Distribution of V1a and V2 vasopressin receptor messenger ribonucleic acids in rat liver, kidney, pituitary and brain. Endocrinology 1992; 131:533–535.
32. Birnbaumer M, Seibold A, Gilbert S, et al. Molecular cloning of the receptor for human antidiuretic hormone. Nature 1992; 357:333–335.
33. Lolait SJ, OCarroll AM, McBride OW, et al. Cloning and characterization of a vasopressin V2 receptor and possible link to nephrogenic diabetes insipidus. Nature 1992; 357:336–339.
34. Dohlman HG, Thorner J, Caron MG, Lefkowitz RJ. Model systems for the study of seven-transmembrane-segment receptors. Annu Rev Biochem 1991; 60:653–688.
35. Thibonnier M, Auzan C, Madhun Z, et al. Molecular cloning, sequencing, and functional expression of a cDNA encoding the human V1a vasopressin receptor. J Biol Chem 1994; 269:3304–3310.
36. Kimura T, Tanizawa O, Mori K, et al. Structure and expression of a human oxytocin receptor. Nature 1992; 356:526–529.
37. Kakar SS, Musgrove LC, Devor DC, et al. Cloning, sequencing, and expression of human gonadotropin releasing hormone (GnRH) receptor. Biochem Biophys Res Commun 1992; 189:289–295.
38. Gorbulev V, Buchner H, Akhundova A, Fahrenholz F. Molecular cloning and functional characterization of V2 [8-lysine] vasopressin and oxytocin receptors from a pig kidney cell line. Eur J Biochem 1993; 215:1–7.
39. Baldwin JM. The probable arrangement of the helices in G protein–coupled receptors. EMBO J 1993; 12:1693–1703.
40. Kojro E, Eich P, Gimpl G, Fahrenholz F. Direct identification of an extracellular agonist binding site in the renal V2 vasopressin receptor. Biochemistry 1993; 32:13537–13544.
41. Rosenthal W, Seibold A, Antaramian A, et al. Molecular identification of the gene responsible for congenital nephrogenic diabetes insipidus. Nature 1992; 359:233–235.
42. De Marco L, Bale AE, Carson E, et al. Nephrogenic Diabetes Insipidus: A novel X-linked dominant inheritance pattern and normal structural V2 receptor gene (abstr). Am J Hum Genet 1993; 53:423.
43. Pan Y, Metzenberg A, Das S, et al. Mutations in the V2 vasopressin receptor gene are associated with X-linked diabetes insipidus. Nature Genet 1992; 2:103–106.

44. Holtzman EJ, Harris HW, Kolakowski LF, et al. A molecular defect in the vasopressin V2 receptor gene causing nephrogenic diabetes insipidus. N Engl J Med 1993; 328:1534–1537.
45. Bichet DG, Arthus MF, Lonergan M, et al. X-linked nephrogenic diabetes insipidus mutations in North America and the Hopewell hypothesis. J Clin Invest 1993; 92:1262–1268.
46. Bichet DG, Birnbaumer M, Lonergan M, et al. Nature and recurrence of AVP2R mutations in X-linked diabetes insipidus. Am J Hum Genet. In press.
47. Davidson FF, Loewen PC, Khorana HG. Structure and function in rhodopsin: Replacement by alanine of cysteine residues 110 and 187, components of a conserved disulfide bond in rhodopsin, affects the light activated metarhodopsin II state. Proc Natl Acad Sci USA 1994; 91:4029–4033.
48. Holtzman EJ, Kolakowski LF, O'Brien D, et al. A null mutation in the vasopressin V2 receptor gene (AVPR2) associated with nephrogenic diabetes insipidus in the Hopewell kindred. Hum Mol Genet 1993; 2:1201–1204.
49. Holtzman EJ, Kolakowski LF, Geifman-Holtzman O, et al. Mutations in the vasopressin V2 receptor gene in two families with nephrogenic diabetes insipidus. J Am Soc Nephrol 1994; 5:169–176.
50. Cooper DN, Krawczak M. Mechanisms of insertional mutagenesis in human genes causing genetic disease. Hum Genet 1991; 87:409–415.
51. Jego N, Thomas G, Hamelin R. Short direct repeats flanking deletions, and duplicating insertions in p53 gene in human cancers. Oncogene 1993; 8:209–213.
52. Wildin RS, Antush MJ, Schoof JM, et al. Reciprocal products of intragenic unequal crossing over in the AVPR2 gene define the mutation mechanism in two patients with X linked nephrogenic diabetes insipidus (abstr). Am J Hum Genet 1993; 53:423.
53. Kawata R, Ohba Y, Yamamoto K, et al. Hyperunstable hemoglobin Koriyama anti-Hb Gun Hill insertion of five residues in the beta chain. Hemoglobin 1988; 12:311–321.
54. Bradley TBJ, Wohl RC, Rieder RF. Hemoglobin Gun Hill: Deletion of five amino acid residues and impaired heme-globin binding. Science 1967; 157:1581–1583.
55. Lo YM, Patel P, Newton CR, et al. Direct haplotype determination by double ARMS: Specificity, sensitivity and genetic applications. Nucleic Acids Res 1991; 19:3561–3567.
56. Newton CR, Graham A, Heptinstall LE, et al. Analysis of any point mutation in DNA: The amplification refractory mutation system (ARMS). Nucleic Acids Res 1989; 17:2503–2516.
57. Jawaheer D, Ollier WE, Thomson W. Multiplex ARMS-RFLP: A simple and rapid method for HLA-DR4 subtyping. Eur J Immunogenet 1993; 20:175–187.
58. Fortina P, Dotti G, Conant R, et al. Detection of the most common mutations causing beta-thalassemia in Mediterraneans using a multiplex amplification refractory mutation system (MARMS). PCR Methods Appl 1992; 2:163–166.
59. Sung CH, Davenport CM, Nathans J. Rhodopsin mutations responsible for autosomal dominant retinitis pigmentosa: Clustering of functional classes along the polypeptide chain. J Biol Chem 1993; 268:26645–26649.
60. Kolodziej PA, Young RA. Epitope tagging and protein surveillance. Methods Enzymol 1991; 194:508–519.
61. Spiegel AM, Weinstein LS, Shenker A. Abnormalities in G protein-coupled signal transduction pathways in human disease. J Clin Invest 1993; 92:1119–1125.
62. Clapham DE. Mutations in G protein-linked receptors: Novel insights on disease. Cell 1993; 75:1237–1239.
63. Khorana HG. Rhodopsin, photoreceptor of the rod cell: An emerging pattern for structure and function. J Biol Chem 1992; 267:1–4.
64. Nathans J. Rhodopsin: Structure, function, and genetics. Biochemistry 1992; 31:4923–4931.
65. Dryja TP, McGee TL, Reichel E, et al. A point mutation of the rhodopsin gene in one form of retinitis pigmentosa. Nature 1990; 343:364–366.
66. Portera CC, Sung CH, Nathans J, Adler R. Apoptotic photoreceptor cell death in mouse models of retinitis pigmentosa. Proc Natl Acad Sci USA 1994; 91:974–978.
67. Rosenfeld PJ, Cowley GS, McGee TL, et al. A null mutation in the rhodopsin gene causes rod photoreceptor dysfunction and autosomal recessive retinitis pigmentosa. Nature Genet 1992; 1:209–213.
68. Deeb SS, Lindsey DT, Hibiya Y, et al. Genotype-phenotype relationships in human red/green color-vision defects: Molecular and psychophysical studies. Am J Hum Genet 1992; 51:687–700.
69. Vollrath D, Nathans J, Davis RW. Tandem array of human visual pigment genes at Xq28. Science 1988; 240:1669–1672.
70. Winderickx J, Sanocki E, Lindsey DT, et al. Defective colour vision associated with a missense mutation in the human green visual pigment gene. Nature Genet 1992; 1:251–256.
71. Tsigos C, Arai K, Hung W, Chrousos GP. Hereditary isolated glucocorticoid deficiency is associated with abnormalities of the adrenocorticotropin receptor gene. J Clin Invest 1993; 92:2458–2461.
72. Weber A, Kapas S, Hinson J, et al. Functional characterization of the cloned human ACTH receptor: Impaired responsiveness of a mutant receptor in familial glucocorticoid deficiency. Biochem Biophys Res Commun 1993; 197:172–178.

73. Weber A, Clark AJL. Mutations of the ACTH receptor gene are only one cause of familial glucocorticoid deficiency. Hum Mol Genet 1994; 3:585–588.
74. Shenker A, Laue L, Kosugi S, et al. A constitutively activating mutation of the luteinizing hormon receptor in familial male precocious puberty. Nature 1993; 365:652–654.
75. Parma J, Duprez L, Van Sande J, et al. Somatic mutations in the thyrotropin receptor gene cause hyperfunctioning thyroid adenomas. Nature 1993; 365:649–651.
76. Brown EM, Gamba G, Riccardi D, et al. Cloning and characterization of an extracellular Ca(2+)-sensing receptor from bovine parathyroid. Nature 1993; 366:575–580.
77. Pollak MR, Brown EM, Chou YH, et al. Mutations in the human Ca(2+)-sensing receptor gene cause familial hypocalciuric hypercalcemia and neonatal severe hyperparathyroidism. Cell 1993; 75:1297–1303.
78. Langley JM, Balfe JW, Selander T, et al. Autosomal recessive inheritance of vasopressin-resistant diabetes insipidus. Am J Med Genet 1991; 38:90–94.
79. Ohzeki T, Igarashi T, Okamoto A. Familial cases of congenital nephrogenic diabetes insipidus type II: Remarkable increment of urinary adenosine 3′,5′-monophosphate in response to antidiuretic hormone. J Pediatr 1984; 104:593–595.
80. Deen PM, Verdijk MA, Knoers NV, et al. Requirement of human renal water channel aquaporin-2 for vasopressin-dependent concentration of urine. Science 1994; 264:92–95.
81. Preston GM, Carroll TP, Guggino WB, Agre P. Appearance of water channels in Xenopus oocytes expressing red cell CHIP28 protein. Science 1992; 256:385–387.
82. Agre P, Preston GM, Smith BL, et al. Aquaporin CHIP: The archetypal molecular water channel. Am J Physiol 1993; 265:F463–F476.
83. Van Hoek AN, Verkman AS. Functional reconstitution of the isolated erythrocyte water channel CHIP28. J Biol Chem 1992; 267:18267–18269.
84. Zeidel ML, Ambudkar SV, Smith BL, Agre P. Reconstitution of functional water channels in liposomes containing purified red cell CHIP28 protein. Biochemistry 1992; 31:7436–7440.
85. Sabolic I, Valenti G, Verbavatz J-M, et al. Localization of the CHIP28 water channel in rat kidney. Am J Physiol 1992; 263:C1225–C1233.
86. Nielsen S, Smith BL, Christensen EI, Agre P. Distribution of the aquaporin CHIP in secretory and resorptive epithelia and capillarty endothelia. Proc Natl Acad Sci USA 1993; 90:7275–7279.
87. Fushimi K, Uchida S, Hara Y, et al. Cloning and expression of apical membrane water channel of rat kidney collecting tubule. Nature 1993; 361:549–552.
88. Sasaki K, Saito H, Saito F, et al. Cloning, expression and chromosomal mapping of human collecting duct water channel (hWCH-CD). J Am Soc Nephrol 1993; 4:858.
89. Grantham JJ, Ganote CE, Burg MB, Orloff J. Paths of transtubular water flow in isolated renal collecting tubules. J Cell Biol 1969; 41:562–576.
90. Woodhall PB, Tisher CC. Response of the distal tubule and cortical collecting duct to vasopressin in the rat. J Clin Invest 1973; 52:3095–3108.
91. Van Der Goot F, Corman B, Ripoche P. Evidence for permanent water channels in the basolateral membrane of an ADH-sensitive epithelium. J Membrane Biol 1991; 120:59–65.
92. Hasegawa H, Zhang R, Dohrman A, Verkman AS. Tissue-specific expression of mRNA encoding rat kidney water channel CHIP28k by in situ hybridization. Am J Physiol 1993; 264:C237–C245.
93. Valenti G, Verbavatz JM, Sabolic I, et al. A CHIP28/MIP26-related protein (BLIP) in basolateral membranes of kidney collecting duct principal cells and gastric parietal cells. Am J Physiol 1994; 267:C812–C820.
94. Ishibashi K, Sasaki S, Fushimi K, et al. Molecular cloning and expression of a new water channel (WCH-3) which expressed selectively in kidney and GI tract. J Am Soc Nephrol 1993; 4:855.
95. Lindshaw MA. Congenital nephrogenic diabetes insipidus. In: Jacobson HR, Striker GE and Klahr S, eds. Principles and Practice of Nephrology. Philadelphia: Decker, 1991:426–430.
96. Knoers N, Verdijk M, Monnens L, et al. Inheritance of mutations in the vasopressin V2 receptor gene in 15 Dutch Families with congenital nephrogenic diabetes insipidus. In: Gross P, Richter D, Robertson GL, eds. Vasopressin, Paris: John Libbey, 1993:571.
97. Pan Y, Metzenberg B, Ravnan B, et al. Molecular and functional analysis of the V2 vasopressin receptor in patients with nephrogenic diabetes insipidus (abstr). Am J Hum Genet 1993; 53:938.
98. Merendino JJ, Thambi NC, Shenkar A, Spiegel AM. Detection of V2 vasopressin receptor gene mutations in X-linked nephrogenic diabetes insipidus by temperature gradient gel electrophoresis. Clin Res 1993; 41:131a.
99. Rosenthal W, Antaramian A, Gilbert S, Birnbaumer M. Nephrogenic diabetes insipidus. A V2 vasopressin receptor unable to stimulate adenylyl cyclase. J Biol Chem 1993; 268:13030–13033.
100. Tsukaguchi H, Matsubara H, Aritaki S, et al. Two novel mutations in the vasopressin V2 receptor gene in unrelated Japanese kindreds with nephrogenic diabetes insipidus. Biochem Biophys Res Commun 1993; 197:1000–1010.

101. van den Ouweland AM, Dreesen JC, Verdijk M, et al. Mutations in the vasopressin type 2 receptor gene (AVPR2) associated with nephrogenic diabetes insipidus. Nat Genet 1992; 2:99–102.
102. Merendino JJ, Speigel AM, Crawford JD, et al. Brief report: A mutation in the vasopressin V2-receptor gene in a kindred with X-linked nephrogenic diabetes insipidus. N Engl J Med 1993; 328:1538–1541.
103. Nathans J, Merbs SL, Sung CH, et al. Molecular genetics of human visual pigments. Annu Rev Genet 1992; 26:403–424.
104. Merbs SL, Nathans J. Absorption spectra of the hybrid pigments responsible for anomalous color vision. Science 1992; 258:464–466.
105. Schlessinger D, Mandel JL, Monaco AP, et al. Report of the Fourth International Workshop on Human X Chromosome Mapping. Cytogenet Cell Genet 1993; 64:147–194.

61

Prospects for Gene Therapy in the Kidney

Vikas P. Sukhatme
Beth Israel Hospital and Harvard Medical School, Boston, Massachusetts

INTRODUCTION

Since this is the concluding essay among these papers on molecular biology of the kidney, it is perhaps fitting to consider possible applications of gene transfer to the study and treatment of renal disease. Literature on this topic is essentially non-existent; therefore much of what follows is in the realm of fantasy.

Prior to a consideration of possible applications to the kidney, however, it will be necessary to review basic terminologies in the area of gene transfer and some of the universal considerations that apply if gene therapy is to be effectively utilized in the clinic (1–3). We begin with a review of general concepts that underlie this form of therapy. This is followed by a discussion of gene delivery methods. Finally, we speculate about the applications of these techniques to renal disease.

GENE THERAPY CONCEPTS

Gene therapy protocols can be operationally divided into two types: somatic cell gene therapy and germ-line therapy. The latter, aimed at altering reproductive cells, is not considered further. In contrast, somatic cell gene therapy is targeted to somatic tissue. Delivery is either in vivo or by ex vivo means. In the in vivo form of gene delivery, the gene is carried in an appropriate vehicle such as a viral vector or is introduced by nonviral means, as by lipofection or direct injection into the body. In ex vivo gene delivery, cells derived either from the patient or from other sources are first genetically modified outside of the body by introduction of a particular gene or genes. These cells are then reintroduced into the body so as to achieve either local, regional, or widespread distribution.

Three major considerations go into any gene therapy protocol. The first is delivery, the ability to introduce the appropriate gene into the cells and tissues of interest. In thinking about delivery systems, two further issues arise. Is the vehicle/methodology under consideration able to introduce the gene into nonreplicating cells? This question is of import, since a variety of target organs (e.g., the kidney) have a very low mitotic index. Second, what is the efficiency with which the gene can be introduced into these cells? (That is, what fraction of cells in a given tissue or organ will receive the gene?) Is this number 50–100% or 1–10% or 0.001–0.1%? A distinction into these three categories has biological significance. Clearly, replacement of an intracellularly acting protein (e.g., a tumor suppressor transcription factor) would require introduction into essentially 100% of target (tumor) cells. (An exception to this statement would occur if there is a "bystander effect," as has been postulated for the herpes simplex virus thymidine kinase gene therapy effects.) A 1–10% efficiency might suffice if the protein functioned extracellularly. Finally, only a very small fraction of target organ cells may need to be transduced to stimulate an immune-mediated reaction. Moreover, in making these assertions, it is critical to ascertain whether the gene therapy acts in a replacement capacity (i.e., to supply a missing factor) or whether it is aimed at countering the action of an existing molecule (protein). In either case, the biological levels of the protein required to produce the desired phenotypic effect also have to be assessed in order to estimate the delivery efficiency needed.

A second key consideration relates to expression. Can the exogenous gene be transcribed and the protein expressed in the target tissue to a high enough level to achieve the desired biological effect for a given delivery efficiency? Are there ways of regulating expression in the tissue of interest? Can tissue specificity of expression be achieved, for example, by incorporation of *cis*-regulatory elements in the transducing vector? And how long does expression last in the delivered cells or tissue?

Safety is the third critical consideration in any gene therapy protocol. Are there concerns about malignancy that can be induced by the introduction of the gene or by utilization of the (viral) vector itself? If delivery and expression are relatively "promiscuous"—i.e. to tissues that are not the intended target—what deleterious effects might be expected in the short or long run in these cells?

These are the three most important questions in any gene therapy protocol. The answers, in turn, will clearly depend on the application in mind—e.g., the severity of the disease or the time frame over which it evolves, on the need for long-term versus short-term expression, on the type and location of target cells and tissues, on the vector used, on the gene being delivered, etc. We now turn to a summary of several possible methods for delivering genes into mammalian cells.

GENE DELIVERY METHODS

Viral Vectors

Several different retroviral vectors have been designed for the transfer of genes into mammalian cells (1,3). The retrovirus system is ideally suited for many ex vivo applications, since retroviruses are able to stably transduce target cells with very high efficiency. Moreover, many "packaging cell lines" exist to generate viruses with enormous host range. These cells are specialized lines that produce replication-defective recombinant viruses, so that cells transduced will not spread virus to other cells. One of the problems with retroviral gene transfer is that relatively low titers of virus are achievable—numbers in the range of 10^4 to 10^6 infectious units per milliliter. Moreover, certain cells, such as, for example, hematopoietic stem cells, have not been efficiently transduced, perhaps due to the lack of appropriate viral receptors on them. Another notable point, an advantage or a disadvantage depending upon the application in question, is that in order for target cells to be productively infected (i.e., achievement of proviral integration), cells have to be in a proliferative state at least for some period of time. This feature may be of advantage for tumor infection. By their very nature, these cells are dividing, and use of retroviral gene transfer may offer a selective targeting advantage.

In general, based on the considerations given above, retroviral vectors will be used primarily in ex vivo gene therapy. Their major advantage is that one can achieve stable expression which, in principle, can last for long periods of time (months to years). Similarly, the above considerations—as well as the facts that retroviral particles tend to be relatively unstable in serum and that they cannot integrate into nondividing cells—have traditionally suggested that their use for in vivo transduction may be rather limited. Recently, several technical advances have occurred which may extend the use of retroviral vectors to in vivo applications. Woo et al. (4) utilized partial hepatectomy, preceding by 1 to 3 days retroviral gene transfer, so as to transduce hepatocytes. The frequency noted was approximately 1%. Two other recent methodologies include the development of a new virus packaging cell line producing 10^6 to 10^7 particles per milliliter following a transient transfection protocol (5). Moreover, in a separate study, a murine leukemia virus–derived vector, in which the envelope glycoprotein has been replaced by the G glycoprotein of vesicular stomatitis virus (VSV), has allowed these vectors to be concentrated to yield titers of $>10^9$/ml (6). These vectors can also efficiently transfer genes into mammalian and nonmammalian cells. These advances broaden the utility of retroviral vectors to in vivo gene therapy applications.

Adenovirus-based vectors have been of particular interest for in vivo gene therapy. High titers of the virus, 10^{10} to 10^{11} plaque-forming units per milliliter, are easily achievable. The virus has a broad tissue host range and there is no need to replicate cells in order to achieve infection. Indeed, adenoviruses can transduce many terminally differentiated cell types, including hepatocytes, skeletal muscle, endothelium, glia, neurons, pulmonary epithelium, and synovial lining cells (7–14). Finally, the adenovirus vector is felt to be relatively safe in that there are no reports of human malignancies associated with adenoviruses and the adenoviral genome is maintained episomally in the target cell. Another notable feature is the duration of expression of the adenovirally delivered gene: typically, a period of weeks to months. Unfortunately the factors that determine this length of time are unknown, though host immunity is likely to be important. Finally, it is possible to incorporate *cis*-regulatory elements into the vector, and these elements do in fact function in the context of the adenoviral genome.

Some of the difficulties with adenoviral vectors include the fact that the generation of recombinants is somewhat tedious, the production of viral stock is fairly labor-intensive, there is a size constraint on the gene being delivered, and adenovirus infection can lead to inflammation. Finally, concern over the mounting of an immune response, especially if repeat therapy is required, may limit the effectiveness of adenoviral therapy.

Other viral vectors include adeno-associated viruses, herpes virus, vaccinia virus, poliovirus, and sindbis and other RNA viruses (1,3). These vectors are not discussed in this minireview.

Nonviral Vectors

Perhaps the best-studied of the "nonviral" approaches to gene delivery include adenovirus-ligand DNA conjugates, lipofection (liposome-mediated gene transfer), and direct injection of DNA (1,3,15). It should be emphasized at the outset that all of these methodologies are best suited for in vivo applications of gene therapy. These methods rely on the ability of mammalian cells to transport macromolecules into the nucleus. Considerable effort is currently being directed to using complexes of DNA and specific ligands (including antibodies) to target gene delivery via recognition of specific receptors on designated cell surfaces. A major limitation of these methods is that, in general, they provide only transient expression of genes. Thus their application may be limited to situations in which intervention over a period of days or weeks is all that is desired. Alternatively, repeat therapy may be required. Of note, direct injection of DNA may produce long-term expression, but so far success has been limited primarily to cardiac and skeletal muscle cells, and that, too, in only a small fraction of cells in the target organ. A recent notable exception to the transient nature of an expressed gene delivered by lipofection is reported by Debs et al. (16), whose work with liposome gene transfer produced long-lived (a few months) gene expression. Why these investigators achieved long-term expression while others have failed is unclear.

APPLICATIONS IN THE KIDNEY

Current Data

Very little literature currently exists on the delivery of genes into the kidney. A literature search reveals the following. Tomita et al. (17) report an efficient method for in vivo gene transfer into the rat kidney. They utilize HVJ (Sendai virus) and liposome methodology. In this protocol, plasmid DNA and a nuclear protein are coencapsulated in liposomes (actually a liposome/red blood cell membrane hybrid) and later cointroduced into cells. In their studies, the reporter gene utilized was the SV40 large T antigen. The gene transfer was conducted by inserting a catheter proximal to the right renal artery with the abdominal aorta clipped distally beneath the left renal artery. The liposome suspension was injected into the kidneys. Four days after injection of this mixture, SV40 large T antigen was detected immunohistochemically in 15% of glomerular capillary cells. The expression of the T antigen declined rapidly over the ensuing 2 to 3 days. In this protocol, the nuclear protein used was the so-called HMG1 protein, a high-mobility group 1 protein that is a nonhistone nuclear protein. It is believed that the success of this method for high-efficiency gene transfer is predicated on the ability of this nuclear protein to enhance plasmid DNA passage into nuclei (18). Interestingly, no expression of the foreign gene was detected outside the glomerulus.

A recent study by Debs et al. (16) reports the use of a particular cationic liposome DNA mixture to deliver genes with high efficiency into a vast number of endothelial cells in a rat. The gene-transfer protocol is initiated by tail vein injection. The authors state that long-term expression is noted in almost all of the endothelial cells of the body as well as in a variety of parenchymal cell types, including the lung, spleen, lymph nodes, and bone marrow. In one of the tables in the paper, the authors note that between 25–50% of endothelial cells in the kidney are transfected. No mention is made of whether these endothelial cells are in glomerular or nonglomerular regions. Also, there is no indication of the duration of expression in these kidney cells. In contrast to the Tomita study (17), no transduction into renal parenchymal cells was obtained.

An abstract presented at the recent American Society of Nephrology meeting indicates that an ex vivo cell-mediated gene-transfer strategy has been tried in the kidney (19). In these investigations, mesangial cells were transduced with a β-galactosidase–expressing plasmid ex vivo. Subsequently, these cells were introduced into the left renal artery. Expression, obtained throughout the kidney and in particular in as many as 40% of glomeruli, was detectable over a 4-week period. Of particular note was the finding that when cells introduced into kidneys were subjected to an anti–mesangial cell antibody, which induces transient mesangial regeneration, the expression of β-galactosidase was dramatically amplified in situ by up to 10-fold, and this high level expression continued for 8 weeks. These findings suggest that a mesangial-cell vector system may provide a useful tool for introducing exogenous genes into the renal glomerulus in vivo. It remains to be seen whether the mesangial cells trapped in the capillary lumen have deleterious effects on kidney physiology.

Recently, in our laboratory, we have begun investigations on the use of adenoviruses to infect the kidney. In preliminary data, we have noted that up to about 10% of endothelial cells can be infected via the arterial route. Currently, we are modifying a variety of parameters—including clamping of the renal vein, infection time, media in which virus is suspended, titer of adenovirus stock utilized, etc.—in an attempt to improve these numbers. We have also shown that adenovirus can be directly injected into the kidney parenchyma. Tubular epithelial cells along the needle track can clearly be transduced, but the efficiency is low.

Possible Applications

We begin by noting certain features of the kidney of relevance to gene therapy. This organ is a particularly complex one, containing many different cell types. Moreover, the architectural organization of the kidney is critical for proper organ function. Thus high-efficiency gene delivery to one particular cell type may be difficult to achieve. A way to circumvent this problem is to aim for more promiscuous delivery but utilize *cis*-regulatory elements to achieve cell-specific expression. Can gene expression be targeted or regulated within the kidney in this manner? Unfortunately, studies aimed at identifying nephron (or better still nephron subregion-specific) *cis* elements are in their infancy. Similarly, we do not yet have in hand enhancers that will direct gene expression to one or another cell type in the glomerulus. It is conceivable that local pH or osmolality might be utilized to modulate gene expression in certain tubular cells.

The kidney has a very low mitotic index. Notable exceptions include a kidney recovering from acute tubular necrosis, in which focal nephron regions may show significant mitoses, or disease states characterized by rapid cell proliferation of mesangial cells or parietal epithelial cells. Similarly, cells lining cystic structures and renal tumors contain dividing cells. These considerations are of importance if one contemplates in vivo retroviral gene transfer therapy. In contrast, the largely nonregenerating population of renal cells may allow for longer-term expression of a gene maintained episomally, as occurs with adenoviral transduction, thus necessitating less frequent repeat therapy.

With regard to delivery routes, gene delivery to the kidney can be achieved by injection into the renal artery or the renal vein, via retrograde injection into the ureter, via direct injection into the parenchyma of the kidney, or perhaps into a subcapsular space. Though these routes of administration may be best suited to in vivo methodologies, they apply to ex vivo gene therapy as well. We turn now to a consideration of specific diseases entities.

Polycystic Kidney Disease (PKD)

When the PKD1 gene is identified, one might consider this disease as a possible target for gene therapy. It is quite clear now that patients with PKD express some of their disease manifestations in the kidney very early in life, perhaps even during fetal development. However, it would still be likely that delivery of the gene product postnatally may be of use. The biggest problem in this regard is gene delivery itself. Since the critical cells affected are those that line the proximal, distal, and collecting tubules, it appears a priori that a rational form of delivery would somehow involve retrograde injection or the use of a vector (agent) filtered in the glomerulus, which would subsequently transduce tubular cells from the luminal side. No data are currently available on whether it is possible, for example, to infect tubular cells with high efficiency. A second concern relates to the mechanism by which the PKD1 gene product functions. If, for example, the mutant protein acts in a dominant negative fashion, high expression levels of an exogenously introduced normal gene may be needed to achieve a phenotypic correction; in contrast, if dosage effect underlies the mutant phenotype, then lower-level expression may be adequate. On the positive side, it is possible that other genes "regulated downstream" by the PKD1 gene product might prove appropriate targets for drug or gene therapy. For example, if PKD1 encoded a transcription factor, some of its targets could be extracellular proteins. Thus, replacement therapy or, better still, therapy to counteract the effects of this factor may not require transduction of every tubular cell. Of course, therapy in the kidney would not ameliorate the extrarenal manifestations of PKD.

Renal Cancer

The area of disseminated renal cancer is one in which the modality of gene therapy may provide considerable advance. The largest group of renal cancers are adenocarcinomas thought to be of proximal nephron origin. The structures tend to be highly vascular and may thus be amenable to gene targeting via the circulation (e.g., by selective arterial catheterization). However, current therapy for this disease when it is restricted to the kidney involves a unilateral nephrectomy and will be hard to supplant by gene therapy methods unless destruction of the tumor vasculature is the goal of therapy. A more likely application for gene therapy would be for metastatic disease, for which current therapeutic modalities are clearly inadequate. In this context, most encouraging is the use of ex vivo gene transfer therapies in a rodent model of renal carcinoma, in which carcinoma cells in culture were transduced with the interleukin-4 (IL-4) cDNA and then reimplanted into the animal (20). A $CD8^+$ T cell response was elicited, which could reject the parental tumor. Such approaches might also be extended to in vivo delivery of the cytokine gene.

Acute Tubular Necrosis (ATN)

The use of gene therapy for the prevention or treatment of ATN is worthy of consideration. It is possible that such therapy could be given in a prophylactic manner in certain clinical situations. For example, it may be desirable to infuse an appropriate growth factor prior to operations known to compromise renal hemodynamics. This factor could be delivered via either subcutaneous or intravenous routes, or endothelial cells in the renal artery could be transduced in vivo by vectors containing the appropriate gene. Such delivery could occur preoperatively or perhaps be given intraoperatively. Admittedly, though, it is unclear whether such intervention might actually protect the kidney from ischemic damage. Recently, antibody to the intercellular adhesion molecule –1 (ICAM-1) has been shown to protect the kidney against ischemia in a rat model (20a). In principle such therapy could also be delivered via antisense oligonucleotides to ICAM-1. A recent thoughtful article (21) discusses the pathophysiology of acute renal failure and is worth reviewing.

The use of gene therapy once either ischemic ATN or nephrotoxic ATN has set in may also be appropriate. One can speculate that delivery of an appropriate growth factor(s) may aid in the recovery process, since such factor(s) may be rate-limiting. Thus, transduction of endothelial cells in the renal arterioles with growth factor genes might provide high local concentrations without systemic toxicity.

Glomerular Disease (Acute/Chronic) and Chronic Renal Disease

Perhaps the most interesting use of gene therapy in the kidney will be in acute or chronic glomerular and chronic interstitial disease. First, in the acute glomerulonephridites, some of which are characterized by an exudative/inflammatory process, it may seem reasonable to intervene by preventing the adhesion of monocytes/macrophages and neutrophils to the glomerular endothelium or to alter their transmigration through endothelium into the mesangium. Alternatively, one could intervene at the level of mesangial cell or parietal cell proliferation by appropriate antagonists to locally produced cytokines. Such therapy might seem most appropriate in the setting of a diffuse proliferative lesion and/or a rapidly progressing crescentic glomerulonephritis. Unfortunately, a major problem here is a clinical one, namely, that the number of patients seen in this acute phase is relatively small. Furthermore, many glomerular disorders, especially those with primarily a nephrotic rather than nephritic presentation, have no overt acute exudative clinical phase and present at a much later stage after the initial insult has subsided. The damaged kidney unfortunately often "progresses" inexorably, typically over several years.

Applications to chronic kidney disease are therefore of great interest from a therapeutic standpoint. This statement is true for several reasons. First, diverse initial events appear to funnel into a common pathway leading to fibrosis. Thus, interventions might be applicable to a variety of disorders. Second, patients are in fact seen in this window sometimes fairly early in the course of their chronic disease, with excellent preservation of renal function. If interventions lead to even a slight slowing in the rate of progression of renal disease, it could be of enormous advantage to the patient, since it might, for example, delay the requirement for dialysis from 10 years to 15 years. Third, there now are beginning to be developed models in which the action of certain cytokines, especially TGF-β, and PDGF are being touted as possible targets for such intervention. Of course, it might be possible to intervene with the activity or production of these molecules by modalities that do not rely on gene therapy, and that is certainly to be encouraged as well. Finally, current therapy for arresting progression is virtually nonexistent.

A few cautionary words are, however, in order with regard to progression (see, for example, Ref. 22). First, by definition, progression is a long-term problem. Thus, evaluation of the efficacy of intervention—whether by conventional drugs or gene therapy—will be expensive and difficult. Animal models must be considered as a reasonable initial alternative. Unfortunately, significant inter- and intraspecies differences are known to exist with regard to progression following the identical initial insult. Finally, the pathophysiology of progression is multifactorial (see below). Thus, intervention to alter the course of chronic renal disease will not be straightforward.

The major pathological lesion in progression is scarring—i.e., increased deposition of extracellular matrix protein (ECM) in diverse locations in the kidney: basement membrane, mesangium, and interstitium. Multiple mechanisms are at play, ranging from metabolic derangements, abnormal production of soluble factor (peptide and nonpeptides such as eicosanoids, nitric oxide, etc.); altered "cell physiology" in normally resident kidney cells and infiltrating ones, including proliferation; secretion of soluble factors; increase in matrix production; change in adhesion molecule expression, etc.; as well as immunological factors (23,24). Interaction among these modalities makes it hard to envision how therapy should best be directed. Below, we focus on attempting to use gene therapy approaches to affect the activity of TGF-β and/or any of the biological functions modulated by TGF-β (25). The rationale is not that TGF-β is the sole effector of renal fibrosis but rather that it provides a concrete example for the discussion of gene therapeutics.

How might one influence the effects of TGF-β acting in the glomerulus or the interstitium? One can view such intervention at a variety of levels. The first question is: Where is the TGF-β produced? It is believed that infiltrating monocytes/macrophages and T lymphocytes are a primary site of TGF-β production. However, the renal tubular epithelium may well be a source for TGF-β after the initial injury. One would desire to reduce the expression of TGF-β by all of these cells. Though this is not impossible, it is difficult to envision how gene therapy could be so directed. A second line of attack would be to try to antagonize the action of TGF-β. A naturally occurring substance such as decorin, a proteoglycan and known TGF-β antagonist, would be ideal, as it might not elicit an immune response (26). It might also neutralize the activity of other members of the TGF-β family (e.g., TGF-β_2 and TGF-β_3) (26). Thus, gene therapy with decorin cDNA could be contemplated. Alternatively, a synthetic protein that would bind TGF-β or would antagonize its action extracellularly at the receptor level could also be envisioned. Finally, perhaps an agent acting postcellularly—that is intracellularly within the "recipient" cell, presumably the mesangial cell, the podocyte, and/or the tubular cell—could be considered. Again at which of these levels one might be able to intervene is at this point highly speculative, but antagonism at the extracellular level is probably the easiest to envision, since it minimizes delivery problems. Other approaches would include methods of inhibiting either the production or action of protease inhibitors such as TIMP. Another modality of action for gene therapy would be to increase production of certain proteases. It is, in general, easier to increase production of a protein rather than to decrease its production by gene therapy methods. Therefore, this approach has a certain straightforward simplicity to it. On the negative side, it is quite clear that the delivery of these proteases would have to be controlled both temporally and spatially, for they are likely to lead to damage if produced in an uncontrollable fashion or over too long a period of time.

A particularly speculative approach to chronic kidney gene therapy would be to use an ex vivo approach to either deliver a gene of interest or to potentially repopulate the kidney with certain cell types that may be multipotent. The studies mentioned above (19) suggest that mesangial cells are able to home into the glomerulus and continue to express a transduced gene for a period of several months. Along these same lines, the ability to introduce cells subcapsularly into the kidney—cells that are secreting a variety of lymphokines or proteins which might act in an antagonistic fashion to other locally made lymphokines—might form the basis of useful therapies, especially in the treatment or the amelioration of interstitial fibrotic processes. Approaches such as these may, for example, be extended to deliver kidney stem cells or nephroblasts (27) (perhaps transduced with an appropriate gene or genes to decrease immunogenicity). Thus reconstituting part of a kidney structure may not be totally in the realm of fantasy. The major concern with regard to these chronic cell-based therapies will be the mounting of a host immune response.

Renal Artery Stenosis

There might be a role for gene therapy for the prevention of renal artery restenosis following angioplasty. This problem is less well studied in the kidney than in the coronaries, but there are considerable data from coronary artery angioplasties. Events identified to date include initial platelet aggregation on denuded endothelium, liberation of growth factor(s) such as PDGF, hyperplasia of vascular smooth muscle cells, and increased extracellular matrix production. Drug therapy directed at one or more or these steps is under investigation. The recent demonstration by Dzau et al. (28) that "postangioplasty" application of antisense oligonucleotides to two cell-cycle–regulated genes prevents restenosis in a rabbit carotid model is most exciting. In fact, application to the kidney may be more straightforward, since the kidney can withstand a longer period of ischemia than the heart. Thus it might be possible, by the use of appropriately shaped catheters (e.g., those containing both distal and proximal balloons), to introduce into endothelial cells agents such as antisense oligos or other constructs that might play a role in preventing restenosis. Of note, in the studies by Dzau, a liposome-based gene therapy was utilized as a single application.

Renal Transplantation

Another application that can be contemplated is the treatment of a renal allograft with an agent delivered to endothelial cells that might help in the postoperative period to decrease the incidence of early transplant rejection. Conceptually, either the organ could be made less immunogenic so as to reduce the number of host T cells generated, and/or the endothelial cells could be altered so as to prevent the adhesion/transmigration of primed immune T cells. These strategies make clinical sense, since it is well known that early rejection episodes lead to reduced long-term graft survival. Therefore, prevention of acute rejection is of particular import. Delivery for this purpose may be straightforward: it would be possible to utilize an adenovirus vector or to transduce, using lipofection, a large proportion of the endothelial cells in an allograft. These vectors could carry antisense constructs to one or more cell adhesion molecules (involved in lymphocyte homing), or dominant negative constructs to these molecules, or antisense constructs to MHC antigens in the transplant, or locally immune-suppressive lymphokines. Chimeric genes encoding CTLA4-Ig and an IL-2-toxin fusion protein are other candidates. Clearly this is an exciting area that merits further investigation, especially since regional delivery could be accomplished pre- or intraoperatively, thus obviating a major problem in most gene therapy protocols. The use of cells injected subcapsularly (intra- or preoperatively) might also provide a source of immunomodulatory molecules, though these cells would themselves be the target of an immune response.

Miscellaneous

Another potential application would be to deliver genes into the peritoneum. The adenovirus vector may be particularly well suited for this purpose, since infection of the mesothelial surface using a peritoneally delivered virus is certainly feasible. On a separate note, applications in the treatment of microangiopathic disease processes can be envisioned. Finally, it should be perfectly feasible to administer erythropoietin via a gene-delivery protocol to either dialysis or predialysis patients. There would be many choices for the recipient cells as well as methods of delivery. Moreover, since EPO levels need not be regulated in a diurnal way, the problem of controlled expression is obviated. Recently, Crystal and colleagues (28a) used an adenovirus containing an EPO gene to raise and maintain the hematocrit in rats for 3 to 4 weeks following a single intraperitoneal or subcutaneous injection.

Applications to Study of Renal Development, Gene Expression, and Models of Renal Disease

If gene delivery seems too far-fetched, there are, however, applications of delivering genes to the kidney that would be of particular use in the study of kidney development in general (29,30)—for example, in defining *cis*-regulatory elements operative in the kidney, in cell lineage analysis, and in the study of models of glomerulonephritis and other kidney disorders. Rather than generating transgenic mice it would, for instance, be simpler to study the effect of *cis*-regulatory elements introduced in vivo using gene-transfer technologies. Similarly, in studying a variety of models of glomerulonephritis, it would be particularly interesting to overexpress one or more growth factors. Such protocols would be more controllable (temporally) and easier to attempt then generating transgenic mice. Gene delivery using ex vivo gene transfer might be of particular interest in trying to understand the role of a particular gene in vivo, especially in a developmental process. For example, cells transduced with a particular cytokine or cytokine "antagonist" could be transplanted subcapsularly, or, to achieve glomerular gene transfer, mesangial cells might provide suitable vehicles (19).

CONCLUSION

This chapter, as emphasized earlier, is of a highly speculative nature, since the gene therapy era with regard to the kidney has barely arrived. It is also by no means exhaustive. However, prior to any further investigation, one will have to achieve a certain data base simply to define which cell types in the kidney can be transduced, by what vehicle, delivered for how long, etc. Moreover, such data will have to be obtained in various disease states, for this information could differ significantly from that noted in normals. For example, in the presence of inflammation, it is possible that liposome-based gene delivery will be particularly efficient, since liposomes are preferentially taken up by phagocytic cells. In conjunction, studies aimed at defining tissue-specific promoter/enhancer elements, so as to enable the targeting of gene expression to specific kidney cell subtypes, must be pursued. Similarly, ex vivo gene delivery is in its infancy. It is hoped that the speculations provided in this paper will whet the appetite of investigators and encourage them to pursue answers to some of these questions as a first step in the realization of possible applications of gene therapy to the study and treatment of renal disease. The beauty of this research is that it necessitates multidimensional expertise—a synergy of cell and molecular biological techniques—with a deep appreciation of kidney physiology in health and in disease.

ACKNOWLEDGMENT

I am grateful to my section colleagues at the Beth Israel Hospital and members of my laboratory for commenting on my flights of fancy. Thanks are also due to S. Nelson and H. Smith for bringing this manuscript to fruition in short order.

NOTE ADDED IN PROOF

Recently, Moullier et al. (31) have reported adenoviral-mediated gene delivery to kidney tubular cells.

REFERENCES

1. Mulligan RC. The basic science of gene therapy. Science 1993; 260:926–932.
2. Miller AD. Human gene therapy comes of age. Nature 1992; 357:455–460.
3. Levine F, Friedman T. Gene therapy techniques. Curr Opin Biotech 1992; 2:840–844.
4. Kay MA, Rothenberg S, Landen CN, et al. In vivo gene therapy of hemophilia B: Sustained partial correction in factor IX-deficient dogs. Science 1993; 262:117–119.
5. Pear WS, Nolan GP, Scott ML, Baltimore D. Production of high-titer helper-free retroviruses by transient transfection. Proc Natl Acad Sci USA 1993; 90:8392–8396.

6. Burns JC, Friedmann T, Driever W, et al. Vesicular stomatitis virus G glycoprotein pseudotyped retroviral vectors: Concentration to very high titer and efficient gene transfer into mammalian and nonmammalian cells. Proc Natl Acad Sci USA 1993; 90:8803–8037.
7. Davidson BL, Allen ED, Kozarsky KF, et al. A model system for in vivo gene transfer into the CNS using an adenoviral vector. Nature Genetics 1993; 3:219–223.
8. Rosenfeld MA, Yoshimura K, Trapnell BC, et al. In vivo transfer of the human cystic fibrosis transmembrane conductance regulator gene to the airway epithelium. Cell 1992; 68:143–155.
9. Jaffe, HA., Danel C, Longenecker G. Adenovirus-mediated in vivo gene transfer and expression in normal rat liver, Nature Genet 1992; 1:372–378.
10. Quantin, B., Perricaudet M, Tajbakhsh S, Mandel JL. Adenovirus as an expression vector in muscle cells in vivo. Proc Natl Acad Sci USA 1992; 89:2581–2584.
11. Roessler BJ, Allen ED, Wilson JM, et al. Adenoviral-mediated gene transfer to rabbit synovium in vivo. J Clin Invest 1993; 92:1085–1092.
12. Lemarchand P, Jones M, Yamada I, Crystal RG. In vivo gene transfer and expression in normal uninjured blood vessels using replication-deficient recombinant adenovirus vectors. Circ Res 1993; 72:1132–1138.
13. Bajocchi G, Feldman SH, Crystal RG, Mastrangeli A. Direct in vivo gene transfer to ependymal cells in the central nervous system using recombinant adenovirus vectors. Nature Genet 1993; 3:229–234.
14. Mastrangeli A, Danel C, Rosenfeld MA, et al. Diversity of airway epithelial cell targets for in vivo recombinant adenovirus-mediated gene transfer. J Clin Invest 1993; 91:225–234.
15. Felgner PL, Rhodes G. Gene therapeutics. Nature 1991; 349:35–36.
16. Zhu N, Liggitt D, Liu Y, Debs R. Systemic gene expression after intravenous DNA delivery into adult mice. Science 1993; 261:209–211.
17. Tomita N, Higaki J, Morishita R, et al. Directed in vivo gene introduction into rat kidney. Biochem Biophys Res Commun 1992; 186:129–134.
18. Kaneda Y, Iwai K, Uchida T. Increased expression of DNA cointroduced with nuclear protein in adult rat liver. Science 1989; 243:375–378.
19. Kitamura M, Taylor S, Shimizu F, Fine LG. Gene transfer into the glomerulus via a mesangial cell vector. Abstracts of American Society of Nephrology meeting, Boston, November 14–17, 1993.
20. Golumbek PT, Lazenby AJ, Levitsky HI, et al. Treatment of establishment renal cancer by tumor cells engineered to secrete interleukin-4. Science 1991; 254:713–716.
20a. Kelly KJ, Williams WW Jr, Colvin RB, et al. Antibody to intercellular adhesion molecule 1 protects the kidney against ischemic injury. Proc Natl Acad Sci USA 1994; 91:812–816.
21. Toback FG. Regeneration after acute tubular necrosis. Kidney Int 1992; 41:226–246.
22. Couser WG. Research opportunities and future directions in glomerular disease. Semin Nephrol 1993; 13:457–471.
23. Nath KA. Tubulointerstitial changes as a major determinant in the progression of renal damage. Am J Kidney Dis 1992; 20:1–17.
24. Neilson EG. The nephritogenic T lymphocyte response in interstitial nephritis. Semin Nephrol 1993; 13:496–502.
25. Border WA, Noble NA. Cytokines in kidney disease: The role of transforming growth factor-beta. Am J Kidney Dis 1993; 22:105–113.
26. Border WA, Noble NA, Yamamoto T, et al. Natural inhibitor of transforming growth factor-beta protects against scarring in experimental kidney disease: Nature 1992; 360:361–364.
27. Burrow CR, Wilson PD. A putative Wilms' tumor–secreted growth factor activity required for primary culture of human nephroblasts. Proc Natl Acad Sci USA 1993; 90:6066–6070.
28. Morishita R, Gibbons GH, Ellison KE, et al. Single intraluminal delivery of antisense cdc2 kinase and proliferating-cell nuclear antigen oligonucleotides results in chronic inhibition of neointimal hyperplasia. Proc Natl Acad Sci USA 1993; 90:8474–8478.
28a Setoguchi Y, Danel C, Crystal RG. Stimulation of erythropoiesis by in vivo gene therapy: Physiologic consequences of transfer of the human erythropoietin gene to experimental animals using an adenovirus vector. Blood 1994; 84:2946–2953.
29. Sukhatme VP. Renal development: Challenge and opportunity. Semin Nephrol 1993; 13:422–426.
30. Avner ED. Renal developmental diseases. Semin Nephrol 1993; 13:427–435.
31. Moullier P, Friedlander G, Calise D, et al. Adenoviral-mediated gene transfer to renal tubular cells in vivo. Kidney Int 1994; 45:1220–1225.

Index

About the Editors

DETLEF SCHLÖNDORFF is Direktor der Medizinischen Poliklinik der Ludwig-Maximilians-Universität München, Germany. Formerly the Abraham Levitt Professor of Medicine and Director of the Nephrology Division at the Albert Einstein College of Medicine of Yeshiva University, Bronx, New York, Dr. Schlöndorff is the author or coauthor of more than 100 professional papers. He serves on the editorial board of numerous scientific journals and is a member of the American Society for Clinical Investigation, the American Society of Nephrology, the International Society of Nephrology, and the American Federation for Clinical Research, among others.

JOSEPH V. BONVENTRE is Associate Professor of Medicine at Harvard Medical School and Associate Director of the Harvard—M.I.T. Health Sciences and Technology Division, Boston, Massachusetts; Associate Professor of Health Sciences and Technology at the Massachusetts Institute of Technology, Cambridge; and Associate Physician at Massachusetts General Hospital, Boston. The author or coauthor of over 120 professional publications and MERIT awardee of the National Institutes of Health, Dr. Bonventre is the Associate Editor of the Renal Fluid and Electrolyte Section of the *American Journal of Physiology*. He is a member of the American Society for Clinical Investigation, the Association of American Physicians, and the International Society of Nephrology Commission on Acute Renal Failure, among others. Dr. Bonventre received the B.S. degree with distinction (1970) in engineering physics from Cornell University, Ithaca, New York, the M.D. degree (1976) from Harvard Medical School, Boston, Massachusetts, and the Ph.D. degree (1979) in biophysics from Harvard University, Cambridge, Massachusetts.